W9-CUO-340

Guide to Good Food

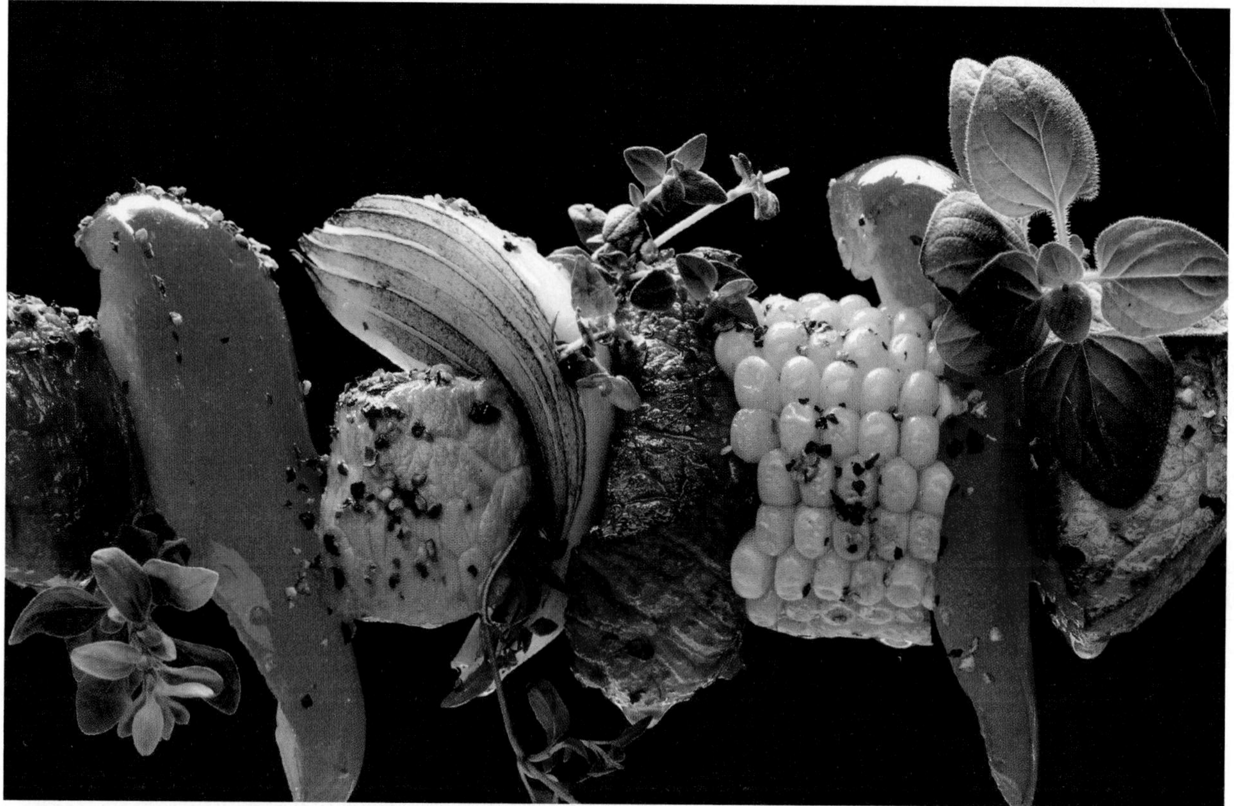

StockFood Munich/Zabert

Velda L. Largen
Author of Family and Consumer Sciences Instructional Materials

Deborah L. Bence, CFCS
Family and Consumer Sciences Author
Reynoldsburg, Ohio

Publisher
The Goodheart-Willcox Company, Inc.
Tinley Park, Illinois

Library of Congress Catalog Card Number 2002033907

ISBN-13: 978-1-59070-517-9
ISBN-10: 1-59070-517-3

3 4 5 6 7 8 9 10–06–11 10 09 08 07 06

Library of Congress Cataloging-in-Publication Data

Largen, Velda L.
Guide to good food / Velda L. Largen, Deborah L. Bence.
p. cm.
Includes index.
ISBN 1-59070-517-3
1. Food. 2. Nutrition. 3. Cookery, International. I. Bence, Deborah L. II. Title.

TX354.L37 2005
641.3--dc22 2004060853

Cover:
StockFood Munich/Zabert

Back Cover:
Courtesy of National Pork Board

Introduction

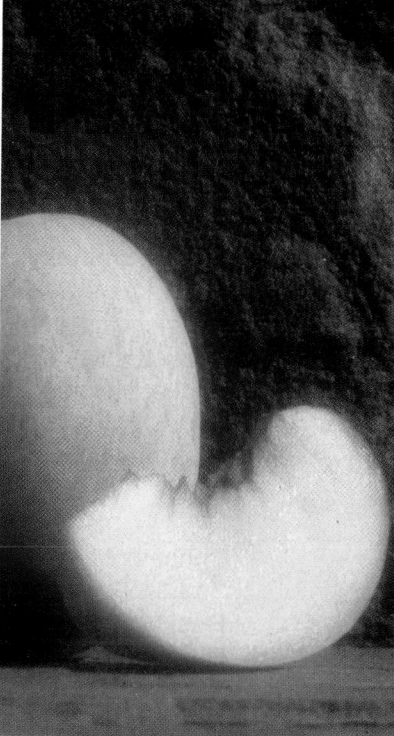
Agricultural Research Service, USDA

Guide to Good Food is designed to give you information about food and nutrition you can use every day. This practical text focuses on the latest advice on diet and physical activity to help you make healthful food and fitness choices. Guidelines for choosing appliances, setting up a food budget, and buying and storing foods will help you make consumer decisions. Tips on using space, time, and energy will help you manage your resources while working in the kitchen. Information on basic cooking methods will give you the background needed to prepare a wide range of foods.

Throughout the text, you will find health, business etiquette, safety, consumer, and environmental tips. Question-and-answer sidelights address common food myths and concerns. Descriptions of food industry careers from the *Dictionary of Occupational Titles* are listed at the beginning of each chapter. Case studies illustrating the need for and use of skills in the workplace appear at the end of every chapter. *Guide to Good Food* also includes several chapters on foods from around the world. These features are intended to show you food is more than just something to eat. Food is at the heart of scientific research. It provides a source of income for millions of people. It is also a part of people's cultural identity.

You will find *Guide to Good Food* easy to read and understand. Hundreds of colorful photos will help you picture the many foods and techniques that are discussed. Numerous recipes will give you the chance to practice food preparation methods covered in the book. Terms are listed at the beginning of each chapter to help acquaint you with vocabulary related to text material. Learning objectives will allow you to key in on important points as you read. Review questions at the end of each chapter will help you assess your understanding of what you read. Learning activities are suggested to give you a chance to further explore topics of interest. Technology applications help you build new skills. All these resources are intended to enhance your experience as you study the interesting and vital topics of food and nutrition.

Reviewers

Teacher Reviewers

Brenda Dumler
Family and Consumer Sciences Teacher
Lee's Summit High School
Lee's Summit, Missouri

Dorothy M. Gunter
Family and Consumer Sciences Instructor
Bartlett High School
Bartlett, Illinois

Ellen Huminsky
Department Chair: Family and Consumer Sciences
Shaker Heights High School
Shaker Heights, Ohio

Belinda Kanis
Family and Consumer Sciences Instructor
West Windsor-Plainsboro High School South
Princeton Junction, New Jersey

Becky Pfeiffer
Regional Occupational Program Instructor, Careers in Hospitality
Duncan Polytechnical High School
Fresno, California

Patricia K. O. Rambo, CFCS
Family and Consumer Sciences Teacher
Tahoka High School
Tahoka, Texas

Nancy Snyder
Family and Consumer Sciences Instructor
Allen High School
Allentown, Pennsylvania

Anne Gerken VanHulst
Family and Consumer Sciences Department Chair
Barron Collier High School
Naples, Florida

Technical Reviewers

Karen Chapman-Novakofski, RD, LD, PhD
Associate Professor and Extension Specialist, Nutrition
Department of Food Science and Human Nutrition
University of Illinois
Urbana-Champaign, Illinois

Barbara Ann F. Hughes, PhD, RD, LDN, FADA
President, B.A. Hughes & Associates
Raleigh, North Carolina

International Food Information Council Foundation
Washington, DC

Jessica Schulman, PhD, RD, LDN
Adjunct Professor and Nutrition Consultant
College of Health Professions
University of Florida
Gainesville, Florida

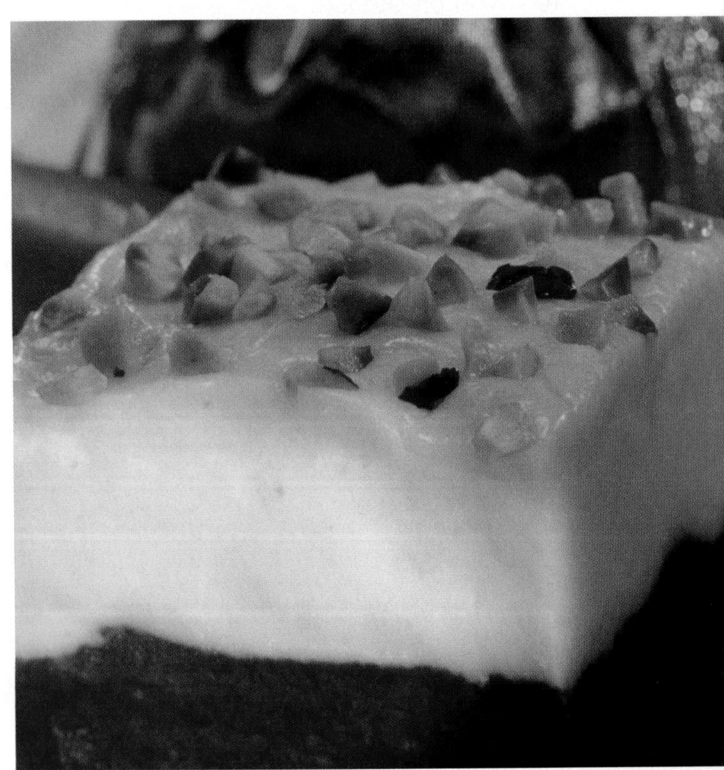

Brief Contents

Part 1
The Importance of Food

Part 2
The Management of Food

Part 3
The Preparation of Food

Part 4
Foods of the World

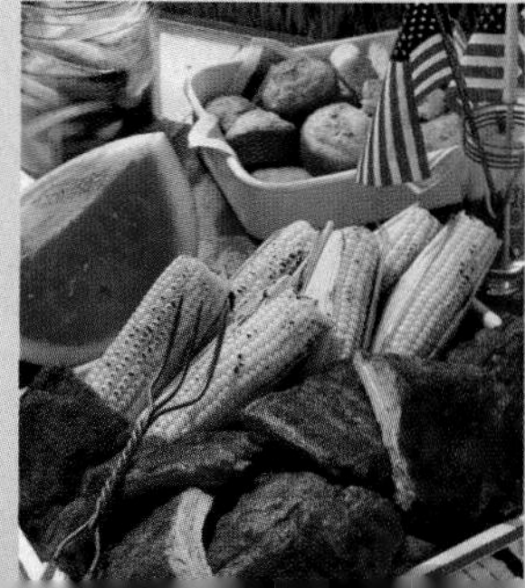
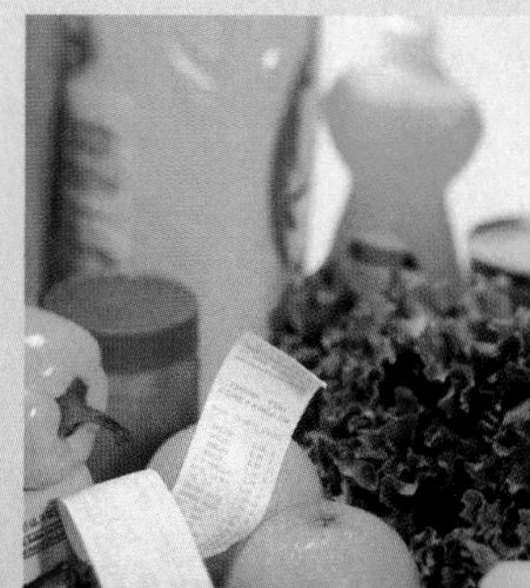
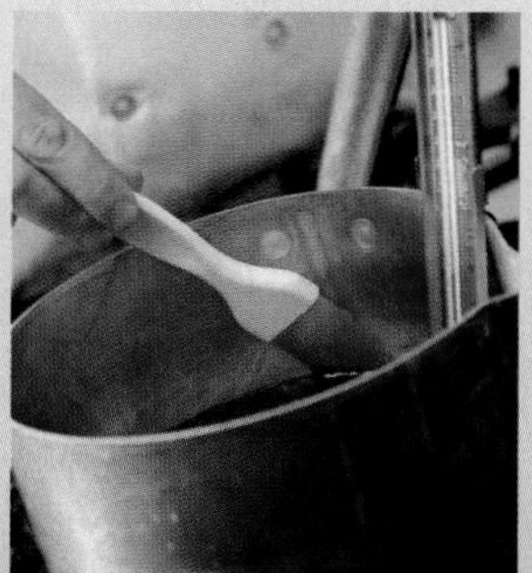
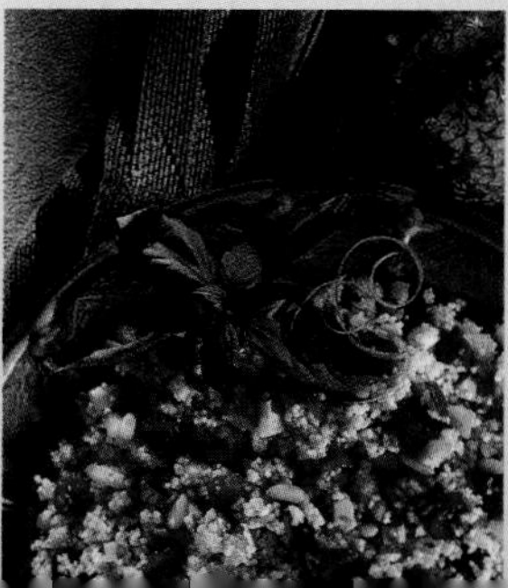

Contents

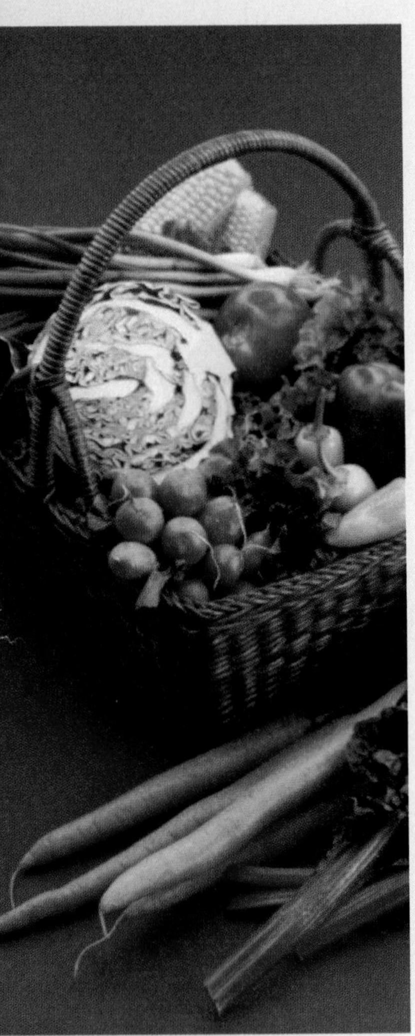

Part 1 The Importance of Food

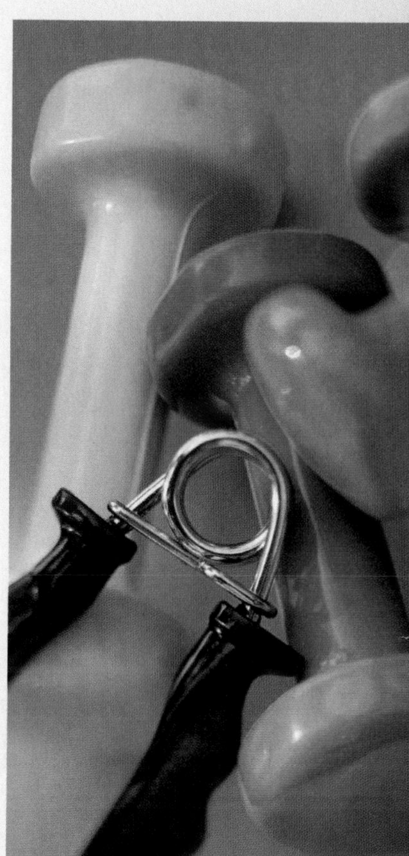

Part 2 The Management of Food

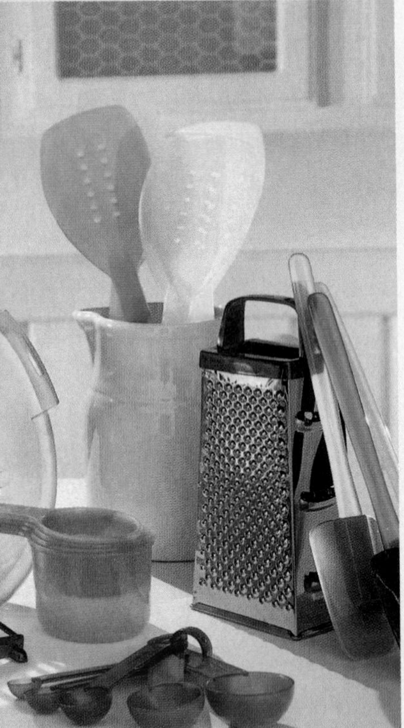

Ekco

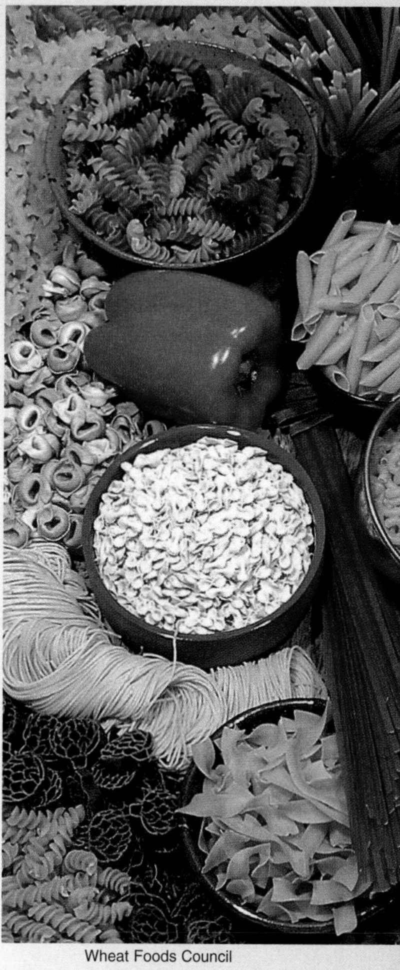
Wheat Foods Council

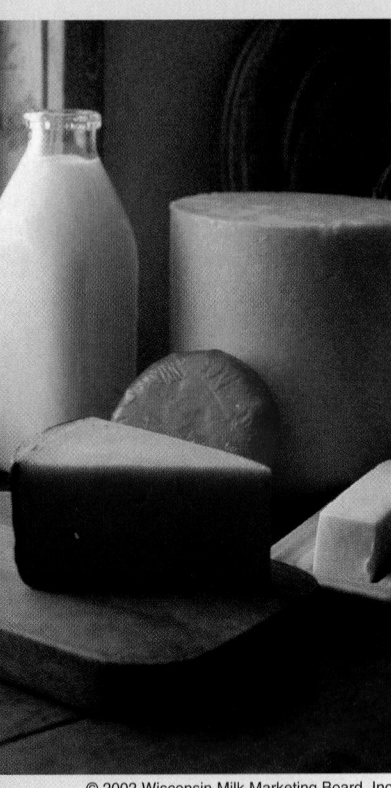

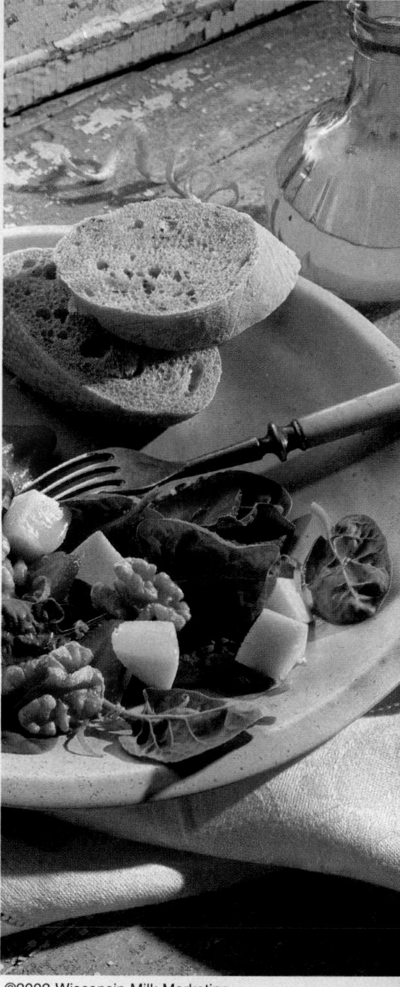

©2002 Wisconsin Milk Marketing Board, Inc.

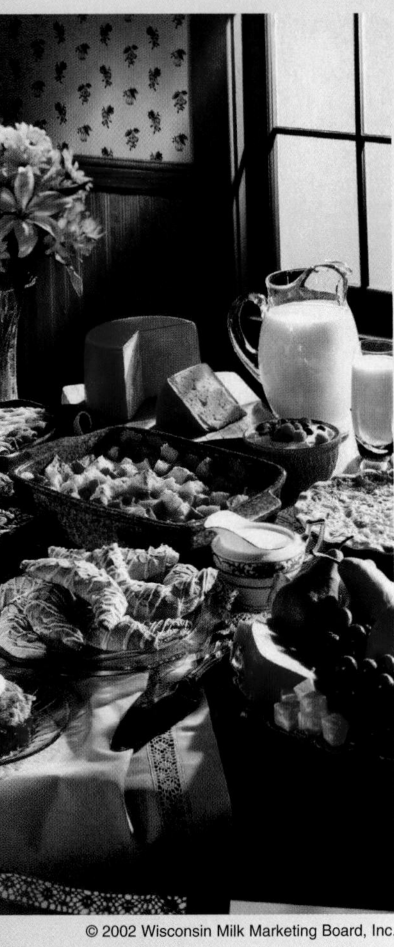
© 2002 Wisconsin Milk Marketing Board, Inc.

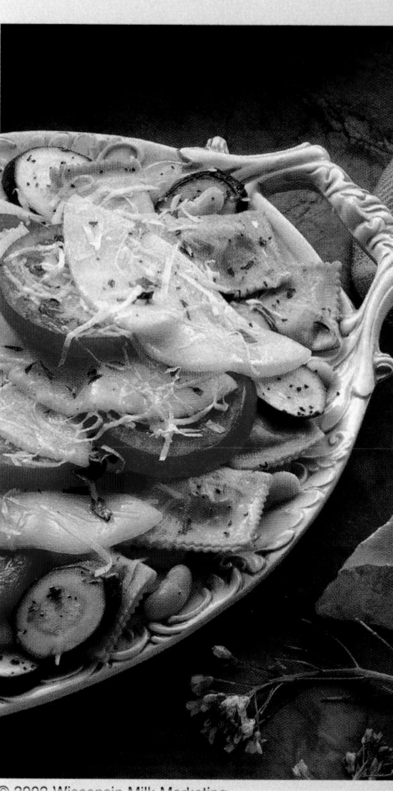

© 2002 Wisconsin Milk Marketing Board, Inc.

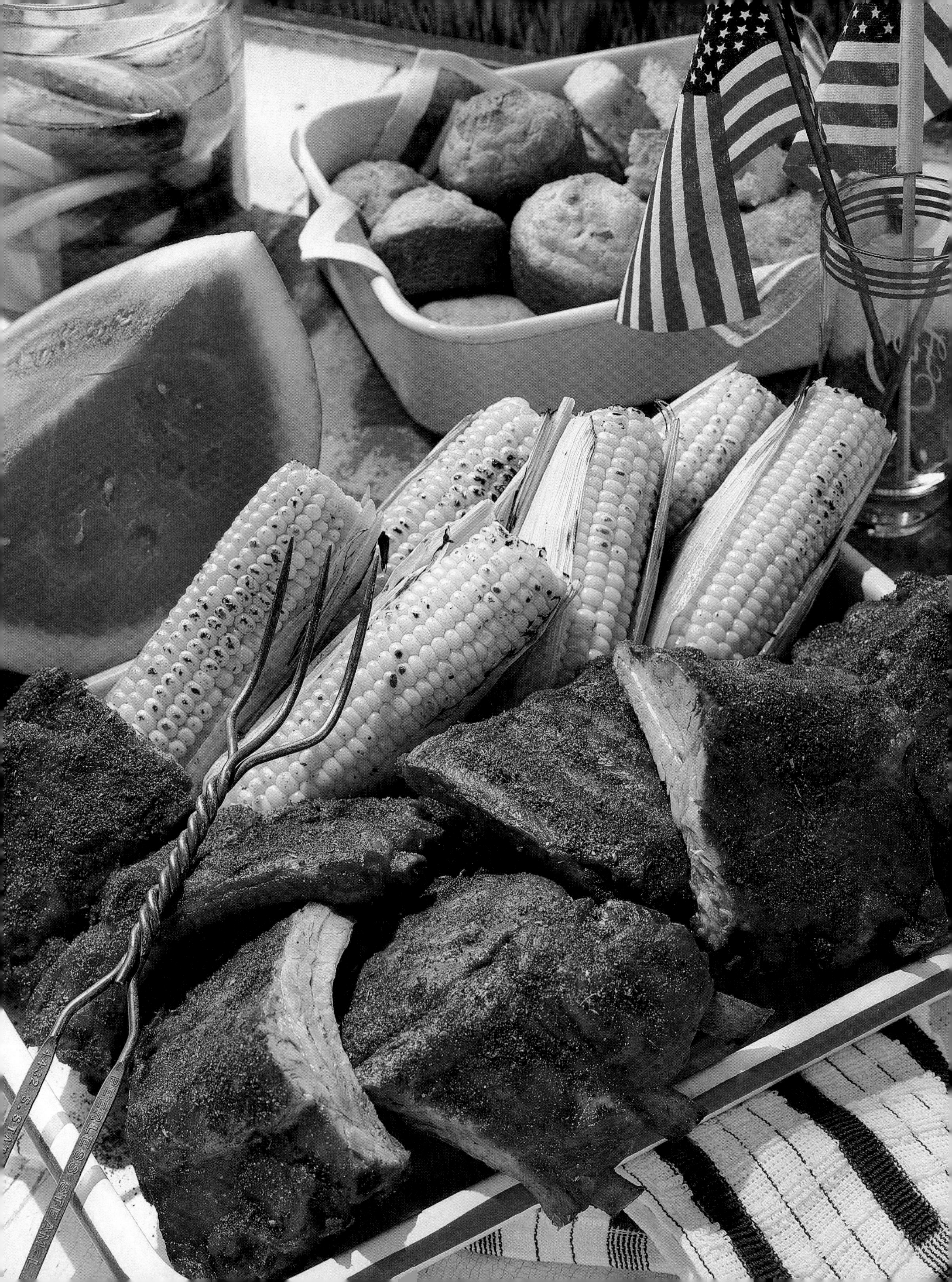
PEERLESS STEAM
4432 S. STA

Part 1
The Importance of Food

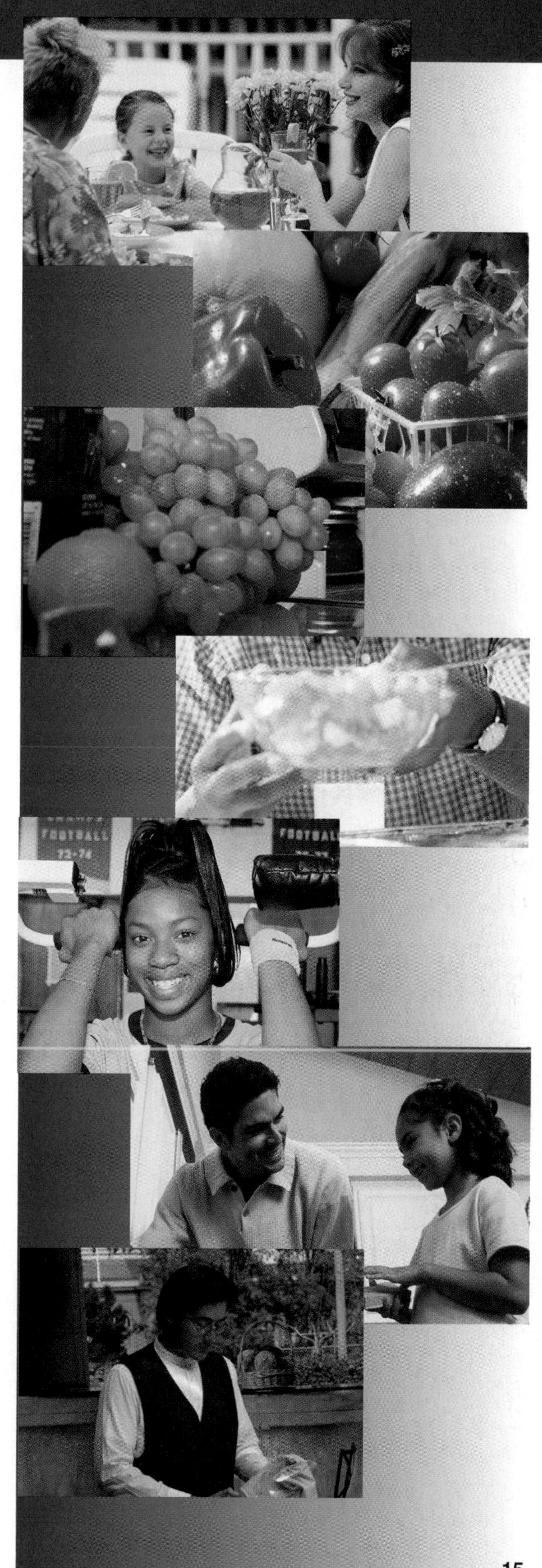

◄ courtesy of National Pork Board

Chapter 1
How Food Affects Life

Food Historian
Prepares a chronological account or record of past or current events dealing with food habits of people within specific social, ethnic, political, or geographic groupings.

Food Photographer
Arranges food and props, adjusts lighting and camera settings, and takes photographs of food for commercial uses.

Food Technologist
Develops and tests new food products in test kitchen and develops specific processing methods in laboratory pilot plant. Also confers with process engineers, flavor experts, and packaging and marketing specialists to resolve problems.

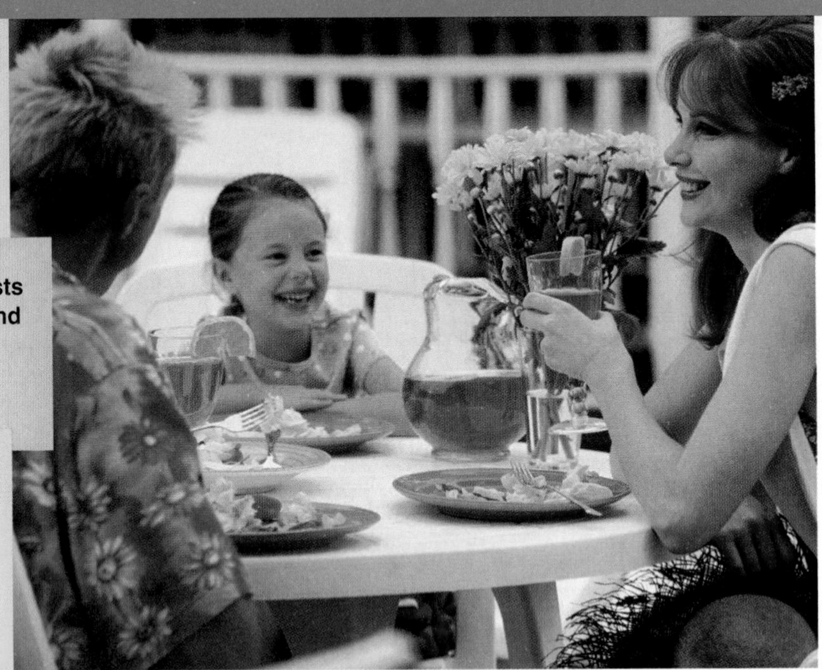

Terms to Know

decision-making process
alternative
hunger
appetite
wellness
stress
culture
fasting
lifestyle
peer pressure
fad
fallacy
functional food
agriculture
environment
United States Department of Agriculture (USDA)
Food and Drug Administration (FDA)
technology
artificial sweetener
fat replacer

Objectives

After studying this chapter, you will be able to

- ❑ explain how the search for food led to the development of civilization.
- ❑ use the steps of the decision-making process to make food choices.
- ❑ describe how food relieves hunger and improves wellness.
- ❑ outline cultural, social, and psychological influences on food choices.
- ❑ list factors that affect the food supply.

Food has different meanings for different people. People who are starving see food as a means of survival. People who are proud of their culture consider traditional foods to be part of their heritage. Members of some faiths regard certain foods as religious symbols. People who are entertaining guests view food as a sign of hospitality.

Clearly, food does much more than meet a basic physical need. It meets emotional, social, and psychological needs as well.

As long as people have walked the earth, they have searched for food and the means to produce it. Efforts to improve food resources are likely to continue as long as life exists.

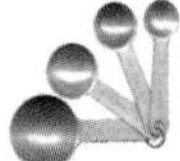

The History of Food

Early people probably ate food raw. At some point, they accidentally discovered cooked food tasted better and was easier to digest. By trial and error, they learned to control fire and use it to prepare food.

Eventually, these early people found they could protect themselves and secure food more easily by living in groups. They formed tribes and began to hunt for food together.

Some hunters became herders when they discovered they could capture and domesticate animals. People also discovered they could plant seeds to produce large amounts of food. This discovery led to the beginning of farming. The advances of herding and farming made the food supply much more dependable.

As food became easier to obtain, not all people had to spend their time hunting and farming. Some were able to learn a craft. Others became merchants. Trading in its simplest form began, and with it came the development of civilization.

The Migration of Food

As civilizations grew and developed, people began searching for food in distant places. By the fifteenth century, Spanish, Portuguese, English, and Dutch sailors were traveling the world in search of tea and spices. These sailors discovered new lands as well as new foods. Thus the search for new food sources fostered European colonization of distant continents and the growth of powerful empires.

European explorers introduced foods they carried with them in the new lands to which they traveled. In North America, Spanish explorers introduced cane sugar and wheat. English explorers brought apples and walnuts, 1-1. The explorers also carried foods from the lands they explored back to their homelands. Therefore, foods that were once native to one place are now found in many places. This type of exchange led to an increased variety of foods throughout the world.

Making Choices About Foods

In the United States, many people are fortunate enough to have a variety of foods available to them. This requires them to make many choices about foods. They must decide when and where to eat. They must choose what to eat and how to prepare it. These choices require some skill in thinking and making decisions.

The Decision-Making Process

You can use a process to make decisions about foods or any other topics. The ***decision-making process*** is a method for thinking about possible options and outcomes before making a choice. It involves the following series of steps:

1. **State the decision to be made.** This helps you define the specific issue you are

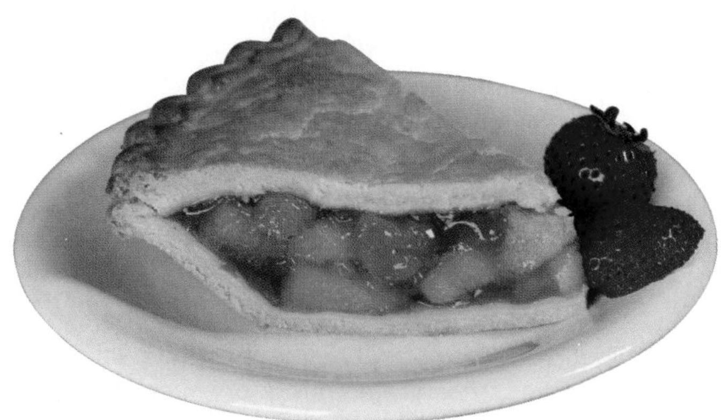

1-1 *Apple pie would not be a U.S. national dish if English explorers had not introduced apples to the New World.*

considering so you can focus your thoughts. You may want to phrase your decision as a question. A decision about food might be What should I do for lunch?

2. **List your alternatives. *Alternatives*** are the various options you might choose. Options for your lunch decision might include making a sandwich, reheating leftovers, and going out for fast food.
3. **Weigh the pros and cons of each alternative.** Each option will generally have some advantages and some disadvantages. Considering these will help you make a choice with which you will be satisfied. For instance, making a sandwich may have the advantage of being convenient if you have the ingredients on hand. It has the disadvantage of requiring some food preparation effort. Reheating leftovers has the advantage of providing a quick, hot, filling lunch. However, it has the disadvantage of lack of variety because you ate the same dish yesterday. Going out for fast food has the advantage of requiring no food preparation effort. On the other hand, this option would cost more money than the other two options.
4. **Make a decision and act on it.** After weighing all the pros and cons, choose the option that best meets your needs. Suppose you do not feel like preparing a sandwich and you do not want to spend money eating out. In this case, reheating leftovers may seem like the best choice.
5. **Evaluate your decision.** Thinking about how happy you were with a decision can help you make decisions in the future. Perhaps after eating the leftovers, you realize you do not like eating the same food two days in a row. You determine making a sandwich would have been worth the extra effort. This will help you make a choice the next time you are deciding what to do for lunch.

Food Meets Physical Needs

Have you ever tried studying for a test when you were hungry? You may have found it hard to concentrate. This is because food is one of your most basic physical needs. The instinct to meet this need is so strong you cannot focus on other issues until this need has been addressed.

Your body needs food to provide the energy required to maintain vital functions, such as keeping your heart beating. You also need energy from food to move your muscles so you can perform tasks like walking, sitting, and climbing, 1-2. Your body needs substances from food to build and repair tissues, too.

Food meets two basic physical needs. First, food eases hunger. Second, it can affect your overall state of health.

Relieves Hunger

A complex system within your body senses when you need a fresh supply of the materials food provides. This system involves your digestive tract, which sends a message to your brain. Your brain receives this message and gives a signal, which you recognize as hunger. ***Hunger*** is the physical need for food. The hunger signal stimulates your stomach to produce hunger pangs. The hunger signal may also stimulate your ***appetite,*** which is a psychological desire to eat.

You can choose how you respond to the sensations of hunger and appetite. If you choose to eat, food relieves your hunger and the pangs in your stomach go away. If you choose not to eat, the pangs are likely to become more intense. You may experience other symptoms as hunger continues, such as a headache or dizziness.

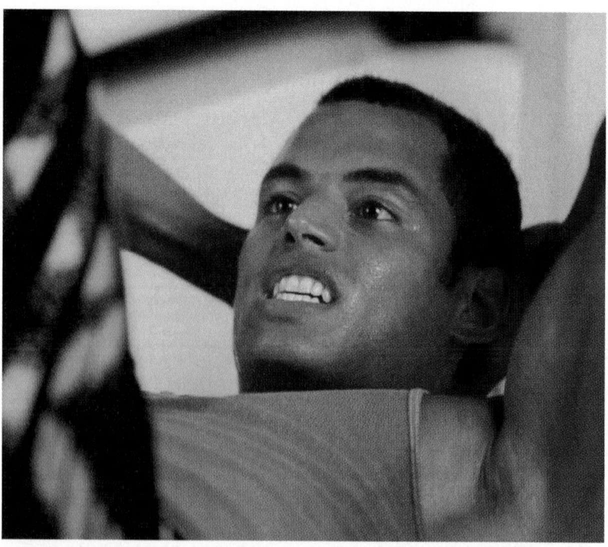

1-2 Food provides the energy needed for physical activity.

Your appetite has a greater influence on your food choices than your hunger. Any food will relieve hunger, but only certain foods will satisfy your appetite. For instance, if you eat meat loaf when you have a taste for pizza, your appetite will not be satisfied.

Q: Do hunger and appetite always go hand in hand?

A: No. For instance, when you are sick, you may be hungry and yet not feel like eating. Conversely, when you smell freshly baked cookies, you may want to eat some even if you are not hungry.

Improves Wellness

Wellness is the state of being in overall good health. It involves mental and social health as well as physical health. Wellness is a goal most people actively try to achieve.

The three areas of wellness—physical health, mental health, and social health—all affect one another. Sensible food choices can help improve all three areas.

In terms of *physical health*, or the health of your body, food does more than relieve hunger. Food helps you grow and develop normally. It can help you avoid developing certain diseases, too. You will read about these functions of food in Chapter 2.

Your *mental health* is the health of your mind. One sign of good mental health and overall wellness is an ability to handle stress. ***Stress*** is mental tension caused by change. For instance, moving to a new community creates many changes. Some of these changes may be positive, such as living in a nicer home. Some of the changes may be negative, such as seeing less of your friends in the old neighborhood. In both cases, the changes can cause stress.

Food can help you manage stress. When you eat the foods your body needs, you are less likely to develop certain illnesses. Illness can be a major source of stress. Therefore, preventing illness through careful food choices can help you avoid stress and improve your mental health. Eating well can also give you the strength to face stressful situations when they arise.

Your *social health* refers to the health of your relationships with other people. Eating healthful foods can help you feel strong and energetic. This strength and energy can give you confidence to be more outgoing as you interact with others. Food also affects the social aspect of wellness by being an important part of many social gatherings. You will read more about this role of food later in the chapter. See 1-3.

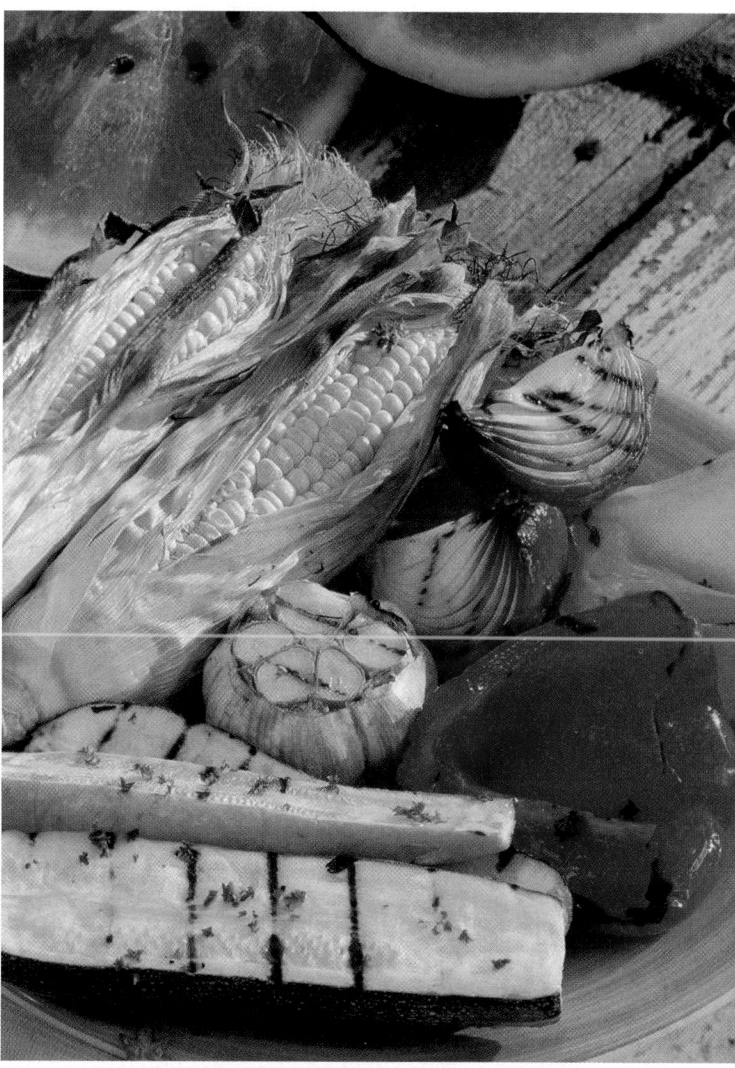

1-3 *A nutritious diet can have a positive impact on physical, mental, and social health.*

Cultural Influences on Food Choices

What do you choose to eat when you are hungry? Where do you usually eat? Who is with you when you eat? When do you eat? How does food make you feel?

Your answers to all these questions reflect your food habits. Chances are, each of your friends would answer these questions a bit differently. This is because the factors that affect food habits are a little different for everyone.

One factor that affects food habits is culture. ***Culture*** is the customs and beliefs of a racial, religious, or social group. People of a certain race form a cultural group. Citizens of a given country and followers of a specific religion are also examples of cultural groups. Many people are part of more than one cultural group.

The United States is a *multicultural society.* The many cultures in this country include those of the Native Americans and the first explorers. The cultures of immigrants from Europe and Asia and slaves from Africa are also part of U.S. culture today. You might think of the United States as a cultural "tossed salad." A tossed salad is a single food item made up of a variety of vegetables. Each vegetable contributes a distinct flavor, color, and texture. In a similar way, each culture that is part of U.S. society contributes unique customs and beliefs to the nation.

In Chapters 27 through 32, you will read more about the native countries of U.S. residents. You will also read about the foods of these countries. As you read, evaluate the variety of foods in the diet of each culture. Also think about how the foods contributed by people who came from other lands have added to the U.S. diet.

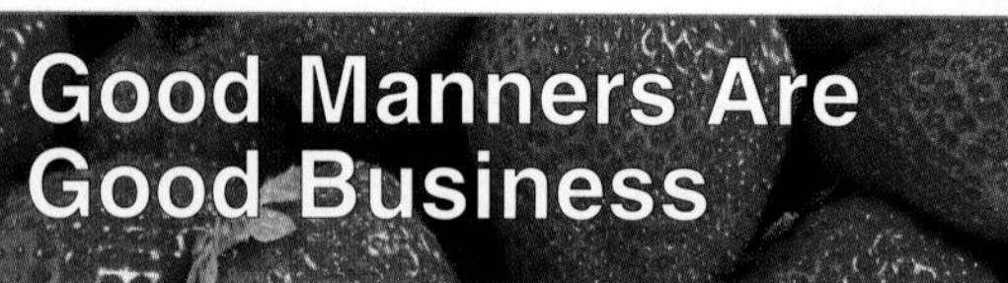

Good Manners Are Good Business

More and more, business is transacted internationally. Even within the United States, dealing with people from different cultures is common. Make a point of learning about the cultures of your business associates. This will allow you to be sensitive to their cultural differences. Your consideration will have a positive impact on your success in the marketplace.

National Origin

The people who colonized various lands brought with them foods from their native cultures. For instance, the French who settled in the United States introduced chowders. The Chinese introduced stir-fried dishes. When the immigrants could not obtain traditional ingredients, they had to adapt their recipes. They incorporated foods that were available locally into their diets.

In the United States, immigrants tended to settle together based on nationality. As a result, many foods are typical of particular regions of the country. For instance, foods of Mexican and Spanish origin are found in the West and Southwest. Asian influence is seen in foods of the Pacific Coast.

Religion

Religion is an important cultural influence on the food habits of many people. Some religions have certain customs regarding food and how people should eat it. For instance, Hindus will not use cattle for food because they consider cattle to be sacred. Muslims can eat only with the right hand.

Through the ages, people have used food for religious offerings. They might place special foods on altars or offer prayers recognizing events symbolized by the foods. The bread and wine used in Christian churches during communion symbolize the sacrifice of Christ's body and blood. Unleavened bread is an important symbol for Jewish people during Passover, the eight-day festival that commemorates their flight from Egypt. Because the Jews had to leave their homes so quickly, they did not have time to allow their bread to rise.

Fasting, or denying oneself food, has long been a religious custom. Some Christians fast during Lent, a 40-day period leading up to Easter. Jews fast on Yom Kippur, the Day of Atonement. At one time, Catholics would not eat meat on Friday. Some Catholics still follow this practice.

Some early people used food as part of their burial ceremonies. For example, the ancient Egyptians buried food with their dead. The Egyptians believed the deceased needed food for their journey into the next world. Some Shintos, Taoists, and Buddhists still offer food

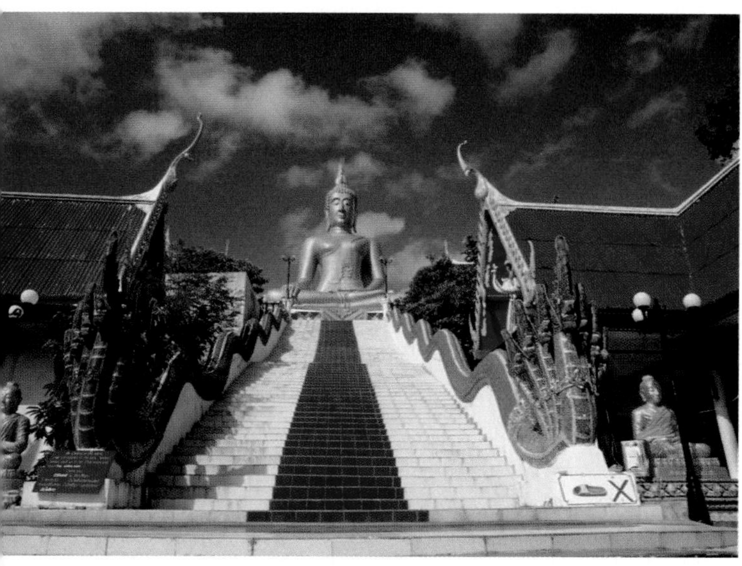

1-4 One food custom of many followers of the Buddhist religion is to refrain from eating meat.

and coins at shrines honoring deceased relatives and friends. See 1-4.

Holidays

People of all cultures have special days set aside each year for celebration. Cultural influences on food choices may be most apparent on these days. Holiday celebrations abound with food traditions. Some holiday foods have special symbolism. For instance, heart-shaped chocolates are given on Valentine's Day as a symbol of love. Other holiday foods have simply become part of the customs connected with the celebration. As an example, many people eat corn on the cob and hot dogs on Independence Day.

Social Influences on Food Choices

For many people, preparing and eating food are social activities. Food can bring people together. It brings family members together at the dinner table. It brings friends together at parties and picnics. When guests come to visit, the host usually offers them something to eat or drink. People often transact business over lunch. In each of these situations, food is part of the social interaction.

Just as food plays a part in social life, social life plays a part in eating habits and food choices. For instance, your family members and friends can affect your meal plans and food preferences. Mass media and current trends may affect your grocery purchases. Are you aware of how these social influences affect the foods you eat?

Q: Isn't fasting a health practice recommended for periodically cleansing the body from the inside out?

A: Health and nutrition experts do not advise depriving your body of nutrients, which is what fasting does. Your liver and digestive system work to remove waste material from your body. Your body does not require any other form of internal cleansing.

Family

Family has a great impact on the foods people eat and how they eat them. For many people, favorite foods are those they grew up eating at home. Foods often play important roles in family traditions and special occasions. Maybe a family night involved spreading a blanket on the living room floor and eating foods picnic-style. Perhaps a special menu was chosen to celebrate family birthdays. Such customs help form a person's preferences and attitudes toward food.

Changing lifestyles have had a tremendous impact on family eating patterns. Your ***lifestyle*** is the way you usually live. Years ago, many families lived on farms, and their lifestyles focused on daily tasks around the farms. Families tended to be large, and children were viewed as economic assets because they could help with farm tasks.

Family eating patterns at that time often involved eating three meals together each day. Family members used mealtime as a chance to share the day's events and discuss problems.

Some families also used this time for spiritual growth. Many of the foods families ate were produced right on the farm. Mothers generally prepared the family meals. Dishes were hearty to provide family members with the fuel they needed to do physical farm work.

Today, relatively few families live on farms. There are more *dual-income families,* or families in which both parents earn a paycheck. Adult family members spend many hours away from home commuting and working. Families are generally smaller, and some parents seem to be more aware of the costs involved in raising children. Lifestyles in many busy households seem to keep everyone running in different directions. Work schedules, after-school activities, and other events keep family members on the go.

Such fast-paced family lifestyles have led to more hectic eating patterns. On average, family members eat fewer meals together. Mothers who work outside the home have less time to cook. Other family members are more likely to share some meal management tasks. However, today's families produce little food, and most people eat fewer home-cooked meals than people in the past. Many meal managers often rely on convenience foods and carryout meals.

Some sociologists feel the move away from daily family meals is unfortunate. When family members do not eat together, they miss an important chance to communicate. Experts who predict trends expect busy lifestyles and current family eating patterns to persist. Nevertheless, a majority of families view family meals as a priority. In the future, family meal managers are likely to continue seeking food products that can be prepared quickly. However, they will try to serve those food items in a family meal setting as often as possible.

Friends

Your friends have an effect on the foods you choose. You may feel a small amount of peer pressure to eat the same foods your friends are eating. ***Peer pressure*** is influence that comes from people in a person's social group. For instance, suppose you are in a restaurant with friends. If they all order pizza, you are also likely to order pizza even if you would really have preferred a sandwich. See 1-5.

Friends may also encourage you to try new foods or preparation techniques. A friend might persuade you to sample a food such as squid, which might have little appeal to you. A friend might convince someone used to eating buttered vegetables to try a vegetable casserole instead.

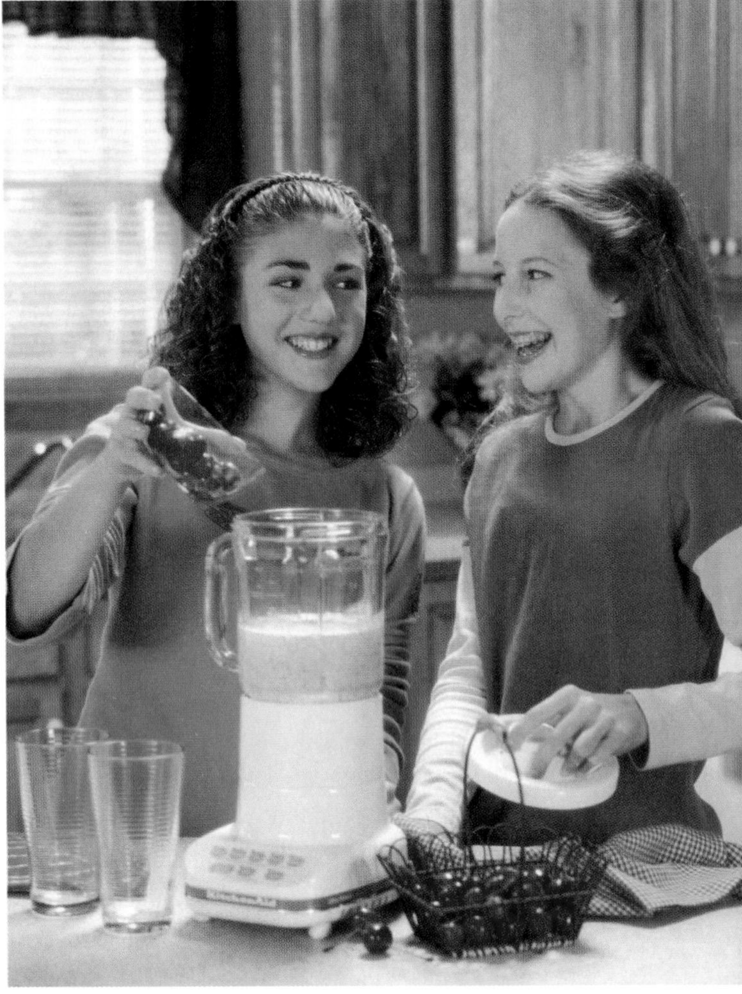

Cherry Marketing Institute

1-5 Friends can influence food choices and eating habits.

Mass Media

Mass media, such as television, radio, magazines, and the Internet, can affect your food choices. The media acquaints you with, reminds you of, and informs you about food products and nutrition issues.

Advertising

A key way the media influence your food choices is through advertising. Advertisements encourage you to try new food products. They also urge you to continue buying products that have been available for years. They do this with a number of techniques. Advertisers may appeal to your curiosity by asking you to try something because it is different. They may appeal to your desire to belong by saying everyone is using the product. They may appeal to your pride by implying the most worthwhile people are those who eat this food. Coupons, rebates, and special offers may also prompt you to use food products.

When you see food advertisements, view them with a critical eye. Try to be aware of how the ad is attempting to sway you. Use the nutrition knowledge you gain in this class to evaluate the advertising message. Does information presented in the ad seem accurate? How would the advertised product help meet your daily food needs? Although an ad can pique your interest in a product, it cannot force you to buy the product. Analyzing food advertisements can help you make wise consumer decisions.

Be a Clever Consumer

Use advertisements as a resource to help you learn about products. However, be aware of the words advertisers use to persuade you to buy. Words such as *delicious, fun*, and *wholesome* are subjective. They have different meanings to different people. You need to evaluate products for yourself to know if they will meet your needs.

Evaluating Information in the Media

News reports and articles in the media can notify you about health issues related to various food products. The media can warn you to avoid products that are found to be unsafe. The media can also inform you about a new finding of a food's special health properties. Learning this information can help you make wise food purchase decisions.

Although news reports are likely to be more fact-based than advertisements, you still need to view them critically. Many news stories about food and nutrition are missing important pieces of information. This may be due to an oversight if the reporter is not an expert on foods and nutrition. It may be because the media source cannot allow enough time or space for all the details. Perhaps omissions occur because reporters do not think their audiences will understand specific facts and figures.

Whatever the reason, you need to realize the usefulness of a report is limited when key points are missing. In reports on food and nutrition, read or listen for answers to the following questions:

- Who conducted the research? Experts in the field of the research are likely to be most knowledgeable about how to interpret findings.
- Where were the results of the research published? A journal reviewed by professionals in the field of the research has more credibility than a popular magazine.
- How was the study set up? A valid study needs to be conducted under carefully controlled conditions. Steps must be taken to keep unplanned variables from affecting the outcomes.
- Who funded the research? You may have reason to be more skeptical if the funding party stands to gain financially from the findings.
- How many people did the researchers study? A study that involves a large group of subjects may be more relevant than one that involves a small group.
- Were the results of this study similar to the results of other studies? Findings are more significant when they match those of a number of research teams. See 1-6.

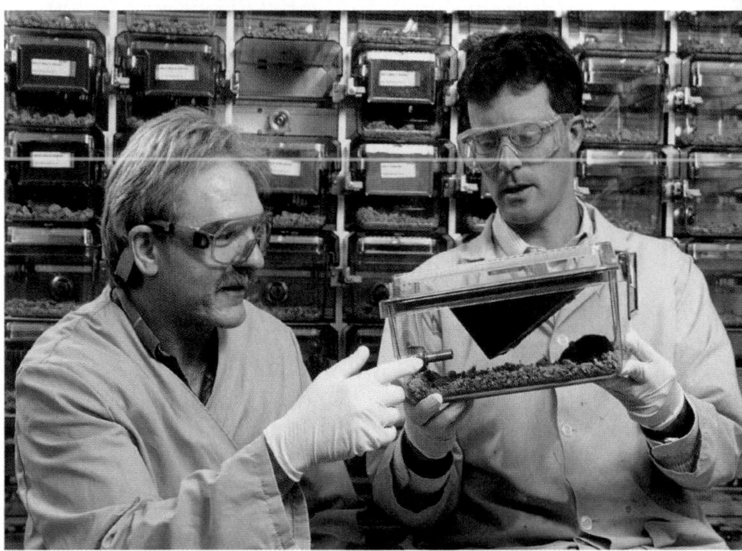

Agricultural Research Service, USDA

1-6 *Researchers compare their study results with those of other scientists to help prove or disprove their theories.*

- How much of the food or nutrient needs to be consumed to experience the benefit or harmful effect? Quantities should resemble what people might normally be expected to consume. Findings are less useful when they are based on very large quantities.
- How often does the food or nutrient need to be consumed? Like the quantity, the frequency of consumption should be realistic.
- Do the beneficial or harmful effects of the food or nutrient build with repeated consumption? This indicates the degree to which the research findings might affect established eating habits.
- Does the food or nutrient have different effects on certain groups of people, such as children or pregnant women? This indicates how much bearing the research has for you and your family members.

Answers to these questions can help you evaluate the information you receive through the media. These answers distinguish a merely interesting story from one that can help you make more healthful food choices.

One other tip applies to food and nutrition information that is available over the Internet. The end of a Web site address gives you a clue about the source of the information. Web sites that end in *.edu* are those of educational institutions. A government agency site ends in *.gov*, and a professional organization site ends in *.org*. These may be the most reliable resources when you are researching a topic. Web site addresses that end in *.com* are sponsored by commercial groups. These sites may provide a wealth of helpful information. However, keep in mind that they exist mainly as a way to promote products.

Food Fads and Fallacies

Incomplete or inaccurate information through the media may be behind many food fads and fallacies. A ***fad*** is a practice that is very popular for a short time. A ***fallacy*** is a mistaken belief. Many food fads and fallacies are related to nutrition, weight loss, and food safety issues. See 1-7.

Some food fads can be harmful to health. For instance, adding raw eggs to milk shakes was a fad among body builders. This fad was based on the fallacy that raw eggs are a superior source of protein for building muscles. The truth is, some raw eggs are contaminated with bacteria that can cause illness. Therefore, eating raw eggs is risky. Cooking eggs will not decrease the quality of the protein, but it will kill harmful bacteria.

Some food fads are not dangerous, but they can lead to disappointment when they do not produce promised results. One such fad that was popular among women was adding gelatin to the diet. This practice was based on the fallacy that gelatin makes fingernails grow better. The truth is, gelatin is a source of protein, which is a main component of fingernails. A diet low in protein may result in weak fingernails. However, most women in the United States consume more than enough protein. Weak fingernails are more likely the result of exposure to water, dry weather, or harsh cleaning agents. Gelatin has not been shown to strengthen weak fingernails.

Before jumping on the bandwagon to try a new trend, find out the facts. Take a little time to research the information on which the fad is based. The time you invest may end up saving you money and possible harm.

Food Product Trends

Consumer demand drives trends for new products in the marketplace. In turn, what products are available influences your consumer choices. When it comes to food products, consumers demand three main qualities. They want foods that are healthful, convenient, and great tasting.

Health

Consumers are becoming increasingly aware of the impact food can have on their health. They are looking for foods that will help them lose excess weight or keep them from gaining it. Consumers are seeking products that will reduce their risks of cancer, high blood pressure, and heart disease.

This consumer concern for health has fueled the trend for functional food products. ***Functional foods*** are foods that provide health benefits beyond the nutrients they contain. Some new food products contain ingredients that give the products certain healthful qualities. For instance, some cereals are made with added fiber to promote heart health.

Many consumers are making more of an effort to read food labels, 1-8. They are using label information to help them choose foods that will meet their goals for good health. This is driving a trend for manufacturers to change the recipes for some food products. Manufacturers

Food Fallacies and Facts
Fallacy: Eating at night causes more weight gain than eating during the day. **Fact:** The time at which a person eats does not affect weight. To avoid gaining weight from excess body fat, the key is to eat no more calories each day than the body needs.
Fallacy: If it tastes good, it must be bad for you. **Fact:** Breads, lean meats, and fruits are among the best-liked foods according to surveys. These are all healthful sources of nutrients that should be part of the daily diet. Sweets and high-fat snack foods should be used sparingly because they contribute many calories and few nutrients. However, they are not "bad," and they do not have to be avoided completely. In fact, studies show that occasionally including such foods in the diet has no negative effects on health.
Fallacy: No fat means no flavor. **Fact:** Fats do contribute to the tastes of foods. However, many foods are deliciously flavored with spices and seasonings, which contribute no fat or calories.
Fallacy: Healthful foods take much time and effort to prepare. **Fact:** Pasta, whole grain breads, fruits and vegetables, and lean meats and poultry can be prepared quickly and easily. Many canned and frozen convenience products that are designed to ease preparation have excellent nutritional value.
Fallacy: Organic fruits and vegetables are free from pesticides and, therefore, do not need to be washed. **Fact:** Organic fruits and vegetables are grown without chemical pesticides. However, organic farmers are permitted to use certain natural pesticide agents. Like all other produce, organic items need to be washed to remove any soil and insect particles that may be present.

1-7 Knowing the facts can help you identify food fallacies when you hear them.

are working to reduce the amounts of fats, sugars, and salt that appear on food labels. For instance, some manufacturers are cutting the amount of sugar in cereals that appeal to children. The manufacturers know this will make their products more attractive to parents.

More and more consumers are looking for organic products. Many people think organic foods are better for them than other foods. Research does not support this belief. However, manufacturers are happy to bring out more organic products to sell to this growing market.

In keeping with the focus on health, consumers have embraced a few key weight-loss diets. A trend related to this is the linking of food products with these diets. Some product labels now claim that foods are approved by the creators of certain diet plans. People following a particular diet plan may be more likely to buy products linked with their plan. Other consumers are also likely to connect these products with goals for a healthy weight.

Convenience

Many consumers say they want to do more cooking at home. However, they do not have a lot of time to spend on food preparation. Therefore, convenience is key to the success of new food products. One-dish meal products

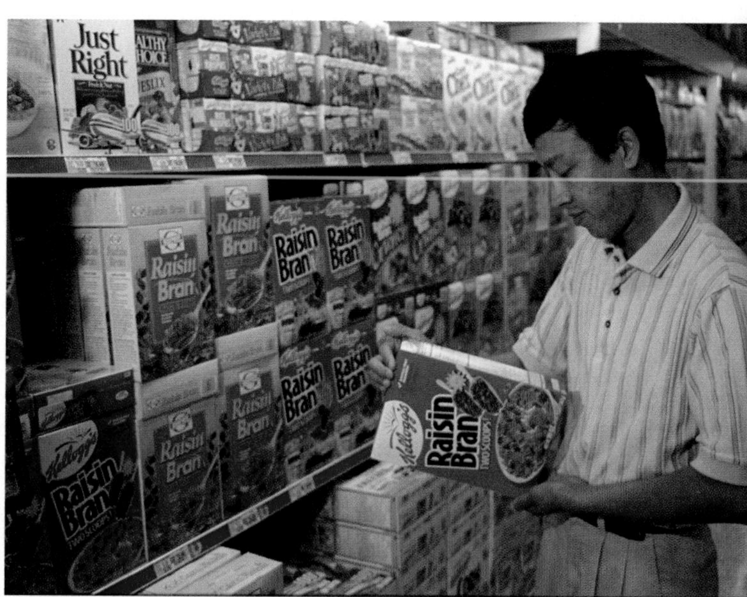

USDA

1-8 Reading labels can help consumers make the most healthful choices when shopping for foods.

have become popular because they reduce the need to spend time preparing side dishes. A number of products have also been introduced to help make tasks easier for home bakers.

Many foods need to be easy to eat as well as easy to prepare. Meals are often eaten on the go, so consumers are looking for foods that are portable. Single servings and packages that prevent spilling are product trends that address this need. Meal shakes that allow consumers to drink breakfast or lunch on the job have also become common.

Great Taste

Consumers are not willing to give up taste for health or convenience. Food manufacturers cannot cheat on taste appeal when creating new products.

One area where this fact is clear is in the ethnic food market. Italian is the most popular ethnic cuisine. However, many consumers are no longer happy with standard Italian foods. It seems consumers are forming more refined tastes. They want ethnic foods that taste authentic. This has led to a growing trend of products that reflect specific regions of Italy. Other cuisines that are on the rise include Turkish and Moroccan.

The desire for great taste is also seen in the appeal of specialty foods, such as fancy desserts. Many consumers have sophisticated tastes. They are willing to pay high prices for flavorful products made with the finest ingredients.

Psychological Influences on Food Choices

People prepare food and eat meals for many psychological reasons. Food can satisfy certain emotional needs. Babies learn to connect food with the warmth and security provided by the people who feed them. Children associate foods with pleasurable experiences, such as cake with birthday parties and popcorn with movies. Adults associate food with times of happiness and security, such as turkey with a family Thanksgiving gathering. Pleasant experiences may cause you to like certain foods. Unhappy experiences may cause you to dislike certain foods.

Children may eat in a certain way because of examples set by family members or friends. If a parent dislikes a food, a child may also claim to dislike it without even trying it. Younger brothers and sisters often follow the examples of older siblings. Have you ever thought you may be influencing others by the way you eat?

Emotions may also cause undereating and overeating. Some underweight people may not eat because of sadness, loneliness, or a deep emotional shock. Some overweight people may find comfort in foods they like. Food psychologically makes up for anger, frustration, or feelings of inadequacy in certain people.

Most people find eating psychologically satisfying. See 1-9. Food appeals to the senses of sight, taste, and smell. It also appeals to people's need for social contact. Enjoying the appearance, flavors, and aromas of a meal in the company of others is a psychologically pleasing experience.

Preparing food can be as satisfying as eating it. Cooking a meal that tastes good and looks attractive can give a person a psychological lift. It can also serve as a creative outlet. Perhaps you have made cookies or baked bread just for a change of pace from your daily activities. Praise for creative cooking can give a boost to the ego. The cook who receives praise for a beautifully prepared dish feels a sense of pride and self-esteem.

Factors That Affect the Food Supply

Many factors affect the supply of foods from which you can choose when you go to the store. These factors include regional agriculture and the environment. The government, economics, and technology also play roles in food choices.

Agriculture and the Environment

Agriculture is the use of knowledge and skill to tend soil, grow crops, and raise livestock. Successful agriculture requires a suitable

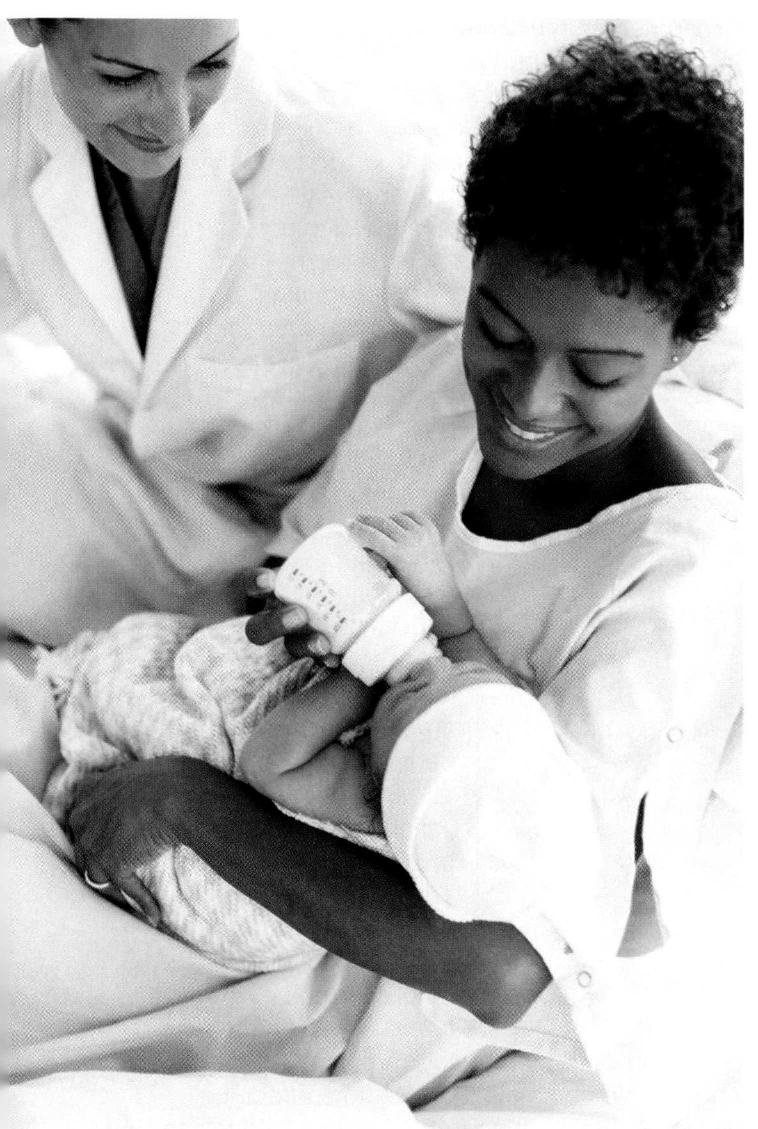

1-9 From the time they are born, most people find eating to be a psychologically pleasing experience.

environment. ***Environment*** refers to such factors as air, water, soil, mineral resources, plants, and animals. The interrelations among these factors ultimately affect the survival of life on earth. Livestock need supplies of food and water. Food crops require the right air temperatures, adequate water, and fertile soil to grow. The specific requirements vary from one type of plant to another. This is why certain crops grow better in some regions than in others.

In the United States, regional agriculture does not affect the availability of foods as much as it affects their costs. This is because foods are routinely shipped from one region to another. You can easily obtain foods even if they do not grow well in your local environment. However, you may have to pay more for them due to transportation costs. The environment also affects food costs when severe weather damages crops. The resulting shortages cause prices to rise.

In some areas of the world, the regional nature of agriculture limits food choices. In these areas, the equipment needed to preserve and ship food from one region to another may not be available. People may not be able to afford food with added transportation costs. Therefore, people's food choices are restricted to crops and livestock that are produced locally.

Just as the environment can affect crop growth, crop growth can affect the environment. Soil that is overworked by farmers can lose its ability to support crops in the future. Watering crops can strain water reserves in areas where there is not enough rain to sustain plant growth. In addition, chemicals used in farming sometimes get into water supplies. Tainted water affects the plants and animals that live in and around it. See 1-10.

Government

The government has a large impact on the food supply. Laws govern the way foods are grown, processed, packaged, and labeled. Government policies affect foods exported to and imported from other countries.

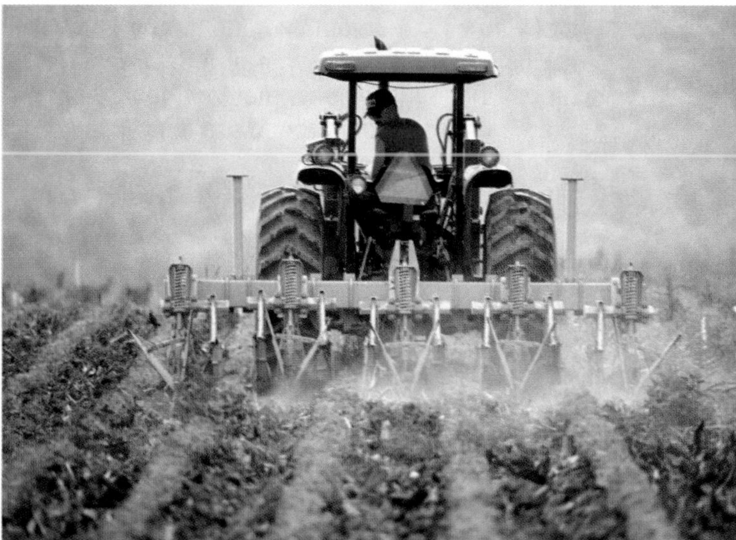

Agricultural Research Service, USDA

1-10 Farmers must use responsible techniques when planting, cultivating, and harvesting their crops in order to sustain the environment.

Two key federal agencies oversee the food supply in the United States. The ***United States Department of Agriculture (USDA)*** enforces standards for the quality and wholesomeness of meat, poultry, and eggs. The ***Food and Drug Administration (FDA)*** ensures the safety and wholesomeness of all other foods. The FDA inspects food processing plants, too. These agencies are responsible only for foods shipped across state lines. Foods sold within the state in which they are produced are controlled by state agencies.

Economics

Economics has a great effect on the food supply. A basic economic concept is the *law of supply and demand*. This means if consumers are willing to pay for a product, producers will provide it. An example of this is a food store in an ethnic neighborhood. Some people in this neighborhood will probably want to buy certain ingredients needed to make ethnic dishes. Therefore, the manager of the neighborhood store will stock these ingredients. In another neighborhood where the people are of a different ethnic group, these ingredients may not be in demand. Stores in this neighborhood are less likely to carry these items.

Consumer demand for some food products affects much more than local stores. Some foods, such as coffee, sugar, and cacao beans (used to make chocolate) are grown in faraway places. Many of the countries where these foods are grown have large populations of poor people. These people often have trouble getting enough food to feed themselves and their families. However, land that might be used to grow nourishing grains and legumes is instead used to raise crops for export. The money made from the exported crops often goes to wealthy landowners. The poor farmers who grow the crops do not earn enough to lift themselves out of poverty. In this way, food choices made by consumers in the United States can have an impact on world hunger.

Many other factors affect the problem of world hunger. People with little money cannot afford to buy quality seeds to grow hearty crops. They are not able to purchase fertilizers and pesticides that will increase the size of their harvests either. They do not own modern farm equipment. They cannot pay for training to learn more productive farming techniques. Without access to education, poor farmers may be unaware that some farming methods can harm the environment. Practicing these farming methods may lead to shrinking crop yields. All these factors work together to limit the amount of food poor people can produce.

A number of organizations are working to deal with world hunger. These organizations want to make an adequate supply of safe and nutritious food available to every person on earth. However, the hunger problem is widespread and complex. Many factors affect the degree to which hunger-relief organizations can meet their goals. See 1-11.

Healthy Living

Good nutrition is important to the healing process when you have been sick. However, if you have been vomiting, do not eat your favorite foods until you are feeling better. This will help you avoid associating these foods with illness. Such an association can make the foods less appealing to you.

This guideline is especially important for people who have chronic illnesses. Cancer patients undergoing chemotherapy and people with AIDS often lose their appetites. However, these people need to maintain healthy weights to help them fight their diseases. Keeping up the appeal of favorite foods can make this task easier.

Technology

Researchers are using the latest technology to expand the food supply. ***Technology*** is the use of knowledge to develop improved methods for doing tasks. Food scientists and technologists are applying what they know to change the composition of certain foods. They are also trying to improve crop yields and ensure the safety of foods.

Nutrient Content

Food technologists are using their expertise to affect the nutrient content of the food supply. They are developing foods that have less of some components and more of others.

For years, consumers have demanded food products that help them meet their goals for slender bodies. More recently, consumers have also become concerned about health issues linked with fat in foods. These consumer factors have created an almost endless market for food products with less sugar and fat.

Food scientists have responded to this market demand. After years of work, they have developed some widely used sugar substitutes called ***artificial sweeteners.*** These are products that sweeten foods without providing the calories of sugar. Artificial sweeteners include aspartame, acesulfame K, sucralose, and saccharin. These products are used in many sugar-free foods and beverages. They are also sold for home use.

Through much research, food scientists have developed a number of ***fat replacers.*** These are products that cut the amount of fat in foods while keeping the flavors and textures fat provides. Some fat replacers are based on carbohydrates, such as grains and starches. Others are based on proteins, such as egg whites or whey protein from milk.

Olestra is a fat replacer made from vegetable oils and sugar. Olestra has no calories because it is specially processed to pass through the body without being digested. Many fat replacers can be used in chilled products, such as salad dressings and ice cream. Some can also be used in baked goods. However, olestra is one of the few fat replacers that can be used for frying. This allows it to be used in snack foods, such as chips and crackers. Olestra has been found to cause digestive problems in some people. Olestra also keeps the body from absorbing some vitamins. To address this concern, vitamins A, D, E, and K are added to products made with olestra.

Another effort to improve the nutritional value of the food supply involves developing

Hunger-Relief Organizations

Bread for the World
50 F Street, NW
Suite 500
Washington, DC 20001
(800) 82-BREAD
www.bread.org

Heifer Project International
P.O. Box 8058
Little Rock, AR 72203
(800) 422-0474
www.heifer.org

OXFAM America
26 West Street
Boston, MA 02111-1206
(800) 77-OXFAM
www.oxfamamerica.org

United Nations International Children's Emergency Fund (UNICEF)
3 United Nations Plaza
New York, NY 10017-4414
(212) 326-7000
www.unicef.org

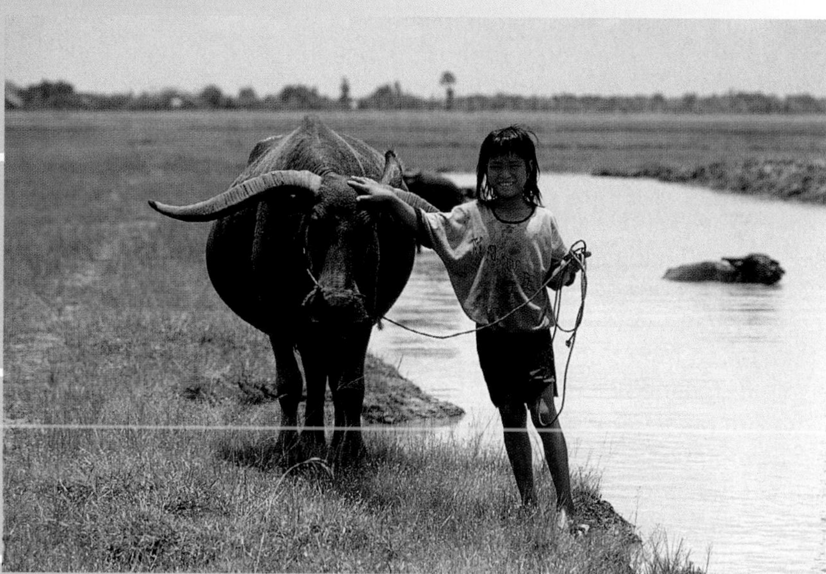

Heifer Project International

Plowing with a water buffalo from an international relief organization will allow this child's family to obtain higher crop yields. The buffalo also provides the family with nutritious milk.

1-11 Organizations such as these are actively working to find permanent solutions to hunger problems throughout the world.

Q: Can't I eat as much of a food as I want as long as it's fat free?

A: You need to choose sensible amounts of all foods and food components. Some fat free products contain extra sugar to help offset flavor and texture differences caused by the lack of fat. These foods may provide as many calories and more sugar than their full-fat counterparts.

crops that are more nutrient rich. Technology is being used to grow grains that are higher in protein. Fruits and vegetables are also being altered. Researchers are finding ways to increase the vitamin and mineral content of these foods.

Availability

Throughout the world, most of the land that can sustain crops is already being farmed. Researchers are studying ways to increase the amount of crops a given piece of land can produce. They are concerned with finding ways to feed the growing number of people on earth. They are also worried about placing added strain on the planet's limited resources.

Food technologists are developing plants that can resist diseases and pests that destroy crops. They are studying plants that grow larger and faster so more food can be produced in less time. Technologists are also growing species of plants that can withstand less favorable environments. All these efforts will help increase the food supply to better meet future needs. See 1-12.

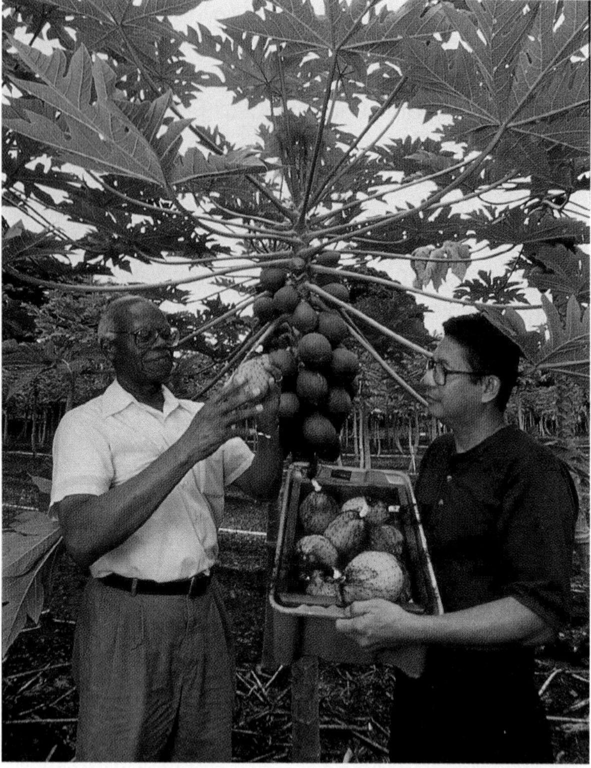

Agricultural Research Service, USDA

1-12 *These scientists are studying ways to control insects that attack papayas.*

Safety

The safety of the food supply is another issue that has attracted the interest of food technologists. Each year, millions of people get sick because of something in the food they ate. Researchers are trying to develop foods that are less likely to transmit diseases. They are working to improve packaging so foods will stay safer longer. They are also developing new preservation methods. Through these efforts, scientists hope to create a safer food supply.

Chapter 1 Review

How Food Affects Life

Summary

In prehistoric ages, people viewed food solely as a means of survival. Early peoples spent most of their time and energy hunting and gathering food. As time passed, people learned to herd and farm. As food resources became more plentiful, people could spend more time in other pursuits. With the development of a more stable food supply came the development of civilization.

You can use the decision-making process to make choices about the foods you eat. Sometimes you will choose foods to relieve hunger. However, your food choices can also affect your state of wellness.

Many factors influence the foods you eat and how you eat them. Cultural factors like national origin, religion, and holidays may affect your food choices. Social factors such as family, friends, mass media, and food product trends also have an impact. Even psychological factors like past events and emotions play a role in your food habits.

A number of factors affect the foods you can buy in the marketplace. The environment affects regional agriculture. Government agencies set guidelines and inspect facilities to be sure foods are safe and wholesome. The economic law of supply and demand directs managers to stock certain products in food stores. Technology influences the nutrient content, availability, and safety of the food supply.

Review What You Have Read

Write your answers on a separate sheet of paper.

1. How did early peoples eat food?
2. What are the five steps of the decision-making process?
3. What is the difference between hunger and appetite?
4. How can food help a person manage stress?
5. The customs and beliefs of a racial, religious, or social group form the group's _____.
6. True or false. Foods of Mexican and Spanish origin are found in the West and Southwest regions of the United States.
7. Give two examples of religious customs regarding food.
8. What are two ways in which family eating patterns differ between farm families of the past and most families today?
9. True or false. Friends can encourage people to try new foods and preparation techniques.
10. Describe two techniques advertisers use to encourage people to buy food products.
11. What are five questions to ask when reading or listening to media reports on foods and nutrition?
12. List two consumer demands that are influencing food product trends and consumer choices in the United States.
13. How can food satisfy some emotional needs of a baby?
14. How does regional agriculture affect the food supply in the United States?
15. What are two key federal agencies that oversee the food supply in the United States?
16. What are two ways researchers are working to increase the availability of the food supply?

Build Your Basic Skills

1. **History/writing.** Research the types of tools used by prehistoric people. Write a report describing some of these tools and noting which ones were used to hunt and prepare foods.
2. **Verbal.** Talk with your grandparents or senior citizens in your community about family food customs they followed as children. Discuss how their family's food customs differed from those of your family.

Build Your Thinking Skills

1. **Determine.** Make a list of all the decisions you make about food in one day. See if you can determine when you have used the steps of the decision-making process.
2. **Analyze.** Analyze food customs in your community. Make a list of cultural, social, and psychological influences that affect the foods available in local restaurants and supermarkets. Compile your list with those of your classmates to prepare a bulletin board about food customs in your community.
3. **Debate.** Participate in a class debate on the advantages and disadvantages of a technological development in the area of foods and nutrition. Conduct research to help support the arguments of your debate team.

Apply Technology

1. Work with a small group of students to write and videotape a commercial for a hypothetical food product. The ad should include nutritional claims about the product. Show your tape in class and ask your classmates to critique the advertising appeal and the information presented.
2. Use the Tufts Nutrition Navigator Web site, navigator.tufts.edu, to find an archived news report on a food or nutrition topic of interest. Evaluate the report using the questions listed on pages 23-24.

Using Workplace Skills

Heldia is a food technologist at Frozen Fresh, Inc. She is helping to develop and test a new line of high-fiber, lowfat frozen entrees. So far, the development process has been discouraging. All the entrées Heldia has tested have an off flavor.

To be an effective worker, Heldia needs skill in applying technology to specific tasks. In a small group, answer the following questions about Heldia's need for and use of this skill:

A. What questions about the frozen entrées might Heldia try to answer using her skill in applying technology?
B. How will Heldia's skill in applying technology affect Frozen Fresh, Inc.?
C. How will Heldia's skill in applying technology affect consumers?
D. What is another skill Heldia would need in this job? Briefly explain why this skill would be important.

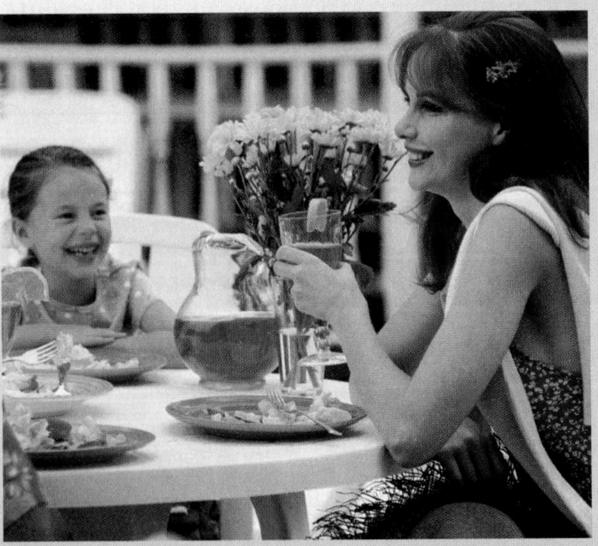

Chapter 2
Nutritional Needs

Research Dietitian
Conducts nutrition research to expand knowledge in dietetics.

Teaching Dietitian
Plans and conducts classes in nutrition and foodservice systems for dietetic interns and medical personnel.

Dietetic Technician
Provides services in assigned areas of foodservice management, teaches principles of food and nutrition, and provides dietary consultation under direction of a clinical dietitian.

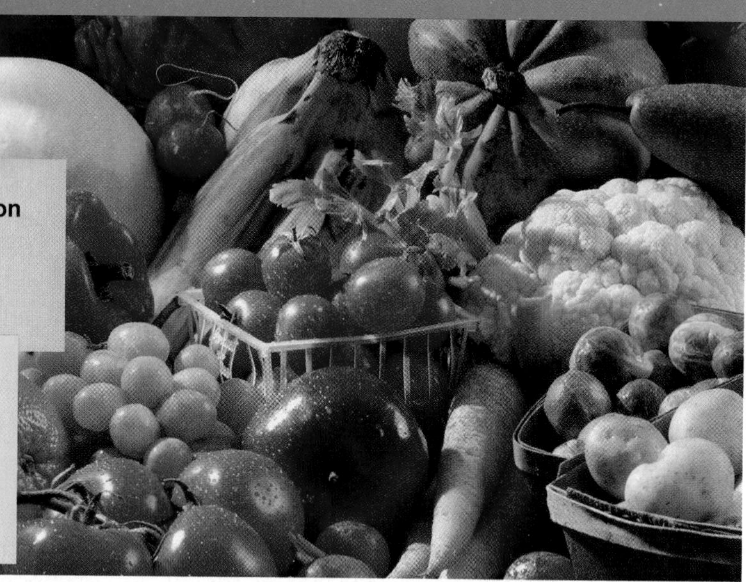

Terms to Know

nutrient
nutrition
malnutrition
deficiency disease
dietary supplement
phytochemical
fortified food
carbohydrate
glucose
fiber
fat
fatty acid
hydrogenation
trans fatty acid
cholesterol
protein
amino acid
protein-energy malnutrition (PEM)
vitamin
fat-soluble vitamin
water-soluble vitamin
night blindness
rickets
dietary antioxidant
scurvy
beriberi
pellagra
anemia
mineral
macromineral
trace element
osteoporosis
hypertension
goiter
digestion
absorption
peristalsis
saliva
metabolism

Objectives

After studying this chapter, you will be able to

- name the key nutrients, describe their functions, and list important sources of each.
- analyze the effects of various nutrient deficiencies and excesses.
- explain the processes of digestion, absorption, and metabolism.

Many people do not know what foods provide the nutrients they need for good health. A ***nutrient*** is a chemical substance in food that helps maintain the body. Children and teenagers often eat too many sweets and fats. These foods may replace breads, cereals, vegetables, fruits, and milk, which are sources of important nutrients. Adults often skip meals or fail to choose a variety of foods. These habits can keep adults from getting the full range of nutrients they need.

Nutrition is the study of how your body uses the nutrients in the foods you eat. If you do not eat the foods your body needs, you may suffer from malnutrition. ***Malnutrition,*** in its simplest form, is a lack of the right proportions of nutrients over an extended period. Besides an inadequate diet, malnutrition can be caused by the body's inability to use nutrients from foods. In either case, the body does not receive all the nutrients it needs. Energy, growth, repair, and the regulation of various body processes can all be impaired.

Eating enough food does not necessarily mean you are eating all the foods you need. The amount of food eaten is not as important as the right variety of foods. A person who is malnourished may be overweight or underweight.

Some of the effects of malnutrition may be long lasting. The foods a teenage girl eats today may affect her pregnancy in later years. The foods a pregnant woman eats may affect her unborn child's growth and development. The foods a child eats may affect his or her growth, development, and resistance to disease. Each person's health and life span may be affected by his or her food choices.

The Nutrients

You need over 50 nutrients for good health. Some of the nutrients supply energy for the body. All the nutrients help build and maintain cells and tissues. They also regulate bodily processes such as breathing. No single food supplies all the nutrients the body needs to function.

You can divide all nutrients into the following six groups: carbohydrates, fats, proteins, vitamins, minerals, and water. A diet that meets the body's needs contains nutrients from all six groups in the right proportions.

Failure to meet your nutrient needs may result in a ***deficiency disease.*** This is an illness caused by the lack of a sufficient amount of a nutrient. Different deficiency diseases are caused by the lack of different nutrients.

Dietary Supplements

In an effort to meet their nutrient needs, some people choose to take ***dietary supplements,*** 2-1. These are purified nutrients that are manufactured or extracted from natural sources. People add supplements to their diets to provide their bodies with greater amounts of nutrients than they get from foods alone.

Supplements usually come in tablet, capsule, liquid, or powder form. Some, such as vitamin C tablets, contain single nutrients. Others, like multivitamin capsules, contain a number of nutrients.

Most health experts agree the best way to get the nutrients you need is to eat a varied diet. However, some people have trouble meeting all their nutrient needs from food alone. Doctors may suggest these people take a dietary supplement to help make up for any shortages in their diets. Seek the advice of a dietitian or a physician before taking any supplements. Avoid supplements that provide large doses of single nutrients.

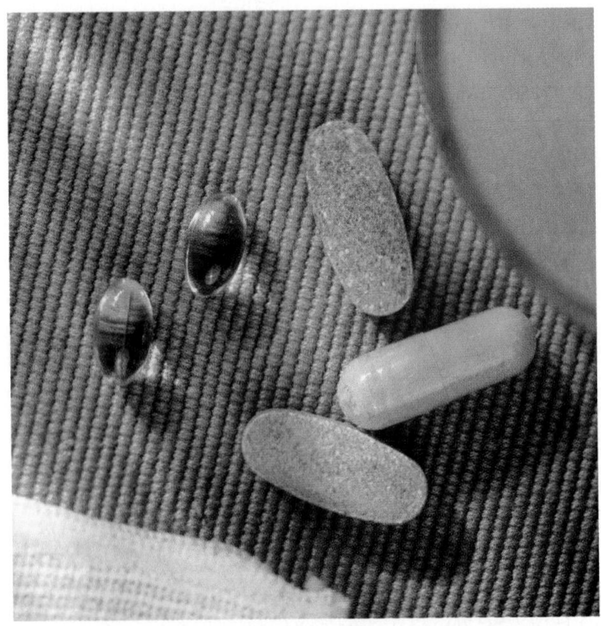

2-1 *Many people take dietary supplements to help meet the need for nutrients that may be lacking in their diets.*

Not all dietary supplements provide nutrients. Some provide nonnutrient substances. Phytochemical supplements are one example. ***Phytochemicals*** are compounds from plants that are active in the human body. They are found in fruits, vegetables, whole grains, herbs, and spices. Researchers have found some of these compounds to have a preventive effect against such diseases as heart disease and cancer.

Scientists still have much to learn about the way phytochemicals work and the health benefits they might offer. Strong evidence exists for recommending that people eat a variety of plant foods. A diet based on plant foods will provide you with a number of phytochemicals. However, most health experts recommend caution in the use of phytochemical supplements until more information is known.

A source of added nutrients in the diet aside from supplements is ***fortified foods.*** These are foods to which nutrients are added in amounts greater than what would naturally occur in the food. For instance, orange juice naturally contains very little calcium. However, calcium-fortified orange juice serves as an excellent source of this important mineral. Fortified foods give people additional options for meeting their nutrient needs through food choices.

Carbohydrates

Carbohydrates are the body's chief source of energy. Three main types of carbohydrates are important in the diet—sugars, starches, and fiber. Sugars are sometimes called *simple carbohydrates.* Starches and fiber are often called *complex carbohydrates.* Most carbohydrates come from plant foods.

Simple carbohydrates include six types of sugars. At the molecular level, glucose, fructose, and galactose are made up of single sugar units. ***Glucose*** is the form of sugar carried in the bloodstream for energy use throughout the body. Therefore, it is sometimes called blood sugar. *Fructose*, which is also known as fruit sugar, is the sweetest of all sugars. See 2-2. A third sugar is *galactose*. It is found attached to glucose to form the sugar in milk.

Sucrose, lactose, and maltose are made up of pairs of sugar units. *Sucrose* is ordinary table sugar. The milk of mammals contains lactose, or milk sugar. Grain products contain *maltose*, or malt sugar.

Complex carbohydrates are made from many glucose sugar units that are bonded together. *Starch* is the most abundant carbohydrate in the diet. It is the storage form of energy in plants. When humans digest starch, they release that energy for use by the body.

Fiber is a form of complex carbohydrates from plants that humans cannot digest. Therefore, it does not provide the body with energy like other carbohydrates. Fiber provides bulk in the diet and promotes normal bowel function.

Functions of Carbohydrates

Carbohydrates have many important functions in the body. They furnish the body with energy. They help the body digest fats efficiently. They also allow the body to use

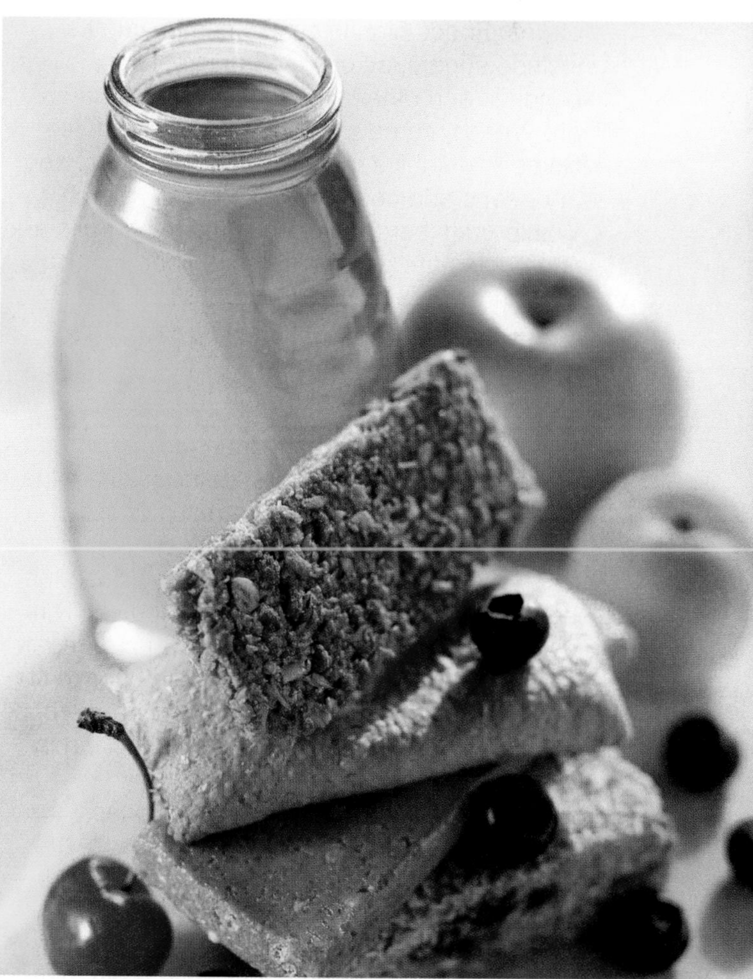

National Honey Board

2-2 Honey and fruit are good sources of fructose, the sweetest of all sugars.

proteins for growth and maintenance instead of energy.

Functions performed by fiber are linked to the prevention of heart disease and some types of cancer. Fiber binds to a compound made from cholesterol and carries it out of the body. This helps lower blood cholesterol levels, which reduces the risk of heart disease. Fiber stimulates the action of the muscles in the digestive tract, helping speed food through the body. The bulk created by fiber may also help dilute *carcinogens* (cancer-causing agents) in food. Experts believe these functions may help reduce the risks of cancer. Therefore, experts advise men through age 50 to consume 38 grams of fiber each day. They advise women to consume 25 grams daily. Recommended intakes drop a bit for older adults.

Sources of Carbohydrates

Many foods are rich sources of carbohydrates. Foods high in simple carbohydrates include sugars, syrups, soft drinks, jams, jellies, candies, and other sweets. Sources of starch are breads, cereals, pasta products, and rice. Some vegetables, such as corn, potatoes, and dry beans and peas, are also high in starch. Whole grain cereal products and fresh fruits and vegetables are good sources of fiber.

Carbohydrate Deficiencies and Excesses

Foods high in carbohydrates are abundant and inexpensive. Therefore, deficiencies in the United States are usually the result of self-prescribed limitations.

A diet low in carbohydrates may cause the body to use protein as an energy source. This can interfere with the normal growth and repair of body tissues. It can also create a chemical imbalance in the body that could be dangerous if it is allowed to continue. If fiber is lacking in the diet, constipation may occur.

Food energy is measured in *calories*. Nutrition experts recommend that most of the calories in your diet come from complex carbohydrates, especially those high in fiber, 2-3. They also recommend limiting the number of calories consumed from fat. Eating a diet high in whole grain breads and cereals will accomplish both goals. These foods are fiber-rich sources of complex carbohydrates. By consuming more calories from these foods, you may consume fewer calories from foods high in fat.

Too many simple carbohydrates in the diet can be a health concern. Foods high in sugars, such as candy and soft drinks, tend to be low in other nutrients. Eating simple carbohydrates in place of other foods may deprive the body of needed nutrients. Eating too many simple carbohydrates in addition to other foods increases the risk of unhealthful weight gain.

Bacteria in the mouth thrive on both types of carbohydrates. As these bacteria grow, they produce acid. This acid can erode teeth, causing tooth decay and gum disease. To help avoid these problems, dentists recommend limiting carbohydrate foods between meals. They also suggest brushing teeth after eating, flossing daily, and getting regular dental checkups.

Q: Does eating too much sugar cause diabetes?

A: People who have diabetes have to monitor their intakes of sugar and all carbohydrates. However, eating sugar does not cause diabetes.

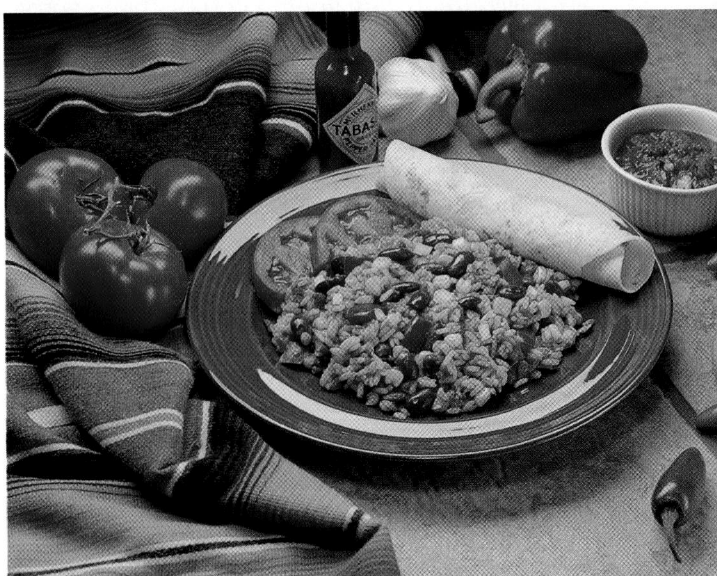

USA Dry Pea & Lentil Council

2-3 *Lentils, beans, and corn are low in fats and high in complex carbohydrates, including fiber.*

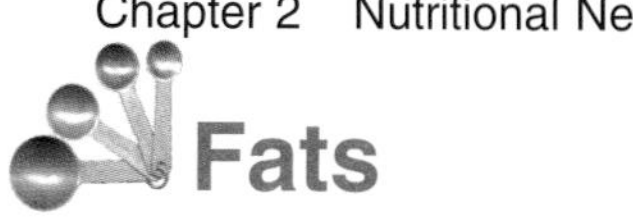

Fats

Like carbohydrates, ***fats*** are important energy sources. Fats belong to a larger group of compounds called *lipids*, which include both fats and oils.

Types of Fats

All lipids contain fatty acids. ***Fatty acids*** are chemical chains that contain carbon, hydrogen, and oxygen atoms. Different types of fatty acids contain different amounts of hydrogen atoms. *Saturated fatty acids* are fatty acids that have as many hydrogen atoms as they can hold. *Unsaturated fatty acids* are fatty acids that have fewer hydrogen atoms than they can hold. Unsaturated fatty acids may be monounsaturated or polyunsaturated. *Monounsaturated fatty acids* are missing one hydrogen atom. *Polyunsaturated fatty acids* are missing two or more hydrogen atoms.

Fats and oils in foods contain mixtures of the three types of fatty acids. However, most fats and oils contain more of one type than the other two types. The fats in meat and dairy products are high in saturated fatty acids. Palm, palm kernel, and coconut oils are also high in saturated fatty acids. Olive and canola oils are good sources of monounsaturated fatty acids. Safflower, corn, soybean, and some fish oils are rich in polyunsaturated fatty acids.

Most fats that are high in saturated fatty acids are solid at room temperature. Most oils that are high in unsaturated fatty acids are liquid at room temperature. A process called ***hydrogenation*** adds hydrogen atoms to unsaturated fatty acids in liquid oils. This turns the liquid oils into more highly saturated solid fats. Most vegetable shortening and stick margarine are made from hydrogenated oils. When oils are partly hydrogenated, **trans *fatty acids*** are created. These are fatty acids with odd molecular shapes. Research suggests the shapes of these fatty acids may create a health concern when they are in the body.

Be a Clever Consumer

When buying oil for cooking, baking, and pouring on salads, choose olive, canola, peanut, sesame, corn, soybean, or safflower oils. Studies show these oils, which are high in monounsaturated or polyunsaturated fatty acids, help reduce cholesterol levels in the blood. However, you should limit your use of even these oils to no more than 8 teaspoons (40 mL) per day.

Cholesterol

Cholesterol is a fatlike substance found in every cell in the body. Cholesterol serves several important functions. It is part of skin tissue. It aids in the transport of fatty acids in the body. The body also needs it to produce hormones.

You need to be aware that health and nutrition experts refer to two types of cholesterol. You consume *dietary cholesterol* when you eat certain foods. It occurs only in foods of animal origin, 2-4. Plant foods do not contain dietary cholesterol. Liver and egg yolks are especially high in dietary cholesterol.

Blood cholesterol circulates through your body in your bloodstream. Your doctor can check your blood cholesterol level. A high blood cholesterol level is a risk factor for heart disease.

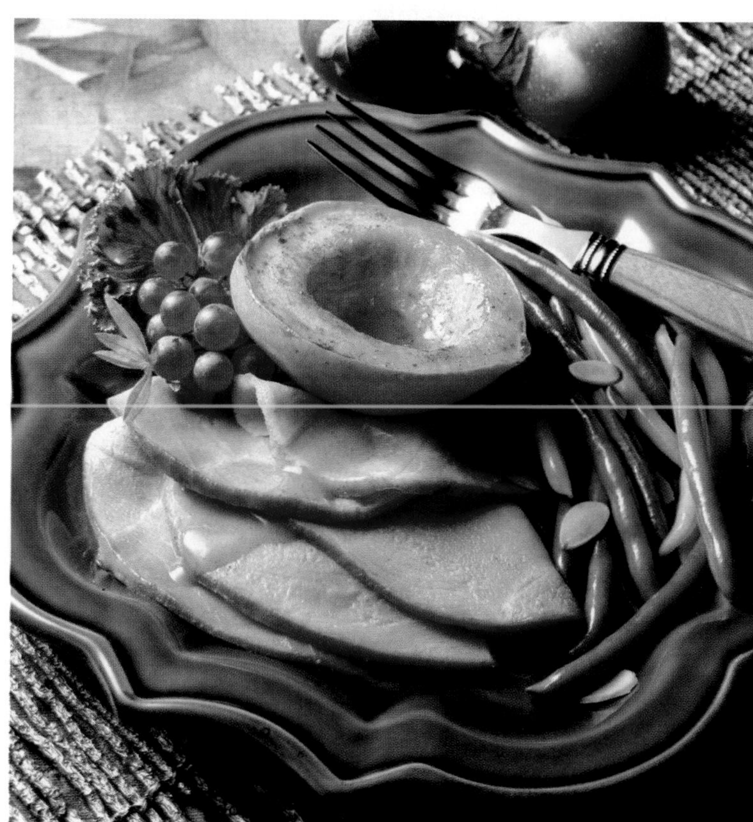

courtesy of National Pork Board

2-4 *Foods like ham that come from animal sources provide dietary cholesterol.*

Doctors urge people to take steps to keep their blood cholesterol levels within a safe range. However, cholesterol in the diet has only a small effect on cholesterol in the blood. A later section describes other factors that have a greater impact on blood cholesterol.

You should note that your body makes the cholesterol it needs. Therefore, you do not need to include cholesterol in your diet.

Functions of Fats

Fats in the diet serve a number of important roles. They provide a source of energy. They carry certain vitamins. Fats also carry flavor substances that make food taste good. They make foods such as meats and baked goods tender, which makes these foods more appealing. Fats help you feel full after eating, too.

Your body needs various fatty acids to make other important compounds, such as hormones. The body can produce some of the fatty acids it needs. However, there are a few fatty acids the body cannot produce. These are called *essential fatty acids*. You must obtain these fatty acids from the foods you eat.

Fats have many other important functions in the body. The body stores energy in fatty tissues. Besides serving as energy reserves, these tissues form cushions that help protect internal organs from injury. Fat under your skin forms a layer of insulation that helps maintain your body temperature. Fats are also part of the membrane that surrounds every cell in the body.

Sources of Fats

Fats can be visible or invisible. You can see butter, margarine, and fat on meat and in chicken and turkey skin. These are *visible fats*. You cannot see fat in foods like eggs, whipped cream, and baked products. These are *invisible fats*. See 2-5.

Many foods contain some fat. Foods that are high in fat include butter, margarine, most salad dressings, oils, and vegetable shortenings. Egg yolks, many dairy products, meats, and avocados are also significant sources of fat.

Fat Deficiencies

Fat deficiencies are rare in the United States. However, a diet too low in fat may result in a loss of weight and energy. Also, too little fat may cause deficiencies of the fatty acids and fat-soluble vitamins carried by fats.

Limiting Excess Fats and Cholesterol

The typical diet in the United States is high in fat. A high-fat diet can contribute to weight problems. This is because fat is a concentrated source of food energy. Fat provides more than twice as many calories per gram as carbohydrates and proteins. Therefore, a diet that is high in fat may also be high in calories. Your body burns calories for the energy needed for movement and the maintenance of body processes. However, if your diet provides more fat or calories than your body needs, your body will store the excess as fat tissue.

Experts recommend no more than 35 percent of the calories in your daily diet should come from fat. No more than 10 percent of total calories should come from saturated fat. You should limit your daily cholesterol intake to 300 mg.

These recommendations are based on more than possible weight problems. Saturated fats and, to a lesser extent, dietary cholesterol can

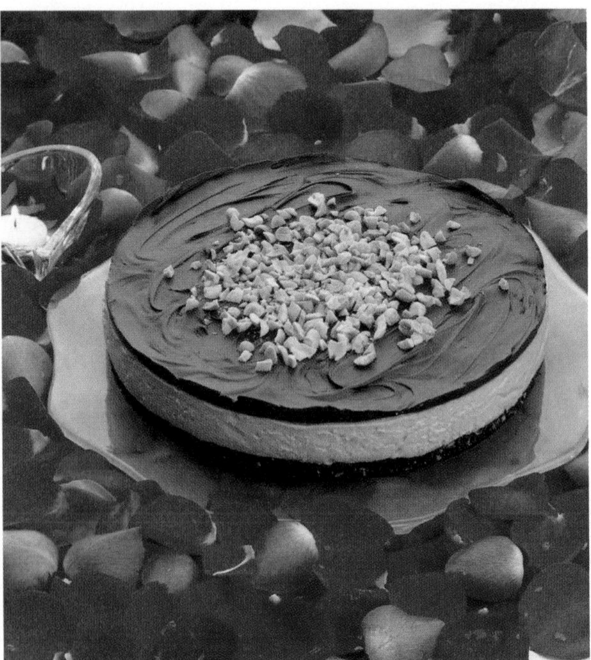

National Peanut Board

***2-5** This rich mousse cake contains whipping cream, peanut butter, cream cheese, and chocolate. These ingredients make the cake high in fat, even though it cannot be seen.*

increase the blood cholesterol level. Another type of fat that raises blood cholesterol is the *trans* fat found in partially hydrogenated vegetable oils. High blood cholesterol is one of several risk factors for heart disease. High-fat diets have also been linked to increased risk of several types of cancer.

Choosing a diet moderate in total fat means eating a variety of fruits, vegetables, legumes, and grain products. You should opt for lean meats, skinless poultry, and fish as well as lowfat and fat free dairy products. For a diet low in saturated fats, limit high-fat meat and full-fat dairy products. Choose fats and oils that have less than 2 grams of saturated fat per serving. Liquid and tub margarine and olive and canola oils meet this guideline. To reduce *trans* fat in your diet, limit foods that list partially hydrogenated oils on their ingredient lists. Such foods include many stick margarines, cookies, chips, and crackers. Commercially fried foods, such as French fries and doughnuts, are also usually fried in these types of oils. To keep dietary cholesterol in check, limit egg yolks and cook with vegetable oil instead of animal fat.

Proteins

Proteins are chemical compounds that are found in every body cell. They are made up of small units called ***amino acids.*** Scientists have found 20 amino acids that are important to the human body. Nine of these amino acids are called *essential amino acids*. The body cannot make some essential amino acids. It can make others, but not at a rate fast enough to meet nutritional needs. Therefore, you must get the essential amino acids from the foods you eat. The other 11 amino acids are called *nonessential amino acids*. You do not have to get these amino acids from foods because your body can make them fast enough to meet its needs.

Animal foods and soybeans have *complete proteins,* 2-6. These proteins contain all nine essential amino acids. Complete proteins will support growth and normal maintenance of body tissues. Most plant foods have *incomplete proteins*. These proteins are missing one or more of the essential amino acids. Incomplete proteins will neither support growth nor provide for normal maintenance.

Incomplete proteins can complement one another. In other words, you can supplement a protein food lacking an amino acid with a protein food containing that amino acid. When combined, the two foods provide a higher quality protein than either would have provided alone. The two foods do not have to be eaten together. They must simply be part of a nutritious diet consumed throughout the day. The proteins in dry beans and grains generally complement each other in this way. Red beans and rice is an example of this combination.

Functions of Proteins

Your body needs amino acids from proteins for growth, maintenance, and repair of tissues. Proteins aid in the formation of enzymes, some hormones, and antibodies. Proteins also provide energy. (Your diet needs to supply enough carbohydrates and fats to meet your energy needs. Otherwise, your body will use proteins for energy before using them to support growth and maintenance.) Regulation of bodily processes, such as fluid balance in the cells, is also a function of proteins.

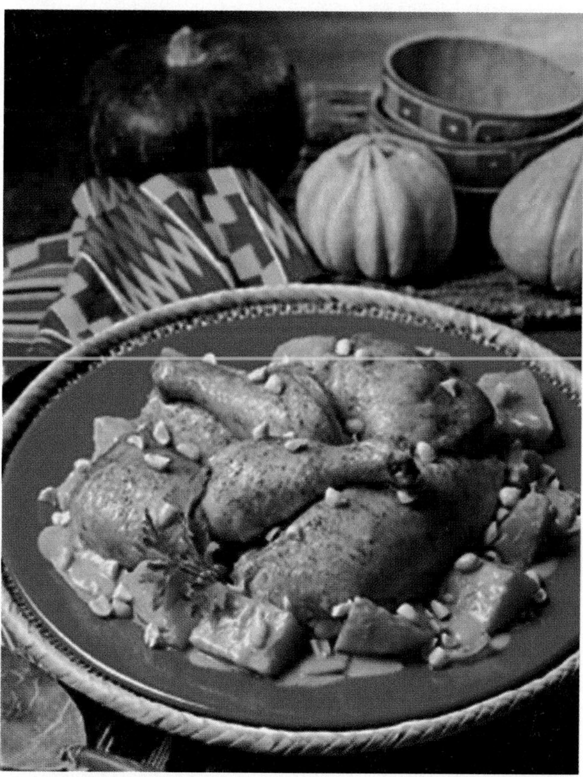

National Chicken Council

2-6 *Meats and other foods of animal origin provide complete proteins.*

Several factors affect a person's need for protein. Age, body size, quality of the proteins, and physical state are four important factors. Children need more protein per pound of body weight than adults because they are growing so rapidly. A larger, heavier person needs more protein than a smaller, lighter person. An injured person needs extra protein for the repair of body tissues.

Sources of Protein

Many animal and plant foods provide proteins. Important protein sources are lean meats, poultry, fish, milk, cheese, and eggs. Dried beans, peas, and nuts are also protein sources. Grain products and vegetables provide smaller amounts of protein.

Protein Deficiencies and Excesses

If the diet does not contain enough protein and calories, a condition called ***protein-energy malnutrition (PEM)*** may result. In adults, symptoms of this condition include fatigue and weight loss. In children, this condition can lead to diarrhea, infections, and stunted growth. PEM is common in many underdeveloped areas of the world. However, even wealthy nations have hungry people who are affected by PEM. People who fail to get enough food for reasons such as drug addictions or eating disorders may also suffer from PEM.

If the diet contains too much protein, the body converts the extra protein to fat and stores it in the fat tissue. The body cannot convert stored protein back into amino acids for use in building tissues. Eating nutritious foods at meals throughout the day will maintain your body's supply of amino acids. See 2-7.

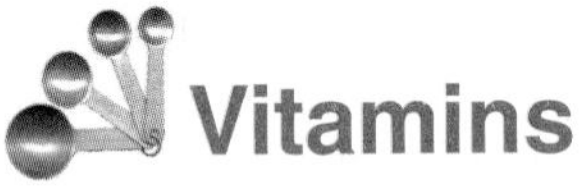

Vitamins

Vitamins are complex organic substances. You need them in small amounts for normal growth, maintenance, and reproduction. Your

Energy Nutrients		
Nutrient	**Functions**	**Sources**
Carbohydrates	Supply energy Provide bulk in the form of cellulose (needed for digestion) Help the body digest fats efficiently Spare proteins so they can be used for growth and regulation	Sugar: Honey, jam, jelly, molasses, sugar Fiber: Fresh fruits and vegetables, whole grain breads and cereals Starch: Beans, breads, cereals, corn, pasta, peas, potatoes, rice
Fats	Supply energy Carry fat-soluble vitamins Insulate the body from shock and temperature changes Protect vital organs Add flavor and satisfying quality to foods Serve as a source of essential fatty acids	Bacon, butter, cheese, chocolate, cream, dressings, egg yolks, marbling in meats, margarine, nuts, olives, salad oils
Proteins	Build and repair tissues Help make antibodies, enzymes, hormones, and some vitamins Regulate fluid balance in the cells and other body processes Supply energy, when needed	Complete proteins: Eggs, fish, meat, milk and other dairy products, poultry Incomplete proteins: Cereals, grains, legumes, lentils, peanut butter, peanuts

***2-7** Carbohydrates, fats, and proteins all supply energy in the diet.*

body cannot produce most vitamins, at least not in large enough amounts to meet your nutritional needs. The best way to get all the vitamins you need is to eat a nutritious diet.

Vitamins are either fat-soluble or water-soluble. ***Fat-soluble vitamins*** dissolve in fats. They are carried by the fats in foods and can be stored in the fatty tissues of the body. Over time, fat-soluble vitamins can build up in the body and may reach dangerous levels. ***Water-soluble vitamins*** dissolve in water. The body does not store them to any great extent. Instead, excess water-soluble vitamins are carried out of the body in the urine.

Although the body does not store large amounts of water-soluble vitamins, consuming large quantities may still be harmful. You are not likely to get harmful quantities of fat- or water-soluble vitamins from the foods you eat. However, taking large doses of vitamin supplements could put you at risk of developing symptoms of *toxicity,* or poisoning.

Vitamins A, D, E, and K are the fat-soluble vitamins. Vitamin C and the B-complex vitamins are water-soluble.

Vitamin A

The body uses vitamin A to make a chemical compound the eyes need to adapt to darkness. Vitamin A promotes normal growth (especially of bones and teeth). The health of tissues such as skin and mucous membranes also depends on the presence of vitamin A.

Sources of Vitamin A

Your body obtains vitamin A in two forms. The first form is the vitamin itself. Vitamin A is in foods like liver, egg yolk, whole milk and fortified dairy products, butter, and fish oils.

The second form of vitamin A is *beta-carotene.* This is a *provitamin,* which is a substance the body can convert into a vitamin. Beta-carotene is in plant foods. Deeper color indicates the presence of more beta-carotene. Therefore, deep yellow and dark green fruits and vegetables normally have a higher vitamin A value than lighter colored produce.

Vitamin A Deficiencies and Excesses

If the diet contains too little vitamin A, the eyes will become sensitive to light. They may develop ***night blindness,*** which is a reduced ability to see in dim light. The skin will become rough, and susceptibility to disease may increase. In severe cases, stunted growth may result.

People seldom get too much vitamin A from food. However, if they take too many vitamin A supplements, fatigue, headaches, nausea, and vomiting may eventually occur.

Q: Will high intakes of vitamin A supplements cure acne?

A: A medicine derived from vitamin A is often prescribed to treat acne. However, high intakes of vitamin A supplements have not been proven to prevent or cure acne. In fact, large doses of vitamin A from supplements can be toxic.

Vitamin D

The major function of vitamin D is to promote the growth and proper mineralization of bones and teeth. Vitamin D performs this function by helping the body use the minerals calcium and phosphorus.

Sources of Vitamin D

Vitamin D occurs naturally in a few foods. These include eggs, liver, and fatty fish. In addition, vitamin D is added to most milk as well as some cereals and margarine, 2-8.

The body can also make vitamin D with exposure to sunlight. Thus, some people call vitamin D the "sunshine vitamin." Sunlight helps convert a substance found in the skin to vitamin D. Advanced age, darker skin color, sunscreen, heavy clothing, and smog all decrease the production of vitamin D in the skin.

Sun exposure is linked to about 30 percent of all cancers. However, you do not have to be in the sun for long periods to manufacture vitamin D. Therefore, you should follow advice for using sunscreens, wearing protective clothes, and avoiding dangerous exposure times. Most people who drink milk and enjoy normal outdoor activities will get enough vitamin D to meet their needs.

Vitamin D Deficiencies and Excesses

If the diet does not contain enough vitamin D, the body will not be able to use calcium and phosphorus as it should. In severe cases, children with vitamin D deficiencies can develop a disease called ***rickets.*** Symptoms of rickets include crooked legs and misshapen breastbones. Adults may develop other bone abnormalities.

If the diet contains too much vitamin D, the body will store the excess. Over an extended period, excesses of vitamin D may result in nausea, diarrhea, and loss of weight. In severe cases, kidneys and lungs may be damaged, and bones may become deformed.

Vitamin E

In humans, vitamin E functions mainly as a ***dietary antioxidant.*** This is a substance in foods that significantly reduces the harmful effects of oxygen on normal body functions. Some cells in the body, such as cells in the lungs, are constantly exposed to high levels of oxygen. Oxygen can destroy the membranes of these cells. When vitamin E is present, however, it combines with the oxygen before the oxygen can react with and harm the cells. Vitamin E also keeps oxygen from reacting with red and white blood cells, fatty acids, carotene, and vitamin A. Cell damage and substance breakdown due to oxygen exposure has been linked to several diseases, including heart disease and cancer.

Sources of Vitamin E

Vitamin E is widely distributed throughout the food supply. Sources include fats and oils, whole grain breads and cereals, liver, eggs, whole milk dairy foods, and leafy green vegetables.

Vitamin E Deficiencies and Excesses

The average diet in the United States supplies sufficient amounts of vitamin E. Therefore, deficiencies are rare. However, premature infants may have deficiencies. Babies that do not reach full term fail to receive enough vitamin E from their mothers before birth. Toxicity from excess dietary vitamin E also seems to be rare. However, people who take

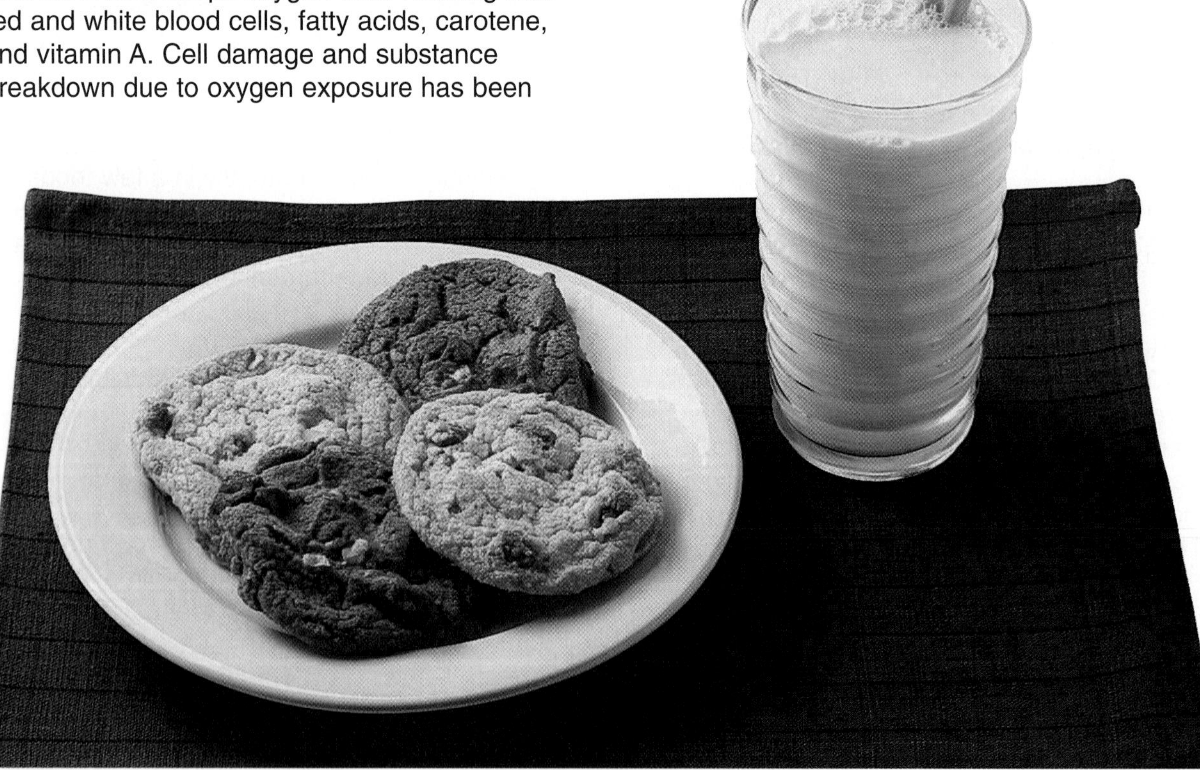

Used by permission of Dean Foods Company

2-8 *Fortified milk is a key source of vitamin D for many people.*

large doses of vitamin E supplements are at increased risk of hemorrhage.

Vitamin K

Vitamin K is known as the blood-clotting vitamin. Vitamin K performs this function by helping the liver make a substance called *prothrombin*. Prothrombin is a protein blood needs to clot. If vitamin K is not available, the liver cannot form prothrombin and other similar substances. As a result, the blood cannot clot properly.

Sources of Vitamin K

Bacteria in the human intestinal tract can make vitamin K. Leafy green vegetables and cauliflower are good dietary sources of vitamin K. Additional sources include other vegetables, organ meats, and egg yolk.

Vitamin K Deficiencies and Excesses

Because vitamin K is in many well-liked foods, most people receive enough vitamin K from the foods they eat. In cases where vitamin K deficiency is severe, however, hemorrhaging can occur due to lack of blood clotting.

The amount of vitamin K consumed in a normal diet is not harmful. However, toxicity can develop through the use of vitamin K supplements. See 2-9.

Vitamin C

Vitamin C, which is also known as ascorbic acid, performs many important functions in the body. It helps in the formation and maintenance of *collagen*, a protein that is part of connective tissue. Collagen is the cementing material that holds body cells together. Vitamin C helps make the walls of blood vessels firm, and it helps wounds heal and broken bones mend. It aids in the formation of hemoglobin (a substance in red blood cells) and helps the body fight infections. It also functions as a dietary antioxidant.

Sources of Vitamin C

Fresh fruits and vegetables are the best sources of vitamin C in the diet. Citrus fruits, strawberries, and cantaloupe are good fruit sources of vitamin C. Leafy green vegetables, green peppers, broccoli, and cabbage are good vegetable sources.

Vitamin C Deficiencies and Excesses

Because vitamin C is a water-soluble vitamin, the body cannot readily store it. Therefore, you need a daily supply. People who smoke face increased oxygen damage in the body and thus need extra vitamin C for its antioxidant effects. Too little vitamin C in the diet can cause poor appetite, weakness, bruising, and soreness in the joints. A

Fat-Soluble Vitamins		
Nutrient	**Functions**	**Sources**
Vitamin A	Helps keep skin clear and smooth and mucus membranes healthy Helps prevent night blindness Helps promote growth	Butter, Cheddar-type cheese, dark green and yellow fruits and vegetables, egg yolk, fortified margarine, liver, whole and fortified milk
Vitamin D	Helps build strong bones and teeth in children Helps maintain bones in adults	Egg yolk; fish liver oils; fortified butter, margarine, and milk; liver; sardines; tuna; the sun
Vitamin E	Acts as an antioxidant that protects cell membranes of cells exposed to high concentrations of oxygen	Eggs; leafy green vegetables; liver and other variety meats; salad oils; shortening, and other fats and oils; whole grain cereals
Vitamin K	Helps blood clot	Cauliflower, leafy green vegetables, and other vegetables; egg yolk; organ meats

2-9 *The fat-soluble vitamins can be stored in the body.*

prolonged deficiency may result in a disease called ***scurvy.*** Symptoms of this disease include weakness, bleeding gums, tooth loss, and internal bleeding.

Vitamin C does help the body fight infection. However, scientists do not agree it will prevent or cure the common cold. Avoid taking vitamin C supplements unless directed to do so by a physician. Excess vitamin C may cause nausea, cramps, and diarrhea.

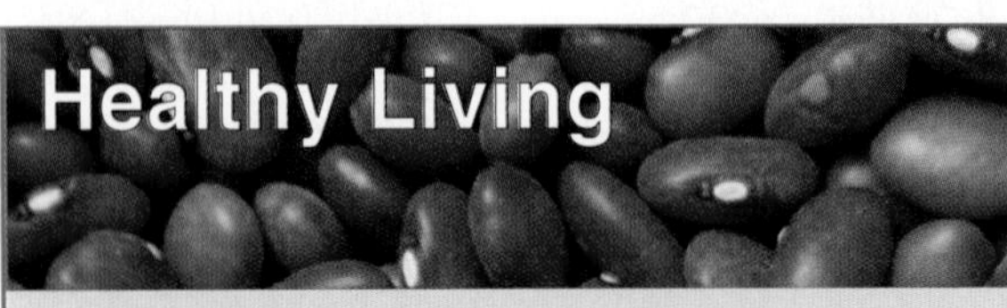

Cooking foods in water can cause a loss of water-soluble vitamins. To preserve the vitamin value of foods, use only a small amount of cooking water. Also, keep the cooking time as short as possible. You can preserve the vitamins lost in cooking liquid by using the cooking liquid in gravies, sauces, and soups.

Thiamin

Thiamin, or vitamin B_1, is part of a larger group of vitamins called the *B-complex vitamins.* All the B-complex vitamins are water-soluble. Each B vitamin has distinct properties. However, they work together in the body.

Thiamin helps the body release energy from food. It forms part of the coenzymes needed for the breakdown of carbohydrates. (*Coenzymes* are chemical substances that work with enzymes to promote enzyme activity.) Thiamin helps promote normal appetite and digestion. It also helps keep the nervous system healthy and prevent irritability.

Sources of Thiamin

Nearly all foods except fats, oils, and refined sugars contain some thiamin. However, no single food is particularly high in this vitamin. Wheat germ, pork products, legumes, and whole grain and enriched cereals are good sources of thiamin, 2-10.

Thiamin Deficiencies

Too little thiamin in the diet will first cause nausea, apathy, and loss of appetite. A severe thiamin deficiency can result in a disease of the nervous system called ***beriberi.*** It begins with numbness in the feet and ankles followed by cramping pains in the legs. The next stage is leg stiffness. If the deficiency is prolonged, paralysis and potentially fatal heart disturbances may result.

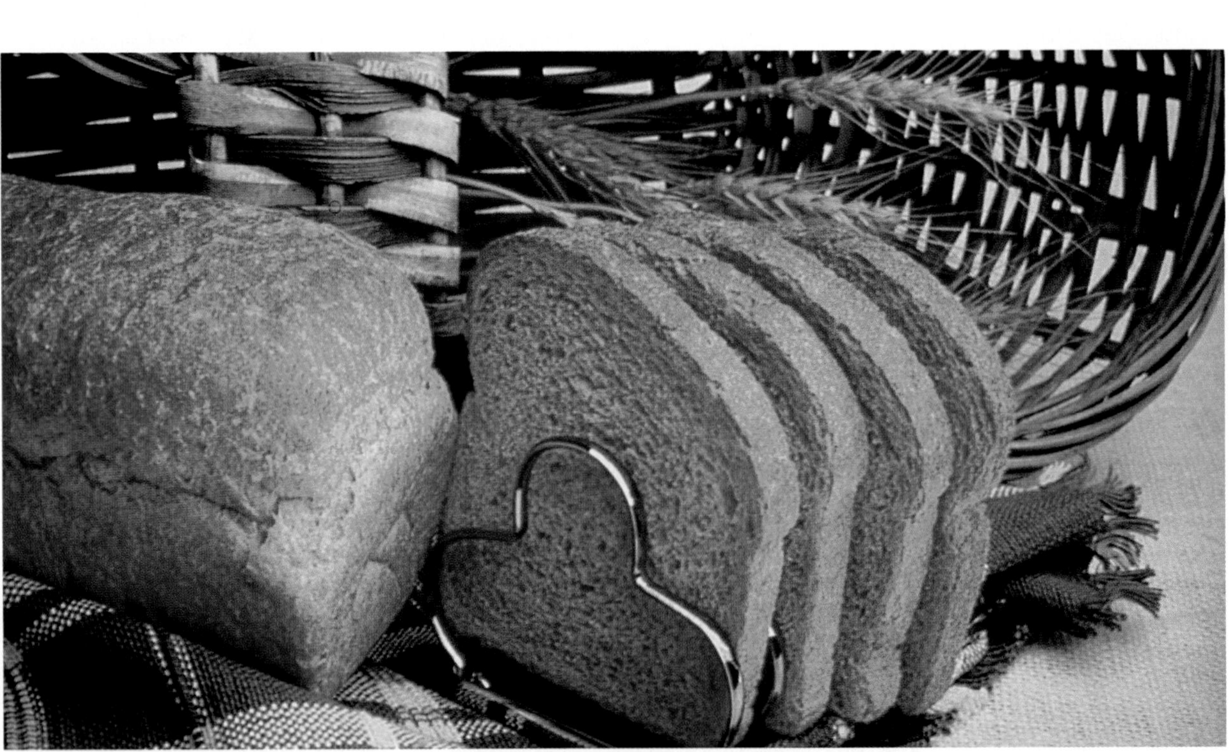

Wheat Foods Council

2-10 *Whole grain breads are good sources of many nutrients, including thiamin.*

Riboflavin

Riboflavin, or vitamin B_2, is the second member of the B-complex group. Riboflavin forms part of the coenzymes needed for the breakdown of carbohydrates. It helps cells use oxygen and helps keep skin, tongue, and lips normal. Helping to prevent scaly, greasy areas around the mouth and nose is also a function of riboflavin.

Sources of Riboflavin

Organ meats, milk and milk products, eggs, and oysters are good sources of riboflavin. Leafy green vegetables and whole grain and enriched cereal products are good sources, too.

Riboflavin Deficiencies

Too little riboflavin in the diet can cause swollen and cracked lips and skin lesions. Later symptoms include inflammation of the eyes and twilight blindness.

Niacin

Niacin forms part of two coenzymes involved in complex chemical reactions in the body. It helps keep the nervous system, mouth, skin, tongue, and digestive tract healthy. Niacin also helps the cells use other nutrients.

Sources of Niacin

The most common sources of niacin include muscle meats, poultry, peanuts, and peanut butter, 2-11. The body can convert *tryptophan*, one of the essential amino acids, into niacin. Milk contains large amounts of tryptophan.

Niacin Deficiencies

Too little niacin in the diet can cause a disease called ***pellagra.*** Skin lesions and digestive problems are the first symptoms. Mental disorders and death may follow if the disease goes untreated. Pellagra normally occurs only when the diet is limited to just a few foods that are not good sources of niacin.

Vitamin B_6

Vitamin B_6 helps nerve tissues function normally and plays a role in the regeneration of red blood cells. It takes part in the breakdown of proteins, carbohydrates, and fats. Vitamin B_6 also plays a role in the reaction that changes tryptophan into niacin.

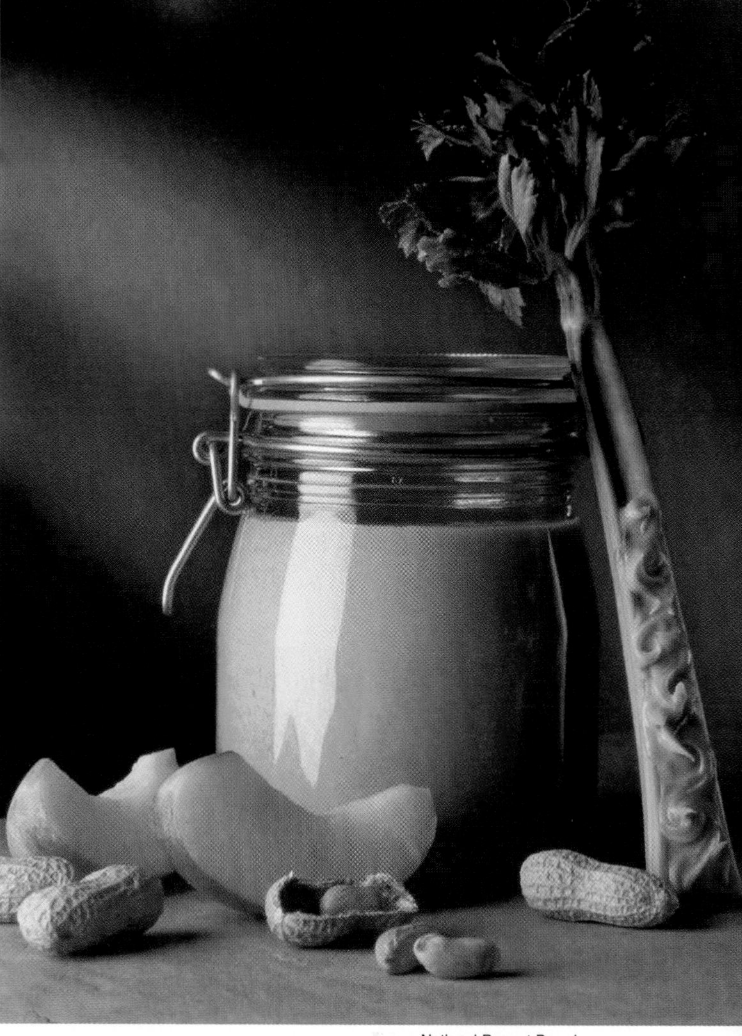

National Peanut Board

2-11 *Peanuts and peanut butter provide niacin.*

Sources of Vitamin B_6

Vitamin B_6 is in many plant and animal foods. The best sources of this vitamin are muscle meats, liver, vegetables, and whole grain cereals.

Vitamin B_6 Deficiencies

Vitamin B_6 is in so many foods that a deficiency rarely occurs naturally. In cases of prolonged fasting, however, a B_6 deficiency can occur. Skin lesions, soreness of the mouth, and a smooth red tongue can develop. In advanced cases, nausea, vomiting, weight loss, irritability, and convulsive seizures may result.

Folate

Folate is another B-complex vitamin. It helps the body produce normal blood cells. It plays a role in biochemical reactions in cells that convert food into energy. Folate is especially important in the diets of pregnant women. It has been shown to help prevent damage to the brain and spinal cord of unborn babies.

Sources of Folate

Food sources of folate include broccoli, asparagus, leafy green vegetables, and dry beans and peas. Liver, yogurt, strawberries, bananas, oranges, and whole grain cereals are good sources, too, 2-12. Most enriched bread and cereal products, including flour, pasta, and rice, are fortified with a form of folate.

Folate Deficiencies

A poor diet, impaired absorption, or an unusual need by body tissues may cause folate deficiencies. Symptoms of folate deficiency include inflammation of the tongue and digestive disorders, such as diarrhea. Folate deficiency can also result in two types of ***anemia.*** This is a condition that reduces the number of red blood cells in the bloodstream. This decreases the amount of oxygen the blood can carry. Symptoms of anemia include weakness and fatigue. People often associate anemia with a deficiency of iron. However, deficiencies of several vitamins and minerals can lead to various types of anemia.

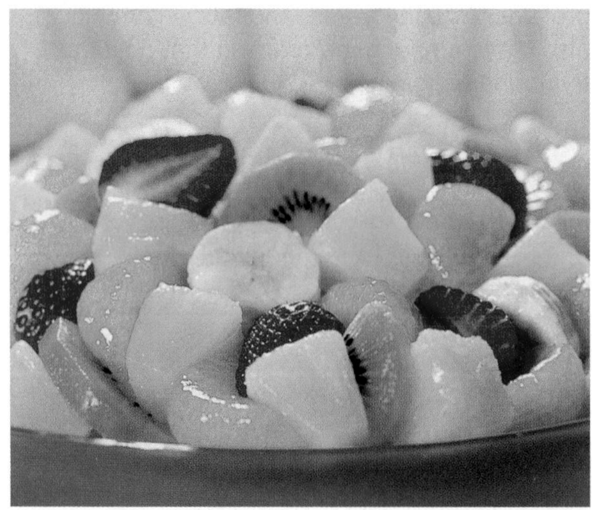

Dole Food Company

2-12 *This fruit salad is a good choice for meeting folate needs. Strawberries, bananas, and oranges are all good sources.*

Vitamin B_{12}

Vitamin B_{12} promotes normal growth. It also plays a role in the normal functioning of cells in the bone marrow, nervous system, and intestines.

Sources of Vitamin B_{12}

Vitamin B_{12} is in animal protein foods and brewer's yeast. Many cereals and breakfast foods are also fortified with this vitamin. A nutritious diet that includes animal foods should supply enough vitamin B_{12}. However, plant foods do not provide vitamin B_{12}. Therefore, strict vegetarians need to eat fortified foods or take a supplement to avoid a deficiency.

Vitamin B_{12} Deficiencies

In simple cases of vitamin B_{12} deficiency, a sore tongue, weakness, loss of weight, apathy, and nervous disorders may result. In extreme cases, *pernicious anemia* can develop. This is a chronic disease typified by abnormally large red blood cells. It also disturbs the nervous system, causing depression and drowsiness. Pernicious anemia can be fatal unless treated.

Pantothenic Acid

Pantothenic acid is part of the B-complex group of vitamins. Its main function is as a part of coenzyme A. The body needs coenzyme A to use the energy nutrients. Pantothenic acid also promotes growth and helps the body make cholesterol.

Sources of Pantothenic Acid

Pantothenic acid is in all plant and animal tissues. Organ meats, yeast, egg yolk, bran, wheat germ, and dry beans are among the best sources of pantothenic acid. Milk is also a good source.

Pantothenic Acid Deficiencies

Pantothenic acid is in so many foods that deficiencies are rare. In cases where a deficiency does exist, symptoms include vomiting, sleeplessness, and fatigue.

Biotin

Of all the B-complex vitamins, biotin is one of the least well known. However, it is as essential in the diet as the other B vitamins. The body needs biotin for the breakdown of fats, carbohydrates, and proteins. It is also an essential part of several enzymes.

Sources of Biotin

Biotin is in both plant and animal foods. Kidney and liver are the richest sources of biotin. Chicken, eggs, milk, most fresh vegetables, and some fruits are also good sources.

Biotin Deficiencies

Because biotin is in most foods, deficiencies are rare. Symptoms of a biotin deficiency are scaly skin, mild depression, fatigue, muscular pain, and nausea. See 2-13.

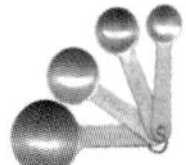

Minerals

Carbohydrates, fats, proteins, and water make up about 96 percent of your body weight. ***Minerals*** are inorganic substances that make up the other 4 percent. Minerals become part of the bones, soft tissues, and body fluids. Minerals also help regulate body processes. Scientists have found the body needs at least 21 minerals for good health. However, they do not yet completely understand the roles of some of these minerals.

The body contains larger amounts of some minerals than others. ***Macrominerals*** are minerals needed in the diet in amounts of 100 or more milligrams each day. Calcium, phosphorus, magnesium, sodium, potassium, and chlorine are macrominerals. *Microminerals,* or ***trace elements,*** are minerals needed in amounts less than 100 milligrams per day. Iron, zinc, iodine, and fluorine are among the trace elements. They are just as important for good health as macrominerals.

Calcium

The body contains more calcium than any other mineral. Most of the calcium is in the bones and teeth. The fluids and soft tissues contain the rest. The body stores a reserve of excess calcium inside long bones.

Calcium combines with phosphorus to build and strengthen bones and teeth. Calcium helps blood clot and keeps the heart and nerves working properly. It also helps regulate the use of other minerals in the body.

Sources of Calcium

Milk and milk products like yogurt and cheese are the best food sources of calcium. Some cereals, fruit juices, and other foods are fortified with calcium. Foods that are labeled "good source of calcium" provide 10 to 19 percent of the recommended daily amount for most people. Foods that are labeled "excellent source of calcium" provide 20 percent or more. Whole fish, green vegetables, and broccoli also provide some calcium in the diet.

Calcium supplements are available. However, most experts agree food sources supply the most beneficial balance of calcium with other nutrients (like phosphorus and vitamin D).

Calcium Deficiencies

Children with severe calcium deficiencies may develop malformed bones. However, these bone disorders are most often the result of a vitamin D deficiency. This is because vitamin D affects the body's ability to use calcium.

Many teens and adults in the United States do not get the recommended daily intake of calcium. If the diet does not supply enough calcium, the body will take the calcium it needs from the bones. This becomes an increasing problem in old age, when bone mass naturally decreases, 2-14. Bones weakened further by the draw on their calcium supply become porous and brittle. This is a condition known as ***osteoporosis.***

Osteoporosis afflicts millions of people in the United States. It causes many fractures of hips and other bones, especially among older women. Resulting complications make osteoporosis a leading cause of crippling and death. Women are most often afflicted because they have less bone mass than men. Osteoporosis is also related to hormone changes that take place in older women. Therefore, women who have gone through menopause are at the greatest risk of developing this disease.

Doctors cannot correct osteoporosis. However, obtaining enough calcium (and phosphorus) can help prevent it. This is especially important during the growth years when bones are developing. Research has shown that being physically active throughout life can also help reduce the risk of osteoporosis. This is because weight-bearing activities, such as walking, helps increase bone mass.

Water-Soluble Vitamins		
Nutrient	**Functions**	**Sources**
Biotin	Helps the body break down the energy nutrients Forms part of several enzymes	Chicken, eggs, fresh vegetables, kidney, liver, milk, some fruits
Folate	Helps produce normal blood cells Helps convert food into energy Helps prevent damage to the brain and spinal cord of unborn babies	Asparagus, bananas, broccoli, fortified bread and cereal products, leafy green vegetables, legumes, liver, oranges, strawberries, whole grain cereals, yogurt
Niacin	Helps keep nervous system healthy Helps keep skin, mouth, tongue, and digestive tract healthy Helps cells use other nutrients Forms part of two conenzymes involved in complex chemical reactions in the body	Dried beans and peas, enriched and whole grain breads and cereals, fish, meat, milk, poultry, peanut butter, peanuts
Pantothenic Acid	Forms part of a coenzyme needed to release energy from carboydrates, fats, and proteins Promotes growth Helps the body make cholesterol	Bran, dry beans, egg yolk, milk, organ meats, wheat germ, yeast
Riboflavin	Helps cells use oxygen Helps keep skin, tongue, and lips normal Helps prevent scaly, greasy areas around the mouth and nose Forms part of the coenzymes needed for the breakdown of carbohydrates	Cheese, dark green leafy vegetables, eggs, fish, ice cream, liver and other meats, milk, poultry
Thiamin	Helps promote normal appetite and digestion Forms parts of the coenzymes needed for the breakdown of carbohydrates Helps keep nervous system healthy and prevent irritability Helps body release energy from food	Dried beans, eggs, enriched or whole grain breads and cereals, fish, pork and other meats, poultry
Vitamin B_6	Helps nervous tissue function normally Plays a role in the breakdown of proteins, fats, and carbohydrates Plays a role in the reaction in which tryptophan is converted to niacin Plays a role in the regeneration of red blood cells	Liver, muscle meats, vegetables, whole grain cereals
Vitamin B_{12}	Protects against pernicious anemia Plays a role in the normal functioning of cells	Cheese, eggs, fish, liver and other meats, milk
Vitamin C	Promotes healthy gums and tissues Helps wounds heal and broken bones mend Helps body fight infection Helps make cementing materials that hold body cells together	Broccoli, cantaloupe, citrus fruits, green peppers, leafy green vegetables, potatoes and sweet potatoes cooked in the skin, raw cabbage, strawberries, tomatoes

2-13 The B-complex vitamins and vitamin C are water-soluble, so you need to eat sources every day.

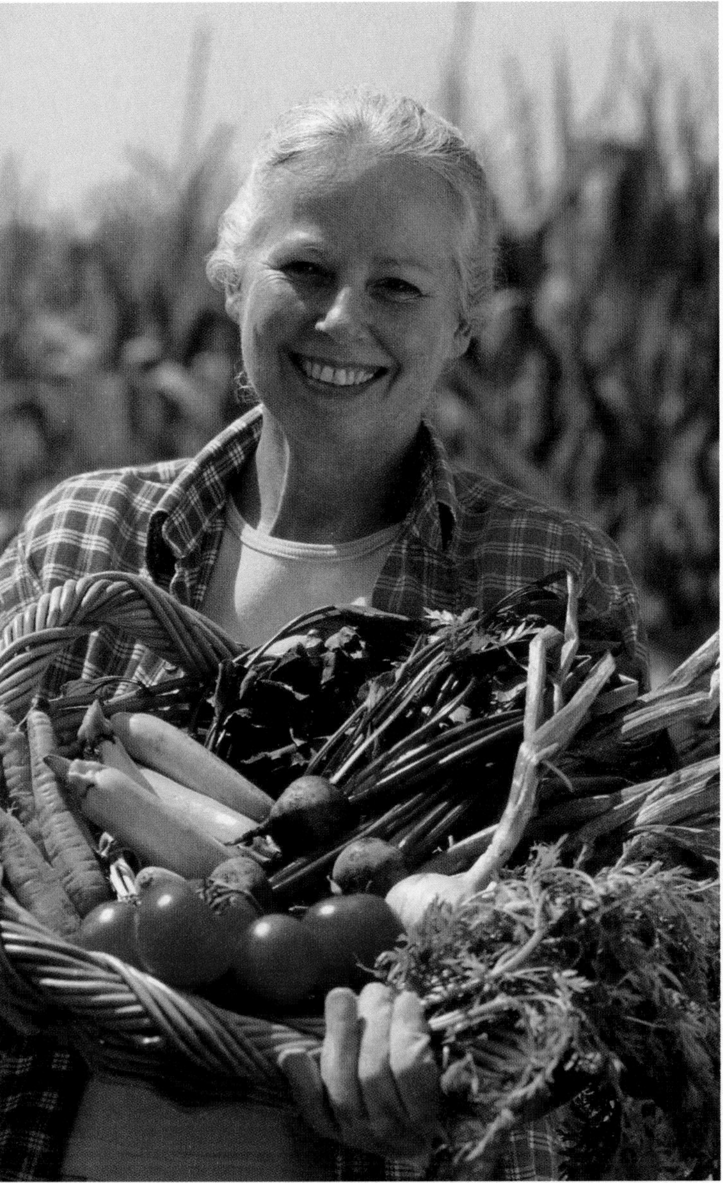

2-14 Older adults need to be sure to include rich sources of calcium in their diets to help protect their aging bones.

Phosphorus

Phosphorus is second only to calcium in the amount found in the body. Phosphorus works with calcium to give strength to bones and teeth. Like calcium, the body stores a reserve of excess phosphorus in the bones.

Phosphorus helps build bones and teeth and aids the body in storing and releasing energy. It helps balance the alkalis and acids in the blood. Phosphorus also helps the body use other nutrients.

Sources of Phosphorus

Meat, poultry, fish, eggs, and milk and other dairy products are good sources of phosphorus. Many soft drinks also supply a large amount of phosphorus. However, they lack the variety of nutrients provided by other food sources. If you eat enough foods that are high in protein and calcium, you should receive enough phosphorus.

Phosphorus Deficiencies and Excesses

Most people have no trouble getting enough phosphorus in their diets. There are no known symptoms for phosphorus deficiency. On the other hand, too much phosphorus in the diet can cause problems. The ratio of calcium to phosphorus in the diet should be no lower than 1:2. However, people who drink a lot of soft drinks and not much milk may have a lower calcium to phosphorus ratio. This can cause calcium to be pulled from the bones to correct the ratio. As mentioned earlier, depleting the bones' calcium supply can lead to osteoporosis.

Magnesium

About half of the body's magnesium is in the skeleton. The other half is in the soft tissues and body fluids.

Magnesium helps cells use proteins, fats, and carbohydrates to produce energy. It helps regulate the body's temperature and keeps the nervous system working properly. Magnesium also helps muscles contract and improves the balance between alkalis and acids.

Sources of Magnesium

Whole grains and grain products are good sources of magnesium. Nuts, beans, meat, and dark green leafy vegetables also supply magnesium, 2-15.

Magnesium Deficiencies

Healthy people who eat a nutritious diet receive enough magnesium. A deficiency, however, can occur in alcoholics. People suffering from malfunctioning kidneys, severe diarrhea, or malnutrition may also form deficiencies. Symptoms include twitching, muscle tremors, an irregular pulse, insomnia, and muscle weakness.

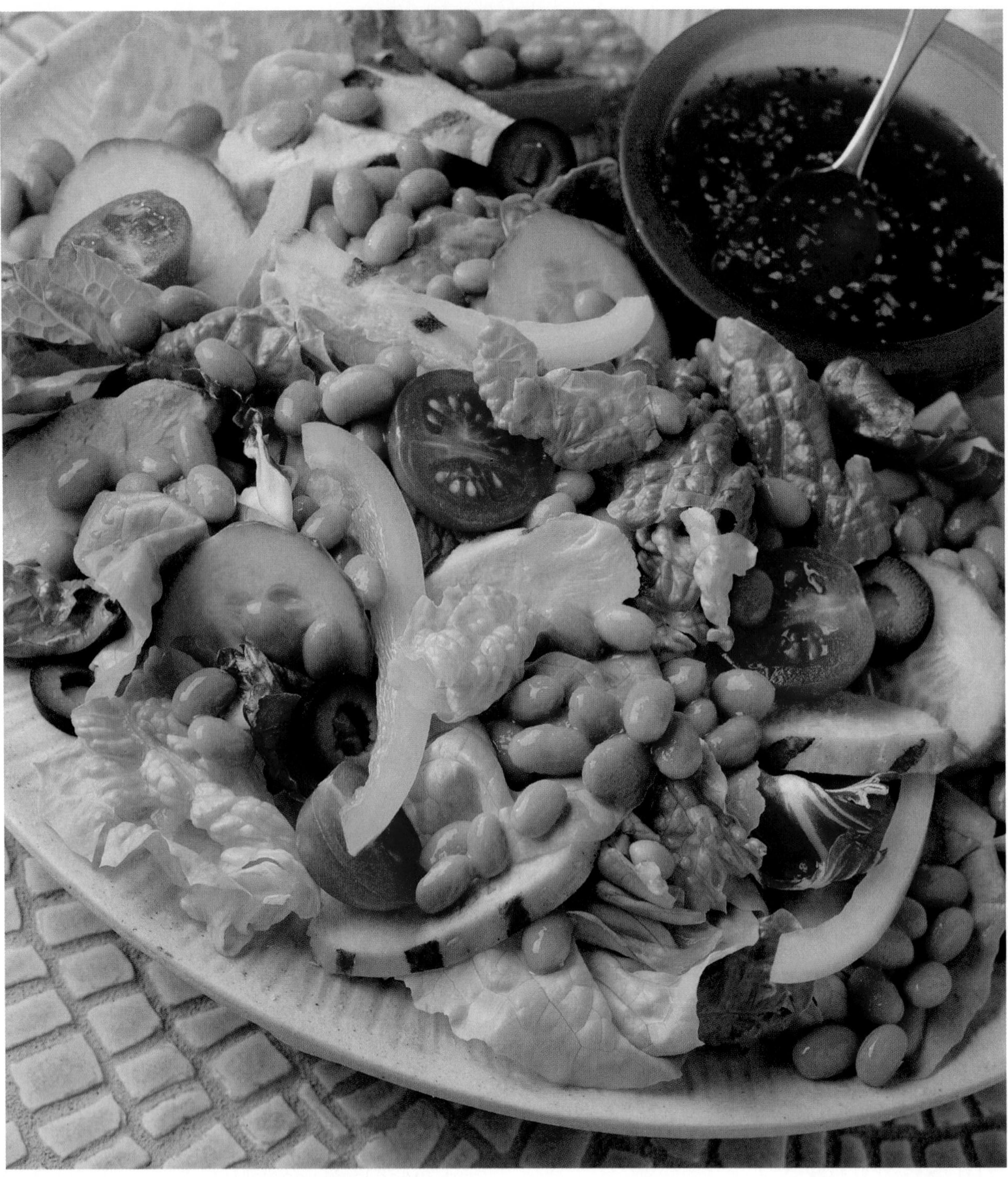

Bush's Baked Beans

2-15 Along with being high in fiber and low in fat, beans are a good source of magnesium.

Sodium, Chlorine, and Potassium

Like calcium and phosphorus, sodium, chlorine, and potassium work as a nutrient team. Blood plasma and other fluids outside the cells contain most of the body's sodium and chlorine. In addition, some sodium is in bones, and some chlorine is in gastric juices. Most of the body's potassium is within the cells.

Sodium, chlorine, and potassium work together to control osmosis. *Osmosis* is the process whereby fluids flow in and out of the cells through the cell walls. These minerals help maintain the acid-alkali balance in the body. They help the nervous system and muscles function properly. They also help the cells absorb nutrients.

Sources of Sodium, Chlorine, and Potassium

Sodium, chlorine, and potassium are in many plant and animal foods. Sodium is in many processed foods. Table salt provides additional amounts of sodium and chlorine. Meat, milk, bananas, citrus fruits, and dark green leafy vegetables are especially good sources of potassium.

Sodium, Chlorine, and Potassium Deficiencies and Excesses

Deficiencies of sodium, chlorine, and potassium are rare in healthy individuals with nutritious diets. Cases of severe diarrhea, vomiting, and burns may require increased amounts of these minerals to replace losses. Persons taking *diuretics* (medications that increase urine output) may need to take additional potassium. Persons who perspire a great deal during heavy work or exercise may lose some sodium. However, normal eating usually replaces these losses.

Normally, you excrete excess sodium through urine. In some cases, however, the body cannot get rid of the sodium, and fluids build up. The resulting swelling is called *edema.* Thus, people with medical problems in which the body retains fluid may have to restrict their sodium intake.

Research has shown there is a link between sodium and ***hypertension,*** or high blood pressure, in some people. Therefore, doctors often prescribe low-sodium diets for people who have hypertension.

People wishing to reduce their sodium intake can begin by limiting their use of salt in cooking and at the table. Sodium is also in many processed foods. Many cured meats, canned foods, frozen entrees, snack items, and condiments like soy sauce and catsup are high in sodium. Reading nutrition labels will help make you more aware of foods containing sodium. Limiting your use of these foods as well as salt can help lower the amount of sodium in your diet. See 2-16.

Q: Will eating a low-salt diet keep me from having high blood pressure?

A: About 10 to 15 percent of people are sodium sensitive. For these people, limiting salt and other sources of sodium may help prevent high blood pressure. A low-salt diet will not protect the rest of the population from this disease. However, health experts advise all people to limit their sodium intake to no more than 2,400 mg.

Trace Elements

The body contains very small amounts of trace elements. Experts have determined some of these minerals are vital for good health. Recommended daily intakes have been set for copper, selenium, manganese, and a number of other trace elements besides those discussed here. However, these minerals have not been shown to pose a great concern in the diets of most people in the United States.

Iron

The human body contains about 4 g of iron. Over half of this iron is in the blood, where it combines with a protein to form hemoglobin. *Hemoglobin* is a protein pigment found in red blood cells. It takes oxygen from the lungs and carries it to cells throughout the body.

Macrominerals		
Nutrient	**Functions**	**Sources**
Calcium	Helps build bones and teeth Helps blood clot Helps muscles and nerves work Helps regulate the use of other minerals in the body	Fish eaten with the bones; leafy green vegetables; milk, cheese, and other dairy products
Magnesium	Helps cells use energy nutrients Helps regulate body temperature Helps muscles and nerves work Improves acid-alkali balance in the body	Beans, dark green leafy vegetables, meat, nuts, whole grains
Phosphorus	Helps build strong bones and teeth Helps regulate many internal bodily activities	Protein and calcium food sources
Sodium, chlorine, and potassium	Work together to control osmosis Help maintain acid-alkali balance in the body Help nervous system and muscles work Help cells absorb nutrients	Sodium: Processed foods, table salt Chlorine: Table salt Potassium: Bananas, citrus fruits, dark green leafy vegetables, meat, milk

2-16 *You need 100 milligrams or more of each of the macrominerals in your daily diet.*

Iron is one mineral the body does not excrete in any quantity. The body stores iron and uses it over and over again. When the body does not have enough iron reserves, anemia can result. Infants, children, and women suffer from anemia more often than men. Loss of appetite, pale skin, and tiredness are general symptoms of anemia.

Women lose varying amounts of iron each month during menstruation. Frequently eating foods rich in iron can maintain iron reserves. If the diet does not supply enough iron, however, a physician may prescribe an iron supplement.

Infants have some iron reserves when they are born. When these reserves are depleted, however, the infant must receive iron from foods, such as iron-fortified cereal. Milk is not a source of iron. Infants kept on a milk-only diet may develop anemia. See 2-17.

Liver is one of the best sources of iron. Other meats, egg yolks, legumes, leafy green vegetables, and enriched breads and cereals are also good sources of this mineral.

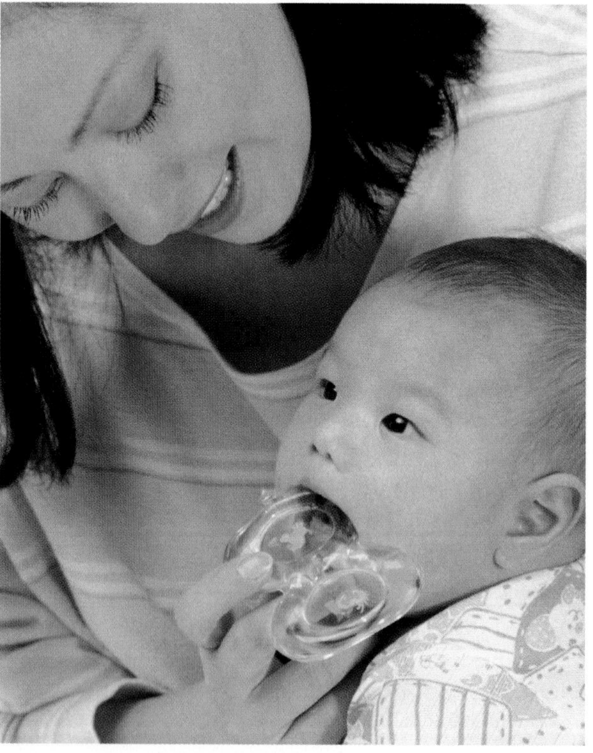

2-17 *Infants are born with enough iron reserves to support them through the first four to six months of life. Iron-fortified cereal is a good source of iron for older infants.*

Zinc

Zinc helps a number of enzymes perform their functions. It helps wounds heal and aids the functioning of the immune system. It promotes normal growth and development in children, too. Lack of zinc can stunt the growth and sexual development of children. Zinc deficiency may also result in poor wound healing and impaired taste and night vision. Large doses of zinc supplements can cause fever, nausea, and vomiting. Over time, heart disease and kidney failure can develop. Meat, poultry, seafood, legumes, and whole grains are good sources of zinc.

Iodine

The thyroid gland stores a third of the body's iodine. This small gland is located at the base of the neck. Iodine is an essential part of *thyroxine,* a hormone produced by the thyroid gland. Thyroxine regulates the rate at which the body uses energy.

If the diet does not contain enough iodine, the cells of the thyroid gland become enlarged. As the gland swells, it forms a lump at the front of the neck. This visible enlargement of the thyroid gland is called a ***goiter.***

Insufficient iodine during the prenatal period and early childhood may cause severe mental retardation. Combined with a slowed growth rate, this deficiency can cause swollen facial features and enlarged lips and tongue. Early treatment can reverse some of these characteristics. Seafood, seaweed, and iodized salt are good sources of iodine.

Fluorine

The greatest quantities of fluorine are in the teeth and bones. The teeth need fluorine for maximum resistance to decay. Fluorine is most helpful during the development of teeth, but it serves a protective function for the life of the tooth. Studies have also shown fluorine may be effective in maintaining the health of bones.

Commonly eaten foods contain little fluorine. In some areas, drinking water contains fluorine naturally. In areas where the natural fluorine level is low, the Food and Nutrition Board recommends adding fluorine to the public drinking water. Many toothpastes also contain fluorine. See 2-18.

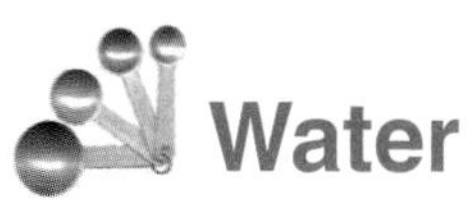

Water

The body must have water to function. People can live more than a month without food. However, they can live only a few days without water.

Functions of Water

Between 50 and 75 percent of your body weight is water. Water is found both inside and outside all your cells. Water aids proper digestion and cell growth and maintenance. All chemical reactions within the body rely on

Trace Elements		
Nutrient	**Functions**	**Sources**
Fluorine	Helps teeth resist decay Helps maintain bone health	Fluoridated drinking water, toothpaste
Iodine	Promotes normal functioning of the thyroid gland	Iodized table salt, saltwater fish and shellfish
Iron	Combines with protein to make hemoglobin Helps cells use oxygen	Dried beans and peas, dried fruits, egg yolk, enriched and whole grain breads and cereals, leafy green vegetables, lean meats, liver
Zinc	Helps enzymes function Helps wounds heal Aids work of the immune system Promotes normal growth	Legumes, meat, poultry, seafood, whole grains

2-18 *Trace elements are needed by the body in very small amounts. However, they are no less important than any other nutrients in your diet.*

water. Water also lubricates the joints and body cells and helps regulate body temperature.

Water Intake and Excretion

Your body takes the water it needs from the liquids you drink and the foods you eat. About 54 percent of your water intake comes from liquids. These liquids include water, milk, broth, coffee, tea, fruit juices, and other beverages. About 37 percent of your water intake comes from the food you eat. Different foods contain different amounts of water. For instance, lettuce contains more water than a slice of bread. Your body also obtains water when it releases energy from carbohydrates, fats, and proteins.

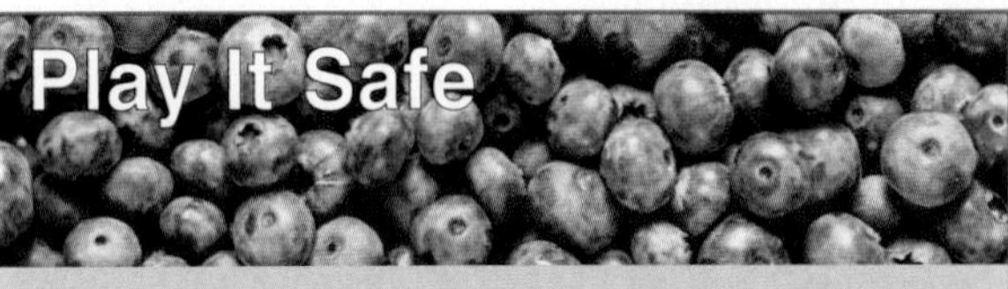

You never know when a disaster, such as an earthquake or flood, might occur. Being prepared can help you cope with an emergency situation.

One way to prepare is to gather supplies you would need in the event of a disaster. Water is one of the basic supplies you should stock. Store three gallons of water for each family member in sealed, unbreakable containers. This is enough water to allow for food preparation and sanitation as well as drinking for a three-day period. Date the containers and replace the water every six months so it stays fresh.

The body excretes most of the water it uses through the kidneys as urine. It excretes the remaining water through the skin and lungs and in the feces.

Water Requirements

Some nutrition experts suggest an easy way to figure your daily water needs. Divide your body weight in pounds by two. The result equals how many ounces of fluids you should drink each day. This means a 150-pound person should drink about 75 ounces of water and other fluids per day (150 ÷ 2 = 75). See 2-19.

Some people need more water. Someone who is in a coma or suffering from fever or diarrhea has increased water needs. People on high-protein diets and those living in hot climates must also increase their water intake.

Diarrhea, vomiting, excessive sweating, or the unavailability of drinking water can deplete body fluids. Thirst is the first symptom of water loss. If water is not replaced, dryness of the mouth, weakness, increased pulse rate, flushed skin, and fever can result.

Digestion and Absorption

Suppose you eat a hamburger for lunch. Before your body can use the nutrients in the hamburger, the hamburger must go through digestion. Then the nutrients must go through absorption. ***Digestion*** is the bodily process of breaking food down into simpler compounds the body can use. ***Absorption*** is the process of taking in nutrients and making them part of the body.

The Digestive Tract

The *digestive* or *gastrointestinal tract* is a tube about 30 feet (9 m) long. It extends from the mouth to the anus. It contains the esophagus, the stomach, the small intestine, and the large intestine. These parts of the digestive tract work together both mechanically and chemically to help the body use food.

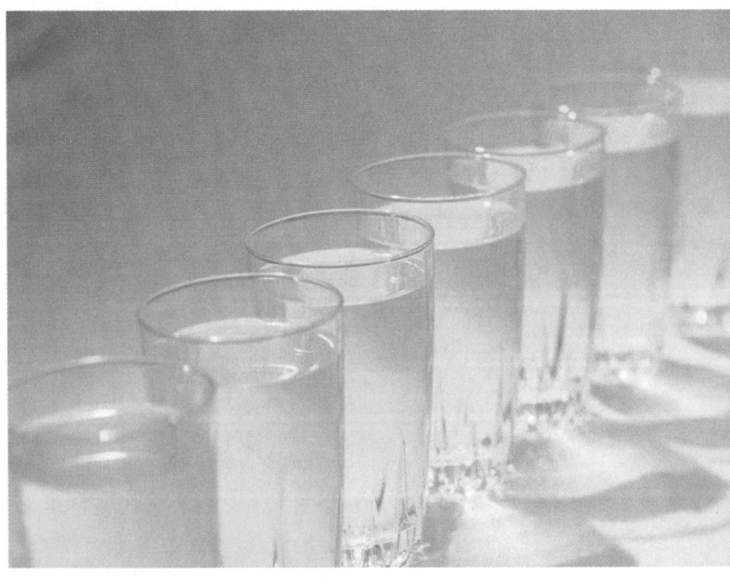

2-19 *Most people need the equivalent of about eight glasses of water a day.*

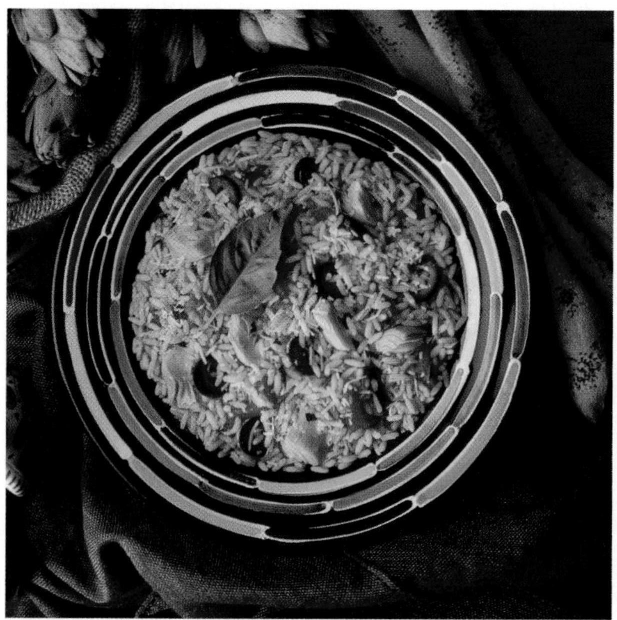

USA Rice Federation

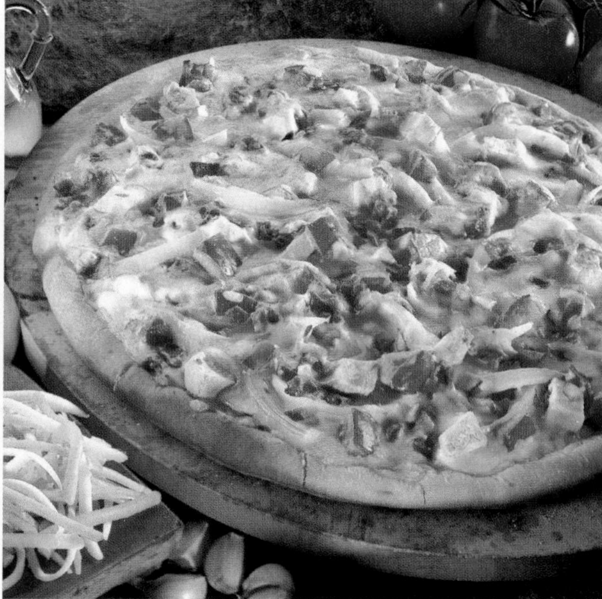

© 2002 Wisconsin Milk Marketing Board

2-20 *This rice dish is higher in carbohydrates and lower in fats and proteins than the pizza. Therefore, you are not likely to feel full as long after eating the rice dish as you would after eating the pizza.*

The Digestion Process

During digestion, the body breaks down complex molecules obtained from food into simple, soluble materials. These simple materials can pass through the digestive tract into the blood and lymph systems. Vitamins and minerals undergo very little chemical change during digestion. However, fats, proteins, and carbohydrates undergo many changes.

The Mechanical Phase

The digestion process involves two phases. The mechanical phase begins in the mouth. Here, the teeth chew the food and break it down into smaller pieces.

Contractions of the muscular walls of the digestive tract carry on the mechanical action. These contractions mix food particles and break them into smaller pieces. With waves of contractions known as ***peristalsis,*** the muscles also push food through the digestive tract. Emotions such as sadness, depression, and fear can slow down peristalsis. Anger and aggression can speed up this process.

The Chemical Phase

Like the mechanical phase, the chemical phase of digestion begins in the mouth. As you chew, food is mixed with ***saliva.*** This is a mucus- and enzyme-containing liquid secreted by the mouth. It moistens food particles, helping them move down the esophagus into the stomach. Saliva also begins to break down starches.

In the stomach, *gastric juices* containing hydrochloric acid and several enzymes are secreted. These juices break down the food further. An ordinary meal usually leaves the stomach in about two to three hours. Carbohydrates leave the stomach first. Proteins are second to leave the stomach, followed by fats. As a result, you will feel hungry sooner after a meal high in carbohydrates than a meal high in proteins and fats, 2-20.

As digestion continues, the semiliquid food mass leaves the stomach and enters the small intestine. Here, intestinal juices, pancreatic juices, and bile act on the food. These secretions contain the enzymes needed to complete the digestion of the proteins, fats, and carbohydrates.

Digestive enzymes help break down carbohydrates, proteins, and fats into simple substances the body can absorb and use. Each type of enzyme has a specific function. An enzyme that breaks down proteins, for example, will not break down fats. Once digestion is complete, absorption can take place.

Indigestible residues, bile pigments, other wastes, and water travel from the small intestine to the large intestine. The large intestine acts as a reservoir, or storage area. Eventually the body will excrete these materials in the feces.

The Absorption Process

The body can absorb water, ethyl alcohol, and simple sugars directly from the stomach. They pass through the stomach walls into the bloodstream. Most absorption, however, takes place in the small intestine.

Millions of hairlike fingers called *villi* line the small intestine. The villi increase the absorptive surface of the small intestine by more than 600 percent. Each villus contains a lymph vessel surrounded by a network of capillaries. Nutrients absorbed by the capillaries pass into the portal vein and travel directly to the liver.

The body absorbs nearly all carbohydrates as *monosaccharides,* or single sugar units. The body absorbs fats and other lipids in two forms: as fatty acids and glycerol and as mono- and diglycerides. (*Glycerol* is an alcohol obtained from the breakdown of fat. *Diglycerides* are compounds formed by the combination of glycerol and fatty acids.) The body absorbs nearly all proteins as amino acids.

Metabolism

Metabolism is the chemical processes that take place in the cells after the body absorbs nutrients. Enzymes cause nearly all metabolic reactions. The body uses some nutrients to replace substances used for growth. It uses some nutrients to carry out bodily processes. The body breaks down some nutrients into simpler substances to release energy. The body uses part of this energy to carry out metabolic reactions. It converts the rest into heat.

Each nutrient follows a distinct metabolic path. The body converts all carbohydrates into glucose for use as an energy source, 2-21. If carbohydrates are not needed for immediate energy, they can be converted to *glycogen.* This is the storage form of carbohydrates in the body. Excess carbohydrates can also be stored in the body as fat tissue.

During fat metabolism, fatty acid chains are shortened. The body uses most fat for fuel.

The body can use amino acids from protein metabolism for cell maintenance or cell growth. It can also use amino acids to make enzymes, antibodies, and nonessential amino acids. The body can use amino acids as an energy source, too.

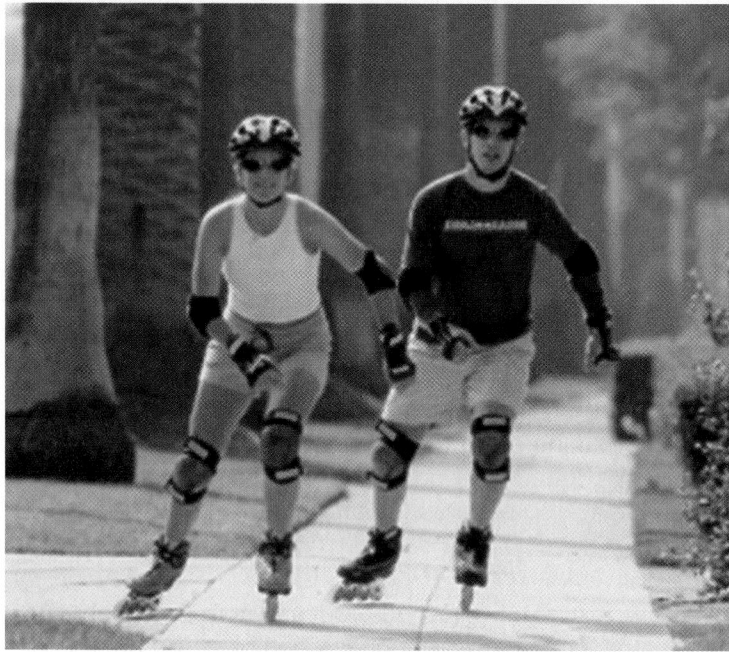

Rollerblade®

2-21 *Carbohydrates provide your body with glucose, which is used as an energy source to fuel physical activity.*

Chapter 2 Review

Nutritional Needs

Summary

Food provides the body with six basic types of nutrients. These are carbohydrates, fats, proteins, vitamins, minerals, and water. Some people choose to get nutrients as well as some nonnutrient substances from dietary supplements.

Individual nutrients within the six basic groups each serve specific functions. No one food supplies all the nutrients the body needs. Health problems arise when there are deficiencies or excesses of various nutrients. Eating a variety of foods is the best way to get appropriate amounts of all the nutrients.

Your body must break down the foods you eat into components it can use. This happens during the digestion process. The digestion process involves both a mechanical and a chemical phase. After foods have been broken down in the digestive tract, the body absorbs the nutrients. Then nutrients are metabolized in the cells to release energy or make other compounds needed by the body.

Review What You Have Read

Write your answers on a separate sheet of paper.

1. True or false. The foods a child eats can affect his or her health as an adult.
2. An illness caused by the lack of a sufficient amount of a nutrient is called a(n) _____.
3. A purified nutrient or nonnutrient substance that is manufactured or extracted from natural sources is a _____.
   A. dietary supplement
   B. fortified food
   C. multivitamin
   D. phytochemical
4. Match the following carbohydrates with their descriptions:
   _____ Blood sugar. A. fructose
   _____ Fruit sugar. B. galactose
   _____ Malt sugar. C. glucose
   _____ Milk sugar. D. lactose
   _____ Table sugar. E. maltose
   F. sucrose
5. What three substances can raise the blood cholesterol level and why is this a concern?
6. List three functions of each of the following nutrients: carbohydrates, fats, and proteins.
7. What type of protein will support growth and normal maintenance?
8. List the fat-soluble vitamins and explain the basic way in which they differ from water-soluble vitamins.
9. Name six of the B-complex vitamins and give a food source of each.
10. Name and describe the calcium deficiency disease that afflicts millions of adults in the United States.
11. What is the process controlled by sodium, potassium, and chlorine whereby fluids flow in and out of cells through the cell walls?
12. Where is most of the body's iron found?
13. How can a person figure his or her daily water needs?
14. In what part of the body does most absorption take place?
15. True or false. Metabolism is the process of breaking food down into simpler compounds the body can use.

Build Your Basic Skills

1. **Math.** Enrico had a glass of orange juice and two pieces of whole wheat toast for breakfast. He had a hamburger, carrot sticks, and an apple for lunch. For dinner, he had a pork chop, mashed potatoes, and fresh broccoli spears. Use Appendix C to calculate Enrico's fiber intake for the day. How does his intake compare to the recommendation given in the chapter?

2. **Writing.** Choose one of the nutrients discussed in this chapter. Write a short story from the point of view of the nutrient. Creatively describe where you live (food sources) and your job (functions in the human body). Share your story in class.
3. **Science.** Make a poster illustrating the digestion process.

Build Your Thinking Skills

1. **Evaluate.** Read the label of a multivitamin supplement. Note the percent Daily Value provided for each of the vitamins in the supplement. Evaluate what this indicates, based on what you learned from the chapter about the effects of excess fat-soluble and water-soluble vitamins in the body. Discuss your findings and conclusions in class.
2. **Plan.** Plan a basic nutrition lesson for a primary school child. Use visual aids that appeal to children, such as magazine pictures, colorful posters, or puppets.

Apply Technology

1. Visit a grocery store and make a list of 10 foods that are enriched or fortified with nutrients. Discuss in class how the technology used to fortify and enrich foods has affected the quality of the U.S. diet.
2. Measure your blood pressure using a blood pressure cuff that gives a digital readout.

Using Workplace Skills

Lupe is a dietetic technician at St. Andrew's Hospital. She consults with patients about how to modify their diets in response to specific health conditions. She has to keep detailed records on each patient for her supervisor to review and for use in follow-up visits.

To be an effective worker, Lupe needs skill in organizing and maintaining files. Put yourself in Lupe's place and answer the following questions about your need for and use of these skills:

A. How would maintaining well-organized files help you when your patients come in for follow-up visits?
B. How would maintaining well-organized files help your supervisor?
C. How might your failure to organize and maintain files affect your patients?
D. What is another skill you would need in this job? Briefly explain why this skill would be important.

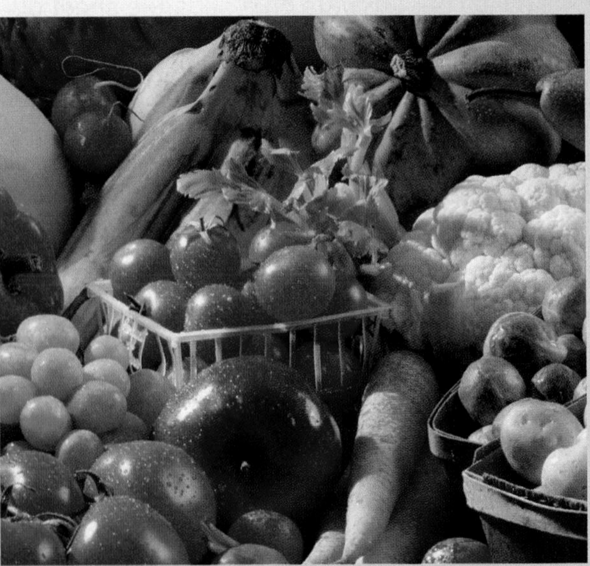

Chapter 3

Making Healthful Food Choices

Nutrition Consultant
Develops, tests, and promotes various types of food products.

Food Columnist
Analyzes news and writes column commentary for publication based on personal knowledge and experience with foods and nutrition.

Family and Consumer Sciences Teacher
Teaches students family and consumer sciences principles, prepares lesson plans, evaluates student progress, maintains discipline, and participates in professional meetings.

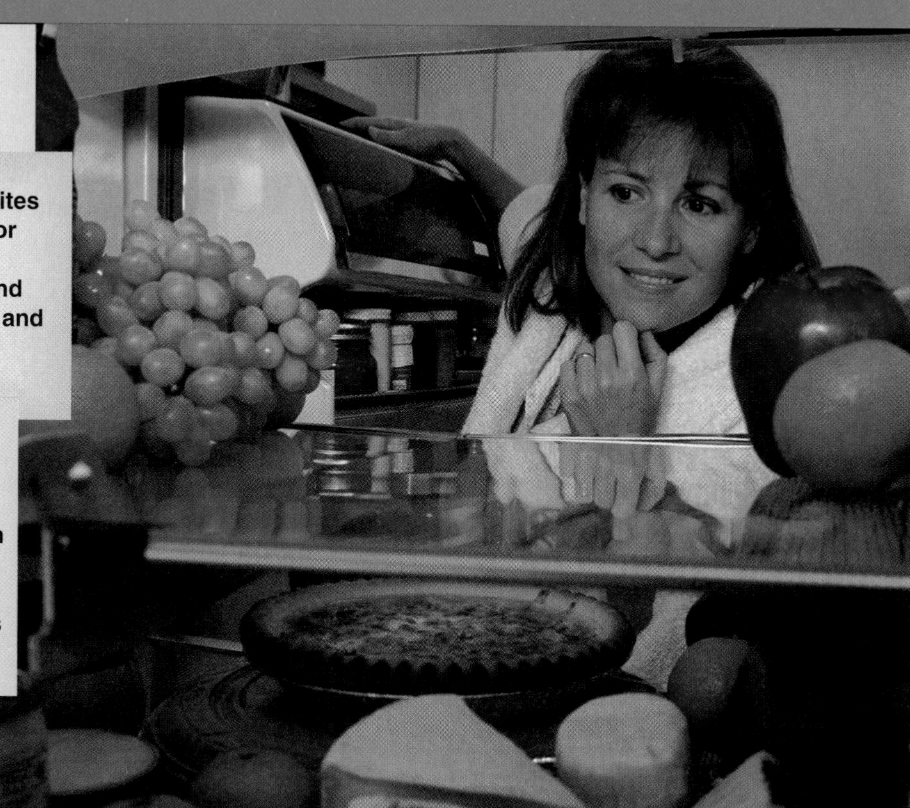

Terms to Know

- Dietary Reference Intakes (DRIs)
- Estimated Average Requirement (EAR)
- Recommended Dietary Allowance (RDA)
- Adequate Intake (AI)
- Tolerable Upper Intake Level (UL)
- USDA Food Guide
- Dietary Guidelines for Americans
- nutrient-dense foods
- processed food

Objectives

After studying this chapter, you will be able to

- ❑ name benefits of making healthful food choices.
- ❑ identify how many daily servings you need from each group in the USDA Food Guide.
- ❑ explain how you can use Dietary Reference Intakes (DRIs), the USDA Food Guide, and the Dietary Guidelines for Americans as diet planning resources to meet your daily needs.
- ❑ list tips to use when shopping for fresh and processed foods.
- ❑ describe suggestions for preparing healthful foods.
- ❑ apply the Dietary Guidelines for Americans when eating out.

Knowing about nutrients gives you an idea of the important role food can play in your health. However, you need to know a bit more to choose foods that will supply adequate amounts of nutrients. Some general guidelines can help you select a nutritious diet. You can use these guidelines when shopping for food, preparing food at home, and eating out.

Benefits of Healthful Choices

Choosing a diet that provides your body with needed amounts of all the nutrients can benefit you in many ways. This important choice can affect your health and appearance. It can have an impact on your job performance and your personal and family life, too.

Making wise food choices can help you maintain good health and may improve your health. An adequate supply of nutrients in your diet will keep you from getting deficiency diseases. For instance, if you consume the recommended amount of vitamin C, you will not get scurvy. Research also indicates some nutrients may lower your risk for certain chronic diseases. As an example, studies show high-fiber, lowfat diets may help protect against cancers of the colon and rectum. Nutrients affect your health in more general ways, too. Carbohydrates provide you with energy, and B vitamins help your body use carbohydrates. When you get enough of these nutrients, you will have the fuel you need to do your daily tasks. If you become injured, vitamin C in your diet helps wounds heal and ample protein helps repair tissue.

You should realize that eating wholesome foods will not guarantee you good health. Your heredity and environment affect your physical well-being. Your personal habits affect your state of health, too. You need to get adequate rest and physical activity. You need to avoid smoking and abusing alcohol and other drugs. These factors all play a part in how you look and feel. They also have an impact on your susceptibility to various diseases.

Getting enough nutrients in your diet can affect your appearance as well as your health. Vitamin A and the B vitamins promote smooth skin. Fluorine and calcium help form strong teeth. Protein is needed to build well-defined muscles. Nutrients also play a role in keeping hair shiny and nails healthy. When you get the nutrients you need, you will look your best.

By affecting your health and appearance, nutrients can affect your job performance. When you are in good health, you have the strength and energy to do top-quality work. You will find it easier to stay focused on tasks. You are better equipped to manage stress, too. When you know you look your best, you have more confidence to accept new challenges. You will be more willing to approach customers to make a sale or to ask supervisors for help. See 3-1.

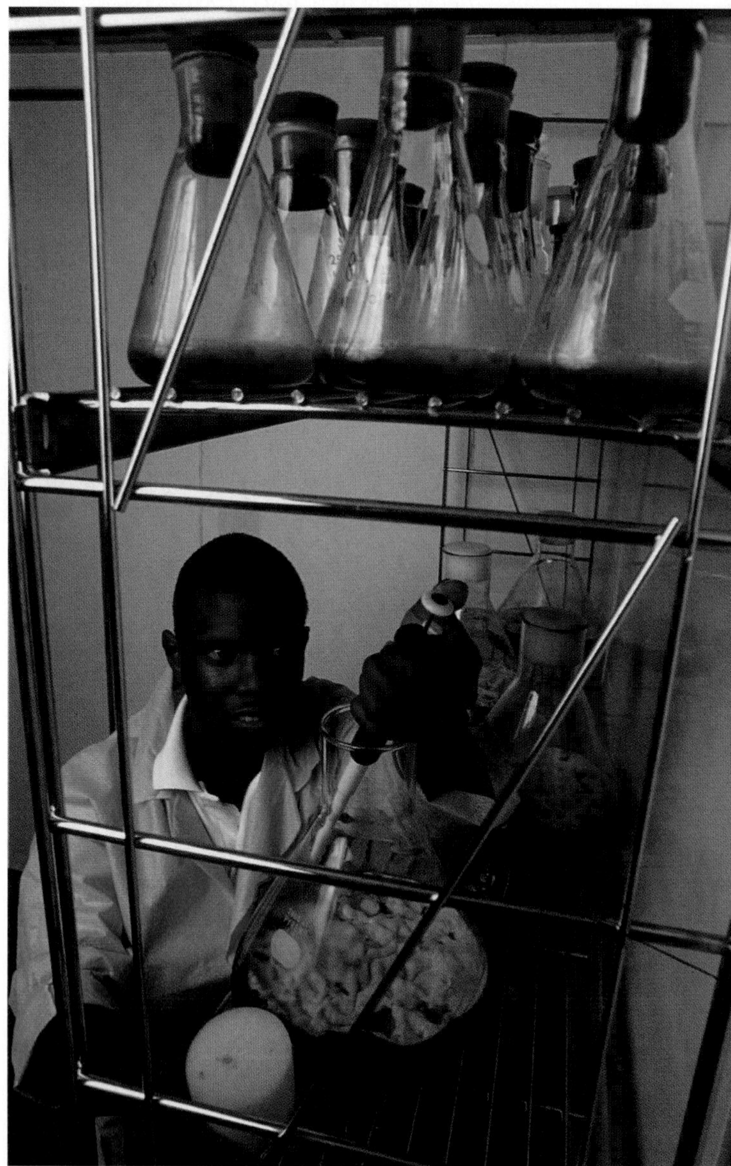

Agricultural Research Service, USDA

3-1 *A healthful diet can give you the energy you need to stay alert and give your job your full attention.*

In similar ways, nutrients can influence your personal and family life. Having good physical health can help you manage all the tasks in your daily schedule. You will have the strength to do household chores. Your ability to concentrate on your schoolwork will improve. You will have a more positive attitude when interacting with family members.

Making healthful food choices will not ensure your future career success. Getting all the nutrients you need will not solve all your personal problems, either. However, when you choose a nutritious diet, you are taking an active role in controlling your total state of wellness.

Diet Planning Resources

Many reports about health issues include links to nutrients. Supermarkets, health food stores, and pharmacies all have shelves lined with bottles of nutrient supplements. Food packages make claims about the nutrient content of products.

You might wish you had some tools to help you sort out all the nutrition information that comes your way. Standards are available to help you know how much of each nutrient you should consume each day. A model has been developed to help you plan nutritious meals. General guidelines exist to help you choose a healthful diet. You can use these resources to help you make healthful food choices.

Dietary Reference Intakes

People need a way to tell if they are meeting their nutrient needs. The Food and Nutrition Board of the National Academy of Sciences developed a set of values to help. This set of values is called the ***Dietary Reference Intakes (DRIs).*** These are estimated nutrient intake levels used for planning and evaluating the diets of healthy people. They are standards against which the nutritional quality of a diet can be measured. The DRIs are designed to help prevent diseases caused by lacks of nutrients. They are also designed to reduce the risk of diseases linked to nutrition. Such diseases include heart disease, some types of cancer, and osteoporosis. See 3-2.

The following four types of values make up the DRIs:

- ***Estimated Average Requirement (EAR).*** This nutrient intake value is estimated to meet the needs of half the healthy people in a group. If your diet does not include at least the EAR of a nutrient, your intake may be insufficient. The EAR value is based on research. There is not enough research available to set an EAR for some nutrients.

DRIs for Teens		
Nutrient	Males 14-18 years	Females 14-18 years
Calories	3,100*	2,300*
Protein	52 g	46 g
Carbohydrate	130 g	130 g
Fiber	38 g	26 g
Vitamin A	900μg	700μg
Vitamin C	75 mg	65 mg
Vitamin E	15 mg	15 mg
Iron	11 mg	15 mg
Calcium	1,300 mg	1,300 mg
Magnesium	410 mg	360 mg
Potassium	4.7 g	4.7 g

*This calorie intake meets the average energy expenditure of healthy, moderately active teens at the reference height and weight of 5′8″ and 134 pounds for males and 5′4″ and 119 pounds for females.

***3-2** Most healthy teens who consume these amounts of nutrients through their daily food choices are eating nutritionally adquate diets.*

- ***Recommended Dietary Allowance (RDA).*** This average daily dietary intake level meets the nutrient needs of nearly all healthy people in a group. This is the amount of a nutrient you should strive to include in your diet. RDAs are based on EARs. Therefore, there are no RDAs for nutrients that do not have EARs.
- ***Adequate Intake (AI).*** This recommended nutrient intake value is set for nutrients for which no RDA can be determined. This value is based on observations or experiments. As future research is completed, the AIs for some nutrients may be replaced by RDAs. Use AIs as guides for daily intake.
- ***Tolerable Upper Intake Level (UL).*** This is the highest level of daily intake of a nutrient that is unlikely to pose risks of adverse health effects. Keep in mind that ULs are not intended to be recommended levels of intake. Health experts have found no advantage to consuming more than the RDA or AI of any nutrient. As intake increases above the UL, the risk of adverse effects increases. Use ULs to check whether you might be consuming too much of any nutrient. See Appendix B, "Recommended Nutrient Intakes."

The USDA Food Guide

The U.S. Department of Agriculture (USDA) prepared an educational tool for selecting nutritious diets. This tool is called the ***USDA Food Guide.*** It is an eating pattern that is based on science. This plan sorts foods of similar nutritive values into groups and subgroups. It also gives recommended daily intakes for each group. Eating the suggested amounts of foods from each group daily will provide you with the nutrients you need. The recommended daily intakes are determined by a person's calorie needs. These needs are based on a person's age, gender, and activity level. See 3-3.

The Food Guide is illustrated by the *MyPyramid* symbol, which includes the Web address MyPyramid.gov. See 3-4. This symbol represents a number of important concepts in nutrition. First, it shows that food intakes require a *personalized approach.* By going to the Web site, each person can find the food group amounts that are right for him or her. Second, MyPyramid uses six color bands to illustrate the importance of *variety* in your daily diet. These bands represent the five food groups and oils. The differing widths of the bands suggest *proportionality* of food choices. This means you need to eat more of some foods and less of others. The narrowing of the bands from bottom to top symbolizes *moderation.* It is a reminder that you should limit forms of foods that are high in solid fats and added sugars. Finally, the person climbing the steps stands for *physical activity.* Being physically active should be part of your daily lifestyle for good health.

As you read about the food groups in the USDA Food Guide, think about your typical food choices. What changes do you need to make to include recommended amounts of foods in your diet? What are some strategies you can use to make these changes?

Fruit Group

The fruit group includes all forms of fruits—fresh, canned, frozen, and dried. Fruit juices are part of this group, too. Fruits (except avocados) are lowfat, high-fiber sources of vitamins and minerals.

Vegetable Group

The vegetable group includes vegetable juices and all fresh (raw and cooked), canned, frozen, and dried vegetables. Like fruits, these foods are good sources of vitamins, minerals, and fiber. The Food Guide divides vegetables into the following five subgroups:

Daily Calorie Needs			
Gender and Age Group	**Inactive**	**Moderately Active**	**Active**
Females, 14-18 years	1,800	2,000	2,400
Males, 14-18 years	2,200	2,400-2,800*	2,800-3,200*

*Lower calorie levels within a range are needed by younger teens; higher levels are needed by older teens.

3-3 Calorie needs are affected by body size as well as age and activity level. These calorie needs are estimates based on median body sizes for 14- to 18-year-old teens.

- dark green vegetables, such as broccoli, spinach, collard greens, and kale
- orange vegetables, such as carrots, sweet potatoes, and winter squash
- legumes, such as dry beans and peas, lentils, and soybean products like tofu
- starchy vegetables, such as white potatoes, corn, and green peas
- other vegetables, such as tomatoes, lettuce, green beans, and onions

Try to select one serving from at least three of the first four subgroups each day. Then choose your remaining daily servings from the other vegetables subgroup. Be sure to include foods from all five subgroups in your diet throughout the week. See 3-4.

Grains Group

The grains group includes such foods as breads, cereals, rice, and pasta. These foods are excellent lowfat sources of complex carbohydrates, which supply energy. They are good sources of B vitamins and iron, too. Whole grain foods are also high in fiber.

The Food Guide divides this group into two subgroups—whole grains and other grains. Whole grains include whole wheat bread, oatmeal, and brown rice. The other grains subgroup is made up of refined grain products. It includes foods like white bread, enriched pasta, and white rice.

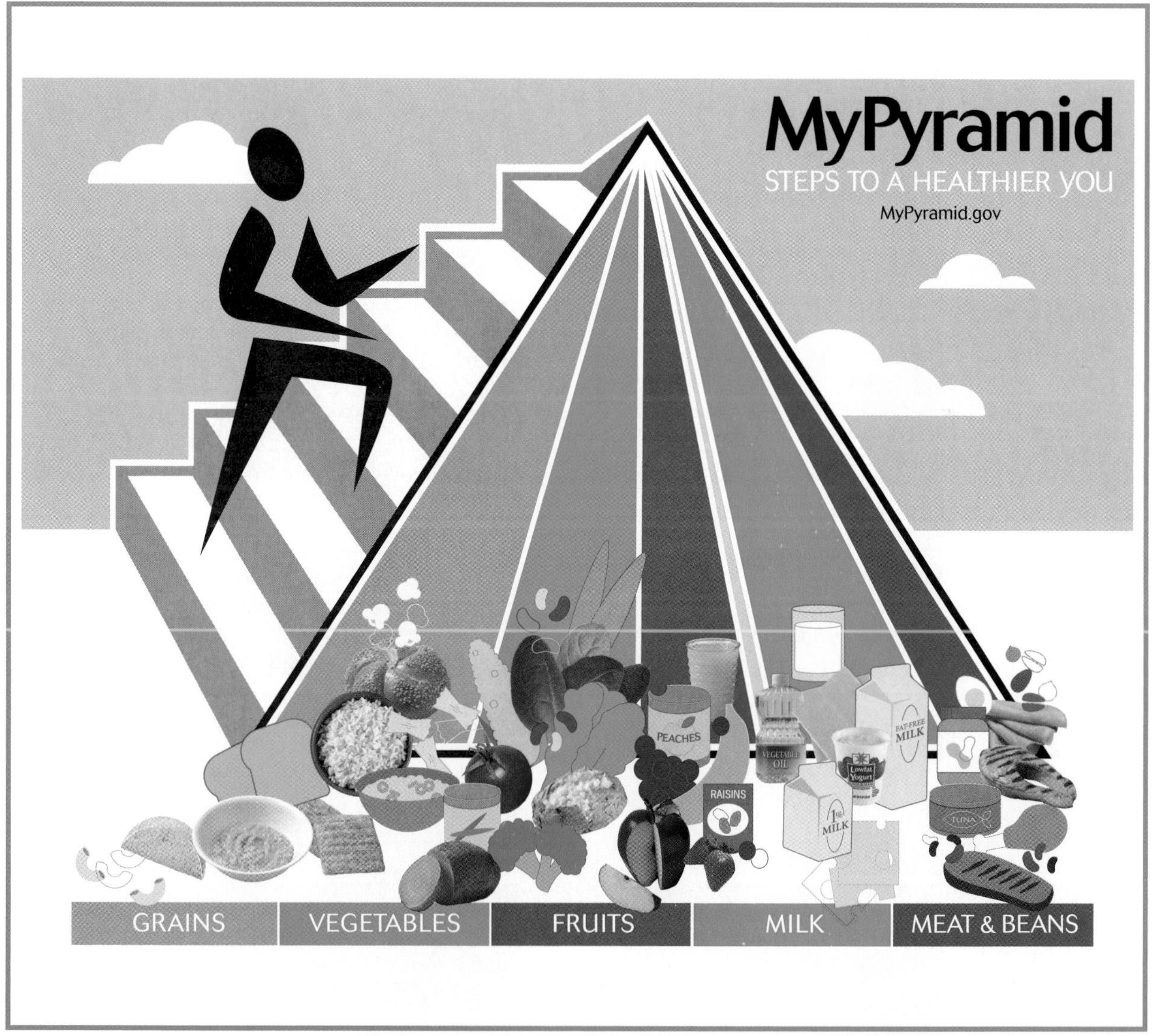

3-4 *Visit the MyPyramid.gov Web site to print out a personalized plan of how much food you need from each food group daily. Then use this information to help you set food and activity goals for good health.*

Meat and Beans Group

Meat, poultry, fish, and such alternates as dry beans, eggs, and nuts are good sources of protein. They also supply vitamins and minerals, including B vitamins and iron. Dry beans and peas are rich in fiber, too. (Note that legumes can be counted as either a meat and beans serving or a vegetable serving, but not both.)

Milk Group

Milk, yogurt, and cheese are your best sources of calcium. They also provide riboflavin, phosphorus, and protein. Whole and fortified milk products provide vitamins A and D, too. Lowfat and fat free dairy products offer the same nutrients as whole milk products while providing less fat and calories.

A number of people avoid foods from this group for health or lifestyle reasons. Yogurt and lactose-free milk may be good alternatives for some people. Extra servings of calcium-rich foods from other food groups can also help meet calcium needs. Such foods include fortified cereals, tofu, canned salmon with bones, and spinach.

Typical foods and serving sizes for each of the food groups are shown in 3-5.

Count Your Servings from the USDA Food Guide		
Food Group	**Serving Size**	**Typical Foods**
Fruit Group	• 1/2 cup fresh, frozen, or canned fruit • 1 medium piece of fruit • 1/2 cup fruit juice • 1/4 cup dried fruit	Apples, apricots, bananas, blueberries, cantaloupe, cherries, figs, fruit juices, grapefruit, grapes, kiwifruit, mangoes, oranges, papayas, peaches, pineapple, plums, raisins, strawberries, watermelon
Vegetable group	• 1/2 cup chopped raw or cooked vegetables • 1 cup leafy green vegetables • 1/2 cup vegetable juice	• Dark green vegetables: broccoli; collard, turnip, and mustard greens; romaine; spinach • Orange vegetables: carrots, pumpkin, sweet potatoes, winter squash • Legumes: kidney, lima, and navy beans; black-eyed peas; chickpeas; lentils; tofu • Starchy vegetables: corn, green peas, white potatoes • Other vegetables: beets, bok choy, cabbage, cucumbers, eggplant, green beans, lettuce, okra, onions, pea pods, peppers, summer squash, tomatillos, tomatoes
Grains group	1 ounce-equivalent • 1 slice bread • 1 cup dry cereal • 1/2 cup cooked cereal, rice, or pasta	• Whole grains: brown rice, bulgur, oatmeal, popcorn, whole grain barley and corn, whole grain cereals and crackers, whole wheat breads, wild rice • Other grains: enriched cereals, crackers, and pasta; white breads, white rice
Meat and beans group	1 once-equivalent • 1 ounce cooked lean meat, poultry, or fish • 1 egg • 1/4 cup cooked dry beans or tofu • 1 tablespoon peanut butter • 1/2 ounce nuts or seeds	Beef; dry beans and peas; chicken; eggs; fish; lamb; lentils; nuts; peanut butter; pork; rabbit; refried beans; seeds; tofu; turkey; veal; venison
Milk group	• 1 cup milk or yogurt • 1 1/2 ounces natural cheese • 2 ounces process cheese	Buttermilk, calcium-fortified soy milk, cheese, cottage cheese, fat free milk, frozen yogurt, goat's milk, ice cream, kefir, lowfat milk, whole milk, yogurt
Oils	4 g = 1 teaspoon	Soft margarines with no *trans* fat, salad dressings, vegetable oils

***3-5** Choose a variety of foods from each group in the USDA Food Guide to get your daily number of recommended servings.*

Solid Fats, Sugars, and Oils

Not all foods fit into the five main groups of the Food Guide. Some foods provide mostly fats, oils, and/or sugars in the diet. Such foods include butter, margarine, jams, jellies, syrups, candies, gravies, salad dressings, and many snack foods. Fats and sugars add flavor and variety to meals. However, foods that are high in these components are often high in calories. They also tend to be low in vitamins and minerals. Therefore, you must use these foods sparingly.

Be aware that many foods in the five main food groups contain solid fats and added sugars. For instance, whole milk is in the milk group. It contains about 8 grams of fat per serving. Pears canned in heavy syrup are in the fruit group. They contain about 2 teaspoons (10 mL) of added sugars per serving. You must consider these contributions along with foods like butter and jam when evaluating the fats and sugars in your diet.

Unlike solid fats, vegetable oils are good sources of vitamin E and essential fatty acids. This is also true of soft margarines with zero *trans* fats. Therefore, the Food Guide recommends including small amounts of oils in the diet each day. See 3-6.

The Food Guide is flexible. People from any ethnic background and economic level can use it to fit their food preferences. For instance, someone who enjoys Mexican food might choose tortillas from the grains group. The tortillas might be filled with tomatillos from the vegetable group and refried beans from the meat and beans group. This tasty entree might be topped with cheese from the milk group. It could be served with papaya from the fruit group. People can choose servings from the five main food groups to form almost any combination of meals and snacks.

Dietary Guidelines for Americans

Another resource can help you plan your diet as part of a healthy lifestyle. This resource comes from the USDA and the U.S. Department of Health and Human Services (HHS). It is the ***Dietary Guidelines for Americans.*** The Guidelines are a set of science-based recommendations that urge people to form healthful diet and activity habits. Making the Guidelines part of your lifestyle can help promote your health. Following them can also reduce your risk for certain diseases. These diseases include heart disease, high blood pressure, some types of cancer, and diabetes.

The Dietary Guidelines for Americans are for people who are over two years of age. They are meant to be used by people of all ethnic backgrounds, regardless of their food preferences.

The Guidelines are revised every five years to reflect current science related to health and nutrition. The present set of guidelines focuses on three key messages for consumers.

- Make smart choices from every food group.
- Find your balance between food and physical activity.
- Get the most nutrition out of your calories.

Recommended Daily Intakes								
Food Group	Calorie Level							
	1,800	2,000	2,200	2,400	2,600	2,800	3,000	3,200
Fruits	1.5 cups	2 cups	2 cups	2 cups	2 cups	2.5 cups	2.5 cups	2.5 cups
Vegetables	2.5 cups	2.5 cups	3 cups	3 cups	3.5 cups	3.5 cups	4 cups	4 cups
Grains*	6 oz-eq	6 oz-eq	7 oz-eq	8 oz-eq	9 oz-eq	10 oz-eq	10 oz-eq	10 oz-eq
Meat and beans*	5 oz-eq	5.5 oz-eq	6 oz-eq	6.5 oz-eq	6.5 oz-eq	7 oz-eq	7 oz-eq	7 oz-eq
Milk	3 cups	3 cups	3 cups	3 cups	3 cups	3 cups	3 cups	3 cups
Oils	5 tsp	6 tsp	6 tsp	7 tsp	8 tsp	8 tsp	10 tsp	11 tsp

*Servings in these groups are ounce-equivalents (oz-eq). See Figure 3-5 for what counts as an ounce-equivalent.

***3-6** The USDA Food Guide is intended to help each person choose the types and amounts of foods that are right for him or her.*

Make Smart Choices from Every Food Group

Each food provides different nutrients, and no one food provides every nutrient. Eating a variety of foods is the best way to get all the nutrients your body needs. Choose a mixture of nutritious foods from each group in the USDA Food Guide. However, make sure you do not go over your calorie needs for the day. A few points can help you meet this goal.

Focus on fruits. The nutrients supplied by the fruit group vary from one fruit to the next. Apricots and mangoes are high in vitamin A. Citrus fruits and strawberries are good sources of vitamin C. Oranges provide folate, and bananas are a source of potassium. Choosing a variety of fruits each day can help you get an array of nutrients.

Vary your veggies. Like fruits, foods in the vegetable group differ in the nutrients they provide. Dark green and orange vegetables are rich in vitamin A. Legumes are high in protein. Starchy vegetables offer complex carbohydrates. Other vegetables supply a variety of vitamins and minerals along with fiber. That is why choosing vegetables from each of the five subgroups in the USDA Food Guide is important.

Get your calcium-rich foods. Do not overlook foods from the milk group. You need three servings of lowfat or fat free milk, yogurt, cheese, or dairy alternatives daily. Getting enough calcium in your diet helps you build and maintain strong bones. Choosing lowfat and fat free foods from this group will help you get the most nutrients for the fewest calories. See 3-7.

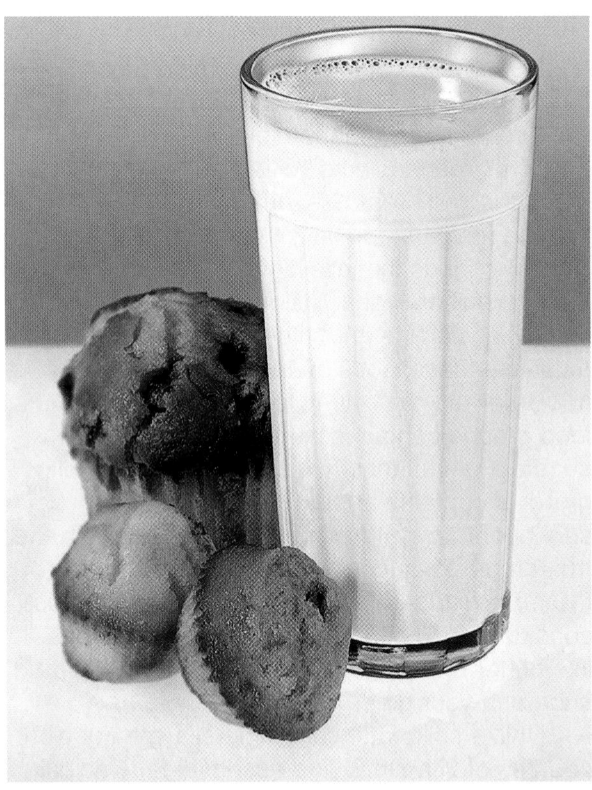

Anchor Hocking

3-7 Getting the three daily servings from the milk group will supply you with the calcium your body needs.

Make half your grains whole. Whole grains, such as brown rice, oatmeal, barley, and whole wheat, are good sources of fiber. Getting enough fiber in your diet helps keep your bowels working properly. Fiber also helps you feel full after eating, so you may be less likely to overeat. At least half your daily servings from the grains group should come from whole grain sources. Read ingredient labels on the bread and cereal products you buy to be sure they are made with whole grains. Choose a variety of grain foods to receive the most health benefits.

Go lean with protein. As you choose foods from the meat and beans group, make sure you are choosing lean cuts of meat. Take the skin off poultry before preparing or eating it to greatly reduce the fat content. Try to include fish in your diet twice a week to get the beneficial types of oils it provides. Avoid fats added during cooking by selecting baked, broiled, and grilled meat, poultry, and fish dishes most often. Choose dry beans and peas frequently as lowfat, high-fiber meat alternates.

Know your fats. Fat is an essential nutrient. However, too much fat in the diet is unhealthful. Saturated fats, *trans* fats, and dietary cholesterol tend to raise blood cholesterol. A high blood cholesterol level is a risk factor for heart disease. All fats provide a concentrated source of calories. A diet that includes too many high-fat foods may not include enough foods that provide all the other needed nutrients. Such a diet may also provide excess calories, which can lead to unhealthful weight gain.

As you choose a variety of foods from each food group, be sure to read the Nutrition Facts panels. This will help you keep your fat intake within recommended limits. Saturated fats should account for no more than 10 percent of your total calories. Keep your intake of *trans* fats as low as possible. Careful food choices will also help you keep your cholesterol intake under 300 mg per day. Your total fat intake should not equal more than 35 percent of your total daily calories.

Reduce sodium (salt), increase potassium. Salt is the main source of sodium in the diets of most people. (A teaspoon of salt provides about 2,000 mg of sodium.) Sodium is a vital nutrient that helps control body fluids and blood pressure. However, too much salt in the diet can promote high blood pressure. Health experts recommend that you keep your intake of sodium below 2,300 mg per day.

Many people in the United States consume more than the recommended amount of sodium. Most of the sodium in the average diet comes from salt that is added to processed foods. Read the Nutrition Facts panel to see how much sodium foods contain. Compare products and choose those that are lower in salt. You also need to limit the amount of salt you add to foods during preparation and at the table.

Besides curbing sodium, be sure to meet your need for 4,700 mg of potassium each day. Potassium helps offset some of the effects sodium has on blood pressure. Foods like sweet potatoes, tomato products, and yogurt are good sources of this mineral.

Don't sugarcoat it. Food products contain two types of sugars—natural and added. *Natural sugars* are found in many nutritious foods, such as fruit and milk. *Added sugars* are ingredients that are put into foods during processing. Foods that contain a lot of added sugars often supply little more than calories. Such foods include nondiet soft drinks, cakes, cookies, ice cream, and candy. Consuming too many of these foods may limit your intake of foods that contain needed nutrients. Excess calories from sugars can lead to weight gain. Sugars also contribute to tooth decay. See 3-8.

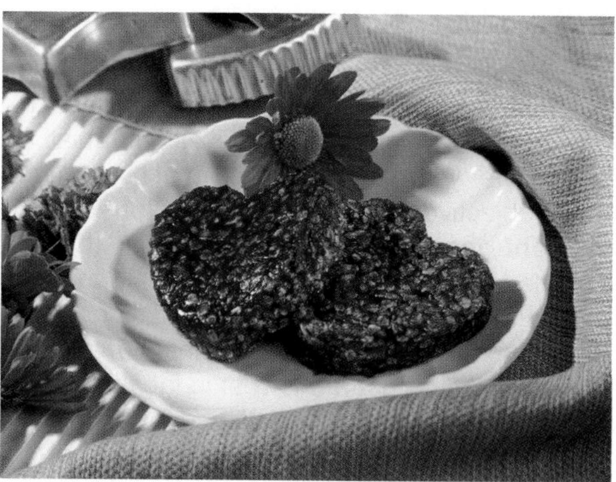

Agricultural Research Service, USDA

3-8 Making smart food choices means limiting foods like cookies, which are high in added sugars and low in nutrients.

The sugars listed on a Nutrition Facts panel include natural and added sugars. You need to read the ingredient list to tell if the food contains much added sugar. Look for such ingredients as corn syrup, fructose, fruit juice concentrate, honey, and molasses. If any of these ingredients appears near the beginning of the list, the food is high in added sugars. You will read more about how to use the information on the Nutrition Facts panel in Chapter 12.

Find Your Balance Between Food and Physical Activity

The goal of the Dietary Guidelines for Americans is to promote health and reduce the risk of disease. In the United States, a main reason for poor health and increased disease risk is overweight. Body weight is not only a result of how many calories you consume through foods. It is also a result of how many calories you burn when you move. Therefore, the Guidelines address more than just food choices. They also focus on physical activity.

A key recommendation of the Guidelines is to maintain body weight in a healthy range. Being overweight is a risk factor for high blood pressure, stroke, arthritis, and many chronic diseases. Weight gain occurs when food and physical activity are not in balance. People who consume more calories through food than they burn through activity will gain weight. To avoid unhealthful weight gain, you may need to eat fewer calories. Choose moderate portions of food. Focus your diet on nutritious foods and limit foods that provide little more than calories.

As you strive to make wiser food choices, take steps to be more active, too. You might choose to exercise or take part in sports. Being physically active will help you burn the calories you consume from foods. It will improve your muscle tone and strengthen your heart and lungs. It will also give you a sense of mental well-being.

The activities you choose should require movement beyond what is needed for your normal daily tasks. You should also limit the amount of free time you spend being inactive. Adults need to get at least 30 minutes of physical activity most, if not all, days of the week. Children and teens need at least 60 minutes of physical activity per day. Spending more time or choosing more intense activities can give you added health benefits. You will read more about managing your weight and being physically active in Chapter 5.

Get the Most Nutrition out of Your Calories

You need to meet your nutrient needs each day. To avoid weight gain, however, you must not go over your calorie needs. To achieve both these objectives, you need to focus your diet on ***nutrient-dense foods.*** These are foods that provide fairly large amounts of vitamins and minerals compared to the number of calories they supply. The most-nutrient dense forms of foods are those that are lowest in fat and free of added sugars, 3-9. Nutrient-dense forms of foods are lower in calories than forms that are less nutrient dense. For instance, fat free milk is the most nutrient-dense form of milk. It is lower in fat and calories than whole milk. Peaches canned in unsweetened fruit juice are a nutrient-dense form of peaches. They are lower in sugar and calories than peaches canned in syrup.

Reading the Nutrition Facts panel on food labels can help you get the most nutrition for your calories. Look at the number of calories a serving of the food provides. Keep in mind that any food providing more than 400 calories per serving is considered high in calories. Use the percent Daily Values to choose foods that are lower in total fat, saturated fat, and cholesterol. A percent Daily Value of 20 percent or more is considered high; 5 percent or less is considered low.

When reading labels, check the serving size and compare it with the amount of food you typically eat. Suppose you eat a portion that is double the serving size listed. You will be getting twice the number of calories listed on the label. You will need to double the amounts and percentages of nutrients listed, too.

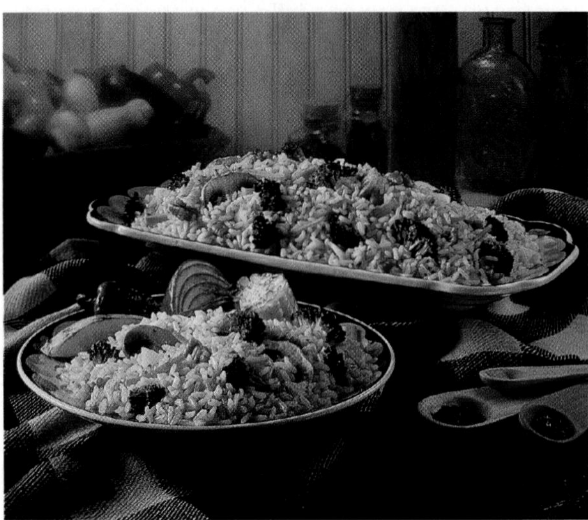

USA Rice Federation

3-9 *A colorful mixture of brown rice and steamed vegetables makes a nutrient-dense side dish.*

Make nutrient-dense choices for all your daily food group servings. This will enable you to have some calories left in your daily allowance. These remaining calories are called ***discretionary calories.*** You may choose to use these calories to eat larger portions of nutrient-dense foods. You could also use them to add small amounts of fats and sugars to your diet.

One use of discretionary calories in the diets of some adults might be alcohol. The Dietary Guidelines advise people who choose to drink alcohol to do so in moderation. This means women should limit their alcohol intake to no more than one drink per day. Men should limit their alcohol intake to no more than two drinks daily. However, many people should stay away from alcohol altogether. Children and teens, as well as people who cannot limit their intake, should not drink alcohol at all. People who will be driving and pregnant and nursing women should not drink alcohol either. Alcohol is an addictive drug. It supplies little more than calories to the diet. Drinking alcohol has been linked with many health problems. These include liver disease, high blood pressure, and some cancers. Excess alcohol also causes many car accidents, suicides, and acts of violence.

Play It Safe with Foods

The main messages in the Dietary Guidelines focus on nutrients, calories, and physical activity. No matter how nutrient dense a food is, however, it can make you sick if it is not wholesome. Therefore, the Guidelines also touch on the topic of food safety.

Q: Won't eating all the recommended daily servings from the USDA Food Guide cause me to consume too many calories?

A: Choosing mainly nutrient-dense foods from each food group will help you stay within your daily calorie needs.

Keeping foods safe involves four basic steps. You can remember these steps by the words *clean, separate, cook,* and *chill.* Be sure your hands, utensils, and work areas are clean before you begin preparing foods. Separate raw foods from cooked and ready-to-eat foods as you shop for, prepare, and store them. Cook foods thoroughly and use a food thermometer to be sure they have reached a safe temperature. Chill perishable foods in a refrigerator or freezer as soon as you can after you buy or prepare them. You will study detailed points for putting these steps into practice in Chapter 6.

Meeting Your Daily Needs

How can you use the various diet planning resources to meet your nutritional needs? An easy way to begin is to plan menus using the USDA Food Guide. Include the recommended number of daily servings in your meals throughout the day. Keep the Dietary Guidelines for Americans in mind as you select foods. See 3-10.

You can use the DRIs to help you evaluate your menu plans. These recommended nutrient intakes can show you whether your menus will provide you with all the nutrients you need. Be sure to consider all beverages, condiments, and snack foods as well as meal items. Use dietary charts, such as those found in Appendix C, "Nutritive Values of Foods," to find each food in your menus. Note the amounts of nutrients supplied by each food. Total the amounts of each nutrient provided by all the foods on your menus. Compare these nutrient totals with the DRIs for your gender and age group.

An easier way to complete this menu evaluation is to use a computer and diet analysis software. You can enter all your food choices into the computer. The software will calculate your nutrient totals. Then it will compare the totals with the appropriate DRIs.

What if your comparison shows that your menu plans are low in some nutrients? You can refer to Chapter 2 to help you identify food sources of needed nutrients. Then you can add these sources to your menu plans.

You can also use this type of analysis to evaluate past food choices. Keep track of all the foods you eat over a three-day period to get an average. After your list is complete, analyze the nutrient content of the food using dietary charts or a software program. If you find your diet is low in some nutrients, you can plan to choose better sources in the future.

Menu Planning with the USDA Food Guide	
Breakfast	2 eggs 2 slices whole wheat toast ½ cup blueberries 1 cup fat free milk
Snack	1 banana 4 whole rye crackers 2 tablespoons peanut butter
Lunch	1½ cups vegetarian chili made with bulgur and lentils 1 piece cornbread 1 cup tossed salad with 1 tablespoon dressing 1 cup fat free milk 1 pear
Snack	1 raisin bagel with 2 teaspoons soft margarine ½ cup orange juice
Dinner	3 ounces broiled chicken 1 cup brown rice ½ cup glazed carrots 1 cup spinach salad with 1 tablespoon dressing 1 whole grain roll with 1 teaspoon soft margarine 1 cup fat free milk ½ cup spiced peaches
Snack	1 cup vegetable juice

3-10 *These menus would provide all the food group servings for a teenage boy needing 2,800 calories per day.*

Choosing Wisely When Shopping for Food

The foods you choose at the grocery store become the foods you will later choose to eat at home. Plan nutritious menus before you go to the store. Then make careful grocery purchases to ensure you stock your shelves with healthful foods. Keeping the Dietary Guidelines for Americans in mind can help you choose wisely when shopping for food. See 3-11.

Fresh or Processed?

When shopping for food, you must consider the time and energy you will have available to prepare it. You must also consider nutrition and your family food budget. Many times, these factors become trade-offs. For instance, you might have to pay more for a frozen dinner in order to

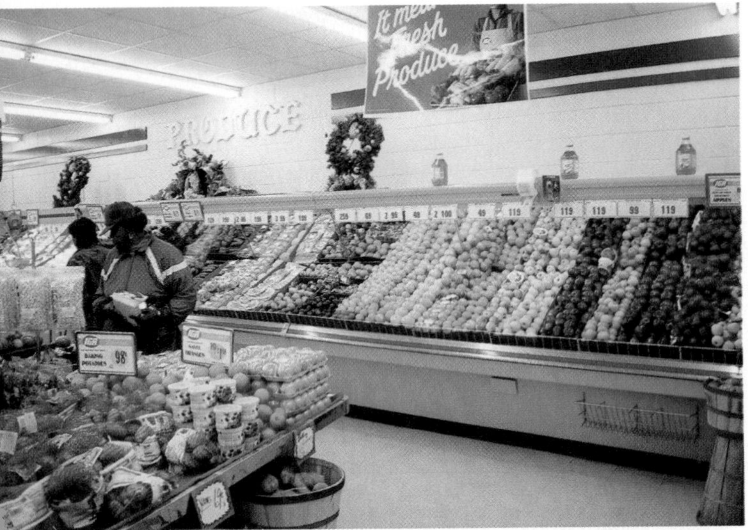
photo courtesy of IGA, INC.

3-11 *Careful shoppers choose healthful foods that will help meet their families' nutritional needs.*

Q: Doesn't it take a lot of time to prepare healthful foods?

A: Some fresh foods take longer to prepare than processed foods. For instance, making spaghetti sauce from fresh tomatoes takes longer than opening a jar of ready-made sauce. On the other hand, you can enjoy many healthful foods with little or no preparation. Fresh fruits and vegetables and whole grain breads are ready to eat as is.

save preparation time. (You will find more shopping guidelines in Chapter 12.)

Processed foods are foods that have undergone some preparation procedure, such as canning, freezing, drying, cooking, or fortification. In most cases, processing adds to the cost of foods. It often decreases the nutritional value of foods, too. For instance, when potatoes are processed into potato chips, they lose nearly all their nutrients. In addition, their fat and sodium contents increase. There are, however, some exceptions to the processing rule. For instance, frozen and canned fruits and vegetables are as nutritious as fresh fruits and vegetables. When whole milk is processed to remove the fat, it becomes more healthful.

Fresh foods, such as fresh meat, poultry, eggs, and produce, have not been processed. In general, the closer a food is to its fresh state, the more nutritious it is likely to be. However, it is important to note that some nutrients in fresh foods can be lost during storage. Fresh foods can also spoil if you keep them too long. Therefore, you should use fresh foods as soon after purchase as possible.

Shopping Tips for Fresh Foods

You will need to evaluate whether fresh foods fit into your food budget and preparation plans. Whenever you feel fresh foods will meet your needs, the following tips can help you buy them:

- Choose a variety of fresh vegetables. They are high in fiber, vitamins, and minerals and low in fat. They are also lower in sodium than most canned vegetables.
- Choose a variety of fresh fruits. They are higher in fiber than fruit juices and lower in sugar than many canned and frozen fruits.
- Stock up on extra fresh fruits to eat as snacks. They can take the place of other snack foods that are higher in fat, sugars, and sodium.
- Look for lean cuts of meats, such as beef round steak, pork tenderloin, and leg of lamb. (For more information on meat cuts, see Chapter 19.)
- Choose meats with little marbling and visible fat. Choose Select grade meats when available.
- Choose fresh chicken and turkey often. Light meat pieces are lower in fat than dark meat pieces.
- Choose fresh fish and shellfish often. Most varieties are low in fat, and fresh seafood is lower in sodium than canned seafood.
- Choose nuts and seeds less often as meat alternates. They are high in fat.

Shopping Tips for Processed Foods

When fresh foods will not fit into your meal management plans, you may decide to buy processed foods. Be aware that some processed foods are more nutritious than others. For instance, applesauce and a fried apple pie are both processed foods. The applesauce has less fiber and more sugar than fresh apples. However, it is lower in fat than the pie, which is more highly processed.

Processed foods have nutrition information on their labels. Reading and comparing package labels can help you get the most healthful products available. Nutrition labeling can help you evaluate how a food fits with the Dietary Guidelines for Americans. You can use calorie information to help you maintain a healthy weight. Look at the calories per serving listed on a label. Consider these calories along with those in your other food choices. Then decide if eating the product will exceed your daily energy needs. See 3-12.

Look at the amounts of fat, sodium, and sugars listed on nutrition labels, too. Remember the Guidelines suggest choosing a diet that is moderate in these substances. Suppose a label shows 18 g of fat, 456 mg of sodium, and 13 g of sugars per serving. This information tells you the food is fairly high in fat, sodium, and sugars. This does not mean you should not purchase the food. However, you will have to choose accompanying foods carefully to stay within recommended limits.

Nutritional labeling can help you compare similar products and different brands of the same product. Suppose you are choosing between three-bean chili and cheese lasagna frozen entrees. Comparing labels can show you which product is lower in calories, fat, sodium, and sugars. Comparing labels can also tell you which product is higher in protein and listed vitamins and minerals. Perhaps you know you want chili, but you cannot decide which brand. Again, comparing the nutrition labels can help you make a healthful choice. (See Chapter 12 for more information on nutrition labeling.)

The following tips can help you choose sensibly when buying processed foods:

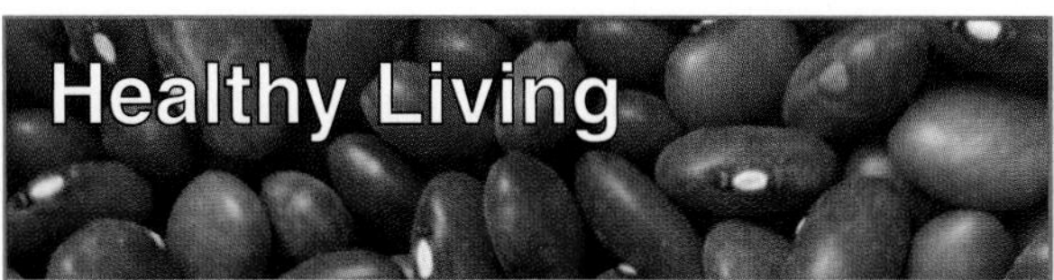

Fat free and reduced fat products can make it easier for you to fit some foods into a healthful diet. As you consider purchasing these foods, however, be sure to read labels carefully. Some products are higher in sodium and sugars than their high-fat counterparts. Also remember that reduced fat products are not dietary cure-alls. Only a fraction of all food products are available in reduced fat versions. Many other foods will continue to supply dietary fat that you cannot ignore.

- Look for whole grain ingredients to appear first on ingredient lists for bread and cereal products. (Be aware that *whole wheat flour* refers to a whole grain ingredient but *wheat flour* does not.)
- Choose bread, English muffins, rice, and pasta often for lowfat complex carbohydrates.
- Choose croissants, biscuits, and muffins less often. They are higher in fat than many other bread products.
- Check the labels on breakfast cereals carefully. Many are good sources of fiber. However, some are high in added sugar and sodium. Granola-type cereals also tend to supply fat.
- Select regular and quick-cooking hot cereals instead of instant products, which tend to be much higher in sodium.
- When buying canned vegetables, choose no-salt-added products, when available.
- Choose fruits canned in juice. They are lower in sugar than those canned in syrup.
- Read labels on fruit juices to be sure they are 100 percent juice. Fruit drinks and punches tend to be high in added sugar and may not contain much juice.
- Choose beans, peas, and lentils often as lowfat, high-fiber alternatives to meats.
- Buy processed meats, like luncheon meats and hot dogs, less often. They are high in fat and sodium.
- Choose canned fish products that are packed in water. They are lower in fat than those canned in oil.
- Choose fat free or lowfat milk and yogurt. They are lower in fat than whole milk products.
- Choose reduced fat versions of dairy products like sour cream and cheese. See 3-13.
- Choose lowfat frozen desserts, such as light ice cream and frozen yogurt, instead of regular ice cream.

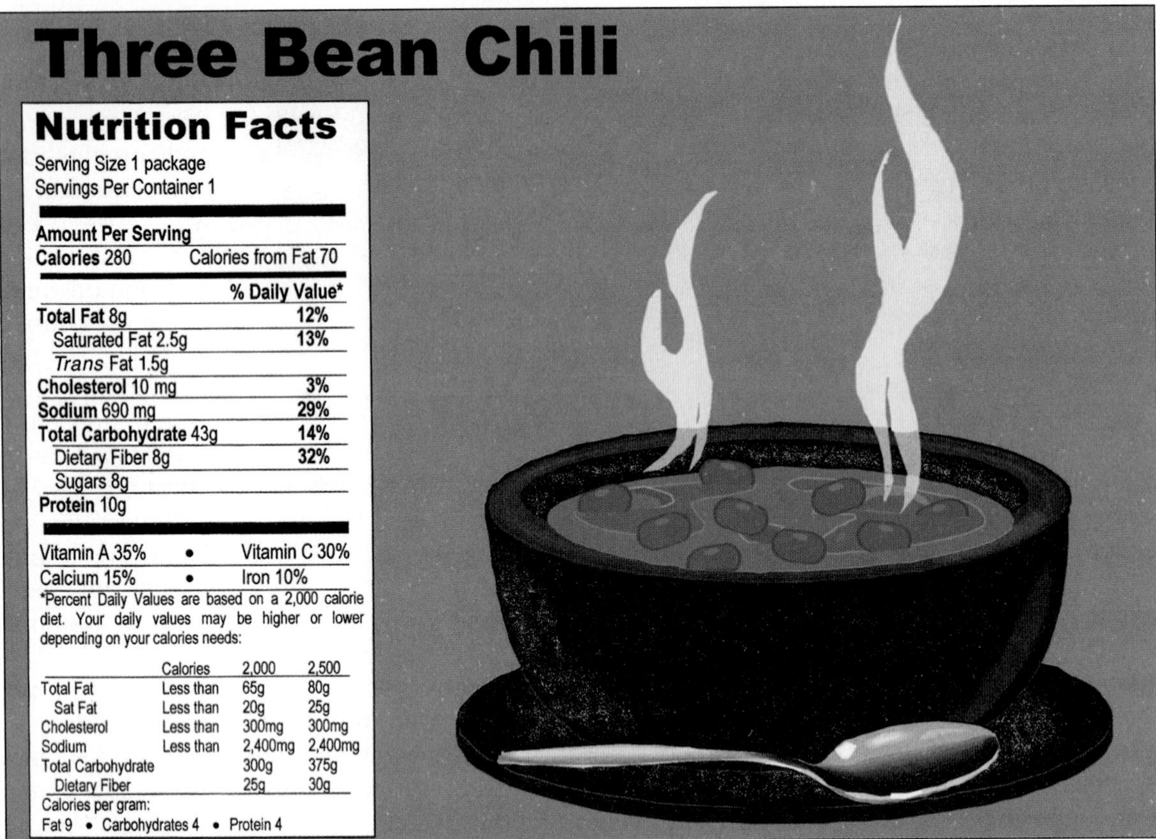

Three Bean Chili

Nutrition Facts

Serving Size 1 package
Servings Per Container 1

Amount Per Serving
Calories 280 Calories from Fat 70

	% Daily Value*
Total Fat 8g	12%
Saturated Fat 2.5g	13%
Trans Fat 1.5g	
Cholesterol 10 mg	3%
Sodium 690 mg	29%
Total Carbohydrate 43g	14%
Dietary Fiber 8g	32%
Sugars 8g	
Protein 10g	

Vitamin A 35% • Vitamin C 30%
Calcium 15% • Iron 10%

*Percent Daily Values are based on a 2,000 calorie diet. Your daily values may be higher or lower depending on your calories needs:

	Calories	2,000	2,500
Total Fat	Less than	65g	80g
Sat Fat	Less than	20g	25g
Cholesterol	Less than	300mg	300mg
Sodium	Less than	2,400mg	2,400mg
Total Carbohydrate		300g	375g
Dietary Fiber		25g	30g

Calories per gram:
Fat 9 • Carbohydrates 4 • Protein 4

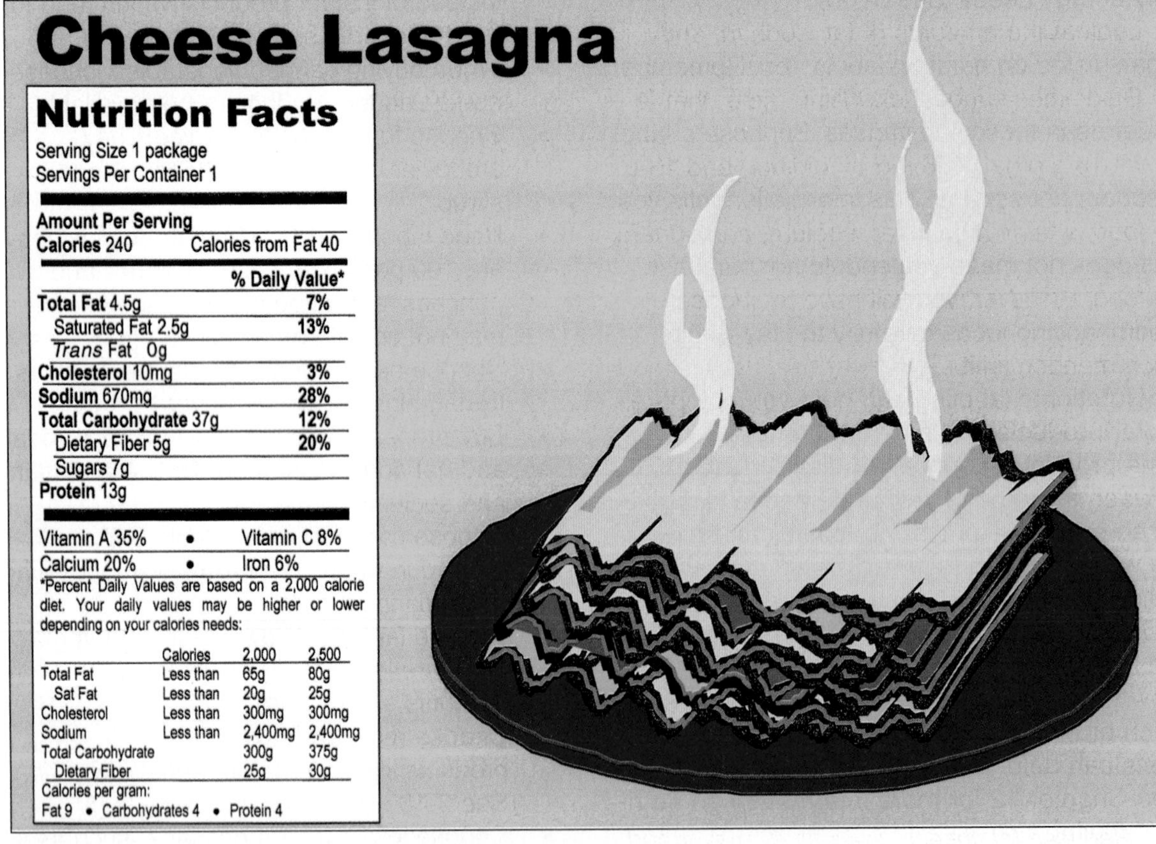

Cheese Lasagna

Nutrition Facts

Serving Size 1 package
Servings Per Container 1

Amount Per Serving
Calories 240 Calories from Fat 40

	% Daily Value*
Total Fat 4.5g	7%
Saturated Fat 2.5g	13%
Trans Fat 0g	
Cholesterol 10mg	3%
Sodium 670mg	28%
Total Carbohydrate 37g	12%
Dietary Fiber 5g	20%
Sugars 7g	
Protein 13g	

Vitamin A 35% • Vitamin C 8%
Calcium 20% • Iron 6%

*Percent Daily Values are based on a 2,000 calorie diet. Your daily values may be higher or lower depending on your calories needs:

	Calories	2,000	2,500
Total Fat	Less than	65g	80g
Sat Fat	Less than	20g	25g
Cholesterol	Less than	300mg	300mg
Sodium	Less than	2,400mg	2,400mg
Total Carbohydrate		300g	375g
Dietary Fiber		25g	30g

Calories per gram:
Fat 9 • Carbohydrates 4 • Protein 4

3-12 *Comparing nutrition information on food labels can help you choose foods that best meet your daily nutrient needs.*

- Consider buying lowfat forms of salad dressings and mayonnaise.
- Read labels on soups, sauce mixes, and packaged entrees carefully. Many are high in sodium.
- Look for lighter versions of snack foods that are high in calories, fat, sugars, and sodium.
- Choose cookies that include fruit and whole grains, such as raisin oatmeal cookies. Avoid those containing more highly saturated fats.
- Choose soft margarine in tubs for use as a table spread. It will be lower in saturated fat than butter and lower in trans fatty acids than stick margarine.

Choosing Wisely When Preparing Food

Making wise food choices at the grocery store is a good beginning to a healthful diet. However, the way you choose to prepare these foods greatly affects their nutritional quality.

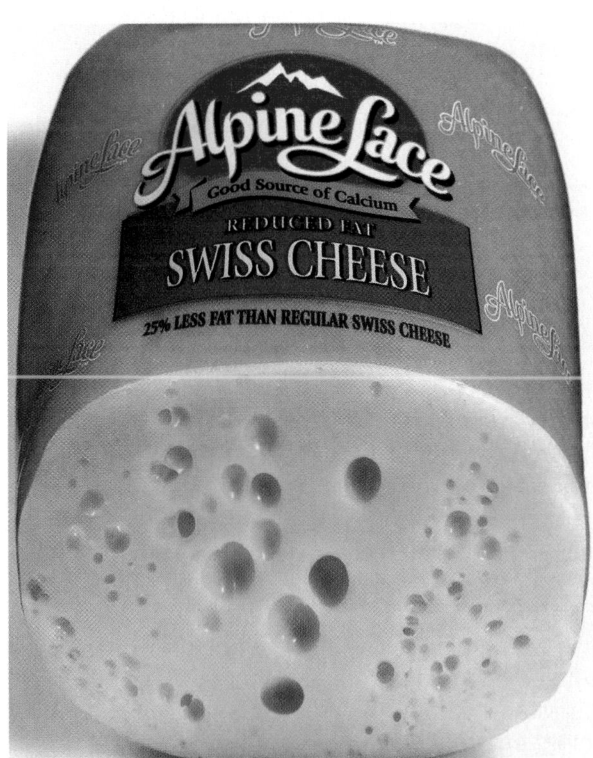

photo courtesy of Land O' Lakes, Inc.

3-13 Reduced fat cheese provides the flavor and nutrients of regular cheese with less fat and fewer calories.

Try to prepare foods from minimally processed ingredients whenever time allows. Preparing foods from scratch gives you more control over what goes into them. You can decide how much fat to use when sauteing vegetables. You can decide when to omit salt or reduce sugar listed in a recipe. The ability to make these decisions can help you prepare foods in keeping with the Dietary Guidelines.

Start with the Main Course

Most meal managers plan meals around a main course, which generally includes a source of protein. A few pointers can help you prepare main courses that will get your meals off to a healthful start.

Remember that your diet should be focused on plant-based foods. Such a diet is likely to be lower in fat and higher in fiber than a diet focused on animal-based foods. A plant-based diet is also rich in substances that may help prevent diseases, including heart disease and some cancers.

To increase your emphasis on plant-based foods, consider preparing meatless entrees on a regular basis. Legumes, such as dry beans, peas, and lentils, are rich in protein and low in fat. You can use them to make hearty soups, stews, and casseroles to serve in place of meat dishes.

Another way to include more plant-based foods in your diet is to let your side dishes become main dishes. Increase the size of your servings from the vegetable and grain groups. Limit the size of your portions of animal protein foods. Remember that you do not need a platter-sized steak or half a chicken to meet your protein needs. A serving of lean, cooked meat, poultry, or fish is just 2 to 3 ounces (56 to 84 g). A 3-ounce (84 g) portion is about the size of a deck of playing cards. If you want to make a moderate portion look bigger, slice it thin and fan it out on your plate. See 3-14.

When your main course does include meat and poultry, start lean. Trim all visible fat from meat. Remove the skin from poultry. These simple steps will reduce fat and calories.

Use lowfat cooking methods when preparing entrees. Such methods include roasting, broiling, grilling, braising, stewing, stir-frying,

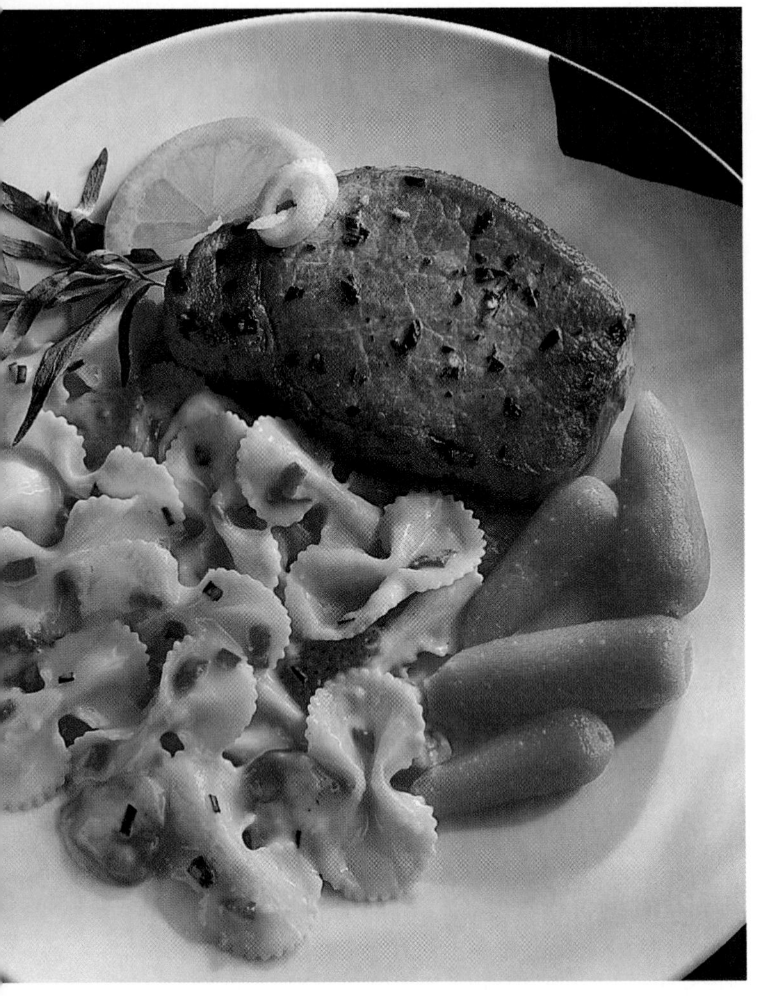

courtesy of National Pork Board

3-14 Choose moderate portions of meat and fill the rest of your plate with grain foods and vegetables.

and microwaving. Use a rack when roasting to allow fats to drain. Avoid using cooking sauces that are high in sugar, fat, or sodium. Add herbs to braising and stewing liquids to season them without salt. Use a nonstick skillet or wok to reduce your need for added fat when stir-frying. Try microwaving to save time as well as fat. (You will find more information about these cooking methods in Chapters 19, 20, and 21.)

Be a Clever Consumer

On a cost per serving basis, meats are among the most costly items you can put in your shopping cart. Legumes can help you stay within your budget when shopping for a main course. Not only are these meat alternates nutritious, they are inexpensive.

You can also stretch your food dollars by mixing meat, poultry, and fish with grain products and vegetables. Casseroles and soups provide more carbohydrates, vitamins, minerals, and fiber than plain meat entrees. Make enough to serve as leftovers. Leftovers save money and heat up quickly for homemade meals in a hurry.

Rounding Out the Meal

After you have planned the main course, you can concentrate on other menu items. Keep in mind not every food you eat must be low in calories, fat, sodium, and sugar. You can balance your food choices to create a total diet that is healthful. For instance, you can balance a high-fat entree, such as spareribs, with lowfat side dishes. Likewise, if you want to serve a rich dessert, you might choose a lighter entree.

Of course, choosing sensible portion sizes will also help you keep your diet in balance. Make a point of actually measuring out servings of some of your favorite foods. See what a serving of cereal looks like in one of your bowls. Become familiar with the appearance of a serving of rice or pasta on one of your plates. See how 6 ounces (175 mL) of juice or 8 ounces (250 mL) of milk looks in one of your glasses. Keeping these portion sizes in mind when you are serving food will help you avoid overeating.

When evaluating your menu, do not forget the items you serve with entrees and side dishes. Toppings and spreads used at the table can affect the nutritional value of foods. Items like sour cream, cream cheese, and jam add fat, sugar, and calories.

Healthful Preparation Tips

Preparation methods can be as important as food choices when it comes to healthful eating. The following tips can help you reduce, replace, or omit ingredients that add fat, sugars, or sodium to foods:

- Cook with liquid oils, such as corn, canola, and olive oil, instead of solid fats, like butter, lard, and shortening, whenever possible, 3-15.
- Avoid adding oil or salt to cooking water when preparing pasta.
- Use only half the amount of butter or

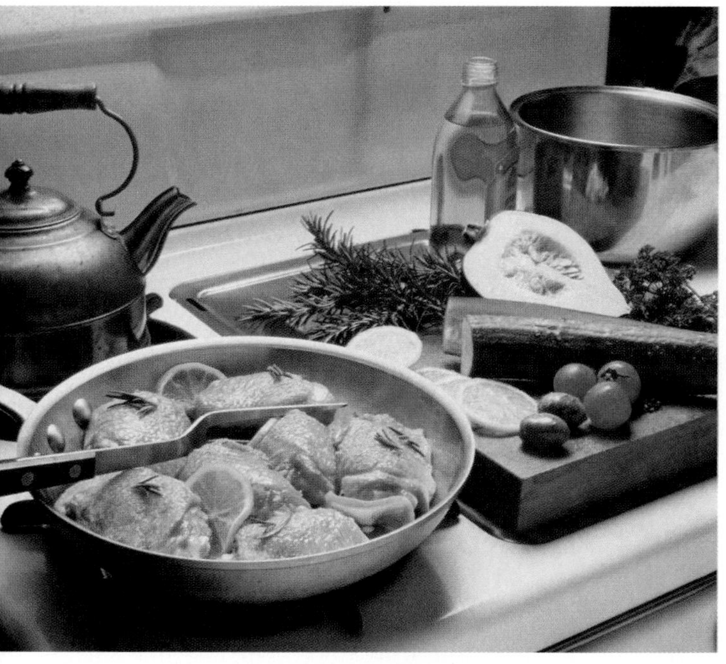

3-15 Cooking with olive oil adds less saturated fat to foods than using shortening or butter.

margarine suggested when preparing packaged pasta, rice, stuffing, and sauce mixes.

- Use salad dressings, mayonnaise, sour cream, and cream cheese sparingly. Try reduced fat versions, or use plain nonfat yogurt in place of these products. You can season yogurt with herbs for tasty dressings and dips.
- Flavor vegetables with herbs and lemon juice instead of salt and butter.
- Omit salt from recipes calling for other ingredients that are high in sodium, such as cheese or condensed soup.
- Reduce the amount of sugar listed in recipes for baked goods. Add vanilla or spices, such as cinnamon, ginger, and cloves, to make these recipes seem sweeter.
- Dust cakes with powdered sugar instead of spreading them with frosting.
- Use fat free or lowfat milk in place of whole milk in recipes. Use fat free evaporated milk in place of cream, except for whipping.
- Use a gravy separator to make it easy to prepare gravies from meat drippings without the fat.
- Chill meat drippings and stocks. Then skim the fat that forms on the top before making gravies and soups.
- Reduce the number of egg yolks used in recipes for baked goods. They are high in cholesterol. Use two egg whites to replace one whole egg. Stretch portions of omelets and scrambled eggs by adding extra egg whites.

Choosing Wisely When Eating Out

Many people choose to eat out when they do not have the time or energy to cook at home. Others eat out as a form of entertainment. In either case, choosing sensibly will allow foods eaten away from home to fit into a healthful diet.

You may not want to worry about nutritional value when you are dining out with friends. There is nothing wrong with occasionally eating a high-fat, high-sodium meal in a restaurant. Simply balance this meal with other meals throughout the day that are lower in fat and sodium. Remember, your *total diet* is what matters.

The more varied a menu is, the easier it is to find healthful food options. You can keep this in mind when choosing a restaurant. Choosing a family restaurant is likely to give you more selection than a fast-food restaurant. However, even the limited menus at many fast-food restaurants offer some health-oriented food options. You might consider ordering a salad with lowfat dressing instead of French fries to accompany your sandwich. You can also cut calories, fat, and sodium from a fast-food meal by choosing regular rather than large-sized items. See 3-16.

In any type of restaurant, menu terms can give you clues about the food you order. Many menu items are high in fat, sugars, and sodium. Watch out for buttered vegetables, fish broiled in butter, and pasta with butter sauce. Be aware of items served with cream sauces, gravy, or cheese. Notice items that are breaded, fried, or wrapped in pastry, too. These items are all likely to be high in fat. Keep in mind that many soups and sauces are high in sodium. Smoked, pickled, and barbecued foods are also likely to be high-sodium items. In addition, foods prepared by these methods have been shown to contain compounds that may cause cancer.

You can control how restaurants prepare your food by requesting that items be made

Fast-Food Comparison			
	Double Cheeseburger Large French Fries Chocolate Reduced Fat Milkshake	Hamburger Regular French Fries Cola	Broiled Chicken Sandwich Side Salad Reduced Fat Milk
Calories	1203	636	560
Total Fat	51 g	22 g	26 g
Saturated Fat	23 g	9 g	7 g
Cholesterol	126 mg	46 mg	112 mg
Sodium	1291 mg	622 mg	971 mg
Carbohydrate	141 g	93 g	46 g
Fiber	6 g	3 g	3 g
Protein	48 g	15 g	36 g
Vitamin A	192 RE	46 RE	411 RE
Vitamin C	21 mg	10 mg	15 mg
Iron	5 mg	3 mg	4 mg
Calcium	539 mg	144 mg	447 mg

***3-16** The calories, fat, saturated fat, and sodium in a fast-food menu can vary greatly, depending on the specific foods ordered.*

according to your preferences. Keep in mind what you have learned about shopping for and preparing food when ordering food in restaurants. For health-conscious menu selections, choose foods prepared with lowfat cooking methods. Ask to have foods prepared without salt or butter. Ask to have high-fat sauces and dressings served on the side. You can add just enough to flavor, rather than smother, your food. Choose whole grain rolls when they are available. Load up on fresh vegetable salads, but go easy on dressing and toppings like bacon bits and cheese. Opt for fresh fruits in place of rich pastries or heavy ice creams for dessert, 3-17.

Remember, the amount of food you eat affects your calorie intake as well as your fat, sodium, and sugar consumption. Ask for a petite or half-sized portion. Consider ordering an appetizer instead of an entree. Split an entree with a friend. Do not feel you have to be a member of the "clean plate club." You can

Q: Isn't a fish sandwich a more healthful fast-food choice than a hamburger?

A: Fish is lower in fat than hamburger. However, most fast-food fish sandwiches are breaded, deep-fried, and served with tartar sauce. This preparation increases the fat content of the fish sandwich, making it a higher-fat choice than the burger. To make informed choices, ask to see nutrition information about menu items before ordering food at a fast-food restaurant.

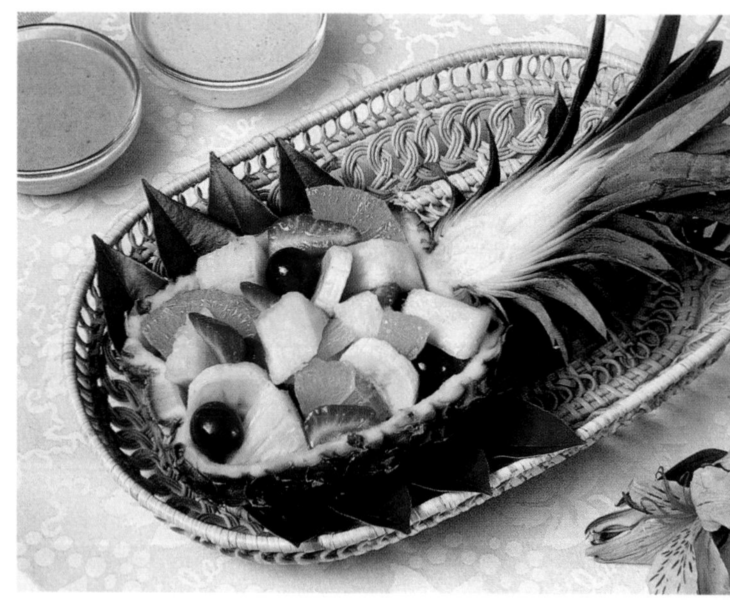

Dole Food Company

***3-17** Fresh fruit makes a delicious, light dessert at the end of almost any meal.*

always ask to have a take-home bag for food you do not finish. You might even want to have half of your entree packed before you begin eating. This will keep you from accidentally eating more than you had intended. These are all ways to help keep yourself from overeating.

Consider having water with your meal instead of ordering a soft drink. Water is a great thirst quencher, and this choice will save you money as well as calories from added sugars.

Keep in mind that foods eaten away from home are not always eaten in restaurants. Use the guidelines given above when choosing foods from vending machines and in the school cafeteria. These guidelines also apply at the snack bar in the mall and the concession stand at ball games.

Eating out, like shopping for and preparing food, requires you to use the principles of variety, moderation, and balance. Follow the Dietary Guidelines for Americans and choose the right number of servings from the USDA Food Guide. Make healthful eating a lifetime habit.

Good Manners Are Good Business

Sharing an entree is an option for light eating when dining with family members or friends. However, it is generally not appropriate at an important business meal. Sharing may be acceptable for casual business dining, but be sure to do it with finesse. Transfer a portion of the food being shared to your dining companion's plate before you begin eating. Eating off the same plate is definitely beyond the bounds of good manners.

Chapter 3 Review

Making Healthful Food Choices

Summary

Making healthful food choices can benefit you in a number of ways. Choosing a nutritious diet can protect and possibly improve your health. An adequate supply of nutrients can help you have healthy skin, hair, and teeth. Having a sound body and healthy appearance can, in turn, have positive effects on your work and family life.

A number of resources can help you make healthful food choices. You can use Dietary Reference Intakes to evaluate the quality of your diet. Use the USDA Food Guide to plan menus that will meet your daily nutritional needs. Follow the Dietary Guidelines for Americans to form good eating and activity habits.

Using these resources, you can make informed choices when shopping for fresh and processed foods. You can also make wise decisions about how you prepare those foods. You can choose sensibly when eating away from home, too.

Review What You Have Read

Write your answers on a separate sheet of paper.

1. What are three factors besides food choices that can affect your health?
2. What is the recommended nutrient intake value set for nutrients for which no RDA can be determined?
   A. Adequate Intake (AI).
   B. Dietary Reference Intake (DRI).
   C. Estimated Average Requirement (EAR).
   D. Tolerable Upper Intake Level (UL).
3. Name the five main food groups in the USDA Food Guide and give the number of servings you should obtain from each group each day.
4. True or false. Foods in all five main groups of the USDA Food Guide may contain solid fats and added sugars.
5. What are the three key consumer messages in the current Dietary Guidelines for Americans?
6. What mineral helps offset some of the effects sodium has on blood pressure?
7. Compare the nutrient density of a baked skinless chicken breast with a fried chicken leg that has the skin.
8. How does processing affect the nutritional value of foods?
9. List five tips to follow when shopping for fresh foods.
10. Name five lowfat cooking methods that can be used to prepare entrees.
11. How can the fat in gravies made from meat drippings be reduced?
12. Which of the following items on a restaurant menu is likely to be your best bet for a lowfat side dish?
    A. Mashed potatoes with gravy.
    B. Steamed broccoli with cheese sauce.
    C. French fries.
    D. Sliced tomatoes sprinkled with fresh herbs.

Build Your Basic Skills

1. **Writing.** Work in a small group to design a pamphlet explaining the key consumer messages of the Dietary Guidelines for Americans. The pamphlet should be geared for a teen audience. The words and design should inspire teens to adopt healthier eating and activity habits. Vote to choose the most creative and effective pamphlet design in your class. Then make copies of the winning pamphlet and pass them out in the school cafeteria.
2. **Math.** Prepare a food item according to a traditional recipe. Then use one of the techniques suggested in the chapter to reduce

the calories, cholesterol, fat, sodium, or sugar in the food product. Use dietary charts or diet analysis software to determine the differences in nutritive values between the two products.

Build Your Thinking Skills

1. **Analyze.** Record all the foods you have eaten in one 24-hour period. Analyze your food record to determine whether you consumed the recommended number of servings from each group in the USDA Food Guide during that day. If you did not, make a list of foods you could add to supply the missing servings.
2. **Summarize.** Bring in two nutrition labels from similar processed foods, such as frozen entrees or breakfast cereals. Prepare a written comparison identifying the nutritional strengths and weaknesses of each product. Summarize your comparison with a paragraph stating which product you would prefer to buy. Give reasons for your choice.
3. **Propose.** Contact a local fast-food restaurant to request nutrition information about its menu items. Use this information to propose an idea for a new health-oriented menu item.

Apply Technology

1. Compare snack chips made with a fat replacer to conventional chips in terms of cost, taste, and nutritional value.
2. Use chapter information to write 30 nutrition tips. Use the tips as daily screen savers on your home or classroom computer.

Using Workplace Skills

Nancy is a family and consumer sciences teacher at Green Valley High School. In her foods classes, Nancy lectures on nutrition, shows videotapes on food safety, and demonstrates preparation techniques. She plans labs and other experiences to help her students learn how to prepare and serve nutritious, appealing meals.

To be an effective worker, Nancy needs skill in teaching others. Imagine you are a student in Nancy's class. Answer the following questions about her need for and use of this skill:

A. What are two characteristics of Nancy's teaching techniques that would most help you learn?
B. How could Nancy's skill in teaching others have an effect on your future?
C. How might Nancy's skill in teaching others affect the number of students who sign up for her class next year?
D. What is another skill Nancy would need in this job? Briefly explain why this skill would be important.

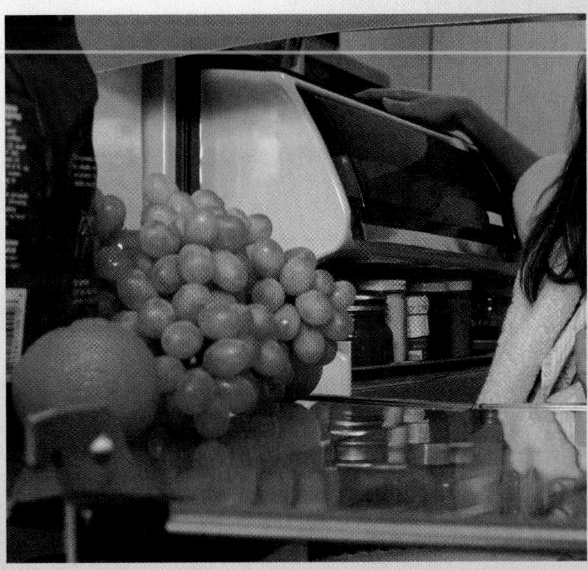

Chapter 4

Nutrition Through the Life Cycle

School Cafeteria Head Cook
Supervises and coordinates activities of workers engaged in preparing, cooking, and serving food in one or more school cafeterias or a central school district kitchen.

Institutional-Nutrition Consultant
Advises and assists personnel in public and private establishments, such as hospitals, health-related facilities, child-care centers, and schools, in foodservice systems and nutritional care of clients.

Dietary Aide
Prepares and delivers food trays to hospital patients, performing any combination of duties on tray line.

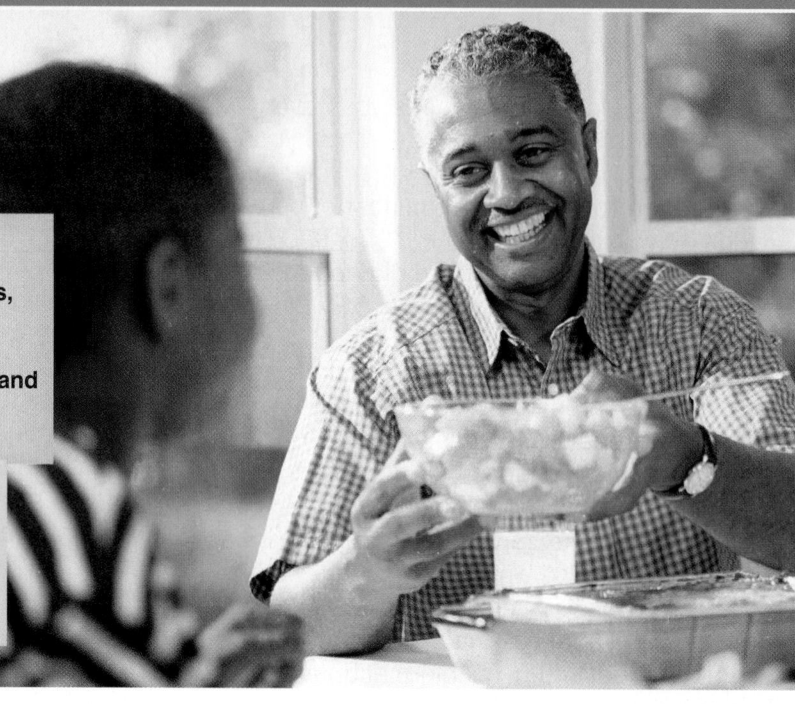

Terms to Know

diet
food allergy
food intolerance
growth spurt
vegetarian diet
medical diet
diabetes mellitus
food-drug interaction

Objectives

After studying this chapter, you will be able to

- describe health and development concerns that affect the nutritional needs of people in different stages of the life cycle.
- list meal-planning tips to meet the nutritional needs of people in different stages of the life cycle.
- plan a nutritious diet for yourself.

A person's ***diet*** is all the food and drink he or she regularly consumes. Each stage of a person's life cycle is affected by his or her diet. From the prenatal period to old age, each stage is associated with nutritional needs. Poor nutrition in any stage may create health problems, shorten the life span, or both.

Nutrition During Pregnancy and Lactation

Diet during pregnancy affects both the mother and the *fetus*, or developing baby. Good nutrition is especially important during pregnancy. This is because the mother nourishes the fetus through her body. The foods the mother eats must supply the nutrient needs of the fetus. Otherwise, nutrients for the fetus may be taken from the mother's tissues. This could cause the mother to suffer deficiencies. See 4-1.

Nutrient deficiencies can be a problem especially in the case of teenage pregnancies. Teen mothers need high levels of nutrients to support their own growth. Deficiencies could negatively affect a teenage mother's development as well as the development of her baby.

Special Needs During Pregnancy

A key nutritional need during the first *trimester* (three month period of pregnancy) is the need for folate. Folate helps prevent *neural tube* damage in the fetus. This is damage to the brain or spinal cord. It can occur in the early weeks of pregnancy before many women even know they are pregnant. This is why all women of childbearing age should meet the RDA for folate each day. Once pregnancy is confirmed, a woman should begin consuming the increased RDA for folate of 600 micrograms daily.

By the beginning of the second trimester, needs for almost all the essential nutrients increase. Some of the extra nutrients are needed to build the child's tissues. Others are needed to protect the mother.

Protein, calcium, and iron are especially important during pregnancy. The mother needs increased amounts of protein to support the growth of the fetus. Most women in the United States eat more than enough protein to meet this increased need.

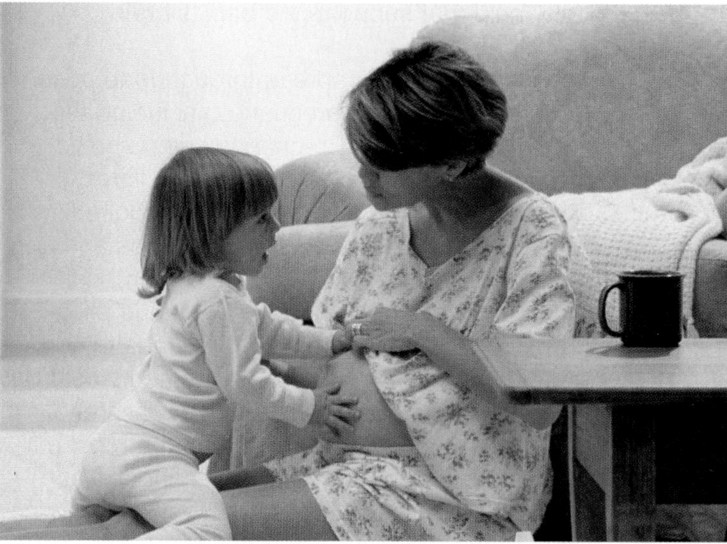

4-1 *During pregnancy, a woman requires extra nutrients to meet the needs of her developing baby.*

The fetus needs calcium for well-formed bones and strong teeth. If the mother's diet does not supply enough calcium, the needs of the fetus will be taken from the mother's bone tissue. This increases the mother's risk of developing osteoporosis later in life.

Iron needs are especially large during the last six months of pregnancy. This is to help the baby build up iron reserves before birth. The baby will need these reserves during the first six months of life. A pregnant woman who does not get enough iron may become anemic as her body works to meet her baby's needs.

Diet During Pregnancy

A pregnant woman should follow a nutritious diet consisting of a variety of foods. She should build the diet around the Food Guide Pyramid. If the woman's diet was adequate before pregnancy, a simple modification is all she should need. During the second trimester, she should add two daily servings from the grains group. She should also add one serving of fruit and one serving of vegetables. In the third trimester, a pregnant woman might add one more serving of grains. These additions will provide extra calories and many needed nutrients. She should limit fats, oils, and sweets. She should also eat fish regularly because they provide a type of fatty acid that supports the baby's brain development.

Some illnesses spread through food pose greater risks during pregnancy, including the risk of miscarriage. Pregnant women should avoid eating foods linked with these illnesses. These foods include raw and undercooked meat, poultry, seafood, and egg dishes and unpasteurized milk and juice. Recommendations about other foods to avoid during pregnancy change based on the latest health and food safety findings. Pregnant women would be wise to check the government's food safety Web site at foodsafety.gov to find the most current advice. Carefully following the food handling guidelines described in Chapter 6 will also help prevent illness.

Q: Isn't a woman supposed to "eat for two" when she is pregnant?

A: A pregnant woman needs to eat enough calories and nutrients to support the growth of her developing baby. However, this is not twice as much food as she normally eats. She requires only an extra 340 calories a day, beginning in the second trimester. By the third trimester, her increased calorie need goes up to 450 calories per day.

Obstetricians often prescribe nutrient supplements for pregnant women. These supplements include iron along with vitamins and other minerals. Many women have low iron reserves, and supplements help them meet the increased demands of pregnancy. Pregnant women should never take supplements without consulting their doctors. Too much of some vitamins and minerals can be harmful to pregnant women and their developing babies.

During pregnancy, the average woman gains about 25 to 35 pounds. However, weight gain and energy needs vary from woman to woman. A pregnant woman should be neither overweight nor underweight. An obstetrician will suggest a suitable weight gain.

Diet During Lactation

During *lactation* (the production of breast milk), a woman has increased energy, protein, mineral, and vitamin needs. The woman needs these extra nutrients to replace the nutrients secreted in the milk. She also needs them to cover the energy cost of producing the milk and to protect her body, 4-2.

The diets of a lactating woman and a pregnant woman are similar. However, the lactating woman's needs for some nutrients are greater.

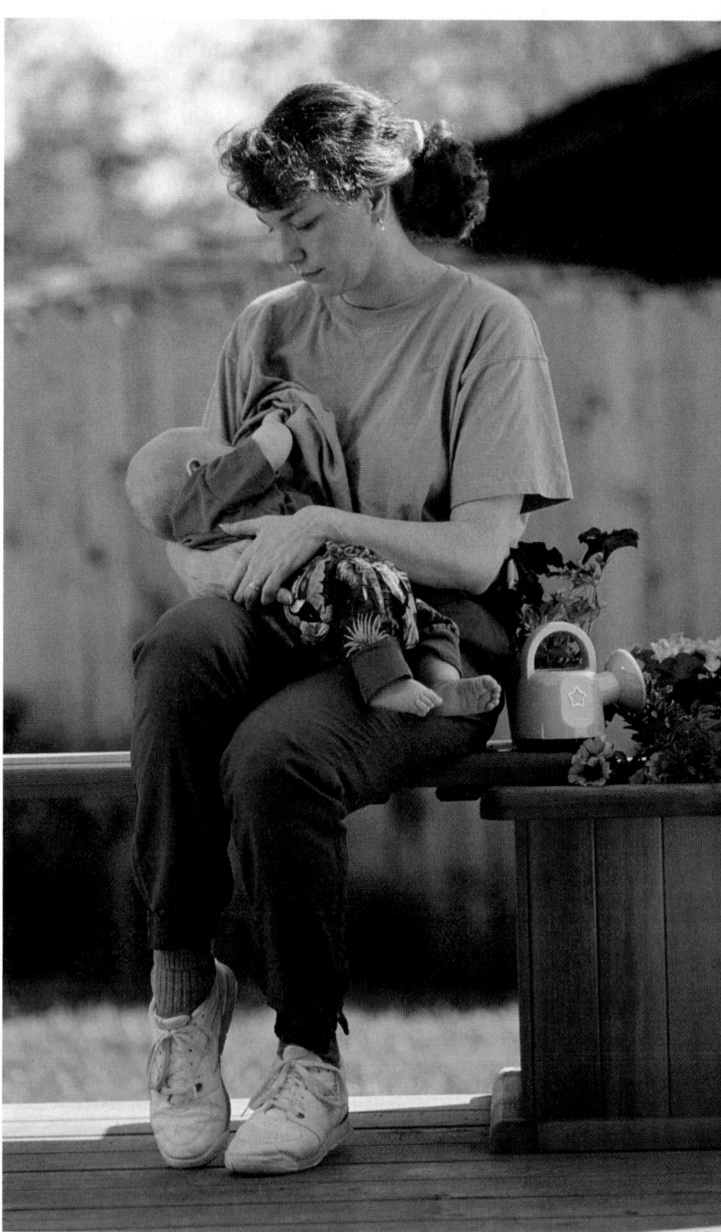

***4-2** Like pregnancy, lactation creates increased nutrient needs for a woman. Her body needs extra nutrients to help it produce milk to feed her baby.*

Lactating women should be sure to get the recommended number of servings from the Food Guide Pyramid each day. Such diets will help them meet their nutrient and energy needs. They should also consume at least 2 to 3 quarts (2 to 3 L) of fluid each day. Lactating women need liquids to provide water in breast milk and to meet their own fluid needs.

Avoiding Drugs During Pregnancy and Lactation

Many drugs can have harmful effects on a developing fetus or nursing baby. This is why pregnant and lactating women should not use alcohol, tobacco, and illegal drugs. Alcohol is a drug, and tobacco contains nicotine, which is a drug. During pregnancy, drugs can pass from the mother's body to the baby through the placenta. (The *placenta* is an organ that nourishes the developing child in the mother's womb.) During lactation, drugs can pass to a baby through breast milk. Pregnant and lactating women should even avoid prescription and over-the-counter medications, such as aspirin, except under a doctor's advice.

Nutrition in Infancy and Early Childhood

Infants and preschool children need good nutrition to grow and develop normally. A healthful diet is more important during the first year of life than at any other time in the life cycle.

Nutritional Needs of Infants

An infant's requirements for all nutrients are higher per unit of body weight than an adult's. Unlike adults, however, an infant has no nutrient reserves. The exception is iron. A full-term baby should have enough reserve iron to last for the first six months of life. A baby needs iron reserves because he or she consumes only breast milk or infant formula during the first few months. Breast milk is not a rich source of iron. Formula may be fortified with iron, but a baby cannot absorb it well.

Infants generally receive injections of vitamin K at birth. This meets their needs for the vitamin until bacteria in their intestinal tracts develop and begin making it. Some breast-fed infants also receive a supplemental source of vitamin D. This helps prevent rickets, the vitamin D deficiency disease that results in malformed bones.

Besides high nutrient needs, an infant has high energy needs to support rapid growth. Growth patterns vary, but an infant's rate of growth is fastest during the first few months of life. During the first three months, a normal, healthy infant will gain about 2 pounds (910 g) a month. The growth rate then slows to about 1 pound (454 g) a month. As growth slows, an infant's energy needs per unit of body weight decrease slightly. By the end of the first year, the infant's weight has almost tripled. His or her length is one and one-half times the birth length.

Feeding Infants

Parents usually need to feed newborns seven or eight times a day. Newborns are just learning to eat, and their small stomachs cannot hold much. Feedings gradually decrease to about five a day by the time the infant is two months old. Although intake varies, most infants will drink about 1 quart (1 L) of breast milk or formula each day. See 4-3.

Breast Milk or Formula

Nutrition experts strongly recommend that mothers breast-feed their infants. Brain development is rapid during the first years of life. Breast milk is recognized as the best food to foster brain development. Breast milk is easy for a baby to digest. It provides nutrients in ratios that

Q: Won't putting some cereal in a baby's bottle help him or her sleep through the night?

A: No data show adding cereal to a baby's bottle will help the baby sleep. A baby's ability to sleep through the night depends on the maturity of his or her nervous system. To protect a baby's developing gums and teeth, a bedtime bottle should contain nothing more than plain water.

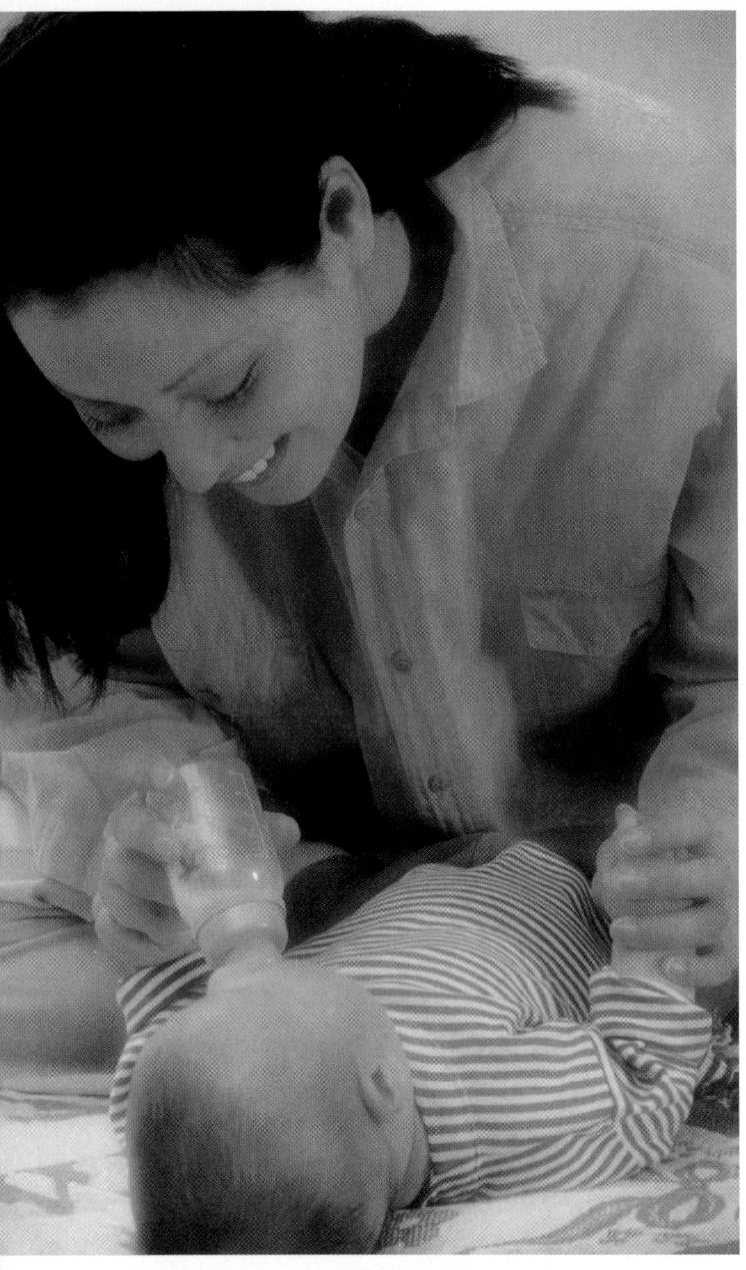

4-3 Infants cannot eat much at each feeding. Therefore, they must eat often to get the nutrients needed to support their rapid growth and development.

are perfectly designed for babies. It contains immune substances that help a baby resist infection. Breast milk also helps protect the baby from developing allergies.

Iron-fortified infant formulas are available for mothers who are unable or choose not to breast-feed their infants. Infant formula contains less carbohydrate and fat and more protein than breast milk. Formula also contains more of many vitamins and minerals. However, babies absorb the lower amounts of nutrients in breast milk better than the nutrients in formula. In addition, too much of some nutrients, such as protein and calcium, can place stress on a baby's immature kidneys.

Cow's milk is difficult for infants to digest and may cause intestinal bleeding. Cow's milk is not a suitable food for babies under 12 months of age. After a baby's first birthday, whole cow's milk can be introduced into his or her diet. Lowfat milk is not recommended for children under 24 months of age because they need fat for normal growth and development.

Solid Foods

The introduction of solid foods into a baby's diet should be gradual. Most infants are ready to begin eating solid foods when they are between four and six months old. The first solid food in most babies' diets is a single-grain, iron-fortified baby cereal. Rice cereal is usually recommended because it is least likely to cause an allergic reaction. Parents may introduce single pureed vegetables and fruits into their babies' diets after cereals. They follow these with strained meats and poultry and then food mixtures.

Most pediatricians tell parents to start with a small amount of just one new food at a time. Parents should feed the baby the same food several times in a row. This will help the parents identify food allergies. A true ***food allergy*** involves a response of the body's immune system to a food protein. Medical tests are required to verify food allergies. Allergy symptoms may include diarrhea, vomiting, skin rashes, and runny nose. Foods to which children are most commonly allergic include peanuts, cow's milk, egg white, orange juice, and wheat. Many experts recommend waiting until babies are a bit older before introducing these foods.

Infants may be sensitive to certain foods without being truly allergic to them. A ***food intolerance*** is a negative reaction to a food substance that does not involve the immune system. Symptoms of food intolerance may resemble allergy symptoms. Whether symptoms are due to allergy or intolerance, they should end when parents stop feeding the baby the problem food. Parents may try reintroducing the food a month or two later. Sensitivities often go away as infants mature.

Sometime between the ages of four and six months, most infants can begin drinking out of a cup. This is when parents often introduce fortified juice, usually apple, as a source of vitamin C.

Parents can add chopped foods from family meals to a child's diet by his or her first birthday.

Nutritional Needs of Preschool Children

Growth is slower between the ages of two and six years than it is during the first year of life. However, growth is still quite rapid. The diet should supply enough calories for a weight gain that fits a child's normal rate of development.

Nutrient needs vary from child to child, depending on growth and activity. A diet consisting of foods from the Food Guide Pyramid should supply sufficient nutrients. Parents should be sure children's food choices include good sources of iron, such as enriched cereals and cooked dry beans.

Meals for Preschoolers

Preschool children often have unpredictable eating habits. Parents can encourage eating by keeping the preschooler's likes and dislikes in mind at mealtime. Most preschool children tend to like foods that are mild flavored, soft, and lukewarm. Finger foods, bright colors, and small portions also appeal to them, 4-4. A pleasant eating atmosphere with a chair, table, and eating utensils that are the right size can encourage good eating. Most pediatricians agree parents should not force children to eat. If children will not eat at one meal, they will often make up for it at another.

When planning meals for a preschooler, follow the Food Guide Pyramid. Some children will not drink the recommended 2 cups (500 mL) of milk. In these cases, parents can feed children more foods prepared with milk. Some toddlers would rather eat five or six small meals than three large meals. Begin with small portions and add more as needed. How and when children consume food is not important. What is important is that each day's diet includes all the necessary nutrients.

Nutrition in the Elementary School Years

During the elementary school years, children grow at a fairly steady rate. Between the ages of 6 and 12, children develop many of the food habits they will follow throughout life. Parents can promote healthy attitudes about good nutrition by setting good examples. They should encourage their children to try new foods. However, parents should refrain from using food as a punishment or reward.

Nutritional Needs of School-Age Children

A 6-year-old child does not need as much food as a 12-year-old child. However, both children need the same kinds of food. The amount

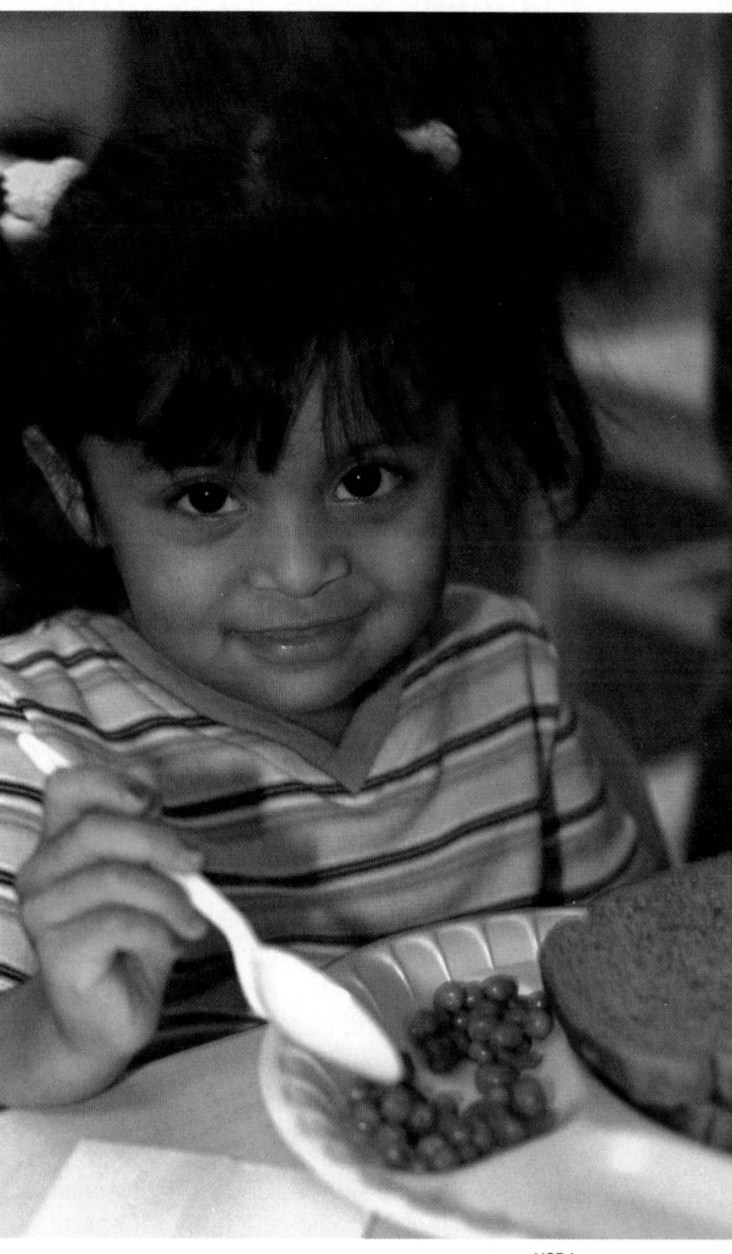

USDA

4-4 Bright colors and small portions help make foods appealing to preschoolers.

of food a child needs depends on his or her growth rate and physical activity. Normally, a child's appetite is a fairly reliable indication of energy needs.

The school-age child should eat foods from all the food groups. Children ages nine and over need a third serving from the milk group each day. All food choices should be nutrient dense to promote growth and development. Many school-age children prefer familiar foods that are mild in flavor. As children grow older, their food tastes gradually change. They will eat larger servings and enjoy a greater variety of foods.

Planning Meals for School-Age Children

Breakfast should supply about one-fourth of the day's total nutrients for a school-age child. Children who skip breakfast do not obtain nutrients when the body needs them most—after a night without food. Studies have shown that children who eat breakfast do better in school than children who skip breakfast.

Children can eat any nutritious food for breakfast. Breakfast does not have to include traditional breakfast foods. Yogurt or a bowl of tomato soup is just as nutritious at breakfast as it is at lunch or dinner.

The basic meal patterns for a school-age child's lunch and dinner are about the same. Each meal should supply about one-third of the day's total nutritional needs. Both meals should contain foods from all the food groups.

Many school-age children have trouble eating enough at meals to meet their nutritional needs. Snacks can provide added nutrients. Most children like fresh fruit, raw vegetables, cheese cubes, yogurt, raisins, and crackers with peanut butter. See 4-5.

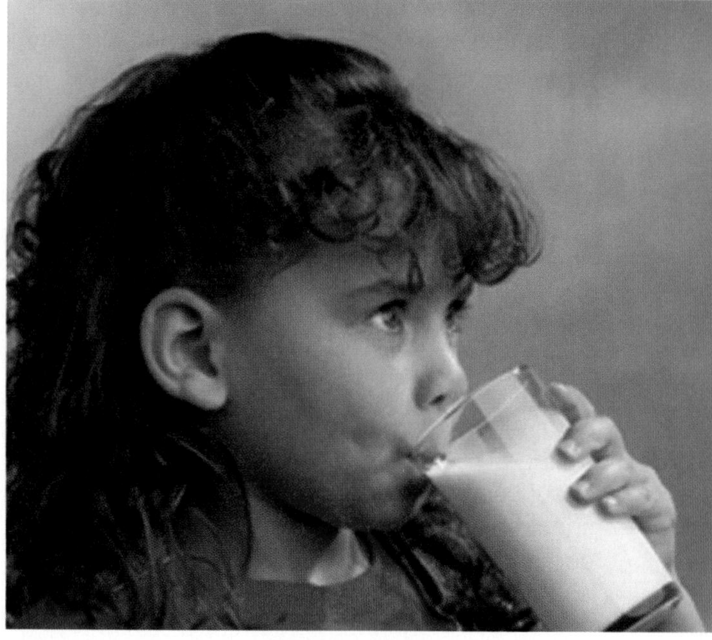

National Fluid Milk Processor Promotion Board

4-5 *Milk is a nutritious accompaniment to a meal or snack for a school-age child.*

Childhood Overweight and Obesity

Overweight and obesity are common among children. An *overweight* child weighs more than what is considered a healthy weight for his or her height. *Obesity* is a condition characterized by excessive deposits of body fat. Children do not have the decision-making skills to make all their own lifestyle choices. Therefore, parents have to help children manage their weight. Otherwise, children are likely to have weight problems as adults.

Parents may begin to address a child's weight problem by encouraging the child to be more active. They can limit the amount of time the child spends watching TV and playing video games. Parents can provide healthful snacks, such as fresh fruit and pretzels. This will help the child avoid snack foods that are simply high in calories. Parents can also help the child learn to use hunger signals to guide his or her eating habits. They might discourage snacking in front of the TV as a routine behavior. They could avoid insisting the child clean his or her plate at mealtimes, too. Instead, parents can provide moderate portions and allow the child to stop eating when he or she is full. These steps will help slow a child's weight gain. In time, his or her growth will catch up to the excess weight.

Parents should consult a registered dietitian before making major changes in a child's diet. Children need a nutritious diet to support growth. Restricting foods may result in a lack of important nutrients.

Nutrition in the Teen Years

All teenagers undergo a period of rapid growth called a ***growth spurt.*** The growth spurt varies from teen to teen. However, girls usually experience it at an earlier age than boys.

During the growth spurt, teens of both sexes need more energy. From ages 14 through 18, active teenage girls need about 2,300 calories per day. Active teenage boys need about 3,100 calories per day. Teens need more of other nutrients, too. They should choose three servings daily from the milk group to meet calcium needs. Teenage girls also need to choose good sources of iron, such as turkey dark meat and whole grain breads.

Many teens have busy schedules, which cause them to skip meals. Foods teens grab on the go are often low in nutrient density. Some teens limit food intake due to weight concerns. All these factors put teens, especially girls, at risk of nutrient deficiencies.

Planning Meals for Teens

The family meal pattern should be satisfactory for teenagers. Teens can increase portion sizes where needed to supply additional energy and nutrients.

Snacks often count for one-fourth of a teen's total daily calorie intake. Thus, nutritious snacks are especially important. Fresh fruits and vegetables, lowfat cheese and yogurt, and sandwiches make nutritious snacks. Cookies made with whole wheat flour, oatmeal, raisins, or nuts add nutrients and satisfy the desire for sweets, 4-6.

Teens should limit their intake of nondiet soft drinks, which are a major source of added sugars in the diet. Instead, teens should most often choose to drink water, fat free milk, and juices.

Q: Do greasy foods, chocolate, and/or cola drinks cause acne?

A: Some people used to think these and various other foods caused teen acne. However, studies have not shown a link between any foods and acne. Of course, eating a nutritious diet can help promote healthy skin.

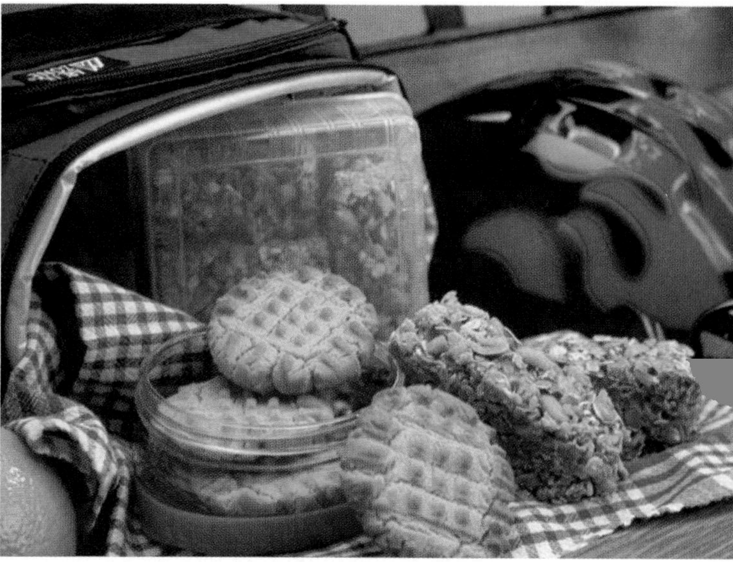

National Peanut Board

***4-6** Cookies made with nutritious ingredients, such as peanuts and peanut butter, can be an occasional snack choice for active teens.*

Adolescent Overweight and Obesity

Overweight and obesity are common among adolescents, just as they are among children. Unlike children, however, teens have the decision-making skills needed to manage their weight. They can learn to make healthful food choices. They can include physical activity in their daily schedules. They can also learn how to handle situations that might prompt them to overeat.

Many adolescents who have weight problems continue to have weight problems as adults. To break this pattern, overweight and obese teens must learn and apply weight management skills. However, teens should note that nutrition experts do not recommend losing weight during the growth years. Teens need energy to support their growth and activity. Instead of restricting calories, experts advise overweight and obese teens to choose calorie sources that are rich in nutrients. They also recommend that teens adopt an active lifestyle that includes at least 60 minutes of moderate activity daily. This is the most important step teens can take to maintain healthy weight all through life. You will read more about weight management in Chapter 5.

Nutrition in Adulthood

Energy needs decrease as people become older. Adults who lead active lives require more calories than adults who lead sedentary lives. However, even active adults require fewer calories than teenagers. The need for most nutrients does not decrease. In fact, the daily need for calcium increases for adults over age 50. Many adults suffer from vitamin and mineral deficiencies.

Jobs, family responsibilities, and other activities make many demands on adults' schedules. As a result, many adults do not take the time to eat properly. Fast-food meals eaten on the run often replace more nutritious meals prepared at home. Snack foods often replace breads and cereals, fresh fruits, and vegetables.

A little planning can improve the nutritional quality of adult diets. An adult can set the alarm 15 minutes early to allow time for a good breakfast. Those who carry their lunches to work can pack sandwiches made on whole grain bread. Packed lunches can also include raw vegetables, a piece of fruit, and a thermos of fat free milk. Adults can prepare nourishing dinner foods in quantity when time is available. They can then freeze the foods for later use. They can keep fresh fruits and vegetables on hand for snacks.

Planning Meals for Adults

Adults should plan their meals around the Food Guide Pyramid. Adults over age 50 need to choose three daily servings from the milk group. Choosing lowfat foods most often will help adults avoid consuming more calories than they need. Eating plenty of whole grain foods, vegetables, and fruits will help adults build a base for healthful eating. As adults grow older, they need to make an effort to remain physically active each day. This will help them stay fit and prevent undesirable weight gain.

Nutrition in the Later Years

As people grow older, they often decrease their physical activity. Their bodies also need less energy to carry on vital processes. Therefore, they require fewer calories. The recommended energy intake for active men 51 years of age is about 2,700 calories. The recommended intake for active women of the same age is about 2,100 calories. See 4-7.

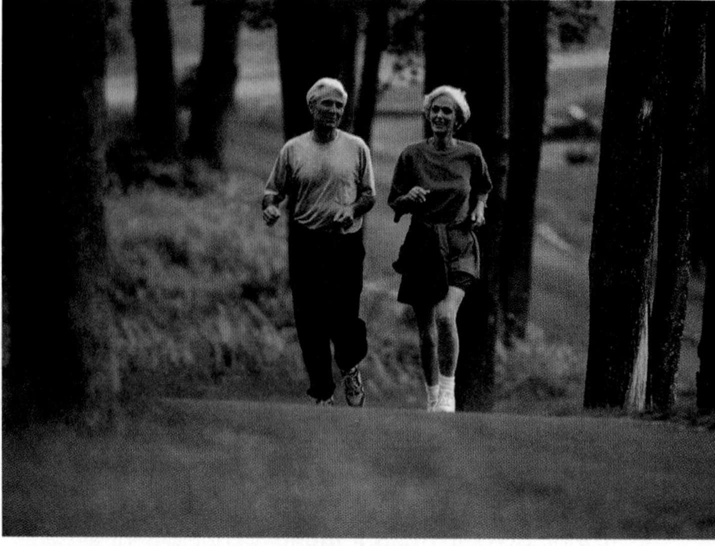

***4-7** Energy needs do not decrease as much for older adults who remain physically active.*

Although energy needs decrease with age, the needs for most nutrients do not decrease. Calorie for calorie, foods eaten by people over 50 need to provide more nutrients than foods eaten by young adults. The diets of many older adults tend to be low in vitamins D, B_6, and B_{12}. Calcium, protein, and fluids are also dietary concerns for many older adults.

Calcium-deficient diets have caused osteoporosis to be a major health problem for older people. The number of older people who suffer from broken bones and curving of the spine reflect this fact. Older women are at the greatest risk of developing osteoporosis. This is because women have less bone mass than men. Earlier in their lives, women are likely to have greater demands made on their calcium stores due to pregnancies. Hormonal changes that take place after menopause also contribute to osteoporosis.

High calcium intake cannot cure osteoporosis once it has developed. People must meet calcium needs and engage in weight-bearing physical activities throughout life to prevent the disease. Older adults need to include three daily servings from the milk group in their diets. Choosing calcium-fortified foods will also help older adults meet calcium needs. Older adults need to include walking, dancing, gardening, or other forms of daily activity in their daily lifestyles. These steps will reduce the natural loss of bone mass that occurs during old age. For those who have osteoporosis, meeting daily calcium needs will keep the disease from worsening.

Be a Clever Consumer

Many products claim to slow the aging process or hide its effects. Keep in mind that aging is a natural part of the life cycle. Products that make dramatic claims can seldom live up to them. There is nothing wrong with buying creams that promote smoother skin or dyes that cover gray hair. However, clever consumers know the keys to a long and healthy life are a nutritious diet and daily physical activity. They also know the importance of avoiding harmful lifestyle behaviors, such as smoking, that increase health risks.

Special Problems of Older Adults

Several factors can affect the diets of older adults. One of these is limited income. Some older people find it hard to afford nourishing foods. They can receive help through federal programs, such as the Food Stamp Program.

Difficulty in shopping is a second factor that can affect the diets of older adults. Those who have this problem can sometimes receive help from church and civic groups. Grocery stores in some areas will deliver groceries for a small fee. Many communities have a service such as Meals on Wheels that delivers nutritious meals to homebound people.

Loneliness makes eating unappealing for some older people. This is because many people view eating as a social activity. Many communities have programs that allow senior citizens to gather for a nutritious noon meal. The older adults may meet at a church or civic center. Social activities sometimes follow the meal. Some schools open their lunch programs to senior citizens for a small fee. Older people who cannot pay may receive their lunches free of charge.

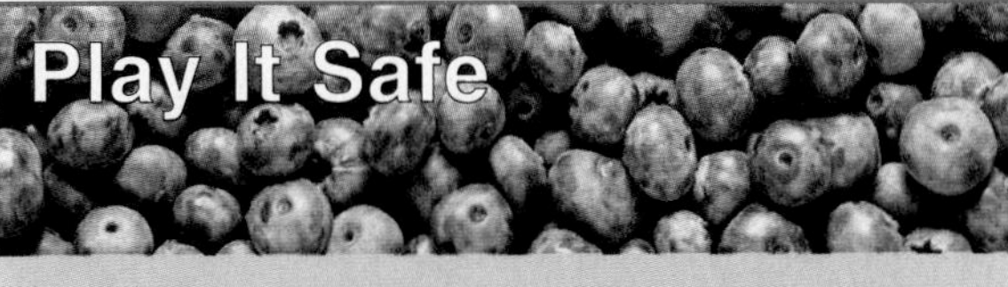

Play It Safe

Foodborne illnesses can be much more serious for older adults than for younger adults. Take extra care to handle food properly when preparing it for older family members. This includes thoroughly cooking any food containing raw eggs. (Some raw eggs are contaminated with illness-causing bacteria.) Consider using egg substitutes in place of fresh eggs. If you do use fresh eggs, cook them until the whites are completely set and the yolks are thickened. Yolks do not need to be hard, but they should no longer be runny.

Planning Meals for Older Adults

Like people in other age groups, older adults should plan their meals around the Food Guide Pyramid. They should eat inexpensive and filling whole grain breads and cereals often. They should choose five or more servings of fruits and vegetables each day for vitamins, minerals, and fiber. Older adults should limit foods that are high in sugars and fats. See 4-8.

Foods from the milk group are especially important in the diets of older people. These foods provide vitamins D and B_{12}, calcium, and protein. People on limited budgets can use nonfat dry milk. Cream soups, puddings, lowfat cheese, and yogurt are alternatives for older people who do not like to drink milk.

Meals should consist of well-liked foods. Food likes and dislikes are hard to change. An older person who needs encouragement to eat is more likely to eat favorite foods.

The way meals are served can also affect their appeal. A fresh flower placed on a table or meal tray can make an ordinary meal seem more special. Older people can carry meals set on trays to the porch or living room for a change of scenery.

During meal preparation, older people who have limited mobility can save physical energy in many ways. They can use convenience products to save preparation steps. They can sit while preparing some foods. They can store frequently used tools and basic food items on shelves within easy reach. Single-handled faucets are easy to use with one hand. Older people can slide heavy objects rather than lifting them. If peeling and chopping vegetables is difficult, precut frozen or canned vegetables can be substituted for fresh. An older person can make some foods ahead of time to reduce preparation tasks at mealtime.

Special Diets

Some people choose to follow special diets. Other people follow special diets on their doctor's advice. A registered dietitian can be a resource to help make sure a special diet meets a person's nutritional needs.

Vegetarian Diets

A ***vegetarian diet*** is a diet built partly or entirely on plant foods. Reasons people choose to follow vegetarian diets include religious beliefs, environmental concerns, and animal rights issues. The types of foods included in vegetarian diets vary. For instance, *lacto-ovo vegetarians* include dairy products and eggs in their diets. *Vegans* eat no animal foods of any kind.

You might think omitting animal foods such as meat, poultry, and fish from the diet would cause a protein deficiency. However, legumes, nuts, and grains are all good sources of protein. By choosing a variety of these plant foods every day, vegetarians can easily meet their protein needs. The types of amino acids lacking in one food will be provided by another. Lacto-ovo vegetarians can also use dairy foods and eggs to increase the protein value of plant foods. Macaroni and cheese is an example of a dish that combines dairy and wheat. See 4-9.

A number of nutrients other than protein are concerns for vegetarians, especially vegans. Shortages of vitamins D and B_{12}, calcium, iron, and zinc are common. Some sources of these nutrients vegetarians might choose are shown in 4-10.

Nutrient deficiencies pose greater risks for certain groups of people. Failure to meet nutrient needs can stunt the growth of infants, children, and teens. Nutrient deficiencies can affect the health of pregnant and lactating women and their babies. Vegetarians in these groups are advised to consult with a registered dietitian. The dietitian can determine whether nutrient needs are being met. He or she can also recommend nutrient supplements when needed.

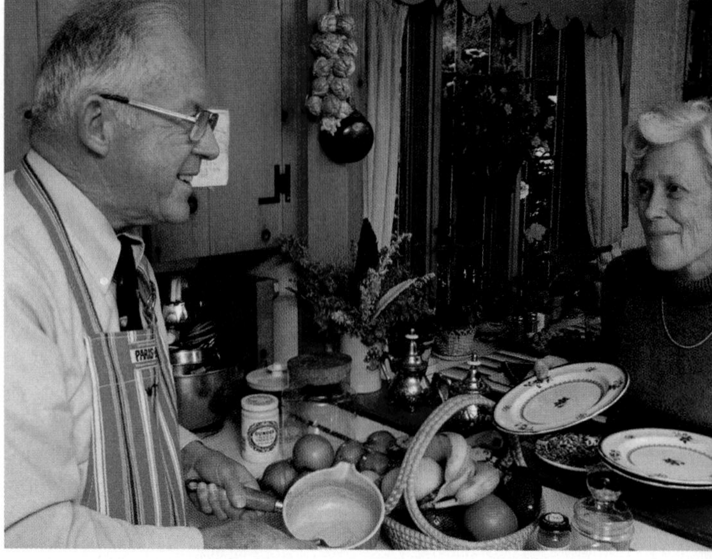

4-8 Eating a nutritious diet is an important factor in maintaining good health during the later years in life.

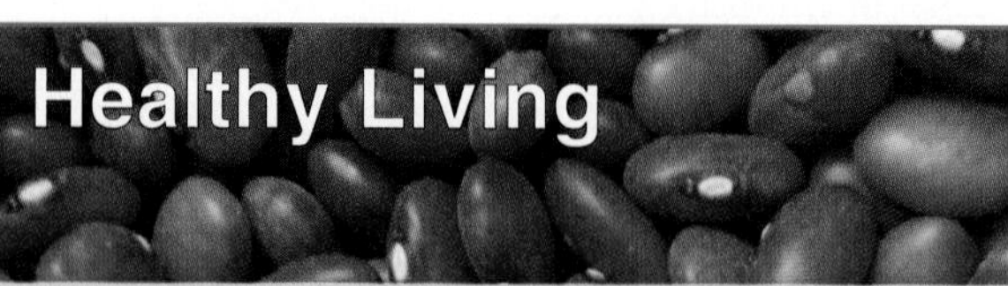

Healthy Living

Some people choose to follow vegetarian diets for health reasons. Vegetarian diets tend to be higher in fiber and lower in saturated fat than diets that include meat. However, the quality of a vegetarian diet, like the quality of any diet, depends on the specific food choices. Remember, all food groups include sources of fat and added sugars. The most healthful vegetarian diets include a variety of foods. They should focus on whole grains, legumes, and fresh fruits and vegetables. Lacto-ovo vegetarians should limit their use of whole eggs and egg yolks and choose lowfat dairy products.

Medical Diets

Medical diets are eating plans prescribed by a physician. They address special needs of people with specific health problems, such as ***diabetes mellitus.*** This is a body's lack of or inability to use the hormone insulin to maintain normal blood glucose levels. Other health problems for which doctors order medical diets include heart disease, cancer, allergies, and HIV/AIDS.

Most people do not have the background needed to plan a medical diet. A registered dietitian can design a diet a patient will be able to follow with success. The dietitian will consider how the medical condition is affecting the patient's body and nutritional needs. He or she will consider the patient's food likes and dislikes. The dietitian will also use the principles of variety, balance, and moderation to outline menus that will meet health goals. See 4-11.

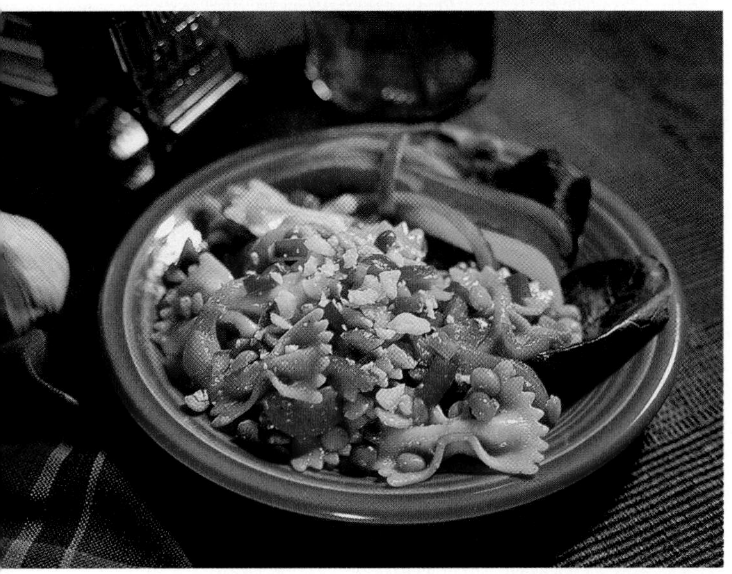

USA Dry Pea & Lentil Council

4-9 The combination of pasta and split peas makes this vegetarian salad a source of complete protein.

Nutrition During Illness

Even people who do not have ongoing health problems get sick from time to time. Knowing how minor illnesses can affect your appetite and nutrient needs can help you handle common ailments.

Drinking liquids is a recommended treatment for many everyday health problems. Warm liquids soothe a sore throat. Chilled liquids help cool a fever. Liquids flush bacteria out of your urinary tract to help prevent infections. They replace fluids lost through diarrhea and through perspiration caused by fever. They help keep sinus and nasal secretions flowing. This provides relief when you have the flu, a cold, or a sinus infection.

A number of common digestive and intestinal disorders are related to food habits. Choose sources of sodium and potassium and avoid greasy, fried, spicy, and high-fiber foods when diarrhea becomes a problem. Eat high-fiber foods, including fresh fruits and vegetables and whole grain breads and cereals, to help prevent constipation.

Nausea, vomiting, and fatigue brought on by illness can often take away your appetite. If a sore throat makes swallowing hard, you may not feel like eating either. However, your body needs nutrients to help the healing process. If you do not feel like eating, try drinking a nutritious beverage instead. Sometimes juice or a nutritious smoothie made with fruit and yogurt goes down easier than solid food.

Food and Drug Interactions

Some drugs can affect the way the body uses nutrients from foods. Similarly, some foods can affect the way drugs are absorbed and used in the body. Such reactions between foods and drugs are called ***food-drug interactions.***

Anytime you must take prescription or over-the-counter medications, be sure to read labels carefully. Follow all directions about consuming foods and beverages. Unless your doctor or pharmacist tells you otherwise, take all medicines with water. Water helps most drugs dissolve quickly, and it does not interfere with absorption. If you must take drugs for an extended period, you may want to consult a registered dietitian. He or she can assess how to best address any nutritional problems the drugs might cause.

Meeting Vegetarian Nutrient Concerns	
Nutrient	**Sources**
Vitamin B_{12}	Fortified cereals and soy milk
Vitamin D	Exposure to sunlight, fortified margarine and milk
Calcium	Fortified cereals, orange juice, and soy milk; leafy green vegetables; legumes; tofu
Iron	Leafy green vegetables, legumes, tofu, whole grains (Eat sources of vitamin C, such as citrus fruits, strawberries, tomatoes, and peppers, with iron sources to improve iron absorption.)
Zinc	Dairy products, eggs, legumes, nuts, tofu, whole grains

4-10 Vegetarians must plan their diets with care to avoid deficiencies of these vitamins and minerals.

Medical Nutrition Therapy		
Medical Condition	**Description**	**Recommended Nutrition Therapy***
Cancer	Uncontrolled cell multiplication, which interferes with normal functioning of body organs	To cope with nausea and vomiting resulting from cancer treatment and medications • Sip cool, clear liquids to prevent dehydration • Choose bland foods that are easy to digest, such as gelatin, crackers, and dry toast • Avoid strong food odors • Avoid greasy, spicy, and very sweet foods
Diabetes mellitus	Lack of or inability to use the hormone insulin, which results in irregular blood glucose levels and can lead to damage of body tissues	Eat regularly scheduled meals Eat a variety of foods Monitor carbohydrate intake, focusing on grain-, fruit-, and milk-group sources Limit fat intake Choose adequate sources of fiber Maintain healthy body weight
Food allergy	A response of the body's immune system to a food protein, which can cause symptoms such as hives and breathing difficulties	Read all food labels carefully to completely avoid the allergy-causing food or ingredient
Gastroesophageal reflux disease (GERD)	Recurrent heartburn caused by stomach acid flowing up into the esophagus	Avoid overeating Eat small, frequent meals Drink liquids between meals rather than with meals Avoid spicy and greasy foods Avoid lying down for at least one hour after eating
High blood cholesterol	Above average amount of cholesterol in the bloodstream, which is a risk factor for heart disease	Moderate total fat intake Limit sources of saturated fats, such as heavily marbled meats and full fat dairy products Choose sources of monounsaturated fats more often, such as olive oil and fish Limit foods containing partially hydrogenated oils, such as margarine, snack foods, and commercially fried foods, to avoid sources of *trans* fats Choose sources of fiber, such as fruits, vegetables, and whole grains
HIV/AIDS	A disorder that causes the body's immune system to shut down and is often accompanied by a loss of appetite leading to wasting	Eat small, frequent meals When feeling well enough to eat, choose high-protein, high-calorie foods, such as cheese, eggs, nuts, and liquid meal replacements Limit liquids with meals to keep from feeling full Strictly follow food safety practices
Hypertension	High blood pressure, which is a risk factor for heart disease	Limit sources of sodium, such as processed foods, salty snacks, and table salt Choose sources of potassium, calcium, and magnesium Moderate fat intake Choose adequate sources of fiber
Lactose intolerance	Inability to produce the enzyme lactase, which is needed to digest the sugar in milk, results in symptoms such as gas, cramps, and bloating after consuming milk products	Choose cheese and cultured dairy products, such as yogurt Eat small amounts of dairy products with other foods Choose lactose-reduced dairy products

** This is a partial list of recommended nutrition therapies and is not intended to replace specific advice of a physician or registered dietitian.*

4-11 Many patients can help control their medical conditions through diet as well as medication.

Chapter 4 Review

Nutrition Through the Life Cycle

Summary

Good nutrition is important at all stages of the life cycle. During pregnancy, a woman must eat a range of foods to supply her developing baby with the nutrients it needs. For the first few months after birth, infants obtain needed nutrients from breast milk or formula. Most parents slowly begin introducing solid foods into their infants' diets when the infants are about four to six months old. Preschoolers and school-age children need help to choose foods that will meet their needs. As children become teenagers, they need more nutrients and calories to support their rapid growth. Adults must select foods carefully to meet their nutrient needs without getting too many calories. Older adults may need to choose foods that will help them counter problems with digestion and mobility. Throughout life, the Food Guide Pyramid can help people choose foods to meet their nutrient needs.

People at any life stage may have special dietary needs. Vegetarians must choose plant foods with care to meet their nutrient needs. People on medical diets must follow a doctor's or dietitian's advice to address specific health problems.

Review What You Have Read

Write your answers on a separate sheet of paper.

1. What can happen if the calcium needs of a fetus are not provided by the foods eaten by the mother?
2. Why should lactating mothers avoid smoking cigarettes, drinking alcohol, and taking medications?
3. True or false. Full-term babies usually need a supplemental source of iron shortly after birth because they have no iron reserves.
4. What is the difference between a food allergy and a food intolerance?
5. List three things a parent can do to encourage a preschooler to eat.
6. How can school-age children who have trouble eating large meals meet their nutritional needs?
7. What are four steps parents can take to help overweight and obese children manage their weight?
8. What are three factors that put teens at risk of nutrient deficiencies?
9. True or false. The need for vitamins and minerals drops dramatically when people reach adulthood.
10. What are two problems that might affect the diets of older adults?
11. True or false. Lacto-ovo vegetarians include dairy products and eggs in their diets.
12. Explain what liquid should generally be used to take medications.

Build Your Basic Skills

1. **Reading/writing.** Visit the government's food safety Web site at foodsafety.gov. Look for advice directed toward pregnant women. Use this information along with food safety guidelines in Chapter 6 to write a food safety brochure for pregnant women.
2. **Verbal.** Choose one medical condition that requires a special diet. Find out as much as you can about that diet and report to the class.

Build Your Thinking Skills

1. **Propose.** Divide a sheet of paper into four sections. Label the sections *Busy Schedules, Skipped Meals, Reducing Diets,* and *Low Nutrient Density Foods.* In each section, write proposals teens could follow to avoid or make up for that particular cause of nutrient deficiencies.

2. **Create.** Create an activity that would encourage school-age children to be more physically active. For instance, you might write a jump rope rhyme or make up an active game. If possible, share your activity with a group of school-age children and discuss the children's reactions in class.

Apply Technology

1. Investigate the features available on two models of baby monitors. Present your comparison in a brief oral report to the class, stating which model you would recommend to an expectant mother.
2. Research the effectiveness of new products containing antioxidant vitamins that are being developed to counter some effects of aging. Summarize your findings in a written report.

Using Workplace Skills

Carmelita is the head cook in the Hayward Heights High School cafeteria. She supervises a staff of seven workers. Each day, they prepare and serve lunch to over 1,500 students during three lunch periods. The staff gets ingredients for the lunch menus from a central warehouse. However, the weekly delivery is often short of some items.

To be an effective worker, Carmelita needs problem-solving skills. In a small group, answer the following questions about Carmelita's need for and use of these skills:

A. What is a specific problem Carmelita has to solve in her position as school cafeteria head cook?
B. How might the other cafeteria workers be affected if Carmelita lacked problem-solving skills?
C. How might the students at Hayward Heights be affected if Carmelita lacked problem-solving skills?
D. What is another skill Carmelita would need in this job? Briefly explain why this skill would be important.

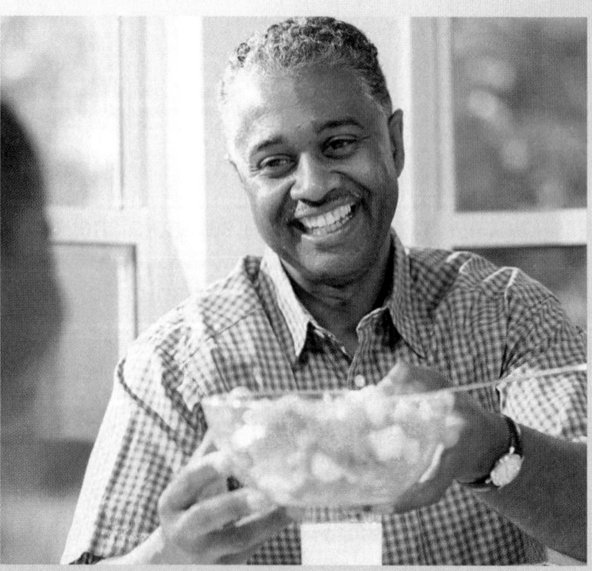

Chapter 5

Staying Active and Managing Your Weight

Exercise Physiologist
Develops, implements, and coordinates exercise programs and administers medical tests, under physician's supervision, to program participants to promote physical fitness.

Athletic Trainer
Evaluates physical condition and advises athletes to maintain maximum physical fitness for participation in athletic competition. Recommends special diets to build up health and reduce overweight athletes.

Reducing-Salon Attendant
Measures, weighs, and records patrons' body statistics; refers information to supervisor for evaluation and planning of exercise program; and demonstrates exercises and use of equipment.

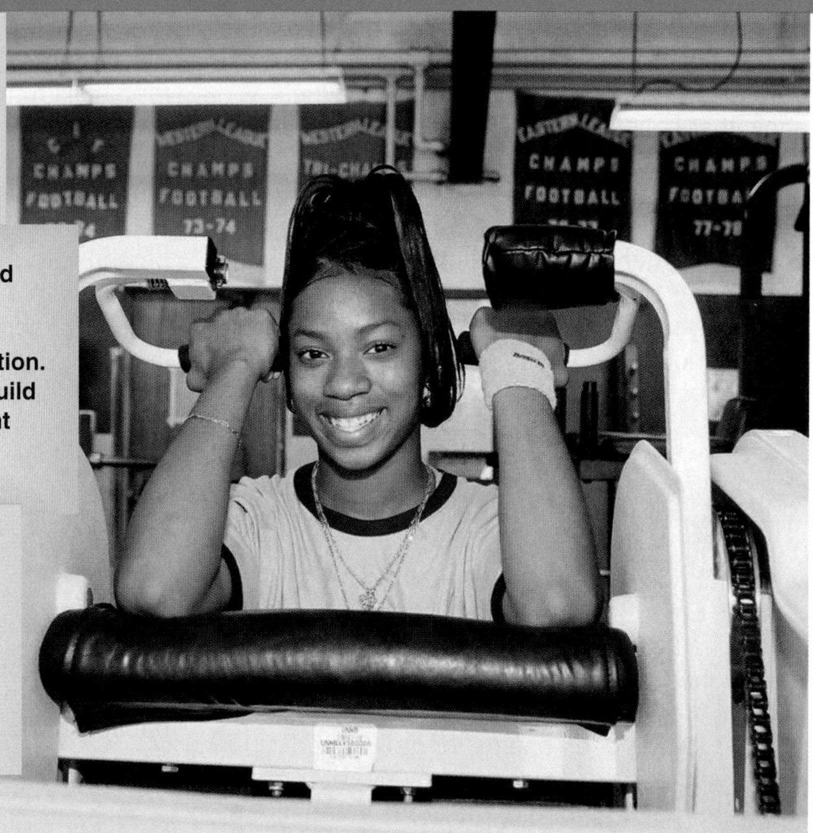

Terms to Know

basal metabolism
calorie
fitness
aerobic activity
dehydration
weight management
body composition
body mass index (BMI)
healthy weight
overweight
underweight
obesity
waist-to-hip ratio
eating disorder
anorexia nervosa
bulimia nervosa
binge eating disorder

Objectives

After studying this chapter, you will be able to

- ❏ identify factors that affect your energy needs.
- ❏ associate physical activity with overall fitness.
- ❏ examine factors that contribute to weight problems and eating disorders.
- ❏ explain the philosophy behind weight management.

Weight problems and lack of physical activity have been pinpointed as major health concerns in the United States today. These concerns are also becoming more and more common among children and teens.

Current health issues are the basis for the Dietary Guidelines for Americans. The Guidelines urge people to maintain body weight in a healthy range. They also advise taking part in regular physical activity. These Guidelines show that eating a healthful diet requires more than choosing foods to meet your nutrient needs. It also involves choosing the right amounts of foods to meet, but not exceed, your body's need for fuel. In addition to what you eat, the Dietary Guidelines focus on how you use the food you consume. Following the Guidelines will help you avoid health problems and enjoy a greater state of wellness.

Energy Needs

What do you know about your body's energy needs? *Energy,* in one sense, is the power to do work. The human body needs energy to move. It needs energy to produce heat and carry on internal processes. During certain periods of life, the body also needs energy for growth and repair. The body produces energy by *oxidizing* (using oxygen to burn up) the foods you eat.

Basal Metabolism

Basal metabolism is the amount of energy the human body needs to stay alive and carry on vital processes. It can be measured as the amount of heat the body gives off when at physical, digestive, and emotional rest.

A person's basal metabolism varies depending on a number of factors. One of these factors is body size. Two people who are the same weight and age, for example, may have different *basal metabolic rates (BMR)*. This is because their body shapes are different. A tall person has a larger body surface area than a short person. Therefore, the tall person has a higher basal metabolism per unit of body weight.

The kinds of tissues that make up the body also affect basal metabolism. Men usually have a larger amount of lean muscle tissue than women. This causes them to require more energy per unit of body weight than women, 5-1.

Age can affect basal metabolism. Children and adolescents have a higher basal metabolism than adults. This is because basal metabolism is greater during periods of rapid growth. After about age 20, basal metabolism gradually declines.

A person's general health can affect basal metabolism. The basal metabolism of a well-nourished person is higher than that of a malnourished person. An increase in body temperature also increases basal metabolism. For this reason, the basal metabolism of a person with a fever is higher than that of a person with a normal body temperature.

Gland secretions can affect basal metabolism. The thyroid gland affects metabolism more than any other gland. Undersecretion of the thyroid gland may lower basal metabolism. Oversecretion can raise it. Adrenaline, which the adrenal glands secrete during times of stress, also increases metabolism.

Physical Activity

When you engage in any physical activity, your energy needs become greater than your basal metabolism. Different activities require

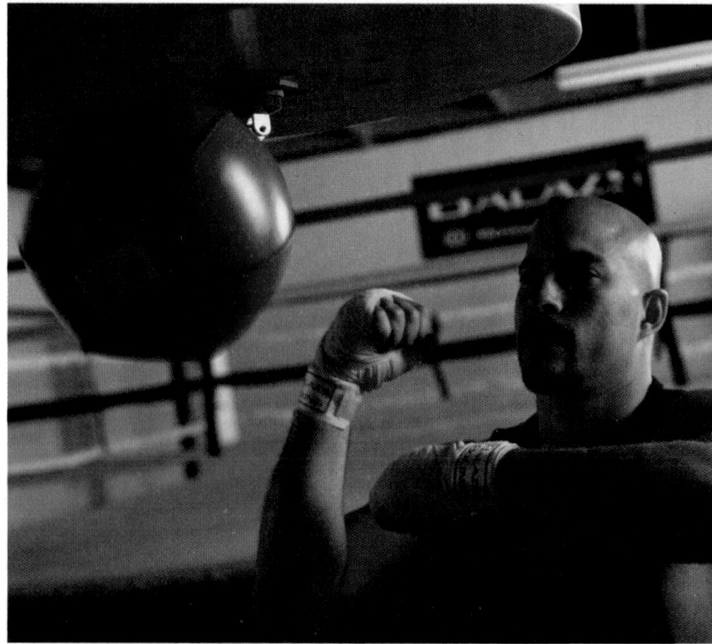

Balazs Boxing (www.BoxingSource.com)

5-1 Men generally have a larger percentage of lean body mass than women, which causes them to have a higher basal metabolism.

different amounts of energy. For instance, it takes more energy to wash dishes than it takes to read a book. It takes still more energy to rake leaves or swim.

Several factors can influence the amount of energy a person needs to perform a physical task. The intensity with which you perform a task can affect energy needs. A person who walks briskly, for example, needs more energy than a person who walks slowly. Body size can affect energy needs. This means a 220-pound (100-kg) student requires more energy to ride a bicycle than a 120-pound (55-kg) student. The temperature of the environment also can affect energy needs. It takes more energy to wash windows when the temperature is 90°F (32°C) than when the temperature is 70°F (21°C).

Meeting Energy Needs with Food

Each food you eat has a particular energy value. Most people refer to the units used to measure the energy value of foods as ***calories.*** Food scientists use the more accurate name for these units—*kilocalories*. One kilocalorie equals the amount of heat needed to raise one kilogram of water one degree Celsius.

The total energy value of a food depends on that food's chemical composition. Placing a food sample inside a device called a *bomb calorimeter* is one way to determine the food's energy value. The food is placed in a special chamber surrounded by water and ignited. As the food burns, it releases energy as heat. You can then determine the energy value of the food by measuring the temperature change of the water.

The three nutrients that provide the body with energy are carbohydrates, fats, and proteins. Carbohydrates and proteins provide the body with 4 calories per gram. Fats provide the body with 9 calories per gram.

Because few of the foods you eat are pure carbohydrates, pure proteins, or pure fats, foods vary widely in their energy values. Foods that are high in fat and low in water have a high energy value. This means a small amount of these foods will provide a lot of energy. Some examples of high energy value foods are nuts, mayonnaise, cheese, and some meats. Foods that are high in water and fiber and low in fat have a low energy value. A serving of these foods provides only small amounts of energy. Most fresh fruits and vegetables have a low energy value. Lean meats, grain foods, and starchy vegetables have an intermediate energy value. See 5-2.

When the energy (calories) you obtain from food equals the energy you expend, your body weight remains the same. When the energy you obtain from food is less than the energy you expend, your body weight decreases. When the energy you obtain from food is greater than the energy you expend, your body weight increases. It takes about 3,500 calories to make up 1 pound (0.45 kg) of body weight. (You will read how to estimate your energy needs later in this chapter.)

Physical Activity and Fitness

Besides affecting your energy needs, physical activity can affect your health throughout life. Physical activity contributes to your overall

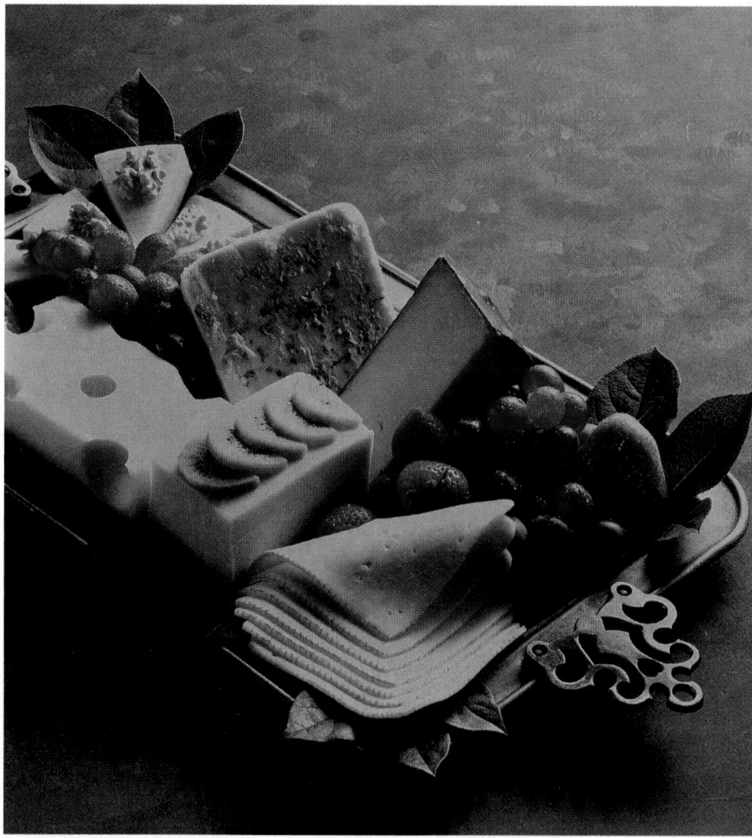

5-2 *Cheese has a high energy value compared to fruits, which contain more water and less fat.*

fitness. ***Fitness*** is your body's ability to meet physical demands. Physical activity has other benefits, too. It speeds metabolism and helps you burn calories so you can reach or maintain a healthy weight. It tones your muscles, builds strong bones, and keeps your skin healthy. It reduces your risk of heart disease, high blood pressure, diabetes, and some forms of cancer. It helps you feel better about yourself. Although you may not have realized it, physical activity can be fun, too.

Amount of Activity

Physical activity cannot give you all these health benefits if you do not do it on a regular basis. The Dietary Guidelines suggest adults get at least 30 minutes of moderate physical activity most, if not all, days of the week. This amount of activity will offer adults some benefits. However, it will not allow adults to maintain healthy body weight and receive all the advantages physical activity provides. To obtain the full benefits of physical activity, some experts recommend adults get 60 minutes of moderate physical activity per day. This advice is for adults of all ages. Older adults who are physically active are less likely to have problems with broken bones and weak muscles.

Experts recommend children and teens also get at least 60 minutes of moderate activity daily. Moderate activity equals the intensity of walking a mile in about 15 minutes. When you are moving at a moderately active level, you should still be able to talk. However, you should not have enough breath to be able to sing. Use these guidelines to help you decide if you need to increase or decrease the pace of your activity.

Maybe you feel like you cannot spare 60 minutes a day for physical activity. If so, look at how you currently use your time. How much time do you spend each day watching television or sitting in front of a computer? How much time do you spend talking to friends on the phone? Consider using some of this inactive time to be more active. Instead of watching television to relax, skate or take a bike ride to unwind after a busy day. Rather than looking up information on the computer, try walking to your local library to do research. Invite friends to join you for a game of tennis or basketball in place of talking to them on the phone.

What if you are already meeting the daily 60-minute activity goal? You could benefit even more by increasing your activity level. You might spend more time being moderately active. You could also try doing more vigorous activities, such as swimming and jogging.

You do not have to set aside a block of time to be physically active. If you prefer, you can accumulate your activity throughout the day. For instance, you might ride your bicycle to and from school, pedaling 15 minutes in each direction. Before dinner, you could spend 20 minutes shooting baskets in the driveway with your friends. Then in the evening, you might take your dog on a brisk, 10-minute walk. By the end of the day, you would have accumulated 60 minutes of activity.

Q: For exercise to be effective, don't I have to "feel the burn"?

A: No. Moderate-intensity activity is just as beneficial as high-intensity exercise. If you are in pain when you are exercising, you are at risk of injury and need to slow your pace.

Types of Activity

Notice that physical activity does not have to mean calisthenics and aerobics classes. These are great forms of exercise. However, everyday tasks such as gardening and climbing stairs also count as physical activity. See 5-3.

Flexibility, strength, and cardiovascular health are all part of fitness. Try to choose activities that target each of these areas. Stretching movements improve flexibility. Lifting weights or heavy objects, such as groceries, infants, and laundry baskets, can help you build strength. ***Aerobic activities,*** which speed your heart rate and breathing, promote cardiovascular health. Jogging, cycling, and skating are good aerobic activities.

Getting Started

Including more moderate physical activity in their lifestyles should not create health concerns for most people. However, people who are

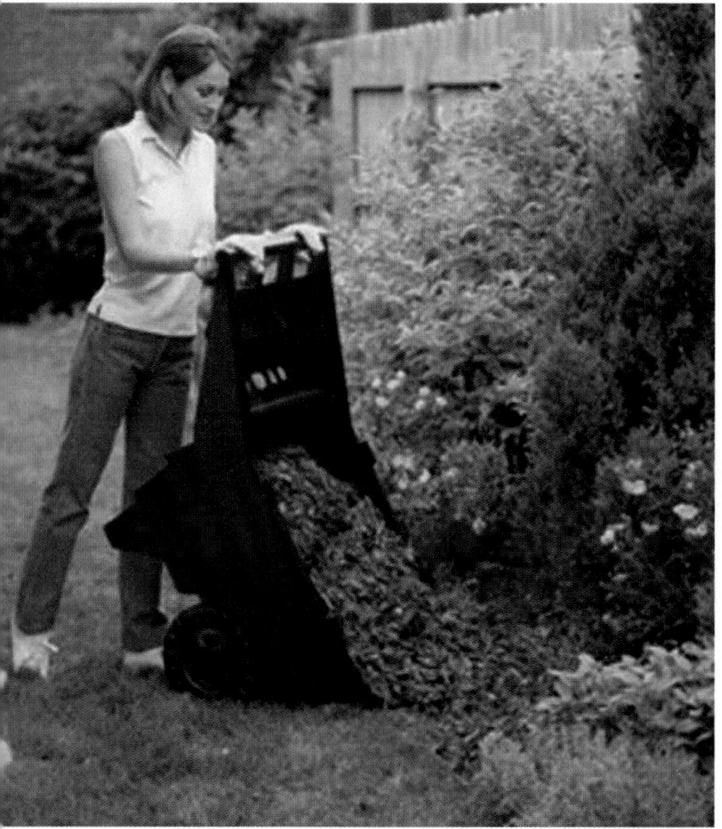

Rubbermaid

5-3 Movement required by some household chores can count as part of your daily physical activity.

starting a new program of vigorous exercise may wish to consult with their doctors first. Consulting a doctor is especially recommended for men over 40, women over 50, and anyone with chronic health problems.

If you have been fairly inactive, you need to begin increasing your activity level slowly. Trying to do too much too soon increases the risk of injury. Setting your initial activity goals too high can also cause you to become discouraged. If you are unable to attain the goals, you are more likely to give up. Starting with a goal to jog 30 minutes every day may be too ambitious. Instead, you might begin with a goal to walk 10 minutes a day three days a week. When you reach your initial goal, you can set a new goal that is more challenging.

Making physical activity a regular part of your day is more important than the types of activities you choose. Vary your activities so you do not become bored. Choose activities that are fun and convenient for you to do. Try making physical activity a social outlet by doing it with family members and friends, 5-4. If you can make physical activity part of your lifestyle, you will enjoy the benefits of fitness for a lifetime.

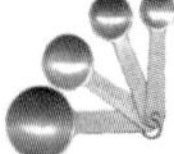

Nutrition for Athletes

Being moderately active each day does not create special dietary needs. Most people can meet their daily nutrient needs by following the Food Guide Pyramid. However, intense physical activity can increase the need for some nutrients. Nutrition also plays a key role in athletic performance. Athletes should be aware of a few specific dietary concerns.

Meeting Fluid Needs

The nutrient that is most likely to affect sports performance is water. Athletes lose much water through sweat when they are training and competing. If an athlete does not replace these fluids, dehydration can set in quickly. ***Dehydration*** is an abnormal loss of body fluids. It can cause headache, dizziness, confusion, and a drop in overall performance. Severe dehydration can even result in death.

To prevent dehydration, athletes should begin drinking fluids before an event. They need to continue drinking ½ to 1 cup (125 to 250 mL) of fluids at 15-minute intervals throughout the event. Athletes need to drink more fluids after working out or competing.

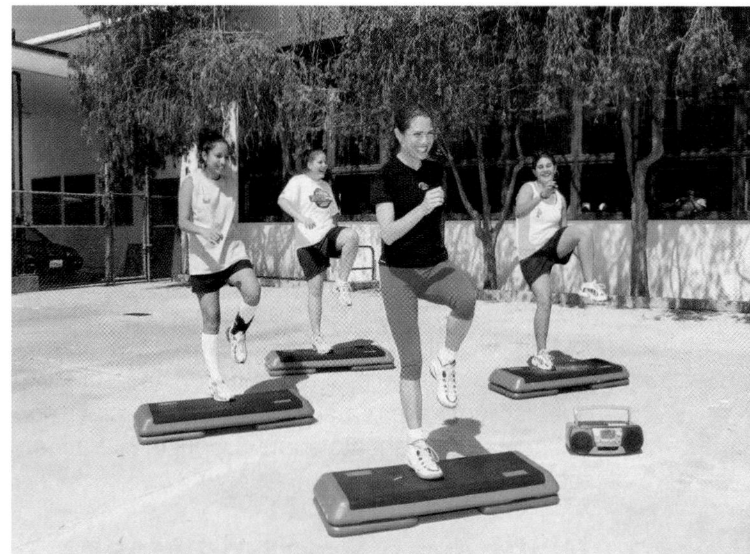

Reprinted with permission from the American Council on Exercise (www.acefitness.org)

5-4 Physical activity is more fun when you ask your friends to join you.

Some athletes choose sports drinks to replace their fluid losses. Sports drinks contain carbohydrates to help athletes replace some of the fuel they are burning through activity. Many sports drinks also contain sodium to replace sodium lost through sweat. This sodium also helps increase fluid absorption. For people who engage in lengthy workouts of 90 minutes or more, sports drinks can be a good choice.

Fluid replacement is equally important for those who take part in less strenuous activities. However, plain water does a fine job of meeting their fluid needs. A normal diet can easily replace sodium and replenish carbohydrates. Although sports drinks offer no special benefits for moderately active people, the taste may encourage them to drink more. This alone makes the choice of a sports beverage worthwhile.

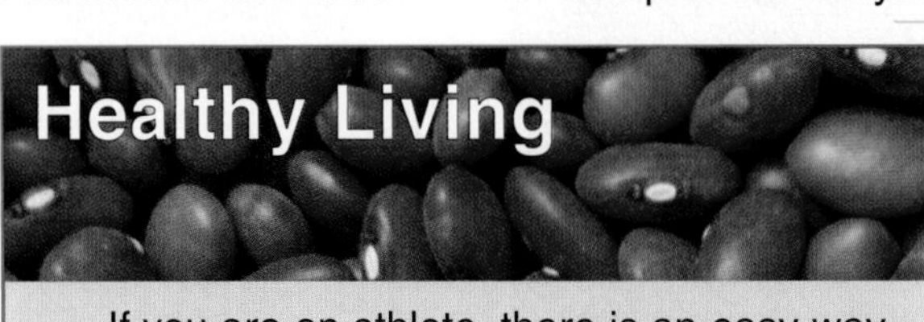

If you are an athlete, there is an easy way to determine your water needs. Weigh yourself before and after workouts. You should drink 2 cups (500 mL) of water for each pound of weight you lose.

Meeting Nutrient Needs

Athletes have some other special nutrient needs besides water. Their high level of activity increases the need for calories. Most of these calories, 55 to 60 percent, should come from complex carbohydrates. Breads, cereals, pasta, rice, and starchy vegetables are all excellent sources of complex carbohydrates. Choosing lean meats, poultry, and fish will supply an athlete's slightly increased need for protein. Lowfat dairy products provide needed calcium. Fresh fruits and vegetables furnish vitamins, minerals, and fiber.

If the above diet sounds familiar, it's not a coincidence. Like less active people, athletes can meet their nutrient needs by following the Food Guide Pyramid. Athletes should avoid nutrient supplements unless they are being taken on the advice of a dietitian. These costly supplements are not always what they claim to be. Tests have shown some products to be ineffective or even harmful.

Planning a Pregame Meal

Gone are the days when many trainers and coaches encouraged athletes to eat big steak dinners before a game. A plate of spaghetti might be more likely on today's training tables. Why the switch? One reason is that trainers once thought athletes needed the protein from the steak for energy. Although athletes do need protein, they need it for growth and repair of muscle tissue—not for energy. Lean meats can easily fit into an athlete's diet at other meals. For a pregame meal, however, the spaghetti makes a better choice. It is an excellent source of complex carbohydrates—an athlete's main energy source. Another reason to choose the pasta before a competitive event is that it is low in fat. Fat stays in the stomach longer than carbohydrates. Avoiding fat before a game keeps energy needed to compete from being used for digestion. See 5-5.

The best time to eat a pregame meal is 2½ to 3 hours before a sports event. An athlete should choose moderate portions so he or she will not feel too full during competition. The athlete should avoid unfamiliar foods, which could cause an upset stomach. He or she should also limit high-fiber foods, such as fruits, vegetables, and whole grains. Fiber is generally beneficial. However, fiber creates bulk in the digestive

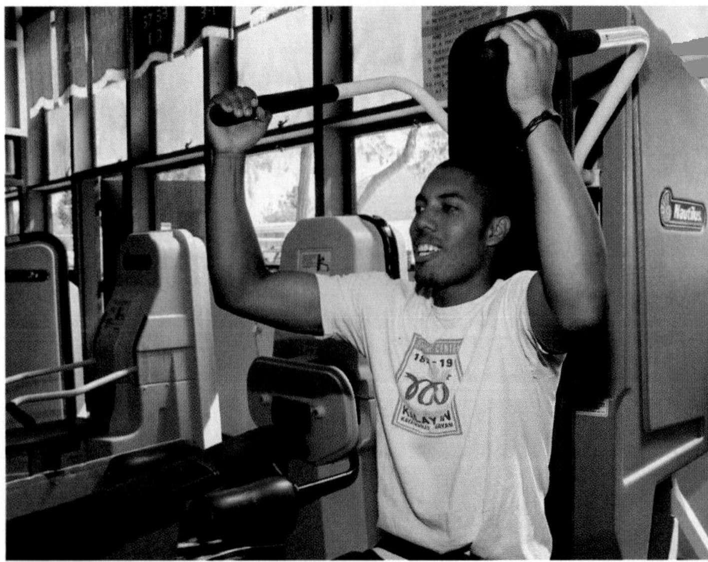

Reprinted with permission from the American Council on Exercise (www.acefitness.org)

5-5 *Athletes need protein to build muscle, but their main source of energy should be carbohydrates.*

system, which can make an athlete feel sluggish during competition.

Meeting Weight Goals

Achieving an optimal performance weight is a critical nutrition issue for many athletes. To compete in lower weight classes, some wrestlers use laxatives to speed food through their digestive systems. They also force themselves to vomit and avoid drinking fluids. To avoid weight gain, some gymnasts skip meals to restrict their calorie intakes. To increase body mass, some football players go on eating sprees. They consume large quantities of high-calorie, low-nutrient foods. To meet weight goals, some athletes in all sports fields have engaged in such unwise, and often dangerous practices. These practices can harm health as well as sports performance.

Be a Clever Consumer

Energy bars and power bars are a big business in the world of sports nutrition. These bars can be tasty, wholesome snacks. Despite their name, however, they may not be your best choice for a mid-event burst of energy. When you eat a bar, some of the energy you need to compete will be diverted to your digestive system. If you consume a sports drink with the bar, the combined amount of carbohydrate may hinder fluid absorption. This could have a negative effect on your performance.

Athletes who want to lose weight need to do so gradually and well before the start of their sports season. They should not try to lose weight while they are training and competing. They should never restrict fluids, force vomiting, or use laxatives, either.

Athletes should not skip meals or otherwise restrict calories. The body needs a steady supply of nutrients throughout the day. It needs energy to fuel activity. Teen athletes also need calories to support normal development. Failing to get enough nutrients and calories can stunt growth.

Athletes who want to gain weight need to add moderate amounts of extra calories to their diets from nutrient-rich sources. They also need to follow a steady program of muscle-building exercise. This will ensure that weight gained is due to lean body mass rather than fat.

All athletes wishing to reach weight goals should seek the advice of a registered dietitian. Many coaches lack sufficient training in sports nutrition to provide guidance about healthful weight loss, maintenance, and gain.

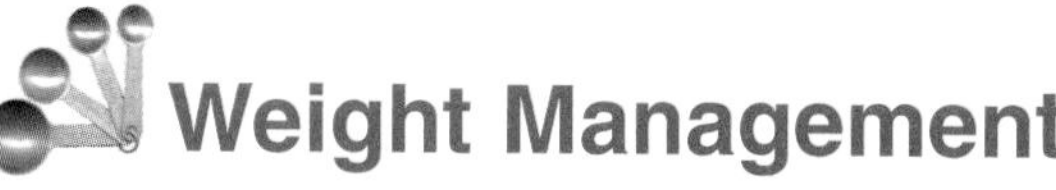

Weight Management

Remember that being physically active is only one of the Dietary Guidelines that focuses on your energy needs. The other guideline is to aim for a healthy weight.

People come in all shapes and sizes. Heredity largely determines bone size and shape. However, maintaining a healthy weight depends mostly on lifestyle. ***Weight management*** means using resources like food choices and physical activity to reach and/or maintain a healthy weight. Weight management is not a short-term program you follow until you lose a few pounds. It becomes part of your way of life.

Determining Healthy Weight

To maintain a healthy weight, you need to be concerned with more than just the numbers on the scale. You need to know the source of your weight. See 5-6.

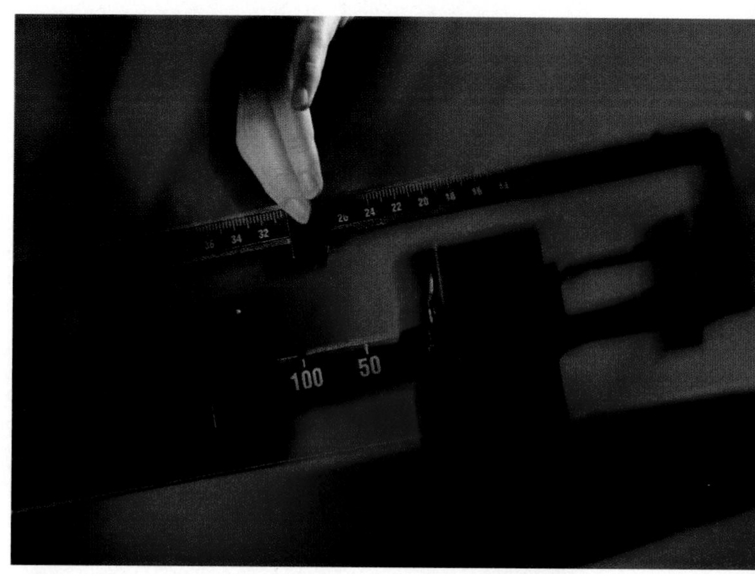

5-6 *Healthy weight is a weight at which your body fat and lean tissue are in an appropriate proportion. It is not a particular number on a scale.*

Body weight includes the weight of bone, muscle, fat, and other tissues. People have different ***body compositions,*** or proportions of these types of tissues that make up their body weights. Muscle and bone tissue weigh more than fat tissue. These factors explain why two people may be the same height but have different weights. The person with greater muscle mass and heavier bones will have the higher weight. However, what concerns health experts most is the amount of weight attributed to fat tissue.

Body Mass Index

Many health professionals assess a person's weight based on his or her ***body mass index (BMI).*** This is a calculation involving a person's weight and height measurements. According to federal guidelines, ***healthy weight*** for adults is defined as a BMI of 18.5 to 24.9. ***Overweight*** is defined as a BMI of 25 to 29.9. An *obese* adult has a BMI of 30 or more. Someone with a BMI under 18.5 is considered ***underweight.***

These BMI cutoffs cannot be used for children and adolescents because their bodies are still growing. Suggested BMI values for evaluating overweight in these younger age groups vary according to age. Table 5-7 can help you find your BMI. Table 5-8 can help you determine whether you are underweight or at risk of being overweight.

The use of BMI in assessing weight has limitations because it does not take body composition into account. For example, consider a football player who has a large proportion of muscle tissue compared to fat. Because muscle weighs more than fat, the man may have a seemingly high weight. His BMI might be in the overweight range. Because his weight is due to muscle, however, it is not a health concern. Therefore, rather than being defined strictly by BMI, ***obesity*** is a condition characterized by excessive deposits of body fat.

Skinfold Test

One way to evaluate whether excess body weight is due to fat or muscle is through a *skinfold test.* This is a measure of a fold of skin using an instrument called a *caliper.* The back of the upper arm, below the shoulder blade, and around the abdomen are common measuring spots. About half the body's fat is located under the skin. Therefore, a skinfold test gives an indication of total body fat.

An inexact variation of a skinfold test you can do yourself is the *pinch test.* Simply grasp a fold of skin at the back of your upper arm between your thumb and forefinger. A fold that measures more than an inch (2.5 cm) thick is often a sign of excess fat.

Body Mass Index

	Weight in Pounds																							
Height	90	95	100	105	110	115	120	125	130	135	140	145	150	155	160	165	170	175	180	185	190	195	200	205
4′11″	18	19	20	21	22	23	24	25	26	27	28	29	30	31	32	33	34	35	36	37	38	39	41	42
5′0″	18	19	20	21	22	23	23	24	25	26	27	28	29	30	31	32	33	34	35	36	37	38	39	40
5′1″	17	18	19	20	21	22	23	24	25	26	26	27	28	29	30	31	32	33	34	35	36	37	38	39
5′2″	17	17	18	19	20	21	22	23	24	25	26	27	28	28	29	30	31	32	33	34	35	36	37	37
5′3″	16	17	18	19	20	20	21	22	23	24	25	26	27	28	28	29	30	31	32	33	34	35	36	36
5′4″	15	16	17	18	19	20	21	22	22	23	24	25	26	27	28	28	29	30	31	32	33	34	34	35
5′5″	15	16	17	18	18	19	20	21	22	22	23	24	25	26	27	28	28	29	30	31	32	33	33	34
5′6″	15	15	16	17	18	19	19	20	21	22	23	24	24	25	26	27	28	28	29	30	31	32	32	33
5′7″	14	15	16	17	17	18	19	20	20	21	22	23	24	24	25	26	27	28	28	29	30	31	31	32
5′8″	14	14	15	16	17	18	18	19	20	21	21	22	23	24	24	25	26	27	27	28	29	30	31	31
5′9″	13	14	15	16	16	17	18	19	19	20	21	22	22	23	24	24	25	26	27	27	28	29	30	30
5′10″	13	14	14	15	16	17	17	18	19	19	20	21	22	22	23	24	24	25	26	27	27	28	29	30
5′11″	13	13	14	15	15	16	17	18	18	19	20	20	21	22	22	23	24	25	25	26	26	27	28	29
6′0″	12	13	14	14	15	16	16	17	18	18	19	20	20	21	22	22	23	24	25	25	26	26	27	28
6′1″	12	13	13	14	15	15	16	17	17	18	19	19	20	21	21	22	23	23	24	25	25	26	26	27
6′2″	12	12	13	14	14	15	15	16	17	17	18	19	19	20	21	21	22	23	23	24	24	25	26	26

5-7 *Body mass index, a calculation based on body weight and height, is used to evaluate how healthy a person's weight is.*

Adolescent Risk for Weight Problems				
Gender	Age	BMI at Risk of Underweight	BMI at Risk of Overweight	BMI at Risk of Obesity
Female	14	15	23	27
	15	16	24	28
	16	16	24	28
	17	17	25	29
	18	17	25	30
Male	14	16	22	26
	15	16	23	26
	16	17	24	27
	17	17	24	28
	18	18	25	28

***5-8** The body mass indexes that identify potential weight problems for an adolescent vary according to age and gender.*

Waist-to-Hip Ratio

Another way to assess healthy weight is to consider the location of excess fat in the body. Some excess fat deposits are more directly linked with health risks than others. People who carry more fat around their middles are sometimes described as having "apple-shaped" bodies. Those who carry their excess weight around the hips and thighs may be described as having "pear-shaped" bodies. An apple shape poses a greater health risk than a pear shape.

A mathematical relationship can help adults evaluate their body shapes. This relationship is called the ***waist-to-hip ratio.*** To figure this ratio, a person needs to measure his or her waist at its narrowest point. Then the person needs to measure his or her hips at their fullest point. Divide the measurement of the waist by the measurement of the hips. Using this formula, a woman with a 28-inch (71-cm) waist and 38-inch (97-cm) hips would find she has a waist-to-hip ratio of 0.74 (28 ÷ 38 = 0.74). Waist-to-hip ratios over 1.0 in men and over 0.85 in women are linked to increased health risks.

Whether you are more likely to carry excess weight around your waist or hips is a matter of heredity. It depends on where fat cells are located in your body. Unfortunately, you cannot shift fat cells from one spot to another. The best advice for someone whose waist-to-hip ratio indicates a health risk is to lose weight. As weight decreases, more inches are likely to be lost from the areas of the body that contain more fat cells. This will improve the waist-to-hip ratio.

Q: Won't doing sit-ups help me lose inches around my waist?

A: No, you cannot spot-reduce. Sit-ups will help tone the muscles in your abdomen. However, exercise that focuses on one area of the body will not cause fat loss from that area. To lose excess fat, you must lose weight.

Hazards of Being Obese

Obesity is a danger to health. High blood pressure, diabetes mellitus, heart disease, some types of cancer, and other diseases are more common among obese people. Records of life insurance companies show obese people die at earlier ages than nonobese people. Some insurance companies view obese people as "high risk" and charge them higher rates.

Too much weight puts a strain on the body's bones, muscles, and organs. A thick layer of fat interferes with the body's natural cooling system. Overweight people use more effort to walk and breathe.

Obese people also face social pressures. The fashion industry focuses little attention on designs for larger sizes. Television and magazines promote the image that being attractive means being thin. Some employers hesitate to hire obese people for certain jobs.

Factors That Contribute to Overeating

People can be overweight for several reasons. Some people inherit a tendency to be overweight. Some people are overweight because of medical problems. However, most people are overweight because they eat more calories than they need for basal metabolism and physical activity.

People overeat for both social and emotional reasons. People associate food with social occasions. Many people keep snacks on hand to serve guests. They go out to dinner with friends. They plan large meals for holidays. See 5-9.

For many people, food marketing triggers a temptation to eat. Ads on billboards, television, and radio and in newspapers and magazines highlight food choices available to consumers. Restaurants, supermarkets, vending machines, and refreshment stands at movie theaters and sports arenas make food easy to get almost everywhere. So many messages about food and eating help keep thoughts about food on many people's minds. Thinking about food often leads to a desire to eat.

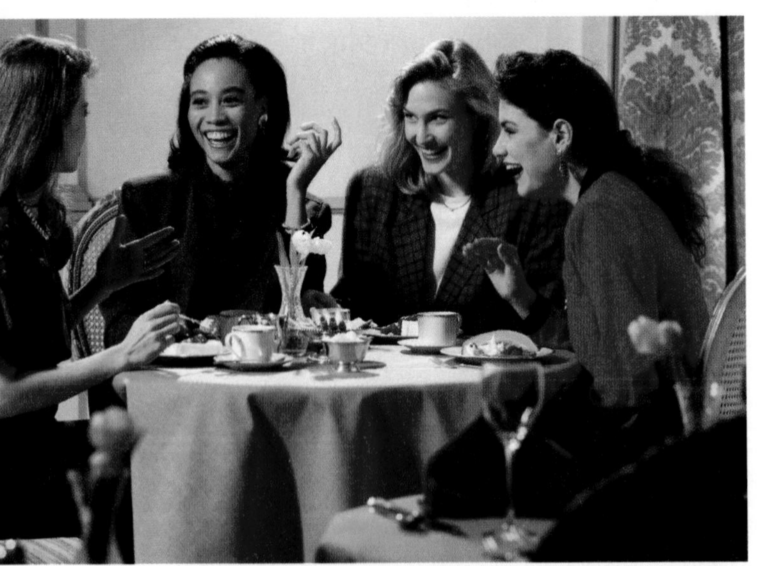

5-9 When celebrating a special occasion or visiting with friends, it is easy to forget about how much food you are eating.

People often eat to fill emotional needs. Strong emotions, such as anger, frustration, depression, boredom, and even happiness, can lead some people to overeat. Some people use food as a reward; others use it as a source of security.

Many people eat out of habit. For example, you may be used to having a snack before bedtime. Even though you are not hungry, habit may prompt you to have a snack.

Deciding to Lose Weight

As an adult, you will need to continue to aim for a healthy weight. If your BMI and a skinfold test ever indicate you have excess body fat, you can take steps to lose weight. Losing weight may allow you to buy clothes in smaller sizes and receive praises from your friends. You are also likely to have more energy and confidence.

These benefits are all worthwhile. To successfully lose weight, however, you must want to lose weight. You should base a desire to lose weight on more than wanting to fit into a new outfit. Efforts to lose weight are most successful when they are part of a lifelong commitment to maintain good health.

Once you have decided to lose weight, you might want to see a registered dietitian. A dietitian can help you design a weight management plan suited to your individual needs. The dietitian might also recommend a vitamin-mineral supplement.

Most successful weight-loss plans involve three main components: changing poor eating habits, controlling energy intake, and increasing physical activity.

Identifying Eating Habits

One of the first steps in losing weight is to keep a *food log*. This is a list of all the foods and beverages you consume. You should also note where you ate, who you were with, and how you felt when eating. Keep this list for at least a week. Studying it will help you discover some of your eating habits. For instance, you may find you often snack in front of the television. You may also learn you eat when feeling sad, frustrated, or nervous. See 5-10.

Once you identify some of your eating habits, you can take steps to change them. If you idly snack while watching television, try keeping your hands busy with an activity instead of with food. If you eat when nervous, try taking a brisk walk when you feel full of nervous energy. If you eat when feeling lonely, call a friend when the urge to nibble strikes.

Controlling Energy Intake

Weight management involves being aware of the energy value of the foods you eat. The amount of energy the body receives from food is measured in calories. The body needs the energy obtained from the foods you eat to function. However, if you eat more calories than your body uses, you will gain weight.

The number of calories your body needs each day to maintain your present weight is called your *daily calorie need.* This need depends on your sex, age, size, body composition, and level of activity. Men usually need more calories than women. This is partly because men generally have a higher percentage of muscle tissue than women. Muscle tissue requires more calories to maintain than fat tissue. Pound for pound, children and teens need more calories than adults. Children and teens need extra energy to support growth. A large person needs more calories each day than a small person. One reason for this is a larger skin surface area allows more heat to be lost from the body. An active person needs more calories to fuel motion than an inactive person.

Your daily calorie need must account for your basal metabolism and your activity level. Your body needs about 10 calories per pound (0.45 kg) to support basal metabolism. You need additional calories to give you energy for activities. Figure about 4 calories per pound (0.45 kg) if you are sedentary; 10 calories per pound (0.45 kg) if you are active. Therefore, an active, 120-pound (55-kg) woman would need about 2,400 calories per day (120 pounds × 20 calories/pound = 2,400 calories). A 170-pound (77-kg), sedentary man would also need about 2,400 calories per day (170 pounds × 14 calories/pound = 2,380 calories).

To lose weight, you must consume fewer calories than your daily calorie need. You will want to remember 1 pound (0.45 kg) of fat equals about 3,500 calories. To lose 1 pound (0.45 kg) a week, you would need to increase the difference between your energy intake and expenditure by 3,500 calories. This is roughly 500 calories a day. You should make this adjustment through a

Food Log

What did I eat?	How much did I eat?	When did I eat?	Where did I eat?	Who was with me?	How did I feel?
Breakfast		7:30 a.m.	kitchen	Christopher	tired
banana	1 medium				
corn flakes	1 1/2 cups				
fat free milk	1/2 cup				
orange juice	3/4 cup				
Lunch		12:10 p.m.	cafeteria	Tanisha	excited
cheeseburger	1			Pilar	
fries	about 15				
lowfat milk	1 cup				
Snack		3:30 p.m.	living room	no one	bored
cookies	2		(watching TV)		

5-10 Keeping track of what, when, where, and with whom you eat can help you identify patterns in your eating behavior.

combination of reduced calories and increased physical activity.

Losing a pound (0.45 kg) a week may not bring you to your goal weight as soon as you had hoped. However, losing weight too quickly can strain your body systems. You may deprive yourself of needed nutrients if you eat too little food. You will also be more successful in maintaining your weight goal if you lose weight slowly. Most experts recommend a steady weight loss at the rate of ½ to 1 pound (0.23 to 0.45 kg) per week. After all, you did not gain your excess weight in a week. Therefore, you should not expect to lose it in a week.

Food labels and recipes can help you keep track of the calories you eat. Packaged food products and many recipes list the number of calories per serving. Be aware of the stated serving size. Many people cannot understand why they do not lose weight when they are following a weight management plan. Often the problem is they misjudge portion sizes. When you begin following your weight-loss plan, you may find it helpful to measure portions. Soon you will become familiar with what a cup (250-mL), half-cup (125-mL), or tablespoon (15-mL) portion looks like.

You should also be aware of the amount of fat in the foods you eat. Health experts recommend that fat make up 20 to 35 percent of your total daily calories. For an active teenage boy, that would be about 70 to 123 grams of fat per day. An active teen girl should consume about 53 to 92 grams of fat daily. Food labels and recipes can help you keep track of your fat intake. A gram of fat contains more than twice as many calories as a gram of carbohydrate or protein. Therefore, calories can add up quickly when you are eating high-fat foods.

Increasing Physical Activity

Watching your food intake is only part of a weight management plan. You also need to get plenty of physical activity. As you read earlier, regular activity speeds up metabolism, promotes good muscle tone, and burns calories. See 5-11.

Check with your doctor to be sure there are no restrictions to the type of activity you might pursue. Then choose an activity you enjoy. You may want to participate in a sport.

Q: Will my stomach shrink if I start to eat less?

A: When you eat, your stomach expands to hold the food you consume. As food passes through your digestive tract, your stomach goes back to its normal size. Reducing your food intake will not reduce the size of your stomach.

Perhaps you would prefer to join an aerobics class. The kind of activity is not as important as its regularity.

Table 5-12 can help you see the effect physical activity can have on weight management. You can burn half of your 3,500-calorie weekly reduction goal with just 30 to 60 minutes of activity each day.

Along with planned activity, try to build extra movement into your daily routine. Take the stairs instead of riding the elevator. Play ball with a friend instead of watching TV.

Weight-Loss Aids

Radio, television, and magazine ads for weight-loss aids are widespread. These aids

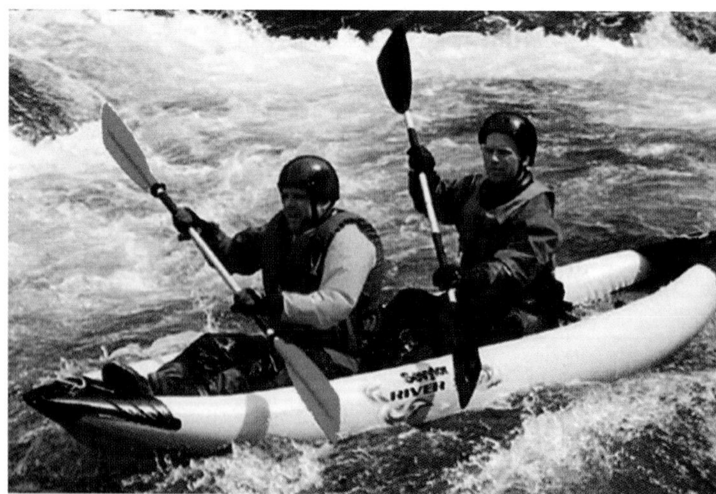

photo courtesy of Sevylor USA, Inc.

5-11 Following a program of regular physical activity is an important part of maintaining healthy weight and overall fitness.

Calories and Activity		
	Approximate Calories Burned per Hour for Person Weighing	
Activity	125 Pounds	150 Pounds
Basketball, recreational	370	450
Bicycling, 10 mph	320	380
Dancing, active	340	410
Golf, carrying clubs	280	320
Horseback riding	200	250
Jogging, 5½ mph	500	600
Racquetball	490	590
Roller skating	320	380
Running, 8 mph	730	880
Skiing, cross-country, 4 mph	490	590
Skiing, downhill	490	590
Soccer	450	540
Swimming, crawl, 35 yd./min.	370	440
Tennis, recreational singles	370	450
Walking, 4 mph	320	380

5-12 An activity chart gives you an idea of how many calories per hour your body burns when doing different activities.

include special pieces of exercise equipment that promise to slim your waist and firm your thighs. They extend to pills promoted to make pounds melt away without any changes in your current exercise or eating patterns. They also include diet plans that claim you will lose weight if you simply eat enough of one kind of food and avoid eating another.

The age-old advice to consumers is certainly valid here: If something sounds too good to be true, it probably is. The problem with most aids that promise quick weight loss is they do not help people develop new lifestyle behaviors. Therefore, as soon as people stop using these products, they go back to their old eating and activity patterns. This causes them to regain the weight.

A few approved prescription drugs are designed to help people lose weight. Some of these drugs work by curbing the appetite. Like all drugs, weight-loss medications have some side effects and cannot be used by all people. Those who take these drugs will find they still need to monitor their food intake and activity levels. With or without drugs, the *only* way to lose weight is to consume fewer calories than you burn.

Tips for Success

If you have a goal to lose weight, your weight management plan should meet several criteria. It should include as many of your favorite foods as possible. It should provide a variety of choices. It should be nutritious and fit into your food budget.

Do not avoid all your favorite high-calorie foods when you are working to lose weight. If you feel as if you are being deprived, you may give up on your weight management plan. Simply learn to enjoy your favorites less often and in smaller portions. Go out for pizza once a week instead of twice a week. Try settling for 5 French fries instead of 10.

Avoid fad diets that focus on just a few foods or omit certain groups of foods. These plans lack variety and are not nutritionally balanced. You are likely to become bored with these diets and stop following them. If you do stick with them, you may be missing important nutrients. In addition, these diets do not help you form good eating habits. Therefore, when you go off these diets you are likely to regain the weight you lost.

A weight-loss plan should include at least the minimum number of servings from each group in the Food Guide Pyramid. This will ensure you obtain needed nutrients. You can choose foods from each group that are lower in fat and sugar. For example, fat free milk can replace whole milk. You can select canned fruits packed in juice instead of fruits packed in syrup. You can substitute whole wheat toast for doughnuts. Plain vegetables can replace creamed vegetables. Lean meats, skinless poultry, and legumes can replace heavily marbled meats. See 5-13.

Protect the Planet

Whenever possible, ride a bicycle or walk to get where you need to go. These activities help you stay in shape and burn calories. They also save energy over taking a car.

When working to reduce weight, try using a smaller plate to make portions look larger. Eat slowly and chew food thoroughly to extend the length of the meal. Use herbs and spices to add variety to foods.

Avoid weighing yourself more than once a week. Your goal is a gradual weight loss. Checking your weight too often may cause you to feel discouraged.

When you are trying to lose weight, the first few pounds may come off rather quickly. (This initial loss is usually due to water loss.) However, weight loss is seldom steady. Plateaus during which you may seem to make little or no progress are normal. Do not be discouraged—be patient!

When working toward a lower weight goal, you should not skip any meal. In fact, you may want to eat extra meals. Eating six small meals each day rather than three large meals will increase your metabolic rate. It will also reduce your chances of overeating.

Do not allow your weight management plan to turn you into a hermit. Skipping holiday meals or trips to the ice cream shop may help you resist the temptation to eat high-calorie foods. However, you may also start to resent your weight management plan and give up completely. When a special occasion arises, feel free to attend. Simply eat moderate portions of the foods that are offered, just as you would at any other meal.

You do not have to avoid eating in restaurants as long as you make sensible food choices. Choose fruit or vegetable juice for an appetizer. Pass up salad dressings, gravies, and rich sauces. Avoid fried menu items and ask to have vegetables served unbuttered. Select fresh fruit for dessert.

You are not a failure if you stuff yourself at the class picnic or eat five candy bars for lunch. Everyone makes unwise choices now and then. Turn your mistake into a learning experience. Continuing to keep the food log you used to identify your eating habits can help you avoid repeating your mistake. Think about what might have caused you to overeat. Then try to avoid that situation in the future.

Reward yourself when you reach intermediate goals in your weight management plan. Set realistic intermediate goals that present a challenge. Choose nonfood rewards that are meaningful to you. For instance, if you meet your physical activity goal for the week, you might reward yourself with a trip to the movies.

Dole Food Company

***5-13** A salad of fresh fruits and vegetables and skinless chicken is a meal option that easily fits into a weight-loss plan.*

If you avoid unplanned snacking, you might reward yourself with a small purchase, 5-14.

Maintaining Healthy Weight

Once you have reached your goal weight, you can begin eating at, rather than below, your daily calorie need. This does not mean you can abandon your weight management plan. Remember, weight management is part of your lifestyle. Maintaining this lifestyle will help you continue to enjoy food in a whole new way.

Keep practicing moderation and balance as you make food choices. You can slightly increase portion sizes or choose an extra food now and then. Follow the Food Guide Pyramid and the Dietary Guidelines for Americans to make healthful selections. Maintain the limit of 35 percent of calories from fat. Continue getting daily physical activity, too.

Underweight

People in some jobs may want to be slightly below healthy weight. Jockeys and fashion models, for instance, often weigh less than their healthy weight. They exercise and watch their calorie intake to maintain their weight.

Unlike jockeys and fashion models, people who are underweight may have a health problem. Not eating enough food to meet the body's needs can cause a person to be underweight. An inability to use food properly or a stressful environment can also cause underweight.

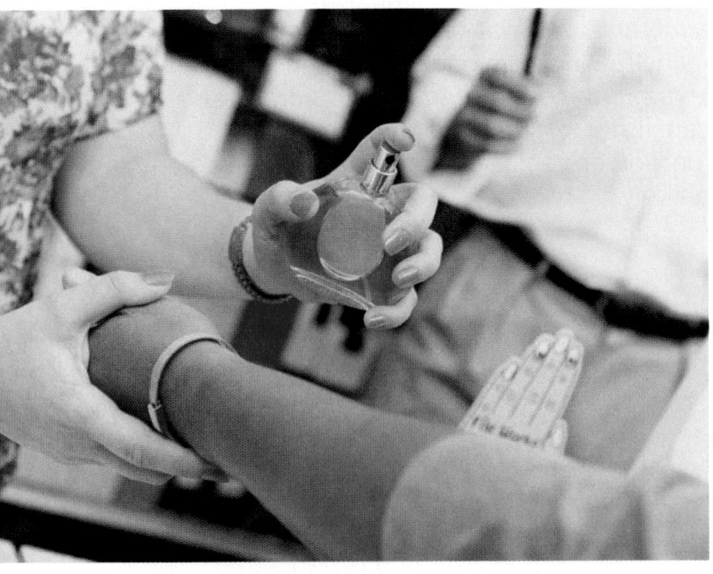

***5-14** A new fragrance or some other nonfood reward can help you celebrate reaching an intermediate goal in your weight management plan.*

People who are chronically underweight often suffer from more infections. They tire easily and feel cold even when the temperature is moderate. Wearing swimsuits and other figure-revealing clothes may embarrass them.

Following a Weight-Gain Plan

Before trying to gain weight, an underweight person should see a physician. The physician will investigate if there are any medical reasons the person's body is not using the food it receives. If emotional problems are causing the weight problems, a physician may be able to recommend a therapist.

The goal of a weight-gain plan should not be a rapid weight gain. Rapid gains usually are the result of increased fat deposits. Instead, people trying to gain weight need to build up muscle tissue. To do this, they need to carefully follow a two-fold plan. First, they need to regularly take part in muscle-building activities, such as weight lifting. This will ensure that weight gain is not due just to added body fat, which would be unhealthful. Second, underweight people need to consume more calories than their bodies need. They should add 700 to 1,000 calories to their daily diets. This will provide enough energy to fuel the added activity plus allow for a gradual weight gain.

Underweight people should continue to follow the Food Guide Pyramid. They can choose more daily servings from each food group. They can also increase portion sizes. Underweight people can increase their calorie intake by eating small meals every few hours throughout the day. Nutritious snacks are also a good way to add calories. Fats should still make up no more than 35 percent of total calories.

Underweight people may have trouble eating large quantities of food. Therefore, they need to consume calories in more concentrated forms. They can choose nutritious, calorie-dense foods from each food group. For instance, dried fruit, cheese, and nuts are concentrated sources of calories. Other ways to add nutrients and calories without adding bulk include stirring nonfat dry milk into soups, casseroles, and cooked cereals. Choosing starchy vegetables, such as peas, potatoes, and corn will add more calories per serving than nonstarchy vegetables.

While eating more of some foods, a person who is trying to gain weight should limit other foods. Drinking beverages with meals and eating high-fiber foods, such as salads, will cause a person to feel full quickly.

An underweight person may do better to consume liquids between meals. Choosing calorie-dense beverages may be a way of increasing energy intake that is easier to swallow than eating solid foods. Some people use nutrient-loaded drinks in place of meals to lose weight. People trying to gain weight can use these drinks in addition to meals. Delicious shakes made with fruit and yogurt can be used in the same way. See 5-15.

Following a weight gain plan can be just as challenging as following a weight loss plan. With continued physical activity and careful food choices, weight will gradually increase. Once a weight goal has been reached, an underweight person can begin eating at his or her daily calorie need. Making good nutrition and physical activity an ongoing weight management program will help maintain healthy weight.

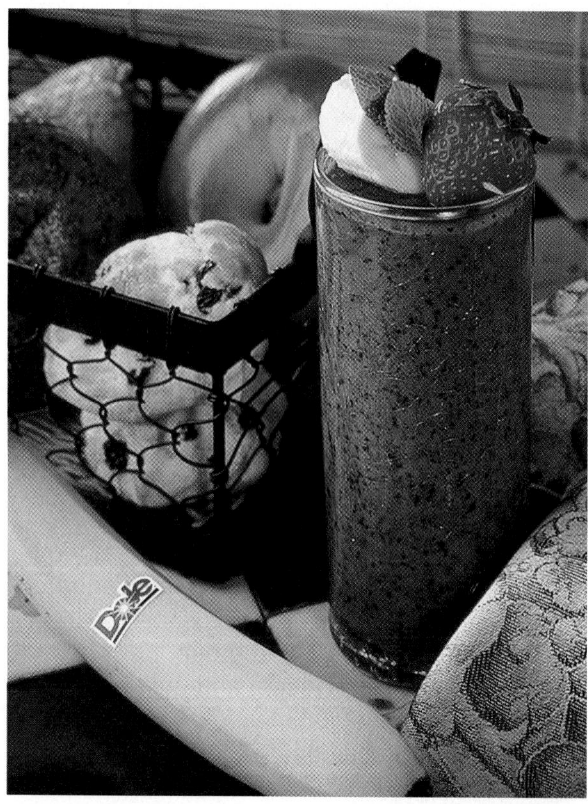

Dole Food Company

5-15 Delicious smoothies made with fresh fruit are easy to drink. They may help people who are trying to gain weight get some extra calories into their diets between meals.

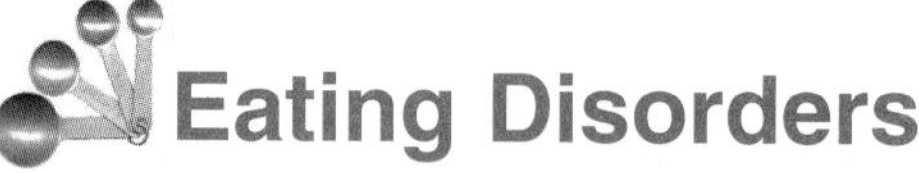

Eating Disorders

An ***eating disorder*** is abnormal eating behavior that risks physical and mental health. Eating disorders can lead to malnutrition, organ damage, or even death. See 5-16.

Doctors do not know what causes eating disorders. However, some type of personal stress often triggers them. The disorders become sources of more stress. They tend to progress until the victims feel unable to handle their problems.

Eating disorders most often affect young women and teenage girls. However, people of both genders and other age groups can also form eating disorders. Three common eating disorders are anorexia nervosa, bulimia nervosa, and binge eating disorder.

Common Eating Disorders

Anorexia nervosa is an eating disorder characterized by self-starvation. The term *nervosa* indicates the disorder has psychological roots. A person with anorexia has an intense fear of weight gain. He or she also has a distorted body image. This person may look like skin and bones, yet he or she may complain of being fat. An anorexic does not realize he or she has an eating disorder.

Starvation causes some body processes to slow down or stop. Blood pressure drops and respiration slows. Hormone secretions become abnormal. This causes anorexic women to stop menstruating. The body cannot absorb nutrients properly. Body temperature drops and sensitivity to cold increases. The heart cannot function correctly. In some cases, it may stop entirely.

Signs of Eating Disorders
abnormal weight loss binge eating self-induced vomiting abuse of laxatives and/or diuretics excessive exercise absent or irregular menstrual periods in females depression

5-16 You should suspect a person has an eating disorder when one or more of these signs is present. Early detection leads to a better chance of recovery.

Bulimia nervosa is an eating disorder that has two key characteristics. The first is repeated eating *binges*. These are episodes during which the bulimic consumes thousands of calories in a short period. The second is an inappropriate behavior to prevent weight gain. For some bulimics, this behavior takes the form of *purging*. This means trying to quickly rid the body of the food. Some bulimics purge by forcing themselves to vomit. Others take laxatives or diuretics to speed food and fluids through their bodies. Bulimics who do not purge may fast or exercise excessively to avoid weight gain. The cycle of bingeing and purging or other countering behavior is repeated at least twice a week. This pattern continues for at least three months.

Bulimics feel a lack of control over their eating behavior. This gives them a sense of guilt and shame. Unlike anorexics, however, they know their behavior is abnormal.

Frequent purging upsets the body's chemical balance. This can cause fatigue and heart abnormalities. Repeated vomiting can harm the teeth, gums, esophagus, and stomach.

Like bulimia nervosa, ***binge eating disorder*** involves repeated episodes of uncontrolled eating. Binge eaters consume large amounts of food. However, they do not take part in an opposing behavior to prevent weight gain. Therefore, many binge eaters are overweight.

Treatment for Eating Disorders

Early treatment of eating disorders improves the chance of recovery with no severe health problems. These disorders require professional care. Treatment centers first on physical effects of the disorder. A person may need to be hospitalized to treat symptoms of malnutrition or other damage to the body.

Once a person's physical health has been addressed, he or she must begin psychological counseling. Counselors often urge family members to take part in therapy. Family members can learn to address issues that may have triggered the eating disorder. They can also learn to offer support as the disordered eater works to change his or her behavior. Group therapy may be used to provide peer support to people with eating disorders, 5-17.

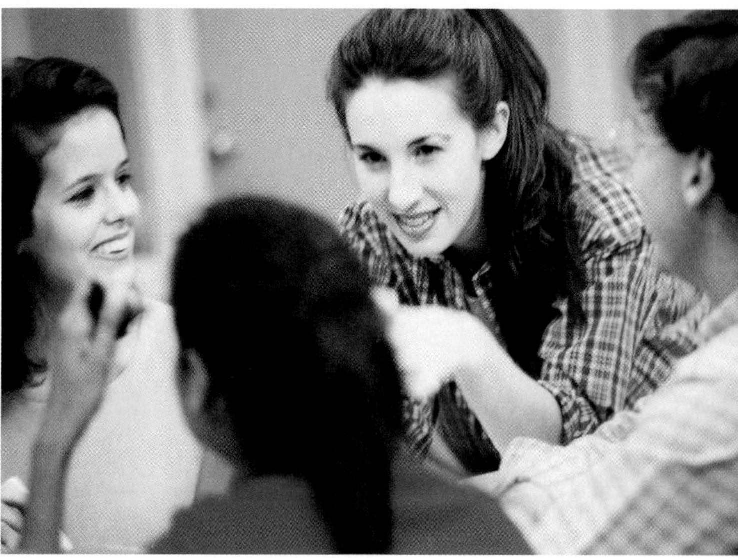

5-17 People recovering from eating disorders can benefit from the support of others who have gone through similar experiences.

Other specialists are often part of the treatment team for someone with an eating disorder. A registered dietitian can help the person learn how to make nutritious food choices. A fitness counselor can aid in setting up a sound program of physical activity. Working as a team, health professionals can help someone with an eating disorder form a healthful relationship with food.

If you think you know someone who has an eating disorder, you should confront the person with your concerns. Speak to the person privately. Be honest as you express care and support. Describe the behaviors that have caused your concern. Use your knowledge of nutrition and eating disorders to counter any excuses the person may offer. Suggest that the person see a professional about these behaviors. Do not threaten or accuse the person, and avoid making promises you cannot keep. If the person seems unwilling to seek help, you should talk to a trusted adult about the situation. A parent, teacher, doctor, or counselor should be able to offer advice. Remember, the sooner someone with an eating disorder gets help, the better his or her chances of recovery are.

Chapter 5 Review

Staying Active and Managing Your Weight

Summary

Your energy needs are based on your basal metabolism and your activity level. The energy value of the foods you eat depends on the amount of carbohydrate, fat, and protein in the food. The way the energy provided by the foods you eat compares with your energy needs affects your body weight.

The energy you use for physical activity plays a vital role in your body's state of fitness. You need to be active every day. Finding a variety of activities you enjoy will help you stay active so you can reap a lifetime of benefits.

Weight management involves balancing the energy you consume from food against the energy you expend through activity. It is a lifestyle that will help you maintain a healthy weight throughout life. Body mass index, a skin-fold test, and waist-to-hip ratio can help determine whether weight is healthy. Being overweight or obese may lead to a number of health problems. People overeat for many reasons. Deciding to lose weight and identifying eating habits are the first steps to reaching healthy weight goals. Weight management involves controlling energy intake and increasing physical activity. A number of weight-loss aids are available. However, the only sure way to lose weight is to consume fewer calories than you expend. After reaching a weight-loss goal, you need to continue to practice weight management to maintain a healthy weight. Weight management principles also apply to people who are trying to gain weight.

Eating disorders could be viewed as the opposite of weight management. They are abnormal eating behaviors that risk health. Anorexia nervosa, bulimia nervosa, and binge eating disorder are three common eating disorders. Treatment requires care of the body and mind to help disordered eaters form a healthful relationship with food.

Review What You Have Read

Write your answers on a separate sheet of paper.

1. True or false. Basal metabolism refers to the amount of energy the human body needs just to stay alive and carry on vital life processes.
2. What are three factors that can influence the amount of energy a person needs to perform a physical task?
3. How many calories are provided by a gram of each of the following: carbohydrates, proteins, fats?
4. How much time do experts recommend adults, children, and teens spend being physically active?
5. What types of physical activities help build flexibility, strength, and cardiovascular health?
6. When should an athlete begin drinking fluids to prevent dehydration?
7. An athlete's main source of energy should be _____.
   A. complex carbohydrates
   B. fats
   C. protein
   D. sugar
8. Why should athletes wishing to reach weight goals seek the advice of a registered dietitian?
9. Explain why the use of body mass index in assessing weight has limitations.
10. Describe three factors that contribute to overeating.
11. Briefly describe a weight management plan for losing 1 pound (0.45 kg) a week.
12. Why are most weight-loss aids ineffective?
13. True or false. In a weight-gain plan, fats should make up no more than 35 percent of total calories.
14. What usually triggers an eating disorder?

15. Identify three health professionals who might be part of a team for treating someone with an eating disorder.

Build Your Basic Skills

1. **Math.** Calculate your daily calorie need for a sedentary lifestyle and an active lifestyle. Also, calculate your daily limit for fat grams.
2. **Writing.** Write a letter to a friend expressing your concern about his or her abnormal eating behaviors. Offer support and suggest a possible course of action your friend might take.

Build Your Thinking Skills

1. **Analyze.** Keep a daily activity log for three days. At 15-minute intervals throughout the day, record how you spend your time. Analyze your activity log to identify how much time you spend being moderately physically active. Write a summary of your analysis stating how you meet the daily goal of 60 minutes of moderate physical activity. If you do not meet this goal, state how you could adjust your daily schedule to be more physically active.
2. **Evaluate.** Evaluate a reducing diet suggested in a popular magazine. Give an oral report comparing the diet with the weight management principles discussed in this chapter.

Apply Technology

1. Visit a health club and note the types of computerized monitors and performance meters that are on the exercise equipment. Report your findings in class.
2. Measure your body fat using a scale with a body fat monitor. If possible, have a trained professional measure your body fat using a caliper. Compare the two measurements.

Using Workplace Skills

Aja is an attendant at New You, which is a weight management salon. She is responsible for recording clients' weights and body measurements. She shows clients how to use the exercise equipment selected for their personalized fitness programs. She also gives clients a menu planning pamphlet prepared by a registered dietitian. Then she suggests ways clients can continue to enjoy their favorite foods while following the guidelines in the pamphlet.

To be an effective worker, Aja needs skill in working well with people from culturally diverse backgrounds. In a small group, answer the following questions about Aja's need for and use of this skill:

A. Why would Aja need to consider the cultural backgrounds of her clients?
B. How could Aja's skill in working with people from diverse cultures affect her clients' success in achieving weight management goals?
C. How would Aja's skill in working with people from diverse cultures affect the salon's business?
D. What is another skill Aja would need in this job? Briefly explain why this skill would be important.

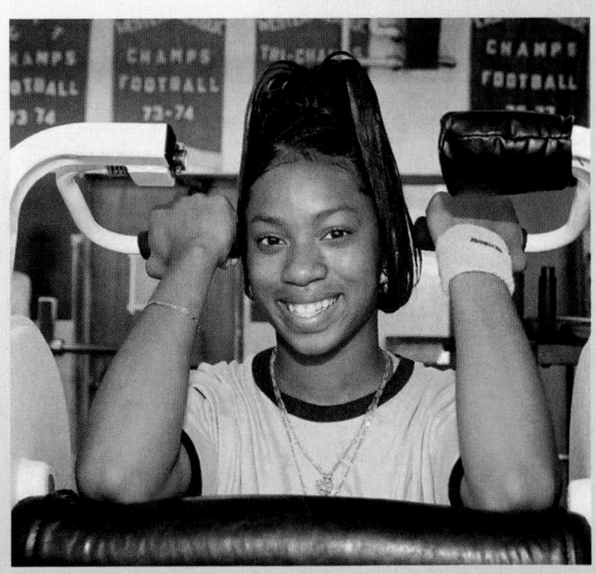

Chapter 6

Safeguarding the Family's Health

Scullion
Performs any combination of tasks involved in cleaning a ship's galleys, bakery, and butcher shop.

Sanitarian
Supervises and coordinates activities of workers engaged in duties concerned with sanitation programs in food processing establishments.

Safety Inspector
Inspects machinery, equipment, and working conditions in industrial or other settings, such as food processing plants, to ensure compliance with occupational safety and health regulations.

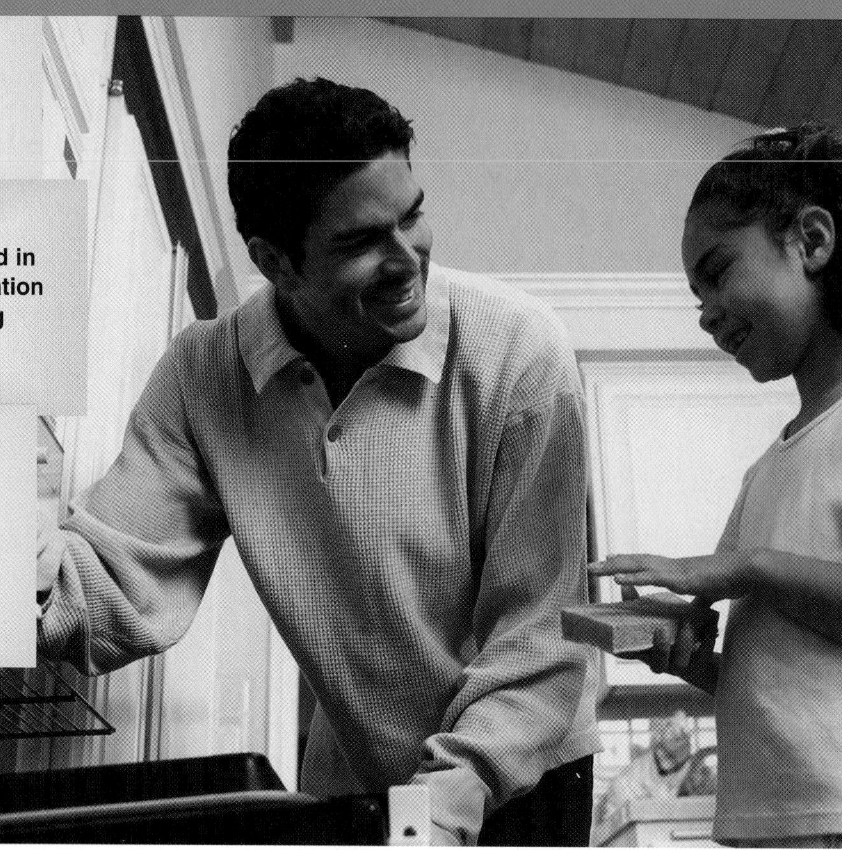

Terms to Know

foodborne illness
contaminant
microorganism
bacteria
toxin
sanitation
cross-contamination
abdominal thrust

Objectives

After studying this chapter, you will be able to

- discuss causes, symptoms, and treatment of common foodborne illnesses.
- list the four key steps to food safety and give examples of each.
- give examples of how following good safety practices can help you prevent kitchen accidents.
- apply basic first aid measures in the home.

Keeping foods safe to eat and making the kitchen a safe place to work are keys to good health. Improper food handling can make you ill. Kitchen accidents can cause severe injuries. You can prevent both illness and accidents by following safety principles.

Foodborne Illnesses

Perhaps you have heard news reports about people getting sick from something they ate. A disease transmitted by food is called a ***foodborne illness.*** Millions of cases of foodborne illness occur in the United States each year. Many of these cases go unreported because people mistake their symptoms for the "flu."

Food Contamination

Most foodborne illnesses are caused by contaminants. A ***contaminant*** is a substance that may be harmful that has accidentally gotten into food. Many contaminants are microorganisms. A ***microorganism*** is a living substance so small it can be seen only under a microscope. Many contaminated foods do not look or smell spoiled, but they can still cause illness.

One type of microorganism that causes many foodborne illnesses is bacteria. ***Bacteria*** are single-celled or noncellular microorganisms. They live almost everywhere. They are not all harmful. Some types of harmless bacteria are normally found in foods.

Food can become contaminated with harmful bacteria at any point from the farm to the table. Soil, insects, humans, and cooking tools can all transfer bacteria to foods. People who produce, process, and consume food must all use care to avoid contaminating it.

Local, state, and federal guidelines define conditions under which foods are to be produced and handled. For instance, federal regulations require some food processors to follow a quality control system called *HACCP*. This stands for Hazard Analysis and Critical Control Point. This system involves looking at food production processes to see where hazards can occur. Processors can then take steps to prevent problems and respond to problems quickly.

Federal laws also ensure that foods sold across state lines are safe. This means foods are processed under sanitary conditions and are honestly prepared, labeled, and packaged. Health inspectors spot-check farms where food is grown and plants where it is processed. Inspectors issue warnings when they find minor violations of health codes. When problems are not corrected or when violations are severe, inspectors may seize foods and close plants.

Raw eggs, poultry, meat, and fish are often contaminated with harmful bacteria, 6-1. Thorough cooking will kill many harmful bacteria. Refrigeration will slow their growth. However, unsafe levels of bacteria can stay in food that is not fully cooked. Food left at room temperature can serve as a breeding ground for bacteria. Improper handling can taint formerly unaffected food.

Bacterial Illnesses

Common foodborne illnesses include *campylobacteriosis, E. coli infection,* and

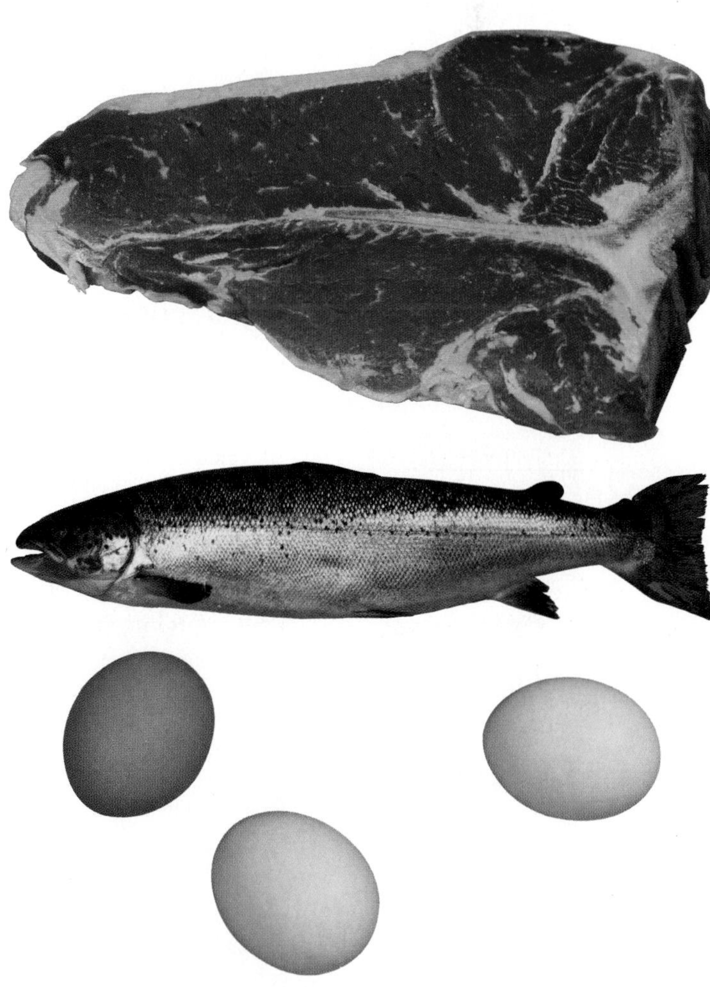

6-1 Raw meat, fish, and eggs can contain harmful bacteria. Careful handling and proper cooking will help prevent foodborne illness.

listeriosis. Perfringens poisoning, salmonellosis, shigellosis, and *vibrio infection* are also on the list. All these diseases are caused by bacteria. Two other foodborne illnesses, *botulism* and *staphylococcal poisoning*, are caused by ***toxins*** (poisons) produced by bacteria.

The bodies of most healthy people can handle small amounts of harmful bacteria. However, when the bacterial count becomes too great, illness can occur. Foodborne illnesses pose a greater risk for some groups of people. These groups include infants, pregnant women, older adults, and people with impaired immune systems.

Symptoms of bacterial foodborne illnesses vary depending on the type of bacteria. Symptoms may appear 30 minutes to 30 days after eating tainted food. The amount of time required for symptoms to develop often makes it hard to pinpoint the source of foodborne illness. Common symptoms are abdominal cramps, diarrhea, fatigue, headache, fever, and vomiting. These symptoms often last only a day or two. In some cases, however, they can last a week or more.

The symptoms of botulism differ from those of most other foodborne illnesses. This disease affects the nervous system. Symptoms include double vision, inability to swallow, speech difficulty, and gradual respiratory paralysis. The death rate for botulism is high. However, a doctor can treat botulism with an antitoxin if he or she diagnoses it in time. See 6-2.

Foodborne Illnesses		
Illness	**Food Sources**	**Symptoms**
Botulism	Improperly processed home-canned low-acid foods, processed meats	Double vision, inability to swallow, speech difficulty, progressive respiratory paralysis that can lead to death Appear: 4 to 36 hours after eating
Campylobacteriosis	Raw poultry and meat, unpasteurized milk	Diarrhea, abdominal cramping, fever, bloody stools Appear: 2 to 5 days after eating Last: 7 to 10 days
E. coli infection	Undercooked ground meat, unpasteurized milk, contaminated water, vegetables grown in cow manure	Bloody stools, stomachache, nausea, vomiting Appear: 12 to 72 hours after eating Last: 4 to 10 days
Listeriosis	Soft cheese, unpasteurized milk, imported seafood products, frozen cooked crabmeat, cooked shrimp, cooked imitation shellfish, luncheon meats	Fever, headache, nausea, vomiting Appear: 48 to 72 hours after eating
Perfringens poisoning	Prepared meat and meat products, gravies, and stuffings kept at improper temperatures	Abdominal pain, diarrhea, possibly nausea and vomiting Appear: 8 to 12 hours after eating Last: 24 hours
Salmonellosis	Raw poultry, meat, eggs, and dairy products	Severe headache, nausea, vomiting, abdominal pain, diarrhea, fever Appear: 8 to 12 hours after eating Last: 2 to 3 days
Staphylococcal poisoning	Meats; poultry; custard; cream pies; egg, chicken, potato, and macaroni salads	Abdominal cramping, nausea, vomiting, diarrhea Appear: 30 minutes to 8 hours after eating Last: 1 to 2 days

6-2 *These are among the many foodborne illnesses that can be caused by improper handling of food.*

Treating Bacterial Foodborne Illnesses

Infants, pregnant women, older adults, and those with chronic illnesses should see a doctor about symptoms of foodborne illness. If you are not in these high-risk groups, you may not need professional treatment for foodborne illness. Resting will help you get your strength back. Drinking liquids will help replace body fluids lost due to diarrhea and vomiting. If you suspect you have botulism, or if your symptoms are severe, you should call your doctor right away.

Other Foodborne Illnesses

Bacteria are not the only microorganisms that can cause foodborne illnesses. Parasites, protozoa, and viruses transmitted by food can cause illnesses, too.

A *parasite* is a microorganism that needs another organism, called a *host,* to live. Hogs and other sources of red meat are often infected with the parasite *Toxoplasma gondii.* This parasite causes the infection *toxoplasmosis,* which can damage the central nervous system. People can become infected with Toxoplasma by eating undercooked meat from animals infected with this parasite.

A couple of foodborne illnesses are caused by *protozoa* (tiny, one-celled animals). *Amebiasis* is caused by drinking polluted water or eating vegetables grown in polluted soil. *Giardiasis* can also be caused by drinking impure water.

Food can transmit a few viruses that cause diseases. (A *virus* is the smallest and simplest known type of microorganism.) For instance, raw shellfish, such as oysters and clams, can transmit *hepatitis A virus.* Symptoms of this virus begin with nausea, vomiting, and fever. However, severe cases can result in liver damage and even death.

The hepatitis A virus is highly heat-resistant. This makes disease prevention difficult because people often eat shellfish raw or just slightly cooked. Contaminated water and sewage are the major sources of this virus. The best way to avoid contamination is to buy shellfish that come only from commercial sources. If you gather fresh shellfish, be sure to stay safely away from any source of pollution.

A few foods have *natural toxins* that can cause illness. Certain varieties of mushrooms and leaves of the rhubarb plant are two such foods. Avoid picking wild mushrooms as well as fruits, roots, and berries unless you are knowledgeable about them. Some varieties can be poisonous.

Q: Can you get worms from eating raw pork?

A: Hogs were once a common host for parasitic roundworms called *trichinae*, which cause the disease *trichinosis*. Improved standards for feeding hogs have all but eliminated this risk in pork. However, trichinae are found in some game meat, and pork may be contaminated with other microorganisms. Therefore, all these meats should be cooked to a safe internal temperature of 160°F (71°C).

Four Steps to Food Safety

Most foodborne illnesses are spread through improper food handling. All the guidelines for keeping food safe to eat can be summed up in four basic steps—clean, separate, cook, and chill. You need to keep these steps in mind when you are buying, preparing, and storing food. This can help you and your family members avoid foodborne illness, 6-3.

Clean

One of the key steps you can take to prevent foodborne illness is to keep yourself and your kitchen clean. You need to follow good sanitation practices. ***Sanitation*** means maintaining clean conditions to prevent disease and promote good health. Encourage family members to abide by the following sanitation guidelines when handling food:

- Wash hands for 20 seconds with soap and warm water before starting to work with food. This may be the biggest step you can take to prevent the transmission of harmful bacteria. Also, wash your hands after

FIGHT BAC!
CLEAN
Wash hands and surfaces often.
SEPARATE
Don't cross-contaminate.
CHILL
Refrigerate promptly.
COOK
Cook to proper temperatures.
Keep Food Safe From Bacteria™

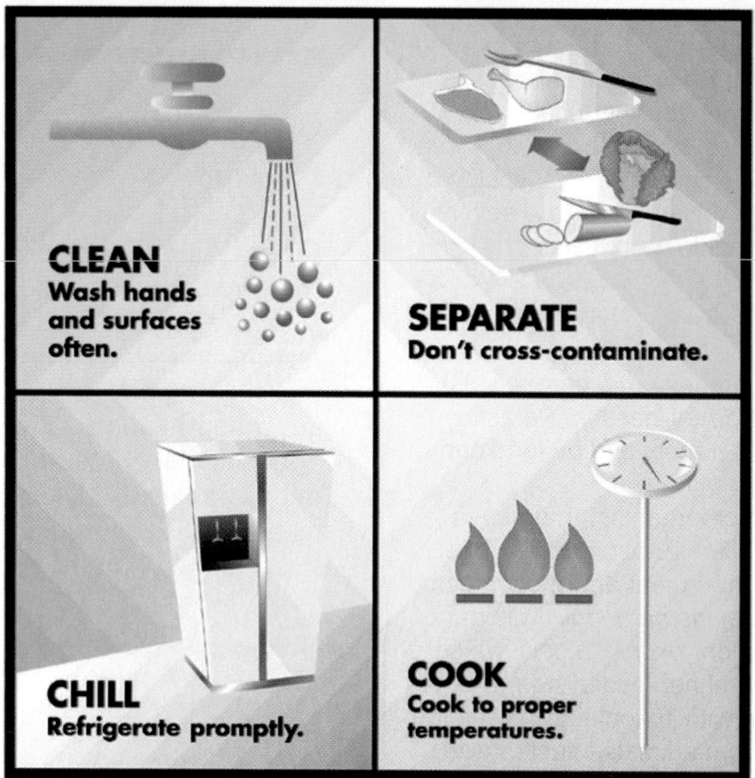

Partnership for Food Safety Education

6-3 Following the four basic steps to food safety—clean, separate, cook, and chill—can help you avoid illness-causing bacteria.

sneezing, coughing, using the toilet, or touching your face, hair, or any unsanitary object. Be sure to clean under your fingernails, too. Dry hands with paper towels or use a clean hand towel.

- Keep long hair tied back and avoid touching hair while you work.
- Wear clean clothes and a clean apron when working around food. Bacteria can accumulate on dirty clothes. Avoid loose sleeves, which can dip into foods.
- If you have an open sore or cut on your hand, put on gloves before handling food. Open sores are a major source of staphylococcal bacteria.
- Designate the kitchen as a nonsmoking area to keep ashes from falling into food.
- Cover coughs and sneezes with a disposable tissue. Wash hands immediately.
- After handling raw meat, fish, poultry, or eggs, wash your hands thoroughly before touching any other foods. This will prevent the transfer of bacteria. See 6-4.
- Keep your work area clean. Wipe up spills as they happen.
- Use paper towels to wipe up juices from raw meat and poultry. Then immediately wash the area on which the juices dripped.
- Remove dirty utensils from your work area before proceeding to the next task. Bacteria grow quickly in spills and on dirty utensils.
- Wash the tops of cans before opening them. Otherwise, dust and dirt could fall into food when you open the can.
- Thoroughly wash cutting boards, counters, and utensils after each use. In addition, regularly clean counters and cutting boards with chlorine bleach solution to kill bacteria.

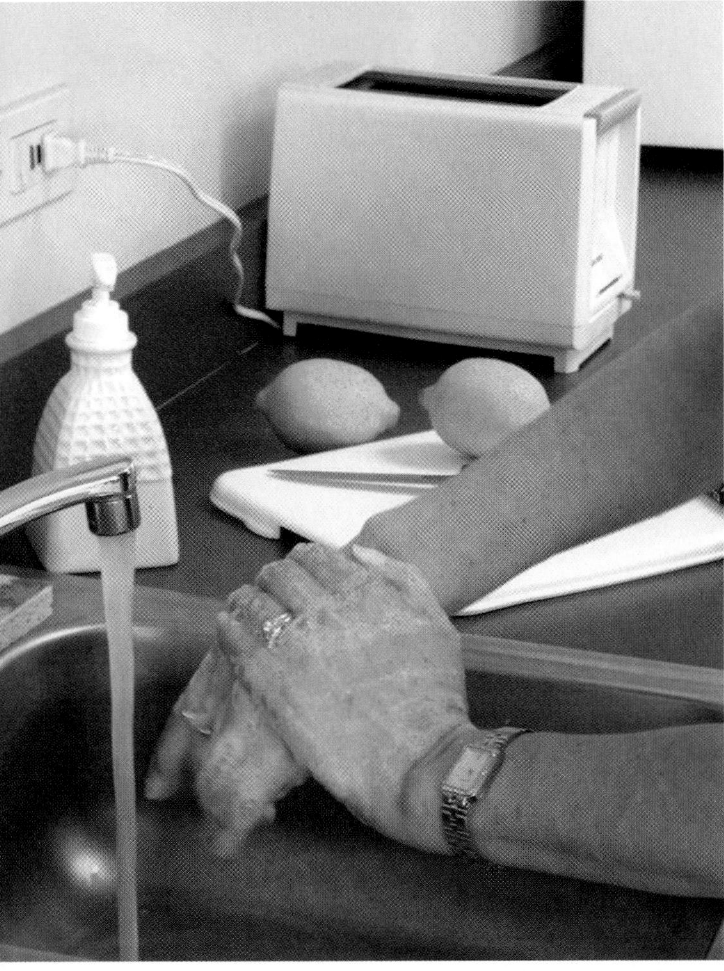

Jack Klasey

6-4 Wash hands before handling food and after touching anything that might be contaminated with bacteria. This may be the biggest step you can take to prevent foodborne illness.

- Wash dishes promptly, using hot water and detergent. Wash dishes in the following order: glasses, flatware, plates and bowls, pots and pans, and greasy utensils. Rinse dishes with scalding water and allow them to air dry. If you must dry dishes, be sure to use a clean dishtowel.
- Dispose of garbage properly and promptly. Frequent washing and air drying of garbage pails prevent odors and bacterial growth.
- Never store sacks of onions or potatoes, canned goods, or any other foods under the kitchen sink. Drainpipes can leak and damage the food.
- Wash dishcloths and sponges daily. (Sponges can be washed in a dishwasher in a covered basket designed to hold small items.) Between uses, rinse dishcloths and sponges well, wring thoroughly, and allow to air dry. This discourages bacteria from breeding on damp surfaces.

Separate

A second step for preventing foodborne illness is to separate cooked and ready-to-eat foods from raw foods. Following this step will avoid the risks of cross-contamination. ***Cross-contamination*** occurs when harmful bacteria from one food are transferred to another food. For instance, juices from a leaky package of raw chicken may contain harmful bacteria. If the juices drip on other foods in your shopping cart or refrigerator, the bacteria will be transferred to these foods. The following guidelines will help you keep foods that may be contaminated separated from other foods:

- Put raw poultry, meat, and seafood in separate plastic bags before placing them in your shopping cart.
- Store raw poultry, meat, and seafood in containers to keep them separate from other foods in the refrigerator. See 6-5.
- Do not taste and cook with the same spoon. Use one spoon for tasting and one for stirring. To taste, pour a little of the food from the stirring spoon onto the tasting spoon. Do not lick your fingers.
- Use clean utensils and containers. Never use the same utensil, cutting board, or plate for both raw and cooked meat, poultry, fish,

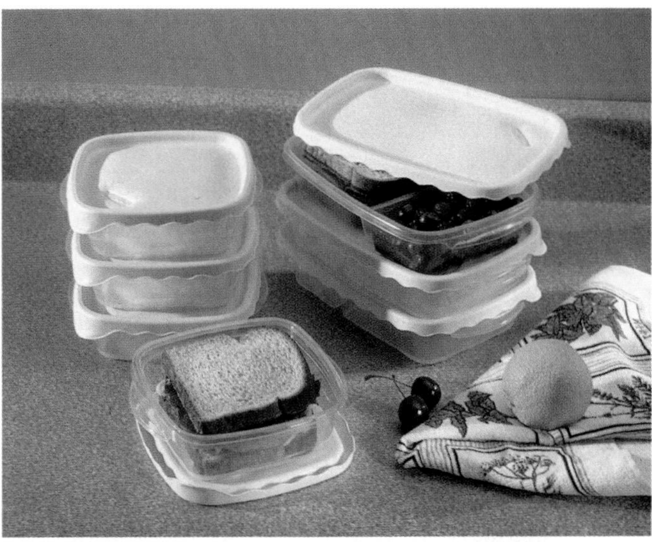

Rubbermaid

6-5 Use food storage containers to keep cooked and ready-to-eat foods separated from raw foods.

or eggs. Utensils can transfer bacteria from raw foods to cooked foods.
- Never use a hand towel to wipe dishes. Dirty towels can transfer bacteria.
- Keep pets and insects out of the kitchen. Do not feed pets in the kitchen or wash their dishes with the family dishes. Remove leftover pet food and dispose of it promptly.
- Never taste any food that looks or smells questionable. Dispose of it promptly.
- Store nonperishables in tightly sealed containers to keep them fresh and free from insects and rodents.

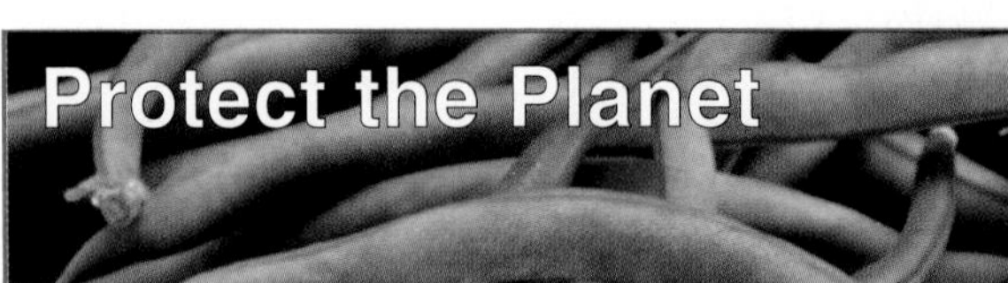

Many commercial cleaning products contain harsh chemicals that damage the environment. Try doing many of your common cleaning tasks with a less toxic cleaner. A low-cost one that you probably already have on hand is baking soda! Sprinkle a little on a sponge dampened with vinegar. Use this vinegar and baking soda mixture for wiping sinks, countertops, and appliances.

Q: Are plastic cutting boards more sanitary than wooden ones?

A: Unlike wooden cutting boards, plastic cutting boards are not porous. This makes them easier to keep clean. However, both types of boards need to be thoroughly cleaned with hot, soapy water after each use.

Cook

Raw meat, poultry, seafood, and eggs can contain harmful bacteria. Cooking these foods to a safe internal temperature is the third step to food safety. High temperatures can kill bacteria. The following guidelines will help you make sure foods are thoroughly cooked:

- Use a thermometer to check food temperatures. Always keep hot foods hot—above 140°F (60°C).
- Cook cuts of meat, such as steaks and roasts, to an internal temperature of 145°F (63°C). Cook foods made with ground meat, such as hamburgers and meat loaf, to an internal temperature of 160°F (71°C). Cook whole poultry to an internal temperature of 180°F (71°C) and breast pieces to 170°F (75°C).
- Stuff raw poultry, meat, and fish just before baking. Stuffing should reach an internal temperature of at least 165°F (74°C).
- Do not partially cook foods and then set them aside or refrigerate them to complete the cooking later.
- Reheat leftovers to 165°F (74°C). When reheating sauces, soups, and gravies, make sure they come to a full boil.
- Boil low-acid, home-canned foods for 10 to 20 minutes before tasting. Dispose of any bulging, leaking, or otherwise damaged container of food.
- Use only clean, fresh, unbroken eggs for eggnog, custard, and other egg dishes. Modify recipes calling for uncooked or partially cooked eggs. Cook eggs until they are firm, not runny.
- Do not eat raw cookie dough or taste partially cooked dishes containing meat, poultry, fish, or eggs.

Chill

Chilling foods is the fourth basic step to food safety. Chilling foods promptly after buying or serving them will keep harmful bacteria from multiplying. The following tips will help you store foods correctly to keep them safe and wholesome:

- Keep cold foods cold—below 40°F (5°C).
- Bacteria multiply fastest at temperatures between 60°F and 126°F (16°C and 52°C), 6-6. This danger zone includes room temperature. This is why you should not allow food to sit out for more than two hours.
- Refrigerate leftovers promptly. Eat or freeze refrigerated leftovers within three days.
- Use a refrigerator thermometer to check the temperature of your refrigerator and freezer

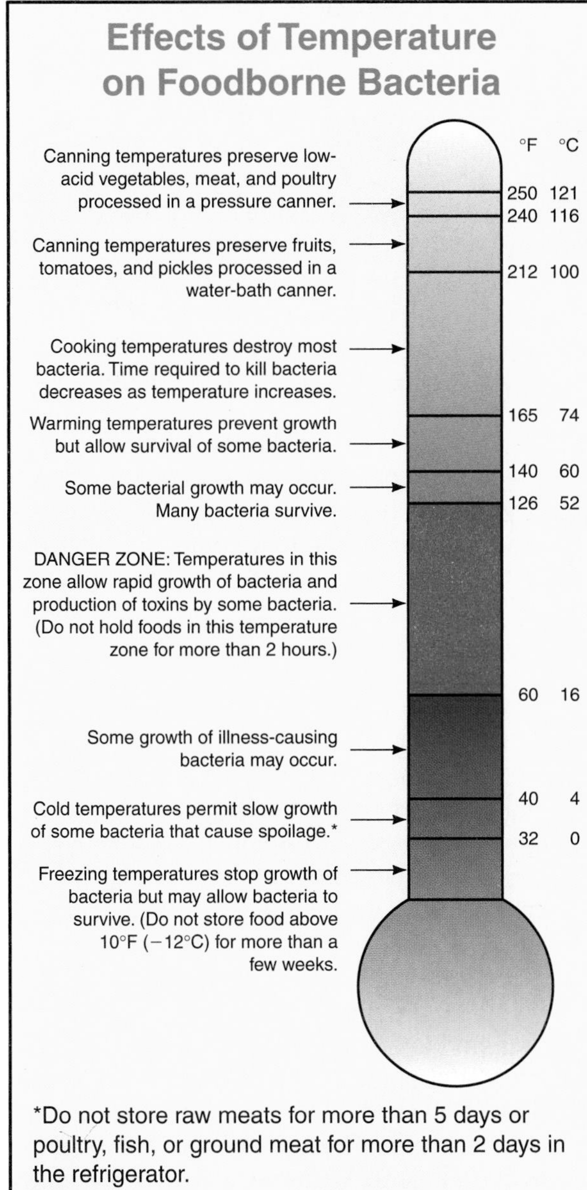

6-6 Bacteria multiply rapidly at moderate temperatures. To prevent this, keep hot foods hot and cold foods cold.

regularly. Refrigerator temperatures should be 40°F (5°C) or just slightly below. Freezer temperatures should be 0°F (-18°C) or below. Also, check the gaskets around the doors to be sure they are tight.

- Thaw foods in the refrigerator or in the microwave oven immediately before cooking. Do not thaw on the kitchen counter or table.
- Keep your refrigerator and freezer clean.
- Package refrigerated and frozen foods properly. Use moistureproof and vaporproof wraps for the freezer. For the refrigerator, cover fresh meats loosely and store left-overs in tightly covered containers. Use foods within recommended storage times.
- Refrigerate custards, meringue, cream pies, and foods filled with custard mixtures when they have cooled slightly.
- Use shallow containers for refrigerator storage to help foods reach safe, cool temperatures faster. You can also hasten cooling by placing containers of food in an ice water bath.
- Remove stuffing from poultry, meat, and fish promptly after serving and refrigerate it separately. Refrigerate gravy, stuffing, and meat immediately after the meal.
- Do not refreeze foods unless they still contain ice crystals. Do not refreeze ice cream that has thawed. Use defrosted foods promptly.
- Make the supermarket your last stop on the way home. Put perishable items in your shopping cart last. Refrigerate or freeze them as soon as you get home.

Cooking for Special Occasions

Cooking for large crowds or cooking outdoor meals requires additional precautions to keep food safe to eat. Before planning any large gathering, be sure the equipment you have can handle large quantities of food. Refrigerators must be large enough to chill increased quantities of warm foods without raising the temperature above 40°F (5°C). Heating appliances must be able to keep hot foods above 140°F (60°C) until serving time.

If using buffet service, put the food in small serving dishes, which you can refill or replace as needed. Another way to keep hot foods hot and cold foods cold is to use heated serving appliances and ice.

Large amounts of food take longer to heat and chill than do small or average amounts. Divide food and place it in small, shallow containers for quicker heating and cooling.

Be sure to thoroughly cook all foods. Then serve them promptly. Refrigerate leftovers immediately after the meal.

Consider preparing some foods several weeks in advance and freezing them. This will help you budget your time. Freezing foods ahead will also prevent overloading your refrigerator the day before the event.

Picnic and barbecue foods present other problems. You may carry these foods some distance before serving them. Use insulated containers to keep these foods at the proper temperature to prevent the growth of bacteria, 6-7. Wrap raw meat, poultry, and fish carefully to keep them from leaking onto other foods. You may want to use a separate cooler for beverages. This will help you avoid repeatedly opening the cooler containing the perishable foods. Do not take perishables from the cooler until you are ready to cook or serve them.

Play It Safe

Pack antibacterial hand cleaner or moist towelettes in your picnic basket. Use them to clean your hands before and after handling food when soap and water are not available.

Use sanitary procedures when preparing picnic foods. Be sure utensils are clean. Do not let hamburgers, hot dogs, or other meats sit next to the grill while the charcoal heats. Keep them in the ice chest. Do not put cooked meat on the same plate that held raw meat.

Eating Safely When Eating Out

Most of the foodborne illness cases reported each year occur in foodservice establishments. Restaurants have strict sanitation guidelines they must follow when preparing food for the public. State health departments inspect foodservice facilities regularly to ensure that guidelines are being met. However, occasional problems still occur.

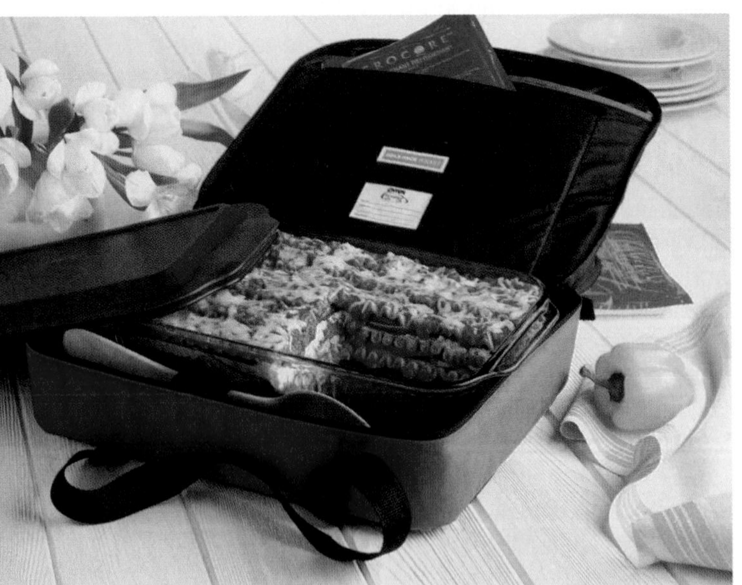

Pyrex

6-7 An insulated carrier can help you transport a hot dish and keep it at a safe serving temperature.

You can take several steps when eating out to protect yourself from foodborne illness. First, look at the surroundings on your way into a restaurant. The parking lot should be free from litter. The way the outside of a restaurant is maintained can give you a clue about how the inside is maintained.

When you enter the restaurant, you should see a concern for cleanliness throughout the establishment. Tables should be wiped. Walls and floors should be clean. Rest rooms should be tidy.

Observe the employees as they wait on you. They should appear to be in good health. Their clothes should be clean. If they have long hair, they should have it tied back. When they serve you, they should not touch the eating surfaces of your tableware.

When your food is served, it should look and smell wholesome. Hot foods should be hot. Cold foods should be cold.

If you have a concern about your food, do not be afraid to speak to your server. If your server cannot answer your questions or correct the problem, ask to speak to the manager.

Most servers will wrap leftovers for you if you wish to take them home. However, be sure you are going directly home and promptly put leftovers in the refrigerator. If you cannot refrigerate food within two hours from the time it was *served*, discard it.

If you choose restaurants with care, you may never have a problem with foodborne illness. However, if you get ill from something you ate at a restaurant, call local health authorities. Others should be warned they may have been exposed to the infected food also.

Storing Food for Emergencies

No one wants to think about hurricanes, floods, tornadoes, and earthquakes. Unfortunately, such disasters can happen.

When they do, people are often stranded in their homes or forced to evacuate for days. Utilities may be cut off, and stores may be closed, unreachable, or out of merchandise. That is why safely storing food and water for emergency situations is important.

The American Red Cross recommends storing at least a three-day supply of food and water for each family member. Be sure to keep special needs of family members such as infants and diabetics in mind. Choose non-perishable foods that do not require cooking. Many canned goods make wise choices. Foods like dried fruits and beef jerky are good choices, too. They are compact and lightweight, so they will be easy to carry if there is an evacuation. Remember to store a can opener and any other tools you might need to prepare the food. Store items in a backpack or a container with wheels and a handle for pulling. This will make it easier to transport your supplies if you have to leave your home. Replace stored food and water every six months so they will be safe and fresh when you need them.

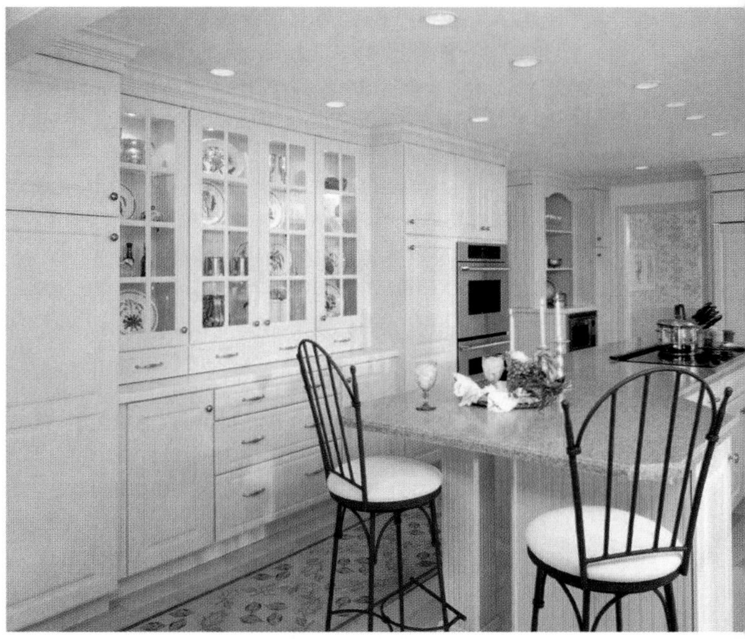

Photo courtesy of Decorá Cabinetry

6-8 Close all kitchen drawers and cabinets when not in use to prevent accidental injuries.

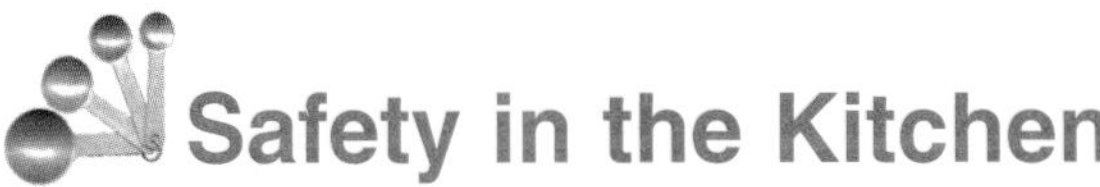

Safety in the Kitchen

Many common kitchen items may seem harmless. However, they can be dangerous if you do not take safety precautions. For instance, people can injure themselves by bumping into open cabinet doors and drawers. Keeping all kitchen cabinets and drawers closed will prevent accidental injuries, 6-8.

Hospital emergency room personnel see the results of thousands of kitchen accidents each year. Some kitchen accidents are due to ignorance. Many result from carelessness. Chemical poisonings, cuts, burns and fires, and falls are the most common of these accidents. Electric shocks, choking, and other types of injury can also occur in the kitchen. You can prevent many accidents by properly using and caring for equipment. Following good safety practices and keeping the kitchen clean will also help you avoid accidents.

Knowledge of basic first aid will help you provide treatment to someone involved in a kitchen accident. A simple first aid kit kept in the kitchen should include the items you need to treat minor injuries.

Preventing Chemical Poisonings

Children are especially susceptible to chemical poisonings. To many children, poisonous household products, such as furniture polishes, cleaners, and bleach, look like food. The following guidelines will help you prevent chemical poisonings:

- Keep all hazardous products in a location where children cannot reach them. In a home with young children, do not store household cleaners under the sink.
- Keep all hazardous products in their original, clearly labeled containers. Do not put them in soda bottles or other food containers. Keep all containers tightly closed.
- Do not rely on containers with safety closures. Some children can open safety caps.
- If the phone or doorbell interrupts you while you are using a hazardous product, take the product with you.
- Pesticides and insecticides used on food can be poisonous. To protect family members, wash all fresh fruits and vegetables thoroughly before use. Cover all food and cooking and eating utensils before using a pesticide in your home.

- Keep medication out of the kitchen and out of a child's reach. Never refer to medicine as candy. Dispose of unused medication promptly where a child cannot reach it.
- Read all warning labels, and keep a poison chart handy. This will help you know what first aid to give if someone is accidentally poisoned. It will also help you know what to tell a doctor.

Treating Poisonings

In a case of poisoning, call the nearest poison control center immediately. Have the poison container with you when you call so you can accurately describe the poison taken. If the label on the poison lists first aid instructions, follow them. Keep the victim comfortable and calm until help arrives.

Preventing Cuts

Knives, sharp appliances, and broken glass cause most kitchen cuts. The following guidelines will help you prevent cuts:

- Keep knives sharp. Dull blades can slip and cause cuts.
- Use knives properly. Move the blade away from your body as you cut. Never point a sharp object at another person.
- Do not try to catch a falling knife in midair. Let the knife fall to the floor, then carefully pick it up.
- Use a knife only for its intended purpose. Do not use it as a screwdriver or to pry open containers. To do so can cause serious injuries.
- Wash and store knives separately from other utensils, 6-9.
- Never put fingers near beaters or the blades of blenders, food processors, or food waste disposers to dislodge foods or objects. Instead, disconnect the appliance and use a nonmetal utensil to remove items that are stuck. If you cannot dislodge an object, call a repair person.
- When opening a can, dispose of the lid immediately.
- Never pick up broken glass with your bare hands. Wear rubber gloves to pick up large pieces. Sweep smaller pieces into a disposable dustpan and wipe up fragments with a damp paper towel. Dispose of broken glass immediately.

Treating Cuts

To treat a cut, cover the wound with a sterile cloth or clean handkerchief. Apply firm pressure to the wound to stop bleeding. If a cut is minor, wash it with soap and water. Apply an antiseptic solution and bandage it with a sterile dressing. If a cut is severe, continue to apply pressure to the wound. Take the victim to the hospital emergency room or family doctor.

Preventing Burns and Fires

Scalding liquids, spattering grease, and hot cooking utensils cause most kitchen burns. The majority of fires are due to malfunctioning electric appliances and carelessness around hot

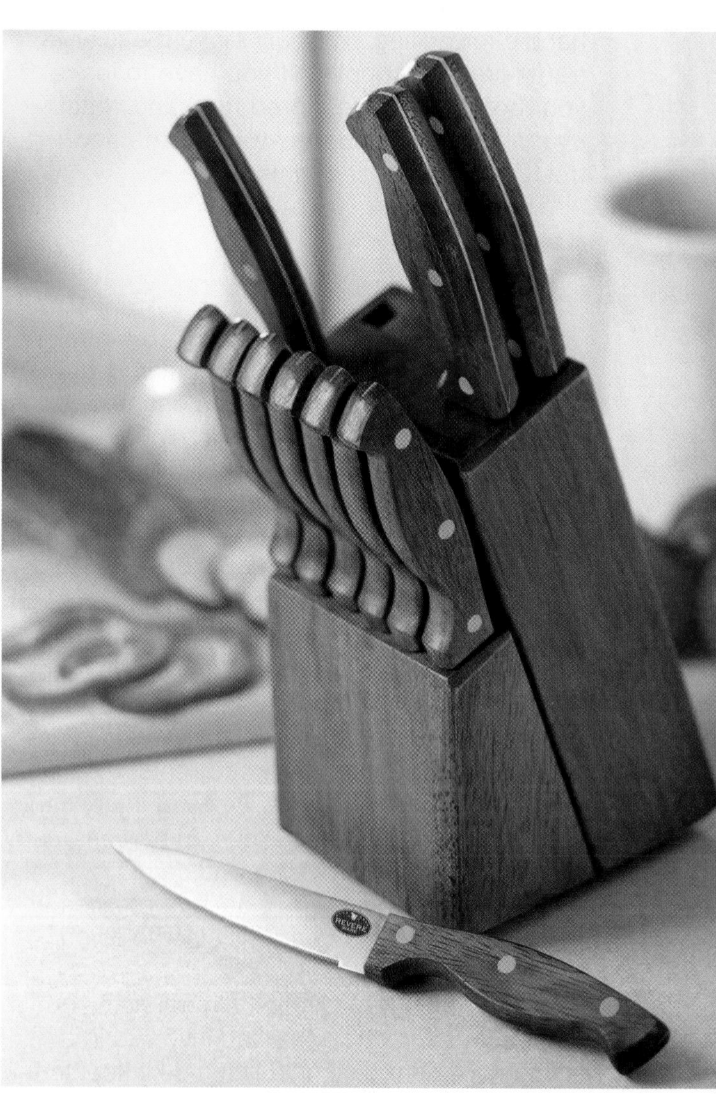

Revere

6-9 Storing knives separately from other utensils can help prevent cuts.

surfaces and open flames. The following guidelines will help you prevent burns and fires:

- Use pot holders to handle hot utensils, 6-10.
- Turn all pan handles inward to prevent accidental tipping.
- To avoid a steam burn, open pan lids away from you so the steam will escape safely.
- Never open a pressure cooker before the pressure has gone down to zero. The pressurized steam within the cooker can rush out and cause a severe burn.
- Do not let children play near the range or cook without help. Teach them proper safety procedures.
- Turn off range and oven controls and disconnect small appliances when not in use.
- Use caution with liquids heated in a microwave oven. The water can reach temperatures over 212°F (100°C) without showing signs of boiling. Adding teabags, beverage mixes, or ice cubes to the water can cause sudden, rapid boiling to begin.

Be a Clever Consumer

When buying a fire extinguisher, choose one that is ABC class rated. This type of extinguisher is a good choice for the kitchen because it is all-purpose. Also, check to be sure the extinguisher has a safety seal. This is an emblem indicating the extinguisher has met the standards of a reputable testing agency.

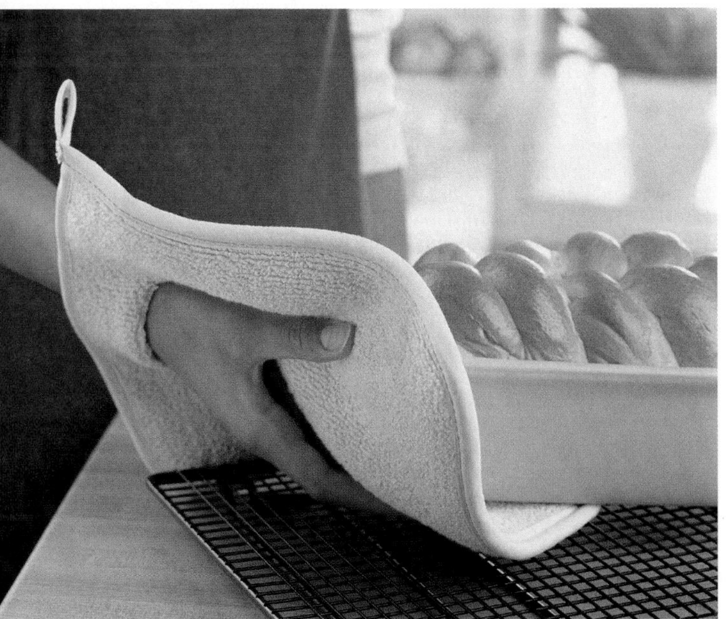

The Pampered Chef®

***6-10** Using pot holders will protect hands from hot cooking utensils.*

- Follow manufacturer's directions for use and care of all electric and gas appliances.
- Be sure to ground all electric appliances. (See Chapter 8.) Avoid using lightweight extension cords and multiple plug adapters.
- When working near the range, wear tight-fitting clothing. Roll up long sleeves.
- Do not hang towels, curtains, or other flammable materials near the range.
- If you must light a gas range manually, light the match first. Then turn on the gas to prevent an accidental explosion. If you smell gas, turn off the controls, open a window, and call the gas company.
- Never leave a pan of grease unattended; it could burst into flames. If grease should ignite, do not pour water on the flames as this could spread the fire.
- Use care around lit candles, canisters of cooking fuel, and other sources of open flames.
- Clean grease from exhaust hoods frequently to prevent grease fires.
- Keep a fire extinguisher handy. Be sure all family members know how to use it. Have it checked periodically. Do not store the extinguisher over the range.
- If your clothes should catch on fire, do not panic and run. Drop to the floor and roll over to smother the flames.
- Install a smoke alarm in the kitchen. Check it monthly to be sure batteries are operating. See 6-11.

Treating Burns

When someone becomes burned, place the burned area immediately under cold running water or in a cold water bath. Do not apply ointments or grease of any kind. Do not break blisters that may form. Call a physician immediately if a burn is severe or if pain and redness persist.

Preventing Falls

Most kitchen falls result from unsteady step stools and wet or cluttered floors. The following guidelines will help you prevent falls:

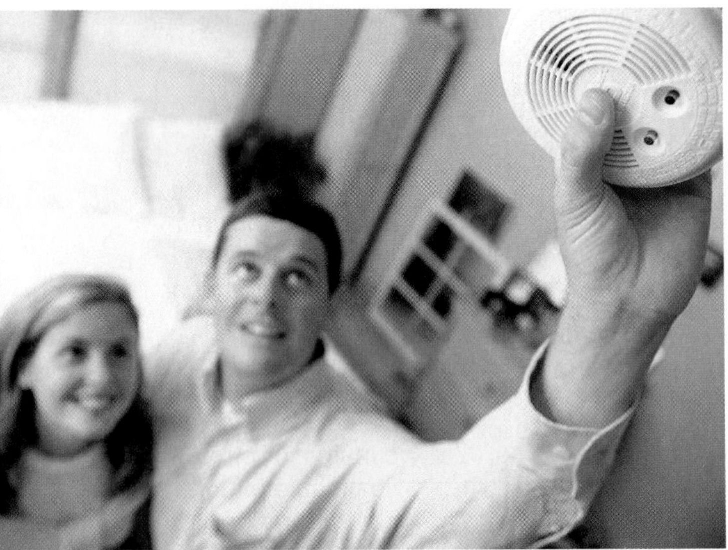

6-11 Test the batteries in a smoke detector regularly to be sure they are functioning.

- Do not stand on a chair or box to reach high places. Use a sturdy step stool or ladder.
- Wait until a freshly washed floor dries before walking across the room.
- Wipe up spills from floors immediately. Be sure no sticky or greasy residue remains.
- Do not let children leave their toys on the kitchen floor. Remove shoes, boots, sports equipment, and other objects from kitchen traffic areas.
- If you use throw rugs, find ones with non-skid backings.

Treating Falls

When someone is injured in a fall, stop bleeding if necessary. Loosen clothing around the victim's neck. If you suspect a broken bone, do not move the victim unless absolutely necessary. Make the victim as comfortable as possible. Do not give the victim anything to eat or drink. Call a physician.

Preventing Electric Shock

Faulty wiring, overloaded electrical outlets, and damaged appliances are common causes of electric shock. Electrical hazards can also be fire hazards. The following guidelines will help you prevent electric shock:

- Never stand on a wet floor or work near a wet counter when using electric appliances.
- Do not touch any electrical plugs, switches, or appliances when your hands are wet.
- Do not run electrical cords under rugs or carpeting.
- Do not use lightweight extension cords with small appliances. If possible, plug appliances directly into electrical outlets. If you must use an extension cord, choose a heavy-gauge one that is designed to carry a heavier electrical load.
- Do not overload electrical outlets by plugging several appliances into the same outlet. See 6-12.
- Place safety covers over unused electrical outlets to prevent children from sticking fingers or objects into them.
- Unplug the toaster before trying to pry loose food that has become stuck.
- When you disconnect appliances, hold onto the plug, not the cord. Replace all cords and plugs when they become worn.
- Do not use damaged appliances.

Treating Electric Shock

If someone receives an electric shock, immediately disconnect the appliance or turn off the power causing the shock. Do not touch the victim if he or she is connected to the power source. If you do, you will receive a shock, too. Use some nonconducting material to pull the victim away from the electrical source. A rope, a long piece of dry cloth, or a wooden pole would be suitable choices. Call for help. Begin rescue breathing.

Q: Will baking soda really put out a fire?

A: Baking soda, when heated, gives off carbon dioxide, which can smother flames. If a pan or skillet is on fire, however, the best step to take is to cover it with a lid and turn off the heat. For oven fires, keep the door closed and turn off the heat.

Preventing Choking

Choking occurs when an object such as a piece of food becomes stuck in the throat. The trapped object blocks the airway, making it impossible for the victim to speak or breathe. Someone who is choking quickly turns blue and

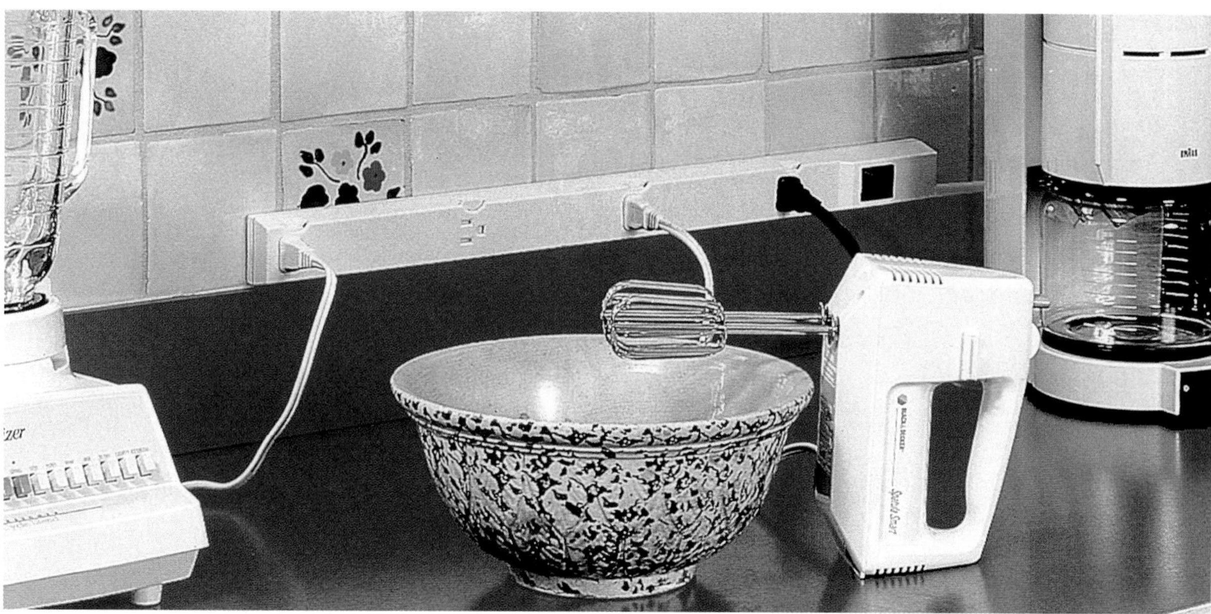

Woods Industries, Inc.

6-12 *An outlet strip with a built-in circuit breaker provides a safe way to plug in a number of electric appliances.*

collapses. The choking victim can die of strangulation in four minutes if the airway is not cleared. The following guidelines will help you prevent choking:

- Chew food thoroughly before swallowing.
- Avoid talking and laughing when you have food in your mouth.
- Do not give children small, round pieces of food, such as slices of hot dogs or carrots. Cut slices in halves or quarters.

Treating Choking

The ***abdominal thrust*** is a procedure used to save choking victims. It involves exerting pressure on the victim's abdomen. This causes the trapped food to be expelled. Being familiar with the steps for performing the abdominal thrust may help you save someone's life, 6-13. If no help is available, you can also perform the abdominal thrust on yourself before losing consciousness.

Be sure a person is choking before using the abdominal thrust. Someone who can cough, breathe, or talk is not choking. If a choking victim losses consciousness, do not attempt to use the abdominal thrust. Instead, call the local emergency number for immediate medical help.

The abdominal thrust can injure a choking victim. Therefore, the victim should see a doctor as soon as possible after the rescue.

The Abdominal Thrust	
1.	If the victim is standing, stand behind him or her. If the victim is sitting, stand behind his or her chair. Wrap your arms around the victim's waist.
2.	With your thumb toward the victim, place your fist against the victim's addomen. Your fist should be above the navel and just below the rib cage.
3.	Grasping your fist with your other hand, use a quick thrust to press upward into the victim's abdomen. Repeat the thrust several times, if needed.

6-13 *The abdominal thrust can save the life of a choking victim.*

Chapter 6 Review
Safeguarding the Family's Health

Summary

Foodborne illnesses are very common in the United States. Although bacteria cause many of these illnesses, people are often at fault for spreading the bacteria. Bacteria can get into food at any point during production, processing, or preparation. Most symptoms of foodborne illnesses affect the digestive system and last only a few days. However, foodborne illnesses can be deadly.

Foods often become contaminated through improper handling. It is important to keep yourself and your kitchen clean when preparing food. You need to separate raw foods from cooked and ready-to-eat foods. You must cook foods thoroughly and chill them promptly after purchase or serving. You need to take special precautions when cooking for a large group or transporting food. You need to be wary when you are eating out to avoid the risk of illness. Storing supplies in a special location will ensure that family members have safe food in the event of an emergency. Following these steps will help you and your family avoid foodborne illness.

Exercising safety is another concern when you are working in the kitchen. Many kitchen injuries are the result of poisonings, cuts, burns, falls, shock, and choking. You can take steps to prevent common kitchen accidents. You should also learn how to provide proper treatment when minor injuries occur.

Review What You Have Read

Write your answers on a separate sheet of paper.

1. True or false. Raw eggs, poultry, meat, and fish are often contaminated with harmful bacteria.
2. For what groups of people do foodborne illnesses pose the greatest risk?
3. What are three microorganisms other than bacteria that can cause foodborne illness?
4. List eight standards for personal and kitchen cleanliness.
5. List five guidelines for keeping foods that may be contaminated separated from other foods.
6. What are the proper temperatures for serving hot and cold foods?
7. How can large amounts of food be heated or chilled quickly?
8. Where do most of the foodborne illness cases reported each year occur?
9. True or false. Older adults are especially susceptible to chemical poisonings.
10. Describe the correct way to pick up and dispose of broken glass.
11. List eight safety precautions that can prevent burns and fires.
12. List three guidelines for preventing falls.
13. What should be used to pull a shock victim away from an electrical source?
14. Briefly describe the steps for performing the abdominal thrust.

Build Your Basic Skills

1. **Verbal.** Write a public service announcement that might be broadcast on radio or television about safe food handling. Include a jingle or slogan to help people remember a specific standard of personal or kitchen cleanliness. Record your announcement on audio- or videotape and play it for the class.
2. **Writing.** Prepare a pamphlet listing simple first aid procedures for poisonings, cuts, burns, falls, and electric shock.

Build Your Thinking Skills

1. **Analyze.** Analyze how food might become contaminated during a specific aspect of food production, processing, or transportation. Make a diagram illustrating this operation and the possible points of contamination. Also note safeguards that

are taken to prevent contamination at these points.

2. **Summarize.** Work in a group of four to research one type of foodborne illness. Prepare a poster to use in giving a presentation to the rest of the class. Each group member should summarize a different one of the following aspects: cause, food sources, symptoms, or prevention.
3. **Create.** Create puppets and a puppet show to present information about kitchen safety to young children. If possible, perform your show at a local preschool or kindergarten.

Apply Technology

1. Make a list of 10 antibacterial personal care and/or kitchen cleaning products that have been introduced to the market in the last five years. Investigate the active ingredient in one of these products and note the pathogens it is designed to remove. Share your findings in class.
2. Develop a segment on food safety and the correct use of food thermometers in different foods to air on your local cable access channel.

Using Workplace Skills

Desmond is a safety inspector at the Tempting Table food processing plant. He inspects the plant's machinery and working conditions to make sure they meet safety and health standards. When Desmond finds a piece of equipment that is not working properly, he helps get it operating safely again. Sometimes plant supervisors have to stop production while equipment is being repaired.

To be an effective worker, Desmond needs skill in maintaining and troubleshooting technologies. In a small group, answer the following questions about Desmond's need for and use of these skills:

A. How might Tempting Table be affected if their plant does not meet health and safety standards?
B. Why would Tempting Table want Desmond to identify potential hazards before problems occur?
C. How might other employees be affected if Desmond fails to identify or correct a problem?
D. What is another skill Desmond would need in this job? Briefly explain why this skill would be important.

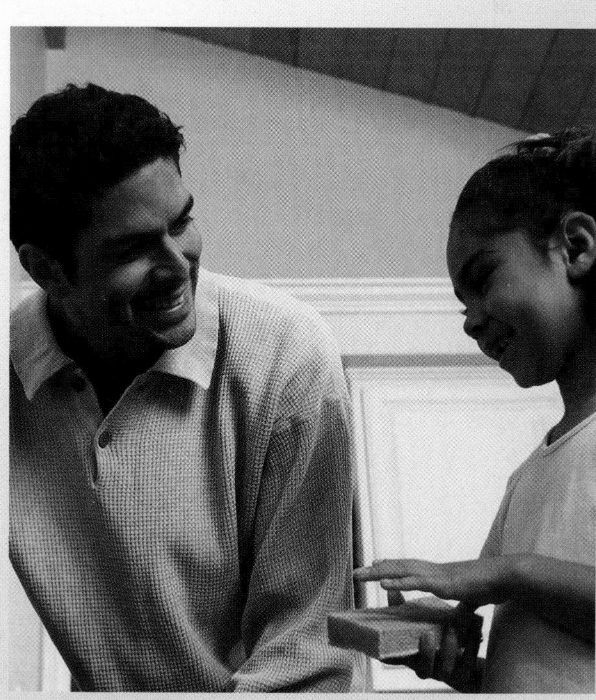

Chapter 7
Career Opportunities

Employment Agency Manager
Manages employment services and business operations of private employment agency.

Personnel Psychologist
Specializes in development and application of such techniques as job analysis and classification, personnel interviewing, ratings, and vocational tests for use in selection, placement, promotion, and training of workers.

Career Placement Services Counselor
Collects, organizes, and analyzes information about individuals through records, tests, interviews, and professional sources, to appraise their interests, aptitudes, abilities, and personality characteristics, for vocational and educational planning.

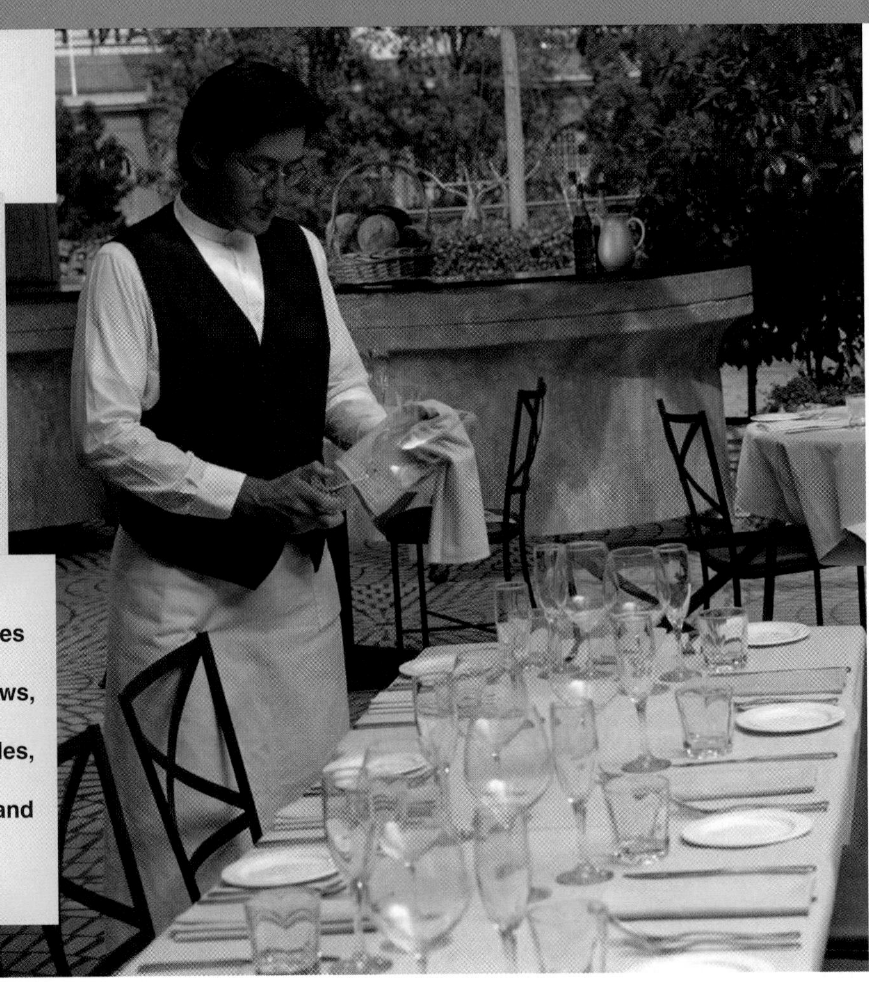

Terms to Know

goal
career ladder
catering
extension agent
dietitian
leader
reference
interview
entrepreneur

Objectives

After studying this chapter, you will be able to

- ❏ analyze your likes, dislikes, interests, and abilities as a preliminary step in choosing a career.
- ❏ describe three general career areas in the field of foods.
- ❏ list the qualifications needed to work in each career area.
- ❏ identify skills and qualities needed for career success.
- ❏ explain the steps involved in finding a job.
- ❏ outline advantages and disadvantages of entrepreneurship.

How will I know which career is right for me? Where will I find a job I will enjoy and that will provide adequate pay? What are my interests? What are my capabilities? Where can I find information to help me make career decisions? These questions are only a few of those you may ask yourself as you begin to plan for the future. Choosing a career is exciting, but it is not always easy.

Choosing a Career

Before choosing a career, you need to do some self-analysis. You can begin by thinking about your likes and dislikes, interests, and abilities.

Do you like working with people, or would you rather work on your own? Are you artistic? Do you like to write? Do you have a special interest, such as creative cooking, music, or sports? Are you a leader, or would you rather have others make the decisions? Do you want to stay in one place, or are you willing to travel? Do you want to continue your education, or are you ready to begin working right after graduation from high school?

Answering these and similar questions can help you find a career in which you can be happy and successful. Once you have a particular career in mind, find out as much as you can about that career.

You can obtain career information from many sources. Talk to your school counselor, teachers, and parents. Find people in your community involved in various careers and ask them questions. Research careers on the Internet. If you know the career of your choice requires further education, research colleges that have the curriculum you will need. Many high school libraries have college catalogs and career manuals.

Q: How can I find out what career areas go with my interests?

A: Your school guidance counselor can give you an interest inventory. This is a computer-scored survey that pinpoints your interests. The computer also matches your interests with those of people who work in various career areas. You can use this information as a guide when choosing which career areas to explore.

Preparing for a Career

Preparing for a career involves setting goals. ***Goals*** are aims you try to reach. They are the endpoints of your efforts. When you decide what career you would like to have 10 years from now, you are setting a career goal. Because this goal will take a number of years to achieve, it is a *long-term goal.* You can set short-term goals that will help you reach your long-term goal. *Short-term goals* can be achieved in a matter of weeks or months. Completing a high school class or getting a part-time job related to your career would be short-term goals.

The classes you take in high school can help you prepare for a career. If you think you would like a career in a particular field, try to take courses related to that field. For instance, some family and consumer sciences classes would help you prepare for a career in the food industry.

The groups you join in high school can also help prepare you for your future career. One organization you may want to think about joining is Family, Career and Community Leaders of America (FCCLA). FCCLA prepares young men and women for future roles at home and in the workplace. FCCLA chapters are often organized through family and consumer sciences classes. See 7-1.

Many careers require education beyond high school. The classes you take now can help prepare you for further education. English, math, communications, social studies, computer training, and science can prepare you for vocational school, community college, or a university.

Another way to prepare for a career is to work part-time while you are still in school. Working during summers and after school can give you valuable experience that can help you later.

Preparing for a career also involves learning about career ladders. A ***career ladder*** is a series of related jobs that form a career. Each job in a career ladder builds on the skills learned in the job below. A career ladder shows

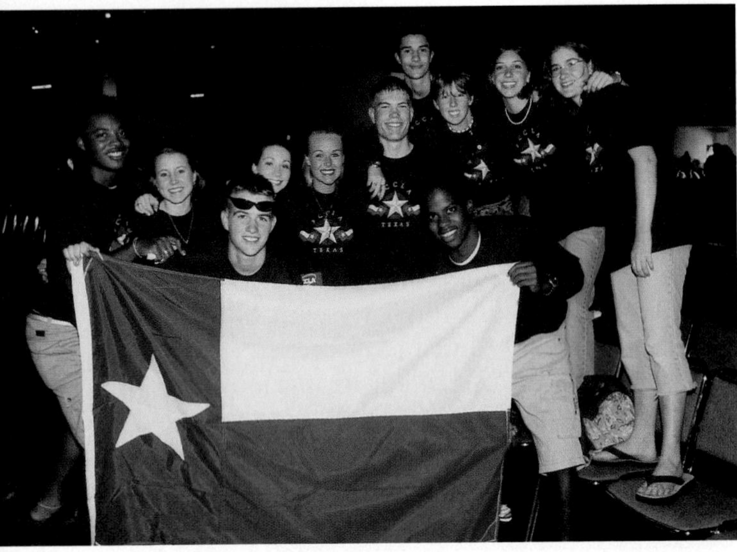

FCCLA

7-1 Through participation in FCCLA, young men and women develop skills they will need in their homes, workplaces, and communities.

you positions into which you can advance. It also gives you an idea of skills you need for advancement. For instance, a produce stocker at a grocery store is an entry-level job at the bottom of a career ladder. Someone in this position might climb the ladder to become the produce manager and then an assistant store manager. The top of this career ladder might be the store manager's job.

Choosing a Career in Foods

Do you think a career in the food industry might interest you? When choosing a career, you need to remember work is only one part of your life. Your personal time to be alone or with family and friends is also a part of your life. These two areas of your life can affect each other. If you enjoy your work, you are more likely to be content when you are not at work. Likewise, if you are happy in your home life, you are more likely to perform well on the job.

Some careers in the food industry can be very demanding. They involve long hours, often at night and on weekends. Some people find this schedule difficult to manage. It prevents them from spending time with family and friends.

Careers in the food industry can also be quite rewarding. They often offer chances for advancement into managerial positions. Many people find the opportunities in this industry well worth the challenges.

If you are thinking about a career in the food industry, find out what specific demands it entails. Also find out what rewards it may offer. Finally, think about how this career would affect your personal and family life. If the job still sounds appealing after you have completed your evaluation, then it may be right for you.

Food-related careers can be divided into three main groups

- the foodservice industry
- the food handling industry
- education and business

The Foodservice Industry

If you are ambitious, hardworking, and friendly, a career in the foodservice industry could be for you. Job forecasters predict job prospects in foodservice will remain bright. The industry will need many people to fill positions for chefs, cooks, and restaurant managers. As people continue to eat many meals away from home, the need for eating establishments and skilled staff will remain strong. See 7-2.

Types of Jobs in the Foodservice Industry

Jobs are available in four areas of foodservice. They are food preparation, customer service, sanitation, and management. Your education, goals, and abilities will help determine which of these areas might be right for you.

Food Preparation

Food preparation jobs are available in coffee shops, snack bars, fast-food chains, and restaurants. Private clubs, school cafeterias, hotels, hospitals, and other large institutions also hire people in this field. Entry-level positions require little, if any, experience.

Usually, you begin working as an assistant to an experienced employee. In small establishments, workers learn how to do many food preparation tasks. For instance, one day you might prepare soups. The next day you might prepare salads or sandwiches or help with breakfast orders. In large establishments, workers specialize in one area. For example, you might become the baker's assistant or the grill cook's assistant.

In many foodservice careers, you can work your way up the career ladder as you gain experience. After learning to be a salad maker, for instance, you might move up to the job of assistant cook. With added experience, you might later become a cook.

Customer Service

Customer service involves working with the people the food establishment serves—its customers. You might work as a waiter serving food to customers. You might work as a busperson setting and clearing the tables. As you gain experience, you could move up to the positions of host, head waiter, cashier, or manager.

Sanitation

Sanitation involves cleaning and maintenance. Jobs in this area of foodservice are for dishwashers, pan scrubbers, and custodians. Their duties are to be sure the kitchen, cooking equipment, serving utensils, and tableware remain safe and sanitary. They must pay special attention to cleanliness to protect the health and safety of both customers and staff. With experience, dishwashers and maintenance people can advance to supervisory positions.

Management

Management positions involve working with both employees and customers. Management positions include owner, manager, and executive chef. Some of these jobs require additional education. Workers may obtain other management positions through training programs, experience, and hard work.

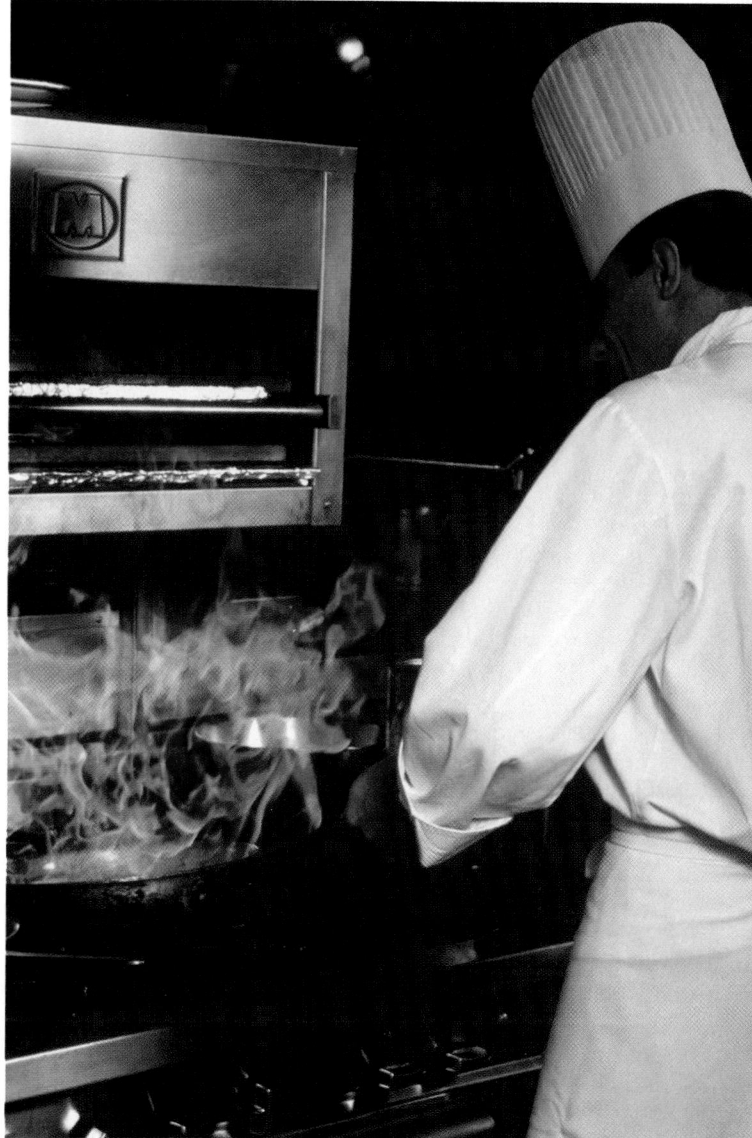

7-2 The growing foodservice industry needs a constant supply of skilled workers to serve the public.

Job Requirements for the Foodservice Industry

Some jobs in the foodservice industry are entry-level positions. Other jobs require special training. Employees can obtain this training in a number of ways.

Many high schools offer work-study programs. In these programs, you can gain on-the-job training while you finish school.

Vocational schools offer courses in food preparation and management. With a vocational school diploma, you may be able to begin your foodservice career at a higher level.

Many foodservice operations have management training programs. These programs vary. Not all of them require a college degree. However, most have specific requirements, which you must meet before being admitted into the program.

Community colleges and universities offer programs that can prepare you for management jobs. Many community colleges have two-year programs in quantity food preparation and hotel and restaurant management. At a university, you can obtain a bachelor's degree in these areas. See 7-3.

Catering

Once you have gained experience in foodservice, you might want to start your own foodservice business. One such business is

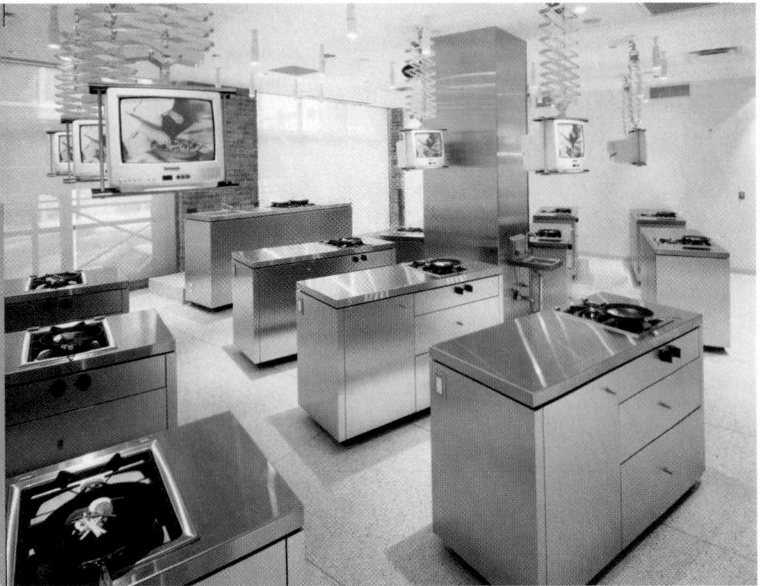

Calphalon

7-3 First-rate college and university programs offer facilities such as these to train future workers in the foodservice industry.

catering. ***Catering*** combines all four areas of foodservice.

Caterers prepare food for parties and other social functions. They plan small parties in private homes as well as banquets and receptions for large groups. Some caterers specialize in baking wedding cakes or preparing fancy hors d'oeuvres. Others prepare complete dinners and supply serving equipment and staff as well.

Caterers may operate out of their homes or from a separate business location. Some caterers work on a large scale and employ other trained people to help them. Other caterers work alone.

The Food Handling Industry

Food production is primarily the job of farmers. However, many people handle the food farmers produce before it reaches consumers.

After harvesting, most food products go to processing plants. Here, skilled workers perform many jobs. Sorting, washing, peeling, slicing, grinding, roasting, and packing are just a few of the many processes food products may undergo.

After processing, food products follow a transportation chain. This chain involves truck, air freight, and train personnel; food brokers; distributors; food wholesalers; and finally food retailers.

At the grocery store, stock personnel help price products and put them on the shelves. The dairy, produce, meat, and bakery managers supervise their particular departments. Meat cutters and butchers cut large wholesale cuts of meat into the smaller retail cuts you buy. Customer service personnel answer your questions, cash checks, and perform other service-related functions. Checkers scan the products you buy or enter product prices on a cash register. Baggers put your groceries into bags. They may also help take groceries to your car and keep shopping carts orderly. In addition, someone must take care of store advertising and displays. Stores also need several people to work in managerial positions. See 7-4.

Job Requirements for the Food Handling Industry

Many people in the food handling industry have entry-level jobs. Such jobs include workers in canning plants and checkers in food stores. In these positions, you would receive on-the-job training. As you become more experienced, your employer might promote you to a supervisory position.

Some workers, such as government inspectors and butchers, require special skills. Acquiring these skills may or may not involve vocational school training or a college degree.

Some managerial positions require a college education. You can achieve others through hard work and experience.

If a career in the food handling industry interests you, try working part-time as a supermarket checker or stock person. This experience could be helpful when you are ready to apply for a full-time job.

Food-Related Careers in Education and Business

Many food-related careers center on informing others about food. Such careers include teachers, extension agents, dietitians, consumer specialists, and researchers. Most of these careers require a bachelor's degree.

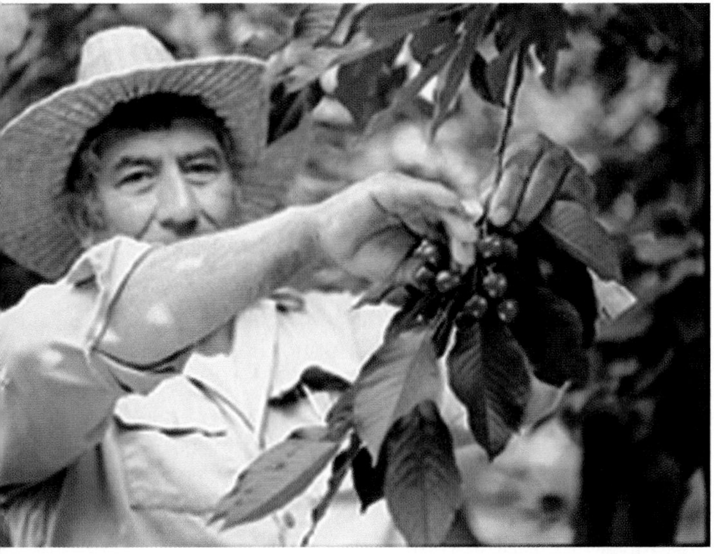

photo courtesy of Northwest Cherry Growers

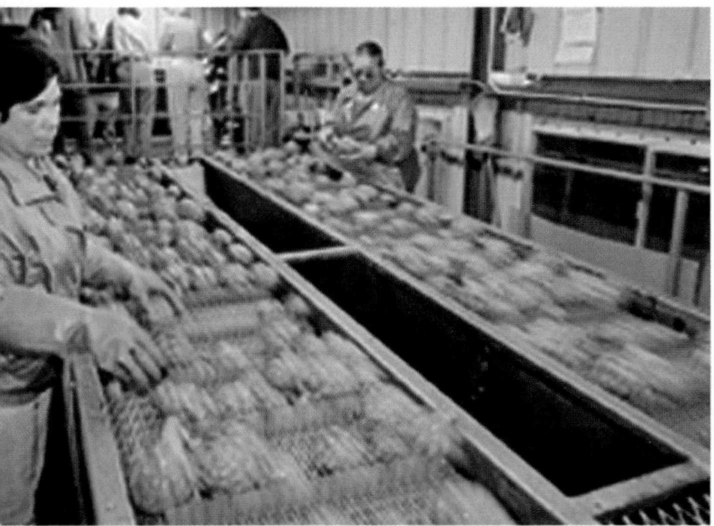

California Artichoke Advisory Board

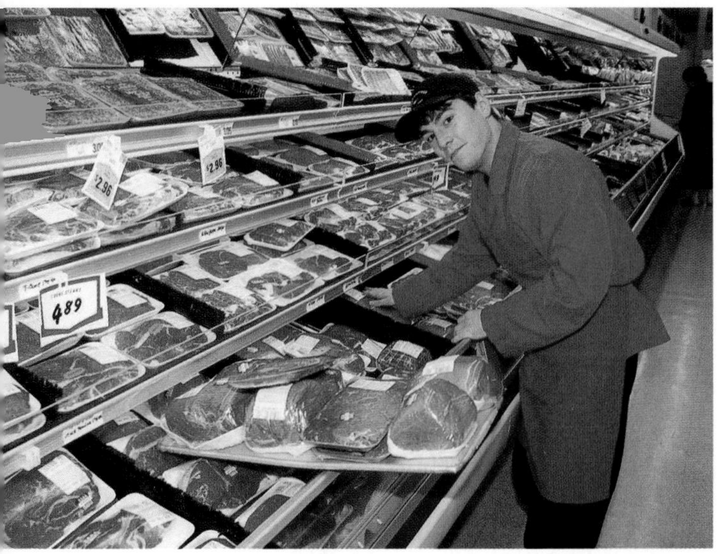

photo courtesy of IGA, INC.

***7-4** Careers in the food handling industry involve harvesting, processing, and selling food products.*

Some require advanced degrees and many years of experience.

Teaching

One career that involves teaching people about foods is family and consumer sciences teacher. These teachers work at all levels—elementary, junior high, high school, college, and adult education. These teachers know about all areas of family and consumer sciences. However, most choose to specialize in one area, such as foods and nutrition. Foods classes focus on nutrition, safety and sanitation, consumer skills, appliances, food preparation, and meal management.

Most schools require teachers to have a bachelor's degree in family and consumer sciences or a similar field. To teach at the college level, teachers generally need at least a master's degree. Many teachers expand their careers and become administrators. Others become consultants or authors of educational materials.

Extension Work

Each state in the United States has at least one *land-grant university*. The three-fold mission of these schools is to promote education, research, and outreach. The outreach part of this mission is handled by ***extension agents.*** This job title comes from the role these workers play in extending knowledge beyond the walls of the university. The extension program is a partnership between state land-grant universities and the Cooperative State Research, Education, and Extension Service (CSREES). CSREES is an agency of the USDA.

Extension agents work with families and youth. They might offer adult classes on such topics as nutrition and health. These specialists might also work with young people in 4-H clubs, 7-5. Some extension agents write educational resources for the people they serve. You may have seen food safety brochures written by a county extension agent.

To be an extension agent, you must have a bachelor's degree in family and consumer sciences. Some positions require a master's degree.

Dietetics and Nutrition

Dietitians are health care specialists who have training in nutrition and diet planning. Most

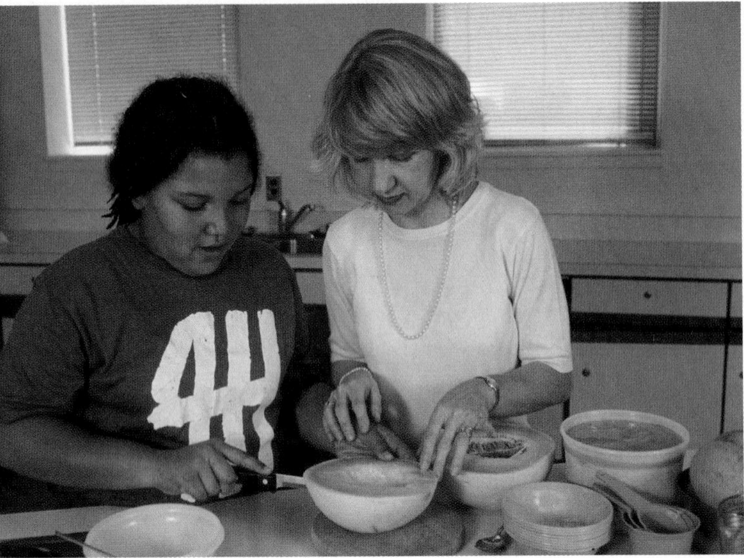

photo supplied by USDA

7-5 Under the guidance of extension agents, youth involved in 4-H learn important life skills.

dietitians become registered because the majority of job openings are for registered dietitians. A *registered dietitian (RD)* is trained to do diet analysis and treatment. Dietitians who are not registered often write and do research. Most dietitians focus their practices on a few specific areas. Such areas include cancer, weight control, vegetarian diets, and eating disorders. Dietitians work in different types of settings.

Nutritional Care

Dietitians in nutritional care work for hospitals, clinics, and nursing homes. These dietitians work with medical personnel to plan diets for patients with special needs. They also oversee the purchase and preparation of food to ensure meals are nutritious.

Administration

Some dietitians work as administrators in the foodservice industry. They plan meals and supervise and train personnel. They also oversee the buying and preparing of food and the purchase of equipment. Hospitals, schools, and other large institutions that serve food hire administrative dietitians.

Education

Dietitians in education may teach courses such as nutrition and diet therapy at the college level. Their students might be men and women studying to be doctors and nurses. Other dietitians lead clinics and workshops for people in the community. Through these programs, they help people form good food habits. Hospitals, medical schools, clinics, and public health agencies hire dietitians in education.

Dietetic Research

Dietitians involved in research study the links between good health and diet. They also help conduct nutritional studies. They may work for the government, private industry, hospitals, and medical schools, 7-6.

Job Requirements for Dietitians

You need a bachelor's degree in dietetics or foods and nutrition to become a dietitian. Also, you must complete an internship before you start working. Depending on your area of interest, you might intern in a hospital, school, or business.

To become an RD, you must graduate from a college or university program approved by the American Dietetic Association (ADA). After graduating, you must pass a national test. To maintain RD status, you must take part in continuing education activities all through your career.

Business

Food professionals in business work in a number of areas to identify food and eating trends. These professionals also make sure consumer needs are considered when food products and services are developed and sold.

Food professionals in business might work for food or appliance companies. Some work

Q: Why might I want to seek the services of a registered dietitian?

A: Diet and health, weight loss, and sports nutrition are among the topics for which you might seek a registered dietitian's advice. A dietitian has specialized training in the study of how your body uses food. He or she can provide you with information that most doctors, coaches, and other professionals are not trained to offer.

in test kitchens to test new food products or develop recipes. Others write ads, consumer brochures, and product directions. Some professionals in this field work for utility companies. They might go to stores and schools to teach about the use and care of cooking appliances. Others work for trade associations, such as the American Egg Board. Their jobs may involve explaining how to select and use specific products.

Many workers in this field focus on one area of business. Such areas include communications, consumer affairs, and research.

Communications

Food professionals in communications often work with the mass media. Some workers in this area are hired by television and radio stations. Others work for food companies and public relations and ad agencies. These workers might inform the public about new food products, food-related appliances, and consumer issues. Food editors and writers at newspapers and magazines work in this area. Food stylists who prepare food to be photographed are also part of this field.

Consumer Affairs

Food professionals in consumer affairs often work for private industries. Many food stores hire professionals in this area. These professionals act as links between the consumer and the store manager. They answer shopper's questions and help promote products and services.

Government agencies also hire food professionals in consumer affairs. For instance, the Federal Trade Commission employs these specialists. Some workers look into consumer complaints. Others carry out follow-up studies. Some write consumer brochures published by the government. Others work as lobbyists involved in passing laws that help consumers.

Research

Universities, the government, and private industries employ researchers, 7-7. Some food professionals in research conduct dietary studies. For instance, they might study the link between obesity and eating habits. Some food researchers work with engineers. They may help develop new equipment like microwave ovens. They also develop new foods, such as grains with higher levels of protein and fruits that ripen more slowly. Others test new products to see if they perform correctly and are suitable for consumer use. Still other researchers find new ways for consumers to use products like cake mixes.

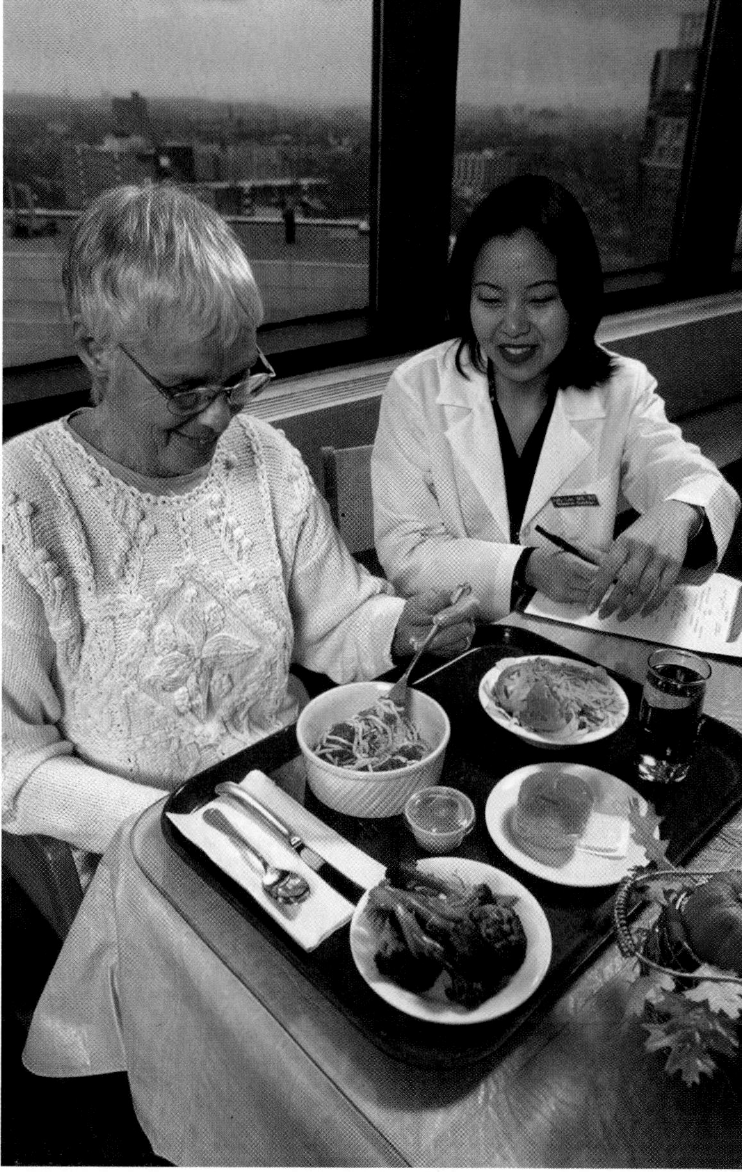

Agricultural Research Service, USDA

***7-6** Some dietitians in research work for the government to help conduct nutrition studies.*

Educational Requirements for Business Careers

To be a food professional in business, you need a bachelor's degree. A degree in family and consumer sciences provides a strong background for going into this field. Most people preparing for this line of work take courses that help them focus on a certain area. For instance, an emphasis on foods and nutrition would help someone who wants to work in a test kitchen.

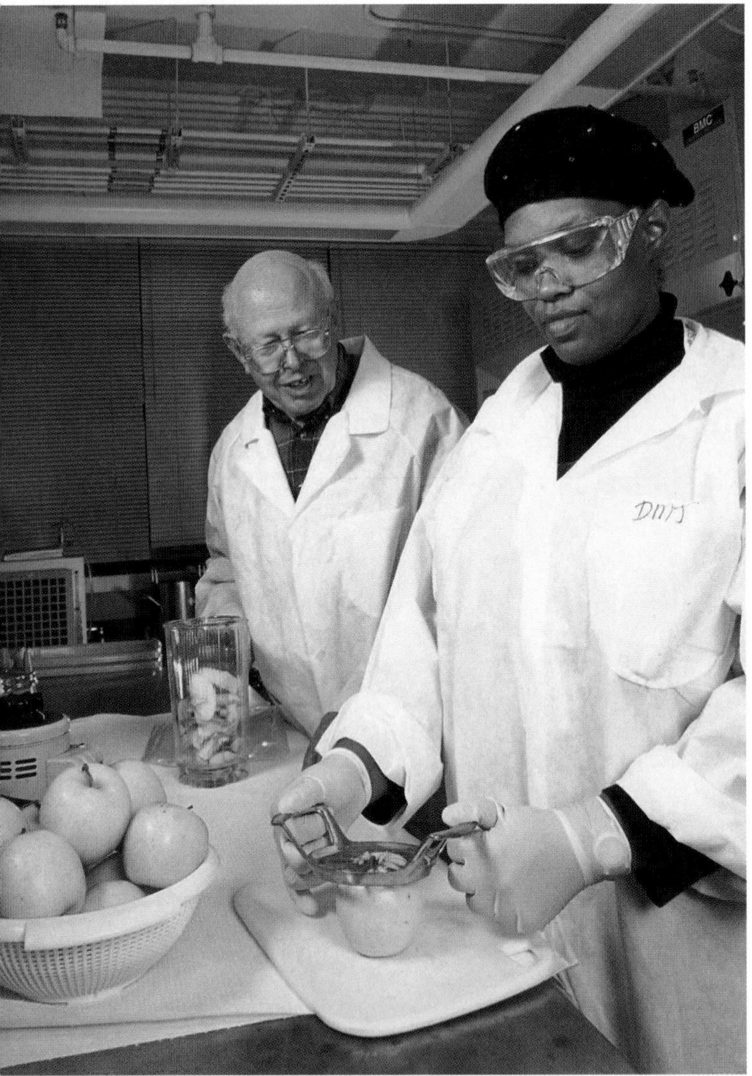

Agricultural Research Service, USDA

7-7 These researchers are gathering data about the microorganisms found on apples.

Extra classes in home equipment would be useful for someone planning to work for an appliance company. A background in journalism would be helpful for someone going into the communications area. Courses in business would aid a future specialist in consumer affairs.

Most researchers have advanced degrees. Some other workers also need advanced degrees.

Getting Ready for Success

To be successful in any job, you need a set of skills. Some of these skills are specific to your particular type of work. However, many skills are needed by all employees, regardless of the fields in which they are working. These skills include basic skills, thinking skills, and technology skills. See 7-8.

You also need certain personal qualities to succeed in the workplace. You need to be the kind of worker others respect. You need to keep developing your skills and improving yourself as a worker, too.

The following sections give many examples of how workers in various food-related jobs need certain skills and qualities. Remember that all workers need each of these skills and qualities to some degree. School classes, volunteer work, and part-time jobs all provide chances for you to develop these resources for job success.

Building Basic Skills

Basic skills are the first subjects you studied in school. They include the ability to do math. A registered dietitian might use math skills to compute a client's nutrient intake. A grocery store manager uses math when planning a budget. A restaurant cashier uses math when making change for customers.

Other basic skills are reading, writing, speaking, and listening. These are skills you need to communicate clearly. Through communication, you can share facts and ideas. Food careers might involve reading recipes, invoices, or research reports. They might require writing menus, sales reports, or consumer brochures. You will need to speak and listen when communicating with customers, coworkers, and employers.

Broadening Thinking Skills

Being able to use thinking skills is a requirement in the modern workplace. Thinking skills include thinking creatively, making decisions, and solving problems. They also involve seeing things in the mind's eye, knowing how to learn, and reasoning. A chef thinks creatively when he or she invents a new dish. A maintenance engineer in a food processing plant must make decisions to solve problems that arise when equipment stops working. A food stylist needs to be able to visualize a photograph before arranging the food and setting up the props. Knowing how to learn is important to dietetic technicians. They are required to complete continuing education activities to maintain their credentials. Food researchers need reasoning skills to interpret the results of studies.

One area where you will use thinking skills is in decisions about use of resources. Resources may include the use of time, money, materials, space, and staff. In any job, employees need to manage their time to complete tasks on schedule. An extension agent may have to manage money and materials to stay within a budget. A restaurant owner needs to manage space. Devoting more space to the kitchen means allowing less space for seating customers. The restaurant owner also needs to manage staff to keep a good balance between customers and waiters. Making careful decisions about the use of resources limits waste and results in the best work output possible.

Using information is another thinking skill. Related skills include acquiring and evaluating data. You will also need to interpret and communicate information based on this data. People in all areas of the food industry are expected to stay alert to important information and respond accordingly. A host in a busy restaurant has to assess where to seat people to keep service consistent. A food editor may have to interpret nutrition facts before writing about them in a newspaper report.

Acquiring Technology Skills

Another skill area you need to develop focuses on the use of technology, 7-9. In today's technological society, computers are

Skills for Job Success	
Skill Area	**Desired Skills**
Basic academics	Read with understanding Write using correct grammar and spelling and logical organization Solve math problems involving addition, subtraction, multiplication, division, fractions, and percents
Communication	Speak, write, and use graphic and electronic forms of communication to send clear messages Listen attentively and respond appropriately
Creative thinking	Propose a variety of solutions to problems Suggest unique ideas
Leadership	Set an example Take responsibility for actions Set and achieve goals
Organization	Make plans Keep resources in order Meet deadlines and complete tasks
Problem solving	Make decisions Resolve difficulties Answer questions
Teamwork	Share responsibilities Cooperate Work toward group goals
Technology	Use a computer Show willingness to learn to use equipment

7-8 Having a basic set of skills desired by employers can help every employee succeed on the job.

used in nearly every job. Therefore, using computers to process information is a critical skill. A related skill is the ability to organize and maintain files. A food wholesaler needs to keep files on the retailers with whom he or she does business.

Technology skills also involve selecting equipment and tools. You need to be able to apply technology to specific tasks and maintain and troubleshoot technologies, too. New knowledge is always being applied to every area of work. For example, people working in food preparation may have more efficient appliances to help them do their jobs. These workers must be familiar with when and how to run these appliances. They also need to know how to care for the appliances to keep them working. When the appliances break down, workers need to know what to do to solve the problem and get their job done.

Understanding systems is another technology skill. It involves understanding social, organizational, and technological systems. It also entails monitoring and correcting performance and designing or improving systems. A *system* is a set of two or more complex parts that interrelate. In the food handling industry, farmers, harvesters, truckers, processors, government inspectors, and distributors form a system. They all play a part in producing food and bringing it to consumers. It is important for each worker to understand the system and his or her part in it. Looking for ways to improve his or her contribution to the system is a duty of every worker.

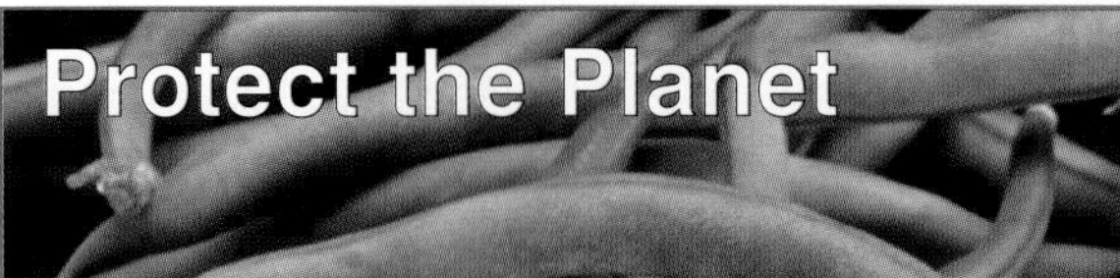

Regardless of what type of career you choose, take steps to care for the earth's environment in your work environment. Carpool to your job. Use a reusable lunch bag to carry your lunch to work. Keep a ceramic mug in your workplace so you will not have to use disposable cups. Recycle office paper and cardboard cartons and reuse manila envelopes. Small efforts made by you and your coworkers can make a big difference!

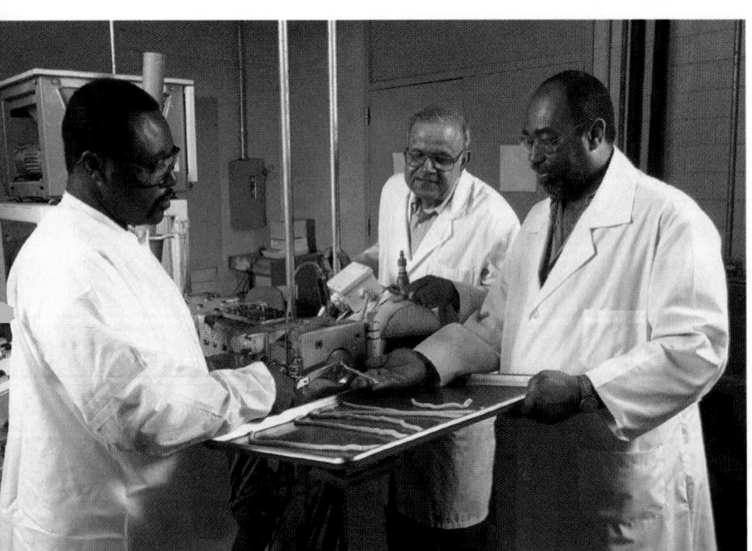

Agricultural Research Service, USDA

7-9 Being able to use computers and other technical equipment is an important skill in many food-related careers.

Developing Personal Qualities

Personal qualities will help you respect yourself and earn respect from others in your workplace. One of these qualities is individual responsibility. This means being ready to answer for your actions. You also need self-esteem to value yourself and your ability to do your job. You need sociability to be friendly and make an effort to get along with others. You should exhibit self-management. This quality allows you to get your job done without always having someone supervise you. In addition, you need integrity. This quality will help you behave in a manner that shows your understanding of and preference for right over wrong.

Personal qualities will help you work on teams, teach others, and serve customers. Members of a fast-food restaurant crew need to be able to work together to reach common goals. Family and consumer sciences teachers need to be able to teach others. Waiters and butchers must fulfill customers' requests.

Other personal qualities are the abilities to lead, negotiate, and work well with people from culturally diverse backgrounds. A bakery manager in a supermarket is just one example of a leader in the food industry. A ***leader*** is a person who has influence over others. A leader has to make decisions. He or she has to set goals and priorities, form plans, and assign work. These duties sometimes call for leaders to help settle differences when conflicts arise. Leaders, like all workers, need to respect the uniqueness of each culture represented in the workplace. This type of attitude will create a positive work atmosphere.

Practicing Workplace Ethics

A worker deserving of other people's respect is one who displays *professional ethics.* These are accepted standards about what is right and wrong in the workplace. Your ethics govern your behavior.

A key ethical practice is to treat other people as you want to be treated. For example, when your boss pressures you to complete a project, you may feel angry. Instead of arguing with your boss, however, you need to show regard for his or her authority. This is the type of treatment you would want to receive if you were the boss.

You should view your treatment of coworkers and customers in the same way. You need to treat coworkers with understanding because this is probably how you would like them to act toward you. You must be patient with customers because you would like to be treated patiently when you are a customer, 7-10.

Honesty is another part of workplace ethics. Being honest means not stealing from your employer. An employee who increases figures on an expense account to get more money than he or she deserves is stealing. An employee who takes home office supplies for personal use is stealing, too.

Another way some employees steal is by not giving an employer a full day's work. They may arrive late to work or go home early. They may take long coffee breaks and lunches. They may spend work time chatting with coworkers. These practices are unethical. They can jeopardize your job if they become habits.

Besides stealing, being honest means using sick leave only when you are sick. When you are not at your job, someone else may have to fill in for you. It is unfair to make your coworkers do extra work if you do not have a valid reason.

You need to discuss your work and offer opinions honestly, too. If you make a mistake, you need to admit it rather than trying to cover it up. If someone asks for your thoughts about an issue, you must express them truthfully. You should not say something you think others want to hear just to win favor with them.

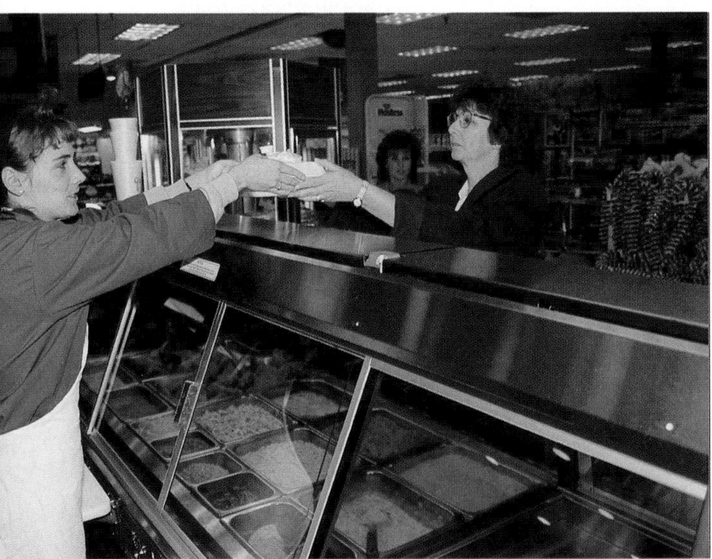

photo courtesy of IGA, INC.

7-10 Treating customers with courtesy and respect is a basic example of practicing professional ethics.

Learning About Professional Organizations

To succeed in your career, you will need to make ongoing efforts to better yourself as a worker. One way to do this is to join a professional organization. This is a group that promotes the field in which its members work.

One professional organization related to the food industry is the ADA. As mentioned earlier, this organization sets standards for registered dietitians. They give approval to college and university programs that meet their goals for training future dietitians. They give the test dietitians have to take to become registered. They sponsor events that help RDs keep up with the latest findings. They make sure RDs complete the required hours of continuing education to maintain their registered status. Through these efforts, they help ensure employers that RDs are experts in their field. A number of other professional organizations related to the food industry are described in Table 7-11.

Organizations use a number of activities and services to promote professions. They may fund research, offer scholarships, and support proposed laws. They may serve as information resources for the public. They may offer benefits like insurance and credit services to their members, too.

Organizations for Professionals in the Food Industry	
Organization	**Functions**
American Association of Family and Consumer Sciences (AAFCS)	Serves family and consumer sciences professionals. Works to improve the quality of individual and family life through education, research, cooperative programs, and public information.
American Dietetic Association (ADA)	Serves dietetic professionals, registered dietitians, and dietetic technicians. Seeks to shape the food choices and impact the nutritional status of the public.
Food Marketing Institute (FMI)	Serves grocery retailers and wholesalers. Conducts educational conferences, seminars, and research programs.
Institute of Food Technologists (IFT)	Serves technical personnel in food industries, production, product development, research, and product quality. Promotes application of science and engineering to the evaluation, production, processing, packaging, distribution, preparation, and utilization of foods.
National Restaurant Association (NRA)	Serves personnel in all areas of the foodservice industry. Supports foodservice education and research.

7-11 People working in every area of the food industry can join an organization to help them grow professionally.

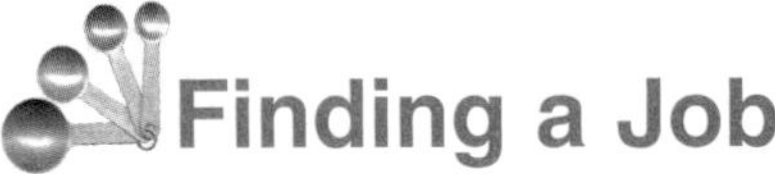

Finding a Job

If a career in the food industry interests you, you can start getting job experience now. Many entry-level jobs are available in restaurants, grocery stores, and other food-related businesses. Getting experience while you are still in high school will prepare you for higher-level positions in the future.

Look for Job Openings

How can you find job openings? The want ads in your local newspaper are a good place to start. Many businesses post signs in their windows when they want to hire someone. Family members, friends, and neighbors may know of businesses that are hiring. Your guidance counselor or school placement office is another source of job information. Many companies post openings for full-time positions on the Internet.

Be a Clever Consumer

One way you might learn about job openings is through an employment agency. Agencies charge a fee to match people with job openings. Sometimes the employer pays this fee. Sometimes the person looking for the job pays it. Carefully read employment agency contracts before signing them. Be sure you understand how much, if anything, you will have to pay.

Apply for a Position

When you hear of a job that interests you, you need to contact the employer to express your interest. Depending on the job, you may make this contact by letter, by telephone, or in person.

If the job is still available, the employer is likely to ask you to fill out an application form. Job applications commonly request certain types of information. If you are ready to relate this information, you will be able to fill out the form quickly and accurately.

You will need to know your Social Security number when filling out an application form. All workers need a Social Security number for tax and identification purposes. You will also need to write your name, address, and telephone number on an application form. You may need to specify the position for which you are applying. The form may ask you to state your expected wages and when you can start working. You will need to list the

Q: Who should I list as a reference on a job application?

A: Most employers do not to view a job applicant's relatives and close friends as suitable references. These people may give biased answers to questions about the applicant. Teachers, coaches, scout leaders, and former employers are better choices when listing references.

names and locations of the schools you have attended. You will have to provide information about any other jobs you have had. You may also have to give the names of references. ***References*** are people employers can call to ask about your capabilities as a worker.

Interview for the Position

If your application form impresses an employer, he or she may ask you to come in for an interview. An ***interview*** is a chance for an employer and a job applicant to discuss the applicant's qualifications.

To make a good impression at an interview, you should be well groomed and neatly dressed. You should speak in a clear voice and have a positive attitude. Be prepared to answer a variety of questions about your skills, interests, and work experiences. See 7-12.

If the interview goes well, the employer may decide to offer you a job. However, the employer is probably interviewing other applicants for the same job. It may take a week or more for the employer to make a hiring decision. You can ask the employer at the interview when you can expect to hear his or her decision.

Receive an Offer or a Rejection

When you receive an offer, let the employer know as soon as possible if you will accept the job. Ask when you should report to work. Find out any necessary information regarding items such as uniforms and training sessions.

If the employer does not offer you the job, ask yourself the following questions:

- Was my application form filled out neatly?
- Did I arrive for my interview on time and appropriately dressed?
- Did I display interest in the job and willingness to work?
- Did I appear friendly and cooperative?
- Did I answer all questions accurately?

If you answer yes to these questions, it may not be your fault that you did not get the job. Perhaps the employer merely felt another applicant was more qualified. Answering no to a question, however, may give you a clue about why you did not receive a job offer. This will help you improve for your next interview.

Changing Jobs

Most workers change jobs at some point during their careers. This may happen for a number of reasons. Some people want new challenges and opportunities that their current jobs do not offer them. Some employees become dissatisfied with the type of work they are doing. Others have disagreements with the people with whom they work. Some people change jobs because they want to move to a new location.

Whatever the reason, you need to take certain steps when you leave a position. Most employers request you give them at least two week's notice that you are resigning. This gives them a chance to begin looking for someone to

Common Interview Questions
In what position are you interested?
Would you be interested in any other positions?
What other jobs have you had?
How many hours a week can you work?
Are you involved in other activities that could cause time conflicts with your work schedule?
What kinds of classes do you take in school?
What class do you like best?
In what activities do you participate at school?
Would you have transportation to and from work?
How much do you expect to earn?
How well do you work with others?
Why should we hire you?

7-12 *Employers ask questions like these to help them evaluate the qualifications of a job applicant.*

replace you. For part-time and entry-level jobs, you can speak to your boss about when you will be leaving. For a professional position, however, you should write a letter of resignation.

You can decide whether you want to tell your supervisor why you are leaving. If you have been unhappy with your job, you may choose to keep your reasons to yourself. Creating hard feelings when you leave will not improve an unsatisfactory work experience. Remember that you may have to use your employer as a reference in the future. Therefore, you should try to leave a job on the best terms possible. Make a point of thanking your supervisor for the opportunities your job has given you.

Good Manners Are Good Business

Arriving late for an interview keeps a busy employer waiting. This is not only bad manners, it is likely to cost you a chance for the job. An employer may assume you will not arrive on time for work if you cannot arrive on time for an interview.

Try to arrive about 10 or 15 minutes before the scheduled time of your interview. This will show the prospective employer that you are punctual. It will also give you time to collect your thoughts before the interview begins.

Entrepreneurship

Some people do not want to work for an employer. They prefer to find opportunities, make decisions, and set schedules on their own. In other words, they prefer to be self-employed. These people are often called entrepreneurs. ***Entrepreneurs*** are people who set up and run businesses.

Many people in food-related businesses are entrepreneurs. Farmers are frequently self-employed, 7-13. Grocers, butchers, and bakers often own their stores. Many restaurateurs and caterers operate their own businesses. Dietitians may go into business as freelance consultants. Food stylists may work alone to set up contracts with clients.

Entrepreneurship holds great appeal for some people. Being their own bosses makes them feel independent. They achieve a sense of satisfaction from setting and reaching business goals.

Entrepreneurship involves risks as well as rewards. Starting a business takes money. The amount depends on the type of business. However, every business has some operating costs and requires the purchase of some equipment and supplies.

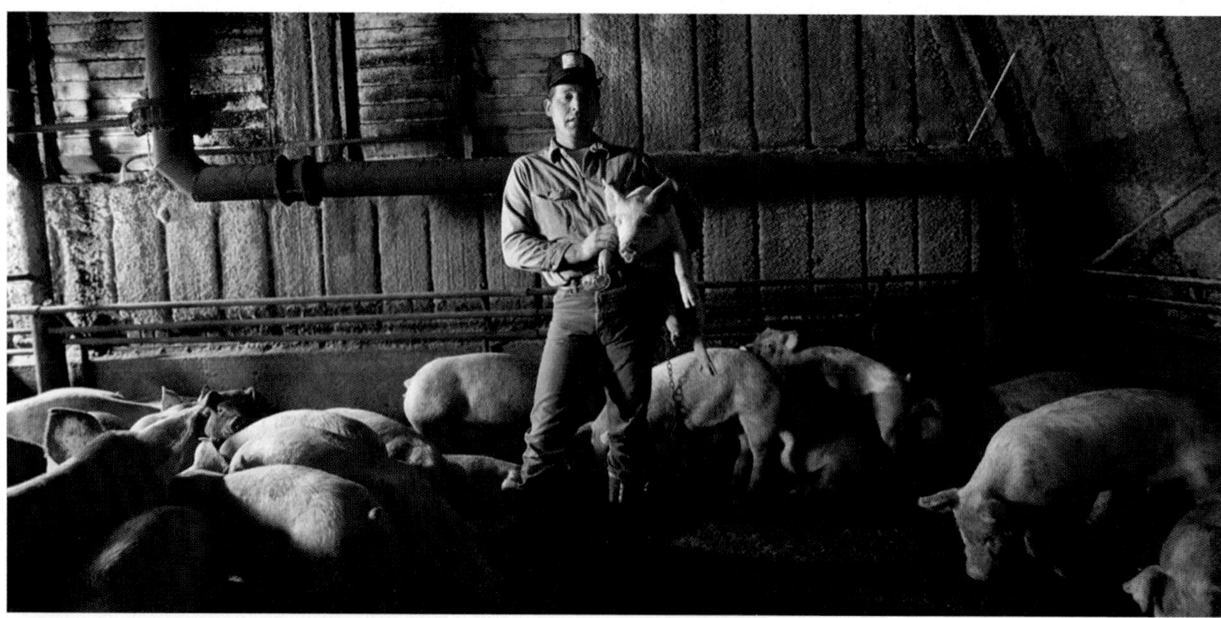

7-13 Many farmers are entrepreneurs.

Starting a business requires responsibility and organization. If a customer is unhappy, an entrepreneur must fix the problem. Entrepreneurs must keep orderly records of the money they take in and pay out. They must also keep track of meetings, customer orders, and employee files.

If entrepreneurship interests you, you should first consider several factors. Think about what kind of business you would like to start. Find out how much need there is for a business of this nature. Be sure it is something you can manage.

Consider working for someone else before starting a business of your own. This will give you work experience and show you some of the points involved in operating a business.

Once you have thought through your business plan, the sky is your limit. Teen entrepreneurs have started such food-related ventures as party planning, pizza delivering, and cookie baking, 7-14. If you are ambitious, you too can be successful in starting a business.

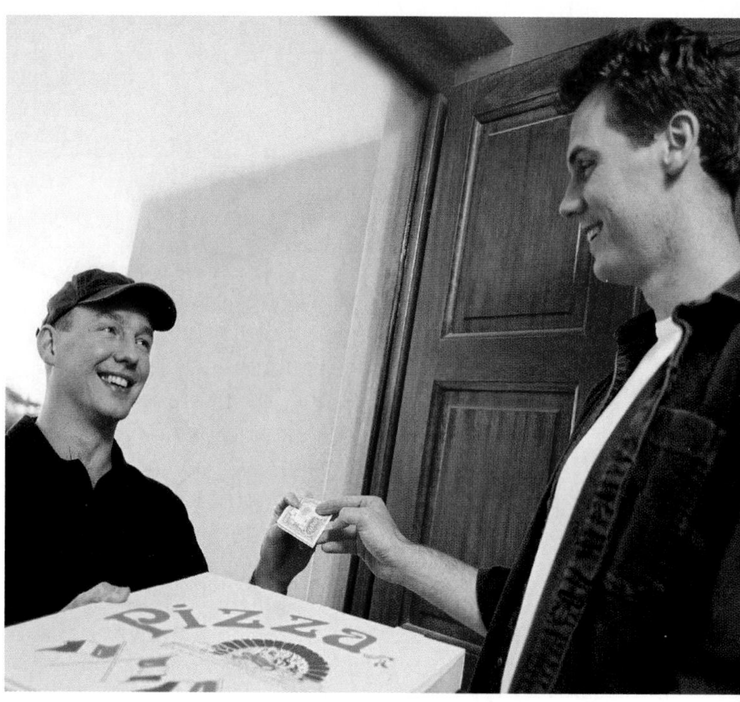

7-14 *One business venture a teen entrepreneur might consider is a pizza delivery service.*

Chapter 7 Review

Career Opportunities

Summary

Thinking about your interests and abilities can help you choose a career. Getting part-time job experience and taking related classes can help you begin preparing for a career.

Careers in the foodservice industry may involve preparing, serving, or cleaning up food. They may also involve managing other people. Many entry-level jobs are open to people with little or no training. Upper-level jobs may require training and/or experience. Catering involves a number of foodservice tasks. It may appeal to people interested in running their own businesses.

Food handling jobs involve growing, processing, transporting, and selling food. Positions in this field are open at a range of levels.

Most food-related careers in education and business require at least a four-year degree. These careers include teaching, extension work, and dietetics and nutrition. Business careers in areas such as communications, consumer affairs, and research may also appeal to people with background in foods and nutrition.

All food-related careers require some common skills. These include basic skills, thinking skills, and technology skills. Personal qualities will help you work with others. To succeed on the job, you also need to practice workplace ethics. Learning about professional organizations is another way to prepare for workplace success.

Finding a job begins with looking for job openings. When you find an opening that interests you, you must apply for it. The impression you make in an interview will help determine whether the employer offers you the job. When you plan to leave a job, be sure to give your employer adequate notice.

If you decide working for someone else is not for you, you may want to become an entrepreneur. Starting your own business can be risky. However, many people feel the rewards are worth it.

Review What You Have Read

Write your answers on a separate sheet of paper.

1. List five questions you should ask yourself before choosing a career.
2. List five sources of information on career planning.
3. Name the four types of jobs available in the foodservice industry. Give an example of each.
4. A career that combines all four areas of foodservice is _____.
5. After harvesting, foods must be processed, transported, and prepared for retail sale. Give an example of a job in each of these areas of the food handling industry.
6. True or false. A person must have a bachelor's degree to fill most family and consumer sciences teaching positions.
7. In what area of business might a food professional look into consumer complaints or work as a lobbyist?
8. Who might employ a food professional in research? Give two examples.
9. List five basic skills needed for success in any career.
10. A person who has influence over others is a(n) _____.
11. Give an example of professional ethics.
12. List three sources of information about job openings.
13. An opportunity for an employer and a job applicant to discuss the applicant's qualifications is called a(n) _____.
14. People who set up and run their own businesses are called _____.

Build Your Basic Skills

1. **Reading.** Check the job advertisements in your local newspaper. What types of job openings are available in the areas of foodservice, food handling, and business and education?
2. **Verbal.** Talk with your school's dietitian or cafeteria manager to learn about quantity food preparation, food purchasing, and foodservice management.
3. **Writing.** Write a one-page paper describing a food-related career that interests you. Explain what qualifications the position demands.

Build Your Thinking Skills

1. **Synthesize.** Form a research team with two of your classmates. As a team, pick a food-related career. Each team member should investigate a different aspect of the career, such as educational requirements, job responsibilities, and salary range. Synthesize information of all team members as you create a poster presentation about the career.
2. **Analyze.** Role-play interview situations between an employer and a job applicant for a foodservice position. Videotape the mock interviews. Play the tape and analyze the behavior of the applicant in order to offer constructive criticism.

Apply Technology

1. Use a computer and word processing software to prepare a professional looking resume.
2. Visit a job search Web site to search for jobs in your region in a food-related career. Note the qualifications employers are seeking for posted positions.

Using Workplace Skills

Sherry is a career placement services counselor at West Barton Community College. Each year she interviews over 100 students who are looking for jobs. She gives them interest surveys and aptitude tests. She also reviews the students' school and employment records. Then Sherry analyzes all this information to help students identify career opportunities for which they would be well suited.

To be an effective worker, Sherry needs skill in using computers to process information. Put yourself in Sherry's place and answer the following questions about your need for and use of this skill:

A. How would having skill in using computers make it easier for you to help each student?

B. How might your lack of skill in using computers to process information affect the students who come to see you?

C. How might West Barton Community College be affected if you cannot adequately use computers to process information?

D. What is another skill you would need in this job? Briefly explain why this skill would be important.

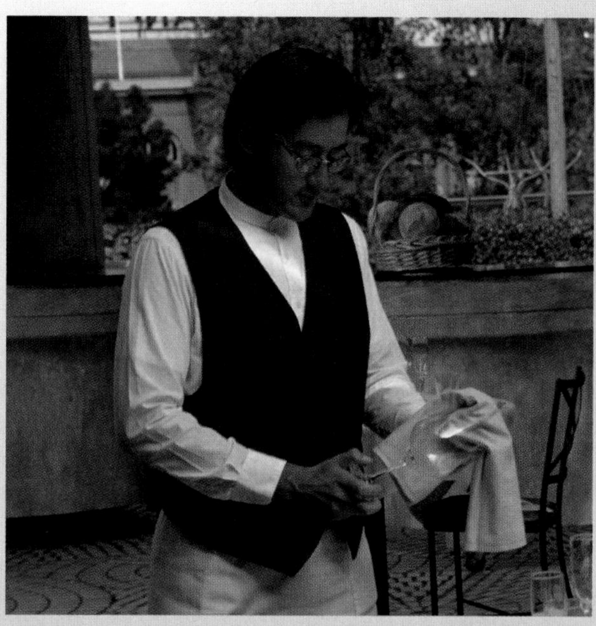

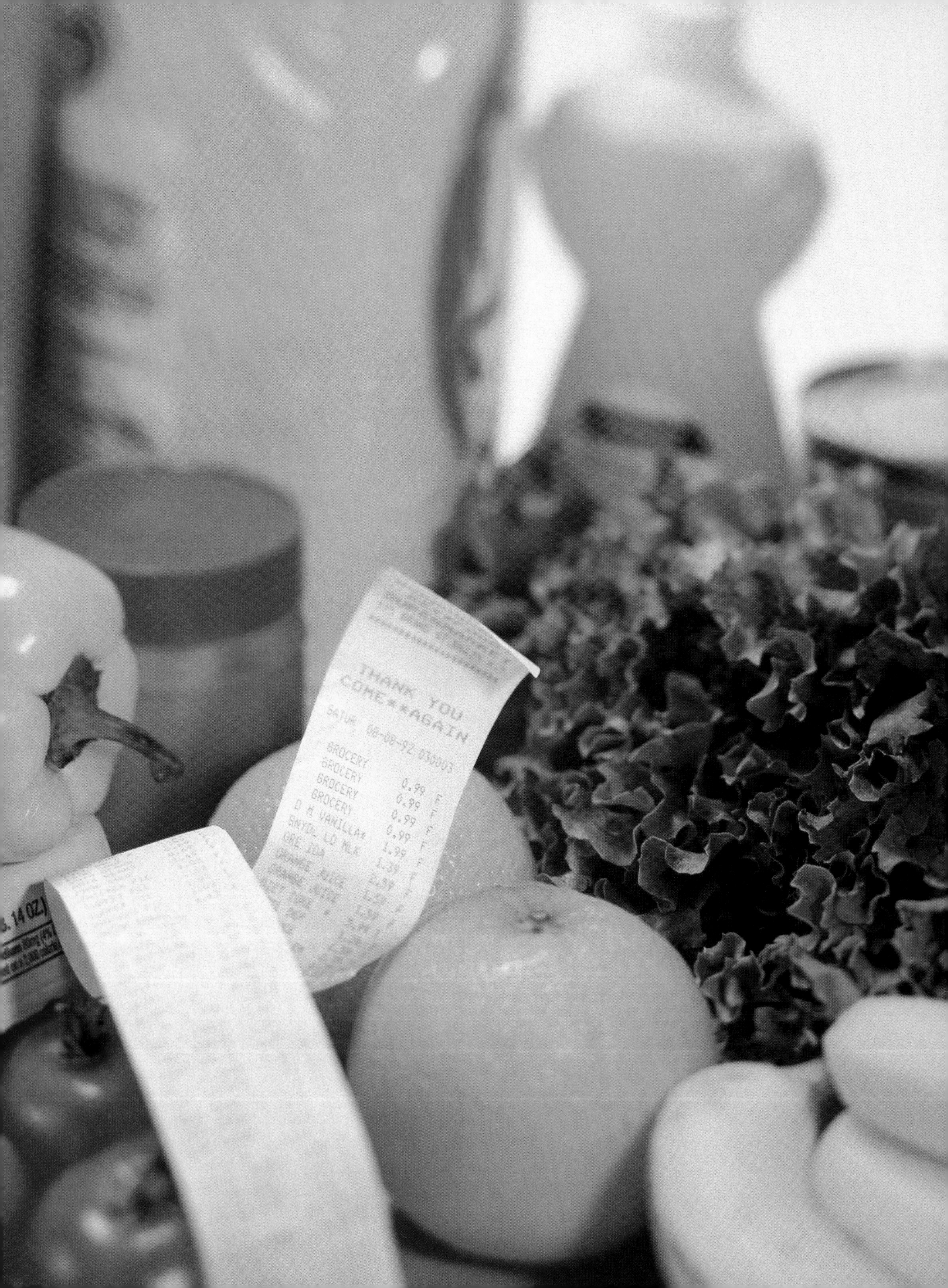
THANK YOU
COME**AGAIN
SATUR 08-08-92 030003
GROCERY
GROCERY
GROCERY
GROCERY
D M VANILLA*
14 OZ)

Part 2
The Management of Food

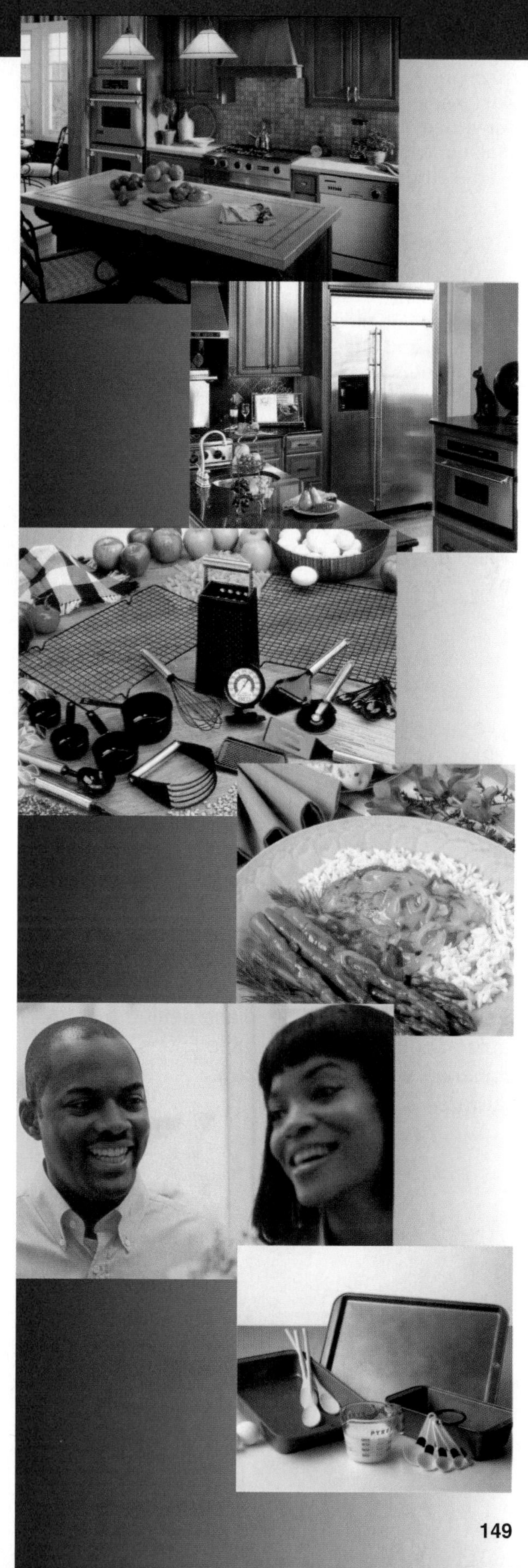

Chapter 8
Kitchen and Dining Areas

Interior Designer
Plans, designs, and furnishes interior environments of residential, commercial, and industrial buildings.

Cabinet and Trim Installer
Outlines installation areas and measures, cuts, and attaches cabinets and trim using hand tools and power tools.

Tableware Salesperson
Displays and sells china, glassware, silver flatware, and holloware.

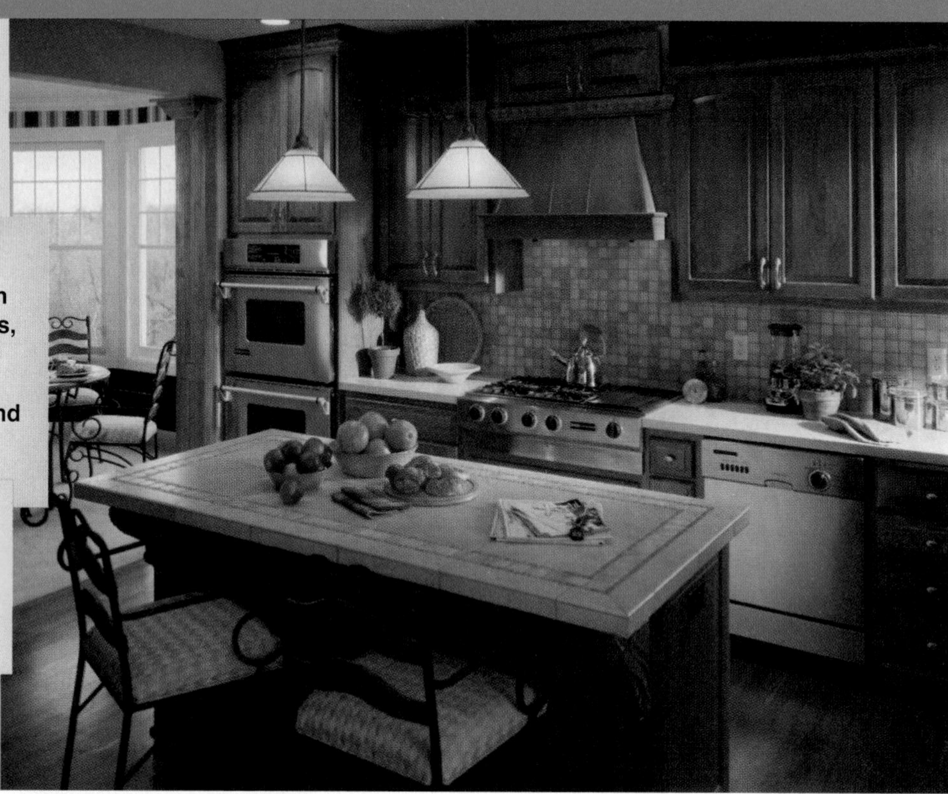

Maytag

Terms to Know

work center
work triangle
universal design
natural light
artificial light
ground
table appointments
dinnerware
flatware
beverageware
tumbler
stemware
holloware
open stock
place setting
table linens
cover

Objectives

After studying this chapter, you will be able to

- describe the three major work centers in a kitchen and the six basic kitchen floor plans.
- explain considerations in kitchen and dining area design.
- identify different kinds of tableware and list selection factors applicable to each.
- set a table attractively.

The kitchen and dining areas are often the busiest areas of the home. Family members spend a lot of time in these areas planning, preparing, and eating meals. Therefore, consider the likes, dislikes, and needs of all family members when designing these areas. Make them comfortable, convenient, and efficient places to work.

Planning the Kitchen and Dining Areas

When planning the design of the kitchen and dining areas, family members should discuss several questions. Do you want to eat your meals in the kitchen, or do you want a separate dining room? How much storage and work space do you need in these areas? How much time will each family member spend in the kitchen and dining areas? What kind of atmosphere do you want these areas to have?

Major Work Centers

Most kitchens have three main ***work centers.*** Each center focuses on one of the three basic groups of kitchen activities—food preparation and storage, cooking and serving, and cleanup.

The focal point of the *food preparation and storage center* is the refrigerator-freezer. This center requires cabinets for food storage. Cabinets also hold containers and tools used to store and serve frozen and refrigerated foods. Sometimes baked goods are mixed in this center. If so, storage space for mixing tools and workspace for mixing tasks will be needed here.

The *cooking and serving center* focuses on the range and oven. One side of the range should have at least 24 inches (60 cm) of counter space. This counter will hold the ingredients when you cook. Cabinets and drawers in this center store utensils, cookware, and serving pieces.

The *cleanup center* always contains the sink. It may also include a dishwasher and food waste disposer. Work done in this center includes dishwashing, cleaning vegetables and fruits, cleaning fresh fish, and soaking pots and pans. Plenty of counter space and storage space are necessities in this work center. Keep coffeepots, teapots, dishwashing detergent, dishcloths, towels, and a wastebasket here. You might also store canned goods and vegetables that require no refrigeration in this center. However, never store food under the sink. See 8-1.

Additional Work Centers

If a kitchen is large, it may include additional work centers. A counter between the range and refrigerator can serve as a *mixing center.* It needs to be at least 36 inches (90 cm) wide. An electric mixer, a blender, mixing bowls, measuring tools, and baking utensils need storage space. Baking ingredients, such as flour and sugar, need to be stored, too.

An *eating center* can have a variety of shapes. A separate table in the kitchen, a built-in breakfast nook, or a counter can serve as an eating area. When planning a counter eating area, provide 18 to 24 inches (45 to 60 cm) of space per person. The counter should be at least 15 inches (38 cm) deep. If the eating area is to be separate, plan to leave at least 30 inches (75 cm) clearance around the table. Add 6 inches (15 cm) more if you place the table in an area where people often walk past it.

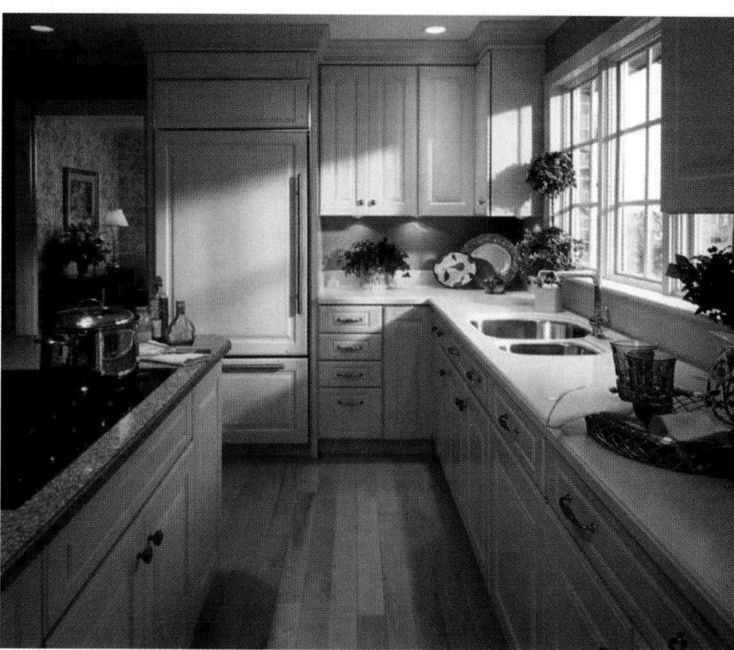

Photo courtesy of Decorà Cabinetry

8-1 *All phases of food preparation center around one of three major work centers in the kitchen.*

Consider tucking a *planning center* into a corner where it can double as a communications center. Use shelves to store cookbooks and phone books. A desk or countertop can hold a computer to be used for meal planning. You might keep a telephone in this area. Hang a bulletin board to post family messages. Keep recipe cards, note pads, and writing utensils in a drawer.

Some kitchens have a *laundry center*. A laundry facility within the kitchen can save steps. However, be sure to locate it away from food preparation areas.

Kitchen Storage Space

As mentioned, you need space in each kitchen work center to store various items. Two points will help you evaluate how much storage space you need and how best to use it. First, you will want to store items where you will be using them. Think about what tasks you are likely to do in each work center. Identify all the supplies you will need to do each task. For instance, you will chop vegetables in the food preparation and storage center. This task requires knives and a cutting board. Store these items in the drawers and cupboards of that center.

The second point to think about when planning your storage space is how often you will use items. Store items you will use often in the most convenient places. For instance, saucepans and a double boiler both belong in the cooking and serving center. You are likely to use the saucepans almost daily. However, you may use the double boiler only occasionally. Therefore, store the double boiler in the back of a cupboard. Store the saucepans in the front of the cupboard, which is easier to reach.

Work Triangle

To make a kitchen as efficient as possible, place the focal points of the major work centers at the corners of an imaginary triangle. This triangle is called a ***work triangle.***

Ideally, the work triangle follows the normal flow of food preparation. You remove food from the refrigerator or freezer and take it to the sink for cleaning. From the sink, you take the food to the oven or range for cooking. After cooking and eating, you return leftovers to the refrigerator.

Kitchen Floor Plans

Work centers fit into a variety of kitchen floor plans. The shape of the kitchen depends largely on the size of the room. See 8-2.

The *U-shaped kitchen* represents the most desirable kitchen floor plan because of its compact work triangle. All the appliances and cabinets are arranged in a continuous line along three adjoining walls.

The *L-shaped kitchen* is popular because it easily adapts to a variety of room arrangements. Appliances and cabinets form a continuous line along two adjoining walls. In a large room, you might use the open area beyond the work triangle as an eating area.

Appliances and cabinets in a *corridor kitchen* are arranged on two nonadjoining walls. This can be an efficient floor plan if the room is not too long and is closed at one end. However, a long room can create a long work triangle that requires many steps. A room that is open at both ends allows traffic through the kitchen, which can interfere with the work triangle.

The *peninsula kitchen* is most often found in large rooms. In this kitchen, a counter extends into the room, forming a peninsula. The peninsula can serve as storage space or an eating area. It can also hold a cooktop or other built-in appliance.

The *island kitchen* is also found in large rooms. In this kitchen, a counter stands alone in the center of the room. An island and a peninsula serve similar functions. In some kitchens, the island also serves as a mixing center.

The *one-wall kitchen* is found most often in apartments. All the appliances and cabinets are along one wall. This arrangement generally does not give adequate storage or counter

Q: Why is a compact work triangle desirable?

A: If the work triangle is large, you will use more energy as you move from one point to another to prepare foods. The total length of the three sides of the triangle should not exceed 21 feet (6.3 m).

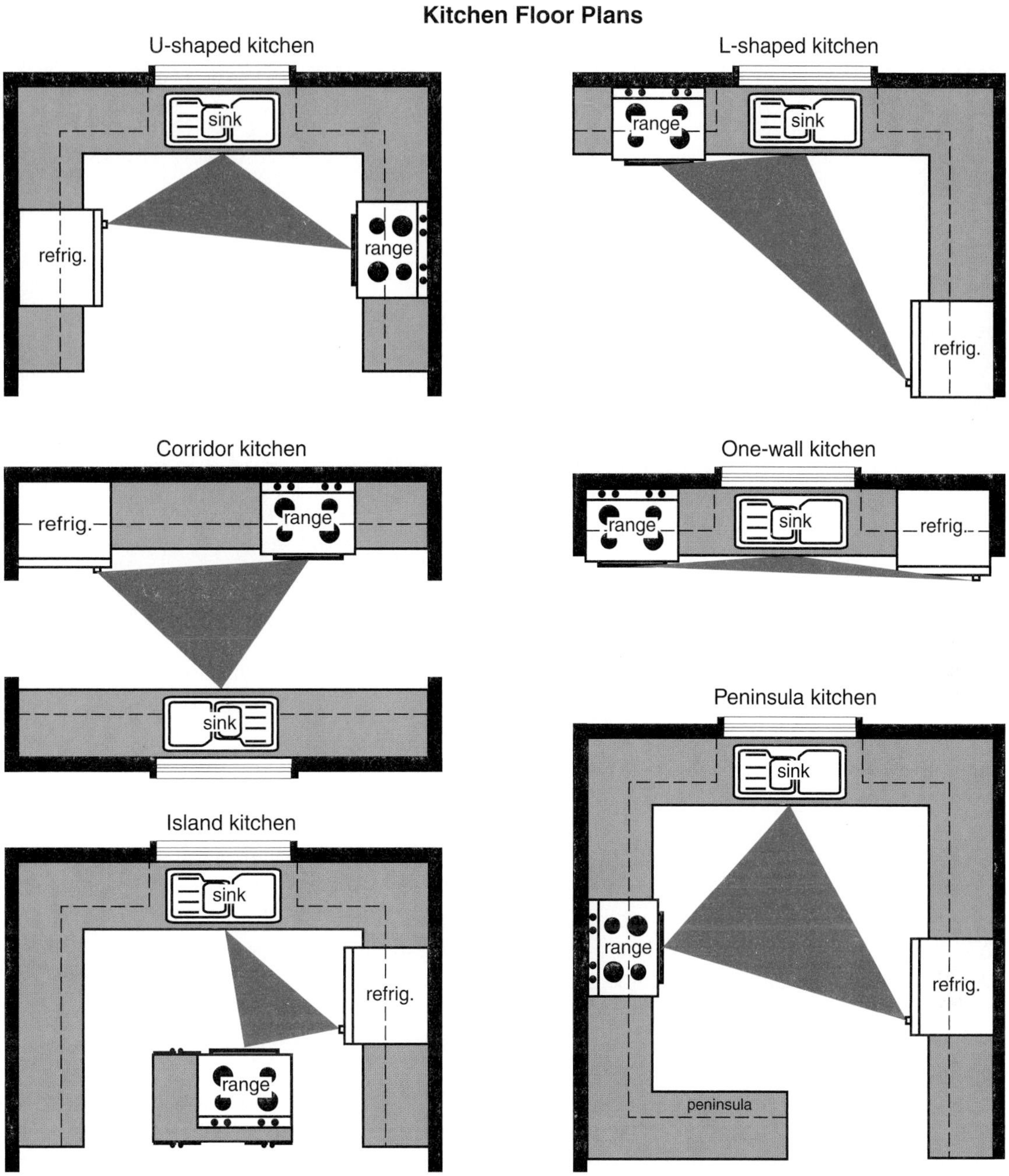

Kitchen Floor Plans

8-2 The size and shape of the work triangle depends on the kitchen floor plan.

space. It also creates a long, narrow work triangle. Often, a folding or sliding door sets off the one-wall kitchen from other rooms.

Meeting Design Needs of People with Physical Disabilities

A well-planned kitchen will help meet the special needs of people with physical disabilities. ***Universal design*** refers to features of rooms, furnishings, and equipment that are usable by as many people as possible. Peninsula, U-shaped, and L-shaped floor plans are examples of universal design. These floor plans provide the fewest restrictions to movement through a kitchen. A floor plan with a compact work triangle also reflects universal design. A compact work triangle prevents household members from using excess energy. This is especially important for people who have limited mobility, such as people who use walkers and crutches.

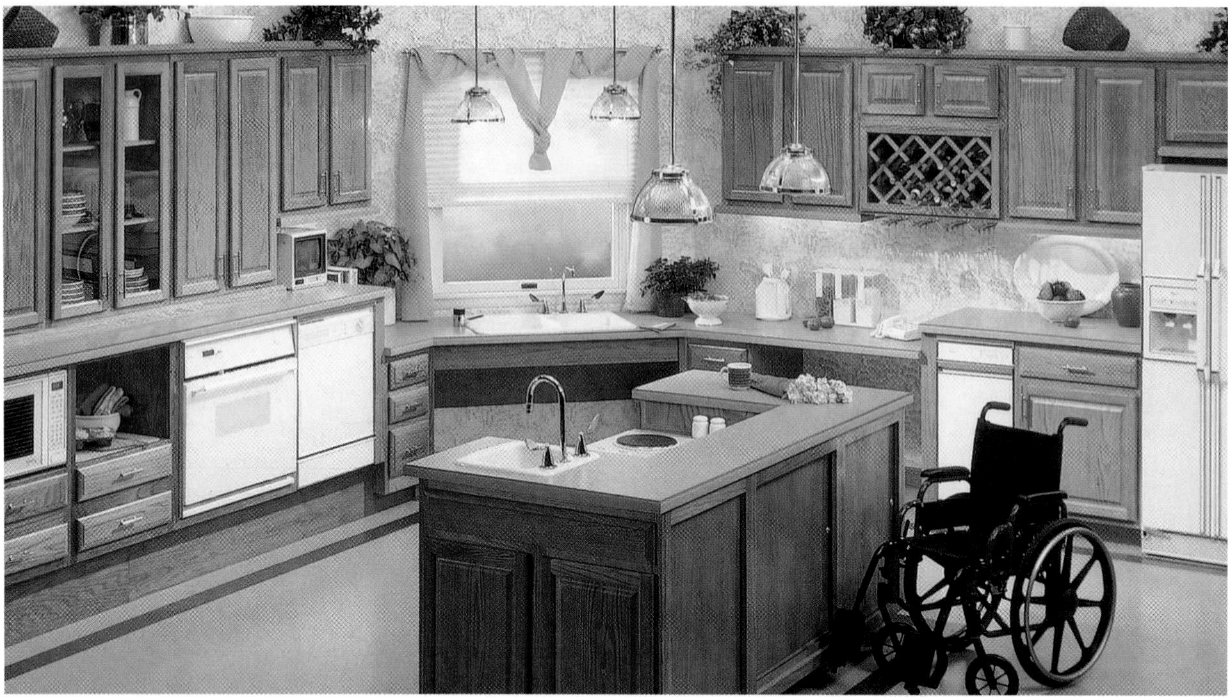

Whirlpool

8-3 The multilevel work surfaces and the contrasting trim on countertops in this kitchen are examples of universal design.

Work surfaces in a universal design kitchen need to be at a variety of levels. This allows family members of all heights to work in the kitchen comfortably. Lower countertops can be reached with ease by children and people seated in wheelchairs. A narrow shelf can be installed above these counters to provide a handy place for items that are used often.

Removing lower cabinets near the sink and cooktop will provide knee space. This will allow someone sitting in a wheelchair or on a stool to move close to these work areas. A shallow sink with a rear drain also allows room for knees. Undercoating the sink and insulating the hot water pipes will protect the legs of people working in a seated position. Mounting a lever-type faucet on the side of the sink will make it easy to reach.

Contrasting trim along counters and around doorways is a universal design feature. Contrasting trim makes edges easier to see. Therefore, people will be less likely to bump into them. This feature is especially helpful for people with limited vision. See 8-3.

Universal design can even be used in kitchen storage spaces. Loop handles on drawers and cabinets are easier to pull open. Adjustable pantry shelves can be placed at heights that allow all family members to reach needed items. Pull-out shelves reduce the need to bend and reach for items stored in the back of lower cabinets. Universal design allows all areas of the kitchen to better meet the needs of each family member.

Planning the Dining Area

The location of the dining area depends on the layout of the home, the size of the family, and the preferences of family members. A kitchen eating area saves steps when serving and clearing meals. However, it may create traffic problems if the kitchen is small. It also lacks the formal atmosphere that may be desired when entertaining guests.

Some homes have space for a separate dining room. A separate dining room offers a more formal setting. It also provides storage for tableware and linens. However, a separate dining room may require extra steps to serve and clear meals.

A dining area attached to the living room provides the attractive decor of a dining room without the space requirements. You may use decorative screens to divide the dining area from the rest of the living room. When entertaining larger groups, you can take the screens down and set up additional tables in the living room.

Patios, porches, and decks may be used as eating areas when weather permits. Meals may also be eaten in the family room, living room, or den. In many homes, these areas are located near the kitchen. If they are not, trays and carts with wheels can help make transporting food and other items easier. Lap trays, tray tables, and card tables can be used to provide impromptu eating space.

Kitchen and Dining Area Design

Kitchen decoration often complements the other rooms in a home. Dining areas are designed to create a comfortable atmosphere for family members and guests. Wall coverings, flooring, counters, cabinets, and lighting are all chosen to create a desired effect.

Wall Coverings

Kitchen wall coverings should be smooth and easy to clean. Wall coverings in the dining area should enhance the mood you are trying to create. Many wall covering materials are available.

Flat finish *paints* are suitable for dining rooms, but eggshell and semigloss finishes are better choices for kitchens. *Ceramic* and *metal tile* are used primarily in kitchens. *Wallpaper* and *vinyl wall coverings* can add to the cheer of a kitchen or the elegance of a dining room, 8-4. *Paneling* can be used to cover rough, unattractive walls in kitchen and dining areas.

Choose wall coverings in colors and patterns to go with your decorating scheme. Consider the cost and care requirements. Also, evaluate how durable the coverings will be when exposed to heat, moisture, and grease from cooking.

Floor Coverings

Like wall coverings, kitchen and dining area floor coverings must be easy to clean.

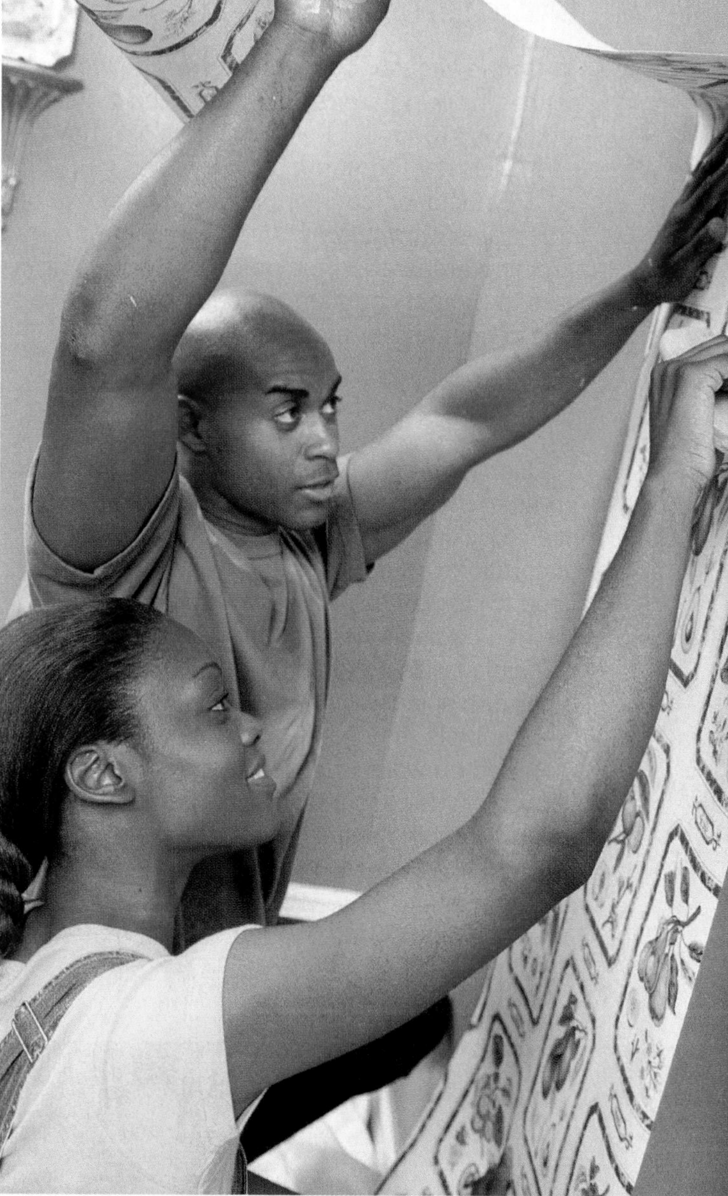

8-4 Wallpaper comes in hundreds of patterns suitable for kitchens. Choose washable wallpaper for easier cleaning.

Floor coverings should also provide walking comfort and be durable. You can choose from several materials.

Vinyl sheets or *tiles* are popular in kitchens. Carpeting especially designed for use in the kitchen is available in many patterns and colors. For dining areas, stain-resistant carpeting is a good choice. *Area rugs* can add to the elegance of a formal dining room. However, avoid rugs in the kitchen, where the danger of tripping causes them to be a safety hazard. Natural wood flooring provides a beautiful and durable alternative to floor coverings.

Countertops

In the kitchen, countertops provide workspace. In dining areas, counter space is used for serving food and holding dishes that have been cleared from the table.

Most kitchen countertops are made of *laminated plastic* or *ceramic tiles*. Counter surfaces in dining areas are often made of *wood*. Use care to protect counter surfaces from damage due to heat and/or moisture.

Cabinets

Cabinets are needed in kitchen and dining areas to store food, appliances, cleaning supplies, cooking utensils, dinnerware, and table decorations. In dining areas, cabinets may be used to display china, crystal, and other items. Kitchen cabinets need to be easy to clean. Cabinets in dining areas should complement other furnishings.

Cabinets may support countertops or be mounted on walls or suspended from ceilings above countertops and appliances. Tall, freestanding cabinets and specialty cabinets, such as corner cabinets with lazy Susans, are also common in kitchens. *Wood, wood veneer,* and *plastic laminates* are popular cabinet materials. See 8-5.

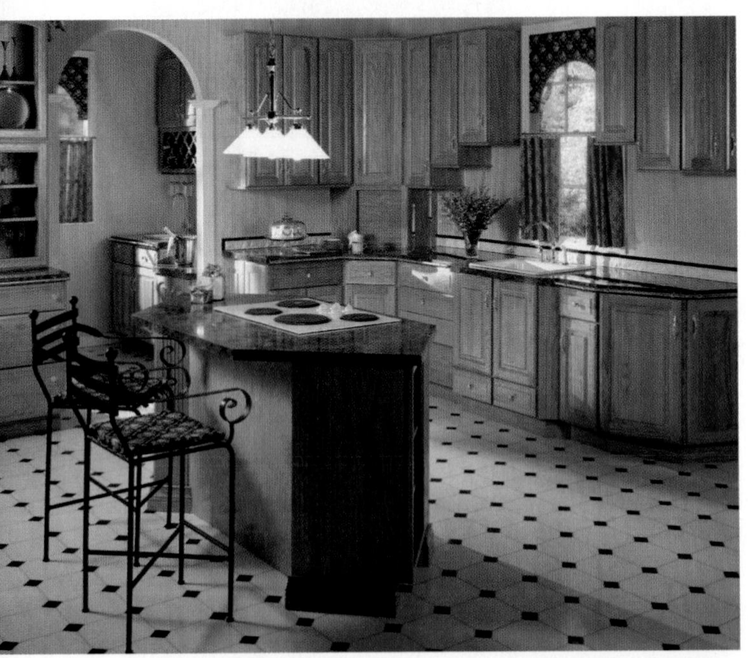

Photo courtesy of Schrock Cabinetry

8-5 *Wood cabinetry creates a warm, inviting atmosphere in a kitchen.*

Lighting

In the kitchen, you need adequate lighting to prevent eyestrain and accidents while performing food preparation tasks. In the dining room, you might use dimmer lighting to create a cozy atmosphere. However, lighting must be sufficient to allow diners to see what they are eating.

Lighting can be classified as natural or artificial. ***Natural light*** comes from the sun. The amount of natural light available during daylight hours depends on the size and placement of windows, doors, and skylights. If natural light is not adequate for performing kitchen and dining tasks, it must be supplemented with artificial light.

Artificial light most often comes from electrical fixtures. Ceiling fixtures provide general lighting for a room. Additional light fixtures are often installed over the range and under cabinets to provide *task lighting* in the kitchen. Accent lamps may be used to achieve softer lighting in dining areas.

Ventilation

You need ventilation in the kitchen to remove steam, heat, and cooking odors. Proper ventilation also helps maintain a comfortable dining atmosphere.

If natural ventilation is not adequate, a fan is necessary. In the kitchen, you can put an exhaust fan in a hood over a cooking surface. You can also install a fan in the ceiling or wall over the range. In the dining area, you might install a ceiling fan to circulate air. Some ceiling fans are combined with light fixtures to provide lighting as well as ventilation.

Electrical Wiring

Kitchens need a large supply of electricity to safely operate food preparation and cleanup appliances. In dining areas, electricity is needed primarily for lighting. You also need electricity to operate serving appliances, such as coffeemakers and warming trays.

When wiring is inadequate, circuits often become overloaded. Be aware of the warning signs of overloaded circuits. Circuit breakers may trip or fuses may blow frequently. Motor-driven appliances, such as mixers, may slow down during operation. Lights may dim when an appliance is being used. Appliances that heat, such as electric skillets, may take a long time to become hot. If any of these signals occurs, call a qualified electrician to check the wiring in your home.

For safety, appliances should be grounded. To ***ground*** an appliance means to connect it electrically with the earth. If a grounded appliance has a damaged wire, the electric current will flow to the earth instead of through your body. Thus you will not receive a severe or fatal shock.

Protect the Planet

Try using compact fluorescent lightbulbs in kitchen and dining areas. They use less energy and last much longer than standard incandescent bulbs.

The National Electrical Code requires all new homes to have Ground Fault Circuit Interrupters (GFCI) as part of the kitchen wiring system. If the outlets in your home have three holes, an equipment grounding wire has been installed. Many appliances have three-pronged plugs that fit into the three holes, thereby grounding the appliances. See 8-6.

ComEd

8-6 *Electrical outlets with three holes indicate that an equipment grounding wire has been installed in the home. The two buttons in the center of this outlet indicate this is a GFCI.*

If the outlets in your home have just two holes, you will need two-pronged adapters for your grounded appliances. Plug an adapter into an outlet. Insert the appliance plug into the other end of the adapter. The adapter has a small wire called a pigtail attached to it. Attaching the *pigtail* to the screw on the electrical outlet plate grounds the appliance.

Low-Cost Redecorating

Most kitchens and dining rooms do not require major remodeling to be efficient and attractive. In many cases, a little redecorating is all you need to update the look of these rooms.

Before beginning any redecorating, analyze the room to decide what you want to improve. Then establish a budget you feel will allow you to affordably reach your goals.

A fresh coat of paint or some new wallpaper can perk up the dullest kitchen or dining area. Painting or refinishing the doors and adding new hardware can do wonders to improve the look of worn cabinets. You may be able to refinish a marred counter surface or replace a stained section.

If storage space is a problem, try hanging inexpensive shelves. Put a freestanding storage cabinet in an unused corner. Use pegboard to hang pots, pans, and other utensils.

Using Design and Decorating Software

You may want to turn to a computer for help when arranging your kitchen and dining areas. A number of software programs are available to assist with design plans and decorating decisions. Interior design software allows you to draw floor plans and place furniture and appliances. Some programs have a three-dimensional format. This feature lets you feel as though you are walking through rooms. It gives you a more realistic perspective than the overhead view provided by a standard floor plan.

Using a computer to design your kitchen and dining area can save time, money, and energy. You can cut shopping time because you will already have in mind what you want. You can avoid the expense of buying items that end up not working in your setting. You can spare yourself the effort of moving furniture and appliances until you are sure you will like the arrangement. Everyone in your family can see how their needs for a comfortable, attractive, functional space will be met.

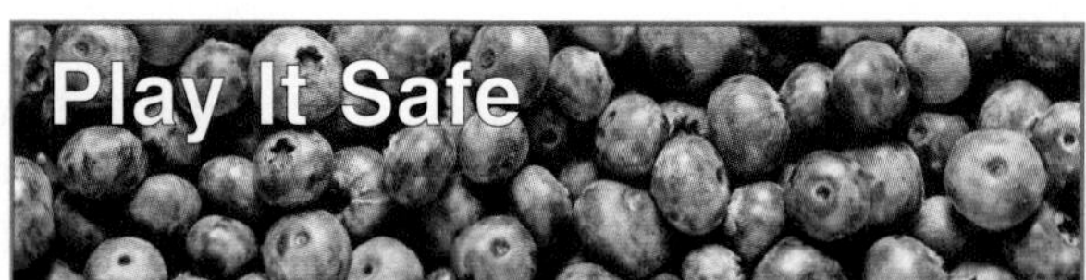

Extension cords can increase your flexibility when you have a limited number of electrical outlets. However, ordinary extension cords are not suitable for use with many appliances. They become too hot and can be fire hazards. Use a heavy-duty extension cord designed for appliance use. A heavy-duty cord uses a heavier wire than a normal cord, and thus can carry a heavier electrical load.

Table Appointments

In the dining area, the table becomes the main focus. You can choose table appointments to make the table an attractive setting for food. ***Table appointments*** are all the items needed at the table to serve and eat a meal. They include dinnerware, flatware, beverageware, holloware, linens, and centerpieces, 8-7.

Dinnerware

Dinnerware includes plates, cups, saucers, and bowls. Many qualities, colors, and patterns are available. The material used to make dinnerware helps determine its durability and cost.

China is the most expensive type of dinnerware, but it is elegant and durable. *Stoneware* is heavier and more casual than china, but it is less expensive. Like stoneware, *earthenware* is moderately priced. However, it is less durable than stoneware. *Pottery* is the least expensive type of ceramic dinnerware. It is thick and heavy, and it tends to chip and break easily. *Glass-ceramic* is strong and durable. *Plastic* is lightweight, break resistant, and colorful, although it may stain and scratch over time. It is most suitable for very casual meals.

Flatware

Flatware, often called "silverware," includes knives, forks, and spoons. It also includes serving utensils (such as serving spoons) and specialty utensils (such as seafood forks). Most flatware is made of sterling silver, silver plate, or stainless steel. As with dinnerware, the material helps determine appearance and cost.

Sterling silver and silver plate require polishing to remove tarnish caused by exposure to air and certain foods. Stainless steel does not tarnish, but like silver, it can be affected by eggs, vinegar, salt, tea, and coffee. To prevent staining, avoid prolonged contact with these foods and carefully rinse flatware as soon as possible.

When selecting flatware, consider the general shape of each piece, its weight, and the way it feels in your hand. A well-designed piece should feel sturdy and well balanced. Look at the finish. All edges should be smooth. Silver plate should be evenly plated.

Q: Where can I find low-cost ideas for redecorating my kitchen?

A: Magazines and home improvement centers can offer many low-cost tips for sprucing up a kitchen. Friends and family members can also be good sources of creative ideas.

Beverageware

Beverageware, which is often called glassware, includes glasses of many shapes and sizes, 8-8. Beverageware can be made of lead glass, lime glass, or plastic. The two basic shapes of beverageware are tumblers and stemware. ***Tumblers*** do not have stems. Juice, highball, and cooler are common tumbler sizes. ***Stemware*** has three parts—a bowl, a stem, and a foot. Water goblets, wine glasses, and champagne glasses are popular stemware pieces.

When choosing beverageware think about how it will look with your dinnerware and flatware. Look to see that the joints between the different parts of stemware are invisible. Examine the

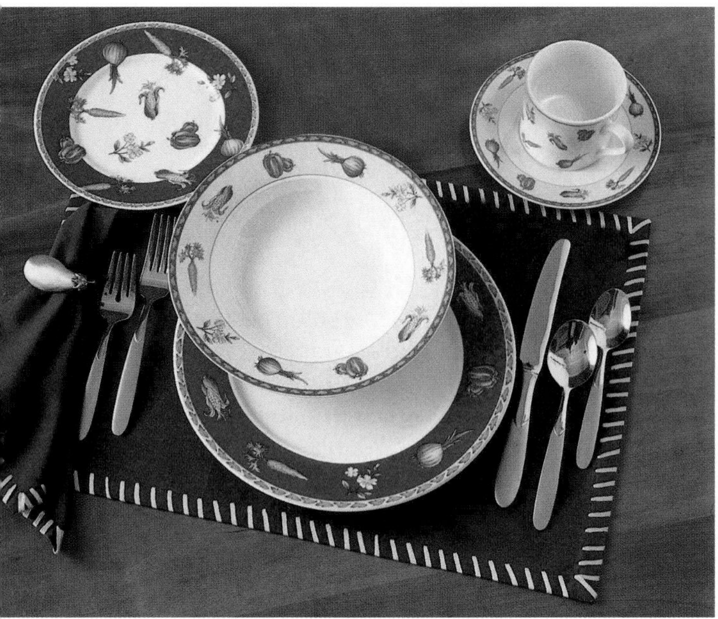

Lillian Vernon

8-7 Dinnerware, flatware, and table linens are among the table appointments used to set an eye-catching table.

edges of beverageware to be sure they are smooth and free from nicks. Glasses should feel comfortable to hold and be well balanced so they will not tip over when filled or empty.

Choose pieces that are multipurpose. For instance, you can use some stemware for serving shrimp cocktails, fruit cups, and ice cream sundaes as well as beverages. Consider plastic beverageware for casual dining and when serving young children.

Holloware

Holloware includes bowls and tureens, which are used to serve food, and pitchers and pots, which are used to serve liquids. Holloware may be made of metal, glass, wood, or ceramic. Some holloware pieces have heating elements.

Holloware tends to be expensive, fragile, and difficult to store. You may purchase holloware pieces to match your dinnerware. However, unmatched holloware that complements other table appointments is less expensive and more popular.

Purchasing Tableware

Dinnerware, flatware, beverageware, and holloware are all referred to as *tableware.* All four types of tableware are available in many patterns and at a variety of prices. When purchasing tableware, you will want to choose items that go well together. You will also want to consider your personal taste, your lifestyle, and the amount of money you have to spend. If you enjoy formal entertaining and can afford the expense, you might select china, sterling silver, and lead glass to grace your table. If you prefer more casual, less expensive tableware, you might choose stoneware, stainless steel, and lime glass for your table.

You can purchase tableware in several ways. You can buy some tableware as ***open stock.*** This means you can purchase each piece individually. Dinnerware and flatware are often sold in place settings. A ***place setting*** includes all the pieces used by one person. For instance, a place setting of dinnerware usually includes a dinner plate, salad plate, sauce dish or bread and butter plate, cup, and saucer. A place setting of flatware usually includes a knife, dinner fork, salad fork, teaspoon, and soupspoon. You can also buy some tableware by the set. A box of four water glasses and a set of dinnerware for eight are examples of sets.

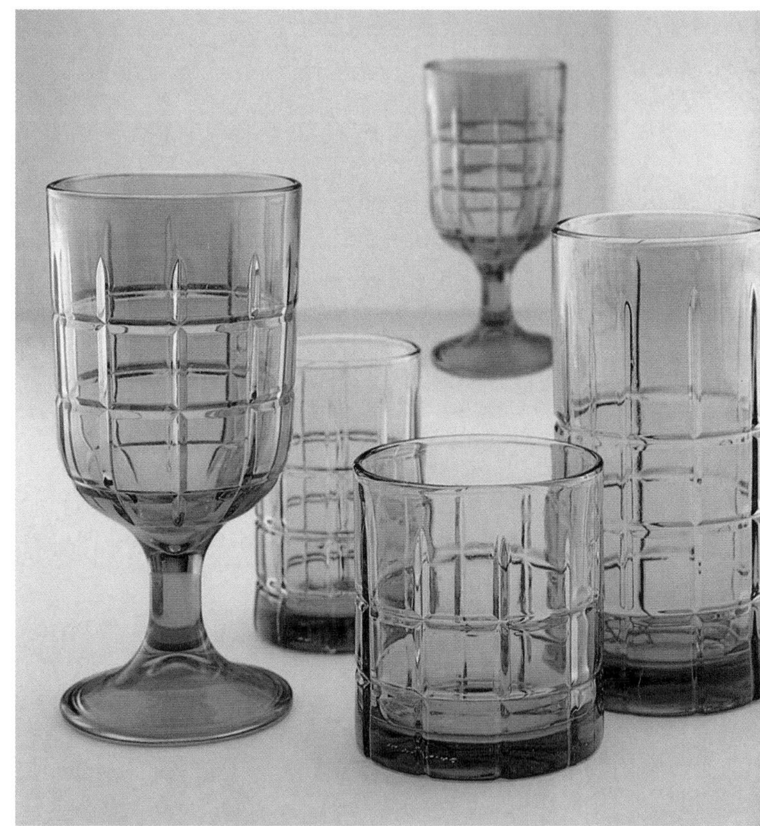

Anchor Hocking

8-8 Different shapes of glasses are designed to hold different types of beverages.

Caring for Tableware

Proper handling and storage will extend the life and beauty of your tableware. Rinse tableware as soon as possible after use. Dried food particles are difficult to remove. You can put most tableware in the dishwasher, but you should check the manufacturer's recommendations.

Store tableware carefully. Handle dinnerware and beverageware with care to prevent chipped, cracked, and broken pieces. Place flatware neatly in a drawer to avoid scratching and bending it.

Be a Clever Consumer

When selecting dinnerware, consider how the color and design will look with food. Pick up a cup to see if it is comfortable to hold. Check the finish of the dinnerware. There should be no chips, cracks, or unglazed spots. China should be translucent, and the glaze should not be wavy or bumpy.

Table Linens

The term ***table linens*** includes both table coverings and napkins. Table linens protect the surface of the table and add to the appearance of the table setting. Many materials are used to make table linens. They are available in a rainbow of solid colors as well as a variety of prints.

Tablecloths provide a background for your table setting. Place mats and table runners are also popular table coverings. *Place mats* come in several shapes and can be used for all but the most formal occasions. *Table runners* are narrower and slightly longer than the table. They are often used with tablecloths or place mats. *Napkins* can match the other table linens or provide a contrast. See 8-9.

The amount of care table linens need depends on the materials used in their construction. Paper tablecloths, place mats, and napkins can simply be thrown away when a meal is over. Vinyl-coated tablecloths and place mats can be wiped clean with a damp cloth. Most fabric cloths can be machine washed and dried. Linen cloths and napkins must be laundered carefully and then ironed while still damp.

The table linens you choose will depend on your other table appointments and your lifestyle. If your dinnerware has a definite pattern, it probably will look best against a plain background. If your dinnerware is very plain, patterned table linens can add interest to the table setting.

Before purchasing table linens, you should consider durability, ease of laundering, colorfastness, and shrinkage.

Centerpieces

You can buy or make centerpieces to add interest to the dining table. Floral arrangements are popular centerpieces. However, avoid using potted plants. Soil and food do not mix.

A centerpiece should be in proportion to the size of the table. Make sure guests will be able to see over the centerpiece while they are seated. If your centerpiece includes candles, light them and be sure they burn above or below eye level. Avoid using candles on the table during the day.

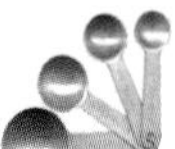

Setting the Table

You should set a table for convenience as well as beauty. There is no "right" way to set a table. The occasion, style of service, size of the table, and menu will help you determine how to set the table.

Begin setting the table with the table linens. A tablecloth should extend evenly on each side of the table. You may lay place mats flush with

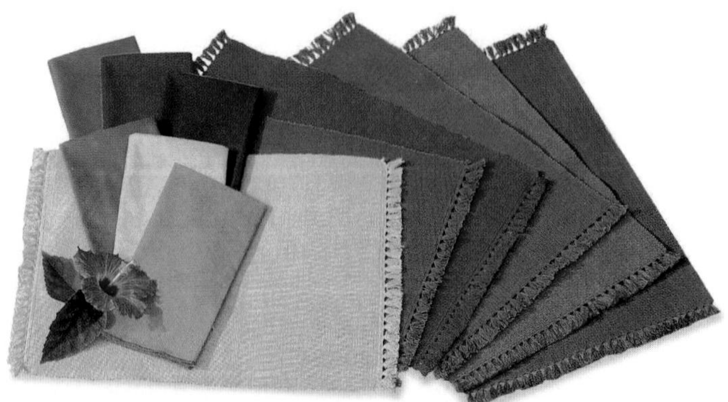

Lillian Vernon

8-9 Table linens in coordinated colors can form the background for an interesting and attractive table setting.

the edge of the table or 1 to 1-1/2 inches (2.5 to 4 cm) from the table edge. Place runners down the center, along both sides, or around the perimeter of the table.

Handle all tableware without touching the eating surfaces. Start by placing the dinner plate in the center of each cover, 1 inch (2.5 cm) from the edge of the table. A ***cover*** is the table space that holds all the tableware needed by one person. If using a salad plate, place it to the left of the dinner plate above the napkin. If using a bread and butter plate, place it just above the salad plate, between the salad plate and the dinner plate. Each guest should be able to tell which appointments are his or hers. See 8-10.

Place flatware in the order in which it will be used, working from the outside toward the plate. Forks go to the left of the plate. Therefore, if you are serving salad before the main course, place the salad fork to the left of the dinner fork. Place the napkin to the left of the forks or on the dinner plate.

Knives and spoons go to the right of the plate. This means a soupspoon goes to the right of the teaspoon if you are serving soup before the entrée. You can place dessertspoons or forks above the dinner plate. The bottom of each piece of flatware should be in line with the bottom of the dinner plate.

Place the water glass just above the tip of the knife. Place other glasses below and to the right of the water glass. If you are serving a hot beverage, place a cup and saucer to the right of the knife and spoon.

Q: Does it matter what direction flatware faces when I place it on the table?

A: When placing flatware, turn knives so the blades are toward the plates. Place forks and spoons with tines and bowls turned upward.

Place salt to the right of pepper when placing shakers on the table. Place rolls, butter, and other foods that will be self-served to the right or left of the host's cover. Place serving utensils needed for foods to the right of serving dishes.

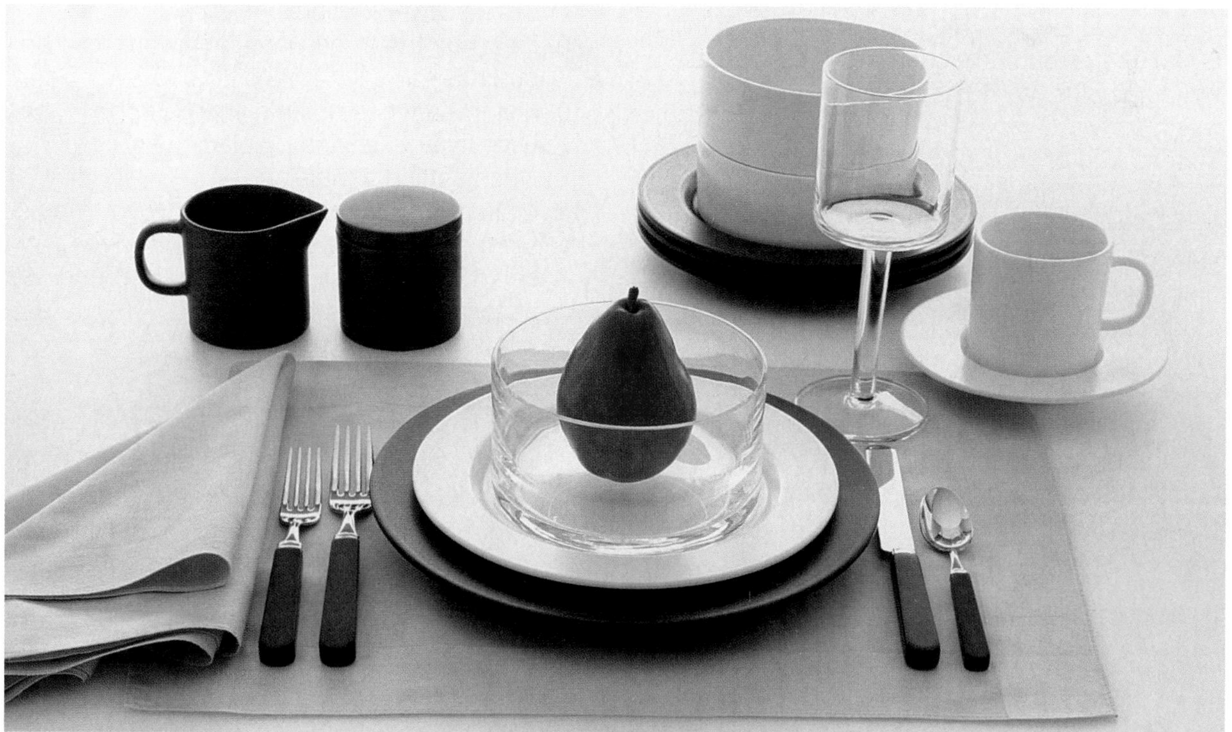

The Calvin Klein Home Collection

8-10 *A properly set table provides each diner with the tableware pieces he or she will need for the meal being served.*

Chapter 8 Review

Kitchen and Dining Areas

Summary

Kitchen and dining areas are heavily used spaces in the home. With careful planning, their design will meet the needs of all family members. Three major kitchen work centers focus on the tasks of preparing and storing food, cooking and serving, and cleanup. If space allows, a home may include additional work centers for such tasks as mixing, eating, planning, and doing laundry. You need space to store supplies required for the tasks you will do in each of these work centers. An imaginary line connects the three major work centers to form a work triangle. This triangle takes on different dimensions in different kitchen floor plans. Peninsula, U-shaped, and L-shaped plans reflect universal design, making the kitchen usable by as many people as possible.

The design of kitchen and dining areas should be both attractive and useful. Choose wall coverings, floor coverings, countertops, and cabinets to suit your family's tastes. Plan ample lighting, ventilation, and electrical wiring to safely meet needs. With planning and creativity, updating the look of kitchen and dining areas will not cost much money. Design and decorating software can help you plan the use and appearance of your kitchen and dining space.

You can find table appointments to suit any taste, lifestyle, and budget. You will want to select dinnerware, flatware, beverageware, and holloware that blend to create the desired dining mood. Use table linens to provide a backdrop for your other table appointments. Choose a centerpiece to add appeal to the dining table. The materials used to make table appointments affect their cost, durability, and care. A few basic guidelines can help you use table appointments to set an attractive table.

Review What You Have Read

Write your answers on a separate sheet of paper.

1. List two items that would be stored in each of the three major kitchen work centers.
2. What is the most desirable kitchen floor plan?
3. True or false. Work surfaces in a universal design kitchen all need to be at a level that can be easily reached from a seated position.
4. What qualities do floor coverings used in kitchen and dining areas require?
5. Name the two classifications of lighting and give sources of each.
6. What are three warning signs of an overloaded electrical circuit?
7. What type of tableware are plates, cups, and saucers and what factor helps determine their cost and durability?
8. What are the two basic shapes of beverageware? Give examples of each.
9. Describe the three ways tableware may be purchased.
10. List three types of table linens.
11. Give five guidelines for placing flatware when setting a table.
12. Make a drawing that shows how you would set the table for a family meal in which the salad is eaten before the main dish and water is the only beverage.

Build Your Basic Skills

1. **Math.** Go to a home improvement store that sells flooring and carpeting. Choose kitchen carpeting and a vinyl sheet design that appeal to you. Figure the cost of covering a 10- by 14-foot (3.0- by 4.3-meter) kitchen floor with each of these products.

2. **Writing.** Find a picture of a table setting in a magazine or catalog. Attach the picture to your written critique of the table setting based on the guidelines given in this chapter.

Build Your Thinking Skills

1. **Analyze.** Pretend to make a cake in your foods lab, following the directions on a packaged mix. While you are doing this, have a partner count the number of times you walk along each side of the work triangle. When you have finished, analyze your motions. Then brainstorm with your partner to come up with ideas for reducing the distance you walked. Share your suggestions with the rest of the class.
2. **Develop.** Develop a checklist of desirable characteristics for kitchen and dining area wall coverings, floor coverings, countertops, cabinets, lighting, ventilation, and electrical wiring. Use the checklist to determine how many of these positive characteristics are found in the kitchen and dining area in your home.

Apply Technology

1. Use a computer and the table function in word processing software to make gridlines. Then open the gridline file in a drawing program to draw the floor plans of your home kitchen according to accurate measurements.
2. Investigate the latest developments in textile fibers for home decorating. Summarize your findings in an oral report, citing possible uses of the fibers in kitchens and dining areas.

Using Workplace Skills

Angelo is a cabinet and trim installer for Kitchen Works. Kitchen Works carries all the latest cabinet materials. They specialize in custom work to suit unusual kitchen designs. Angelo goes to customers' homes to measure where cabinets will go. Then he measures and cuts the materials and attaches the cabinets and trim using hand tools and power tools.

To be a successful employee, Angelo needs to know how to learn. Put yourself in Angelo's place and answer the following questions about your need for and use of this skill:

A. What new information might you need to learn to continue to perform your job well?

B. How might Kitchen Works' customers be affected if you were unable to learn and apply new knowledge and skills?

C. How might Kitchen Works be affected if you were unable to learn and apply new knowledge and skills?

D. What is another skill you would need in this job? Briefly explain why this skill would be important.

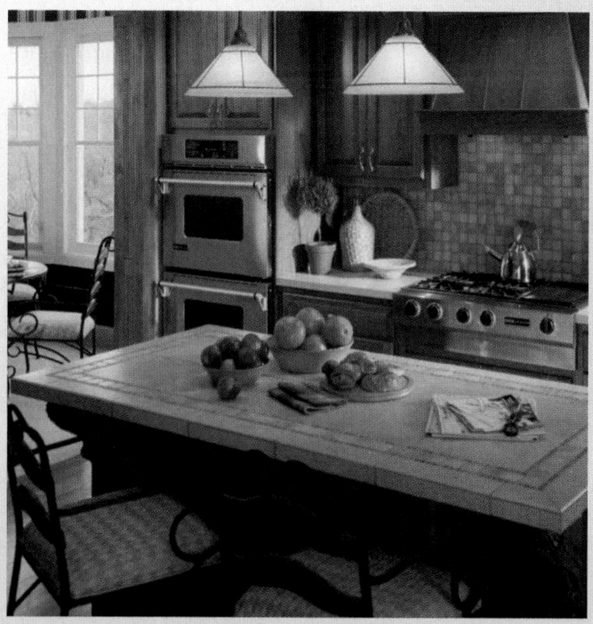

Chapter 9

Choosing Kitchen Appliances

Appliance Line Assembler
Assembles major household or commercial appliances, such as ranges, ovens, refrigeration units, and dishwashers, using hand tools.

Wholesale Appliance Sales Representative
Sells household appliances to retail businesses for manufacturers. May train dealers in operation and use of appliances.

Household Appliance Inspector
Inspects and tests electrical household appliances, such as ranges and food mixers, for appearance and mechanical and electrical characteristics, using testing devices and hand tools.

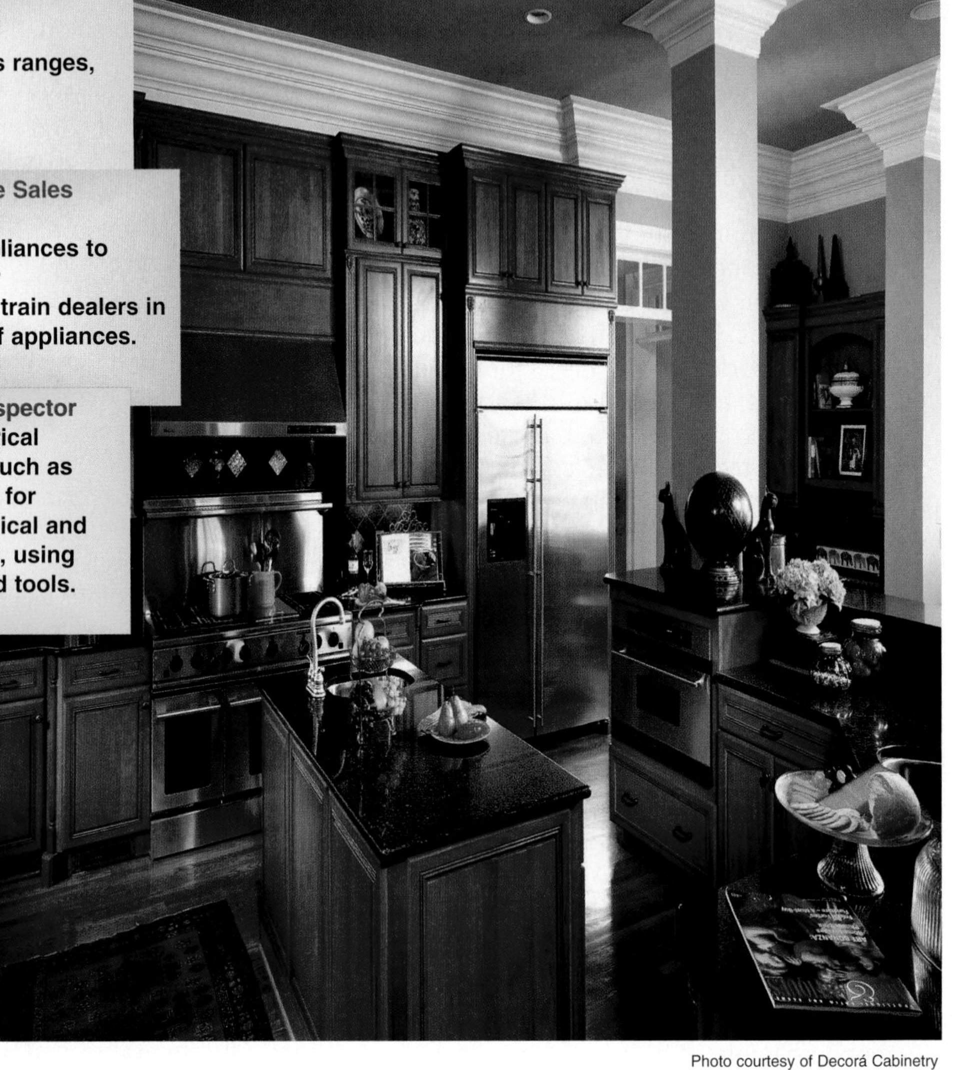

Photo courtesy of Decorá Cabinetry

Terms to Know

warranty
service contract
EnergyGuide label
ENERGY STAR label
combination oven
convection cooking
downdraft vent
microwave
wave pattern

Objectives

After studying this chapter, you will be able to

- ❑ evaluate safety seals, warranties, and energy labeling to help you make purchase decisions when buying kitchen appliances.
- ❑ describe styles and features of major kitchen appliances.
- ❑ list points to consider when purchasing portable kitchen appliances.

Today's appliances make food preparation and cleanup easier. Major appliances are available in a range of styles and offer a wide variety of features. Portable appliances perform a multitude of kitchen tasks. Keep in mind that kitchen appliances are an investment. You can spend a lot of money for appliances. You will probably be using the appliances you choose for many years. Therefore, you will want to plan your appliance purchases carefully.

Safety and Service

Information is available when you buy an appliance to help you know what you can expect from your purchase. Using this information can help you buy safe, efficient products. Safety seals, warranties, and energy labeling can help you get your money's worth when you shop for appliances.

Safety Seals

Most appliance manufacturers hire independent agencies to test their appliances for safety. These agencies ensure that appliances meet standards of the industry. One such agency that has been testing appliances for years is Underwriters Laboratories (UL). Appliances that pass safety tests carry a safety seal. This seal indicates the appliance has the testing agency's certification of safety. See 9-1.

When shopping for appliances, look for those made by well-known manufacturers. Buy appliances from reputable dealers. Look for safety seals on the appliances. These steps are your best defense against appliances that fail to meet safety standards.

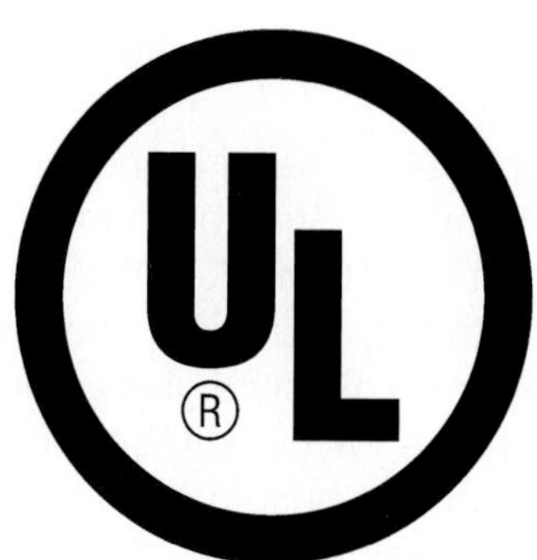

9-1 Electrical appliances carrying the Underwriters Laboratories (UL) mark have been carefully tested for safety.

Warranties

A ***warranty*** is the seller's promise that a product will be free of defects and will perform as specified. A warranty can be full or limited. A *full warranty* states the issuer will repair or replace a faulty product free of charge. The warrantor may also opt to give you a refund for the product. A *limited warranty* states conditions under which the issuer will service, repair, or replace an appliance. For instance, you may have to pay labor costs, or you might have to take the appliance back to the warrantor.

Carefully check the warranty and be sure you understand the terms before you buy an appliance. Both limited and full warranties must state how and where you can fulfill them. They must also give other details about coverage. Review the warranty to see if it covers the entire item or just parts. Find out if it includes labor costs. Note how long the warranty is in effect.

Terms of a warranty should be stated clearly so you can understand them. If you have any questions, call or write the manufacturer.

Service Contracts

A ***service contract*** is like an insurance policy for major appliances that you can buy from an appliance dealer. Service contracts cover the cost of needed repairs for a period after the warranty has expired. However, if your appliance does not need repairs, you receive no service for the money you spent on the contract.

Most warranties cover the period during which you are most likely to need service. If you are thinking about buying a service contract, be sure you know what you are getting. Read the terms of the contract carefully. Find out if it covers both parts and labor. Ask if the coverage will be good if you sell the appliance or move out of the service area. Check to see if there is a limit to the amount of service you may receive. Be sure you understand all the terms fully before you buy the contract.

Energy Labeling

The amount of energy appliances require can vary widely from model to model. As a consumer, you must pay for the gas and electricity your appliances use. Energy also has an environmental cost because natural resources are used to produce it. Therefore, you should look into how much energy appliances will use when you are making buying decisions.

To help consumers, the Federal Trade Commission (FTC) requires ***EnergyGuide labels*** on many major appliances. These yellow tags show an estimate of yearly energy use for major appliances. This estimate is shown on a scale in kilowatt-hours. The ends of the scale show the highest and lowest energy usage of similar models. An estimate of the yearly operating cost is also given for the model on which the label appears. This cost is based on national average energy costs.

EnergyGuide labels are required on refrigerators, freezers, and dishwashers as well as a number of nonkitchen appliances. You can use these labels when you shop. Compare EnergyGuide labels on appliances of the same size. This will tell you which model is the most energy efficient and least costly to operate. See 9-2.

A second type of label you can use to find appliances that are energy efficient is the ***ENERGY STAR label.*** The U.S. Environmental Protection Agency (EPA) and the U.S. Department of Energy (DOE) run this labeling program. The ENERGY STAR label can appear on refrigerators, freezers, and dishwashers. Unlike EnergyGuide labeling, ENERGY STAR labeling is not required. Appliances that have the ENERGY STAR label must exceed federal minimum energy standards by a certain amount. These appliances perform as well as similar appliances, but they use less energy. Therefore, they are better for the environment. They also save consumers money. See 9-3.

Based on standard U.S. Government tests

ENERGYGUIDE

Dishwasher
Capacity: Standard

Model(s) Maytag
MDB9100 MDB9150
MDBD880

Compare the Energy Use of this Dishwasher with Others Before You Buy.

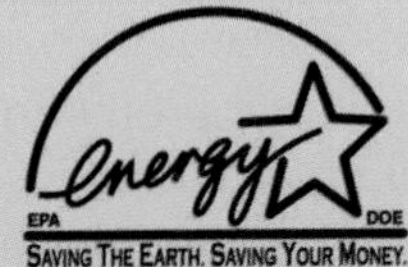

This Model Uses
555 kWh/year

ENERGY STAR
A symbol of energy efficiency

Energy use (kWh/year) range of all similar models

Uses Least Energy 344 **Uses Most Energy 699**

kWh/year (kilowatt-hours per year) is a measure of energy (electricity) use. Your utility company uses it to compute your bill. Only standard size dishwashers are used in this scale.

Dishwashers using more energy cost more to operate. This model's estimated yearly operating cost is:

$46 When used with an electric water heater

$31 When used with a natural gas water heater

Based on six washloads a week and a 1997 U.S. Government national average cost of 8.31¢ per kWh for electricity and 61.2¢ per therm for natural gas. Your actual operatin cost will vary depending on your local utility rates and your use of the product.

Important: Removal of this label before consumer purchase violates the Federal Trade Commission's Appliance Labeling Rule (16 C.F.R. Part 3

courtesy of Maytag Appliances

9-2 Consumers can use EnergyGuide labels to compare the energy efficiency of various models of an appliance.

Major Kitchen Appliances

Every part of kitchen activity involves major appliances. You use them to cook and store food and to clean up after preparing food. Today's appliances have many convenience features that reduce the time and effort needed to do these tasks.

When shopping for an appliance, consider how your family will use it. You should also think about your space limitations and your budget.

The size of appliance you need depends on the size of your family. For instance, a family of eight will probably need a larger range than a single person.

Look for appliances with universal design styles and features. Such appliances will allow all family members to work in the kitchen with ease. For instance, you might choose a side-by-side refrigerator. This style gives wheelchair users and children access to both refrigerated and frozen foods. A built-in oven can be installed in the wall at a level that is easy to reach while seated. Front- or side-mounted appliance controls are a good choice for some families. These controls can assist people who have trouble seeing or reaching rear-mounted

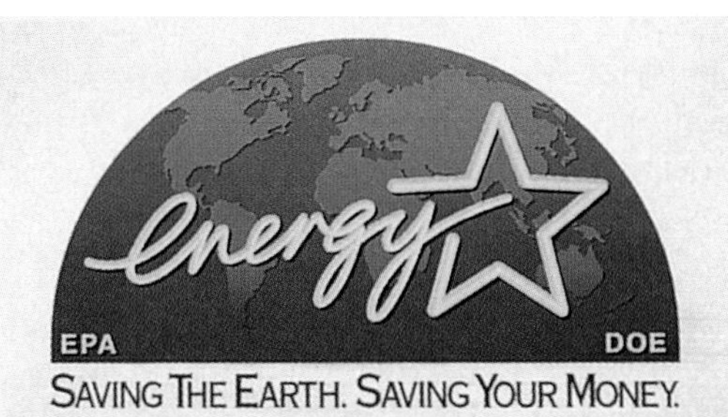

9-3 Look for the ENERGY STAR label on refrigerators, freezers, and dishwashers as an indication of energy efficiency.

controls. An oven with a window and an interior light can help family members who have limited vision. Audible signals on appliances can aid people who have trouble seeing. Indicator lights assist those who have difficulty hearing. See 9-4.

Size is an important factor to consider when buying an appliance. Measure the appliance to find out if it will fit in the area where you want to put it. There must be adequate space for servicing and ventilation. Also measure the doors in your home. They must be wide enough to move the appliance into the room where you plan to install it.

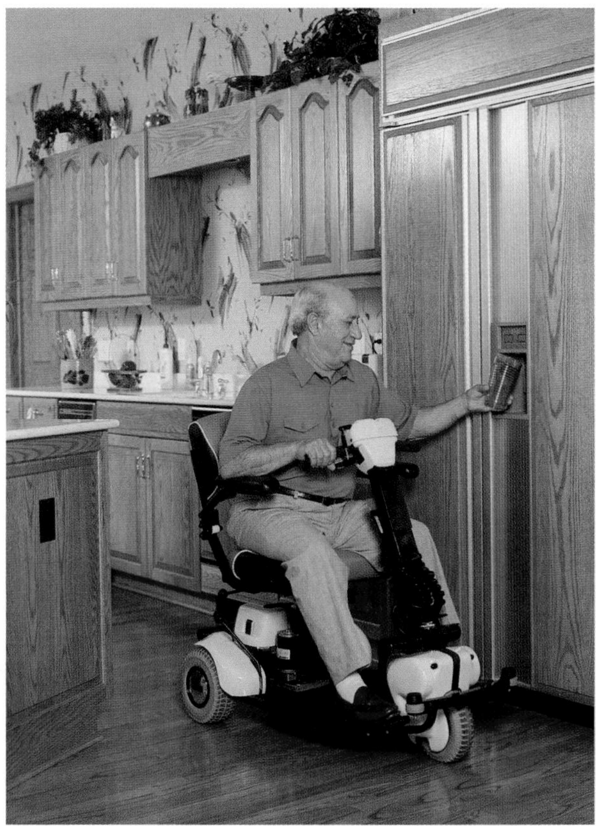

Bruno Independent Living Aids, Inc.®

9-4 The universal design of a side-by-side refrigerator allows all family members to easily reach both chilled and frozen foods.

Major appliances require a large financial investment. You must plan their purchase just like any other major household purchase. However, do not buy strictly on the basis of price. Service is also an important consideration. A bargain appliance may not seem to be such a good buy if no one in your area will service it.

Read the use and care manuals that come with your major appliances. Using the information in the manuals will help you get the best service from your kitchen equipment.

Trends and Technology in Major Kitchen Appliances

Consumers today are looking for appliances that perform a range of functions. They want appliances that are easy to clean and require little effort from the user. Consumers in smaller homes and apartments want compact models to conserve space. Some other consumers are looking for appliances with extra capacity, such as ovens with more racks. Consumers also want features that help reduce gas and electric bills. The latest technology has allowed current appliance designs to meet all these needs.

Energy efficiency is a leading trend in today's appliances. The latest models do more tasks with less energy than appliances of the past. Better insulation and temperature sensors are among the features that allow new appliances to be more efficient.

Another trend in the appliance industry is the use of high-tech electronics. Electronics allow consumers to use touch pad controls and programmable settings for specific tasks. Some appliances have graphic displays and/or voice modules. These features tell the user what settings he or she has selected on the appliance. They can show how a programmed cycle is progressing. They can also point out when something is not working right. See 9-5.

Some appliances are being made to connect to the Internet. They allow consumers to quickly send questions and requests for service to the manufacturer or a local dealer. Internet appliances also let consumers receive recipes and messages about their appliances.

Today's consumers want appliances that reflect the latest trends in kitchen design. Smooth, stainless steel surfaces and gourmet features give appliances a professional look. Some consumers want their appliances to have an integrated look. They can use customized trim kits to make appliances mesh with the style of kitchen cabinets. Each year, new appliances are offered in the latest fashion colors. However, white is always in style because it fits into almost any decor.

Be a Clever Consumer

When appliance hunting, visit several dealers to compare prices. Inquire about installation and delivery costs and any other costs not included in the purchase price. These items vary from dealer to dealer. They can significantly add to the price of an appliance.

Ranges

Ranges are available in several types and styles with a variety of features. Before purchasing one, carefully analyze your cooking and baking needs. Then study the many models available.

Fuel

You first need to choose the type of fuel you wish to use—gas or electricity. Consider fuel costs, cooking needs, safety issues, appliance performance, and personal preferences when making your choice. Many times, you may decide based on the type of fuel hookups in your home.

Electric ranges require a 240-volt electrical circuit for operation. Electric current flows through coils of wire called heating elements. The current produces heat. Coils can be visible or hidden under a smooth, glass-ceramic top. Some smoothtop electric ranges feature *radiant* elements and *halogen* elements, which heat much faster than traditional electric coils. See 9-6.

Gas ranges require both a gas line and a 120-volt electrical circuit. The ignition system and range accessories, such as timers, clocks, and lights, require electricity. Gas ranges can use bottled manufactured gas (liquefied petroleum or LP gas) or natural gas.

In some gas ranges, the broiler is a separate unit located under the oven. In other gas ranges and electric ranges, the broiler is in the oven.

A few appliance manufacturers make dual-fuel ranges and cooktops that allow consumers to cook with both gas and electricity. One range model has a gas rangetop with an electric oven. A modular cooktop allows consumers to place gas burners and electric elements side by side.

Range Styles

Ranges come in three basic styles. *Freestanding ranges* have finished sides, so you can place them at the end of a counter. However, they have a built-in look when placed between two counters. Freestanding ranges are the most popular style. They offer the widest selection of colors and features. Besides the oven below the cooktop, some models have a second oven above the cooktop.

Both slide-in and drop-in ranges fit snugly between two cabinets. *Slide-in ranges* sit on the floor. *Drop-in ranges* sit on a cabinet base. Both styles have the oven below the rangetop.

Ranges are available with several oven arrangements. Some have a single gas or electric oven. Some have two ovens, one of which may be a convection or microwave oven.

Some ranges have ***combination ovens,*** which can do two types of cooking. Many combination ovens provide a choice of conventional

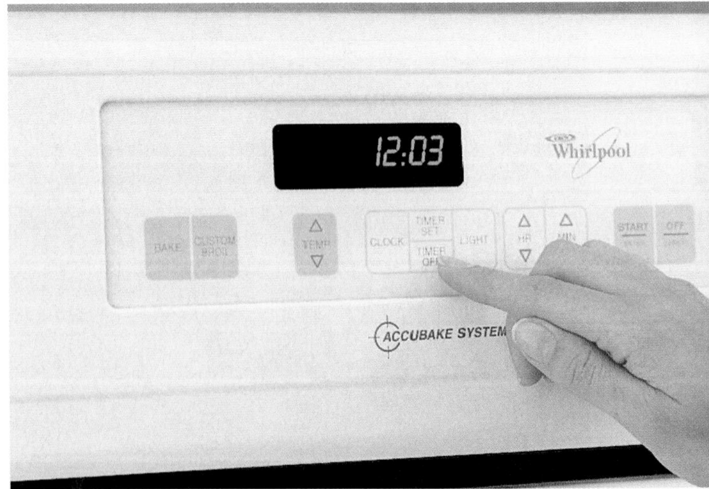

Whirlpool® Home Appliances

9-5 *Along with convenient programming, electronic touch pad controls give appliances smooth surfaces that can be wiped clean with ease.*

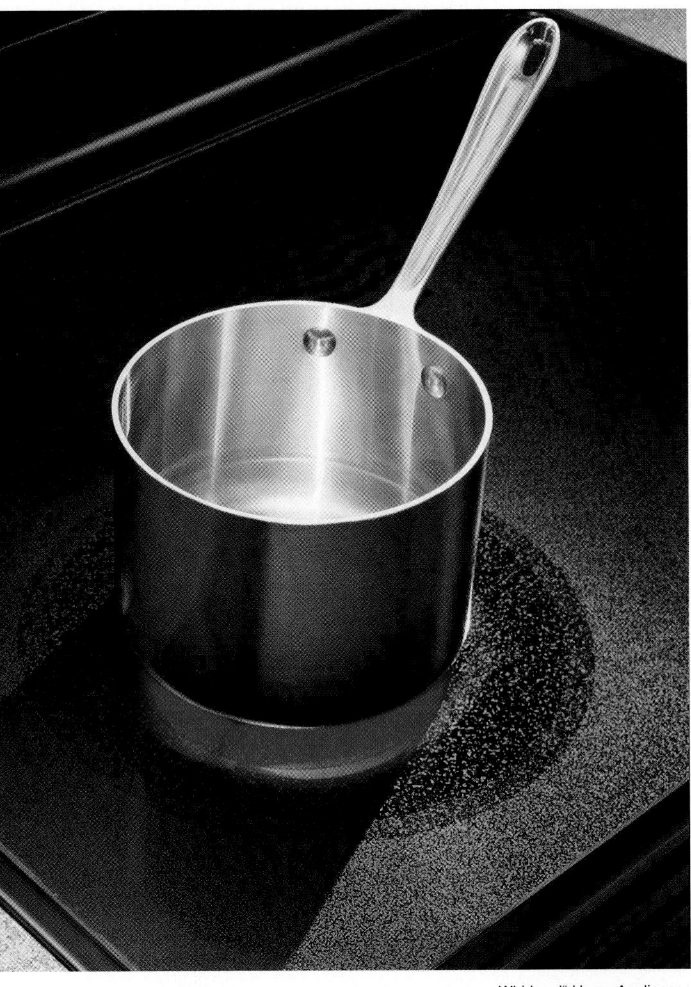

Whirlpool® Home Appliances

9-6 Radiant elements provide quick, even heat for rangetop cooking.

or convection cooking. ***Convection cooking*** uses a stream of heated air to bake and roast foods. This saves energy, reduces cooking time, and promotes more even cooking than conventional cooking. Smaller combination ovens most often provide a choice of microwave or convection cooking.

Ovens and cooktops are also available as separate built-in units. An oven may be built into a wall or specially designed cabinet. A built-in cooktop is installed in a countertop along a wall or in an island or peninsula. These separated units offer great flexibility in kitchen design.

Range Features

Ranges offer many special features. *Griddle, grill,* and *rotisserie units* are available on some ranges. These usually snap in place over a portion of the cooking surface. *Thermostatically controlled cooking units* keep food at a constant temperature, which you select.

Some ranges offer *super-hot ovens.* This feature offers the browning of a conventional oven in cooking times that are comparable to a microwave oven.

Many ranges are available with a hood mounted over the cooktop. The hood contains an exhaust fan to draw away heat and odors as they rise from food. An alternative to an overhead hood is a ***downdraft vent.*** This ventilation system has a fan mounted under the cooktop. It draws cooking fumes away from food before they have a chance to rise through the room. See 9-7.

Automatic cleaning features allow consumers to avoid the chore of cleaning the oven. *Self-cleaning ovens* use very high temperatures (750°F to 1,000°F or 400°C to 540°C) to burn away oven spills. The consumer must wipe away a small amount of ash after cleaning. Self-cleaning ovens cost more than conventional ovens. However, the cost of cleaning is less than that of commercial oven cleaners.

Continuous cleaning ovens have specially coated walls. Food spills oxidize over time during normal operation. Continuous cleaning ovens cost less than self-cleaning ovens. However, some people find them less effective.

Using and Caring for Ranges

Always practice good safety habits when using a range. Place pans on surface units before turning on the units. This will prevent accidents and also save energy. Turn all pan handles inward to prevent accidental tipping. Avoid wearing loose-fitting clothes when working around the range. They are a fire hazard.

Be careful not to drop heavy objects on the rangetop. Most ranges have a porcelain-enamel coating, which can crack or chip if struck. Wipe up spills immediately with a damp cloth. Do not use cold water when the range is hot. Porcelain can crack from severe temperature changes.

Wash the surface of the range regularly. Wash removable parts in warm, soapy water. Then rinse and dry them carefully. Clean the oven regularly using a commercial oven cleaner or the self-cleaning feature. Also, wipe up spills when they occur to keep the oven neat between cleanings.

Microwave Ovens

Microwave ovens vary widely in price, size, and features. When buying a microwave oven,

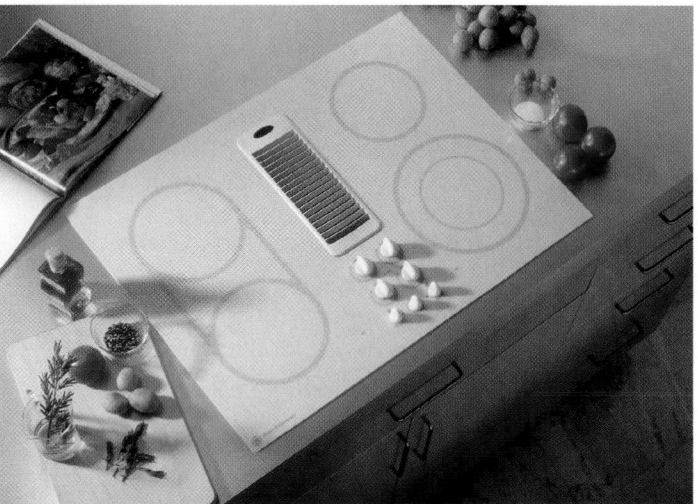
GE Appliances
downdraft vent

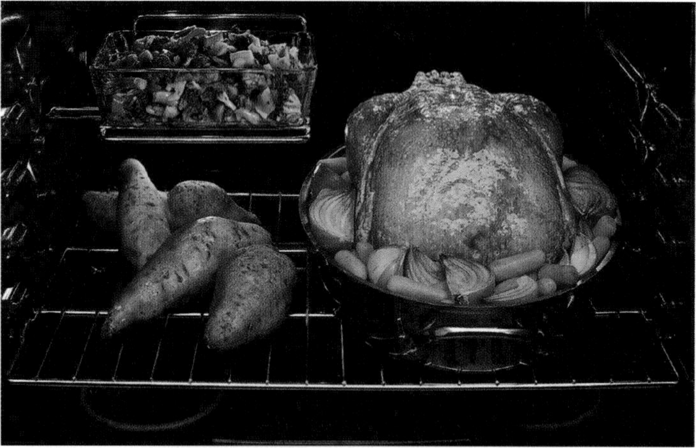
courtesy of Maytag Appliances
flexible oven racks

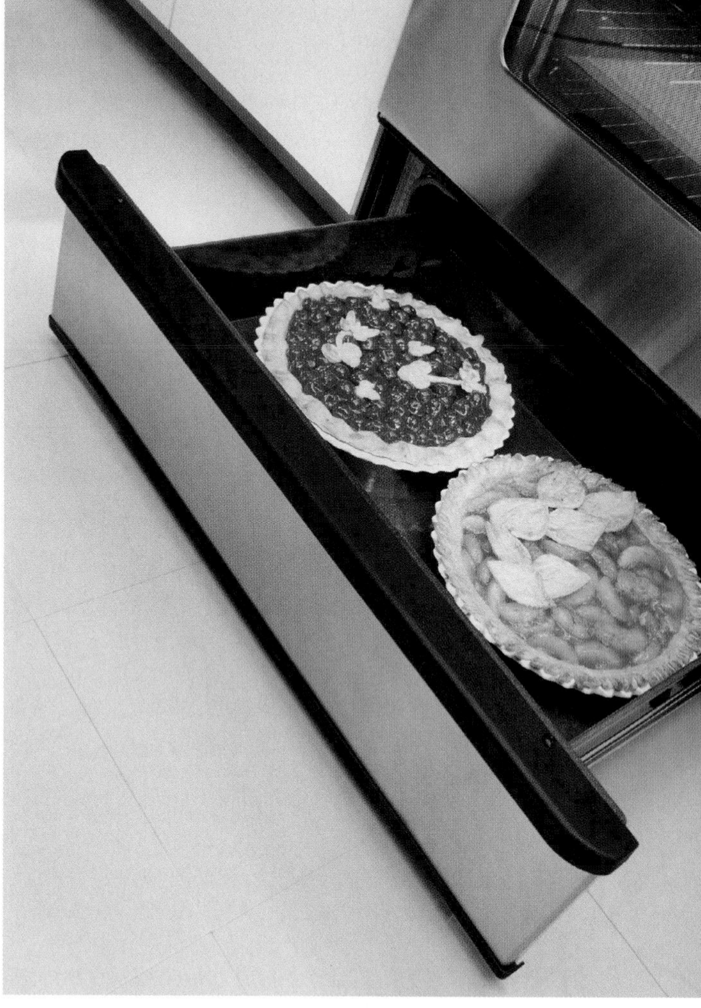
Whirlpool® Home Appliances
warming drawer

9-7 *Range features include downdraft vents that remove heat and cooking odors without an overhead hood. Other convenient features include racks that make oven space more flexible and warming drawers for holding cooked foods at serving temperatures.*

you need to consider what best fits your needs. Do you want to use your microwave oven for full cooking procedures, or will you mainly use it to defrost and reheat prepared foods? Do you need several levels of power, or will a simple model with one power level meet your needs?

Microwave ovens can defrost, cook, or reheat food in a fraction of the time required by conventional ovens. Microwave cooking can also save up to 75 percent of the energy used by conventional ovens.

Microwave cooking is done by high-frequency energy waves called ***microwaves.*** Energy in a microwave oven is produced by the *magnetron tube*. The repeated cycle in which this energy is emitted is called the ***wave pattern.*** A *stirrer fan* in the oven distributes the microwaves throughout the oven cavity. The oven walls, floor, and door liner are made of metal. The metal confines the microwaves and reflects the energy toward the food. This allows the microwaves to penetrate the food from the top and all sides. The energy from the microwaves causes the molecules of the food to vibrate. The friction of the vibrating molecules creates heat, which cooks the food.

Microwave Oven Styles

Two main styles of microwave ovens are available. *Countertop microwave ovens* are the most popular and offer the greatest choice of features. With a manufacturer's kit, you can mount some models under cabinets instead of taking up counter space, 9-8.

Two types of *over-the-range microwave ovens* are available. One type has a light and exhaust vent located underneath it. This type hangs over the range in place of a standard range hood. The other type is the upper oven on a two-oven range. These are available with both gas and electric ranges. Both types of over-the-range microwaves are similar to countertop models. However, they often have less capacity and offer fewer options.

Both styles are available as combination microwave/convection ovens. This type of oven allows you to cook with microwaves only, convection heat only, or both methods simultaneously.

Microwave Oven Features

Basic model microwave ovens may have only one to three power levels and a dial timer. More sophisticated models have 10 power levels. These microwaves generally have electronic touch pad controls and a digital display. This display shows a precise time and power setting and may also include a clock and a kitchen timer.

You will need to decide what special features you want when you shop for a microwave oven. Most microwave ovens come with *turntables,* which slowly revolve food throughout the cooking period. This eliminates the need to periodically interrupt the cooking cycle and turn food by hand.

Automatic settings allow you to program the type and sometimes the amount of food. The oven determines cooking times and correct power levels for you. Many microwave ovens have automatic settings for defrosting foods and making popcorn. On some ovens, this is a one-touch feature.

An *add time* feature allows you to add 30 or 60 seconds of cooking time with one touch. You do not have to reprogram the microwave or press the start pad to extend cooking time.

A *child lock* allows an adult to program in a code so a child cannot operate the microwave oven. This safety feature reduces the risk of accidental injury to the child or damage to the appliance.

Using and Caring for Microwave Ovens

Do not plug a microwave oven into an extension cord. Plug it into a 120-volt grounded electrical outlet. The microwave oven should be the only appliance on the electrical circuit. Sharing the circuit with another appliance can reduce the amount of electrical power to the microwave oven. This can affect the cooking time and may harm the oven itself.

Take care not to turn on a microwave oven when it is empty. This could damage the interior.

The door seal on a microwave prevents radiation leakage. Do not let anything become caught between the sealing surfaces. Immediately clean up any food spills to keep the seal intact. If the door or hinges should become damaged, do not use the oven until you have it repaired.

To clean the interior and exterior of the oven, use a damp cloth and mild detergent. Never use an oven cleaner or abrasive cleansers.

Refrigerators

A refrigerator's main job is to keep foods cold and retard food spoilage. Refrigerator space is measured in cubic feet (cubic meters). Fresh food storage compartments should provide about 3.5 cubic feet (0.11 cubic meters) of space for each adult family member. Freezers

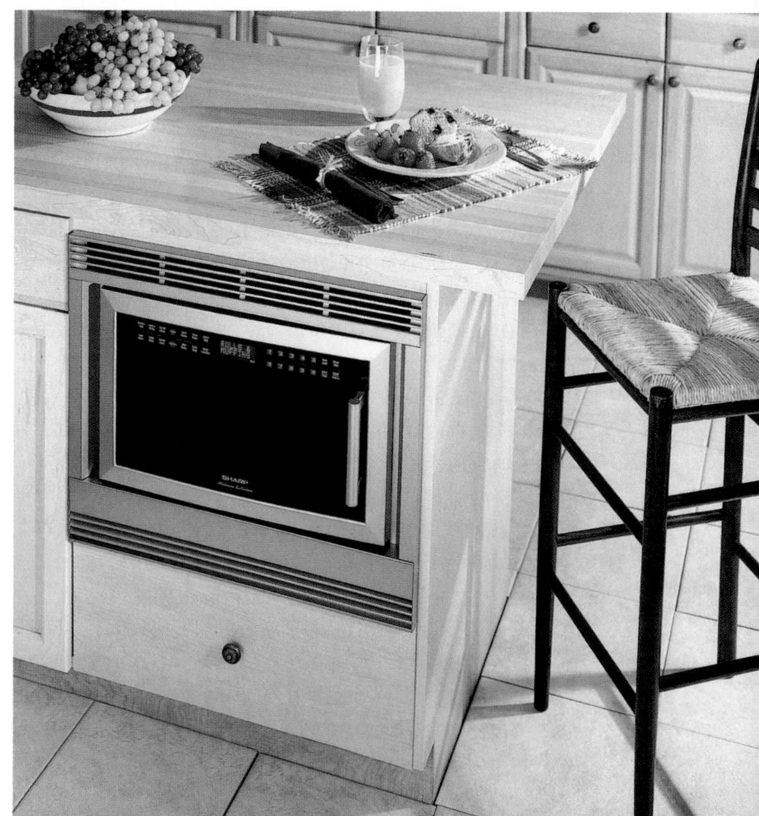

Sharp Electronics

9-8 A trim kit allows this countertop microwave oven to be installed as a built-in appliance.

should provide about 1.5 cubic feet (0.04 cubic meters) of space per person. If you shop less than once a week, you may need additional storage space.

Refrigerator Styles and Features

Refrigerators come in four basic styles, which are based on the placement of the freezer. *Top-mount refrigerators* have the freezer above the refrigerator. They are the most common and energy efficient style. *Side-by-side refrigerators* have the freezer beside the refrigerator. They provide more freezer space, but the narrow compartments may make it hard to store large food items. *Bottom-mount refrigerators* have the freezer below the refrigerator. This style places refrigerated foods at a height that is easier to reach, but fewer models are available. *Single-door refrigerators* do not have true freezers. Instead, they have frozen food storage compartments, which are sealed by an inner door. These compartments are cold enough to freeze ice cubes and store frozen foods for up to one week. However, these compartments are not cold enough to thoroughly freeze fresh foods.

Most refrigerator models are *frost free*. This means frost does not accumulate in either the refrigerator or the freezer. You can save on purchase and operating costs by buying a *manual-defrost* model. However, to avoid wasting energy, you should defrost them when frost reaches a thickness of 1/4 inch (0.6 cm).

Refrigerators can have many special features. Choose those that meet your family's needs. Refrigerators can have *automatic ice-makers* in the freezer section. They can have *ice and water dispensers* in their doors, too. Some refrigerators have *pullout shelves* to give easier access to foods. *Temperature-controlled compartments* for meat and other foods are also among the features available in some models. See 9-9.

Using and Caring for Refrigerators

For food safety and energy efficiency, keep the fresh food compartment at 37°F to 40°F (3°C to 4°C). Keep the freezer at 0°F to 5°F (-18°C to -15°C). Keep foods covered to hold in moisture and prevent unpleasant odors in the refrigerator. Try to take out all the items you need from the refrigerator at one time. Each time you open the refrigerator door, warm air enters. The refrigerator then has to use more energy to lower the temperature again.

To ensure food safety, keep both the inside and the outside of the refrigerator clean. Refrigerator parts and accessories also need regular cleaning. Wash ice cube trays, door gaskets, crisper drawers, and shelves with warm, soapy water. Rinse and dry carefully.

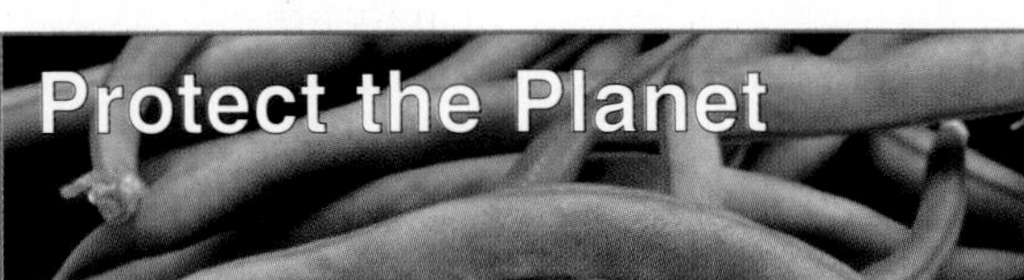

The condenser is the long, folded tube on the back of the refrigerator. You need to keep the condenser clean for the refrigerator to operate efficiently. To clean the condenser, use the crevice tool or long brush attachment of your vacuum cleaner. (Refer to your vacuum cleaner's instruction manual.)

Freezers

Some families find they need 2 to 4 cubic feet (0.06 to 0.11 cubic meters) more freezer space per adult than that provided by a refrigerator-freezer. A separate freezer allows you to take advantage of supermarket specials and seasonal food buys by making quantity purchases.

Freezer Styles

Freezers are available in two styles. *Chest freezers* allow you to easily store large, bulky packages. In contrast, *upright freezers* are easier to organize for quick storage and removal of frozen foods. They also have in-door storage. However, upright freezers cost more to operate because they are less energy efficient.

Many freezer models require manual defrosting. Others have automatic, frostless systems. Frostless models are more expensive to buy and operate.

Regardless of which style you choose, your freezer should have a lock and a safety alarm or light. The lock prevents curious children and pets from accidentally becoming trapped inside the freezer. The safety alarm or light tells you when the temperature has become too high or if the freezer is not operating.

Using and Caring for Freezers

Place your freezer in a cool, dry, well-ventilated area to reduce energy use and operating costs. Wrap foods in moistureproof

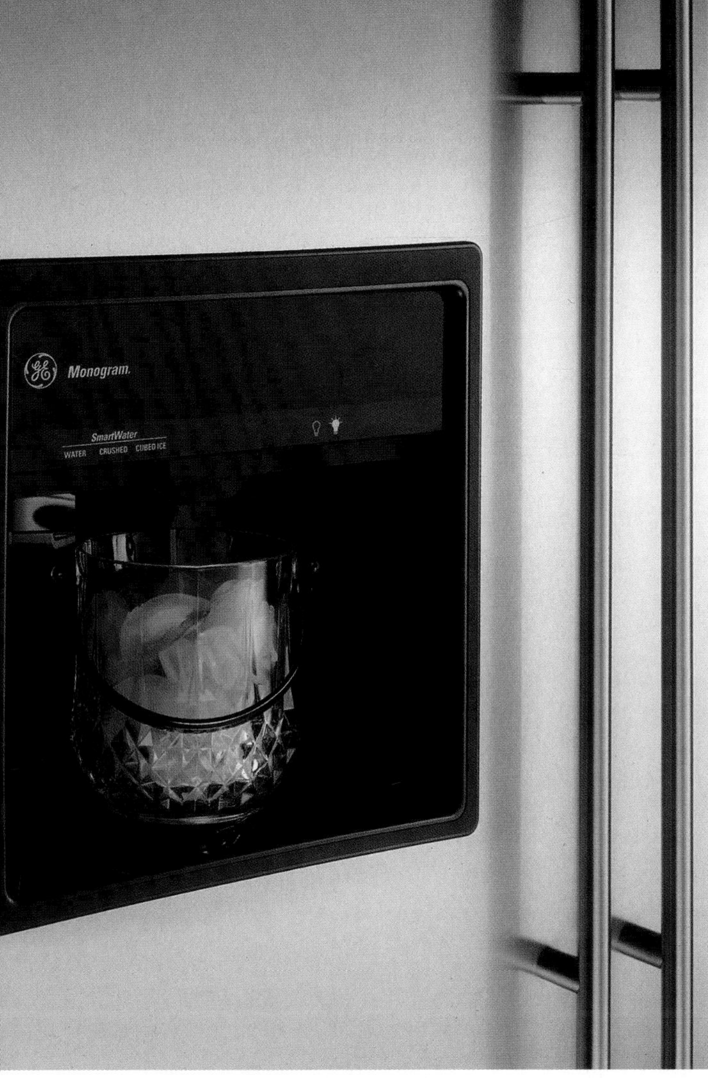

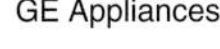
GE Appliances

ice and water dispenser

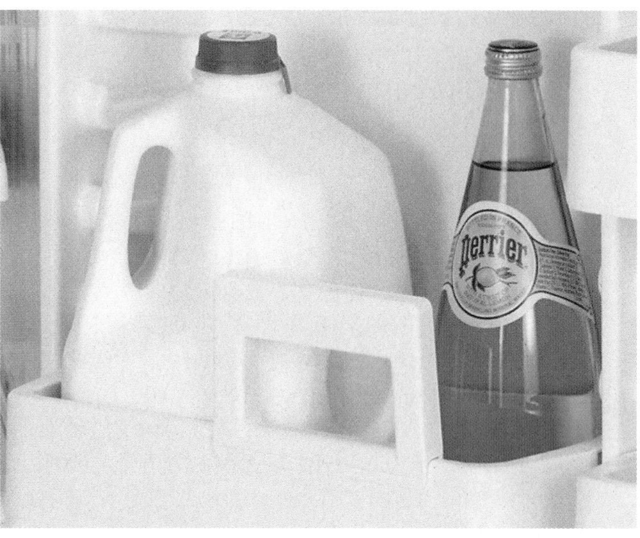

courtesy of Maytag Appliances

extra-wide door storage

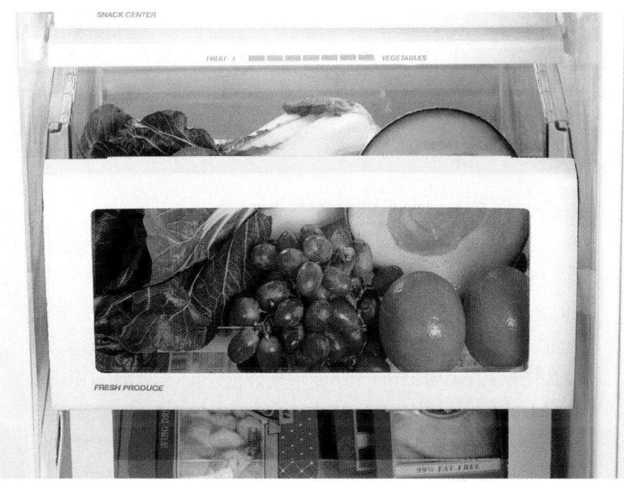

courtesy of Maytag Appliances

humidity-controlled crisper drawer

***9-9** Through-the-door ice and water dispensers, extra-wide door shelves, and humidity-controlled crisper drawers are refrigerator features designed to meet specific consumer needs.*

and vaporproof materials and date them for freezer storage. Be sure the freezer temperature remains at 0°F (-18°C). You can use a special freezer thermometer to check the temperature.

Clean the exterior of the freezer when needed. Use a damp, soapy cloth. Rinse and dry well. Do not use abrasive cleansers. They can scratch the finish.

Dishwashers

Dishwashers have a number of advantages. They can save time and personal energy. Dishes washed in a dishwasher are more sanitary. This is because the water is hotter and the detergent is stronger than the water and detergent used in hand washing. In addition, air drying is more sanitary than drying with a dish towel.

Dishwasher Styles

Two basic types of dishwashers are available. *Built-in* models are the most popular type. They fit between two cabinets and load from the front. Built-in dishwashers are permanently connected to a drainpipe, hot water line, and electric circuit.

Portable dishwashers are the second type. They are designed to be rolled to a sink for use. A portable dishwasher connects to the sink faucet with a hose and drains into the sink. You can convert some portable models to built-ins. Apartment dwellers and families who

Q: Will food stored in a freezer remain safe to eat if there is a power failure?

A: During a power failure, keep the freezer door closed to prevent warm air from entering the freezer. Normally, food in a fully loaded freezer will remain frozen for two days. If the freezer is only half full, food should stay frozen for one day. Even if food is fully thawed, it is safe to immediately cook or refreeze if it is below 40°F (4°C).

move frequently often purchase portable dishwashers.

Dishwasher Features

Dishwashers offer a choice of wash cycles. Cycles differ in the number and length of washes and rinses, amount of detergent used, and water temperature. Basic models offer three cycles for cleaning dishes with light, normal, or heavy soil. Higher-priced models offer more cycles, such as a china cycle and a pots and pans cycle. Models that have a *soil sensor* feature automatically adjust the wash cycle to provide the needed level of cleaning.

Dishwasher models come with a number of other features to meet consumer needs. *Adjustable racks* accommodate dishes of all sizes. A *delay-start* feature allows you to program the dishwasher to start at a later time. This keeps the noise and hot water use of the dishwasher from disrupting family activities. A *hard food disposal* grinds food particles, so you do not need to rinse dishes before putting them in the dishwasher. A *water-heat booster* raises the temperature of the wash water to 140°F (60°C), which is needed for effective cleaning. This energy-saving feature allows you to turn down your home water heater. A *timer* shows how much time is left in the wash cycle. Some models are also designed with extra *sound insulation* to provide quieter operation. All new dishwashers have a *no-heat drying* option. Use of this feature can save as much as one-third of the energy used for heat drying. See 9-10.

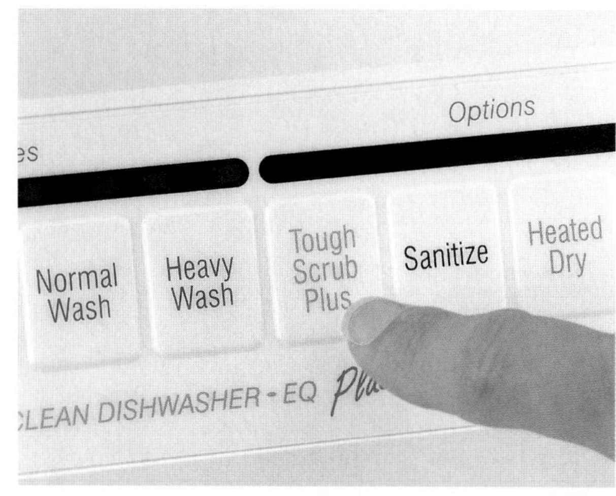

courtesy of Maytag Appliances

multiple wash cycles

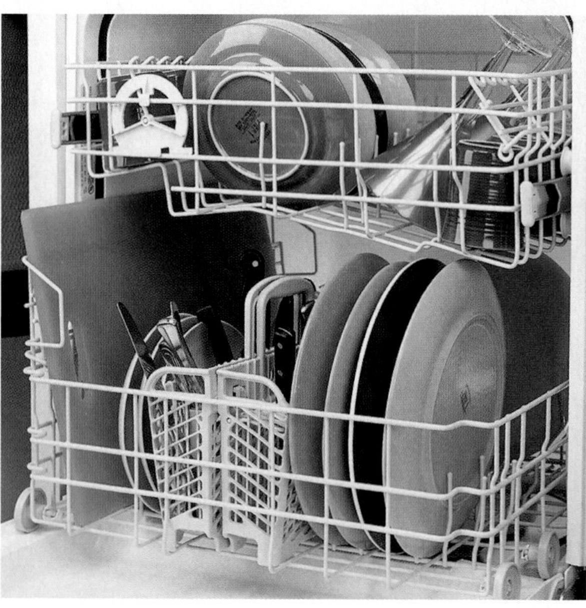

courtesy of Maytag Appliances

adjustable racks

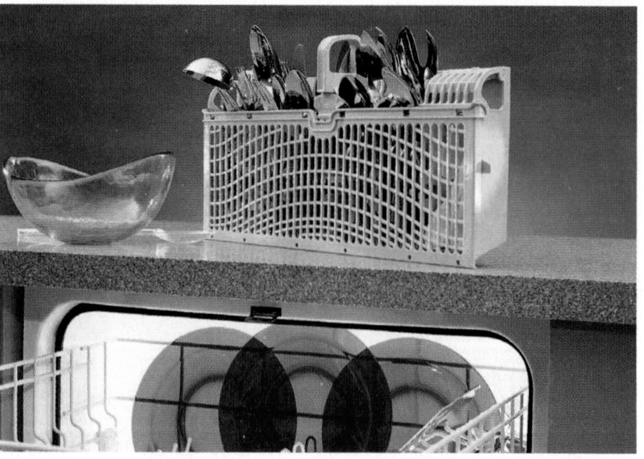

Whirlpool® Home Appliances

flatware basket

9-10 *When buying dishwashers, consumers must choose options in wash cycles and rack arrangements that best suit their cleaning needs.*

Using and Caring for Dishwashers

Scrape dishes carefully before loading the dishwasher. If food hardens on dishes, it will be harder for the dishwasher to remove. Food left on dishes will also create odors in the dishwasher.

When loading the dishwasher, place dishes so they face the water source and avoid crowding them. Point knives, forks, and spoons down into the flatware basket. Angle pieces with recessed bottoms so water will run off.

To use a dishwasher most efficiently, run it only when there is a full load. Use an automatic dishwasher detergent. If the water in your area is high in some minerals, spots may form on glassware. Using a rinse agent will help reduce spotting.

To maintain water temperature and pressure needed for proper cleaning, you should not use the washing machine while using the dishwasher. You should also avoid watering the lawn and taking a bath or shower.

Periodically empty the drain screen of any food particles that have collected. Occasionally wipe the outside of the machine with a soapy cloth, then rinse and dry.

Other Major Appliances

Some people choose to buy other major appliances to help with food preparation and cleanup tasks. *Warming drawers* are useful for holding prepared foods at serving temperatures for a few hours. *Food waste disposers* use sharp blades to grind food scraps into tiny particles, which wash down the drain. *Trash compactors* compress food and nonfood waste to about one-fourth its initial size.

Before purchasing any of these appliances, consider your needs and the styles and features available. Be sure the appliances will fit in your kitchen without taking away needed storage space. Look at your budget and be sure the benefits you receive from the appliances will be worth their costs.

Portable Kitchen Appliances

Major appliances are needed for basic kitchen functions. However, they cannot do many of the individual preparation tasks meal managers must perform. For these tasks, meal managers often rely on the time and energy savings provided by portable appliances. These small appliances can do many tasks faster and better than you could do them by hand.

Trends and Technology in Portable Kitchen Appliances

Consumers want portable appliances that simplify their work in the kitchen. However, today's appliances are used far beyond the kitchen. Coffeemakers, for instance, may be found anywhere from the office to the garage. Several models are available that will even plug into the cigarette lighter in a car.

The biggest advance in appliance technology in recent years is the development of *smart appliances*. These are appliances that communicate with one another. For instance, an alarm clock in the bedroom might be designed to communicate with a coffeemaker in the kitchen. Such an alarm clock would automatically reprogram the start time on the coffeemaker whenever the alarm setting is changed. You are likely to see a variety of smart appliances hit the market in the coming years. See 9-11.

Smart appliances are intended to compete with other appliances in terms of price. They are also designed to be easy to operate. Smart appliances all over the home may be controlled

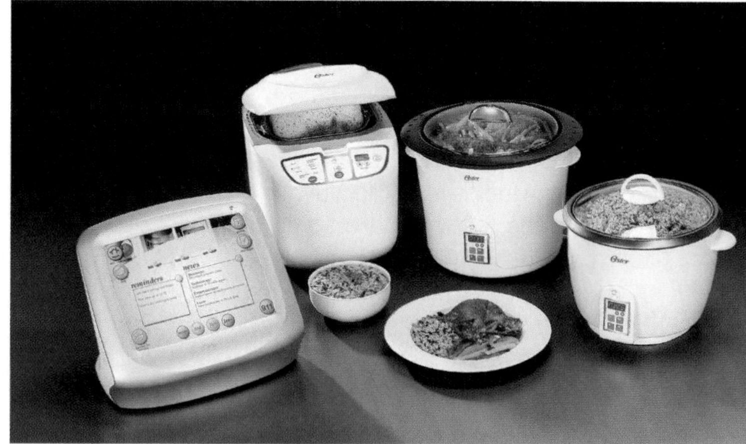

Oster

9-11 *In the future, more portable kitchen appliances may operate like these smart appliance prototypes. They are designed to communicate with one another through the programming console on the left.*

from a central countertop console or handheld unit. Proposed appliances will communicate using electric wires that already exist in the home. Battery-operated smart appliances may communicate with radio frequencies.

A number of needs have set the pace for all of today's portable kitchen appliances. Consumers require appliances that perform quickly and safely. Sensors that turn off appliances when not in use are one safety feature found on many of today's portables. Appliances should be easy to clean. Many appliances have dishwasher-safe parts to address this need. Modern appliances also need to take up a minimum of room. Cordless and under-the-cabinet appliances are conveniently sized to help consumers maximize limited space in the kitchen.

Modern portable appliances are designed with smooth, sleek shapes in trim sizes. Most appliances are available with white, black, or metal finishes. They are neutral enough to blend with any kitchen decor. However, many portable appliances also come in a range of popular colors to reflect the latest kitchen decorating trends.

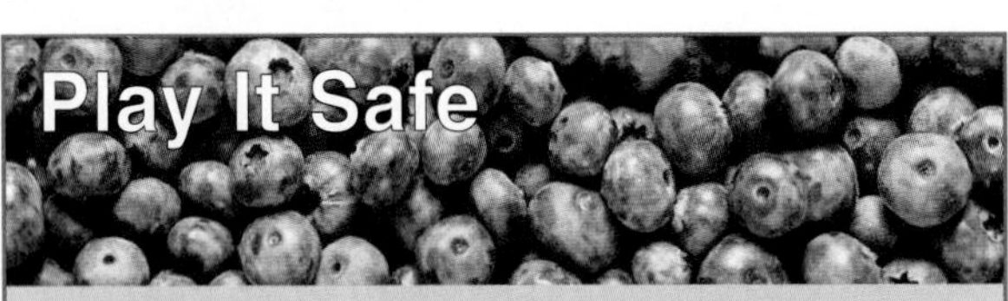

Never use a fork, knife, or other metal object to dislodge a piece of food while the toaster is plugged in. You could receive an electrical shock or damage the heating elements. Instead, unplug the toaster before trying to dislodge stuck food.

Purchase Considerations for Portable Appliances

When purchasing small appliances, select those that give the most satisfaction for the money spent. Consider what the appliance does, its limitations, and its special features. Then decide what to buy.

The following are some questions to consider:

- Is the appliance made by a reputable manufacturer and sold by a reputable dealer?
- Does the appliance come with a warranty?
- Who provides servicing when the appliance needs repairs?
- Will you use the appliance frequently?
- Does another appliance you already have do the same job?
- Do you have adequate, convenient storage space for it?
- Does the appliance have adequate power to perform its intended tasks?
- Does it have a convenient size and shape for your needs?
- Is it sturdy and well balanced? (Motor-driven appliances should not tip or "walk" during use.)
- Are parts easy to assemble for operation and easy to disassemble for cleaning?
- Does it have quality construction features? See 9-12.
- Does the appliance have built-in safety features?
- Does it have a safety seal to guarantee that it meets electrical safety standards?

General Use and Care for Portable Appliances

Before using any portable appliance, you should carefully read the manufacturer's instruction booklet. The booklet will give directions for proper use that will help your appliance last for years. Do not allow children to use portable appliances without supervision.

The manufacturer's booklet will tell you how to clean your appliance. You should clean most portable appliances after each use. Allow hot appliances to cool before cleaning. Wash most removable parts in warm, soapy water. Some parts may be safely cleaned in a dishwasher. You should not immerse most appliance motor bases and heating elements. You can wipe them clean with a damp cloth.

Toasters and Toaster Ovens

Toasters are one of the most common kitchen appliances. You can choose between two- and four-slice models, depending on the size of your family. Look for a model with extra wide openings if you like to toast bagels and thick slices of bread.

Toaster ovens bake and broil small food items in addition to toasting bread. These appliances are handy for dorm rooms and other

durable materials
comfortable handles
sufficient number of heat or power settings
heat-resistant legs, handles, and controls
clearly marked, conveniently located controls

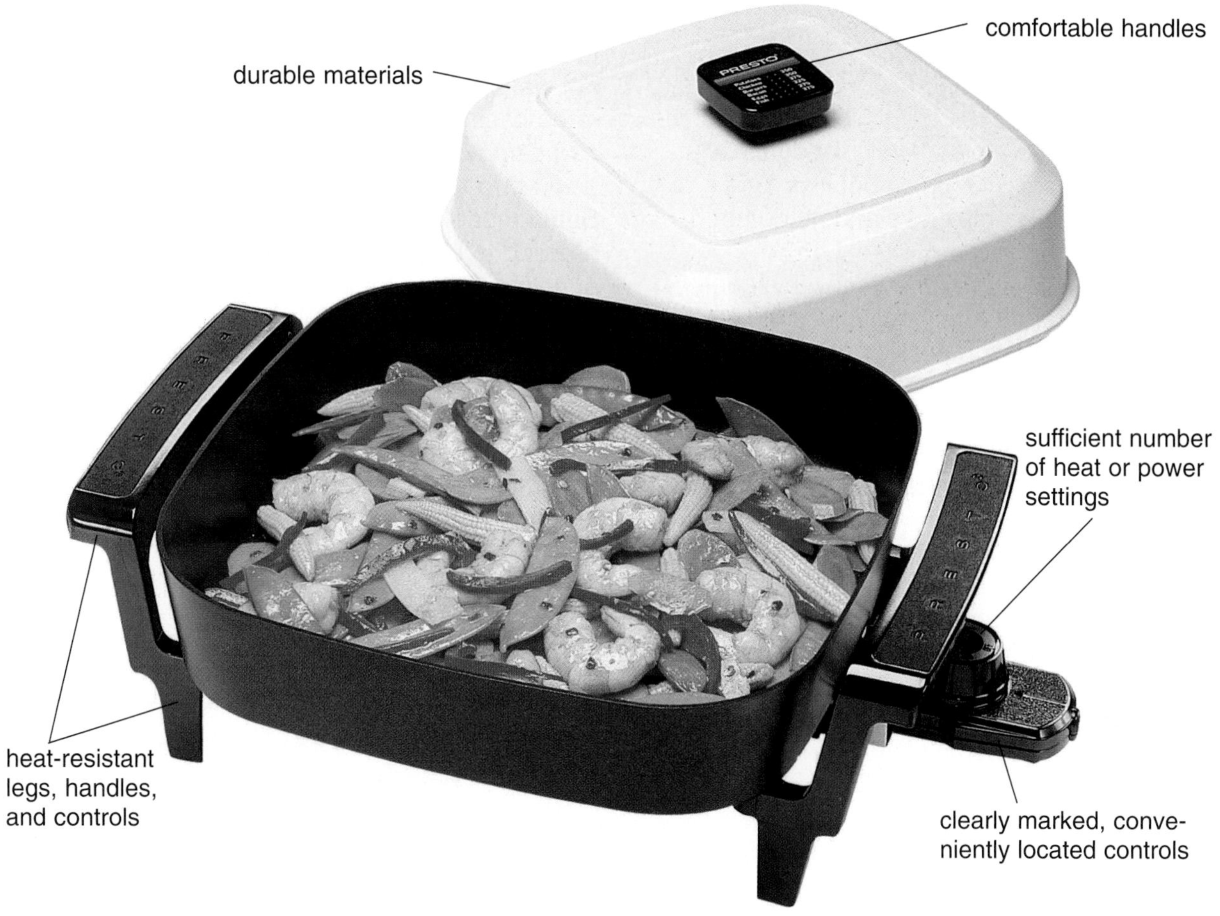

National Presto Industries, Inc.

9-12 Quality construction features help ensure that your portable kitchen appliances will perform well for years.

small quarters. They use less energy and create less heat in the kitchen than full-sized ovens.

When using a toaster, allow toast to rise automatically. Do not push up the lever yourself. Be sure to clean crumbs out of the toaster regularly. Many models have a snap-out crumb tray to make this easier.

Electric Mixers

Electric mixers are popular among home bakers for blending ingredients, beating egg whites, and whipping cream. These appliances are available in stand and handheld styles. Unlike hand mixers, *stand mixers* leave your hands free. They are also better for heavy-duty mixing jobs. Many have attachments, such as choppers and juicers. Some models feature a display that shows elapsed mixing time and speed, too. You can remove some stand mixer heads from the stand and use them as hand mixers.

The motor on a stand mixer should be strong enough to beat stiff mixtures without overheating. Some models have a gradual start feature that slowly increases speed to eliminate splatters. Otherwise, the mixer should provide even, constant mixing at every speed. The beaters should be easy to insert and remove. They should cover the full bowl diameter for thorough mixing of small or large amounts of food.

Hand mixers are smaller, lighter, and less expensive than stand mixers. However, they are not as versatile. You must hold them during the entire mixing operation. They should have stable heel rests or other means of support for standing on the counter when not in use.

For safety, turn the mixer off before inserting or removing beaters. If the cord is detachable, remove it from the wall outlet before removing it from the appliance.

Blenders

You might use a blender to blend milk shakes, puree soup, or crush cookies for a crumb crust. Unlike mixers, blenders do not incorporate air into foods.

A blender should have a removable container, molded of heat-resistant glass or plastic. The container should have a wide opening, a handle, a pouring spout, and measurement markings on the side. Also look for a self-sealing vinyl cover that resists odors and stains. A removable center cap makes it easy to add ingredients.

Do not overload the blender. Make sure the blender container and lid are firmly in place before starting the appliance. Always stop the motor before scraping the sides of the container. Use a rubber scraper rather than a metal one. Do not remove the container until the motor has stopped completely.

Food Processors

The food processor performs many time-consuming jobs quickly and easily. Figure 9-13 compares the tasks it performs with the tasks performed by mixers and blenders.

When buying a food processor, look for one that meets your needs for features. A safety interlock switch ensures that you have locked the cover in place before starting the processor. A dishwasher-safe container and cutting disks or blades will ease cleanup. You may want a food pusher that adapts to processing small or slender foods. Also make sure the control panel is easy to operate.

For best results, do not overload a food processor. Medium-sized loads process more evenly than large ones. Before processing, make sure you lock the cover into place and put the food pusher (if chopping, slicing, or shredding) in the feed tube. When processing is complete, turn the control switch to off. Wait until the blade or disc comes to a complete stop before removing the cover.

Coffeemakers

Coffeemakers have thermostatic controls that brew coffee without boiling it and then keep it at drinking temperature. The two types of automatic coffeemakers are the percolator and the drip coffeemaker. In an *electric percolator,* hot water is repeatedly pumped over a perforated basket holding ground coffee. In an *automatic drip coffeemaker,* hot water slowly drips down through ground coffee into a pot below. Some models have automatic timers that allow brewing to begin at a preset time. Special types of coffeemakers are available for brewing espresso and cappuccino.

Never let an empty coffeemaker remain turned on, as this could ruin the appliance and create a fire hazard. Carefully clean the coffeemaker after each use. Oils and sediment that accumulate in the coffeepot can affect the flavor of future pots.

Q: What type of coffee filter should I use?

A: Coffee experts suggest using a reusable gold filter or an oxygen-bleached paper filter. Chemically bleached filters and unbleached brown filters can affect the flavor of coffee.

Electric Can Openers

An electric can opener quickly and easily cuts lids off metal cans. A magnet holds the lid for easy removal. Some models adjust to accommodate cans of different heights. Most have removable cutting assemblies for easy cleaning. Many can openers also sharpen knives.

Always wash the tops of cans before opening cans. This prevents dust on the tops of cans from getting into the food. Clean the cutting assembly with hot, soapy water after each use. Food residue left on the cutting blade can serve as a breeding ground for bacteria. If the blade is not cleaned, these bacteria could contaminate other foods the next time you use the appliance.

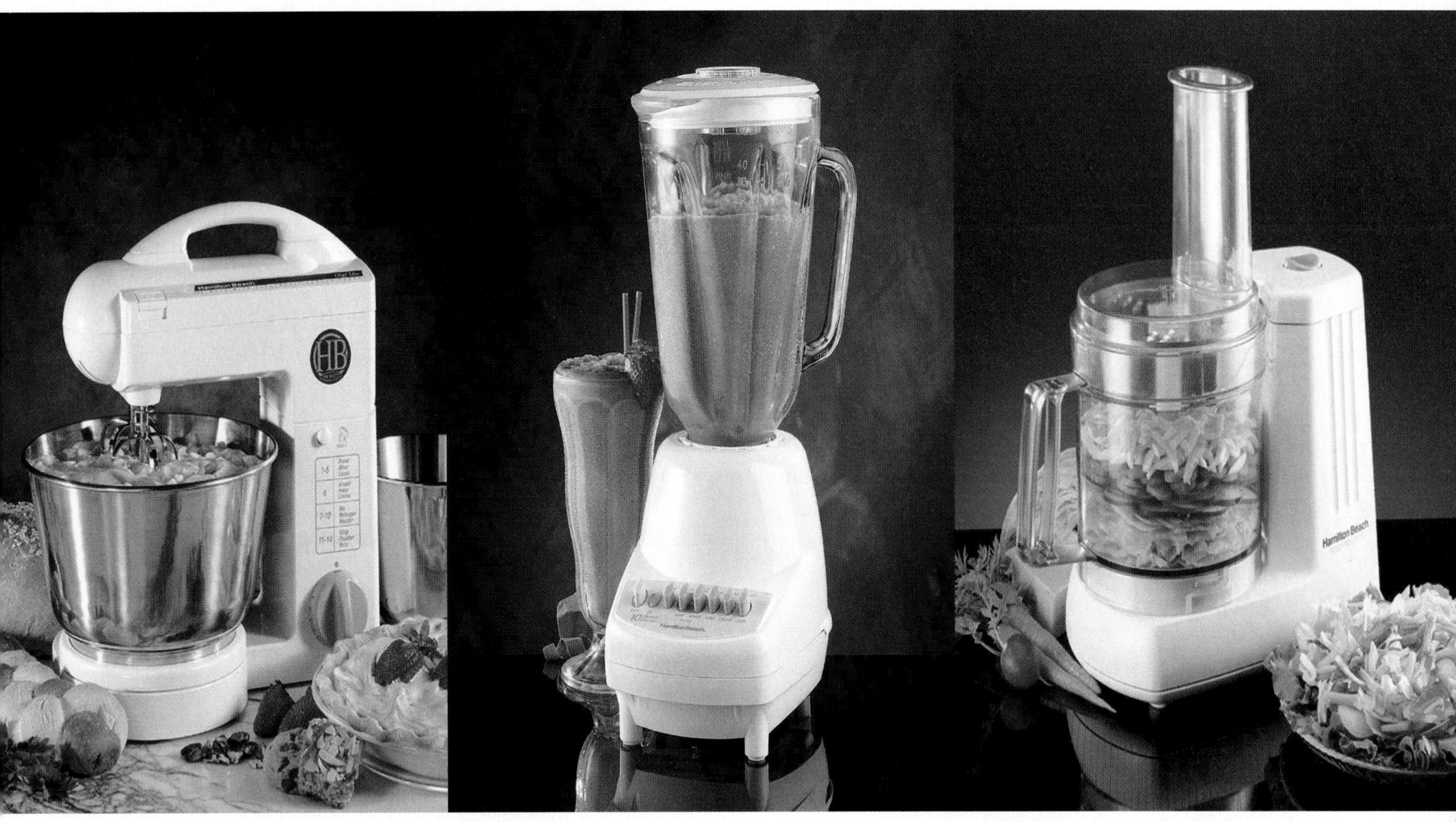

Hamilton Beach

Comparing Appliance Functions			
Task	**Stand Mixer**	**Blender**	**Food Processor**
Beat egg whites	X		
Blend liquid mixtures	X	X	X
Chop foods			X
Crush ice		X	
Grate cheese			X
Grind dry ingredients (nuts, crackers)		X	X
Grind raw meat			X
Knead stiff dough	X		X
Mash potatoes	X		
Puree foods		X	X
Shred vegetables			X
Slice meats and vegetables			X
Whip cream	X		

9-13 *Mixers, blenders, and food processors perform some overlapping functions, but one appliance cannot completely replace another.*

Electric Skillets

A thermostat controls the temperature throughout the entire cooking process in an electric skillet. The electric skillet can take the place of the oven in some instances, thus saving energy. You can use it to fry, roast, pan-broil, stew, or simmer foods. You can also use it to bake casserole dishes, quick breads, cakes, custards, and desserts.

An electric skillet should have a high dome cover to provide maximum capacity and versatility. The cover should have a vent. Also look for a clearly visible heat indicator light and a cooking surface that suits your needs. Aluminum is least expensive, stainless steel is durable, and a nonstick coating provides easy cleaning.

Be sure the heat control is off before connecting or disconnecting the skillet. Remove acidic foods immediately after cooking to prevent discoloration of the pan. Be sure to allow the skillet to cool to room temperature before cleaning it. Running cold water in a hot pan can cause warping.

Q: Do long cooking times cause a loss of nutrients in foods prepared in a slow cooker?

A: No. Low cooking temperatures used in a slow cooker help preserve heat-sensitive vitamins. In addition, water-soluble nutrients are retained in the cooking liquid that is served with meals from a slow cooker.

Slow Cookers

Slow cookers are versatile, timesaving appliances. You can use them to prepare pasta sauces, roasts, and a range of one-dish meals, such as soups and stews. You can combine ingredients in a slow cooker in the morning. At the end of the day, you will have a meal that is ready to eat without much additional preparation time. See 9-14.

Most slow cookers have at least two heat settings for cooking. Some also have a setting for keeping cooked food warm during serving. The cooking vessel on some models can be placed on a rangetop. This saves dishes when browning meat is the first step in a slow-cooker recipe. It also allows leftovers to be stored and reheated in the same container in which they were cooked. The heating base of some slow cookers doubles as an electric griddle for extra versatility. Some models feature a glass dome cover that can also serve as a casserole or serving dish.

Look for a model with a removable cooking vessel that has a nonstick surface for easy cleaning. Some cooking vessels and lids are dishwasher safe. Use care not to use abrasive cleaners, which can scratch glass covers and nonstick surfaces. Use a damp, soapy cloth to wipe the heating base clean. Avoid immersing it in water.

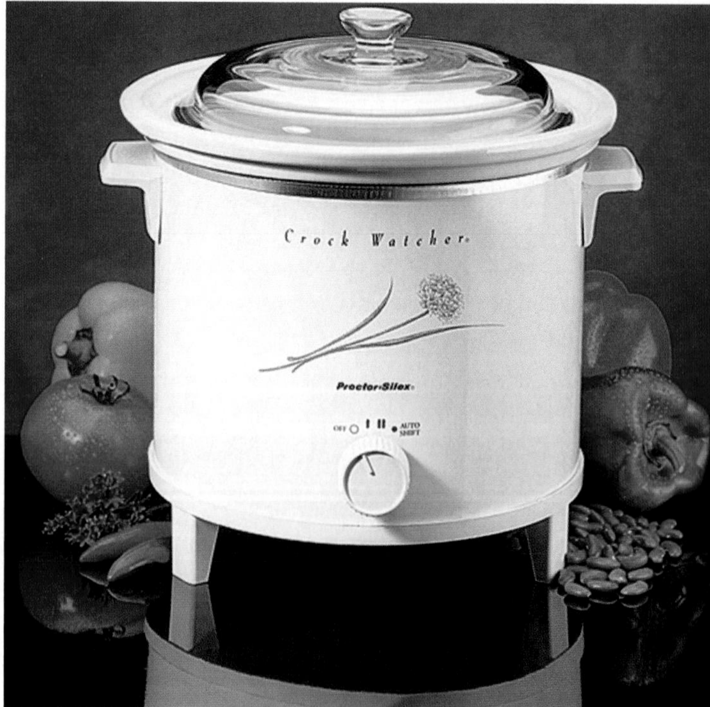

Proctor-Silex

9-14 Slow cookers allow you to serve hot, home-cooked meals without a lot of last minute preparation.

Bread Machines

Bread machines mix and knead bread dough. They allow the dough to rise, and then they bake the bread. See 9-15. Some machines feature a viewing window so you can see how

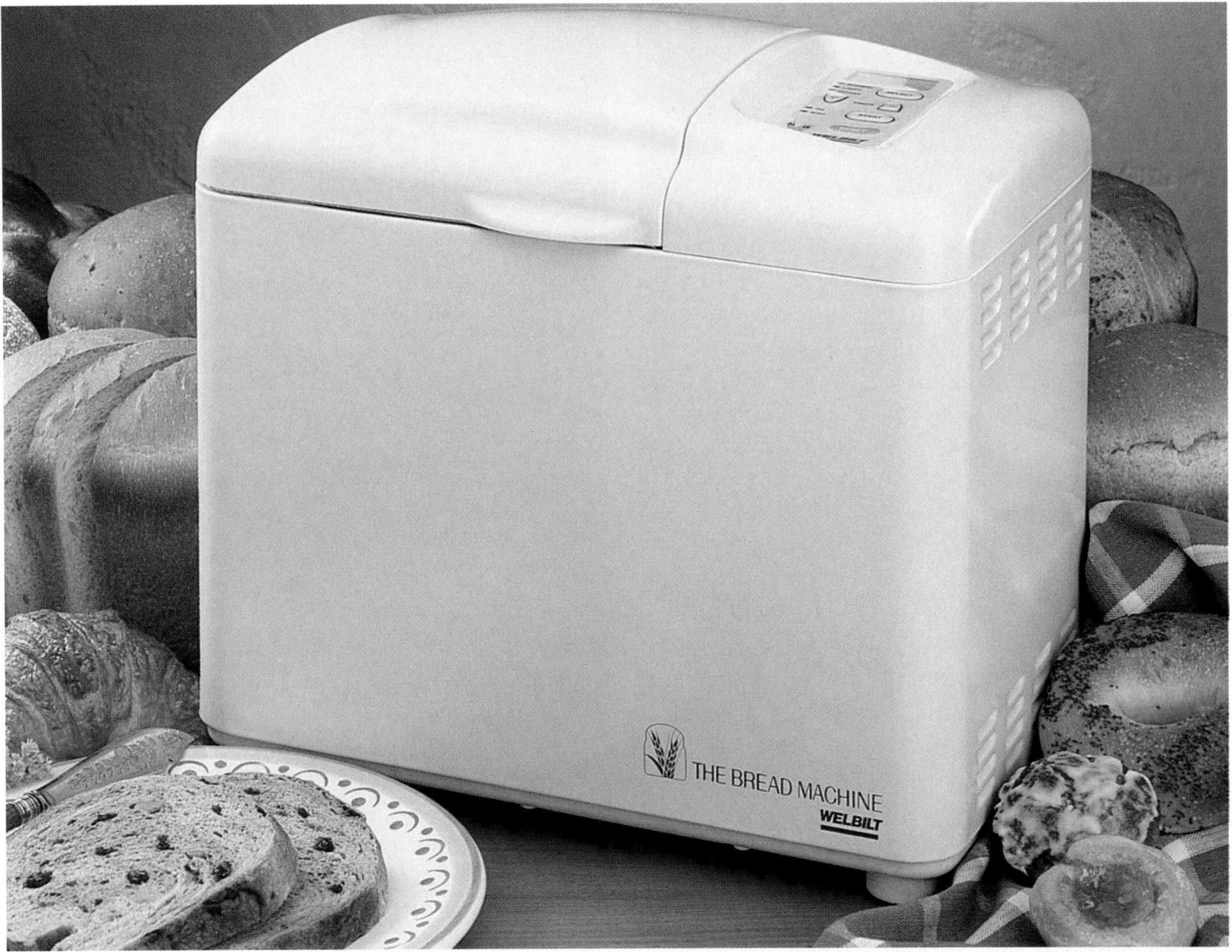

Welbilt

9-15 A bread machine does everything needed to prepare homemade bread except measure the ingredients!

the dough is progressing. A manual setting allows you to use a bread machine to prepare dough for pizza, rolls, and other yeast products. You must then shape these products by hand and bake them in a conventional oven.

Many models feature a timer. This allows you to preset the bread machine to begin baking at a later time. You should not use this feature if you are preparing a recipe that includes perishable ingredients like milk and eggs.

When shopping for a bread machine, consider the loaf size you want. Different machines produce different sizes, and some machines produce more than one size loaf.

Do not unplug the appliance during kneading or baking. This may cause the bread to bake improperly. Wait for the appliance to cool down before touching or cleaning it. Be aware that some parts of the bread machine may have nonstick surfaces that can be scratched by metal utensils.

Other Portable Kitchen Appliances

In addition to the small appliances discussed, there are many others available on the market. These include pasta makers, cappuccino makers, electric tea kettles, and iced tea makers. Electric woks, knives, coffee grinders, ice cream makers, waffle bakers, and grills are also among the variety of portable appliances offered. See 9-16.

Many portable appliances are versatile, performing several functions. Others do just one task. These single-function appliances are often fad items that appear on the market one year and disappear the next. Others meet real

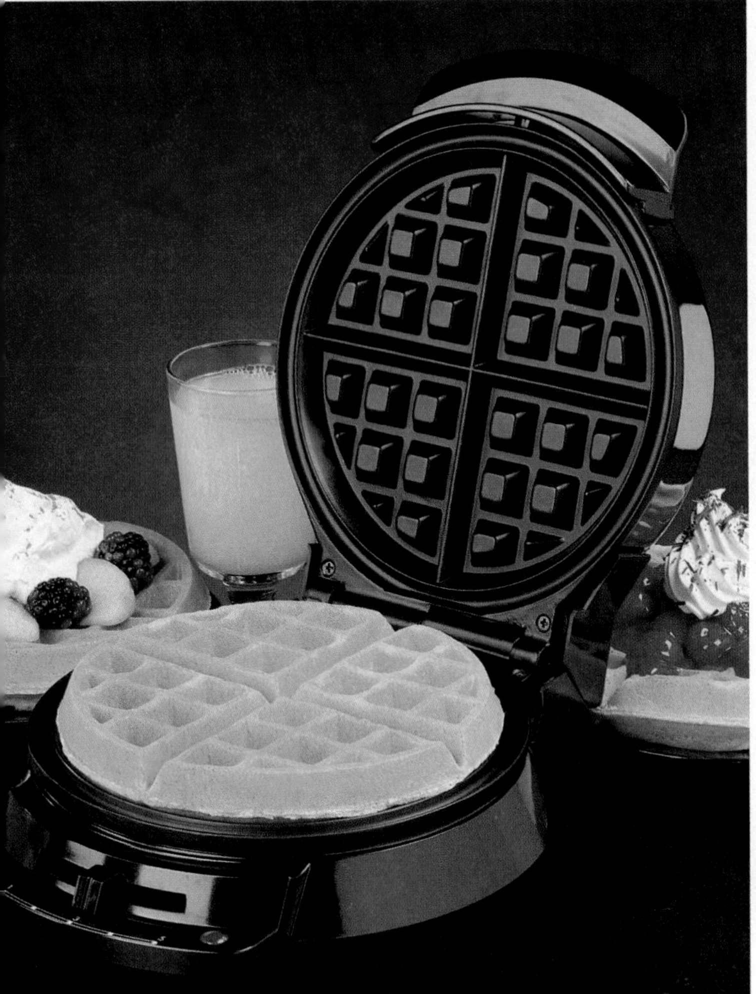

Hamilton Beach

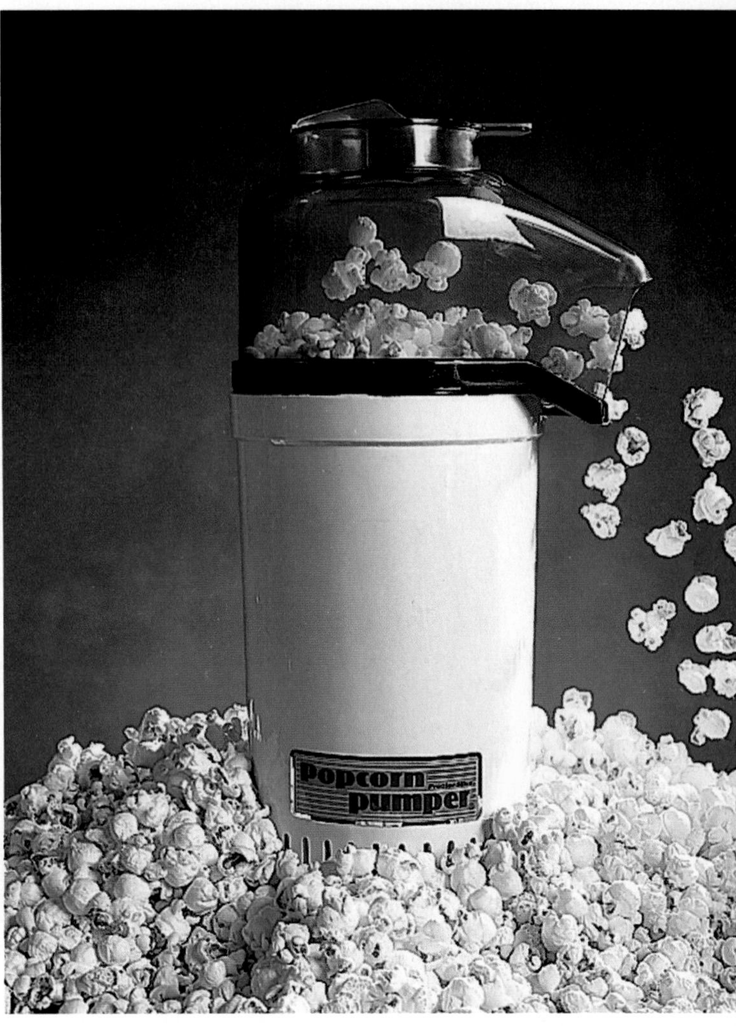

Proctor-Silex

9-16 From making golden brown waffles to popping fresh, hot popcorn, portable appliances are available to perform a broad range of kitchen tasks.

consumer needs and become lasting options for appliance buyers.

When choosing a more specialized appliance, consider your storage space. Think about how often you will use the appliance. Also check to see if you have another appliance that will perform the same task. As with all appliances, make your selections based on need, available features, quality construction, and ease of use and care.

Chapter 9 Review

Choosing Kitchen Appliances

Summary

You can do nearly every kitchen task more easily with the help of appliances. Use available information to help you make wise consumer choices. Safety seals on appliances assure you the appliances have been tested to work safely. Warranties state what you can expect from a manufacturer if an appliance does not perform as intended. EnergyGuide and ENERGY STAR labels help you choose appliances that are energy efficient.

Major kitchen appliances handle the basic tasks of cooking, storage, and cleanup. Cooking appliances include gas and electric ranges and microwave ovens. Refrigerators and freezers store perishable foods; dishwashers ease cleanup.

All major appliances come in several sizes and styles. Different models offer different features. Major appliances are expensive. You must weigh your options carefully to choose the appliances that best meet your family's needs. Following manufacturers' recommendations for use and care will help your appliances work properly and last for a long time.

There are many portable appliances available to help do food preparation tasks. These include toasters, mixers, blenders, food processors, coffeemakers, can openers, electric skillets, slow cookers, and bread machines. When choosing portable appliances, choose those that are convenient to use and store. Look for well-built models that provide the features you desire.

Review What You Have Read

Write your answers on a separate sheet of paper.

1. Give two suggestions for buying appliances that have met safety standards.
2. Explain the difference between a full warranty and a limited warranty.
3. List three examples of the trend toward the use of high-tech electronics in new major appliances.
4. What types of fuel hookups are required to run electric and gas ranges?
5. Explain the difference between self-cleaning ovens and continuous cleaning ovens.
6. Which style of microwave oven offers the greatest choice of features?
7. List three basic styles of refrigerators.
8. What two safety features should consumers seek when buying freezers?
9. Describe two energy-saving features available on some dishwasher models.
10. What are smart appliances?
11. List five questions to consider when purchasing portable appliances.
12. What is the advantage of using a toaster oven over using a full-sized oven when baking small food items?
13. Which type of mixer is best for heavy-duty mixing jobs?
14. True or false. Blenders can be used to whip cream.
15. True or false. For most efficient operation, food processors should be filled to capacity before processing.
16. Why should a coffeemaker be thoroughly cleaned after each use?
17. What are five cooking methods that can be done using an electric skillet?
18. Name two features that would make a slow cooker easy to clean.
19. What is the advantage of a timer feature on a bread machine?
20. What are three factors consumers should consider when thinking about buying a specialized portable appliance?

Build Your Basic Skills

1. **Writing.** Investigate appliance testing at Underwriters Laboratories or another testing agency. Find out what kinds of tests appliances must pass in order to meet safety standards. Write a brief report of your findings.
2. **Verbal.** Visit an appliance or department store. Compare the prices and features of several models of the major or portable appliance of your choice. Ask about the warranties that come with each model. Find out if service contracts are available. Check safety features and energy ratings. Use your findings to give an oral report in class.

Build Your Thinking Skills

1. **Compare.** Bake equal portions of a casserole, such as macaroni and cheese, in a conventional oven and a microwave oven. Compare the cooking times and the quality of the dishes. If possible, also compare the results using a convection oven.
2. **Evaluate.** Look through a catalog or an Internet site that offers a variety of portable appliances. Evaluate the functions of each appliance. Make a three-column table on a sheet of paper. In the first column, list all the types of portable appliances that are available. Place a check in the second column beside appliances that perform a variety of functions. Place a check in the third column beside appliances that perform a function another appliance can do. Use your list as the basis for a discussion of how portable appliances meet consumer needs.

Apply Technology

1. Work in a small group to prepare a poster illustrating the features and advantages of smart kitchen appliances that are linked to a home computer and/or the Internet.
2. Use a kitchen appliance with programmable features. Then evaluate whether these features would truly save a meal manager time and effort.

Using Workplace Skills

Gary works on the assembly line at the CookCraft appliance factory. He uses hand tools to mount clocks on ranges. Gary has seen many of his coworkers quickly tire of doing this routine task day after day. Some workers quit; others pay little attention to their work and are eventually fired for failing to meet quality standards.

To be a successful employee and avoid the fate of his coworkers, Gary needs positive personal qualities. Put yourself in Gary's place and answer the following questions about your need for and use of these traits:

A. What positive personal qualities would you find useful as an appliance line assembler?
B. How will having each of these personal qualities help you deal with the routine nature of your work?
C. How could you use your personal qualities to have a positive influence on your coworkers?
D. What is a skill you would need in this job? Briefly explain why this skill would be important.

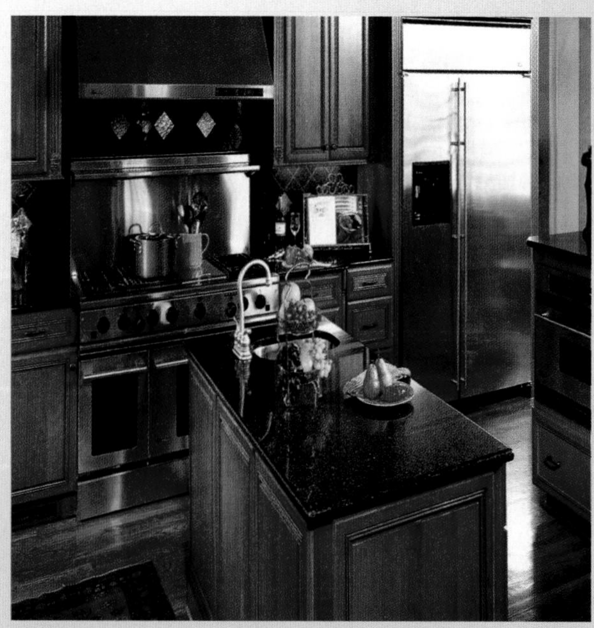

Chapter 10
Kitchen Utensils

Housewares Designer
Originates and develops ideas to design the form of manufactured housewares products.

Wholesale Housewares Demonstrator
Demonstrates use, care, and features of kitchen utensils to encourage retail business owners to carry products in their stores.

Cutlery Grinder
Sharpens knives, cleavers, and other fine-edged cutting tools, using whetstone and grinding and polishing wheels.

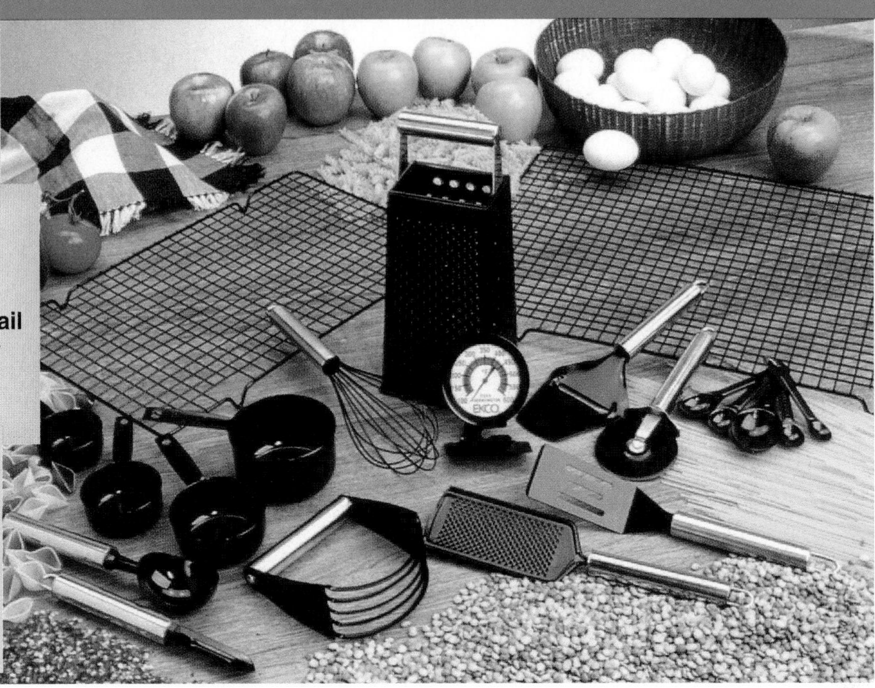

EKCO

Terms to Know

whisk
stockinette
serrated blade
tang
French knife
colander
pitting
porcelain enamel
nonstick finish
saucepan
pot
double boiler
pressure saucepan
springform pan
casserole

Objectives

After studying this chapter, you will be able to

- identify various small kitchen utensils and discuss their functions.
- explain how to select and care for cooking and baking utensils.
- demonstrate the use of various pieces of small kitchen equipment, cookware, and bakeware.

Small equipment can do much to save time and increase efficiency. Housewares departments in many stores carry a wide variety of kitchen gadgets. You need many of these small tools for meal preparation. You may not really need others, but they are helpful.

Small Equipment

Choose tools that best meet your needs and budget. Before buying small equipment, ask yourself the following questions.

- What kinds of kitchen tasks do I perform and how often do I perform them? You may not need to buy a specialized piece of equipment for a task you seldom perform.
- How is the equipment designed and how does it work? Avoid complicated equipment that is hard to assemble. Choose well-designed tools that are easy to operate.
- What quality of materials are used to make the equipment? For example, many tools are made of stainless steel, a rustproof and durable material.
- How are the handles constructed? The handles should fit your hand comfortably. They should be sturdy enough to withstand frequent use.

To receive the most satisfaction from your small equipment, select tools wisely. Follow manufacturers' directions for their use and care. Also, store your small equipment in a convenient location.

Small kitchen utensils can make many food preparation tasks easier. You can group utensils according to the types of tasks they perform.

Measuring Tools

Measuring tools are essential for baking. Failing to measure ingredients accurately can result in poor quality food products.

Liquid measures are made of glass or clear plastic. Use them to measure liquid ingredients, such as milk, water, and vegetable oil. They should have handles, pouring lips, and clearly marked measurements. The most common sizes available are 1 cup, 2 cup, and 4 cup. (Metric liquid measures are 250 mL, 500 mL, and 1 L.)

Dry measures are made of metal or plastic. Use them to measure dry ingredients, such as flour and sugar, and solid ingredients like shortening and peanut butter. They are commonly sold in sets containing ¼-cup, ⅓-cup, ½-cup, and 1-cup sizes. (Metric dry measures are 50 mL, 125 mL, and 250 mL.)

Measuring spoons are also made of metal or plastic. Use them to measure small amounts of liquid and dry ingredients. A typical set includes ¼-teaspoon, ½-teaspoon, 1-teaspoon, and 1-tablespoon sizes. (Metric measures are 1 mL, 2 mL, 5 mL, 15 mL, and 25 mL.) See 10-1.

Mixing Tools

Virtually every recipe requires you to mix ingredients together. You can use spoons for many mixing tasks. *Wooden spoons* are available in many sizes and shapes for stirring and mixing. They will not scratch pan surfaces, and their handles remain cool. Use *slotted spoons* to remove pieces of food from a liquid. Use *heavy metal spoons* to stir thick mixtures.

Use a *rotary beater* to beat, blend, and incorporate air into foods. When you manually turn the crank, the beaters rotate. Beating speed depends on how fast you turn the crank.

Use a ***whisk*** to incorporate air into foods. Use them for eggs, soufflés, and meringues. When preparing sauces, use a whisk to prevent

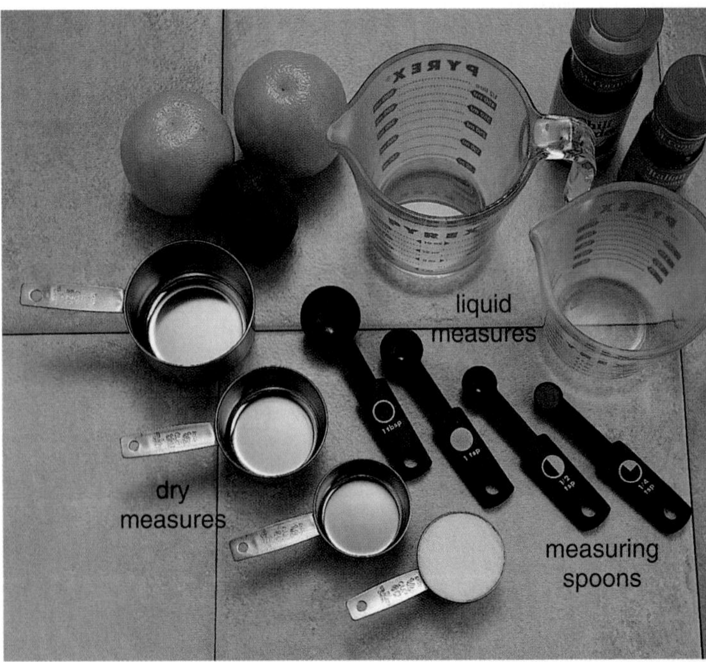

EKCO

10-1 Using the proper tools to accurately measure ingredients helps ensure the outcome of a recipe.

lumps from forming. Most chefs prefer a whisk to a rotary beater. See 10-2.

Baking Tools

A number of tools are used just for preparing baked goods. One such tool is a *sifter.* Use a sifter to blend dry ingredients and remove lumps from powdered sugar.

A *pastry blender* is made of several thin, curved pieces of metal attached to a handle. Use it to blend shortening with flour when making pastry. You can also use it to blend butter and cheese mixtures.

Use *pastry brushes* to brush butter or sauces on foods. You can also use them to remove crumbs from a cake before frosting it and to baste foods in the oven. For basting, the pastry brush must be heat-resistant.

Protect the Planet

Use handheld kitchen utensils instead of electrical appliances whenever possible. Items like electric cheese graters and power potato peelers may seem like nifty gadgets, but they use energy unnecessarily.

Use a rolling pin, pastry cloth, and stockinette when rolling dough or pastry. Place dough on the *pastry cloth* and roll it with the *rolling pin.* The cloth keeps the dough from sticking to the counter while it is being kneaded or rolled. The ***stockinette*** covers the rolling pin and prevents the dough from sticking to the rolling pin.

Spatulas can be made of plastic or metal. They come in various widths and lengths. All spatulas should be somewhat flexible. Use *bent-edged spatulas* to remove cookies from a baking tray. You can also use them to turn meats, fish, pancakes, eggs, and omelets.

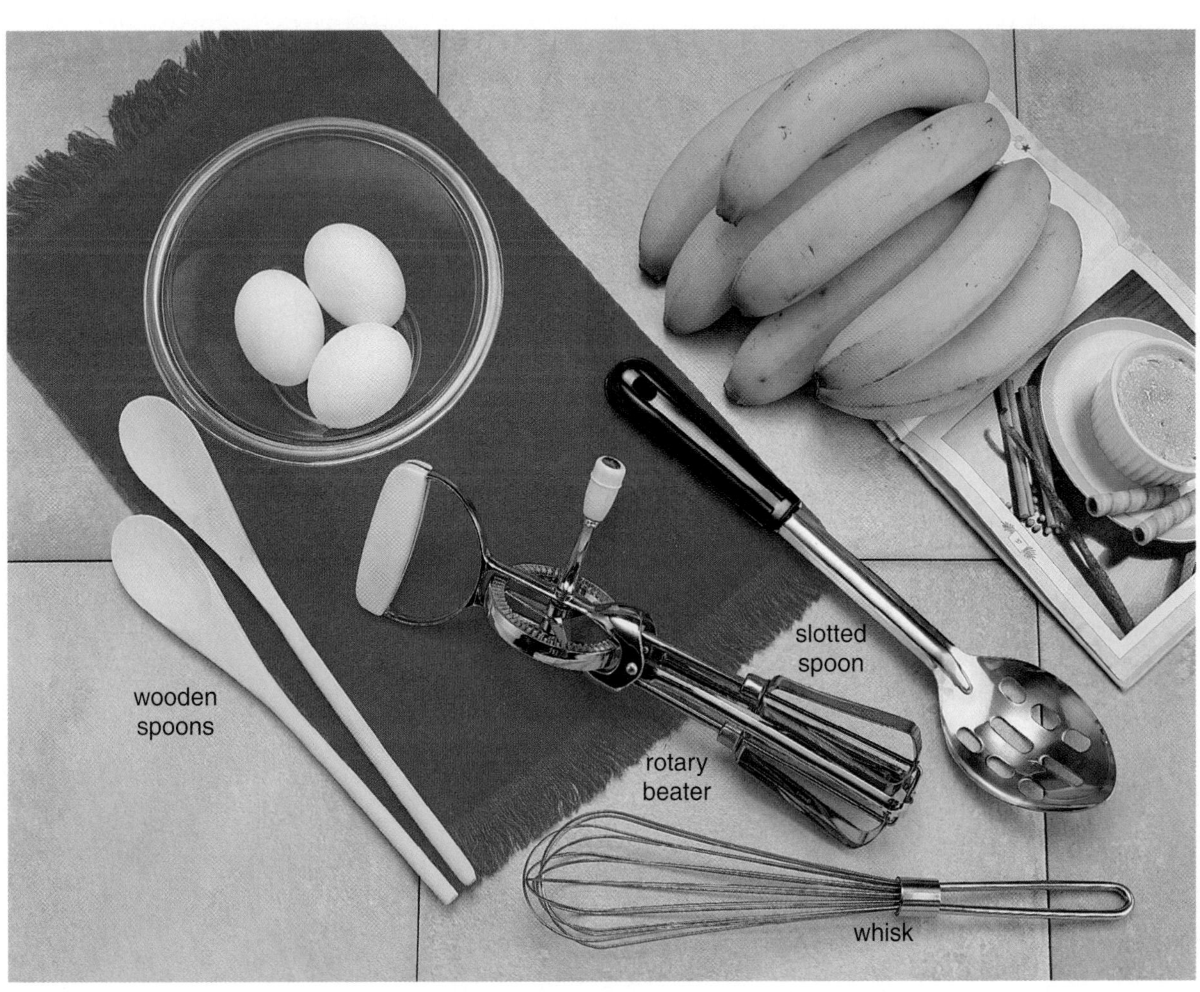

10-2 *Choose the best tool for each mixing task—stirring, blending, beating, or incorporating air.*

Use *straight-edged spatulas* to spread cake icings and meringues and to level ingredients in dry measures. Use *rubber spatulas* to scrape bowls and saucepans and to fold one ingredient into another. See 10-3.

Thermometers

Being able to accurately measure the temperature of a food product can improve your cooking success. It can also help you reduce your risk of foodborne illness. Many foods contain harmful bacteria that can be killed by thorough cooking. Use a thermometer when cooking protein foods, such as meat, poultry, fish, egg dishes, and casseroles. Be sure these foods have reached recommended internal temperatures.

Several types of thermometers are available. *Oven-safe thermometers* are designed to be placed in a food while it is cooking. *Instant-read thermometers* are inserted into a food at the end of cooking time. This type of thermometer will provide an accurate reading in a matter of seconds.

Special thermometers are available for candy making and deep frying. *Candy thermometers* clip to the side of a pan. They are marked with the temperatures needed for different kinds of candies. *Deep-fat thermometers* also clip to the side of a pan. They register oil temperatures for deep frying foods like doughnuts and French fries.

Two other types of thermometers are important pieces of kitchen equipment. Use a *refrigerator-freezer thermometer* to keep track of the temperatures at which you store foods. The refrigerator should not be more than 40°F (4°C). Keep the freezer at no more than 0°F (-18°C). An *oven thermometer* can help you make sure your oven heats to the temperature for which you set it. An oven that overheats can cause

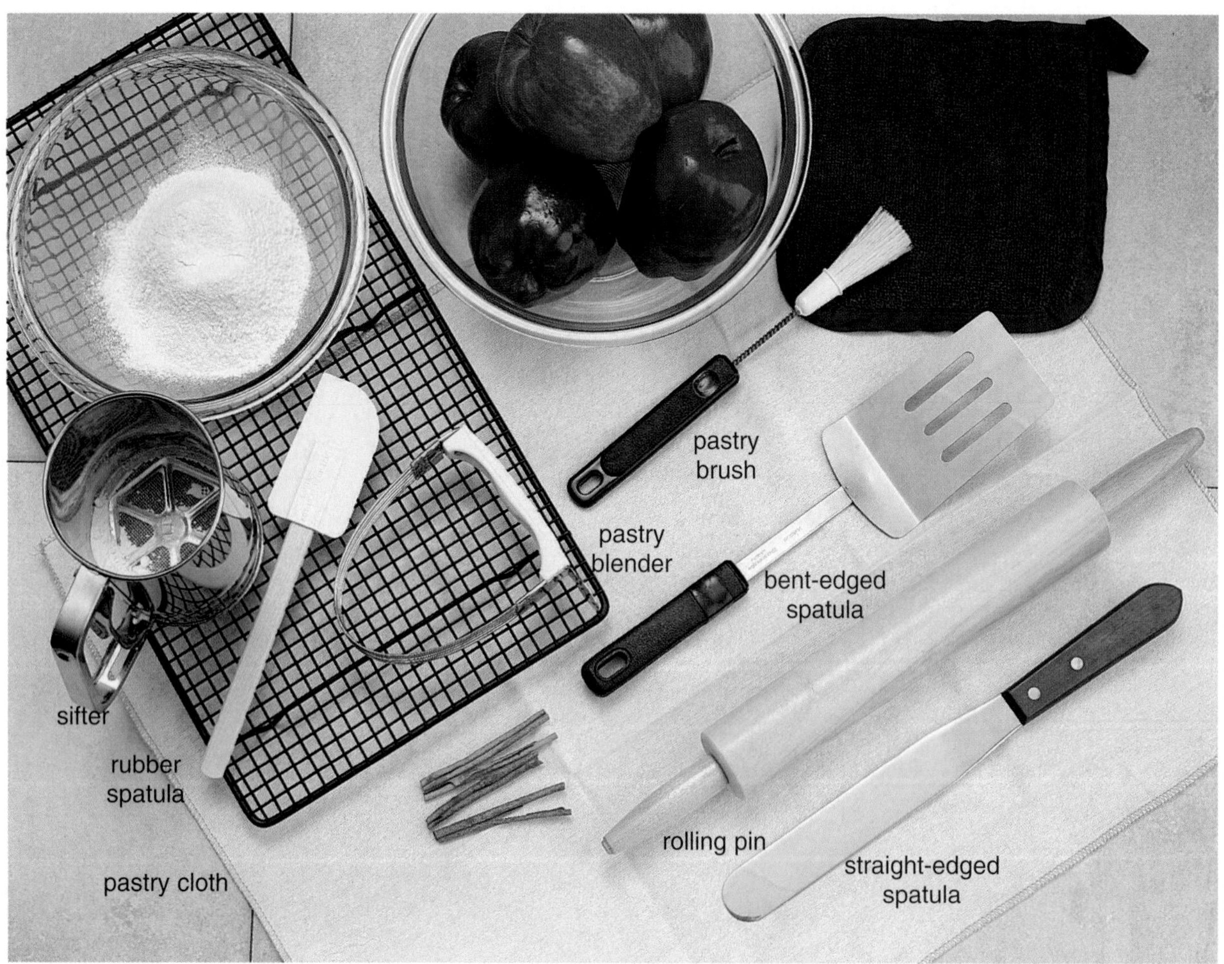

***10-3** Using the correct tools can affect the quality of baked products.*

foods to burn, whereas an oven that underheats can lengthen cooking times. See 10-4.

Cutting Tools

Preparing ingredients often involves a variety of cutting tasks. You can use *kitchen shears* to snip herbs and trim vegetables. You can also use them to cut meat, dough, cookies, and pizza. *Poultry shears* are heavier and sharper than ordinary kitchen shears. You can use them to cut through fowl and fish bones. Use kitchen shears for food preparation tasks only.

Use a *peeler* to remove the outer surface of fruits and vegetables. A peeler removes only a thin layer, so nutrients lying near the surface are preserved. You can also use peelers to make decorative carrot, chocolate, and cheese curls for garnishes.

A *shredder-grater* is a four-sided metal tool used to shred and grate foods such as cheese and cabbage. Openings of different sizes make it possible to grate and shred food into small or large pieces.

Cutting boards can be made of a variety of materials and are usually rectangular in shape.

Q: Why do some of the foods I prepare seem to be undercooked even when I check them with a thermometer?

A: A thermometer is only helpful if it reads temperatures correctly. The directions that come with your kitchen thermometers should tell you how to test their accuracy. The directions should also tell you how to *calibrate,* or adjust, your thermometers if they are not precise.

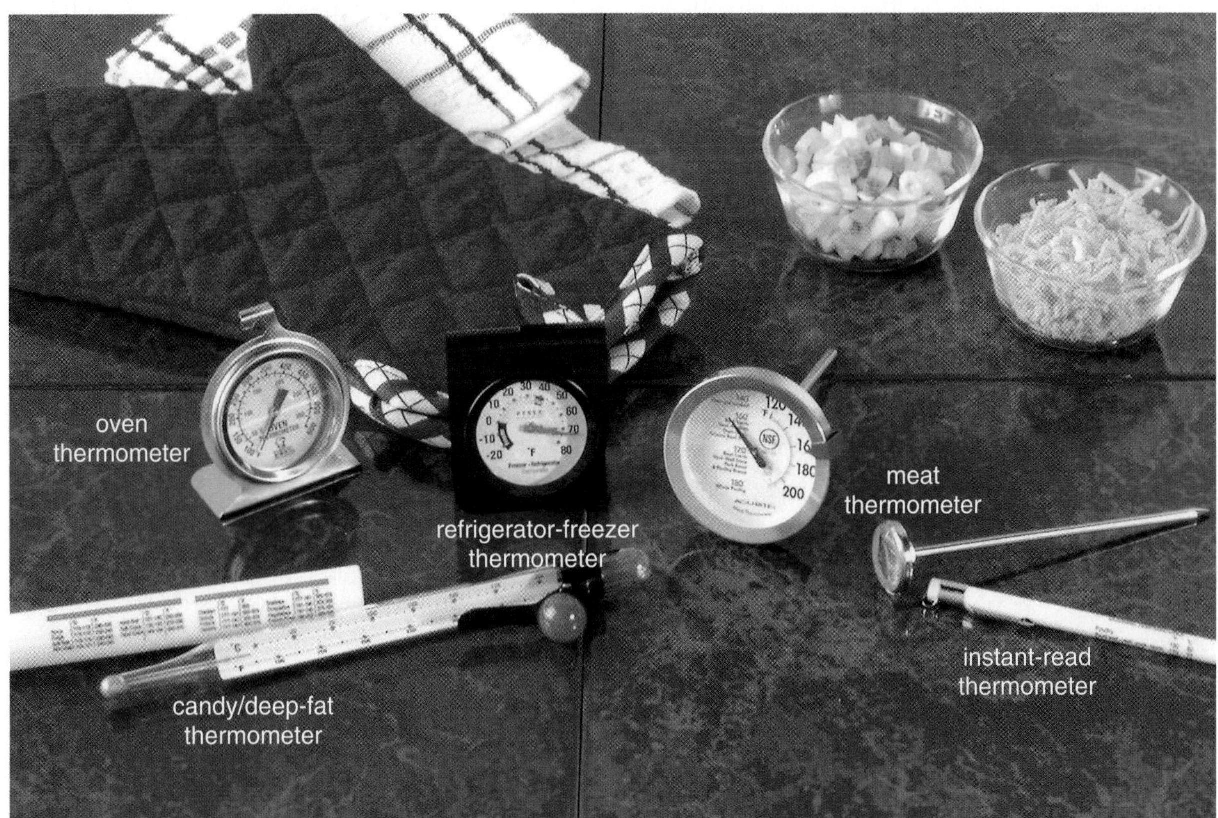

Jack Klasey

***10-4** A variety of kitchen thermometers will help you accurately measure food and appliance temperatures to assure safe, quality food products.*

They are sometimes built into a cabinet or counter. Use a cutting board when cutting and chopping foods to protect tables and countertops. See 10-5.

Knives

You will use knives for many kitchen tasks. You can use them to cut, slice, chop, and bone. Different types of knives are used for different cutting tasks.

Knife blades can be smooth or serrated. A ***serrated blade*** has a sawtooth edge. This type of blade is especially helpful for cutting bread without flattening the air cells. Knives are made of carbon steel or stainless steel. Carbon steel is easy to sharpen because it is soft. However, it will stain and rust easily unless you wash and dry the knife soon after each use. Stainless steel is durable and will not rust, but stainless is so hard that sharpening is difficult. (Some manufacturers, however, produce a type of stainless steel that is soft enough to sharpen easily.)

Knife handles can be made of wood, plastic, or bone. High-quality knives usually have hardwood handles. A knife handle should fit your hand comfortably. It should also be properly balanced and constructed for maximum safety. For safety, the ***tang*** (prong of the blade that attaches to the handle) should extend at least one-third of the way into the handle. At least two rivets should join the blade and handle. Three rivets should join larger knives. Never soak a knife, as soaking can cause the handle to loosen.

The most popular kitchen knives are French knives, slicing knives, utility knives, and paring knives. A ***French knife,*** also known as a chef knife, is the most versatile of all kitchen knives. Use it to cut, chop, and dice fruits and vegetables. You might choose a *slicing knife* for cutting meat, poultry, bread, and soft vegetables, such as tomatoes. A *utility knife* is a good all-around knife. You can use it to trim fat from meat and cut tender vegetables, cheese, and cold cuts. A *paring knife* is the smallest knife used in the kitchen. Use it to peel fruits and vegetables. See 10-6.

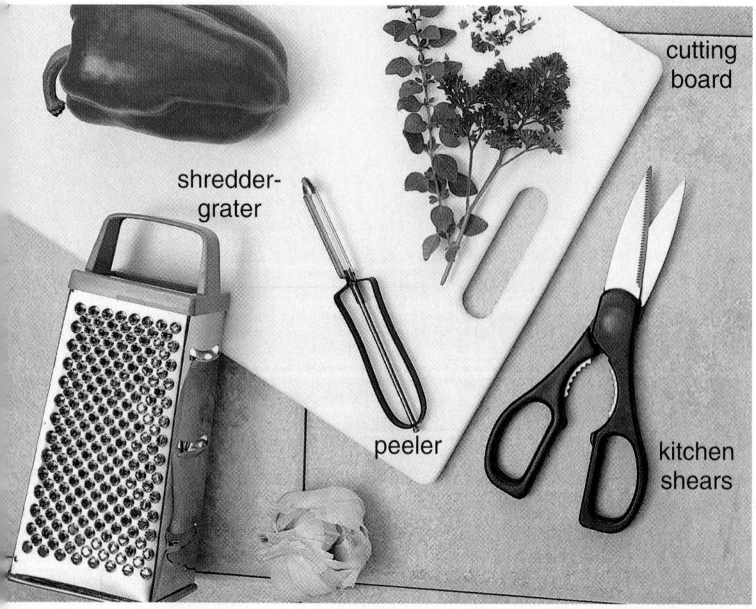

__10-5__ A number of cutting tools are available so food can be cut into pieces of just the right size and shape for any recipe.

Other Preparation Tools

Tongs usually are made of metal. They are helpful for turning meats and fried foods. You might also use them for handling such foods as corn on the cob, hard-cooked eggs, and baked potatoes.

Kitchen forks are made of heavy-duty metal. Use them when transferring heavy meats and poultry. You can also use a kitchen fork to turn heavy foods.

Ladles are round cups attached to long handles. They come in different sizes for different purposes. Use a ladle for dipping and pouring. You might use a ladle to serve punches, soups, sauces, gravies, and salad dressings.

A *baster* is a long tube attached to a flexible bulb. A baster uses suction to collect juices from meat and poultry for basting (covering foods with liquid). You can also use it to skim fat from soups and gravies.

Colanders are perforated bowls used to drain fruits, vegetables, and pasta. A colander should have heat-proof handles.

Strainers are available in several sizes. Use them to separate liquid and solid foods. See 10-7.

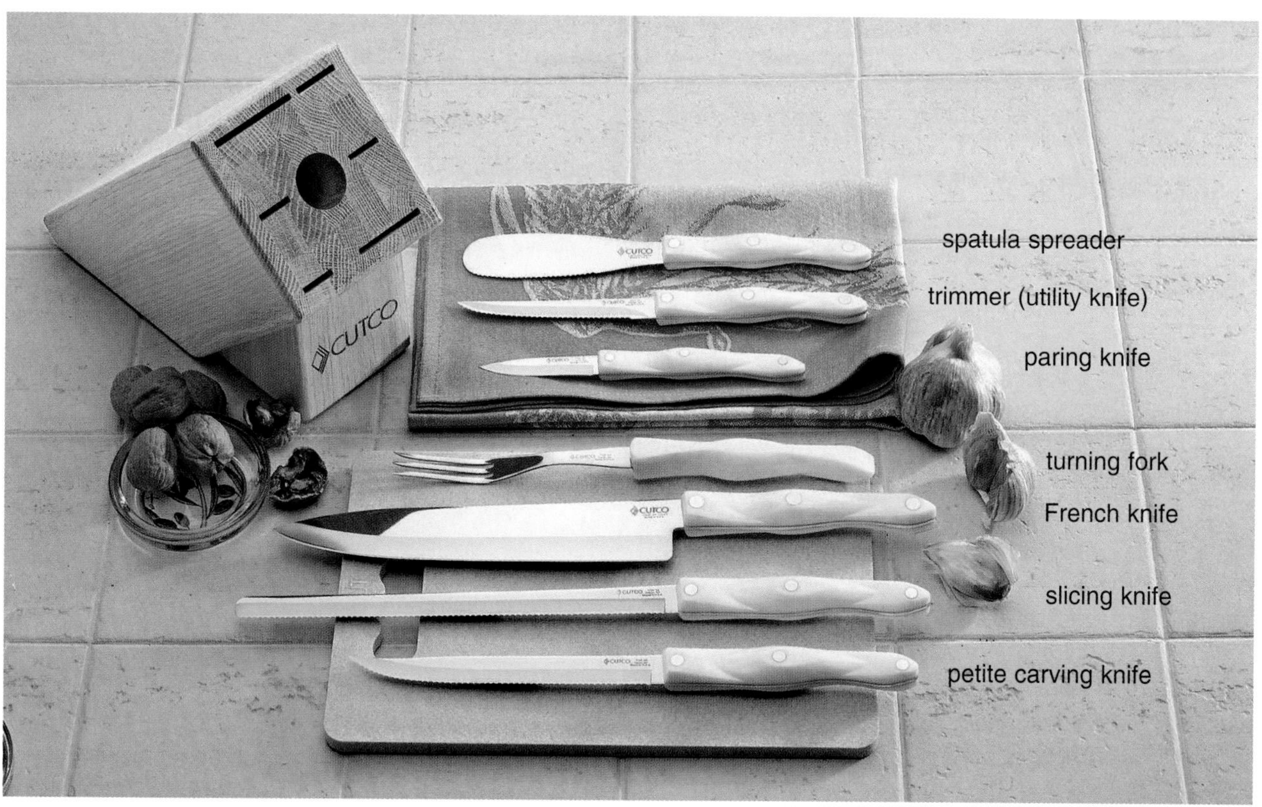

Cutco

10-6 Choose different knives for different cutting needs.

Can openers have round blades that puncture the tops of cans. Most can openers have handles that you squeeze to keep the blade in the proper position. Then you turn a key on the side of the can opener. This causes the blade to turn and cut around the edge of the can.

Cooking and Baking Utensils

Before buying cooking and baking utensils, consider your needs and the special features each utensil offers. All cooking and baking utensils should be durable. They should conduct heat evenly and be easy to clean. They should last a long time and maintain their appearance with normal care.

You can buy cooking and baking utensils separately or in sets. Cooking utensils include pots, pans, skillets, double boilers, griddles, and omelet pans used on top of the range. Baking utensils include cookie sheets, cake pans, bread pans, muffin pans, pie plates, casseroles,

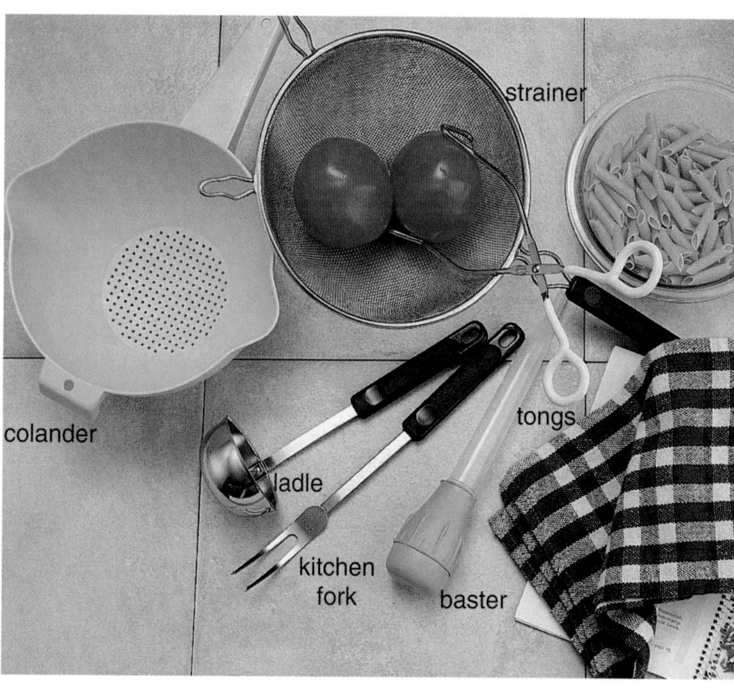

10-7 Small utensils are designed to perform a variety of food preparation tasks.

and roasters. Many conventional bakeware pieces can also be used in a microwave oven.

Cookware and Bakeware Materials

Cooking and baking utensils are made from a number of materials. Metal, glass, ceramic, and plastic materials are the most popular of these materials.

Metal Materials

Several metals are used for conventional cookware and bakeware. Cast iron is a cookware material that distributes and holds heat well. Its porous surface holds oils that help prevent sticking. Iron is heavy, however. It can also rust, retain food flavors, and lose its nonstick qualities unless you care for it properly.

Aluminum is a lightweight, corrosion-resistant cookware and bakeware material. It conducts heat rapidly and is reasonably priced. It comes in several thicknesses. Cast aluminum is used for heavier utensils, such as skillets. Sheet aluminum is used for lighter utensils, such as cookie sheets. Aluminum is susceptible to scratches, dents, and detergent damage. Food and minerals can cause ***pitting*** (marking with tiny indentations). Hard water, eggs, and alkalis, such as baking soda, can cause darkening.

Copper is a good heat conductor. However, you cannot use pure copper utensils for cooking. When heated, copper reacts with food and forms poisonous compounds. Copper cooking utensils must be lined with another material to make them safe for cooking. You must clean copper with a special cleaner to keep it from discoloring.

Stainless steel is an alloy of steel, nickel, and chromium. It resists stains, does not discolor, and is strong and durable. However, it does not distribute heat evenly, so hot spots can occur. Stainless steel may darken if overheated. It is relatively expensive.

Some stainless steel pieces have a copper or aluminum bottom to improve heat distribution. Other pieces may have a core of copper, carbon steel, or other heat-conducting metal. These materials help conduct heat across the pan bottom and up the sides. A heat-conducting core prevents scorching, conserves fuel, and allows low temperature cooking.

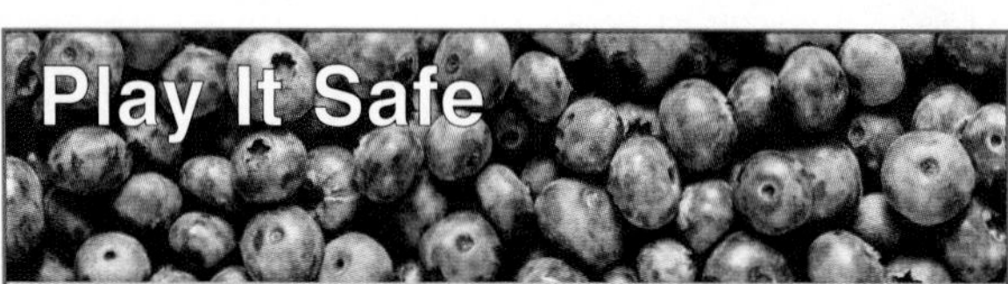

Be sure to wash the tops of cans before opening them. This prevents any dust that might be on the cans from getting into the food. Also, wash the blade of the can opener, whether manual or electric, after each use. Food residue left on a can opener blade provides a medium for bacterial growth.

Glass and Ceramic Materials

Glass and ceramic materials are used for a range of cookware and bakeware pieces. These materials are attractive. However, you must handle them with care to avoid cracking, chipping, and breaking.

Transparent glass utensils allow you to see food while it is cooking. Glass does not react with the flavors or colors of food. However, glass is a poor heat conductor. See 10-8.

Glass-ceramic is strong and durable. It can withstand a wide range of temperatures. This property allows you to take glass-ceramic utensils from the freezer and put them directly in the oven. This material has the drawbacks of developing hot spots and heating unevenly.

Porcelain enamel is a glasslike material. It is fused to a base metal at very high temperatures. The outer surfaces of metal cookware and bakeware are often coated with porcelain

Q: Does cooking foods in cast iron affect their nutritional value?

A: The iron content of some foods can be increased slightly when the foods are cooked in cast iron cookware. This is especially true of acidic foods, such as those containing tomatoes or vinegar, that simmer for an extended period. The acid dissolves small amounts of iron, which you consume when you eat the food.

enamel. This makes the utensils colorful and easy to clean.

Ceramic materials are made from nonmetallic minerals that are fired at very high temperatures. Ceramic materials include earthenware and terra-cotta. These materials are not suitable for rangetop cooking. However, they can retain heat well. This makes them good choices for many bakeware pieces.

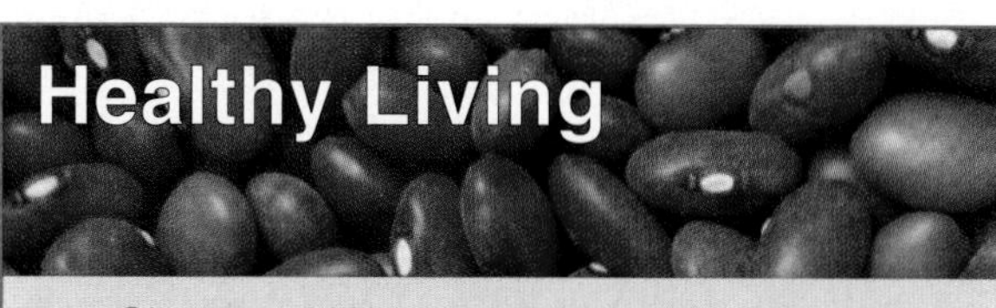

Choose skillets with a nonstick finish for frying. Because foods won't stick to the surface, you can reduce or eliminate added fat when you cook. This will help you reduce fat and calories in your diet.

Plastic Materials

Plastic utensils are dishwasher safe, stain-resistant, break-resistant, and easy to clean. However, plastic utensils cannot withstand oven temperatures above 350°F to 400°F (175°C to 205°C), depending on the type of plastic. They cannot withstand direct heat, either. This makes plastics impractical for broiling or rangetop cooking. Plastic bakeware, however, is excellent for use in microwave ovens.

Nonstick Finishes

Nonstick finishes prevent foods from sticking to utensils. They may be applied to both the inside and outside of cookware and bakeware for easier cooking and cleanup. The effectiveness of a nonstick finish depends on the type of finish and how it is applied. Take care to avoid damaging these finishes. Metal utensils and scouring pads can scratch them.

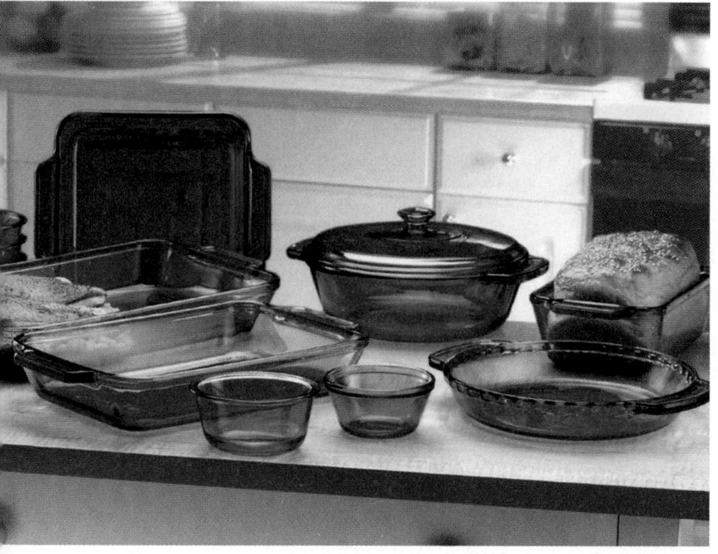

Anchor Hocking

10-8 Glass bakeware can be used to serve foods as well as prepare them.

Microwavable Materials

The main requirement for a microwave cookware material is that microwaves must be able to pass through it. Otherwise, the microwaves will not be able to reach the food. Microwaves can pass through materials such as ceramic, plastics, glass, wood, and paper. These materials can all be used for cooking in a microwave oven.

Metal cookware reflects microwaves and prevents them from cooking food in a microwave oven. Therefore, metal cookware is generally not recommended for microwave cooking. However, some cookware containing metal is specially designed for microwave use. Some microwave griddles and browning dishes use metal cooking surfaces to achieve the desired browning of foods. When considering these and other metal items for use in a microwave oven, refer to the manufacturer's directions.

Not all containers made from microwavable materials are microwave safe. For instance, you should not use cookware made from microwavable material if it has bands of metal trim. The trim can cause arcing. Disposable plastic containers from margarine and whipped toppings are not recommended for microwave cooking. They are made of soft plastics that may melt when they come in contact with hot food. This can cause chemicals from the plastics to get into the food. You should not use containers that absorb liquid, such as wooden bowls, when microwaving liquids. The moisture absorbed by such a container will attract microwave energy away from the food.

Cooking Utensils

You probably use saucepans and pots for cooking foods in water or other liquids over direct surface heat, 10-9. ***Saucepans*** generally have one handle. ***Pots*** have two handles. Sizes range from a 1 pint (0.5 L) saucepan to a 12 quart (12 L) stockpot. For maximum

Q: Do I have to purchase special cookware for use in my microwave oven?

A: No. Some cookware is specially designed for the way microwave ovens cook. You may have seen molded plastic pieces for microwaving foods like bacon, muffins, and popcorn. However, most conventional cookware made of materials other than metal can be used in microwave ovens.

cooking efficiency, the bottoms of pots and pans should be about the same diameter as the surface unit. Handles should be heat-resistant and comfortable to hold. You can buy some pots and pans with matching lids.

A ***double boiler*** is a small pan that fits into a larger pan. You put food into the smaller pan. Then you put a small amount of water in the larger pan. As the water simmers, the heat produced by the steam gently cooks the food.

Pressure saucepans cook foods more quickly than conventional saucepans. This is because as pressure increases, temperature increases. Choose a pressure saucepan that carries a safety seal. Be sure to read manufacturer's directions carefully before using a pressure saucepan.

Skillets are available in a variety of sizes with and without lids. Skillets have wide bottoms and low sides. They are generally heavier than saucepans. Use skillets for panbroiling foods or for cooking foods in a small amount of fat.

Griddles and omelet pans are variations of skillets. A *griddle* is a skillet without sides. It often is coated with a nonstick finish. Use it for grilling sandwiches and making foods like French toast and pancakes. An *omelet* or *crepe* pan is an uncovered skillet with a narrow bottom and sloping sides. Use it to make omelets and delicate French pancakes.

Baking Utensils

When selecting baking utensils, it is important to consider whether the utensil's surface is shiny or dull. The outer surface of a pan affects the amount of heat the pan absorbs. A shiny or bright surface reflects part of the heat away from the food. A dull or dark surface absorbs heat. Products baked in bright, shiny pans will have softer, lighter crusts. Products baked in dull, dark pans will have darker and crisper crusts.

Insulated bakeware is made from two sheets of metal. An air space between the two sheets creates a layer of insulation. This layer helps protect baked goods from overbrowning.

Cookie sheets are often made of aluminum. They are flat sheets of metal with a low rim on one or more sides for strength. Use them for baking cookies, toasting bread, and supporting small utensils, such as custard cups.

Cake, angel food, springform, jelly roll, pizza, muffin, and loaf pans are usually made of aluminum. Cake and loaf pans are also available in glass and ceramic materials. Many bakeware pieces are available in several sizes. See 10-10.

Cake pans can be round, square, or oblong. You can make angel food, sponge, and chiffon cakes in an *angel food cake pan.* It is a deep, round pan, narrower at the bottom than at the top. It has a tube in the center, and the bottom may be removable. A ***springform pan*** is also round and has a removable bottom. Its sides hook together with a latch or spring. Use springform pans for making cheesecakes, tortes, and

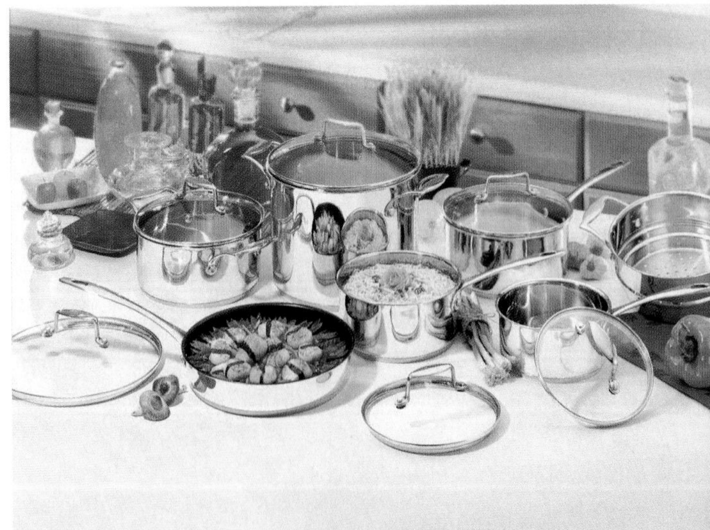

Revere

10-9 *Cookware comes in a variety of sizes and shapes for preparing all types of foods on top of the range.*

other desserts that are delicate and difficult to remove from the pan. A *jelly roll pan* is a large, shallow oblong pan. Use it to make sheet cakes and to bake the sponge cake for cake rolls. *Pizza pans* are large and round. They may have a narrow rim around the edge. *Muffin pans* are oblong pans with round depressions. Use them for baking muffins and cupcakes. Loaf pans are deep, narrow, oblong pans. You will use them most often for breads and loaf cakes.

Pie plates are round with sloping sides. They are generally made of glass or aluminum. Use them when making dessert and main dish pies.

Casseroles are baking dishes with high sides. They can be made of glass, glass-ceramic, or earthenware. Some casseroles are designed for freezer-to-oven use. *Soufflé* dishes are a variation of a casserole. They have high, steep sides.

Roasting pans can be oval or oblong. They are larger and heavier than pots, pans, and skillets. Most have high, dome lids, and many have racks or trivets.

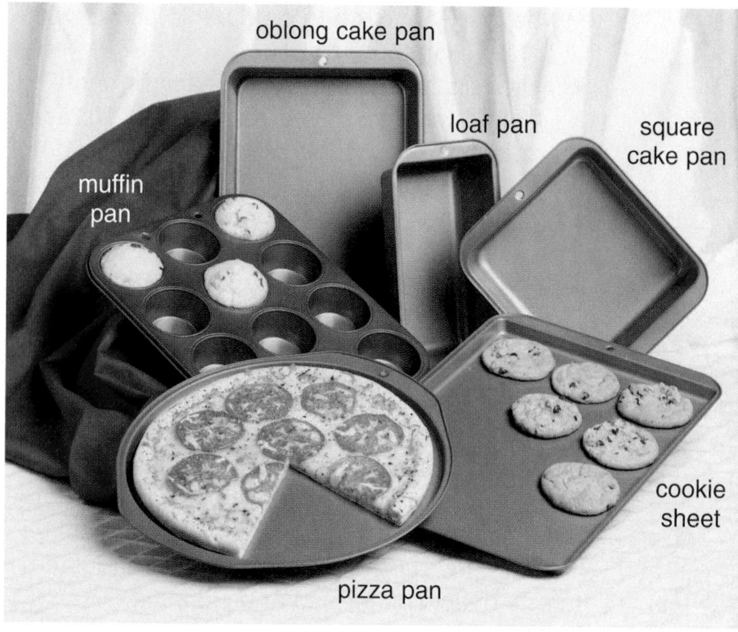

Baker's Secret

***10-10** Each piece of bakeware is designed for preparing specific kinds of food items in an oven.*

Microwave Cookware

Check use and care information to be sure cookware is designed for use in a microwave oven. The shape of cookware can affect how evenly foods cook in a microwave oven. Cookware shapes can also affect cooking time.

Round-shaped containers allow microwaves to hit food evenly. Microwaves can overlap in the corners of square cookware pieces. This causes food in the corners to overcook.

Ring-shaped pans give great results when microwaving cakes, meat loaves, and other foods. This shape accounts for the fact that foods tend to cook slower in the center of a microwave oven. The circular arrangement allows foods to cook more evenly. Ring shapes also allow microwaves to hit foods from the center as well as the top, bottom, and sides. This increased microwave penetration speeds cooking time. (You can improvise a ring-shaped pan by placing a microwavable glass in the center of a round container.)

Cookware pieces should correspond to the amount and kind of food you are microwaving. Choose single-serving pieces when cooking for one. They work well for quickly reheating leftovers. Try custard cups for poaching eggs one at a time. Use a rack with a slotted or raised surface when cooking meats so fats and juices can drain. Select deeper containers when cooking foods like milk that may boil over.

Select microwavable cookware in a variety of sizes and shapes to meet all your cooking needs. Pieces that nest together provide easy storage. Pieces with lids allow you to cover foods in the refrigerator and hold in steam in the microwave oven. See 10-11.

Choosing Cooking and Baking Utensils

Consider the following features when buying cooking and baking utensils:

- Utensils should be sturdy and well balanced to prevent tipping. All edges should be smooth. Pan bottoms should be flat for good heat conduction. Beware of crevices where food particles can collect.
- Handles should be heat-resistant, sturdy, and securely attached.
- Lids should be well constructed and should fit tightly. Handles on lids should be heat-resistant and easy to grasp with a pot holder.
- Utensils should be light enough for you to handle comfortably and safely. They should

be heavy enough to be durable and to withstand warping.
- Utensils should be able to stack or hang from a wall rack if you have limited storage space.

Use and Care of Cooking and Baking Utensils

To maintain your cooking and baking utensils, proper use and care are essential. Some materials only tolerate certain temperatures. You must condition some utensils before you use them. You must use special cleaning compounds to clean some utensils. Always read the use and care information that accompanies cooking and baking utensils. Follow manufacturer's directions for use and cleaning.

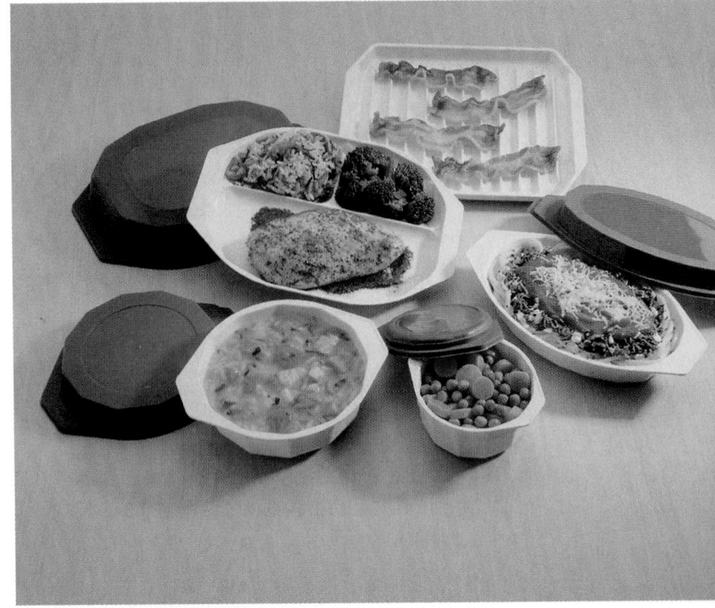

Nordic Ware

10-11 *Microwave cookware allows microwaves to pass through to the food. Lids speed cooking by holding in steam.*

Chapter 10 Review
Kitchen Utensils

Summary

Small kitchen equipment includes measuring, mixing, baking, and cutting tools as well as thermometers and other preparation tools. When selecting these items, think about the types of tasks you perform. Also consider the quality and cost of the tools.

Cookware refers to items used on top of the range. Bakeware includes items used in the oven. Cookware and bakeware are commonly made from metal, glass, ceramic, and plastic materials. In addition to the material, the shape and size of microwave cookware can affect its performance. When buying cookware and bakeware, look for pieces that are well made and that are easy to handle and store. Follow manufacturers' use and care directions.

Review What You Have Read

Write your answers on a separate sheet of paper.

1. What types of ingredients are measured with measuring spoons?
2. True or false. Most chefs prefer a rotary beater to a whisk.
3. Which type of spatula would be used to level ingredients in dry measures?
   A. Bent-edged spatula.
   B. Rubber spatula.
   C. Straight-edged spatula.
   D. None of the above.
4. What type of thermometer is inserted into a food at the end of cooking time?
5. List four uses for kitchen shears.
6. What is the smallest knife used in the kitchen?
   A. French knife.
   B. Paring knife.
   C. Slicing knife.
   D. Utility knife.
7. A perforated bowl used to drain fruits, vegetables, and pasta is a _____.
8. What are the four most common types of materials used to make cooking and baking utensils?
9. True or false. Pure copper cannot be used for cooking because it reacts with food and forms poisonous compounds.
10. Explain why certain utensils should be avoided when using cookware that has a nonstick finish.
11. Which of the following cookware materials is not recommended for use in a microwave oven?
    A. Ceramic.
    B. Metal.
    C. Paper.
    D. Plastic.
12. What is the difference between a saucepan and a pot?
13. What baking utensil is used to make sheet cakes?
14. True or false. Round containers cook foods more evenly than square containers in a microwave oven.
15. List three features to consider when buying cooking and baking utensils.

Build Your Basic Skills

1. **Writing.** Make a display of small kitchen tools for a showcase in your school. Write a brief description of each tool and explain its use in the kitchen.
2. **Math.** Make a list of cooking and baking utensils a single person would need in his or her first apartment. Then visit the cooking and baking utensil section of a department store. Figure how much it would cost to equip this hypothetical kitchen.

Build Your Thinking Skills

1. **Analyze.** Make a poster chart to help you analyze different materials used for cooking and baking utensils. List the characteristics, uses, care requirements, advantages, and disadvantages of each material.
2. **Compare.** Bake some cookies on a cookie sheet with a shiny finish and on one with a dull finish. Compare results and explain any differences.
3. **Propose.** Make a list of the small equipment, cookware, and bakeware found in the kitchen labs in your classroom. Propose uses for any utensils you did not read about in the chapter. Then investigate the functions of these utensils to see if your suggested uses were on target.

Apply Technology

1. Compare the speed and accuracy of a digital food thermometer and a dial food thermometer.
2. Investigate how the various materials used as nonstick finishes on cookware and bakeware have been improved in the last 20 years.

Using Workplace Skills

Regina is a housewares designer for Top Chop Company. She develops ideas for kitchen utensils. Lately, Regina has been working on a line of utensils for people with limited ability to use their hands.

To be a successful employee, Regina needs skills in thinking creatively. In a small group, answer the following questions about Regina's need for and use of these skills:

A. What is one of the questions about utensil design Regina must creatively answer as she plans the new product line?
B. How will Regina's ability to think creatively affect consumers with manual limitations?
C. How will Regina's ability to think creatively affect Top Chop?
D. What is another skill Regina would need in this job? Briefly explain why this skill would be important.

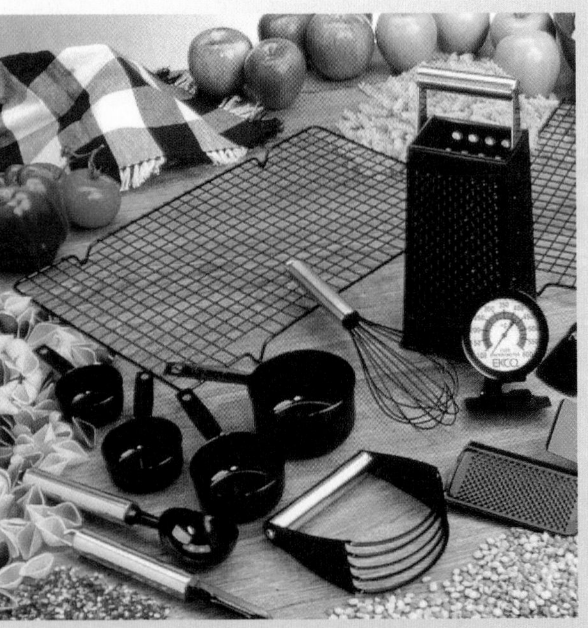

Chapter 11
Planning Meals

Domestic Cook
Plans menus, orders ingredients, prepares food, and cleans kitchen and cooking utensils in private home. May also serve meals and perform seasonal cooking duties, such as canning.

Caterer
Prepares and serves food and refreshments at social affairs.

Head Banquet Waiter
Plans details for banquets, receptions, and other social functions. Hires extra help, directs setting up of tables and decorations, and supervises wait staff.

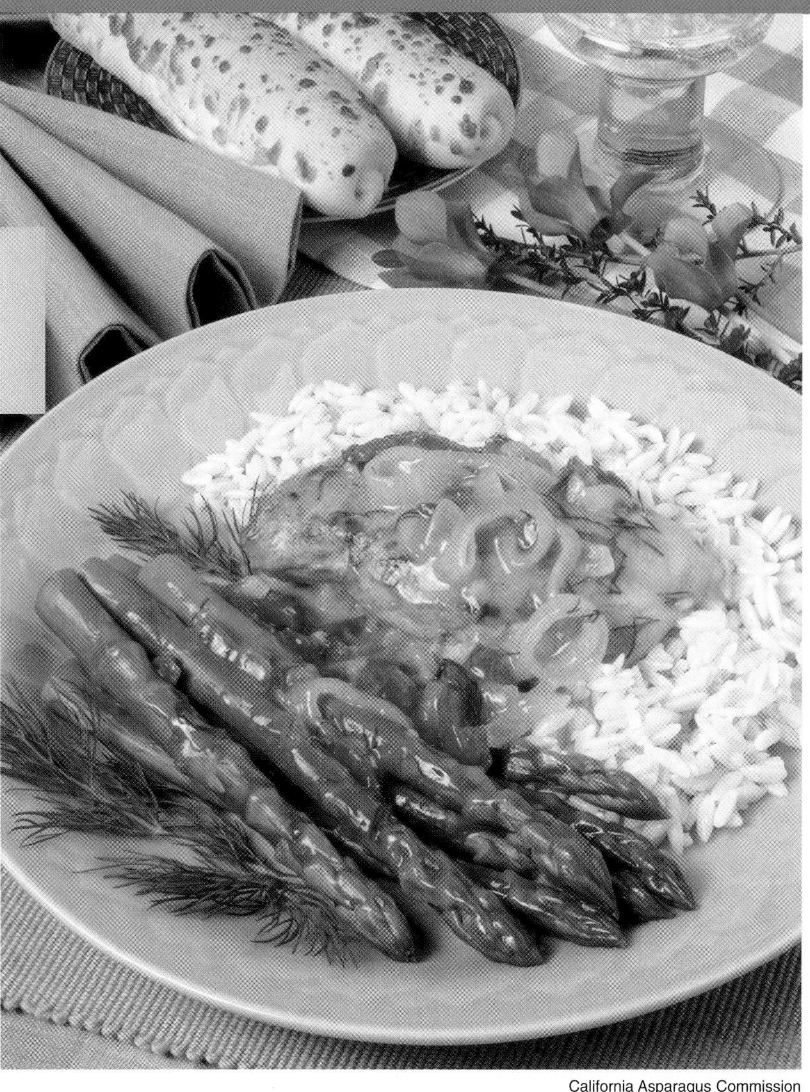

California Asparagus Commission

Terms to Know

meal manager
menu
course
convenience food
budget
income
fixed expense
flexible expense
taste buds
finished food
semiprepared food
work simplification
prepreparation
conservation
recycling

Objectives

After studying this chapter, you will be able to

- ❑ plan nutritious menus using meal patterns based on the Food Guide Pyramid.
- ❑ prepare a family food budget.
- ❑ plan menus with an appealing variety of flavors, colors, textures, shapes, sizes, and temperatures.
- ❑ describe resources a meal manager can use as alternatives to time and energy.

A ***meal manager*** is someone who uses resources to reach goals related to preparing and serving food. A meal manager's resources include money, time, energy, knowledge, skills, and technology. Food and equipment are resources, too. Meal managers must make many decisions based on these resources. They must decide how much time and money they are willing to spend planning and preparing meals. This will affect their decisions about what foods to serve and how to prepare them.

A meal manager will use available resources to reach the following four goals:

- Provide good nutrition to meet the needs of each family member.
- Use planned spending to make meals fit into the family food budget.
- Prepare satisfying meals that look and taste appealing.
- Control the use of time and energy involved in meal preparation. See 11-1.

The meal manager is responsible for seeing these goals are reached. However, he or she may not be the only one working to reach them. The meal manager may assign various tasks to other family members.

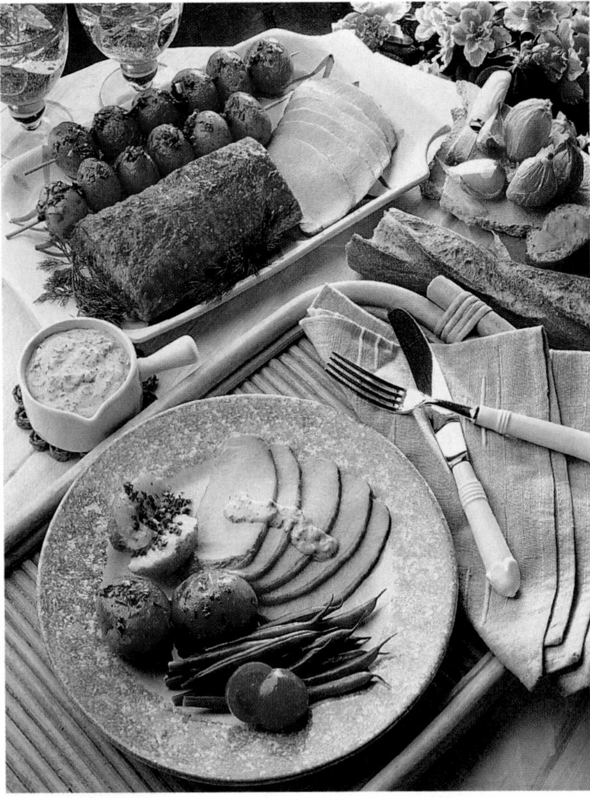

courtesy of National Pork Board

11-1 *A meal manager must use available resources to plan nutritious, affordable meals that look and taste appealing.*

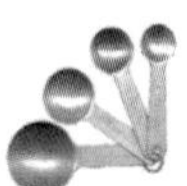

Provide Good Nutrition

People tend to eat foods they like. However, foods people like may not always be the foods they need to stay healthy. For good health, the foods people eat must supply their bodies with the right amounts of proteins, carbohydrates, fats, vitamins, minerals, and water. Everyone needs the same nutrients, but not in the same amounts. For instance, pregnant women need more of some nutrients than other adults. Active people need more of some nutrients than inactive people.

Meal Patterns

A diet that follows the USDA Food Guide can provide all the nutrients. Meal managers can use a meal pattern based on the Food Guide to plan nutritious meals. A *meal pattern* is an outline of the basic foods normally served at each meal. A Food Guide meal pattern includes one or two servings each from the fruit and vegetable groups. It includes two ounce-equivalents from the grains group. This pattern includes two ounce-equivalents from the meat and beans group. It also includes one serving from the milk group.

A meal manager can follow this basic pattern when planning each meal. It works equally well for breakfast, lunch, and dinner. The meal manager can use snacks to fill in added food group servings needed by individual family members. He or she can also add servings to one meal to make up for a shortage in another meal. For instance, some people may want to skip the vegetable group at breakfast. An extra vegetable serving for lunch, dinner, or snack can easily accommodate this preference. The point is to be sure family members consume the recommended number of servings from each group throughout the day. See 11-2.

Careful planning allows the meal manager to make sure foods served throughout the day meet each family member's nutritional needs. Breakfast generally supplies one-fourth of the day's total needs. Lunch and dinner each supply one-third, and snacks supply the remaining needs.

Breakfast

Eating breakfast helps prevent a mid-morning slump. A good breakfast should be rich in complex carbohydrates for energy. Enriched or whole grain toast and cereals are popular carbohydrate choices for breakfast. The morning meal is a good time to work a source of vitamin C into your diet. Many people choose fruit or juice as a rich source. Breakfast should provide a small amount of fat to help the meal stay with you throughout the morning. Children and teens should include a lowfat choice from the milk group for breakfast. Foods from the meat and beans group are optional at breakfast. Remember, you need only the equivalent of 5 to 7 ounces (140 to 196 g) of lean, cooked meat from this group each day.

Lunch

Many meal managers make good use of leftovers at lunchtime. They use leftovers to prepare nutritious salads, casseroles, and sandwiches. For instance, you could use leftover roast beef in two ways. Family members who carry their lunches to work or school could take hearty roast beef sandwiches. Those who eat their lunches at home could add strips of roast beef to a chef's salad.

In cold weather, hot foods are popular for lunch. Those who must take their lunches can carry soups, stews, and casseroles in wide-mouthed vacuum containers. In warmer weather, you can use the same containers to carry fruit juice, milk, or cold main dish salads.

Food Guide Meal Patterns					
Meal	Fruit Group (1-2 servings per meal)	Vegetable Group (1-2 servings per meal)	Grains Group (2 oz-eq per meal)	Meat and Beans Group (2 oz-eq per meal)	Milk Group (1 serving per meal)
Breakfast	Apple, cranberry, grapefruit, and orange juices Papayas, mangoes Melon Strawberries	Hash browns Onions, peppers, broccoli, mushrooms in omelets Tomato juice	Bagels English muffins Grits Oatmeal Pancakes Plantains	Eggs Canadian bacon Ham	Cheese in omelets Hot chocolate
Lunch	Applesauce Bananas Cherries Fruit salad Grapes Plums	Lettuce and tomato on sandwiches Coleslaw Vegetables in soups	Sandwich bread and rolls Pasta in soups and salads Pita bread Tortillas	Beans in soups Luncheon meat Ham, chicken, tuna, and egg salad Peanut butter Refried beans	Cheese on sandwiches Cottage cheese
Dinner	Baked apples Cranberry sauce Fruit desserts Grilled pineapple Poached pears Spiced peaches	Baked and mashed potatoes Broccoli, green beans, spinach, squash Stir-fried vegetables Tossed salad	Biscuits, cornbread, dumplings Bulgur, kasha, couscous Cassava Rice, pasta	Baked beans, lentils Beef, lamb, pork, veal Chicken, turkey Fish, shellfish Tofu	Milk Pudding
Snacks	Dried figs, dates, and apricots Raisins	Carrot and celery sticks Cauliflower	Crackers Matzos Popcorn	Hard-cooked eggs Nuts Sunflower seeds	Yogurt Kefir

***11-2** Foods within each group can be served for any meal to provide the recommended number of servings throughout the day.*

Dinner

Dinner is the one meal of the day many people can eat leisurely and share with family members. Dinner is often a heavier meal than lunch.

The meal manager can add variety to dinners in many ways. Occasionally serving a new dish is an easy way to add interest to family meals. The meal manager can also try serving common foods in new ways. For instance, instead of serving chicken, peas, and biscuits separately, you can combine these foods and serve them as chicken and dumplings. A tossed salad, dessert, and beverage would complete the meal.

In hot weather, appetites often become sluggish. You might replace a filling hot entree with a cool, refreshing salad. Hot rolls and a fresh fruit dessert would complete the meal.

Varying preparation methods is another way to add variety to meals. For instance, you can use ground beef to make meat loaf, sloppy joes, or Swedish meatballs. You can bake, boil, mash, oven-brown, fry, or cream potatoes. See 11-3.

Healthy Living

Research has shown that going to work or school without breakfast has a negative impact on work and studies. If you never seem to have time for breakfast, set your alarm 15 minutes earlier. If getting up earlier does not appeal to you, try starting breakfast preparations before you go to bed. Peel an orange, wrap it tightly in plastic, and put it in the refrigerator. Prepare a hard-cooked egg or place a bowl and spoon next to the cereal box. In the morning, you can eat your fruit and cereal (or egg) while making toast.

If traditional breakfast foods do not appeal to you, try eating nonbreakfast foods that you like. Hamburgers, soup, pizza, or yogurt provide many important nutrients and may appeal to you more than cereal and milk.

Snacks

With planning, the meal manager can make sure between-meal snacks satisfy nutritional needs as well as hunger. Fresh fruits and vegetables, cheese and crackers, milk shakes, and hard-cooked eggs are good snacks. They supplement other foods eaten during the day by adding important nutrients to the diet.

Planning a Meal

A written menu can be a useful tool in helping a meal manager reach the goal of providing good nutrition. A ***menu*** is a list of the foods to be served at a meal. Daily menus can help meal managers assess whether family members are getting the recommended servings from the USDA Food Guide.

Some menus are planned with several courses. A ***course*** is a part of a meal made up of all the foods served at one time. At an elaborate dinner, appetizer, soup, salad, main course, and dessert may each be served as separate courses. At an informal supper, the salad, main dish, and dessert may all be served at the same time. An appetizer and soup may be omitted from the menu.

Generally, the best menus center on one food. In the Food Guide meal pattern, grain foods are often the largest portions on the plate. However, plain grain foods have mild flavors that can be seasoned to blend with almost any other food. Therefore, meal managers usually center their menus on a protein food instead. Foods from the meat and beans group often call certain menu combinations to mind. For instance, roast turkey calls to mind stuffing and yams. Baked ham may make you think of scalloped potatoes and green beans.

Q: Aren't you more likely to gain weight if you eat a heavy meal late in the day?

A: Timing of meals does not trigger weight gain, consuming excess calories does. Therefore, you will not gain weight if the heavy meal is within your daily calorie needs. However, if the meal puts you over your daily calorie needs, you will gain weight no matter how early in the day you eat it.

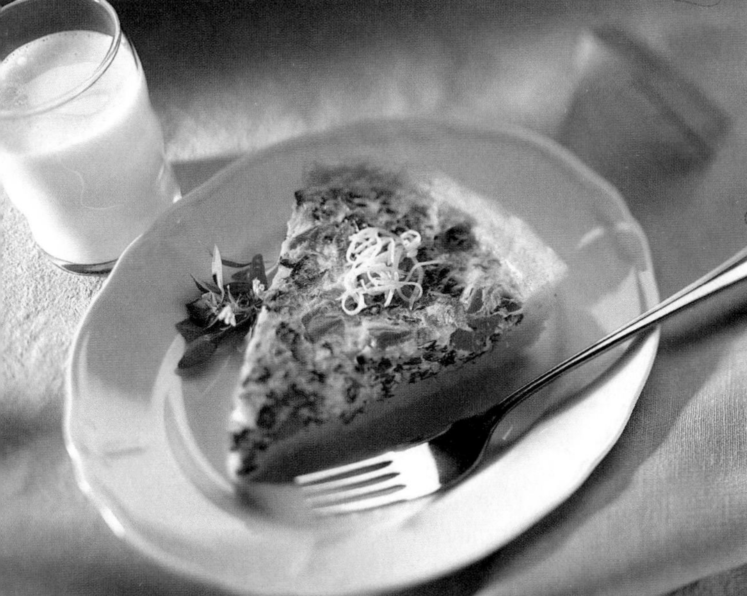

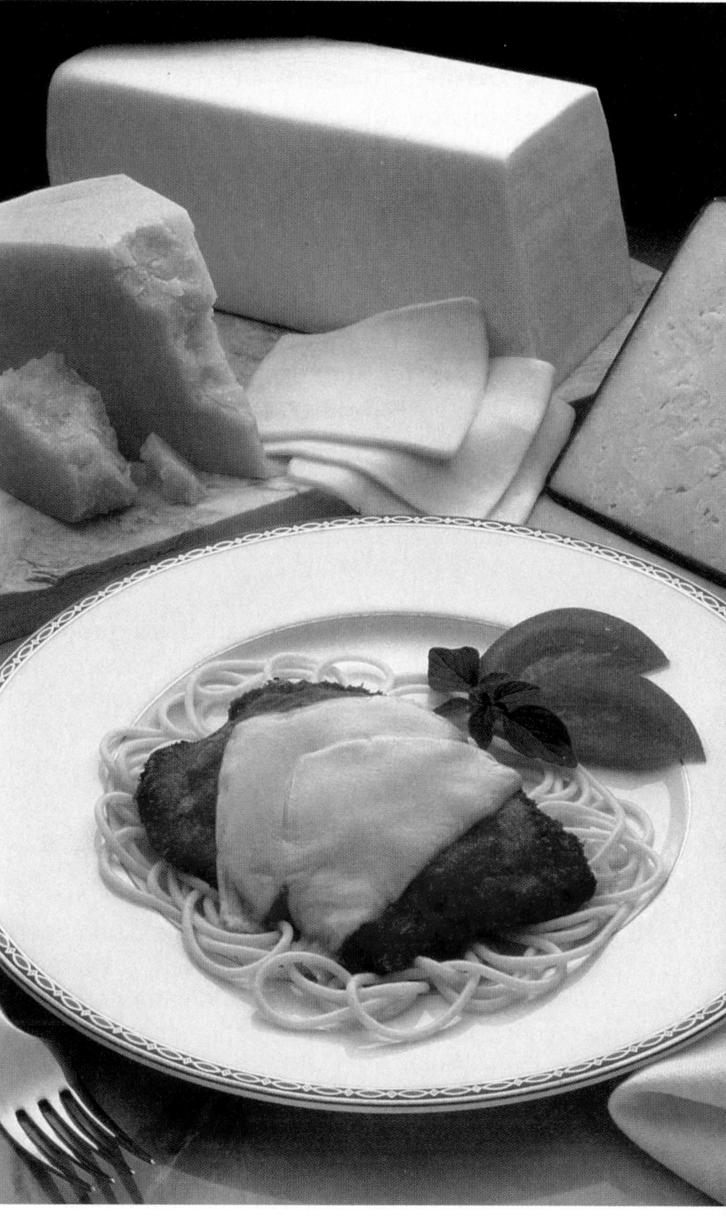

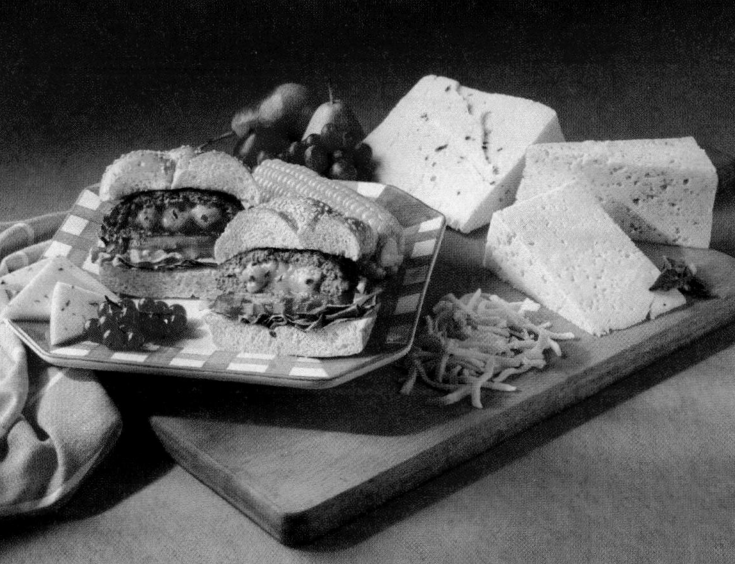

***11-3** Foods served at breakfast, lunch, and dinner generally supply the majority of nutrient needs.*

When planning a meal, you may find it easiest to make your menu selections in the following order:

1. Choose the main dish of the main course.
2. Select the grain foods, such as rice, pasta, or stuffing, that will accompany the main dish. You may serve bread or rolls along with or in place of other grain foods.
3. Select one or two vegetable side dishes that will complement the main dish. (Vegetables and grain foods may also be part of the main dish rather than side dishes. Casseroles and hearty soups often include vegetables and grains in this way.)
4. Choose the salad.
5. Select the dessert and/or first course. Desserts and appetizers are often good places to work a serving from the fruit group into your menu.
6. Plan a beverage to go with the meal. Fat free milk is often a good beverage choice. Serving milk is an easy way to include a food from the milk group in your menu, 11-4.

Q: Won't snacking between meals offset my efforts to lose weight?

A: Snacks won't interfere with weight loss as long as the calories they provide are considered in the daily meal plan. In fact, a snack between meals can keep you from feeling overly hungry. This could prevent you from overeating at mealtime—a practice that can definitely offset weight loss efforts.

Later sections in this chapter will give you other points to keep in mind as you choose individual menu items. Following these guidelines will help you serve meals that are appealing as well as nutritious.

Planning for Special Needs

Some people have health problems that affect their food needs. For instance, someone with heart disease may be advised to eat a diet low in sodium, cholesterol, and saturated fat. When planning meals, a meal manager must consider such special needs.

Initially, the meal manager and the family member with unique needs should work with a registered dietitian. The dietitian can offer guidance in meal planning. He or she can also assess whether nutrient needs are being met.

A meal manager could plan separate meals for a family member with unique needs. In most cases, however, other family members can adapt their eating habits to follow the special diet. For example, all family members can follow a lowfat, high-carbohydrate diet prescribed to someone with diabetes mellitus. Adapting family eating habits has two key advantages. First, it keeps the family member with special needs from feeling isolated. He or she will not feel deprived of foods other family members are enjoying. Second, it saves the meal manager the time and effort of planning and preparing two sets of meals. Special diets often have a third advantage of being more healthful than the family's typical diet.

Use Planned Spending

The second goal of meal management is planned spending. Nearly all families find they need to establish a spending plan for food. Families in the United States spend, on the average, about 20 percent of their incomes for food. Families must consider a variety of information when determining the amount of money they can spend for food.

Factors Affecting Food Needs

The activity, size, sex, and age of each member affect a family's food needs. It costs more to feed some people than it does to feed others because people's nutrient needs differ. It costs more to feed an athlete, for example, than

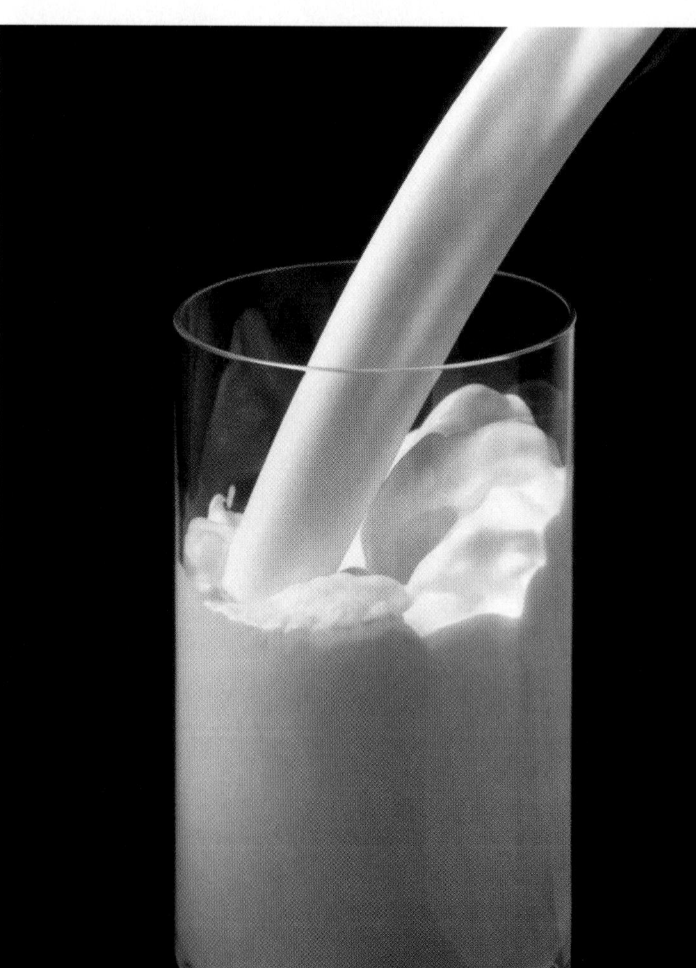

11-4 An ice cold glass of milk goes well with almost any meal.

it does to feed an office worker. It costs more to feed a person who weighs 250 pounds (112 kg) than a person who weighs 110 pounds (49 kg). After the age of 12, it costs more to feed boys than it does to feed girls. It also costs more to feed a teenager than it does to feed a senior citizen.

Health problems also influence food needs. A family member who is allergic to wheat or milk, for example, might need special foods. These special foods are often expensive.

Factors Affecting Food Purchases

You might think all families with similar food needs would spend about the same amount of money for food. However, this is not always true. You can acquire similar quantities of nutrients at very different costs, depending on the foods purchased.

Think of two baskets of food. One basket contains a beef rib roast, fresh asparagus, fresh oranges, bakery bread, and a frozen cake. The other basket contains ground beef, canned green beans, frozen orange juice concentrate, store brand bread, and a cake mix. Both baskets provide similar nutrients. However, the second basket will cost quite a bit less. See 11-5.

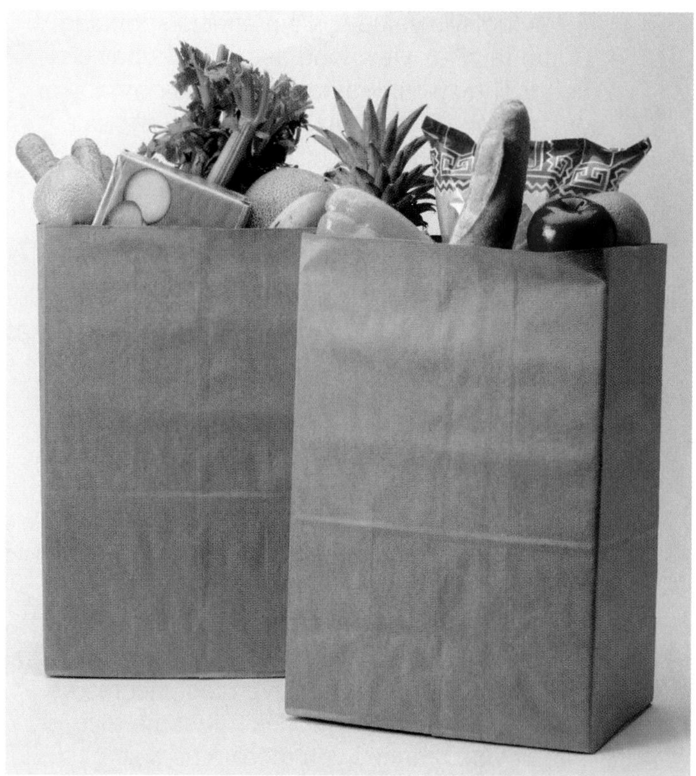

11-5 *Two bags of groceries can have similar nutritive values at very different costs.*

The following factors determine the amount of money a meal manager spends for food:

- family income
- meal manager's ability to choose foods that are within the family food budget
- meal manager's shopping skills and knowledge of the marketplace
- amount of time the meal manager has to plan and prepare meals
- food preferences of family members
- family values

Income is a major factor in determining the amount of money a family spends for food. Generally, as income increases, a meal manager spends more money for food. As income increases, the use of dairy products, better cuts of meat, and bakery goods tends to increase. Meanwhile, the use of less expensive staple foods, such as beans and rice, tends to decrease.

Knowing how to choose the tastiest, most nutritious foods for the money spent is an important meal management skill. A meal manager needs to know how similar products differ in quality and nutrition. He or she needs to know when buying a brand name is important. He or she should be able to identify products that contain hidden service costs. A meal manager also needs to know how to compare prices on a per serving basis. Recognizing seasonal food values and choosing quality meats and produce are other meal management skills.

The meal manager's available time and energy affect the family food budget. If these resources are limited, the meal manager will have to spend more money on convenience foods. ***Convenience foods*** are foods that have had some amount of service added to them. For instance, a meal manager who has ample time and energy could buy ingredients to make homemade lasagna. However, a meal manager who has little time and energy might purchase frozen lasagna instead. The frozen entree costs more, but it cooks quickly and requires no preparation.

Food likes and dislikes affect spending on food purchases. A family that eats steaks and fresh produce will spend more than a family that eats casseroles and canned goods.

A family's value system affects spending. Some families view food as merely a basic need. They would rather spend their money on other goals. Other families value meals as a source of entertainment. These families are likely to spend more money for food.

Preparing a Food Budget

Most families have a set amount of money that must cover many expenses. To keep from overspending in one area, such as food, they establish a household budget. A ***budget*** is a plan for managing how you spend the money you receive, 11-6. The meal manager has a responsibility to stay within the budget. The following steps will help you prepare a budget:

1. On a piece of paper, record your average monthly income. ***Income*** is money received. You will probably receive most income as wages earned by working. Income also includes money you receive as tips, gifts, and interest on bank accounts. Unless you can count on receiving a set amount from these sources, however, do not include them in your budget. Also, be sure to list only your take-home pay. Money deducted from your paycheck for taxes and other payments is not available for you to use for household expenses.
2. List your monthly fixed expenses and the cost of each. A ***fixed expense*** is a regularly recurring cost in a set amount. Fixed expenses include rent or mortgage payments, car payments, insurance premiums, and installment loan payments. You should also list savings as a fixed expense. Otherwise, you might end up spending money you intended to save.
3. List your flexible expenses and their estimated monthly costs. ***Flexible expenses*** are regularly recurring costs that vary in amount. Flexible expenses include food, clothing, utility bills, transportation, and entertainment.
4. Figure the total of your fixed and estimated flexible expenses. Compare this amount

Monthly Budget		
Income		$1600
Fixed expenses		
Rent	$495	
Car payment	250	
Insurance premium	100	
Savings	80	
Flexible expenses		
Food	160	
Nonfood items	40	
Clothing	80	
Utility bills	120	
Gasoline/oil	75	
Entertainment	120	
Gifts and contributions	80	
Total expenses		$1600

11-6 *Figuring your monthly budget will help you decide how much you can afford to spend for various items, including food.*

with your income. If your income equals your expenses, you will be able to provide for your needs and meet your financial obligations. If your income is greater than your expenses, you can put the extra money toward future goals. If your expenses are greater than your income, however, you will need to make some adjustments.

Reducing Food Expenses

You can handle a budget shortage in two ways: increasing income and decreasing expenses. Working overtime or getting another job would provide you with extra income. Looking at your current spending patterns will help you see how you can reduce expenses.

Although you cannot do much to change your fixed expenses, you can adjust your flexible expenses, including food. Save your grocery store receipts for a few weeks to see what kinds of foods you are buying.

You already know the cost of food has little bearing on its nutritional value. Each group of the USDA Food Guide includes both expensive and inexpensive foods. Protein foods are the most costly, but prices of foods in this group vary widely. T-bone steak, for example, costs more than ground beef. Both, however, provide similar nutrients. Milk, eggs, and cheese also are protein foods. Dried milk costs less than fluid fresh milk. Medium eggs usually cost less than large eggs. Domestic cheeses cost less than imported cheeses. Dried legumes are an inexpensive source of protein that can help stretch food dollars. See 11-7.

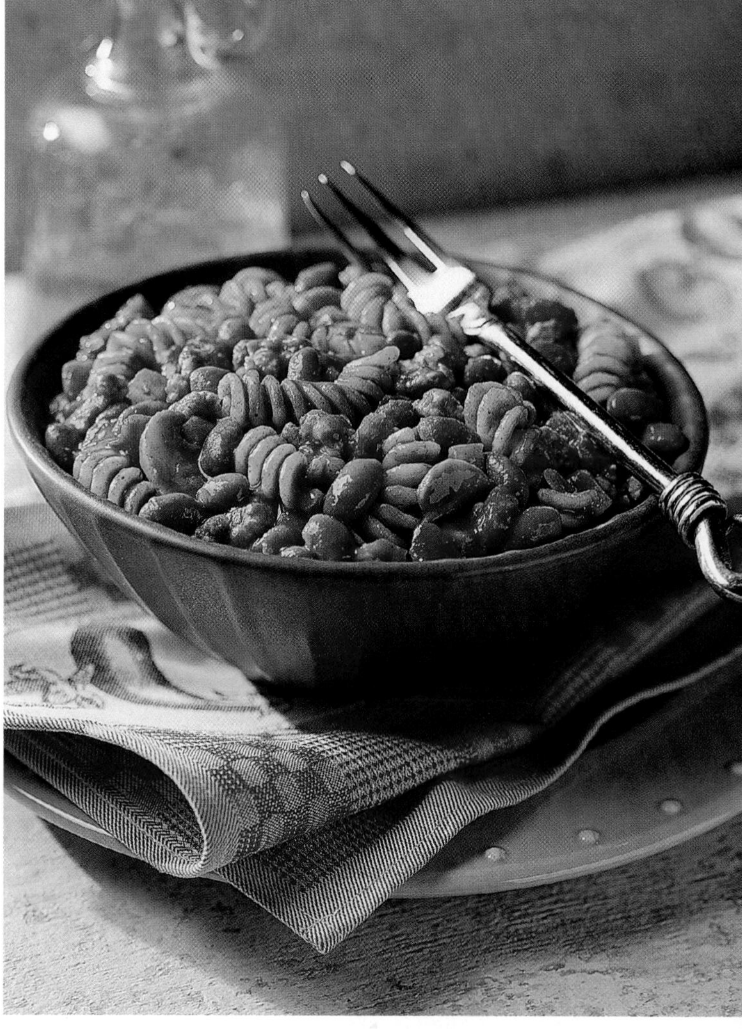

Bush's Chili Magic Chili Starter

11-7 Beans and pasta are lowfat sources of plant protein that help make the ground turkey in this hearty dish go further.

The fruit and vegetable groups are the next most costly food groups. However, foods in these groups vary widely in price, too. Before you buy, compare prices of fresh produce with frozen and canned products. Fresh fruits and vegetables are usually economical when they are in season. During off-seasons, however, canned and frozen products usually are cheaper. Grocers often price small pieces of fresh produce lower than larger pieces. Store brand and generic canned and frozen fruits and vegetables cost less than national brands.

The skillful meal manager also knows margarine usually costs less than butter. Unsweetened ready-to-eat breakfast cereals usually cost less than presweetened cereals. Cereals you cook yourself cost even less. Store brand bread usually costs less than brand name bread or bakery bread. Large packages usually are better buys than small packages. However, wise shoppers compare prices on a per serving basis before buying one size over another.

Convenience products and snack foods are often costly. You may be able to save money by preparing more foods from scratch and buying fewer snack foods. Using coupons and taking advantage of store specials will also help you cut costs.

Remember the grocery store is not the only place you buy food. Restaurants, concession stands, and vending machines also take a portion of your food dollar. You will need to evaluate these purchases in relation to your overall budget.

After identifying ways you can reduce food costs, determine a realistic figure for your monthly food budget. If you do your shopping weekly, divide this amount by four. Then keep careful track of your food purchases for a few weeks to see whether you are overspending. Sometimes your records may show you have spent more than your weekly budget. For instance, stocking up on sale items one week may cause you to spend more than your estimated amount. However, this may enable you to spend less money the following week.

Food is only one of the flexible expenses in your budget. You can take similar steps to reduce other spending areas, such as clothing, transportation, and entertainment.

Be a Clever Consumer

If you are like most people, your grocery purchases include more than just food. It may be convenient to pick up items like shampoo, lightbulbs, and film when you are at the grocery store. However, these items generally cost less at discount stores. Therefore, unless they are on sale, you might be smart to leave these items off your grocery list.

Prepare Satisfying Meals

The third goal of meal management is to prepare satisfying meals. All family members should find a meal appealing. This goal can be one of the most difficult to accomplish.

Food Preferences

Studies have shown people like some groups of foods better than others. People find vegetables, salads, and soups least appealing. They like breads, meats, and desserts best, 11-8. Studies also show wide ranges of preferences within a liked class of foods. In the meat class, for instance, respondents listed grilled steak, fried chicken, and roast turkey among their favorites. The least-liked foods in the same group were lamb, liver, fish, and creamed and combination dishes.

The foods you prefer to eat usually are familiar foods that taste good to you. Many factors affect your food preferences, including sight, smell, and touch. As a result, the flavor, color, texture, size, shape, and temperature of foods help determine how well you like them.

Flavor

Flavor is a mixture of taste, aroma, and texture. Information about the taste of food is conveyed to your brain by nerves at the base of your taste buds. ***Taste buds*** are flavor sensors covering the surface of the tongue. The four basic tastes recognized by human taste buds are sweet, sour, salty, and bitter.

Some foods have one distinct flavor. Sugar, for example, is sweet. Other foods have a blend of flavors. Sweet and sour pork has the sweetness of sugar. It also has the sourness of vinegar and the saltiness of pork.

Aroma is closely associated with flavor. When you like a food, it will taste even better to you if it has a good smell. For example, if you

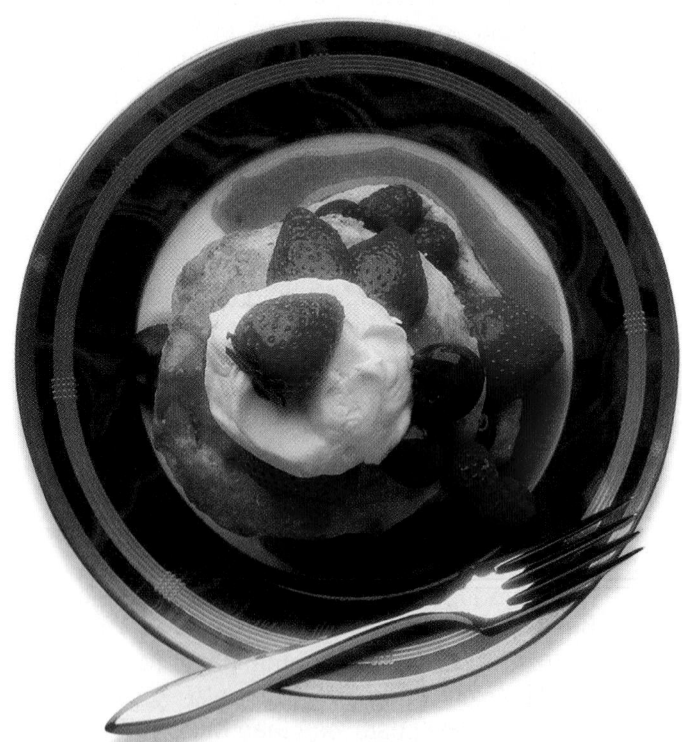

11-8 *Not surprisingly, desserts are one of the most popular food categories.*

like coffee, the smell of coffee brewing will stimulate your appetite and taste buds.

Flavor should be an important consideration when planning meals. Some flavors seem to go together. Turkey and cranberry sauce, peanut butter and jelly, and apples and cinnamon are popular flavor combinations. Other flavors seem to fight one another. For instance, you should not serve rutabagas and Brussels sprouts together. Their strong flavors do not complement each other.

When planning meals, do not repeat similar flavors. For instance, avoid serving tomatoes on a salad that will accompany pasta with tomato sauce. Your menus should not include all spicy foods or all mild foods. Plan to serve foods with different flavors.

Color

When used correctly, color not only appeals to the eyes, but also stimulates the appetite. The colors of a meal should provide a pleasing contrast, but they should not clash. For instance, the colors of tomatoes or carrots would not be pleasing with red cabbage.

Garnishes can add color to a meal. A sprinkling of nutmeg on custard or paprika on cheese sauce adds a touch of color. Meal managers can use lemon wedges, green pepper strips, and parsley sprigs to add color to a plate. Spiced peach halves, orange twists, and cucumber slices are also simple garnishes. They can add eye appeal to many foods.

Presentation

Presentation refers to the way food looks when it is brought to the table and presented to a diner. Along with colors, the arrangement of foods on a plate affects their presentation. Some restaurant chefs put much emphasis on the presentation of foods. They carefully fan out meat slices to make a moderate portion look bigger. They artistically sprinkle snipped herbs or grated cheese over pasta. They skillfully drizzle dessert sauces to write words or draw pictures.

If you are preparing a fancy meal, you may want to try some of these creative techniques. For everyday meals, however, two simple guidelines will help you present food attractively. First, avoid heaping foods on top of one another. Place foods side by side and spread them slightly to fill most of the space on the plate. Second, be careful not to smear or splash food on the edge of the plate. If you happen to drip, use a paper towel to wipe the edge of the plate before serving it.

Q: Are people born with natural preferences for some flavors?

A: Research indicates that babies seem to have a natural preference for sweet flavors over other flavors. However this is not true of salty flavors. People who decrease their use of salt will soon find they have less of a taste for salt.

Texture

Texture is the feel of food in the mouth. Familiar food textures are hard, chewy, soft, crisp, smooth, sticky, dry, gritty, and tough. A meal made up of foods that are all soft or all crisp lacks interest. A meal made up of a variety of textures is much more appealing.

Serve foods in combinations that have texture contrasts. Crisp cookies and soft, smooth pudding is one example. Tossing toasted, slivered almonds into a pan of green beans adds a pleasing difference in texture.

When planning meals, work for a balance between soft and solid foods. Be sure to consider chewy versus crunchy, dry versus moist, and smooth versus crisp. Avoid serving two or more chopped, creamed, or mashed dishes together.

Shape and Size

The size and shape of food items affect how appetizing they look. Avoid serving several foods made up of small pieces. For instance, spears of broccoli would be a better choice than peas to accompany a chicken and rice casserole. When choosing a salad to serve with the casserole, a lettuce wedge would be more appealing than coleslaw. Choose foods with various shapes and sizes when planning meals. See 11-9.

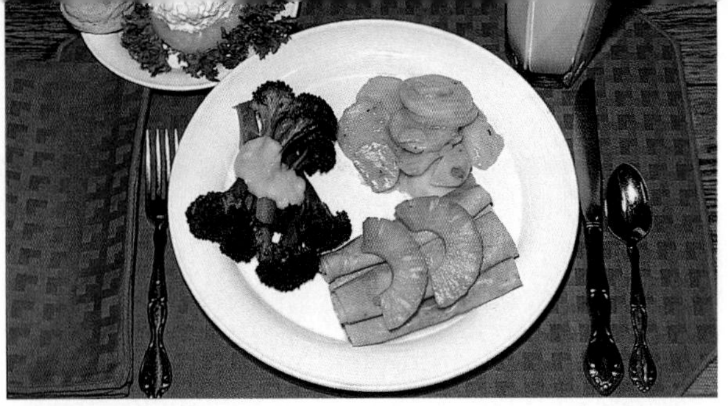

This meal repeats the flavor of cheese in the cottage cheese salad, au gratin potatoes, and cheese sauce. It also repeats the flavor of pineapple in the salad and garnish.

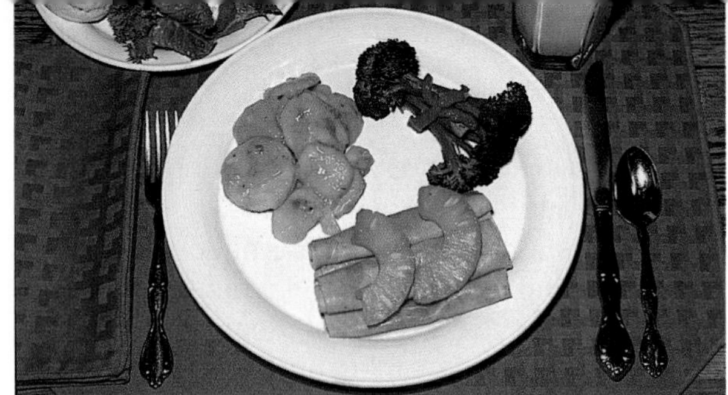

By changing the salad to lettuce with dressing and topping the broccoli with pimento, important flavor contrasts are made.

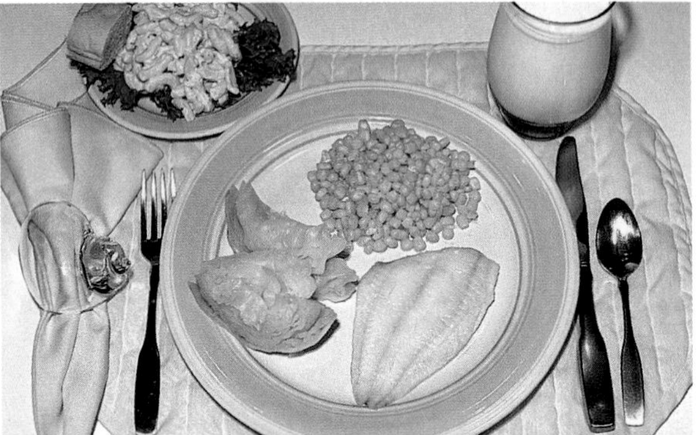

Everything in this meal is pale in color.

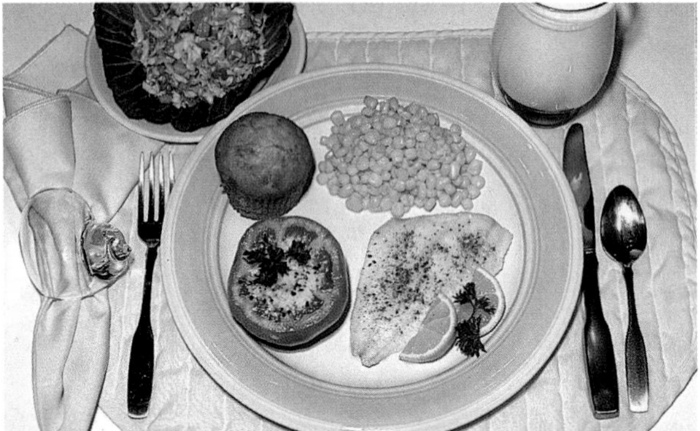

Add color by garnishing the fish and replacing the macaroni salad with a colorful slaw. Then switch the steamed cabbage for a baked tomato.

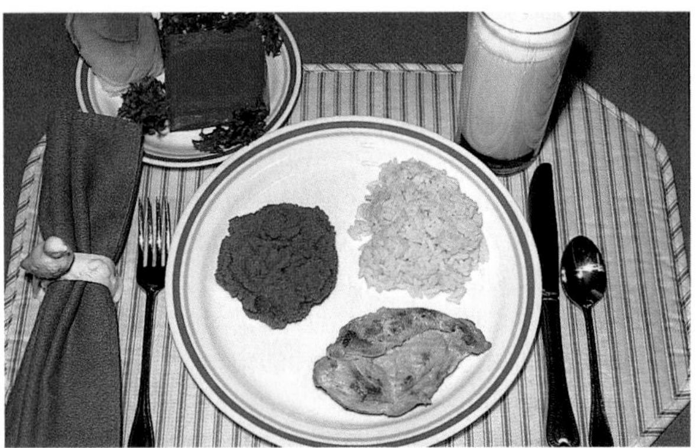

All the foods in this meal have soft textures.

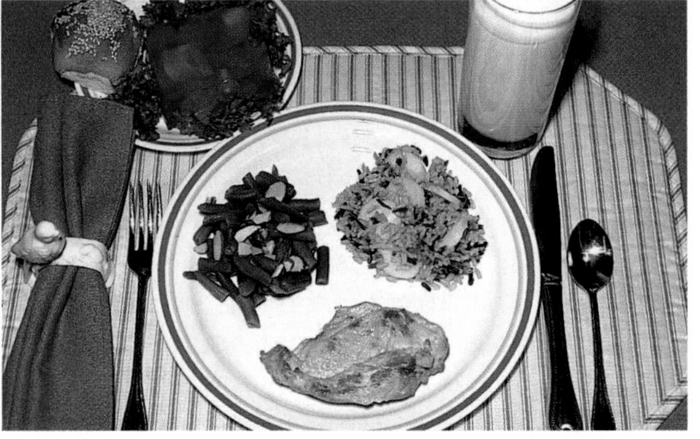

The soft yams have been replaced with crisp-tender green beans. Almonds in the green beans and water chestnuts in the wild rice add crunch. Seeds on the roll and fruit in the gelatin also add texture variation.

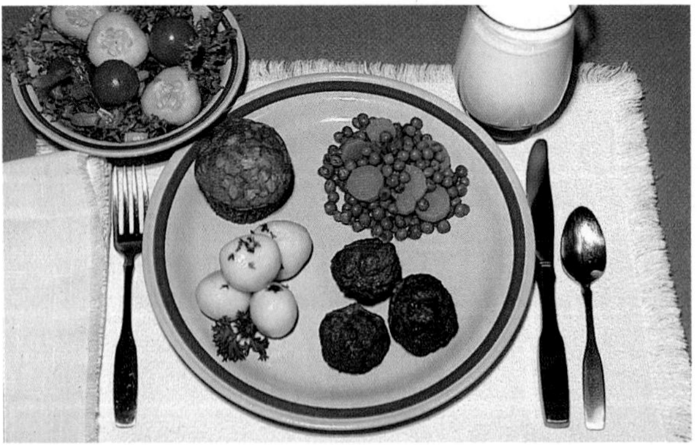

The use of so many round shapes makes this meal look boring.

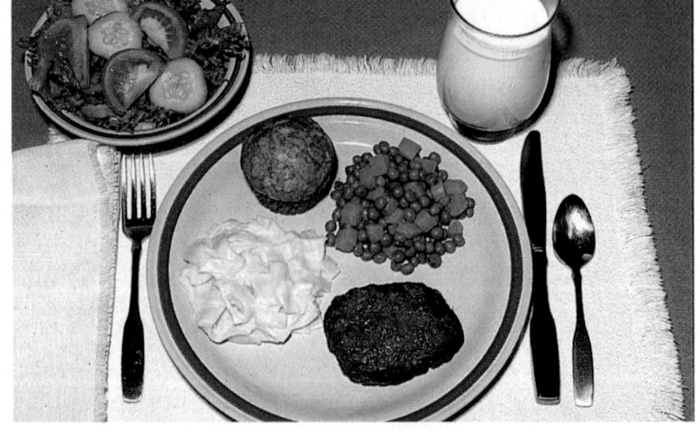

Substituting noodles for the potatoes and changing the shapes of other foods make this meal look much more appealing.

Dianne Debnam

***11-9** The most appealing meals include foods with a variety of flavors, colors, textures, shapes, and sizes.*

Temperature

The temperature of foods can also affect appetite appeal. A cold salad, for example, provides a pleasing temperature contrast to a piping hot entree. Icy cold sherbet cools the sensation created by steaming chili.

Hot foods should be hot and cold foods should be cold. Imagine a steaming bowl of soup and the same soup barely warm. Picture a cold, crisp tossed salad next to a room temperature salad bowl filled with wilted greens. Foods served lukewarm do not usually stimulate the senses of taste and sight.

Control the Use of Time and Energy

The fourth goal of successful meal management is controlled use of time and energy. Many meal managers think of this goal before any of the others. A meal manager's lack of time for planning and preparing meals can affect decisions involving the other management goals. For example, the meal manager with little time may have to choose convenience foods. This will cause him or her to spend extra money.

Several factors help determine the amount of time the meal manager needs to plan and prepare meals. These include family size, food preferences, meal standards, budget, and the efficiency of equipment. The meal manager's knowledge and skills will affect his or her use of time, too. A meal manager will spend more time preparing meals for a large family than for a small family. A meal that provides enough leftovers to feed a small family two meals would feed a large family only once. Preparing complex dishes and five-course dinners requires more time than using convenience foods to make one-dish meals. When convenience products do not fit into the budget, a meal manager will spend more time preparing foods from scratch. Likewise, a lack of equipment can cause a meal manager to spend more time doing preparation tasks. An inexperienced meal manager may spend more time preparing meals than someone who has learned shortcuts and developed speed.

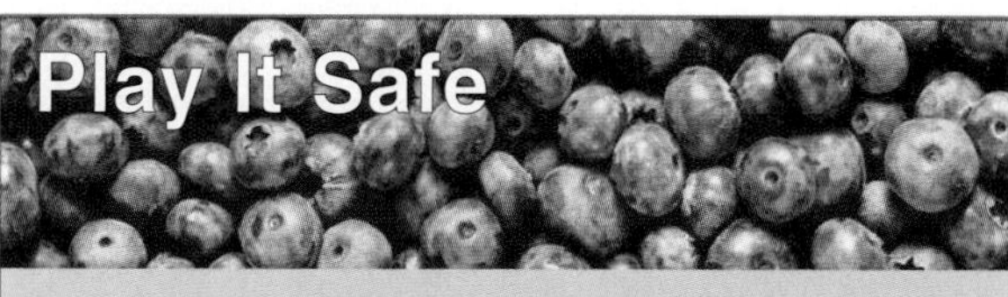

Lukewarm foods are not only unappetizing, they may be unsafe. Keep foods above 140°F (60°C) or below 40°F (5°C). Foods kept between these temperatures provide an excellent medium for the growth of microorganisms that can cause foodborne illness.

Alternatives to the Use of Time and Energy

The meal manager uses time and energy to plan menus, buy and store food, and prepare and serve meals. He or she also needs time and energy to care for the kitchen and dining area.

A meal manager can use several alternatives to time and energy. These include eating out, money, knowledge, skills, technology, and time itself.

Eating out helps many busy meal managers meet their goal to control the use of time. With a little thought, eating out can meet the other three meal management goals, too. Meal managers can help family members choose items from the menu that meet the goal of good nutrition. They can limit the frequency of dining out to meet the goal of planned spending. They can choose restaurants with varied menus to meet the goal of satisfying meals.

Money is a good alternative to time and energy for some families. However, many families find money too limited to use often as a time alternative. When money is available, the meal manager can buy time by purchasing ready-made foods. Buying efficient kitchen appliances and hiring help are other ways a meal manager can use money as an alternative.

A meal manager's *knowledge* and *skills* can be alternatives for both time and money. A meal manager's assets include knowing when, where, or how to shop to gain the most value. Knowing how to creatively prepare a variety of foods and efficiently organize the kitchen are also assets. A meal manager obtains many of his or her skills through experience. He or she gains other skills by studying and asking questions.

Technology can be an alternative to time and energy in the kitchen. You can use a computer to help you plan menus. Menu-planning software programs often come with preplanned menus. You can use these menus as is or adapt them to reflect your personal preferences. Saving menus for favorite meals will reduce planning time in the future. You can also save recipes and shopping lists that go with the menus. When you do not have time for meal planning, you can call up a favorite menu on the computer. See 11-10.

A meal manager can use *time* itself to save time. Successful meal managers are aware of how they use time, and they look for ways to save it. Using time to organize the kitchen for efficiency can save time later when preparing meals. Using time to plan menus can save time later by helping you shop more efficiently. You can make the most of the time you spend cooking by preparing extra food to freeze for later use.

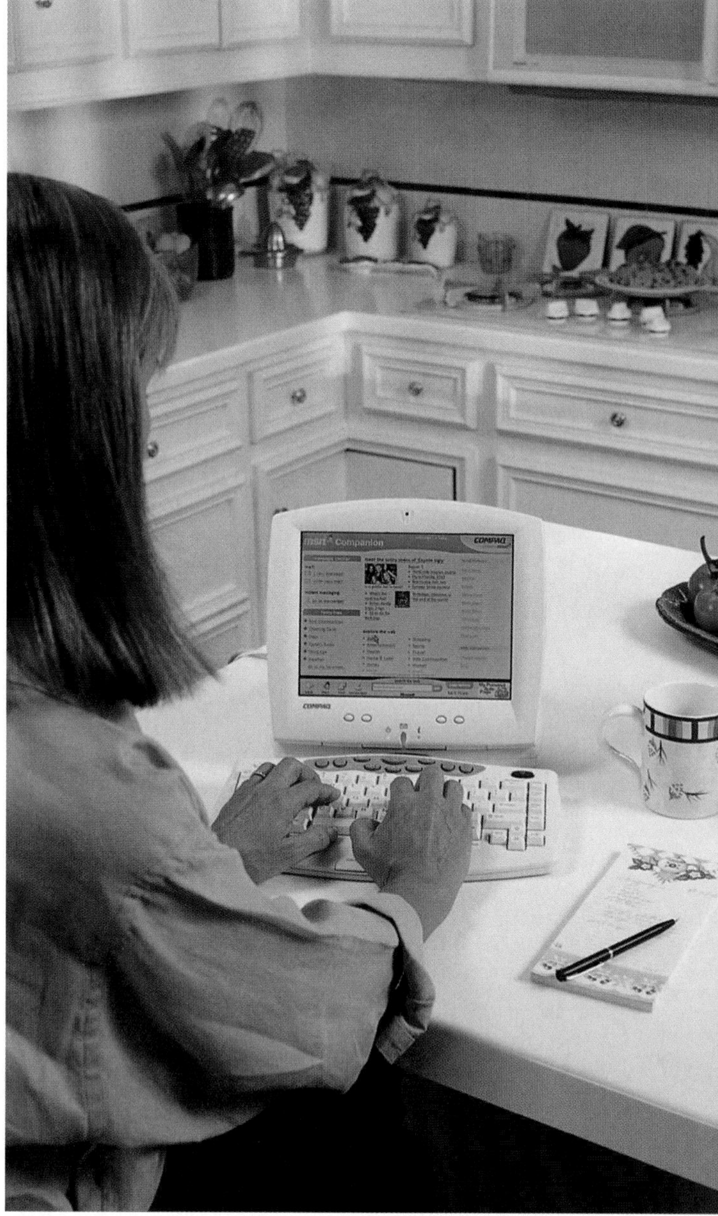

Compaq

11-10 *Using a computer to find recipes, plan menus, and write shopping lists can save meal managers time and energy in the kitchen.*

Using Convenience Foods

Some meal managers use convenience foods to reduce or eliminate food preparation and cooking time at home. Some ready-made foods are so commonly used, people do not think of preparing meals without them.

You can group convenience foods according to the amount of service they contain. ***Finished foods*** are convenience foods that are ready for eating either immediately or after simply heating or thawing. Packaged cookies, canned spaghetti, and frozen fruits are examples of finished foods. ***Semiprepared foods*** are convenience foods that still need to have some service performed. Cake mixes are semiprepared foods. The meal manager beats in eggs and liquid, pours the batter into pans, and bakes it for a specified time.

The cost of convenience depends on the amount of service a product contains. Generally, the more built-in service a product contains, the higher the product's price will be. A product that contains more service reduces the amount of time the meal manager spends measuring, mixing, and cooking. Most convenience foods cost more than their homemade counterparts. However, there are some exceptions. Frozen orange juice concentrate and some commercial cake mixes cost less than their homemade counterparts.

Convenience foods have both advantages and disadvantages as explained in 11-11. Before buying a convenience product, ask yourself the following questions:

- How does the convenience food help meet my family's daily nutrient needs?
- Does buying convenience foods fit into my food budget? (Is the time I save worth the extra cost?)
- How does the cost of the convenience product compare with the cost of the homemade product?
- How costly are any additional ingredients I must add? (Some convenience mixes require the addition of foods like meat, eggs, or sour cream.)

Convenience Foods	
Advantages	**Disadvantages**
Time and energy are saved because the meal manager does not have to measure, mix, peel, and slice. The inexperienced cook can prepare meals confidently. The meal manager who does not like to cook can prepare nutritious meals for the family without spending hours in the kitchen.	Many mass-produced foods do not taste as good as home-prepared foods. Frequent use of convenience foods is expensive. Some convenience foods are high in fat and sodium.

11-11 Before buying a convenience food, a meal manager should consider both the advantages and disadvantages.

- How much do I need to feed my family? (The cost of a convenience product may seem reasonable if you are feeding one or two people. However, it may seem costly if you are feeding three or more.)
- How do the appearance and flavor of the convenience product compare with those of its homemade counterpart?

Work Simplification

Work simplification is the performance of tasks in the simplest way possible to conserve time and energy. Work simplification techniques can help meal managers reach their goal for controlling the use of time. The meal manager can simplify tasks by minimizing hand and body motions. He or she can organize workspace and tools. Changing the product or the method used to prepare the product can also simplify some tasks.

You can minimize hand and body motions in many ways. Performing a task repeatedly can eventually result in reduced preparation time. This is because the person performing the task develops a skill. A professional cook who chops celery every day soon learns an efficient method for chopping celery.

Another way to minimize motions is to rinse and soak dishes. This simplifies the task of washing dishes.

Saving yourself steps in the kitchen is a method of work simplification, too. Try not to walk back and forth across the kitchen while preparing a meal. Instead, get all your equipment ready first. Then go to the cabinets and then to the refrigerator to get the ingredients you need.

An organized kitchen simplifies work. Store tools in the area where you most often use them. For instance, you can store pots and pans in a cabinet close to the range. Many experienced meal managers buy duplicates of inexpensive tools like rubber spatulas, wooden spoons, and measuring utensils. They store these tools in different parts of the kitchen where the tools will be easy to reach. By using the correct tool for each task, the meal manager can also simplify work. Measuring flour in a dry measure is much more efficient than measuring it in a liquid measure.

You can simplify work by changing the food product or the method used to prepare it. For instance, if the meal plan calls for biscuits but time is short, you can opt for store bought bread instead. Making dropped biscuits instead of rolled biscuits would be another way to save time.

Prepreparation is another work simplification technique. ***Prepreparation*** is any step you do in advance to save time when you are getting a meal ready. Chopping onions and shredding cheese might be prepreparation tasks. After completing these steps, you can put the onions and cheese in bags in the freezer. When preparing a recipe calling for these ingredients, you can quickly measure the portion you need from the freezer bag. Washing and trimming chicken, peeling oranges, and cooking rice may be other prepreparation tasks you could do.

Conserving Resources in the Kitchen

Conservation refers to the planned use of a resource to avoid waste. Human energy is not the only type of energy meal managers need to conserve in the kitchen. They also need to conserve fuel energy, such as gas and electricity. Steps you can take to conserve energy include using the oven to cook more than one food at a time. Cover pans on the range to keep in heat, 11-12. Avoid unnecessarily opening the oven door and letting out heat while using the appliance. Likewise, avoid opening refrigerator and freezer doors, which lets in heat.

Water is another resource you need to conserve in the kitchen. Avoid letting the water run while washing dishes. Run the dishwasher only when it is full.

You can also conserve resources in the kitchen by ***recycling.*** This means processing a material so it can be used again. Many communities collect empty metal cans, plastic bottles, and glass containers for recycling. The metal, plastic, and glass can be made into new products. Collection facilities often take cardboard from cereal, cracker, and convenience mix boxes, too. Recycling these items keeps them from taking up space in public garbage landfills. It also lessens the need for raw materials to make new products. A meal manager can easily take these steps to help care for the environment while meeting meal planning goals.

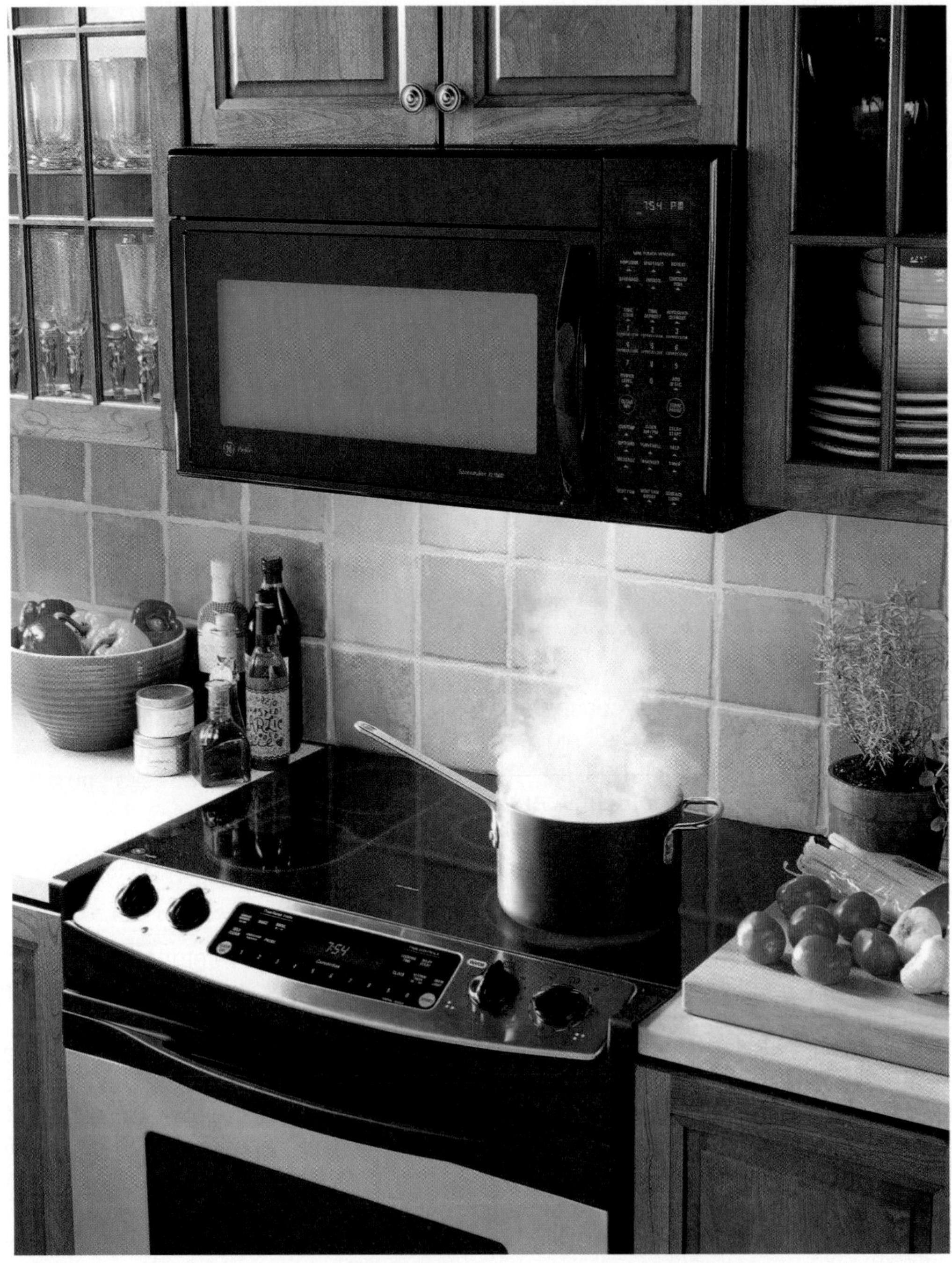

GE Appliances

11-12 *Covering pans on the range helps save energy by holding in heat.*

Chapter 11 Review

Planning Meals

Summary

Meal managers have four main goals in planning meals for their families. The first goal is to provide good nutrition for all family members. Meal managers can use a meal pattern based on the USDA Food Guide as a resource to help meet this goal.

The second goal is to use planned spending. A family must consider factors that affect food needs and food purchases when preparing a household budget. A meal manager can use his or her consumer skills to reduce food expenses and stay within the established budget.

The third goal of meal management is to prepare satisfying meals. Meal managers must be mindful of family food preferences to achieve this goal. They must also consider flavors, colors, textures, shapes, sizes, and temperatures of foods. This will help them plan menus that are varied and appealing.

The fourth meal management goal is to control the use of time and energy. Meal managers can use a number of resources as alternatives to time and energy. They can use convenience foods and work simplification techniques to reduce the time they spend planning and preparing meals. Meal managers can use appliances efficiently and recycle to conserve fuel energy and other resources in the kitchen.

Review What You Have Read

Write your answers on a separate sheet of paper.

1. Name six resources a meal manager can use to reach goals related to preparing and serving food.
2. What portion of a day's total nutrient intake do breakfast, lunch, dinner, and snacks generally supply?
3. What is usually the first step in planning a menu?
4. True or false. All families with similar food needs spend about the same amount of money for food.
5. List four factors that help determine the amount of money a meal manager spends for food.
6. Describe the steps you would take to estimate the amount of money you could spend for food each week.
7. Which of the following statements about food costs is not true?
   A. Dried milk costs less than fluid fresh milk.
   B. During off-seasons, canned fruits and vegetables cost less than fresh.
   C. Store brands cost less than national brands.
   D. Presweetened cereals cost less than unsweetened cereals.
8. List the six elements that affect the sensory appeal of a meal. Give examples of foods that show contrast for each element.
9. List four resources a meal manager can use as alternatives to time and energy.
10. Convenience foods that are ready for eating either immediately or after simply heating or thawing are called _____.
11. Describe three ways a meal manager can simplify tasks.
12. Give two suggestions for conserving fuel energy and one suggestion for conserving water in the kitchen.

Build Your Basic Skills

1. **Math.** Compare the costs of foods with built-in convenience with their less convenient counterparts. Examples might include shredded cheese and bulk cheese, instant rice and long grain rice, and ready-made juice and frozen concentrate.
2. **Verbal.** Visit the school cafeteria or a nearby foodservice operation and observe employees involved in food preparation. What work simplification techniques do you see employees using? How could employees make better use of work simplification techniques? Share your findings in a brief oral report to the class.

Build Your Thinking Skills

1. **Evaluate.** Keep track of all the meals you have eaten for one week. Evaluate the meals according to the USDA Food Guide. If each day's meals were not nutritionally balanced, suggest where you could have added or subtracted menu items to provide the recommended number of daily servings.
2. **Analyze.** Write menus for your family's meals for a week. Attach the menus to a report analyzing how they meet the four goals of meal management.

Apply Technology

1. Use a computer and menu-planning software to plan meals for one week.
2. Use a computer and a spreadsheet program to prepare a monthly budget. Then use the budget to analyze your family's food spending.

Using Workplace Skills

Emilio owns a catering business. People hire him and his staff to prepare food and bring it to their homes or rented banquet halls. Many people also ask Emilio to stay and serve the food to their party guests. Many of Emilio's clients order fancy foods, such as shrimp cocktail and exotic fruits. They want the foods to be expertly seasoned and beautifully garnished. They often insist on ordering more than enough food to feed the expected number of guests. All these factors add to the catering bill. However, most of the clients have limited budgets.

To be an effective worker, Emilio needs skill in making good use of money. Put yourself in Emilio's place and answer the following questions about your need for and use of this skill:

A. What are four expenses you must consider when deciding how much to charge your clients?
B. How might your clients react if you exceed their budgets?
C. What would happen if you underestimate your expenses when billing clients?
D. What is another skill you would need in this job? Briefly explain why this skill would be important.

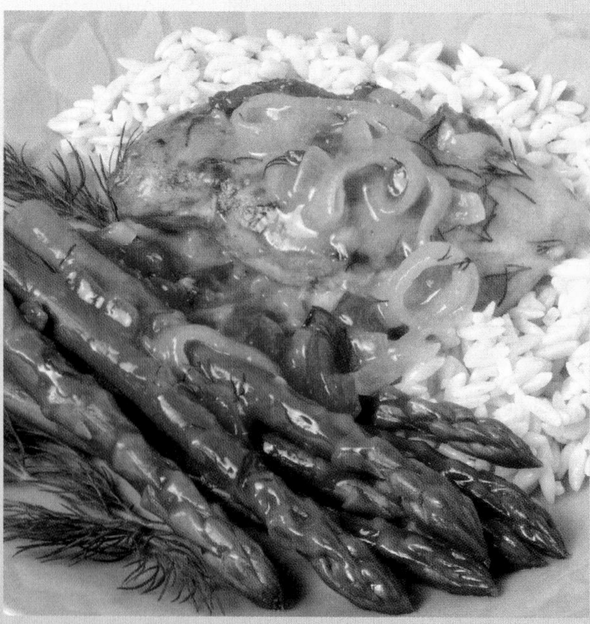

Chapter 12
The Smart Consumer

Comparison Shopper
Compares prices, packaging, physical characteristics, and styles of merchandise in competing stores.

Retail Food Demonstrator
Prepares samples of food products for grocery store customers in order to promote sales; answers customer questions.

Nutrition Aide
Advises low-income family members about how to plan, budget, shop, prepare balanced meals, and handle and store food following prescribed standards.

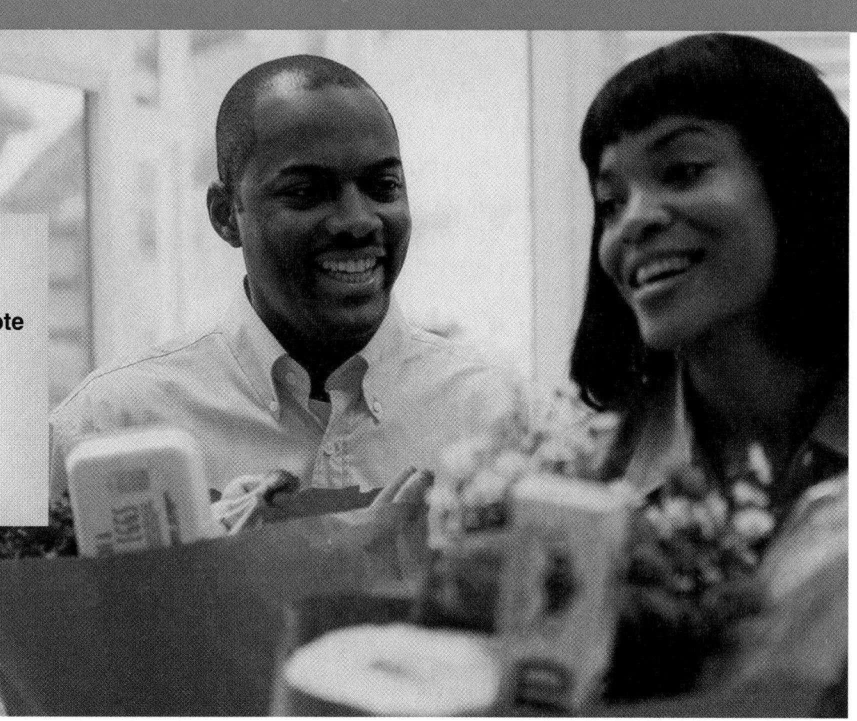

Terms to Know

- produce
- comparison shopping
- impulse buying
- grade
- brand name
- store brand
- national brand
- generic product
- precycling
- unit pricing
- organic food
- pesticide
- food additive
- GRAS list
- nutrition labeling
- Daily Value
- universal product code (UPC)
- open dating

Objectives

After studying this chapter, you will be able to

- ❑ evaluate store features to decide where to shop for food.
- ❑ identify factors that affect food costs and comparision shop to decide what foods to buy.
- ❑ use information on food product labels to make informed decisions about the foods you buy.
- ❑ list sources of consumer information.

To be a smart consumer at the grocery store, you need to know how to read labels and compare prices. You need to be able to choose foods that will give you the most nutrition for your money. You also need to understand basic marketing techniques.

Making wise decisions about where to shop and what to buy takes knowledge and practice. As you develop consumer skills, you will be able to plan appealing, nutritious meals while staying within the family budget.

Choosing Where to Shop

Consumers can choose between many kinds of food stores. Some large stores stock thousands of items. Other stores are small and stock just a few specialty items. Some stores sell only food, whereas others also sell drugs, cosmetics, toys, and clothing.

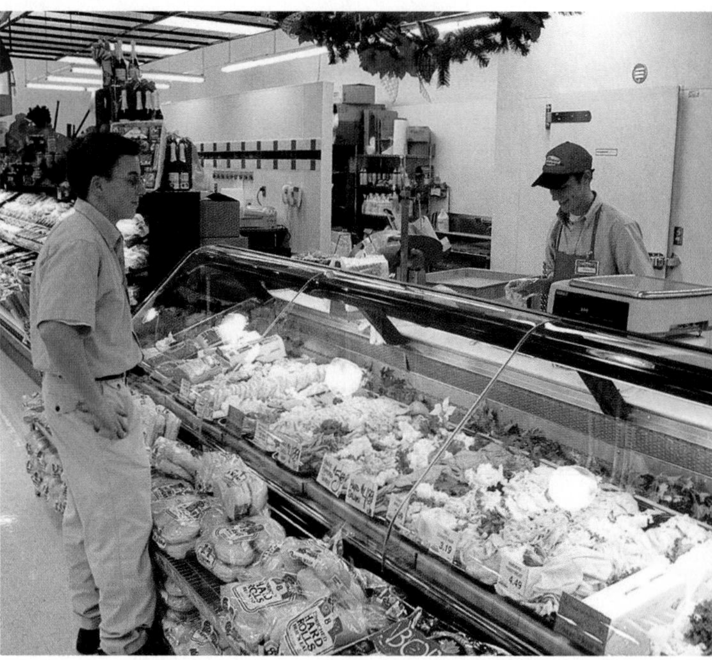

photo courtesy of IGA, INC.

12-1 Many supermarkets have deli departments that sell party trays, freshly sliced meats and cheeses, and ready-to-eat salads and entrees.

Types of Stores

Being familiar with the different types of stores will help you know what to expect when you shop. You may find one store that meets all your needs, or you may shop in several stores.

Supermarkets vary in size. They are self-service stores, and they carry both food and nonfood items. Many supermarkets have specialty food sections, such as delis and bakeries, 12-1. Some offer customer services, such as home delivery, check cashing, and credit. A number of supermarkets offer consumers such conveniences as in-store pharmacy and banking services, too.

Discount supermarkets sell food in large quantities at reduced prices. You may be able to buy some items by the case or in restaurant-sized containers. Discount supermarkets often sell the same products as other stores. However, they may not carry fresh meat or ***produce*** (fresh fruits and vegetables). At some discount supermarkets, shoppers must pack their own groceries in bags or boxes.

Twenty-four hour convenience stores can be large or small. They are always open for their customers' convenience. However, customers may pay higher prices because of the increased cost of longer business hours.

Specialty stores carry one specific type of product. Dairies, bakeries, butcher shops, and ethnic markets are specialty stores. *Delicatessens* are also a type of specialty store. They sell ready-to-eat foods like cold meats, salads, and rolls. Foods sold in specialty stores are generally high in quality, but they are often high in price, too.

Outlet stores offer reduced prices on products from individual food manufacturers. Some items in an outlet store may not meet the manufacturer's quality standards for retail sale. However, the foods are nutritious.

Food co-ops are owned and operated by groups of consumers. They keep prices low by buying foods in bulk, leaving off profits, and requiring volunteer labor of their members. Most co-ops have limited hours and are open only to their members.

Farmers' markets sell food directly from the farm to the consumer. You may be able to get fresher produce at lower prices by shopping at a farmers' market. However, to make wise purchases, you need to recognize signs of quality and know retail prices. See 12-2.

Roadside stands are open near farms during the growing season. They are much smaller than farmers' markets. Usually just one

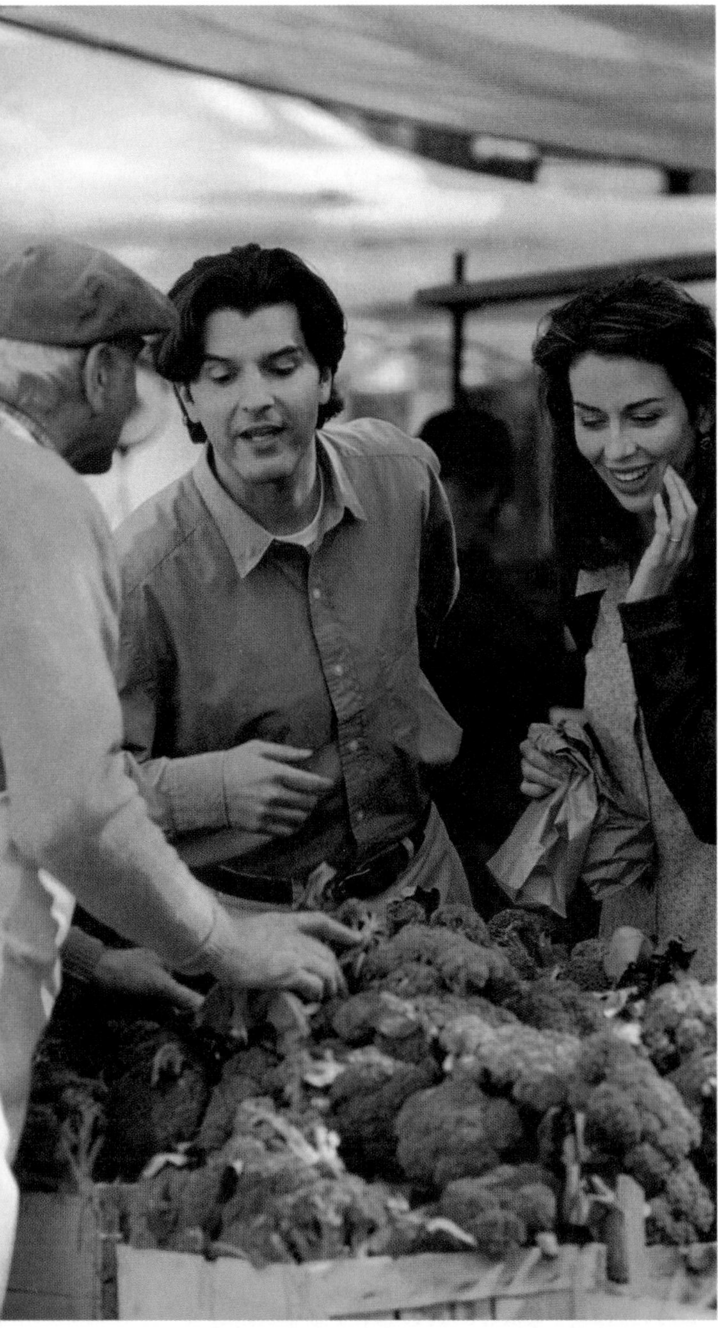

12-2 Freshness and low prices prompt some consumers to shop for their produce at farmers' markets.

family runs them. Roadside stands specialize in homegrown fruits and vegetables, often at a considerable savings.

Store Features

You may shop at a particular food store because it is the only store near you. If you have the opportunity to choose among several stores, however, you might want to ask yourself the following questions:

- What services does the store offer?
- Is the store neat and clean? Are the shelves and cases well stocked?
- Are the store's hours convenient?
- Are the employees courteous and helpful?
- Does the store stock a variety of foods, brands, and sizes?
- Are the prices for both advertised and non-advertised items comparable to those of other area stores?
- Are the dairy and meat cases cold and clean?
- Is the produce fresh? Is it well chilled? Is the variety good?

Supermarket Trends

Today's fast-paced lifestyles are the force behind many supermarket trends. Busy consumers are looking for answers to meal problems, and food stores are responding. Many grocery stores have gone beyond selling standard convenience foods. They now offer fresh, refrigerated, ready-to-eat meal items, such as sandwiches and complete lunch kits. Supermarkets are also offering take-out foods, such as hot side dishes, entrees, and complete meals. These meal items may save consumers time and money over restaurant take-out foods.

Another supermarket trend is a new twist on an old selling technique—*cross merchandising.* This technique involves pairing items from different grocery sections to prompt consumers to buy and use the products together. For instance, shortcakes might be paired with fresh strawberries. Cross merchandising is now being used to encourage consumers to think about buying meal items together. For example, ready-made salads and loaves of garlic bread might be displayed near fresh pastas and sauces.

A third supermarket trend to meet the needs of busy consumers is self-checkout. Self-checkout saves time by reducing long lines. Shoppers can check out at their own pace and make their purchases with greater privacy. Self-checkout stations have touchscreens that guide consumers through the process of scanning and bagging their own groceries. The stations accept coupons and payment with cash or credit or debit cards. See 12-3.

Electronic Shopping

Some Internet-using consumers are choosing to shop for groceries electronically. An online grocery shopping service provides a consumer with the computer software needed to use the service. The consumer logs on to the service. Then he or she creates a grocery list from menus of items on the computer screen. When the list is complete, the consumer electronically sends the order and arranges for delivery. Professional shoppers fill the order and deliver it to the consumer's door.

Online shoppers can be nearly as selective as if they were in a store. Consumers choose from a wide variety of brands and sizes displayed on the computer screen. They can specify how they want fresh produce to look. They can read product nutrition and pricing information on the packages shown on the screen. They may be able to use coupons, too.

Online shopping services are not free. Consumers usually pay subscription fees, delivery charges, and a percentage of their total grocery bills. However, many people feel avoiding traffic, crowded stores, and heavy grocery bags is worth the cost.

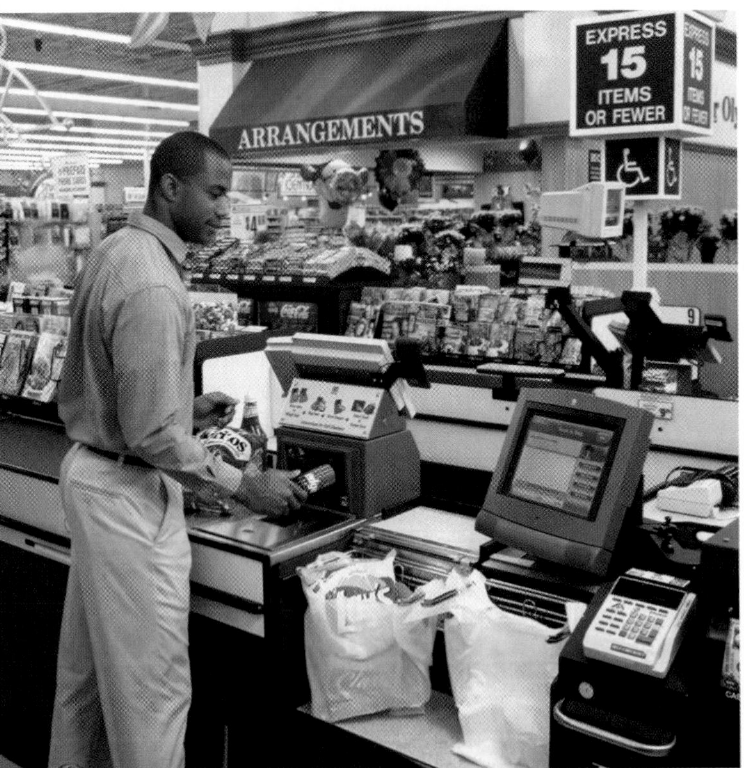

NCR Corporation

12-3 Self-checkout stations offer supermarket shoppers speed, privacy, and control when making grocery purchases.

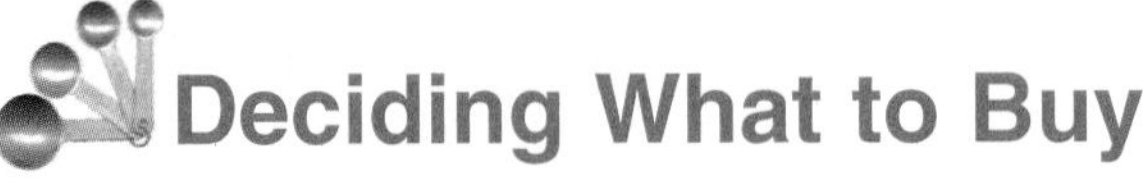

Deciding What to Buy

You can make most of your decisions about what to buy by writing weekly menus before you go shopping. Try to plan meals around advertised specials. For example, if ham is a good buy, plan to serve it in several ways during the week. Keep your menus flexible. Suppose you wanted to serve zucchini for one meal, but you find out yellow squash is on sale. You might want to eliminate the zucchini from your menu and add the yellow squash.

Using a Shopping List

A shopping list can help you save time, avoid extra trips for forgotten items, and stick to your food budget. Keep a list handy in your kitchen so you can jot down items when you find you need them. Before going to the store, check the recipes you plan to prepare during the week. Be sure you have all needed ingredients on hand. Check for staples such as flour, sugar, and milk. Add any needed items to your list. Also add advertised specials if you need them and if they really are bargains.

Organize your list according to categories, such as produce, dairy, meat, and frozen foods. Place the categories in the same order as the store aisles.

Carry your shopping list with you and stick to it. You will be less tempted to buy groceries you do not need.

Factors That Affect Costs

A number of factors affect the costs of food products. You can get the best buys if you learn to comparison shop and avoid impulse buying. ***Comparison shopping*** involves evaluating different brands, sizes, and forms of a product before making a purchase decision, 12-4. ***Impulse buying,*** on the other hand, is making an unplanned purchase without much thought.

You can cut costs by using coupons for items you need. However, avoid buying a product you do not need just because you have a coupon for it. Most coupons have expiration dates. Some require you to buy more than one

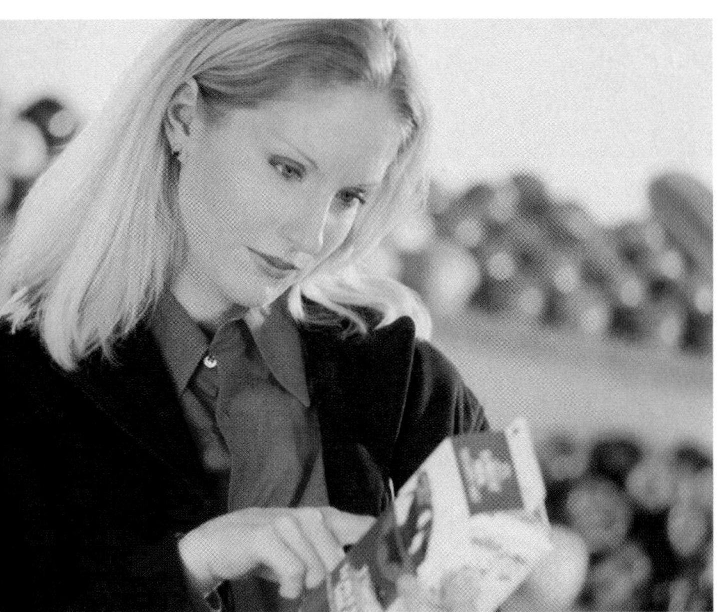

12-4 Reading labels helps consumers compare products to be sure the items they choose will be the ones that best meet their needs.

item. Be sure you have met all the qualifications before you try to redeem coupons.

Promotions affect the costs of food products. For instance, stores sell some items in multiples, such as three boxes of macaroni and cheese for five dollars. In a case such as this, determine what you would pay for one box. This will help you decide if the multiple price is a good value.

Grades, brands, and packaging are other factors that affect how much you pay for food products. Understanding these factors can help you be a smart consumer.

Grades

Many food products are given a ***grade,*** which is an indication of quality. Foods with higher grades usually cost more than those with lower grades. Grades are based on factors that affect the appeal of a food rather than its wholesomeness. For instance, a lower-grade peach may not have a uniform shape or a characteristic color. However, it is nutritious and safe to eat. In many cases, only products with the highest grades are sold in fresh form. Lower-grade products are often used as ingredients in processed foods.

Brands

A product's cost is affected by its ***brand name.*** This is the name a manufacturer puts on products so people will know that company makes the products. A ***store brand,*** also called a *house brand*, is a brand sold only by a store or chain of stores. A ***national brand*** is a brand that is advertised and sold throughout the country. Manufacturers of national brands often package some of their products with store brand labels. However, because the store brands are not promoted with big advertising budgets, they often cost less than national brands.

Q: How can product grades help me make purchase decisions?

A: When choosing foods for dishes where appearance is important, you may want to look for higher grades. However, keep in mind that foods are graded before shipping. Shipping sometimes causes damage that reduces product quality.

In many grocery stores across the country, consumers can choose generic products. A ***generic product*** is a plain-labeled, no-brand grocery product. Generic products generally cost quite a bit less than national and store brands. The prices are lower because manufacturers spend less money on packaging and advertising. In addition, a generic product may be made of lower-quality ingredients.

Generic food products usually are nutritionally equivalent to brand name items. However, they may not be of the same quality as brand name products. For instance, generic fruits and vegetables may have uneven sizes and shapes. Their colors and textures may vary. You may find generic products to be a good value, especially when uniform appearance is not essential.

Packaging

Another factor that affects the cost of food products is the amount and type of packaging material. Packaging affects the environment as well as product costs. As a smart consumer, you need to make a habit of precycling when deciding what to buy. ***Precycling*** is thinking about how packaging materials can be reused or recycled before you buy a product. For instance, you might plan to use a resealable plastic container to store leftovers. You might choose a product in a glass jar instead of a plastic container because you can recycle the glass. You might avoid buying a single-serving product because of the excessive packaging.

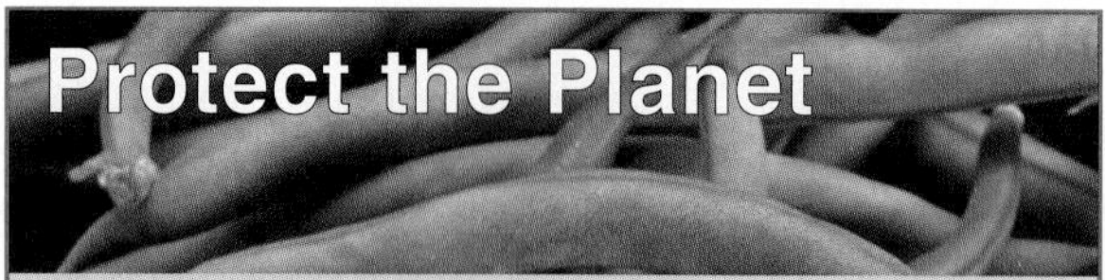

Protect the Planet

Avoid buying individually packaged products, such as one-serving juice containers and single-portion entrees. These smaller packages not only tend to cost more per serving, they also require more packaging material. Choose larger packages instead. You can use small, reusable containers to divide large items into single servings at home.

Using Unit Pricing

Many, but not all, grocery stores use unit pricing. ***Unit pricing*** is a listing of a product's cost per standard unit, weight, or measure. Examples are the cost per dozen, pound (.45 kg), or quart (L). Unit prices generally appear with selling prices on shelf tags underneath the products to which the prices refer, 12-5.

With unit pricing, you can compare the cost of different forms of products quickly and easily. For example, you can purchase green beans fresh, canned, and frozen. Suppose the unit price labels told you the canned green beans cost $.06 per ounce (28 g). Frozen green beans cost $.09 per ounce (28 g), and the fresh green beans cost $.11 per ounce (28 g). Obviously, the canned green beans would be the most economical.

Unit pricing can also help you compare different package sizes and different brands. For example, unit pricing may tell you that 1 ounce (28 g) of strawberry jam from a small jar costs $.16 while the same amount of jam from a large jar costs $.11. Unit pricing may also tell you that Brand X canned pears costs $.06 per ounce (28 g), whereas Brand Y canned pears costs $.07 per ounce (28 g).

As a smart consumer, you need to be aware of foods' per serving costs as well as their unit costs. The reason for this can be illustrated by comparing two boxes of breakfast cereal. A 20-ounce box of raisin bran cereal costs $3.19. A 20-ounce box of toasted oat cereal costs $3.69. The raisin bran has a lower unit cost. However, by looking on the product label, you can find the number of servings in each package. The box of raisin bran contains only 9 servings, whereas the box of toasted oats contains 18 servings. To figure the cost per serving, divide the total product price by the number of servings in each package. This calculation tells you the raisin bran costs about $.35 per serving. The toasted oats cost about $.21 per serving. If your family likes both types of cereal, the toasted oats are a better buy.

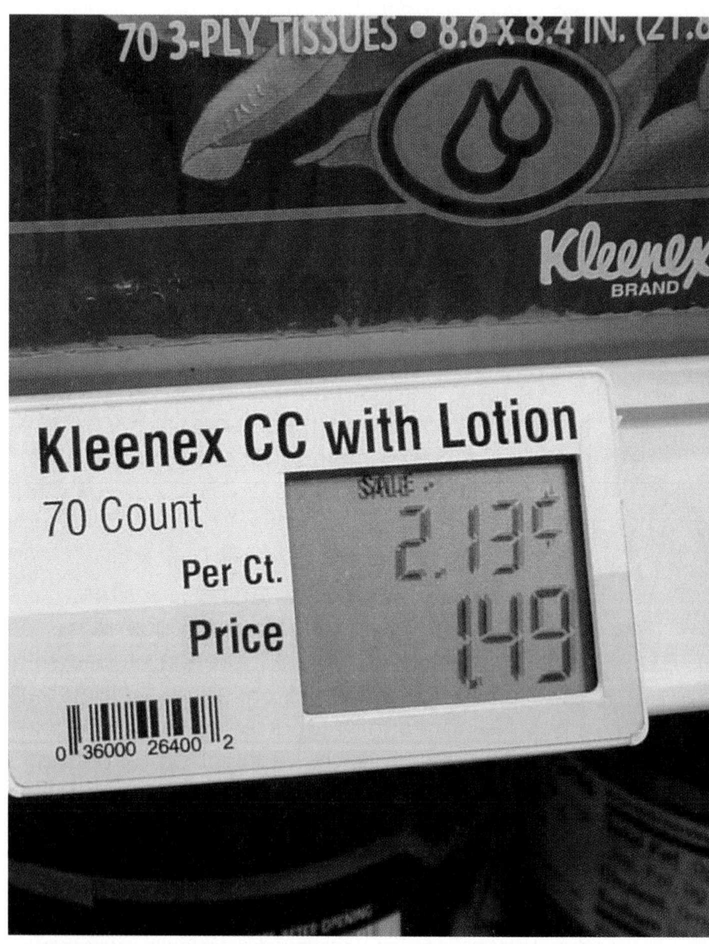

NCR Corporation

12-5 *Some supermarkets use electronic shelf tags, which readily reflect changes in unit prices due to store sales and price adjustments.*

Organic Foods

As you decide what to buy, you may think about choosing some ***organic foods.*** These are foods produced without the use of synthetic fertilizers, pesticides, or growth stimulants. Genetic engineering methods and ionizing radiation are also banned in the production of organic products.

The United States Department of Agriculture (USDA) has set standards for organic foods. Organic plant foods must be grown on land that has been free of chemical pesticides for at least three years. (***Pesticides*** are agents used to kill insects, weeds, and fungi that attack crops.) Organic standards also limit the types of fertilizers farmers can use to help plants grow. Organic meats and poultry must come from animals raised without the use of antibiotics or hormones to promote growth. Drugs may be used only to treat sick animals. See 12-6.

Along with fresh organic foods, you can buy processed foods that have organic ingredients. Look for the exact percentage of organic ingredients in a product to be stated on the label.

Organic foods often cost quite a bit more than nonorganic products. Many consumers are willing to pay higher prices for organic foods. These consumers often say they are concerned about the effects standard farming methods may have on foods or the environment.

Be a Clever Consumer

Consider the impact of coupons on unit cost. Small packages often have a higher unit cost than large packages of the same product. When using a coupon, however, the small package often becomes the better buy. For instance, suppose a 10-ounce (284 g) box of cereal costs $2.49 and a 20-ounce (568 g) box costs $4.39. The small box would have a unit cost of $.25 per ounce (28 g). The large box would have a unit cost of $.22 per ounce (28 g). With a $.75 coupon, the small box would cost $1.74; the large box would cost $3.64. With the coupon, the unit cost of the small box would be $.17; the unit cost of the large box would be $.18.

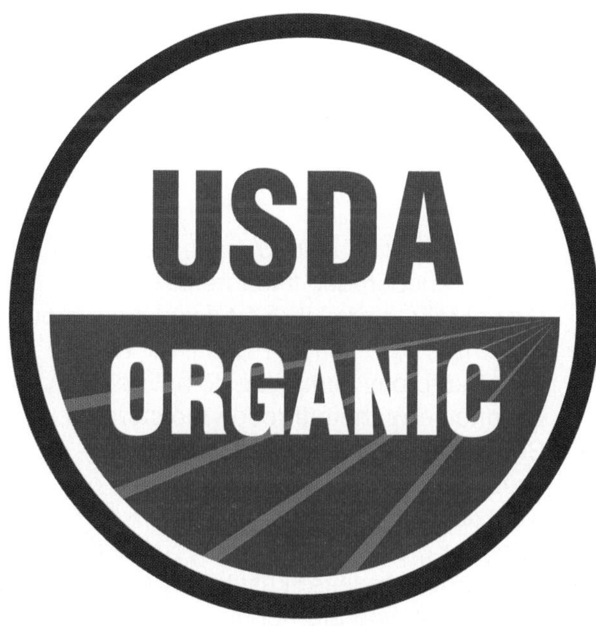

12-6 The USDA organic seal assures consumers that organic foods have been produced according to national standards.

Food Additives

Another factor that may affect your decisions about what to buy in the supermarket is ***food additives.*** These are substances that are added to food for a specific purpose, such as preserving the food. Although over 3,000 additives are in use today, they all fill one of the following four basic purposes:

- add nutrients
- preserve quality
- aid processing or preparation
- enhance flavors or colors

The Food and Drug Administration (FDA) and the USDA rigidly control the kinds and amounts of additives manufacturers can use in foods. Food scientists test foods and food additives to ensure their safety.

Before the government passed rigid food additive laws, about 600 additives were in use. The FDA placed these additives on the "Generally Recognized as Safe" or ***GRAS list.*** The FDA has retested the additives that appear on this list to make sure they are safe according to today's standards. Food manufacturers can use any additive that appears on the GRAS list without permission. However, they must obtain permission from the FDA for use of additives that are not on the GRAS list.

Q: Aren't organic foods more nutritious than foods grown by conventional methods?

A: Tests have not shown organic foods to be more nutritious or safer than nonorganic foods. Consumer panels have found the look and taste of organic and nonorganic foods to be similar, too.

Shopping Tips

Following some shopping guidelines will help you decide what to buy when you shop for food. These tips will also help you save money without sacrificing nutrition, quality, or taste.

- Read labels to be sure you know what you are buying.
- Compare brands and then select the brand that best meets your needs.
- Compare prices on a cost per serving basis.
- Buy foods that are in season when possible. Foods that are in season are generally low in price and high in quality.
- Take advantage of advertised specials, but be sure advertised prices are sale prices. Some stores feature regular prices in their advertisements.
- Compare the costs of different forms of the same food, such as canned, fresh, and frozen.
- Prepare foods from scratch if you have the time. Most convenience foods cost more than homemade ones.
- Use nonfat dry milk and margarine in cooking instead of fluid milk and butter to stretch dairy dollars.
- Avoid higher costs for cubed and sliced meats and cheeses. Buy large pieces and cut them at home.
- Plan meals that focus more on plant foods, such as dried legumes, which cost less than meat. See 12-7.

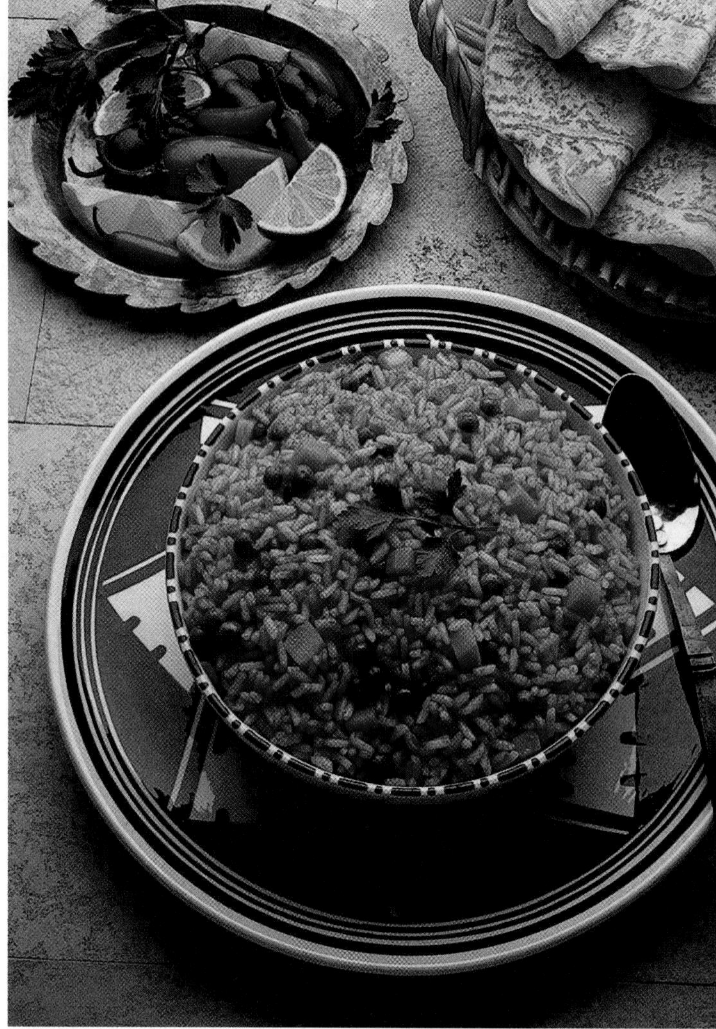

USA Rice Federation

12-7 Meatless entrees, such as this hearty, nutritious rice dish, are economical alternatives to main dish meats.

- Resist the temptation to make impulse purchases encouraged by store displays.
- Do not take a grocery cart if you plan to buy just one or two items. You will be less tempted to buy items you do not need if you have to carry them through the store.
- Shop when stores are least crowded—usually midmorning or midafternoon on weekdays.
- Shop for groceries just after you have eaten. You are less likely to buy unneeded items when you are not hungry.
- Do your grocery shopping by yourself. Shopping with another person makes some people more likely to buy foods they do not need.

Using Food Labeling

Food labels provide a wealth of information that can be helpful to consumers. Federal law requires the following items on food labels:

- the common name and form of the food
- the volume or weight of the contents, including any liquid in which foods are packed
- the name and address of the manufacturer, packer, or distributor
- a list of ingredients, in descending order according to weight. For instance, suppose a label lists "chicken, noodles, and carrots." The product would need to contain, by weight, more chicken than noodles and more noodles than carrots.

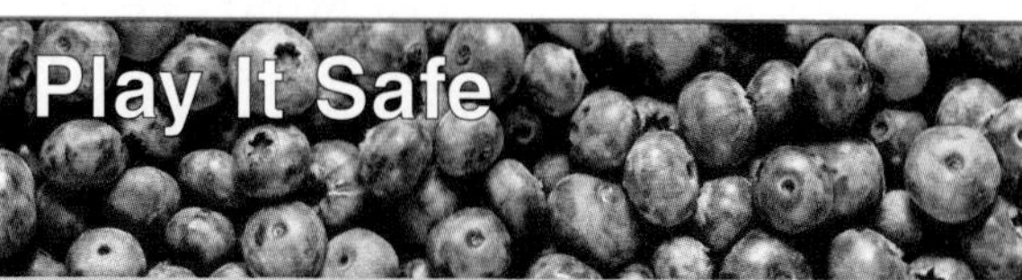

Organisms that cause foodborne illnesses multiply quickly at temperatures above 40°F (5°C). Put refrigerated and frozen foods in your grocery cart last to prevent the growth of these organisms. Store all food properly when you arrive home. If you will not be going directly home after grocery shopping, take an insulated cooler to the store with you. Use it to keep perishable foods cool until you can store them properly.

Nutrition Labeling

Another type of information the FDA requires on almost all food packages is ***nutrition labeling.*** This is a breakdown of a food product's contributions to an average diet. You can identify this labeling by the heading "Nutrition Facts." See 12-8.

The first item that appears under the heading on a nutrition label is the *serving size.* This is stated in both household and metric measures. The number of *servings per container* appears next. Serving sizes are the same for similar food products to help consumers make comparisons between products.

Calorie information includes the number of calories per serving along with the number of calories from fat. This can help you limit fat to no more than 35 percent of your total calories.

Nutrients found in each serving of food products also appear on nutrition labels. The nutrients listed are those that are most directly linked to the health concerns of today's consumers. The list must include the amount of total fat, saturated fat, *trans* fat, cholesterol, sodium, total carbohydrate, dietary fiber, sugars, and protein. Vitamin A, vitamin C, calcium, and iron are listed as well. Information about other nutrients, such as thiamin and monounsaturated fat, is optional. However, foods about which manufacturers make nutritional claims and foods with added nutrients must include additional information on the label.

At the bottom of larger nutrition labels, standard information about Daily Values is shown for 2,000- and 2,500-calorie diets. ***Daily Values*** are dietary references that appear on food labels. They are designed to help consumers use label information to plan healthy diets. The reference of Daily Values includes maximums for fat, saturated fat, cholesterol, and sodium for both calorie levels. Daily minimums for total carbohydrate and fiber are also given. This reference information is the same on all nutrition labels that include it.

Percent Daily Values based on a 2,000-calorie diet are given for each of the nutrients listed on the label. Your daily calorie needs may be higher or lower than 2,000 calories. Therefore, your Daily Values may also be higher or lower. You will need to keep this in mind when reading the percent Daily Values on food labels.

Many manufacturers make health and/or nutritional claims about their food products on product labels. Health claims link the effect of a nutrient or food to a disease or health condition. For instance, a can of unsalted vegetables might have a claim linking a diet low in sodium with a reduced risk of high blood pressure. The FDA regulates the conditions under which these claims can be used. The FDA has also set standard definitions for terms used in nutritional claims, such as *lowfat, high fiber,* and *reduced calories.* You can use claims on product labels to help you find foods with the nutritional qualities you want. See 12-9.

Universal Product Code

Another item found on food labels is the ***universal product code,*** or ***UPC.*** This is a series of lines, bars, and numbers that appears on packages of food and nonfood items.

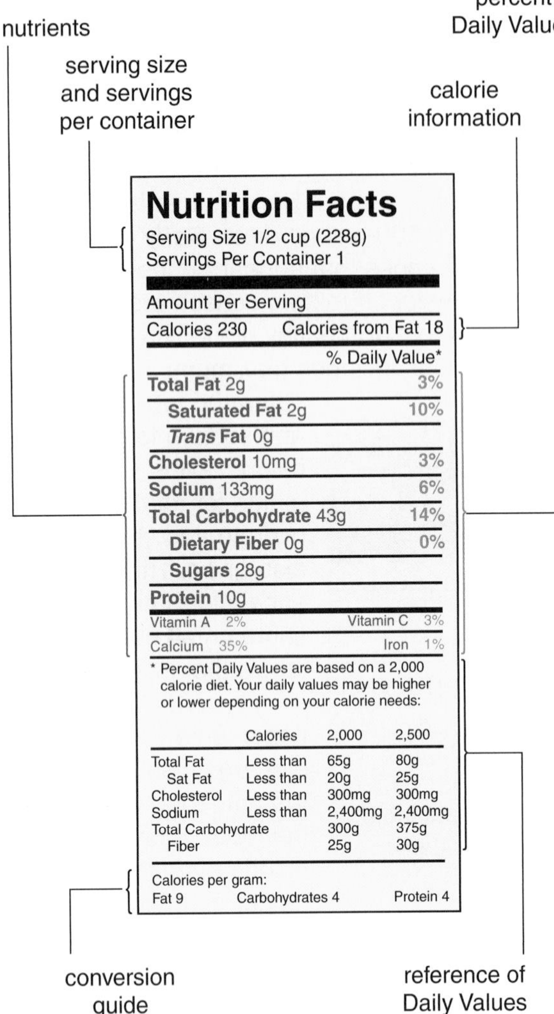

Nutrition Facts

Serving Size 1/2 cup (228g)
Servings Per Container 1

Amount Per Serving

Calories 230	Calories from Fat 18
	% Daily Value*
Total Fat 2g	3%
Saturated Fat 2g	10%
***Trans* Fat** 0g	
Cholesterol 10mg	3%
Sodium 133mg	6%
Total Carbohydrate 43g	14%
Dietary Fiber 0g	0%
Sugars 28g	
Protein 10g	

Vitamin A 2%	Vitamin C 3%
Calcium 35%	Iron 1%

* Percent Daily Values are based on a 2,000 calorie diet. Your daily values may be higher or lower depending on your calorie needs:

	Calories	2,000	2,500
Total Fat	Less than	65g	80g
Sat Fat	Less than	20g	25g
Cholesterol	Less than	300mg	300mg
Sodium	Less than	2,400mg	2,400mg
Total Carbohydrate		300g	375g
Fiber		25g	30g

Calories per gram:
Fat 9 Carbohydrates 4 Protein 4

***12-8** Some food products may carry a simpler version of the nutrition label. However, all nutrition labels provide consumers with valuable information.*

Grocery checkers pass the UPC on items over a laser beam scanner. As the items pass over the scanner, the store's computer reads the codes. The correct prices are then rung up on the computer terminal at the clerk's counter. The computer prints a description of the items and their prices on the customer's receipt.

Open Dating

Many products have dates printed on their labeling. Some of these dates are printed in codes that are used mostly by manufacturers. However, ***open dating*** uses dates consumers can clearly recognize on perishable and semi-perishable foods. It can help you obtain products that are fresh and wholesome. Dates also help you know which product to use first. Manufacturers use four types of dates.

A *pack date* is the day a food was manufactured or processed and packaged. It tells you how old the food is at the time you buy it. Canned foods often have this type of date.

A *pull* or *sell date* is the last day a store should sell a product. The pull date allows for some storage time in your refrigerator. Milk, ice cream, and cold cuts often have pull dates stamped on their containers or packages.

An *expiration date* is the last day a consumer should use or eat a food. Yeast and baby food have expiration dates.

A *freshness date* is often found on bakery products like bread and rolls. A product with an expired freshness date has passed its quality peak. However, you can still use it.

Q: Does "no sugar added" on a label mean the same thing as "sugar free"?

A: No. Added sugars refer to sugars manufacturers put in foods during processing. However, many foods, such as milk, fruits, and juice products, contain natural sugars. The number of grams of sugar shown on a Nutrition Facts panel includes both added and naturally occurring sugars.

Help with Consumer Problems

From time to time, you may have problems with food products or the businesses that sell them. Many sources of consumer help exist. The source that will best be able to assist you will depend on your particular problem.

Food stores can help you with a quality problem caused by the way they handled a food product. For instance, you might discover a loaf of bread you just purchased is moldy. If you return the bread, most store managers will

Nutrient Content Claims	
cholesterol free	Fewer than 2 milligrams of cholesterol and 2 grams or fewer of saturated fat per serving.
fat free	Fewer than 0.5 grams of fat per serving.
fresh	Food is raw, has never been frozen or heated, and contains no preservatives.
high fiber	5 grams or more fiber per serving. (Foods making high-fiber claims must also meet the definition for low fat, or the level of total fat must appear next to the high-fiber claim.)
light/lite	A nutritionally altered food product that contains one-third fewer calories or half the fat of the "regular" version of the food. This term can also be used to indicate the sodium of a low-calorie, lowfat food has been reduced by 50 percent. In addition, labels may state that foods are light (lite) in color or texture.
*low calorie	40 calories or fewer per serving.
*low cholesterol	20 milligrams or fewer of cholesterol and 2 grams or fewer of saturated fat per serving.
*low fat	3 grams or fewer fat per serving.
*low sodium	140 milligrams or fewer sodium per serving.
reduced calories	At least 25 percent fewer calories per serving than the "full-calorie" version of the food.
sodium free	Fewer than 5 milligrams of sodium per serving.
sugar free	Fewer than 0.5 grams of sugar per serving.

*Foods with a serving size of 30 grams or fewer or 2 tablespoons or fewer must meet the specified requirement for portions of 50 grams of the food.

***12-9** Manufacturers must adhere to these definitions when making nutrient content claims about food products.*

refund your money or give you a new loaf. See 12-10.

Product manufacturers can help you with a food quality problem that is due to a processing error. Suppose when you open a package of rice mix, you find the seasoning packet is missing. Look on the package for a toll-free telephone number, Web site, or address you can use to contact the manufacturer. Keep the package handy so you can refer to it for specific product information the manufacturer might need. Be polite as you make a brief complaint and reasonable request for what action you would like the manufacturer to take. For instance, you might ask for a coupon for a free package of rice mix.

The *Food Safety and Inspection Service (FSIS)* can help you with a food safety problem involving meat, poultry, or egg products. The FSIS is the branch of the USDA that handles product *recalls,* or removal of products from the market. If you found metal shavings in a can of beef stew, the FSIS might contact the manufacturer to recall the product.

The *FDA* is the agency that handles food safety complaints linked to products that do not contain meat or poultry. If you found a piece of glass in a box of cereal, the FDA would handle the investigation. Be prepared to provide

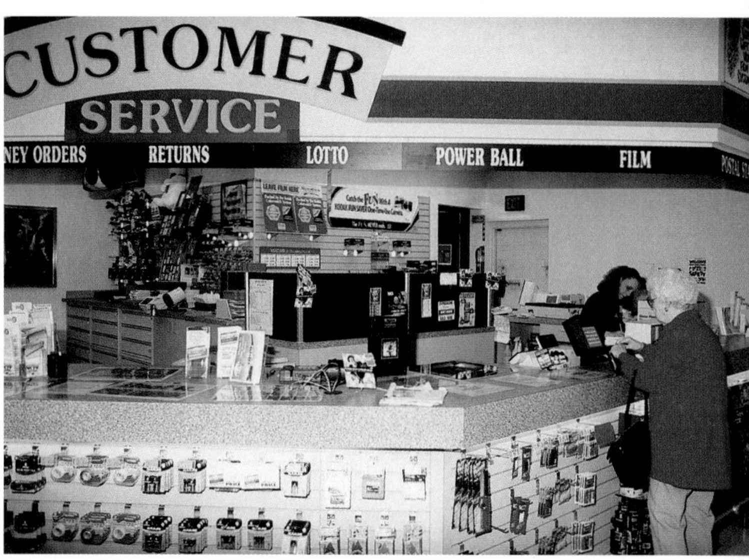

photo courtesy of IGA, INC.

***12-10** Most food stores have a customer service counter to help address shoppers' questions and problems.*

detailed product information when you call. See 12-11.

City, county, or state health departments address safety problems you might have with food from restaurants. They inspect facilities, issue warnings and fines, and close businesses when needed.

Better Business Bureaus (BBBs) can help you when you have a problem with the way a food store or restaurant conducts business. BBBs promote honest advertising and selling practices. Imagine the prices at a food store checkout regularly ring up higher than the shelf tags. If the store manager does not give you a satisfactory response, a BBB can contact the store on your behalf. The BBB can also offer to resolve your complaint by other means, if necessary.

These sources of help do more than handle consumer complaints. They can answer questions and provide a variety of consumer information. Some also do testing, grading, and inspecting to ensure the quality and safety of the food supply.

What Do You Need When Making a Product Complaint?	
•	Your name, address, and telephone number
•	Brand name, product name, and manufacturer of the product
•	Size and type of package
•	Codes and dates from product package
•	Name and location of store and date you purchased the product
For food safety complaints, you will also need	
•	Original package or container
•	Foreign object found in the food product (if applicable)
•	Any uneaten portion of the food

12-11 *Having all the necessary information available will make it easier for the appropriate agency to process your product complaint.*

Chapter 12 Review

The Smart Consumer

Summary

Smart consumers must shop carefully to get the most from their food dollars. They can choose from many types of stores. Evaluating store features can help them decide where to shop. Busy lifestyles are driving many trends in supermarkets and are also the force behind an increase in electronic shopping.

Using a shopping list and comparing costs can help consumers know what to buy. Many factors can affect costs, including product grades, brands, and packaging. Unit pricing makes it easy to compare costs of different brands, forms, and sizes. Knowing about organic foods and food additives can help consumers make purchase decisions, too.

Food labeling provides consumers with information about the food products they buy. Nutrition labeling helps them get the most nutritional value for the money they spend. The UPC speeds checkout. Open dating helps consumers select foods that are fresh and wholesome.

Various resources can help consumers who have problems with food products. These resources can also provide information and other consumer services.

Review What You Have Read

Write your answers on a separate sheet of paper.

1. At what type of food store might consumers have to pack their own groceries in bags or boxes?
2. True or false. Brands and sizes of food products are much more limited for electronic shoppers than for store shoppers.
3. How can a shopping list help a meal manager?
4. A 16-ounce (473 mL) can of green beans usually costs $.69. This week, a large supermarket chain is advertising 2 cans for $1.29. Is this a bargain? Explain why or why not.
5. Why do generic products cost less than national and store brands?
6. Consumers can easily compare the cost of different brands, sizes, and forms of the same or similar products with _____.
7. What are two reasons consumers often give for being willing to pay higher prices for organic foods?
8. What are the four basic purposes of food additives?
9. List eight tips to help consumers save money when shopping for food.
10. True or false. The net weight shown on canned foods includes the liquids in which the foods are canned.
11. Why might food products provide people with different percents of their Daily Values than those listed on labels?
12. Describe how the UPC works at the checkout stand in a grocery store.
13. The last day a product should be sold is called the _____.
    A. expiration date
    B. freshness date
    C. pack date
    D. pull or sell date
14. Name four sources of help with consumer problems.

Build Your Basic Skills

1. **Math.** Do a price comparison study of the cost of different forms of a food product. For example, compare the cost per serving of a chocolate cake made from scratch, a chocolate cake made from a mix, a frozen chocolate cake, and a bakery chocolate cake. (All of these cakes should be two-layer, 8-inch (20-cm) cakes with chocolate frosting.)
2. **Reading.** Mount the entire label from a can of food in the center of a sheet of paper. Label each of the points of information required on food packages. Also label the UPC and each part of the Nutrition Facts panel.

Build Your Thinking Skills

1. **Evaluate.** Visit several supermarkets of comparable size. Using the criteria for choosing a food store given in the chapter, evaluate each store. Write a report summarizing your findings and identifying the store at which you would most like to shop. Explain the reasons for your choice.
2. **Organize.** Organize your family's weekly grocery shopping list to match the order of the food aisles in the store where you shop. Use the list to do the shopping. Share with the class how the list affected the shopping process.

Apply Technology

1. Investigate the lab procedures used to determine the nutritional values of food products itemized on Nutrition Facts panels.
2. Make a list of ways UPC and scanner checkout benefit consumers and food stores.

Using Workplace Skills

Carine is a retail food demonstrator at Johnsen's Supermarket. She tells store customers about food products and answers their questions as she offers them samples she has prepared. The store manager expects Carine to help boost sales of the products she demonstrates.

To be a successful employee, Carine needs basic speaking skills. Put yourself in Carine's place and answer the following questions about your need for and use of these skills:

A. What are three specific speaking skills that will help you communicate with your customers?
B. How might store customers respond if you do not have adequate speaking skills?
C. How might the store manager respond if you do not have adequate speaking skills?
D. What is another skill you would need in this job? Briefly explain why this skill would be important.

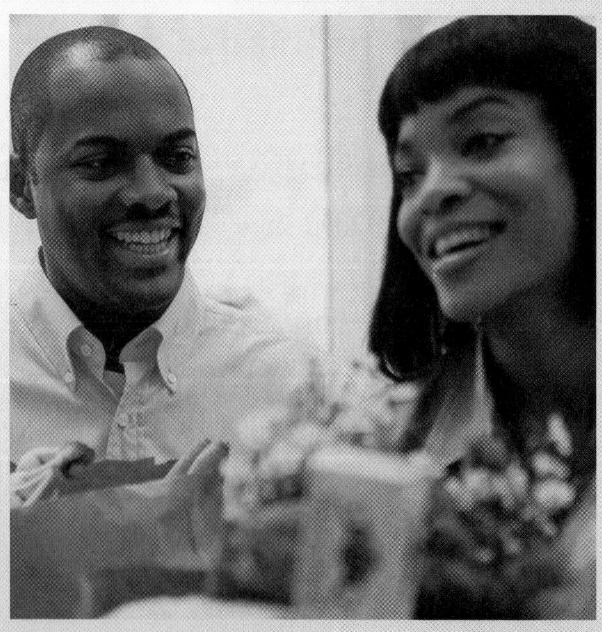

Chapter 13
Getting Started in the Kitchen

Coffee Roaster
Controls gas-fired roasters to remove moisture from coffee beans.

Time-Study Engineer
Develops work measurement procedures and directs time-and-motion studies to promote efficient and economical utilization of personnel and facilities.

Food Tester
Performs standardized tests to determine physical or chemical properties of food or beverage products or to ensure compliance with company or government quality standards.

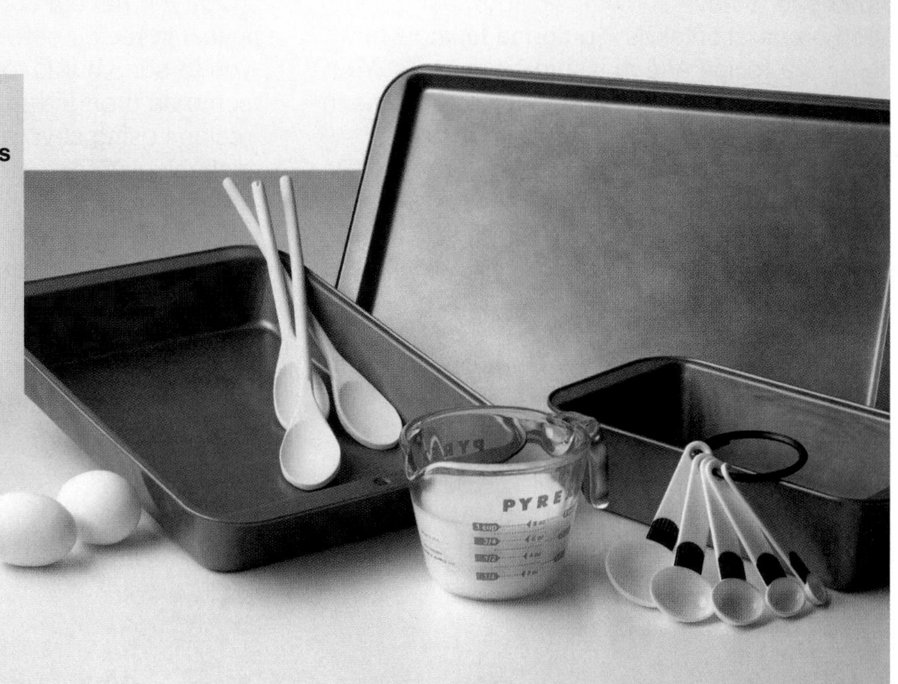

Baker's Secret

Terms to Know

recipe
yield
cooking time
watt
dehydration
standing time
hot spot
arcing
time-work schedule
dovetail
blend
decaffeinated
caffeine
tea

Objectives

After studying this chapter, you will be able to

- ❏ identify abbreviations and define cooking terms used in recipes.
- ❏ measure liquid and dry ingredients and fats for use in recipes.
- ❏ change the yield of a recipe.
- ❏ plan time-work schedules.
- ❏ follow a recipe to prepare a sandwich, snack, or beverage.

You do not have to have cooking skills to satisfy hunger. You can eat convenience foods that require little or no preparation. However, you can add unlimited variety and interest to meals when you know how to prepare foods from scratch.

Before you can begin working in the kitchen, you need to have some basic knowledge and food preparation skills. You need to know how to read a recipe and measure ingredients. You also need to be able to plan your use of time in the kitchen.

Choosing a Recipe

A ***recipe*** is a set of instructions for preparing a specific food. Many basic cookbooks provide menu ideas as well as recipes. Specialty cookbooks contain many ideas and recipes for international foods and unusual dishes. Magazines, newspapers, and appliance manuals can also be good sources of recipes. The meal manager can use these resources to help plan and prepare daily meals.

If you have a computer, you may wish to invest in recipe software. Most programs allow you to add your favorite recipes to those that come on the software. You can search for recipes using several factors, such as type of dish, cuisine, and preparation method, 13-1. You can easily adjust the number of servings and make a printout of any recipe. Many programs also allow you to prepare food budgets, shopping lists, and nutritional analyses. You can also explore numerous recipe Web sites on the Internet. Many sites offer the same search features as software programs. You can often

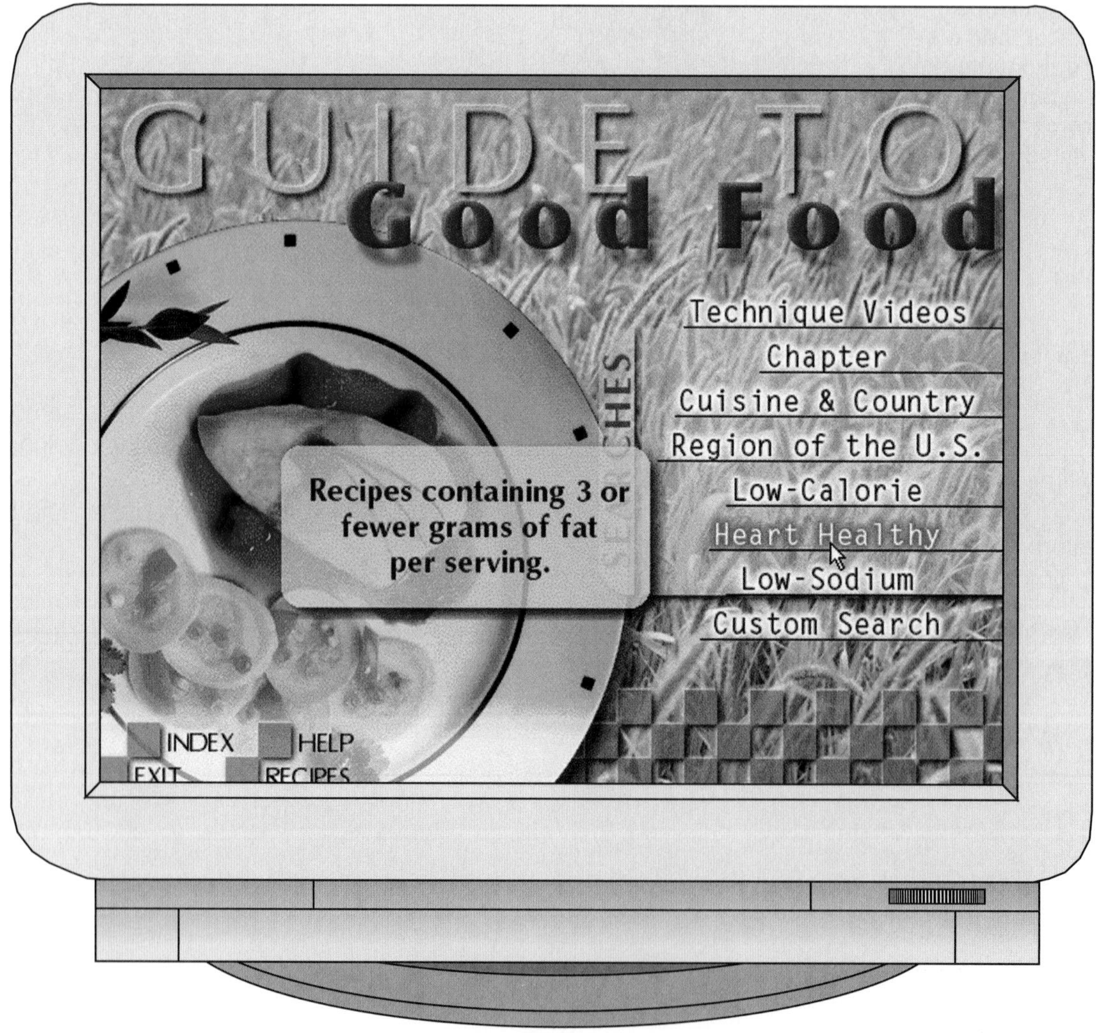

13-1 Recipes software allows you to search for recipes by categories.

save favorite recipes in a personal online recipe file, too.

Good recipes are written in a clear, concise manner. A recipe should list ingredients in the order in which you will be combining them. Amounts should be easy to measure. Directions for mixing and/or handling procedures must be complete. Baking or cooking times and temperatures and pan sizes need to be accurate. The recipe should state the ***yield,*** which is the number of average servings the recipe makes. Many recipes also include a nutritional analysis to help you evaluate how the food will fit into a healthful diet. See 13-2.

A recipe is your work plan for the food you are going to prepare. You will want to read through the recipe before you begin to prepare it. This will allow you to be sure you understand the directions and have all the ingredients you will need. When you are ready to begin, reread the recipe. Follow the directions carefully as you prepare the product.

Abbreviations

The amounts of ingredients listed in recipes are often given as abbreviations. You need to be able to interpret these abbreviations. This will help you make sure you include ingredients in the right proportions. See 13-3.

Q: If I follow recipes carefully, do I need to be concerned about food safety?

A: Be aware that not all recipes are developed by people who know safe food handling methods. As you read through a recipe, remember the four basic steps for keeping foods safe to eat—clean, separate, cook, and chill. You would be wise to avoid recipes that include unsafe practices, such as marinating meat at room temperature.

Cooking Terms

Recipes use a variety of terms to describe exactly how you are to handle the ingredients. For instance, a recipe that includes carrots is not likely to tell you to cut the carrots. This term is too general to let you know how the carrots should look in the finished product. Instead, the recipe might tell you to *slice, dice, shred,* or *julienne* the carrots. Becoming familiar with specific

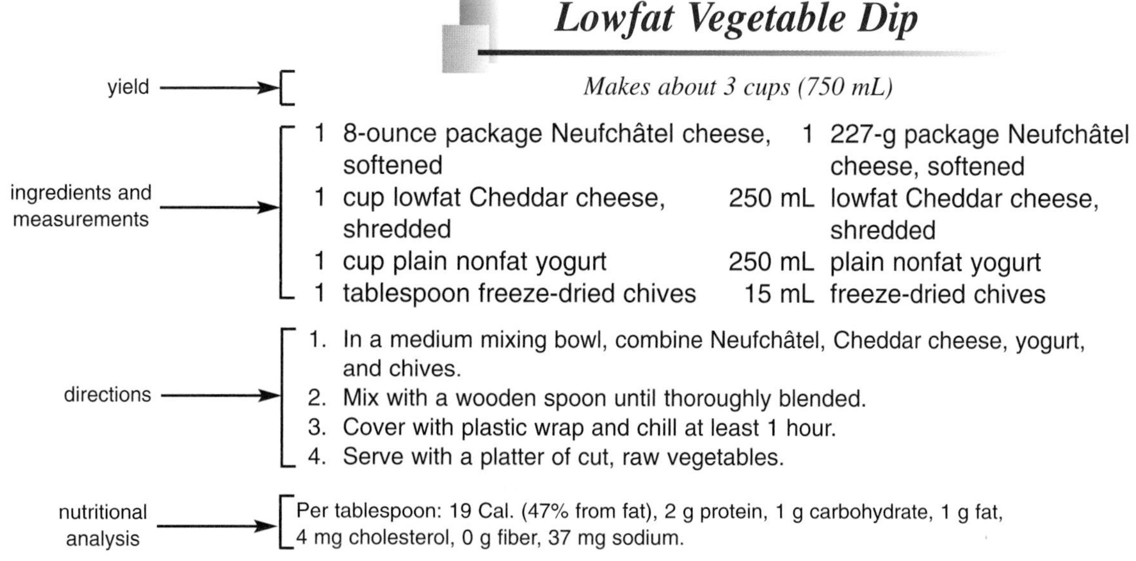

***13-2** A well-written recipe should include all the information you need to prepare a particular food.*

cooking terms will help your food products turn out as expected. See 13-4.

Using Microwave Recipes

Cooking foods in a microwave oven is not hard. However, microwave cooking does differ from conventional cooking. Therefore, using microwave recipes requires some specific knowledge.

Cooking Time

Cooking time in a microwave recipe refers to the total amount of time food is exposed to microwave energy. Microwave cooking time for most foods is much shorter than conventional cooking time. Some foods can be heated in a matter of seconds. Microwave cooking time is often divided into two or more intervals. Between cooking intervals, the recipe may tell you to stir the food, add ingredients, or change the oven's power setting.

Knowing how powerful your microwave oven is can help you decide how long to cook foods. Microwave cooking power is measured in ***watts.*** Most new models produce a maximum of 600 to 1,100 watts. More watts means faster cooking. Check microwave recipes to see if they give the wattages at which they were tested. If your microwave oven has a higher wattage, you may need to use less time or a lower power setting. If your recipe does not list a wattage, you may have to prepare some foods by trial and error. Start with the shortest time stated in the recipe. Then check to see if more time is needed.

Q: Doesn't microwave cooking reduce the nutritional value of foods?

A: Some vitamins are heat sensitive, and some vitamins and minerals are water-soluble. These nutrients can be lost through any cooking process. However, fewer nutrients tend to be lost through microwave cooking. This is because cooking times are short and only small amounts of water are used to cook foods.

Just a few minutes of overcooking can cause ***dehydration,*** or drying out. Dehydration may occur when microwave cooking continues until foods are fully cooked. This is because many foods will continue cooking after the allotted time in the oven. To account for this tendency, many microwave recipes specify ***standing time.*** This is the time during which foods finish cooking by internal heat after being removed from a microwave oven. For instance, a recipe for baked potatoes may specify four minutes of cooking time and five minutes of standing time. Wrapping foods in aluminum foil will help hold in heat during standing time.

Abbreviations Used in Recipes	
Conventional	
tsp. or t.	teaspoon
tbsp. or T.	tablespoon
c. or C.	cup
pt.	pint
qt.	quart
oz.	ounce
lb. or #	pound
Metric	
mL	milliliter
L	liter
g	gram
kg	kilogram

13-3 Recipes often include these abbreviations.

Covering Foods

Many microwave recipes state you should cover foods during cooking. Covering foods in a microwave oven serves several purposes. Covering distributes heat more evenly and helps foods retain moisture so they will not dry out. The steam held in by the cover can help speed cooking time and tenderize foods. Covers are also useful for preventing spatters inside the microwave oven.

You can use a number of materials to cover foods in a microwave oven. Tight fitting casserole lids are excellent for foods that require steam for

Glossary of Food Preparation Terms

bake. To cook in the oven with dry heat.

barbecue. To cook on a rack or spit over hot coals or some other source of direct heat.

baste. To spoon pan juices, melted fat, or another liquid over the surface of food during cooking to keep the food moist and add flavor.

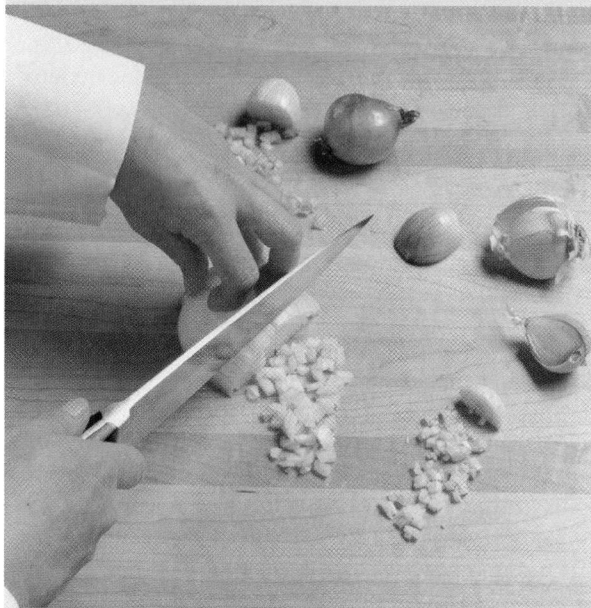

Chop

beat. To mix ingredients together with a circular up-and-down motion using a spoon, whisk, or rotary or electric beater.

bind. To thicken or smooth out the consistency of a liquid.

blanch. To scald or parboil in water or steam.

blend. To stir ingredients until they are thoroughly combined.

boil. To cook in liquid at 212°F (100°C).

bone. To remove bones from fowl or meat.

braise. To cook in a small amount of liquid in a tightly covered pan over low heat.

bread. To coat with dry bread or cracker crumbs.

broil. To cook uncovered under a direct source of heat.

brown. To turn the surface of a food brown by placing it under a broiler or quickly cooking it in hot fat.

brush. To apply sauce, melted fat, or other liquid with a basting or pastry brush.

candy. To cook in a sugar syrup until coated or crystallized.

caramelize. To heat sugar until a brown color and characteristic flavor develop.

chill. To make a food cold by placing it in a refrigerator or in a bowl over crushed ice.

chop. To cut into small pieces.

clarify. To make a liquid clear by removing solid particles.

coat. To thoroughly cover a food with a liquid or dry mixture.

coddle. To cook by submerging in simmering liquid.

combine. To mix or blend two or more ingredients.

cool. To let a food stand until it no longer feels warm to the touch.

core. To remove the center part of a fruit such as an apple or pineapple.

cream. To soften solid fats, often by adding a second ingredient, such as sugar, and working with a wooden spoon or an electric mixer until the fat is creamy.

crush. To pulverize.

cube. To cut into small squares of equal size.

cut. To divide into parts with a sharp utensil.

cut in. To combine solid fat with flour using a pastry blender, two forks, or the fingers.

deep-fry. To cook in a large amount of hot fat.

devein. To remove the large black or white vein along a shrimp's back.

dice. To cut into very small cubes of even size.

dissolve. To cause a solid food to turn into or become part of a liquid.

dot. To place small pieces of butter or another food over the surface of a food.

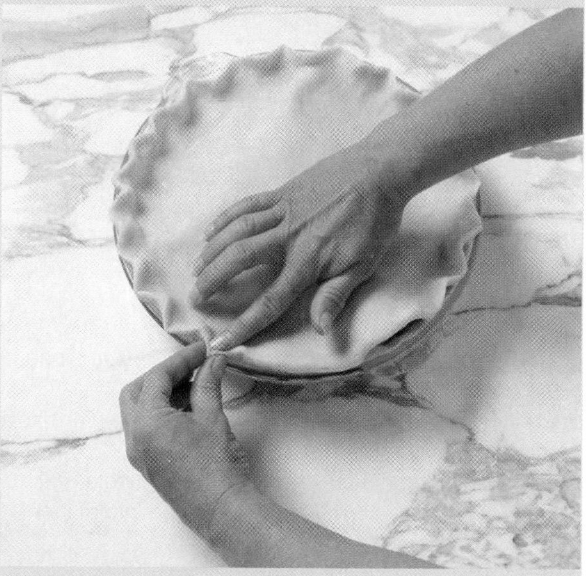

Flute

drain. To remove liquid from a food product.

dredge. To coat a food by sprinkling it with or dipping it in a dry ingredient such as flour or bread crumbs.

dress. To prepare a food for cooking.

dust. To lightly sprinkle the surface of a food with sugar, flour, or crumbs.

elevate. To lift a food off the floor of a microwave oven to allow microwaves to penetrate the food from the bottom as well as from the top and sides.

(Continued)

13-4 *Being able to interpret these terms will help you prepare recipes successfully.*

flake. To break fish into small pieces with a fork.
flour. To sprinkle or coat with flour.
flute. To make grooves or folds in dough.
fold. To incorporate a delicate mixture into a thicker, heavier mixture with a whisk or rubber spatula using a down, up, and over motion so the finished product remains light.

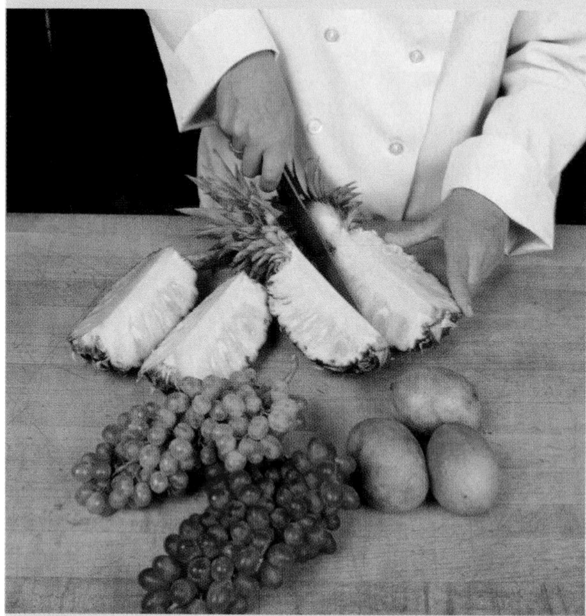

Quarter

fricassee. To cook pieces of meat or poultry in butter and then in seasoned liquid until tender.
fry. To cook in a small amount of hot fat.
garnish. To decorate foods by adding other attractive and complementary foodstuffs to the food or serving dish.
glaze. To apply a liquid that forms a glossy coating.
grate. To reduce a food into small bits by rubbing it on the sharp teeth of a utensil.
grease. To rub fat on the surface of a cooking utensil or on a food itself.
grill. To broil over hot coals or to fry on a griddle.
grind. To mechanically break down a food into a finer texture.
hull. To remove the outer covering of a fruit or vegetable.
julienne. To cut food into thin, stick-sized strips.
knead. To work dough by pressing it with the heels of the hands, folding it, turning it, and repeating each motion until the dough is smooth and elastic.
marinate. To soak meat in a solution containing an acid, such as vinegar or tomato juice, that helps tenderize the connective tissue.
mash. To break a food by pressing it with the back of a spoon or masher or forcing it through a ricer.
melt. To change from a solid to a liquid through the application of heat.
mince. To cut or chop into very fine pieces.
mix. To combine two or more ingredients into one mass.
mold. To shape by hand or by pouring into a form to achieve a desired structure.
panbroil. To cook without fat in an uncovered skillet.
panfry. To cook in a skillet with a small amount of fat.
parboil. To boil in liquid until partially cooked.
pare. To remove the stem and outer covering of a vegetable or fruit with a paring knife or peeler.
peel. To remove the outer layer.
pit. To remove the seed(s) of a fruit or vegetable.
poach. To cook over or in a simmering liquid.
preheat. To heat an appliance to a desired temperature about 5 to 8 minutes before it is to be used.
punch down. To push a fist firmly into the top of risen yeast dough.
puree. To put food through a fine sieve or a food mill to form a thick and smooth liquid.
quarter. To cut into four equal pieces.
reconstitute. To return to a previous state by adding water.
reduce. To decrease the quantity of a liquid and intensify the flavor by boiling.
refresh. To quickly plunge blanched vegetables in cold water to stop the cooking process.
roast. To cook uncovered in the oven with dry heat.
roll. To shape into a round mass; to wrap a flat, flexible piece of food around on itself; to flatten dough to an even thickness with a rolling pin.
rotate. To turn food in a microwave oven one-quarter to one-half turn at one or more intervals in the cooking period to allow microwaves to hit it in a more even pattern.

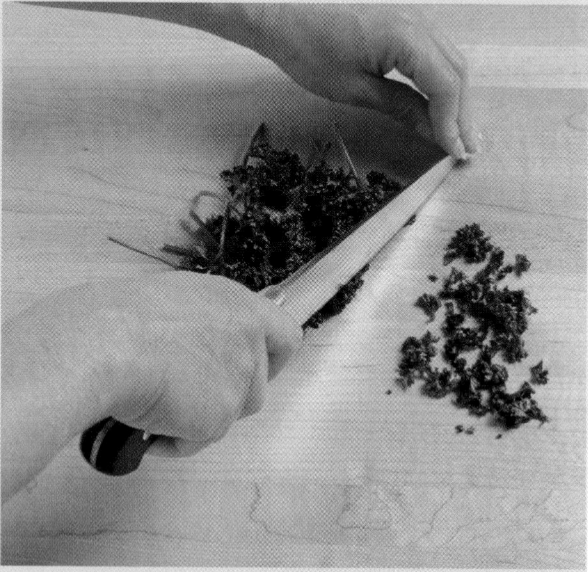

Mince

saute. To cook food in a small amount of hot fat.
scald. To heat liquid to just below the boiling point; to dip food into boiling water or pour boiling water over the food.
scallop. To cover with sauce and bake.

(Continued)

score. To make small, shallow cuts on the surface of a food.
sear. To brown the surface of a food very quickly with high heat.
season. To add herbs, spices, or other ingredients to a food to increase the flavor of the food; to prepare a cooking utensil, such as a cast iron skillet, for cooking.
section. To separate into parts.
separate. To remove one part from another, as the yolk from the white of an egg.
shape. To form.
shell. To remove from an outer covering.
shield. To use small pieces of aluminum foil to cover areas of a food that might become overcooked in a microwave oven.
shred. To cut or break into thin pieces.
sift. To put through a sieve to reduce to finer particles.
simmer. To cook in liquid that is barely at the boiling point.
skim. To remove a substance from the surface of a liquid.
slice. To cut into thin, flat pieces.
sliver. To cut into long, slender pieces.
snip. To cut into small bits with kitchen shears.
sprinkle. To scatter drops of liquid or particles of powder over the surface of a food.
steam. To cook with vapor produced by a boiling liquid.
steep. To soak in a hot liquid.
sterilize. To make free from microorganisms.
stew. To cook one food or several foods together in a seasoned liquid for a long period.
stir. To mix with a circular motion.
stir-fry. To cook foods quickly in a small amount of fat over high heat while stirring constantly.
strain. To separate solid from liquid materials.
thicken. To make a liquid more dense by adding an agent like flour, cornstarch, or egg yolks.
toast. To make the surface of a food brown by applying heat.
toss. To mix lightly.
truss. To prepare fowl for cooking by binding the wings and legs.
unmold. To remove from a form.
vent. To leave an opening through which steam can escape in the covering of a food to be cooked in a microwave oven.
whip. To beat quickly and steadily by hand with a whisk or rotary beater.

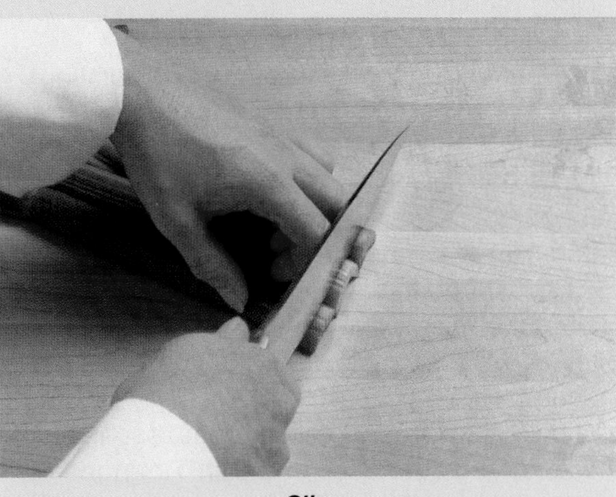

Slice

cooking. Waxed paper works well as a loose covering, 13-5. Covering foods with paper towels will help absorb spatters. (Choose paper towels designed for microwave use, as they are free of materials not approved for food contact.)

Covering food with plastic wrap or placing it in a plastic cooking bag will help retain moisture. (Plastic wraps designed for the microwave oven work best because they will not melt during cooking.) However, pressure from steam can build up inside containers that are tightly covered with plastic. Therefore, recipes often recommend venting the plastic wrap. This means turning back a corner of the wrap to form a steam vent.

Not all foods require a cover in the microwave oven. You may leave some foods uncovered to allow excess moisture to evaporate. You may need to cover other foods for only part of the cooking time. For best results, follow the directions in your recipe.

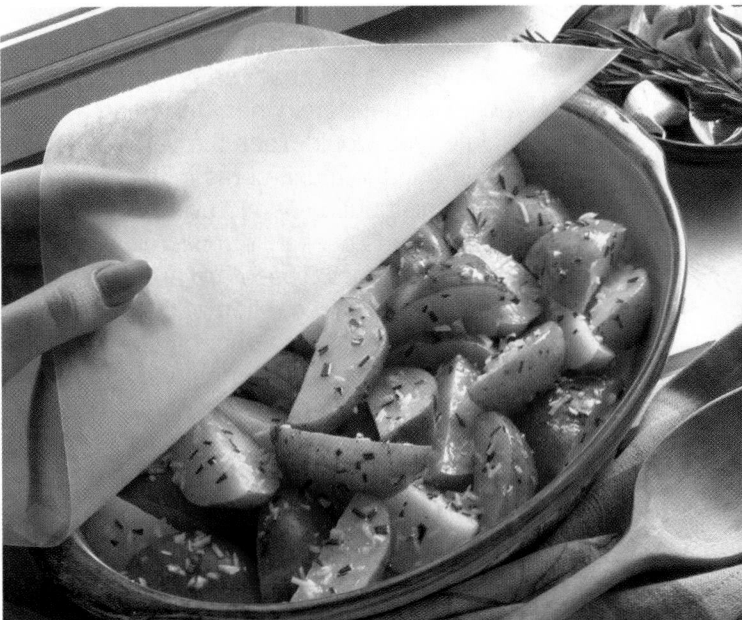

photograph courtesy of The Reynolds Kitchens

13-5 *Waxed paper is a good choice for loosely covering vegetables in a microwave oven.*

Evenness of Cooking

Microwaves are not always distributed evenly throughout the microwave oven cavity. This tends to be more of a problem in older models. Uneven distribution of microwaves can cause foods to cook unevenly. The shape of food pieces can also affect how evenly they cook. Microwave recipes use a number of techniques to promote more uniform cooking.

Many microwave recipes recommend rotating food at one or more intervals in the cooking period. Rotating food one-quarter to one-half turn allows microwaves to hit it in a more even pattern. (*Turntables* included in many microwave ovens or bought as separate accessories rotate food automatically during the entire cooking cycle.)

Foods tend to cook more slowly in the center of a microwave oven. Therefore, recipes often suggest arranging individual foods, such as potatoes, in a circular pattern. They recommend placing large or dense foods, such as meats, around the edge of a dish. Arrange unevenly shaped foods, like chicken legs, with the thicker parts toward the outside of the container. Place quicker-cooking foods in the center, where they will receive less microwave energy. For instance, mushrooms will cook faster than carrots because the mushrooms are more porous. Therefore, when arranging a vegetable plate, you would place the carrots around the outside and the mushrooms in the center.

Uneven distribution of microwaves may cause some foods cooked in a microwave oven to develop ***hot spots.*** These are areas that absorb a greater concentration of microwaves and, thus, reach a higher temperature than surrounding areas. Stirring foods partway through cooking will redistribute the heat and promote more even cooking. You can rearrange foods you cannot stir by switching pieces on the outside with those in the center.

Unevenly shaped foods can overcook in the areas most directly exposed to microwaves. For instance, the outer edge of a pie may finish cooking before the center. Some recipes recommend *shielding* areas that might overcook with small pieces of aluminum foil. You will often use shields only during the last part of the cooking time. The foil will reflect the microwaves so the covered areas will not continue to cook. However, microwaves will penetrate the uncovered areas, allowing them to finish cooking. Thus the food product as a whole will cook more evenly.

Play It Safe

Take care when removing plastic and all coverings from microwaved foods. Lift covers away from you to avoid the danger of steam burns.

Take care to keep foil shields at least one inch from the oven walls. When metal meets oven walls, ***arcing,*** or sparking, can occur. The presence of narrow bands of metal, such as wire twist ties and metal-trimmed china can also cause arcing. Arcing is not dangerous, but it can mar oven walls. Be sure to check manufacturer's directions before using any type of metal in a microwave oven.

Some microwave recipes recommend elevating foods to promote faster, more even cooking. *Elevating* means lifting a food off the floor of a microwave oven. This allows microwaves to penetrate the food from the bottom as well as the top and sides. Some microwave ovens have a glass tray on the oven floor that provides elevation. You can also place foods on a rack or an inverted glass dish to achieve the same results.

Browning Techniques

Many foods cook so quickly in a microwave oven they do not have time to brown. Browning does not affect the quality and flavor of food. However, browning does affect appearance, which in turn affects appetite appeal.

Some microwave recipes suggest techniques to compensate for a lack of browning. Some meat recipes suggest using browning agents to give the appearance of browning. You can use gravies and sauces to cover many dishes. For baked goods, lack of browning is less noticeable on dark-colored items, such as chocolate or spice cakes. Use frostings and toppings to cover lighter items. See 13-6.

High-Altitude Cooking

Atmospheric pressure decreases at high altitudes. At an altitude of 3,000 feet (914 m), this decrease begins to affect the outcome of food products. As the altitude increases, so does the effect on food. If you are cooking at high altitudes, you may need to make some adjustments to your recipes.

Water boils at a lower temperature at high altitudes. Therefore, most foods cooked in liquid will require more cooking time. Liquids also evaporate faster at high altitudes. You may need to add extra liquid when preparing some foods. You may need to reduce the temperature of deep fat to keep foods from overbrowning before they are thoroughly cooked.

Breads and cakes tend to rise more during baking at high altitudes. To account for this, you may need to increase oven temperature. This will help set the batter before air cells formed by leavening gases have a chance to expand too much. You may need to decrease baking time to keep foods from overcooking at the higher oven temperatures. Reducing the amount of leavening agents used in recipes will help compensate for excess rising. Using larger baking pans will also keep baked goods from overflowing the pans as they rise.

For best results when cooking at high altitudes, choose recipes designed for high-altitude cooking. Many commercial mixes include high-altitude directions on the package.

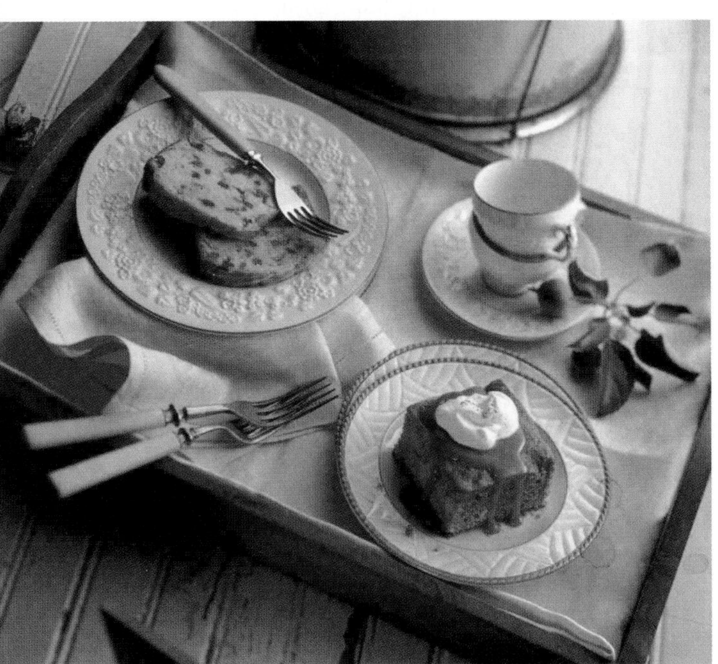

photo courtesy of Land O'Lakes, Inc.

13-6 Whole wheat flour and spices give this cake a darker color. This, along with the caramel sauce, would help hide the lack of browning that would result from baking the cake in a microwave oven.

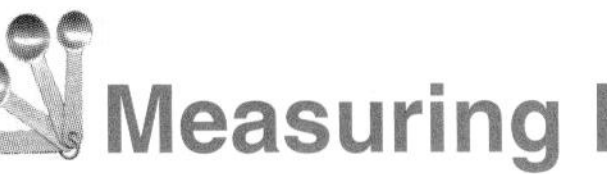

Measuring Ingredients

When preparing foods, you will need to measure different types of ingredients in different ways. Knowing how to measure ingredients correctly will help your food products turn out right.

Measuring Dry Ingredients

Dry ingredients include sugar, flour, baking powder, baking soda, salt, and spices. Measure these ingredients in dry measuring cups. Spoon the ingredient into the correct measuring cup until it is overfilled. Do not shake or tap the measuring cup. Hold the measuring cup over the ingredient container or a sheet of waxed paper. Then use a straight-edged spatula to level off any excess. The ingredient should be even with the top edge of the measuring cup, 13-7.

Some older recipes call for *sifted flour*. Sifting before measuring is unnecessary because flour is thoroughly sifted during the milling process. You can generally just stir flour lightly and then measure it like other dry ingredients. However, you should not skip the sifting step when a recipe tells you to sift flour with other dry ingredients. In this case, sifting helps combine the ingredients.

Brown sugar is a dry ingredient, but you measure it a bit differently. As you spoon brown sugar into a dry measuring cup, press it down firmly with the back of the spoon. This is called *packing*. Overfill the measuring cup, then level it off with a straight-edged spatula. The brown sugar should hold the shape of the measuring cup when you turn it out into a mixing bowl.

Use measuring spoons to measure small amounts (less than ¼ cup [50 mL]) of dry ingredients. Dip the correct measuring spoon into the ingredient container and bring it up heaping full. Level off the top with a straight-edged spatula.

Measuring Liquid Ingredients

Liquid ingredients include milk, water, oil, juices, food colorings, and extracts. Measure these ingredients in liquid measuring cups. The handle and spout on liquid measuring cups make it easy to pour liquid ingredients. The extra room at the top of the cup will help you avoid spilling.

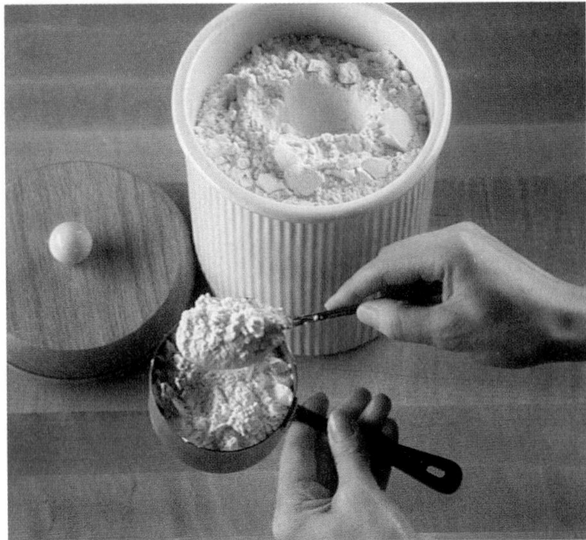

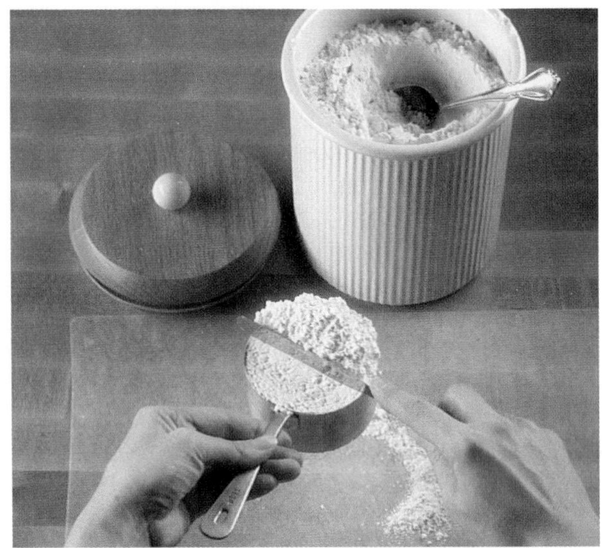

Fleischmann's Yeast, Inc.

13-7 Carefully spoon dry ingredients into a dry measuring cup and level off any excess with a straight-edged spatula.

You cannot get an accurate measurement when you look through a measuring cup at an angle. Therefore, set the liquid measuring cup on a flat surface. Then bend down so the desired marking on the measuring cup is at eye level. Slowly pour the liquid ingredient into the measuring cup until it reaches the mark for the desired amount.

Use measuring spoons to measure small amounts (less than ¼ cup [50 mL]) of liquid ingredients. Carefully pour the ingredient into the correct spoon until it is filled to the edge.

Measuring Fats

Butter, margarine, shortening, and peanut butter are fats used in recipes. You can measure them in three basic ways. Markings on the wrapper of stick butter or margarine can help you measure the amount you need. A stick of butter or margarine equals 8 tablespoons or ½ cup (125 mL). Use a sharp knife to cut through the wrapper at the marking for the desired number of tablespoons.

You can measure shortening and peanut butter in dry measuring cups. Use a rubber spatula to press these ingredients into the measuring cup, making sure you eliminate any air pockets. Overfill the measuring cup, then level it with a straight-edged spatula. See 13-8.

You can also use the *water displacement method* to measure solid fats. Fill a 2-cup (500 mL) liquid measuring cup with 1 cup (250 mL) of cold water. Then carefully spoon in the solid fat until the water level rises by the amount you need. For instance, suppose you need ½ cup (125 mL) of shortening. You would spoon the shortening into the measuring cup until the water level reached 1½ cups (375 mL). Make sure the fat is not clinging to the side of the measuring cup. Drain off the water before using the fat.

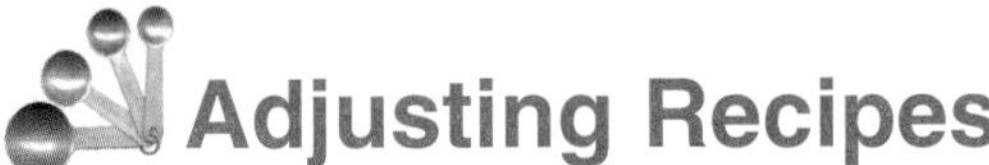

Adjusting Recipes

You may need to adjust some recipes before you can use them. You may want to change the amount the recipe makes. You may want to adjust a conventional recipe for microwave cooking. Knowing some basic information can help you make these adjustments with success.

Changing Yield

Some recipes will make more or less of a food product than you want. For instance, a recipe might make four dozen chocolate chip cookies. When making them for a family reunion, you may want twice that many. A recipe for a chicken and rice casserole might make eight servings. When preparing dinner for four, you might want only half that amount. Being familiar with *measuring equivalents* will help you adjust the yield of a recipe.

Conventional units of measure used in recipes are teaspoons, tablespoons, and cups. Changing the yield of a conventional recipe can be tricky. You may have to convert from one unit to another. For instance, 3 teaspoons is the equivalent of 1 tablespoon. Suppose you are doubling a recipe that calls for 1½ teaspoons of baking soda. Two times 1½ teaspoons equals 3 teaspoons, or 1 tablespoon. Likewise, ¼ cup equals 4 tablespoons. Suppose you are halving a recipe that calls for ¼ cup sugar. You can easily figure half of 4 tablespoons is 2 tablespoons. Figure the adjusted amounts of each ingredient before you begin cooking. Write the adjusted amounts on your recipe so you will remember them as you work.

The main metric unit of measure used in recipes is the milliliter. Changing the yield of a metric recipe is easy. You do not have to convert from one unit to another. Chart 13-9 gives common equivalents for conventional and metric measurements.

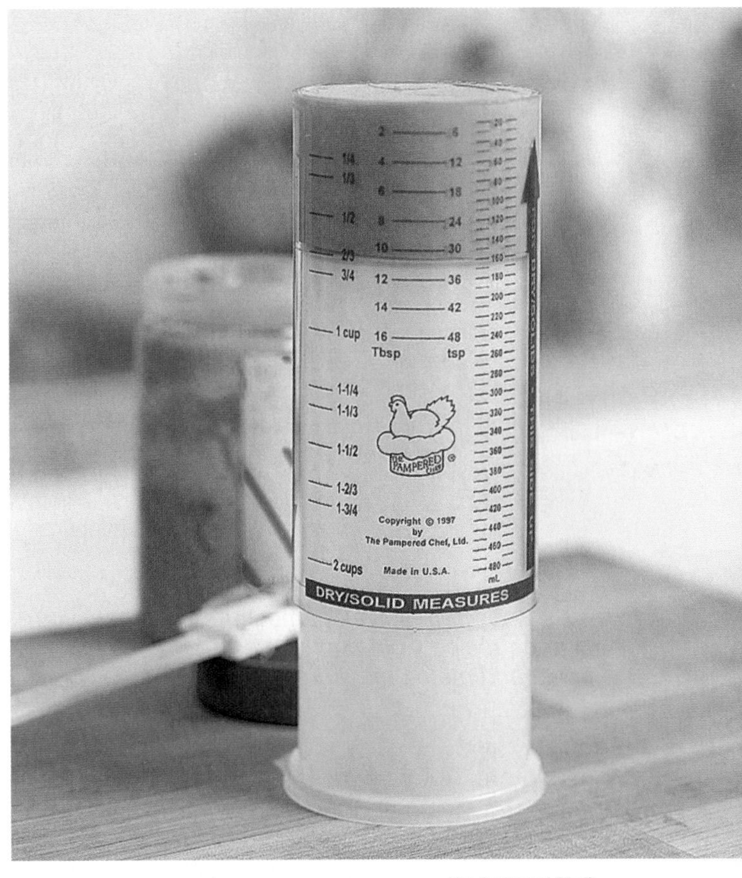

The Pampered Chef®

13-8 *Firmly press ingredients such as solid fats and peanut butter into a measuring cup before leveling with a straight-edged spatula.*

Converting Recipes for Microwave Use

You can convert most conventional recipes for use in a microwave oven by adjusting the proportions of some ingredients. Reduce the amount of liquid used in recipes by one-third. This will account for the lack of evaporation inside a microwave oven. Eliminate cooking oils and fats from recipes unless they provide flavor or consistency. Halve the amount of seasonings, as their flavors intensify with microwave cooking. If needed, you can add more seasonings after cooking.

Choose the power setting according to the type of food you are preparing. Most foods are microwaved on high power. Cook delicate foods, such as cheese, eggs, and milk products, on medium-high power.

For guidelines on cooking times, look in a microwave cookbook for a recipe similar to the one you are preparing. As a rule, start with one-fourth of the conventional cooking time. Check food and add time as needed. Remember that some foods will continue cooking after you remove them from the microwave oven. Remove these foods just before they finish cooking to allow for this standing time.

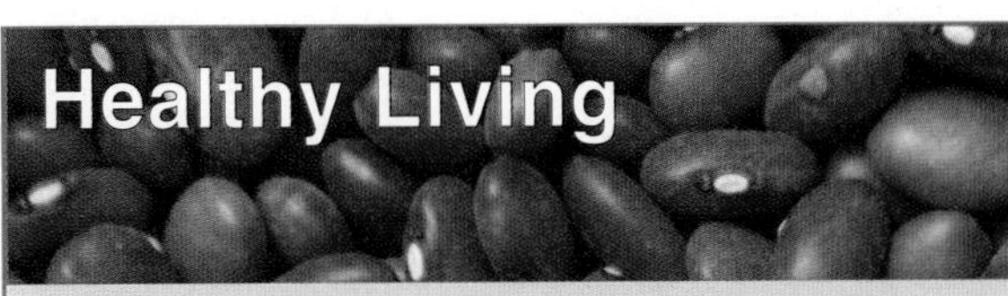

Changing the amounts of some ingredients in recipes can allow you to make more healthful food products. For instance, you may be able to reduce the amount of fat, salt, sugar, and eggs in baked goods. Such reductions are in keeping with the Dietary Guidelines for Americans. Follow standards for basic ingredient proportions to produce quality food products.

Common Equivalent Measures		
Conventional Measure	Conventional Equivalent	Approximate Metric Equivalent*
1/4 teaspoon	—	1 milliliter
1/2 teaspoon	—	2 milliliters
1 teaspoon	—	5 milliliters
3 teaspoons	1 tablespoon	15 milliliters
2 tablespoons	1/8 cup	30 milliliters
4 tablespoons	1/4 cup	50 milliliters
5 1/3 tablespoons	1/3 cup	75 milliliters
8 tablespoons	1/2 cup	125 milliliters
10 2/3 tablespoons	2/3 cup	150 milliliters
12 tablespoons	3/4 cup	175 milliliters
16 tablespoons	1 cup, 1/2 pint	250 milliliters
2 cups	1 pint	500 milliliters
4 cups	1 quart	1 liter

* Based on measures seen on standard metric measuring equipment.

13-9 *Knowing equivalent measures can help you change recipe yield and convert between conventional and metric measures.*

(Chapters 14 through 25 include additional tips for microwaving various foods.)

Ingredient Substitutions

You should read through a recipe to be sure you have all the needed ingredients before you begin cooking. If you are out of a needed ingredient, you may be able to make a substitution. See 13-10.

Using a Time-Work Schedule

When serving a meal, you would not want the vegetable to finish cooking 20 minutes after you serve the main course. As a meal manager, you are responsible for making sure all the food is ready at the same time. You can accomplish this goal by using a ***time-work schedule.*** This is a written plan that lists times for doing specific tasks to prepare a meal or food product.

A time-work schedule should be specific enough to identify the order and timing of all the critical preparation steps. On the other hand, it should be flexible enough to allow you to make adjustments. If you underestimate your speed or need to substitute an ingredient, you may need this flexibility.

Preliminary Planning

Before you are ready to write your time-work schedule, you need to think about the tasks involved in preparing your meal. You will also need to gather a few basic tools. You need recipes for each menu item. You need paper and a pencil to write the schedule. (Using a pencil makes it easier to revise the plan, if needed.) You may also want a calculator to help you figure the total time required to prepare each food.

The following steps outline how to do some preliminary planning. Examples on the next page show how completed plans would look for the meal shown in 13-11.

1. On a piece of paper, set up a food preparation time chart as shown in 13-12. List your menu items in the first column. Add table setting to this list because you need to reserve time for this task.
2. Use your recipes to identify preparation tasks you will need to do as you make each menu item. Then list estimates in the chart for the time required to prepare, cook, and serve each food. (Some recipes give estimated preparation and cooking times, which will help you with this task.)
3. Add the total time required to prepare each item and list these totals in the chart.
4. In the last column, rank menu items in order of the total time required to prepare them. The item ranked number 1 should be the food requiring the most time. This step will help you decide which menu items to prepare first.

Making a Schedule

You can use your completed food preparation time chart to help you plan your actual time-work schedule. The first decision you need to make when writing a time-work schedule is what time you want to begin eating the meal. You will need to think about your daily activities and the activities of other diners when making this decision. Allow yourself enough time to prepare the meal so you will not feel rushed. Allow family members enough time to come to the

Substituting One Ingredient for Another	
You may use these	**For these**
1 whole egg, for baking or thickening	2 egg yolks
1/2 cup (125 mL) evaporated milk plus 1/2 cup (125 mL) water	1 cup (250 mL) fluid whole milk
1 cup (250 mL) reconstituted nonfat dry milk	1 cup (250 mL) fluid fat free milk
3/4 cup (175 mL) milk plus 1/3 cup (75 mL) butter	1 cup (250 mL) heavy cream
1 tablespoon (15 mL) vinegar or lemon juice plus milk to make 1 cup (250 mL) (Allow this mixture to stand several minutes before using.)	1 cup (250 mL) sour milk or buttermilk
1 cup (250 mL) margarine	1 cup (250 mL) butter
3 tablespoons (45 mL) unsweetened cocoa powder plus 1 tablespoon (15 mL) butter or margarine	1 ounce (28 g) unsweetened chocolate
1 1/4 cups (300 mL) sugar plus 1/4 cup (50 mL) liquid used in recipe	1 cup (250 mL) corn syrup
2 tablespoons (30 mL) flour	1 tablespoon (15 mL) cornstarch
7/8 cup (220 mL) all-purpose flour	1 cup (250 mL) cake flour

***13-10** You can sometimes make substitutions for ingredients you do not have on hand.*

meal leisurely. You may want to plan your serving time at least 15 minutes after a guest's intended arrival time. This will allow a time cushion for any unexpected delays.

Once you have decided when to begin eating the meal, the following steps will help you write your time-work schedule:

1. Set up a chart like the one in 13-13. Write the time you plan to begin eating at the bottom of the time column.
2. Look at the *serving time* column of your food preparation time chart. Work backward from your eating time to determine when you need to begin serving.
3. Look at the *cooking time* column of your food preparation time chart. Identify the time at which you need to begin cooking each item.
4. Use your recipes to help you list all the preparation tasks you need to do. Refer to the *preparation time* column of your food preparation time chart. It will help you decide how much time to allow for these tasks.

To keep your schedule flexible, avoid listing specific times for every task. Instead, group tasks in 5- or 10-minute blocks of time. Plan to do related tasks together. For instance, you can

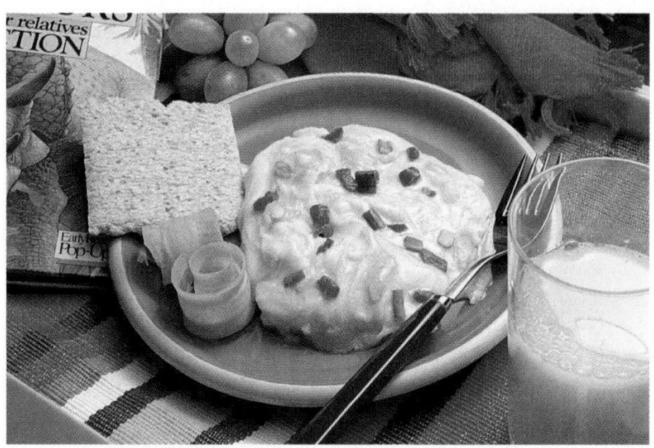

American Egg Board

Menu
Peppered Egg Scramble Crisp Bread
Grapes Orange Juice

***13-11** You can prepare and serve this nutritious breakfast in just 20 minutes.*

Food Preparation Time Chart					
Menu Item	**Preparation Time**	**Cooking Time**	**Serving Time**	**Total Time**	**Rank**
Peppered egg scramble	7 minutes	5 minutes	1 minute	13 minutes	1
Crisp bread	—	—	1 minute	1 minute	5
Grapes	1 minute	—	1 minute	2 minutes	4
Orange juice	3 minutes	—	1 minute	4 minutes	2
Table setting	3 minutes	—	—	3 minutes	3

13-12 Charts showing preparation, cooking, and serving times for each menu item can help meal managers plan their work.

wash the grapes at the same time you are washing the pepper and onions.

Remember to dovetail your meal preparation tasks as you plan your schedule. ***Dovetail*** means to overlap tasks to use your time more efficiently. You can often dovetail during cooking time. For example, while keeping an eye on the cooking eggs, you can mix the orange juice.

Another point to keep in mind is you do not have to prepare food items ranked number 1 first. Sometimes it is helpful to get simple tasks, such as setting the table, out of the way. You may also want to prepare foods that do not need to be served hot ahead of time. This will prevent hot foods from cooling while you prepare other menu items.

Even a complete schedule is no guarantee that plans will go smoothly from start to finish. Sometimes one dish might cook in more or less time than you estimated. In these cases, you might have to keep some foods warm while you finish preparing the other foods.

As you become more skilled in the kitchen, you will be able to use less detailed schedules. Until that time, however, a schedule that is both detailed and flexible will be helpful.

Time-Work Schedule	
Time	**Tasks**
7:40	Set table. Wash red pepper, green onion, and grapes.
7:45	Place grapes in serving bowl. Chop pepper and onion. Grate cheese.
7:50	Beat together eggs, milk, pepper, onion, and cheese. Begin cooking eggs. Mix orange juice concentrate.
7:57	Place crisp bread in a lined basket. Pour juice. Serve eggs.
8:00	Eat.

13-13 A time-work schedule lists actual times for doing specific food preparation tasks.

Cooperation in the Kitchen

You will not always work alone in the kitchen. At home, family members may help you prepare meals. At school, you will work with classmates to prepare food products. The kitchen can become crowded when several people are working together. Therefore, you will need to cooperate in order to make the best use of your time, space, and skills. See 13-14.

Consider each person's skills when assigning meal preparation tasks. If you are in a hurry, you may not want someone with little baking experience to make biscuits. If you have the time, however, you might want this person to help you with the biscuits. This will give him or her more baking practice.

Your time-work schedule should indicate who will do each task listed. Be sure to rotate tasks from one time to the next to give everyone a range of kitchen experience.

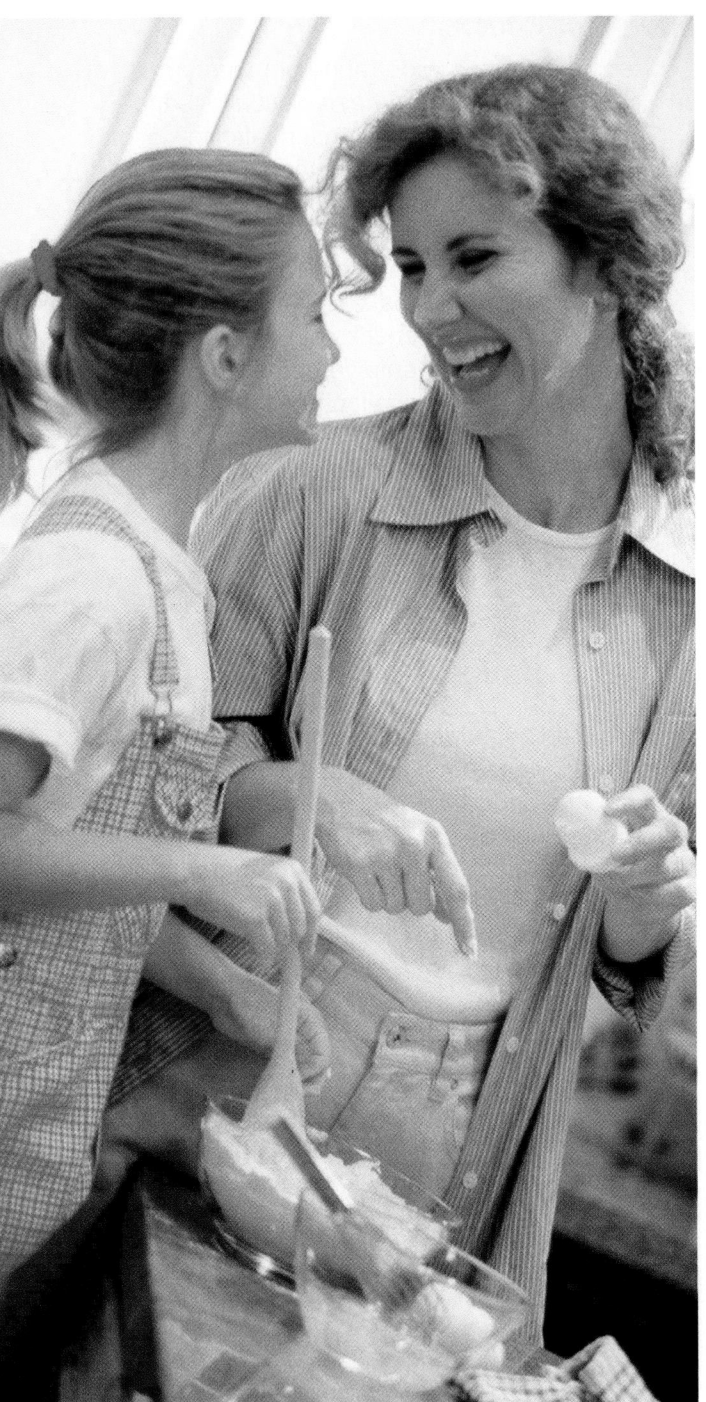

13-14 Learning to cooperate when sharing kitchen space and equipment with others is an important food preparation skill.

Preparing Simple Recipes

You can put your basic food preparation knowledge to work by making a simple recipe. While you are developing your cooking skills, choose recipes with just a few ingredients and a short list of directions. As you gain experience, you can move on to recipes that require more advanced preparation techniques.

Sandwiches

Many sandwich recipes are simple to prepare. Sandwiches are a common choice for packed lunches because they travel well and can be eaten without utensils. Sandwiches are also popular party and picnic foods because they are convenient to serve to a group.

Sandwich Ingredients

All sandwiches are made with some type of bread and a filling. You can use many different kinds of breads and rolls to make sandwiches. Rye, whole wheat, pumpernickel, French, Italian, potato, and raisin are just a few of the many breads you might choose. Pita bread, tortillas, bagels, and other ethnic breads and rolls add still more variety. The bread or roll chosen should be fresh and either whole grain or enriched.

Sandwich fillings are often protein foods. Leftover meats and poultry are good choices. Cheese, hard-cooked eggs, peanut butter, and canned fish also make good fillings.

Lettuce, pickles, tomatoes, and other vegetables complement some sandwiches. Bacon curls, ripe olives, and spiced fruits complement others. First choose the filling; then choose the extras.

Preparing Sandwiches

The following guidelines will help you prepare nutritious, attractive, and flavorful sandwiches:

- Use a variety of breads and fillings.
- Spread a thin layer of soft butter, margarine, or mayonnaise to the edge of the bread. This will keep the filling from soaking into the bread.
- Cut sandwiches into halves or quarters to make them easier to eat. For party sandwiches that are extra interesting and attractive, cut bread into shapes, such as circles, diamonds, and hearts.
- Garnish sandwiches attractively. Garnishes can improve the appearance and food value of a sandwich.

- Keep sandwiches refrigerated until serving time. Bacteria grow quickly above 60°F (16°C). Therefore, pack sandwiches in a cooler when transporting them. Use ice, frozen gel packs, or chilled drinks to keep perishable ingredients safe. Wrap sandwiches well to prevent staling. Pack lettuce, pickles, tomatoes, and other relishes separately to keep sandwiches from getting soggy.
- Make hot sandwiches just before serving. Serve them hot, not lukewarm. See 13-15.
- Use freshly toasted bread for sandwiches served on toast.

Be a Clever Consumer

Take advantage of sale prices on sandwich ingredients. Then prepare sandwiches and freeze them. (Do not use mayonnaise, hard-cooked egg white, jelly, or lettuce or other raw vegetables. These foods do not freeze well, and you can add them to sandwiches later.) Wrap all sandwiches for the freezer in moistureproof and vaporproof wrapping and label them.

Microwaving Sandwiches

Most sandwiches can be microwaved in under a minute. However, the size of most microwave ovens makes it hard to heat more than a few sandwiches at a time. Therefore, you may wish to use a conventional oven if you are serving hot sandwiches to a crowd.

Follow a few tips when microwaving sandwiches. Because the bread is porous, it will warm faster than the filling. Using frozen bread will keep the bread from drying out before the filling is warm. Using several thin slices of meat will allow sandwiches to heat faster and more evenly than using one thick slice. Wrapping sandwiches in paper towels will help absorb excess moisture during heating.

Snacks

Like sandwiches, many snack foods are easy to make. Some require no cooking. Others can be quickly heated in a microwave oven. Even someone who is just learning his or her way around the kitchen can make simple snacks with ease.

Foods for Snacks

People choose a wide range of foods for snacks. Some snacks are hearty, such as sandwiches and leftover pizza. Other snacks are light, such as fruit and popcorn. With a little imagination, you can make a variety of snacks out of ingredients you probably have available.

With a bit of planning, you can have snacks on hand that are nutritious and simple to prepare. Stock up on foods like yogurt, whole grain crackers, and cheese slices to grab in a hurry. Store a bag of cut up fresh vegetables in the crisper of your refrigerator. Make a healthful snack mix out of raisins, nuts, and ready-to-eat cereal. Your snack food choices can help meet your daily serving needs from the five main food groups. When nutritious snack foods are convenient, you will be less likely to choose foods that provide empty calories. See 13-16.

courtesy of National Cattlemen's Beef Association and Cattlemen's Beef Board

13-15 *Make sure hot sandwiches are hot when you serve them.*

Beverages

People drink beverages with meals and throughout the day. Beverages can quench thirst and help meet your body's need for water. Some beverages also provide other nutrients. For instance, milk is a good source of calcium, and many fruit and vegetable juices are high in vitamin C.

Many beverages require no preparation. Those beverages that have recipes are usually simple enough for even the most inexperienced cooks to prepare.

Cold Drinks

Milk, bottled water, carbonated beverages, fruit and vegetable juices, lemonade, punch, smoothies, and milk shakes are popular cold drinks. Be aware that nondiet soft drinks are the number one source of added sugars in the U.S. diet. Many fruit drinks and punches also supply little more than sugar. Follow the Dietary Guidelines for Americans by balancing these beverages with more nutritious beverage choices, such as milk and juices. Also, be sure to choose pure water often.

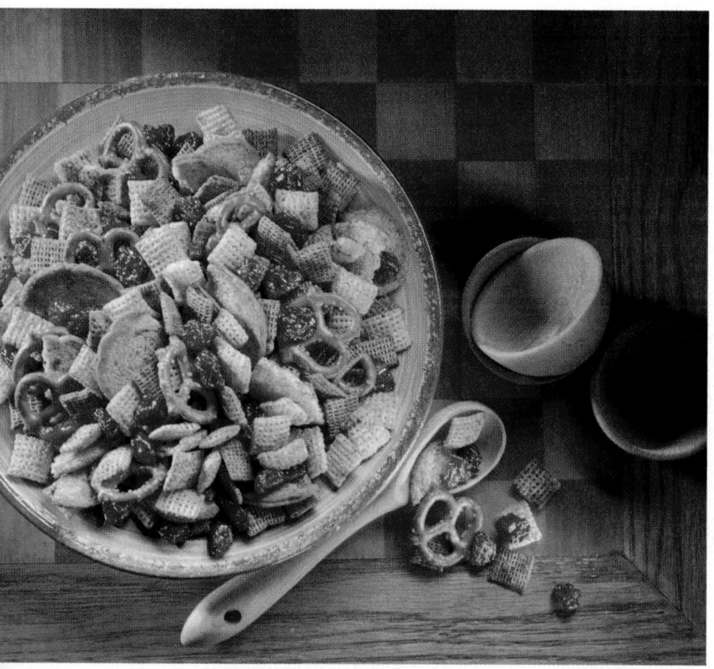

Cherry Marketing Institute

***13-16** Ready-to-eat cereals are the key ingredient in many tasty, nutritious snack mixes that are easy to prepare.*

Many drinks are ready to enjoy, right from the refrigerator. Make sure to serve drinks icy cold. Have plenty of ice on hand to keep drinks chilled.

When preparing cold drinks for a party, you can freeze fruit juices in ice cube trays. These ice cubes will not dilute drinks. You can also use fruit juices to make ice rings to float in punch bowls. Ice rings take longer to melt than ice cubes, so they keep punches cold longer. For outdoor events, pack canned beverages and drink boxes in coolers. Use insulated picnic jugs to hold large amounts of cold beverages.

When preparing sparkling punch for a party, make the punch base ahead of time and chill it well. Chill the soda for the punch separately. Make the base by mixing all ingredients except the soda. Just before the party, pour the punch base over an ice ring in a punch bowl. Add the soda at the last minute to keep the punch from getting "flat."

Smoothies and milk shakes are thick, frosty treats. Ingredients can vary, but smoothies are often made with yogurt and fruit; milk shakes contain milk and ice cream. When preparing these beverages, have all ingredients as cold as possible. Using frozen fruit in a smoothie will help make the drink extra thick and cold. Combine all ingredients in a blender. Adding the liquid ingredients first will help the solid ingredients become thoroughly blended. Blend for about 20 to 30 seconds until the mixture is smooth. Pour it into tall glasses and serve with straws. See 13-17.

Coffee

Coffee is a popular beverage at breakfast and with desserts. However, many people drink coffee all day long.

Coffee is made from the beans of the coffee plant. The beans are dried, roasted, and packaged for shipment. The flavor of coffee beans depends on the variety, growing conditions, and roasting technique.

You can buy a single variety of coffee beans. You can also buy coffee ***blends,*** which are mixtures of several varieties of coffee beans. Coffees that have added flavorings, such as hazelnut or French vanilla, are available, too.

You can choose ground or whole bean coffee. Ground coffee comes in different *grinds* for use with different preparation methods. If

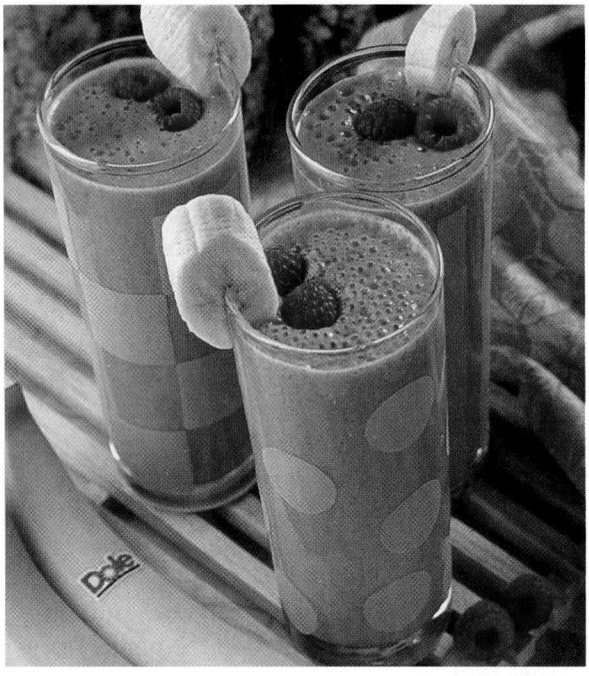

Dole Food Company

13-17 Fresh fruit and yogurt make smoothies tasty, nutritious cold drinks.

you choose whole bean coffee, you can have it ground at the store. For freshness, however, you might prefer to grind it yourself just before brewing. Coffee stales quickly when exposed to moisture and air. Buy only enough coffee to last a week or two. To help maintain freshness, store both ground and whole bean coffee in opaque, airtight containers at room temperature.

You can purchase coffee in instant form. *Instant coffee products* are dry, powdered, water-soluble solids made by removing the moisture from very strong, brewed coffee. Some brands are freeze-dried. Prepare instant coffee by adding freshly boiled water to the coffee granules according to the manufacturer's directions.

Decaffeinated coffee is made by removing most of the caffeine from coffee beans before roasting. ***Caffeine*** is a naturally occurring compound in coffee and some other plant products that acts as a stimulant. Decaffeinated coffee is available in several grinds and in instant form.

Preparing Coffee

When you brew ground coffee, be sure to start with fresh, *cold* water and a clean pot. Thoroughly wash the inside of your coffeepot with hot, soapy water and rinse it well after each use. Oily film that collects on the inside of a coffeepot can cause coffee to be bitter.

Most homemakers use *drip coffeemakers* to make coffee. These appliances have water reservoirs, baskets, and serving pots. Measure water for the desired amount of coffee and pour it into the water reservoir. Place a filter in the basket and add the appropriate amount of coffee. Coffee packers generally recommend 1 to 2 tablespoons (15 to 30 mL) ground coffee per 6-ounce (175 mL) serving. You may use more or less, depending on your taste preferences. Put the basket in place, with the serving pot below. When the water becomes hot, it filters through the coffee into the empty pot below.

Q: Can you become addicted to caffeine?

A: People who consume caffeine on a daily basis can become physically dependent on it. Headaches are a common withdrawal symptom for people who suddenly stop consuming caffeine. Many health experts suggest limiting daily caffeine intake to no more than the amount in two small cups of coffee.

Serve coffee as soon as possible after brewing it. Heating coffee too long can cause it to become bitter. This is because bitter substances present in coffee become more soluble at high temperatures. Correctly prepared coffee is clear and flavorful. It is piping hot and has a pleasing aroma.

In addition to plain coffee, a number of coffee drinks have become popular in the United States. These drinks are made with a base of plain coffee or a strong type of coffee called espresso. A special type of coffeemaker is available for brewing espresso at home. See 13-18.

Popular Coffee Beverages

espresso. A strong coffee brewed by forcing very hot water under pressure through finely ground, darkly roasted coffee beans. Espresso is typically served as a 2-ounce (50 mL) portion in a small cup called a *demitasse.*

cappuccino. A coffee beverage comprised of one part espresso, one part steamed milk, and one part frothed milk. It is often served with a sprinkling of cocoa or cinnamon.

iced cappuccino. A chilled coffee beverage prepared by pouring 1½ ounces (45 mL) of espresso over ice and adding 3 ounces (90 mL) of cold milk. Frothed milk is spooned on top and the beverage is sweetened to taste.

caffé latte. A coffee beverage prepared in a mug by adding 6 to 8 ounces (175 to 250 mL) of steamed milk to 1½ ounces (45 mL) of espresso. Syrups in flavors like hazelnut and almond are often added.

café mocha. A coffee beverage prepared by mixing chocolate syrup or powder and 5 ounces (155 mL) of steamed milk with 1½ ounces (45 mL) of espresso. This beverage may be topped with whipped cream.

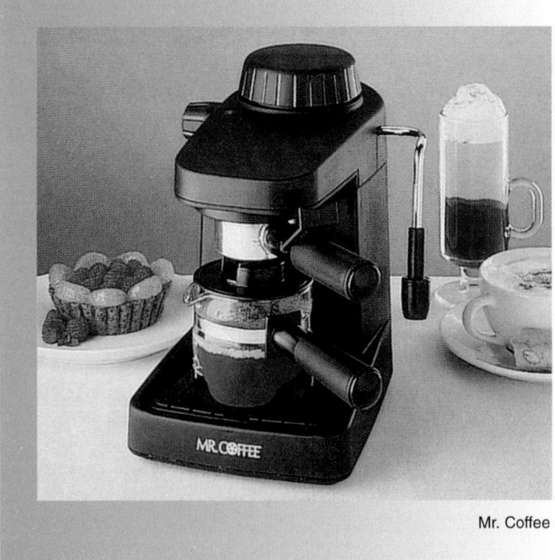

Mr. Coffee

13-18 These are just a few of the many popular beverages you can make with coffee.

Tea

Hot tea may be served in place of or in addition to coffee at brunches, dinners, receptions, and other occasions. Iced tea is popular at picnics and other warm-weather get-togethers.

Tea is made from the leaves of a small tropical evergreen. Teas vary according to the age of the tealeaves and the way they are processed. *Black teas* are made from tea leaves that are fermented and dried. When brewed, black teas are amber in color and have a rich aroma and flavor. *Green teas* are made from tea leaves that are not fermented. When brewed, green teas are a greenish-yellow color. They have a delicate flavor and little aroma. *Oolong teas* are made from partially fermented tea leaves. The appearance and flavor of the beverage made from oolong teas falls between that of the black and green teas. All three varieties of tea are available decaffeinated.

Other Forms of Tea

Tea is available in instant form. Instant teas may be sweetened and flavored with lemon or other flavors. You can dissolve them in cold or freshly boiled water.

Tea can be flavored. Spices like cinnamon, herbs like mint, and floral fragrances like jasmine are popular flavorings.

Herbal teas are made from a variety of plants. These teas have become popular because they come in many interesting flavors and they do not contain caffeine. Fennel seeds, chamomile flowers, ginger root, and blackberry leaves are just a few of the ingredients commonly found in herbal teas.

Some people have allergic reactions to some of the plants used in herbal teas. When purchasing herbal teas, it is best to choose from among commercial brands. Avoid herbal mixtures that claim to have special health or medicinal properties.

Preparing Tea

You can purchase tea in filter paper teabags or in loose form. To prepare either form of tea, begin by rinsing a clean teapot or cup with boiling water to preheat it. Place a teabag or loose tea in the preheated pot or cup. (Place loose tea directly in the bottom of the pot or cup, in a cheesecloth bag, or in a tea ball. A *tea*

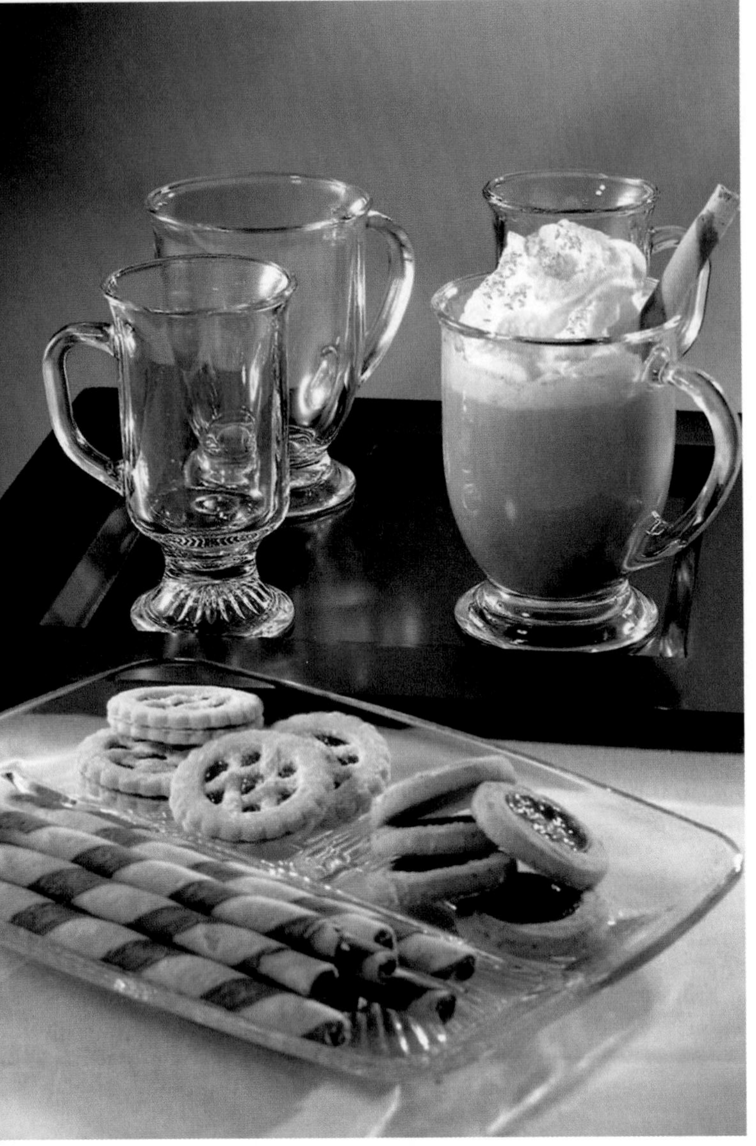

Anchor Hocking

13-19 Hot chocolate is a delicious complement to a plate of cookies at a winter get-together.

ball is a perforated ball made of silver or stainless steel.) Then pour freshly boiled water over the tea. Allow the tea to steep two to six minutes, until it reaches the desired strength. Remove the tea leaves from the pot before serving. If the tea leaves stay in contact with the water too long, the tea can become bitter. Serve cream, sugar, and lemon with tea.

Prepare iced tea by first making strong hot tea. If desired, dissolve honey or sugar in the tea. Then pour the tea over ice and stir until chilled. Making the hot tea stronger than you usually drink it will keep the ice from diluting the iced tea too much.

Chocolate and Cocoa Beverages

Hot chocolate is made from unsweetened chocolate. Cocoa is made from cocoa powder. Both of these beverages contain milk. This means you must use low temperatures to prevent scorching. See 13-19.

To prepare hot chocolate, combine unsweetened chocolate in a heavy saucepan with water. Stir over low heat until chocolate is melted. Then stir in sugar and a dash of salt and simmer for two to three minutes to form a syrup. Add heated milk and heat the beverage to the proper serving temperature.

Begin preparing hot cocoa by combining cocoa with sugar and a dash of salt in a heavy saucepan. This will prevent the cocoa from lumping when you stir in the hot water, which is the next step. After adding the hot water, bring the mixture to a boil over medium heat. Stir constantly for two to three minutes. Add heated milk and heat to the proper serving temperature.

Do not allow hot chocolate or cocoa to boil after adding milk. Beating these beverages with a rotary beater until foamy will keep the milk from forming a scum layer. If desired, you may flavor either beverage with vanilla extract and top with marshmallows or whipped cream.

Chapter 13 Review

Getting Started in the Kitchen

Summary

To prepare meals, you need to know how to choose and read recipes. You need to be familiar with abbreviations and cooking terms used in recipes. If you live in a high-altitude area, you should be aware of how the atmospheric pressure can affect food products. You should also know the correct way to measure dry and liquid ingredients and fats.

Knowing how to adjust recipes is another basic food preparation skill. Being familiar with measuring equivalents will help you easily adjust the yield of a recipe. Following a few guidelines can help you adjust conventional recipes for microwave cooking. Knowing how to substitute one ingredient for another will come in handy when you run out of something you need.

As a meal manager, you will need to know how to make a time-work schedule. This will help you plan your use of time in the kitchen. It will also help you when working with others, such as in a school foods lab.

You can put basic cooking skills to use when preparing simple recipes. Sandwiches, snacks, and beverages are good foods for beginning cooks to make. Using a variety of ingredients, you can easily prepare many hot and cold sandwiches and healthful snack foods. With a little effort, you can learn how to make cold drinks, coffee, tea, and chocolate and cocoa beverages. When you pair these beverages with sandwiches and snacks, you will be ready to serve unexpected guests or hold off hunger between meals.

Review What You Have Read

Write your answers on a separate sheet of paper.

1. What are the components of a well-written recipe?
2. Give the unit of measure for which each of the following abbreviations stands:
   A. c.
   B. oz.
   C. t.
   D. tbsp.
3. Complete each of the following statements.
   A. To stir ingredients until they are thoroughly combined is to _____.
   B. To cut into very small cubes of even size is to _____.
   C. To rub fat on the surface of a cooking utensil or on a food itself is to _____.
   D. To heat an appliance to a desired temperature about 5 to 8 minutes before it is to be used is to _____.
4. How can dehydration occur during microwave cooking?
5. Why should plastic wrap used to cover food in a microwave oven be vented?
6. What happens to the boiling point of water at high altitudes?
7. True or false. Dry ingredients should be spooned into a dry measuring cup until the cup is filled just to the edge.
8. Double and halve each of the following amounts:
   A. 2 tablespoons
   B. 1½ teaspoons
   C. ¾ cup
   D. 1⅔ cups
9. Explain why time-work schedules for preparing meals need to be flexible.
10. What is the first decision that needs to be made when writing a time-work schedule?
11. Give two tips for microwaving sandwiches.
12. How can you prevent cold drinks from being diluted by ice cubes?
13. Why should coffee be served as soon as possible after brewing?
14. Teas made from partially fermented tea leaves are called _____.
   A. black teas
   B. green teas
   C. herbal teas
   D. oolong teas

15. When preparing hot cocoa, why must the cocoa powder be combined with sugar before adding hot water?

Build Your Basic Skills

1. **Geography.** On a photocopy of a map of the United States, color in the areas where high-altitude cooking principles would apply.
2. **Math.** Find a sandwich recipe with a yield of 8 servings or fewer. Copy the recipe and calculate how much of each ingredient would be needed to serve 40 party guests.

Build Your Thinking Skills

1. **Analyze.** Select two types of cookbooks from your school or local library. Analyze the strengths and weaknesses of each cookbook. Write a critique stating which one you prefer and why.
2. **Plan.** Select a breakfast or luncheon menu. Collect recipes for the foods you have selected. Plan a time-work schedule for the members of your lab group. Prepare the menu following your schedule.
3. **Evaluate.** Prepare several coffee blends. Evaluate the color, aroma, and flavor of each blend. Identify the blend you prefer and explain why you prefer it.

Apply Technology

1. Use a computer and a spreadsheet program to develop a spreadsheet with a formula that will calculate measurements when doubling and halving recipes.
2. Use a computer and the table function in word processing software to create a time-work schedule.

Using Workplace Skills

Suda is a time-study engineer. Food product manufacturers hire her to study the way their assembly line workers perform tasks. The manufacturers want Suda to help them find ways to increase production. Suda analyzes the placement of equipment and supplies. She also looks at the physical motions involved in doing each job. Then she improves the system or designs a new system that will eliminate wasted and nonproductive motions.

To be an effective worker, Suda needs skill in designing and improving systems. In a small group, answer the following questions about Suda's need for and use of these skills:

A. How will Suda's skill in designing and improving systems affect the manufacturers who hire her?
B. How will Suda's skill in designing and improving systems affect assembly line workers?
C. Why might manufacturers hire Suda to analyze their production systems instead of doing it themselves?
D. What is another skill Suda would need in this job? Briefly explain why this skill would be important.

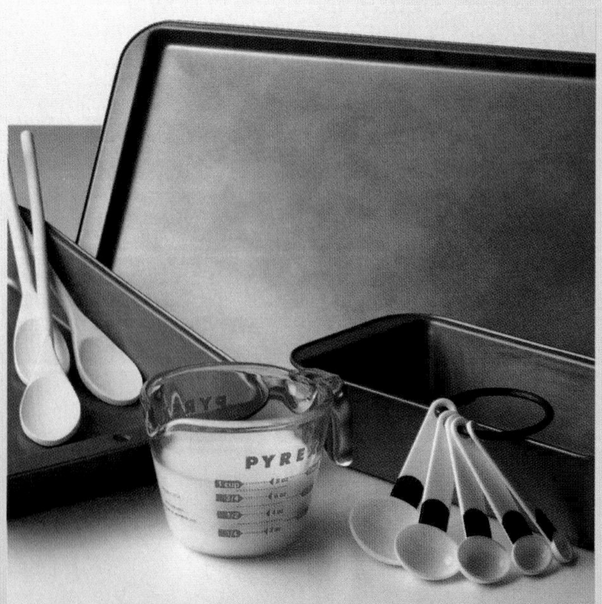

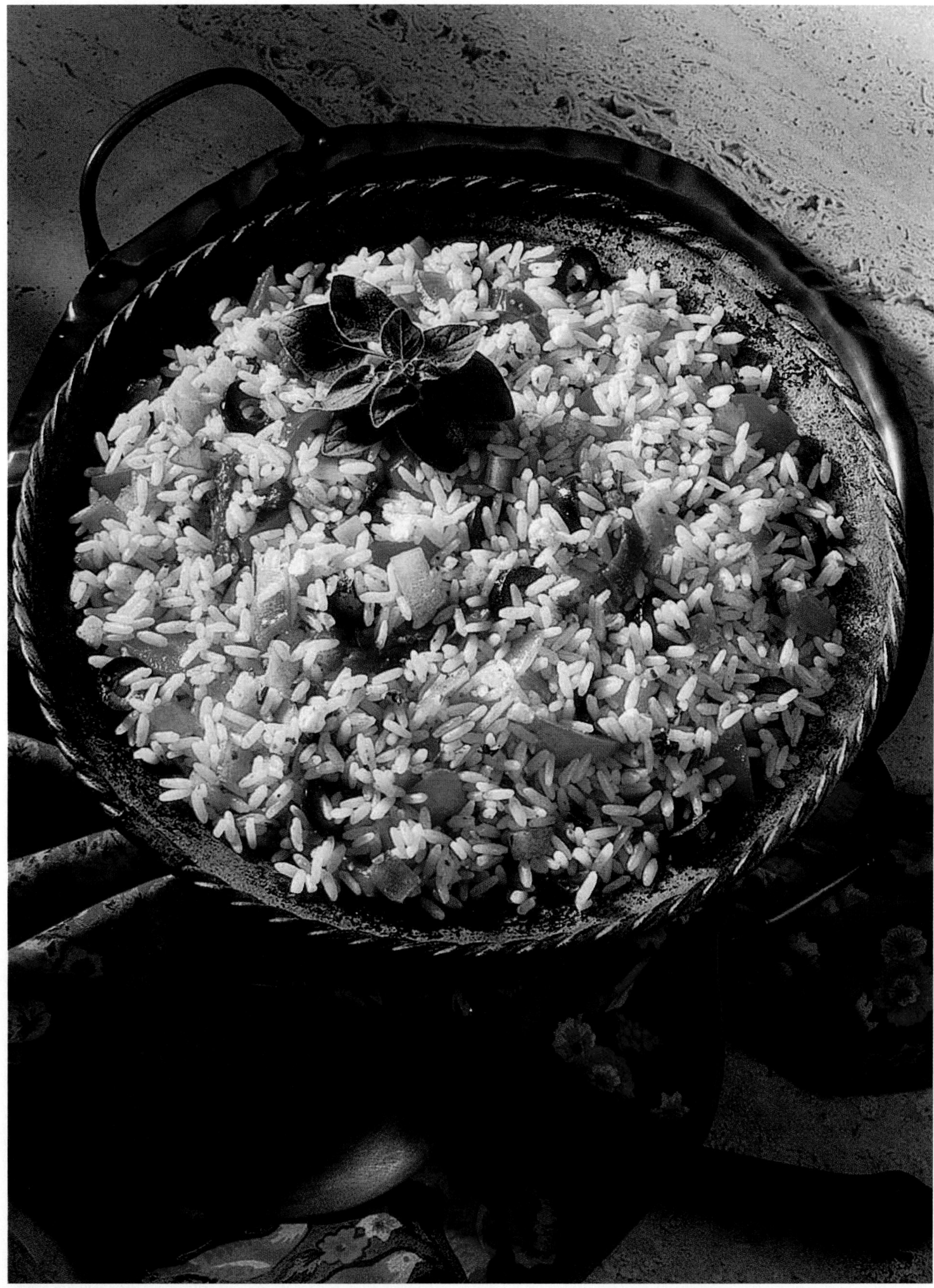

USA Rice Federation

Practice using abbreviations, cooking terms, and measuring techniques to prepare simple recipes. Soon you will be ready to move on to more advanced dishes like this.

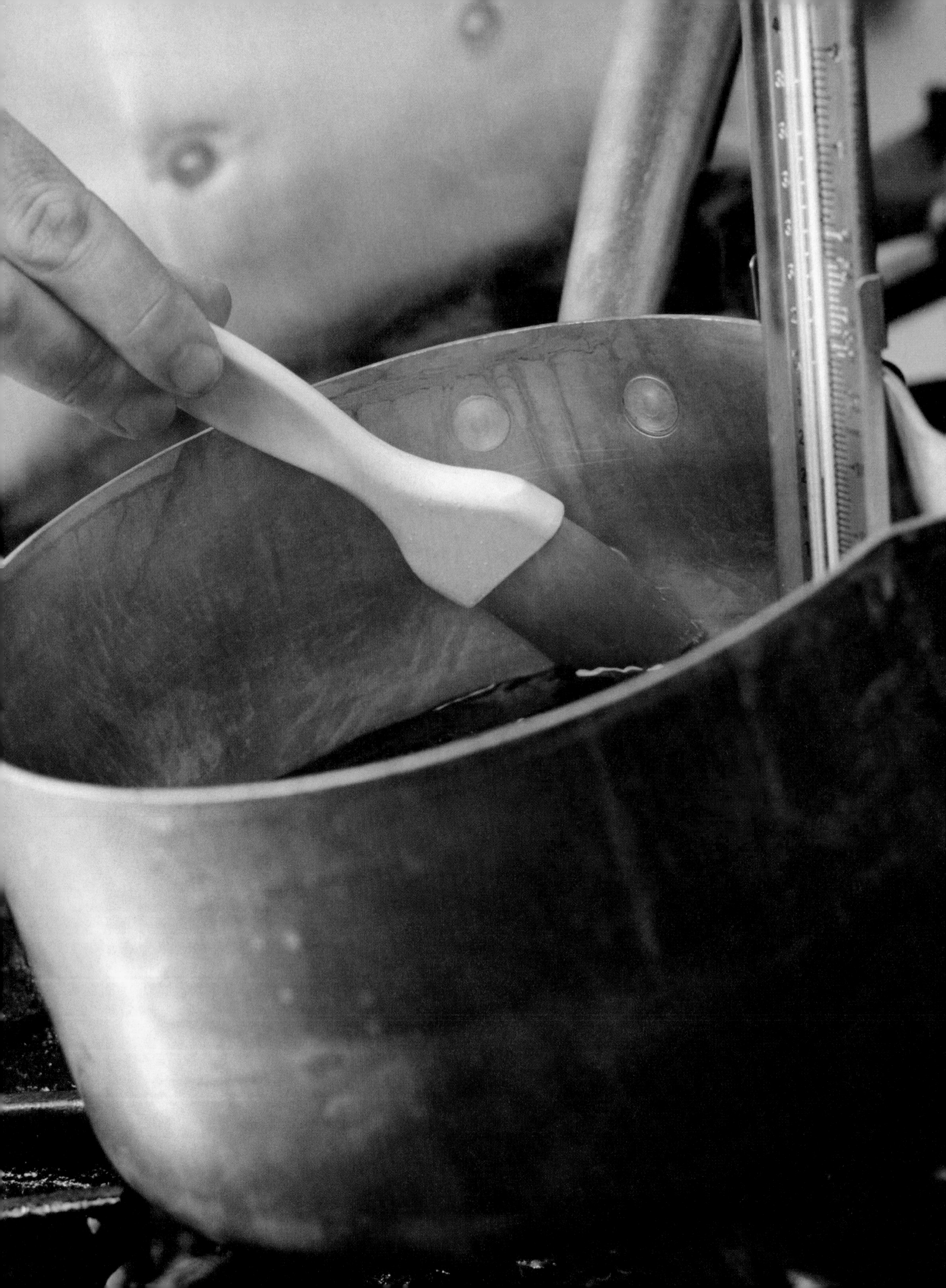

Part 3

The Preparation of Food

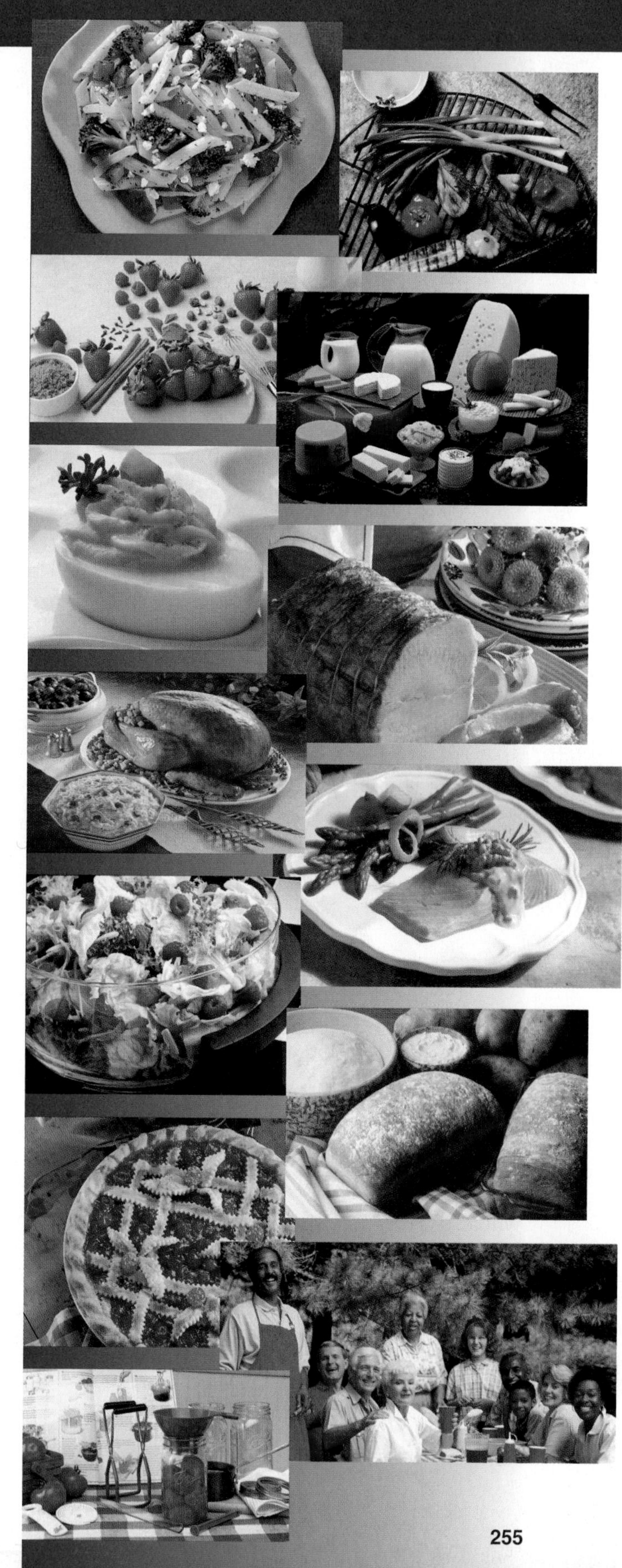

Chapter 14
Grain Foods

Cash Grain Farmer
Plants, cultivates, and harvests one or more grain crops, such as barley, corn, rice, and wheat, for cash sale.

Cereal Popper
Controls pressure cylinders to expand or puff whole grain to produce breakfast cereal.

Miller
Supervises and coordinates activities of workers engaged in cleaning and grinding grain and in bolting flour to ensure milling according to specifications.

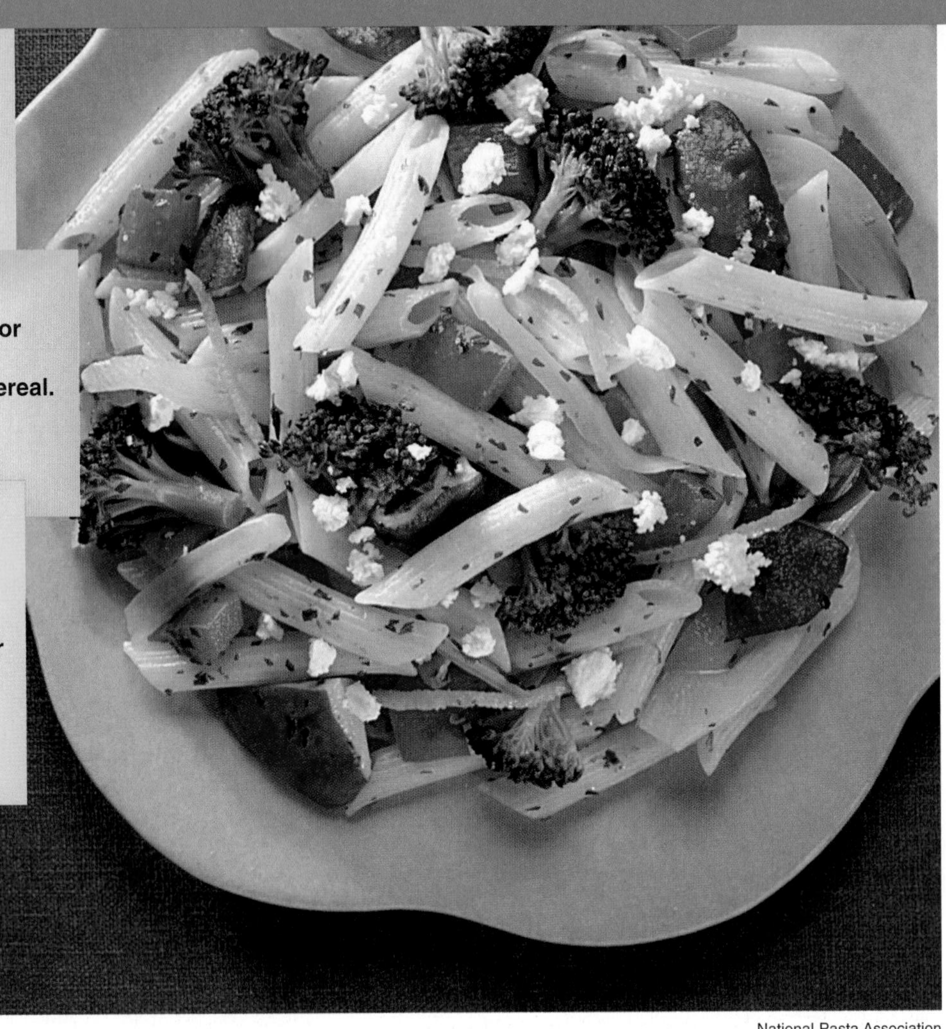

National Pasta Association

Terms to Know

cereal
kernel
bran
endosperm
germ
whole grain
refined
pasta
enriched
starch
gelatinization
syneresis

Objectives

After studying this chapter, you will be able to

- list a variety of cereal products.
- describe how heat and liquids affect starches.
- prepare cooked breakfast cereals, rice, and pasta.

Cereals are major staple foods for people throughout the world. This is because they are easy to grow and store. They are also low in cost and have high energy value.

Types of Cereal Products

Cereals are starchy grains that are suitable to use as food. Corn, wheat, rice, oats, barley, and rye are the cereals most often used as food in the United States. They are used to make a wide variety of products, including breakfast foods, flours, meals, breads, pasta products, and starches.

Grain Structure

Grains differ in size and shape, but they all have kernels with similar structures. A ***kernel*** is a whole seed of a cereal. It has three parts: the bran, the endosperm, and the germ.

The ***bran*** is the outer protective covering of the kernel. It is a good source of vitamins and fiber (cellulose).

The ***endosperm*** makes up the largest part of the kernel. It contains most of the starch and the protein of the kernel, but few minerals and little fiber. It holds the food supply the plant uses to grow.

The ***germ*** is the reproductive part of the plant. It is rich in vitamins, minerals, protein, and fat. It makes up the smallest part of the kernel. See 14-1.

Whole grain cereal products contain all three parts of the kernel. ***Refined*** products have had the bran and germ removed during processing.

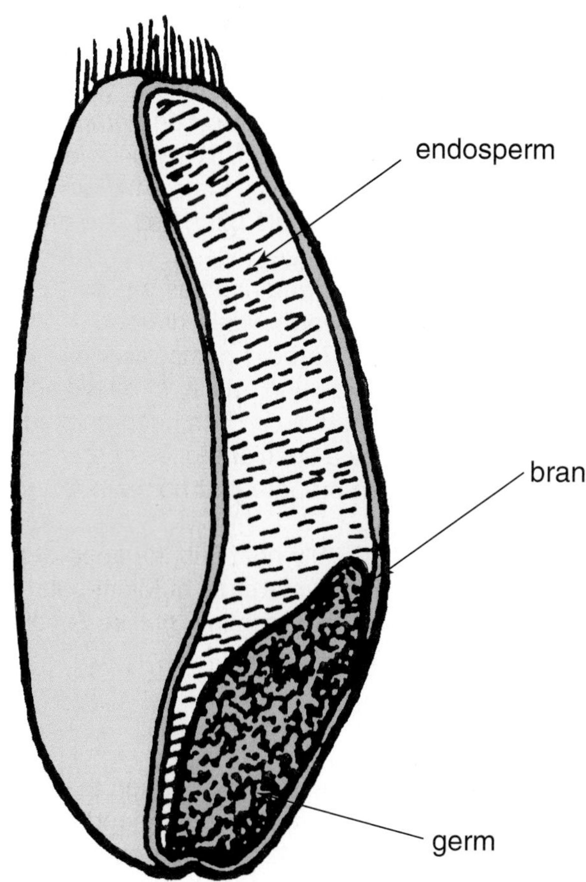

14-1 Each part of a kernel of grain contains different nutrients.

Breakfast Foods

Corn, rice, wheat, and oats are made into popular breakfast foods. Breakfast foods can be made from whole grain, enriched refined grain, or a combination of both. They can be presweetened or unsweetened. Some have added ingredients, such as raisins or nuts.

Cereals may be ready-to-eat, or they may require some amount of cooking. *Ready-to-eat cereals* may be puffed, shredded, flaked, granulated, rolled, or formed into shapes. You can pour them into a bowl and eat them without any preparation.

Cereals that require cooking are available in cracked, crushed, granular, and flaked forms. They require the addition of liquid and heat. *Quick-cooking* or *instant cereals* are partially cooked and require little time to prepare. *Raw* or *old-fashioned cereals* require longer cooking times. Oatmeal and oat bran are examples of these types of cereals.

Flour

Any grain can be made into flour. However, most homemakers use wheat flours for baking because the gluten in wheat flours is superior. (*Gluten* is an elastic protein substance that provides the structure in baked goods.)

You can buy many different kinds of wheat flour. *All-purpose flour* is made from a milled and sifted blend of different varieties of wheat. It is made up primarily of the endosperm. You can buy all-purpose flour bleached or unbleached.

Bleached flour is whiter than *unbleached flour,* but there is no nutritional difference between the two. People use both types at home for general baking and cooking.

Cake flour is made from a class of wheat called soft wheat. Cake flour feels soft and satiny. People use it for making cakes and other baked products with delicate textures.

Instant or *quick-mixing flour* is all-purpose flour that has been specially treated to blend easily with liquids. People use it to make gravies and sauces.

Self-rising flour is all-purpose flour with added leavening agents and salt. You must adjust your recipe when using this type of flour. See 14-2.

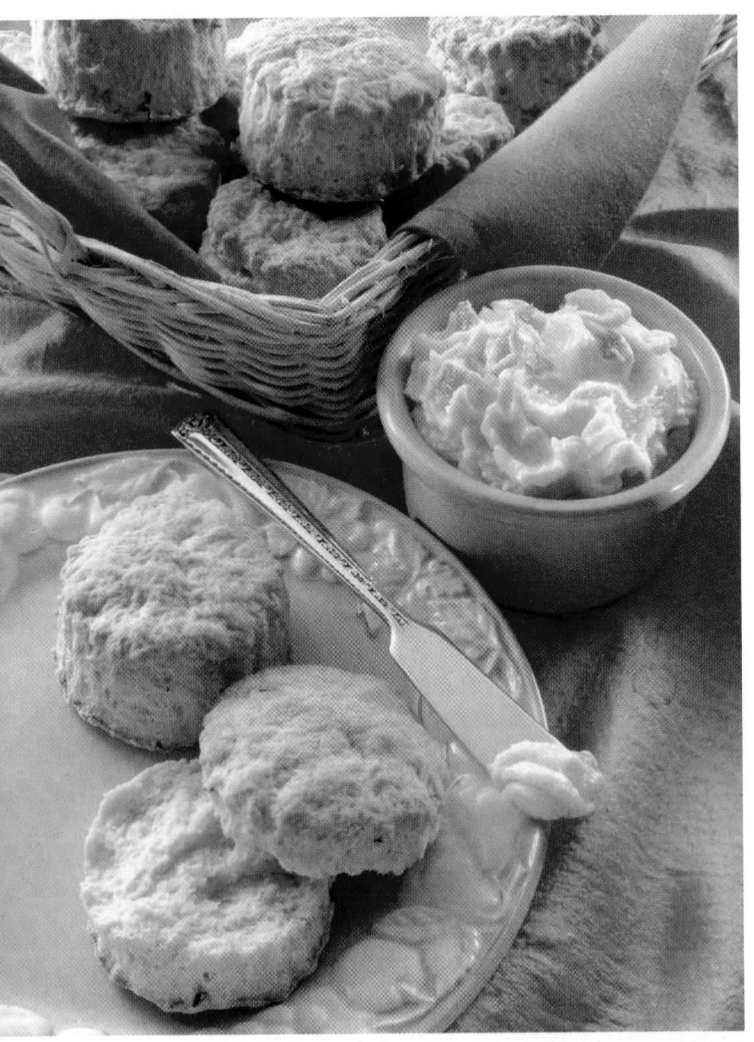

photo courtesy of Land O'Lakes, Inc.

14-2 These biscuits are made with all-purpose flour, baking powder, and salt. Some biscuit recipes call for self-rising flour in place of these ingredients.

Whole wheat flour is made by milling the entire wheat kernel so it contains the bran, germ, and endosperm. Whole wheat flour gives baked products a nutlike flavor and coarser texture than does all-purpose flour.

Potato flour is made from cooked potatoes that have been dried and ground. People on wheat-free diets often use potato flour.

Sifting buckwheat meal produces *buckwheat flour.* It is finely ground and often used to make pancakes.

Rye flour is a finely ground whole grain flour made by sifting rye meal. It is popular for making breads.

Soy flour is made from ground soybeans. It has a strong flavor and must be combined with wheat flour for use in baked products.

Rice flour is made by milling white rice. It is a white and starchy flour popular in Asia and the Far East.

Rice

Rice (also called *white rice*) is the white, starchy endosperm of the rice kernel. *Brown rice* has had the hull removed but contains the bran and germ as well as the endosperm.

Rice can be classified according to grain length or method of processing. *Long grain rice* is dry and fluffy when cooked. Many people use it as a side dish. *Short grain rice* is small and sticky when cooked. People often use it in puddings, croquettes, and rice rings.

Parboiled or *converted rice* has been steeped (soaked) in warm water, drained, steamed, and dried. Parboiling improves the nutritive value and keeping quality of milled rice.

Precooked or *instant rice* has been cooked, rinsed, and dried by a special process before packaging. You can prepare it at home in a matter of minutes.

Wild rice is not really rice. It is the seed of a grass that grows in the marshes of Minnesota and Canada. It has an appealing, nutlike flavor and is rather expensive. See 14-3.

Pasta

Pasta is a nutritious, shaped dough that may or may not be dried. Macaroni, noodles, and spaghetti are all pastas. Pasta dough is made from *semolina,* which is produced from *durum wheat.* Durum wheat is specially grown for pasta making. It gives pasta products a nutty

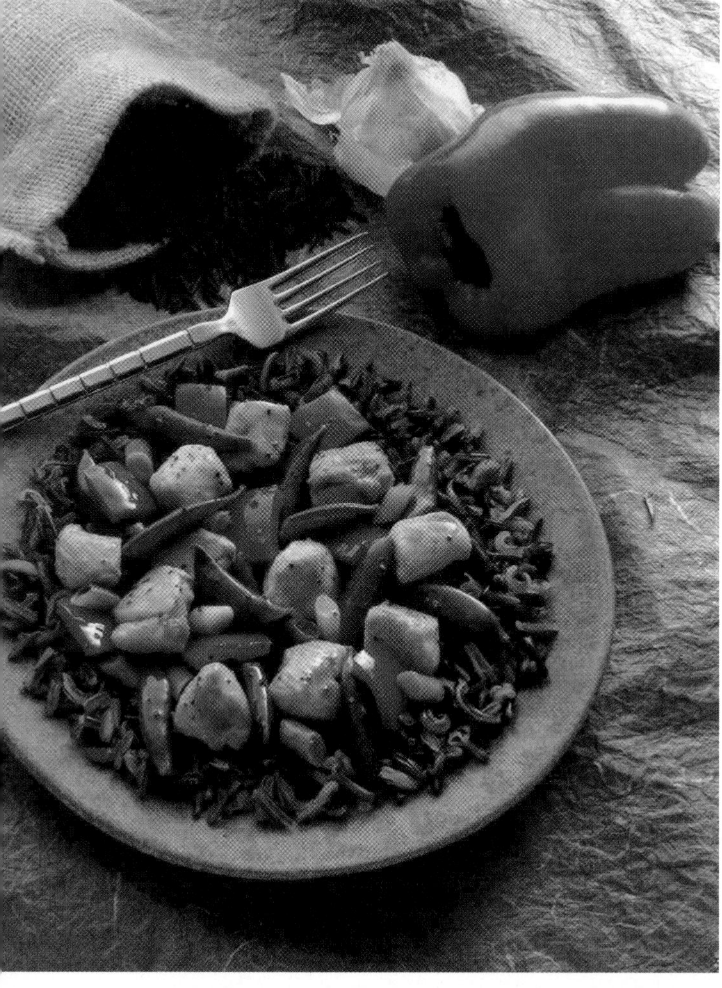

photo courtesy of Land O'Lakes, Inc.

14-3 The firm texture and nutlike flavor of wild rice make it an appealing accompaniment to this chicken and vegetable dish.

flavor and firm shape. Noodles are made by adding egg to the pasta dough.

Pasta comes in many shapes and sizes. Commercially, pasta is made by machine. Some people, however, enjoy making homemade pasta either by hand or with a pasta-making appliance.

Other Grain Products

Cereals are used to make a variety of other products. *Cornmeal* is made from ground white or yellow corn. It is often enriched.

Hominy, a popular food in the South, is corn minus the hull and germ. When broken into pieces, it is called *hominy grits.*

Cornstarch is the refined starch obtained from the endosperm of corn. People use it as a thickening agent in cooking.

Pearl barley is the whole barley grain minus the hull. It is high in minerals, and people often use it in soups.

Bulgur wheat is whole wheat that has been cooked, dried, partly debranned, and cracked. It is a popular Middle Eastern side dish.

Wheat germ is the germ portion of the wheat kernel separated during milling. Wheat germ is high in vitamins and minerals. You can add it to foods for flavor and nutrition.

Farina is a wheat product made by grinding and sifting wheat that has had the bran and most of the germ removed. People use farina as a thickener and as a cooked breakfast cereal. Cream of Wheat® is a popular brand of farina.

Couscous is granules of precooked, dried semolina, which is the same wheat product used to make pasta. Couscous cooks quickly, so it is a convenient choice for meal managers on a tight schedule. You can use it as a side dish or as a base to top with stews or stir-fried dishes. See 14-4.

Selecting and Storing Cereal Products

Cereal products are nutritious, economical, and versatile enough to serve at any meal. You can store them for extended periods without refrigeration. Therefore, you will want to keep a variety of cereal products on hand at all times.

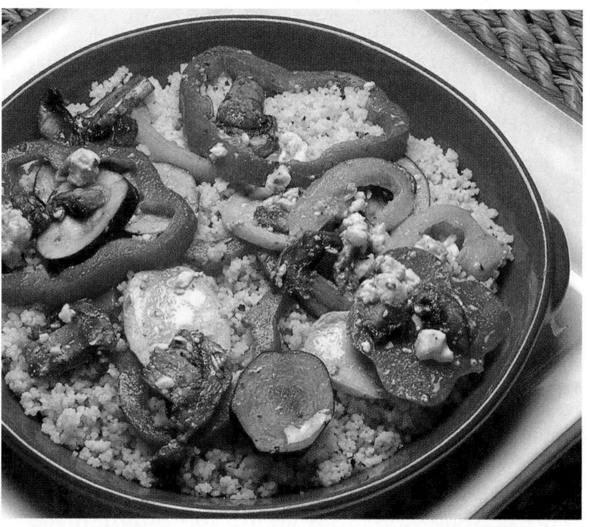

Wheat Foods Council

14-4 Couscous can be used in place of rice or pasta to form the foundation of a meal.

Nutritional Value of Cereal Products

According to the Food Guide Pyramid, you should eat 6 to 11 servings from the grains group each day. A serving equals 1 ounce (28 g) of ready-to-eat cereal or ½ cup (125 mL) cooked cereal, rice, or pasta. Cereals and cereal products are excellent sources of complex carbohydrates. They are also important sources of protein. Sprinkling a little cheese on your pasta or pouring milk on your breakfast cereal can enhance the protein quality.

Choosing a variety of cereal products, including some whole grain products, will provide you with the greatest nutritional value. Whole grain cereals contribute important amounts of B vitamins, iron, magnesium, and zinc. Refined cereals furnish only calories and protein unless they are enriched. ***Enriched*** products have added nutrients to replace those lost through processing. Enriched cereals contain added thiamin, niacin, riboflavin, folic acid, and iron in specified amounts. Federal law requires white flour, white rice, pasta, cereal, and most bakery products shipped across state lines to be enriched.

Most cereals are naturally low in fat, sodium, and sugar. However, these ingredients are added to many breakfast cereals and rice and pasta mixes. Use the Nutrition Facts panel to help you assess the nutritional value of the products you buy.

Good Manners Are Good Business

Eating spaghetti (or other long pastas) with grace can be a bit tricky anywhere. At a business dinner, however, you will want to make a special effort to be neat while you eat. The proper way to eat long pastas is to wrap them around your fork. Capture a few strands of pasta between the tines of the fork. Hold the fork against your plate or a spoon. Rotate the fork slowly until you have shaped the pasta into a small ball.

Cost of Cereal Products

Cereal products are generally inexpensive, but costs vary according to the type of item. Convenience products and products with added ingredients tend to cost more.

Breakfast foods can be costly or economical. Ready-to-eat cereals are more expensive than those that require cooking. Presweetened cereals and cereals with added ingredients cost more than plain cereals. Small boxes often cost more per unit of weight than large boxes. Single serving boxes cost the most per serving.

All-purpose flour is generally the least expensive type of flour. Specialty flours, such as cake flour and instant flour, are usually higher in price.

Most pasta products, regardless of shape or size, are low in cost, 14-5. Fresh-made, gourmet pastas are more expensive. Packaged pasta dishes with special sauces and seasonings also cost more.

Long grain and short grain rice are the lowest priced rice products. The convenience of converted or instant rice adds to the cost. Wild rice and seasoned rice mixes also carry higher price tags.

Storing Cereal Products

Store flours, breakfast foods, pasta products, and rice in tightly covered containers in a cool, dry place. Grain products stored uncovered will attract dust and insects. Some may also pick up moisture, which will cause them to lose their characteristic texture. Breakfast foods will keep well for two to three months. Brown and wild rice will keep for six months. White rice and pasta will keep for a year.

Q: Are enriched grain products as nutritious as whole grain products?

A: Enriched products contain added vitamins and iron to replace nutrients lost when the bran and germ are removed from the grain kernel. However, whole grains provide fiber and other healthful substances, which are not found in enriched products.

Cooking Starches

Starch is a complex carbohydrate stored in plants. Cereal grains contain plant cells that are the sources of starch granules. Wheat flour, cornstarch, and tapioca are starches commonly used in cooking.

Uses of Starch

Cooks use starches primarily as thickening agents. Mixtures thickened with cornstarch or tapioca are translucent, whereas mixtures thickened with flour are opaque. Therefore, cooks use flour to thicken gravies and unsweetened sauces. They use cornstarch and tapioca to thicken puddings and sweet sauces. They also use cornstarch and tapioca to thicken unsweetened sauces in which they want a translucent appearance.

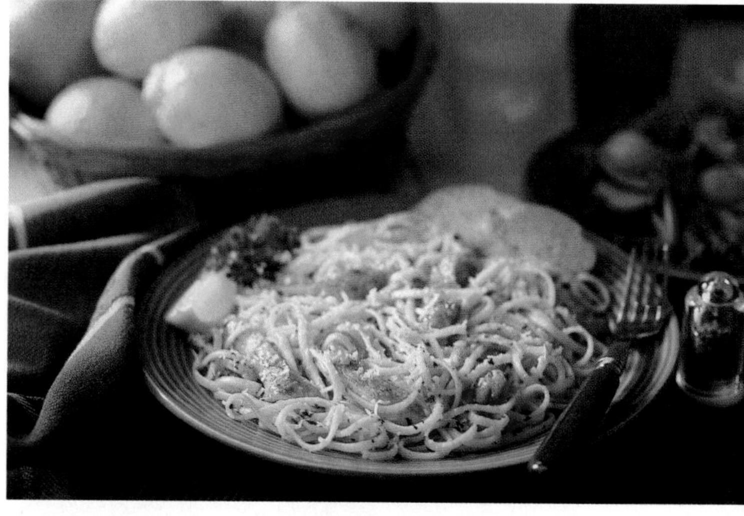

courtesy of American Italian Pasta Company

14-5 Pasta makes a filling and inexpensive entree that can be served in a variety of ways.

Food Science Principles of Cooking Starches

Starches differ in chemical structure and composition. Thus, different starches behave differently. Some starch mixtures form gels; others do not. Some starches form firm gels; others form weak gels. Some cooked starch mixtures are clear; some are semiclear; others are opaque.

Effects of Heat and Liquids on Starch

Granular starch is completely *insoluble* (unable to dissolve) in cold water. The granules need heat to become *soluble* (able to dissolve). Both dry and moist heat affect starch.

Dry heat causes starch to become slightly soluble and to lose some of its thickening power. This is why gravy made from browned flour is thinner than gravy made from unbrowned flour. Dry heat also causes color and flavor changes. The effect of dry heat on starch causes the dark crust of baked goods, toast, and some ready-to-eat breakfast cereals. See 14-6.

Mixing starch granules with water and heating them causes them to become soluble. They absorb water and swell. As starch granules swell, the starch mixture thickens. As heating continues, the starch mixture becomes thicker until it reaches a maximum thickness. This process is called ***gelatinization.*** It is basic to cooking all starches.

During cooling, bonds form between the starch molecules. Because of this bonding, most starch mixtures form gels. The spaces of the gel network hold water. If you cut the gel, or if it stands too long, water may leak out. This is called ***syneresis.*** You may have seen this leakage in a lemon pie filling.

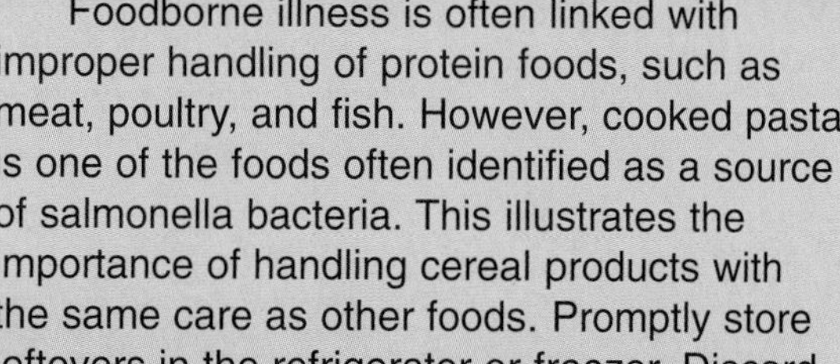

Foodborne illness is often linked with improper handling of protein foods, such as meat, poultry, and fish. However, cooked pasta is one of the foods often identified as a source of salmonella bacteria. This illustrates the importance of handling cereal products with the same care as other foods. Promptly store leftovers in the refrigerator or freezer. Discard foods that have been kept at room temperature for more than two hours.

Factors Affecting Starch-Thickened Mixtures

The temperature, time, agitation, and mixing method used when cooking with starch can all

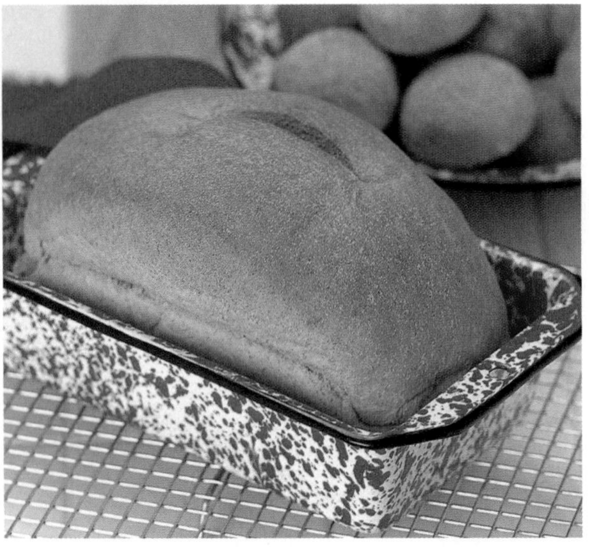

Wheat Foods Council

14-6 The golden brown crust on a loaf of bread is the result of dry heat on the starch in flour.

affect the outcome of the mixture. You must control these factors during cooking.

The *temperature* used to cook starch mixtures must be warm enough to make the starch molecules swell uniformly (the same amount). It should not be so hot that it causes uneven swelling or lumping. When lumping occurs, the molecules in the middle of the lump do not swell. They stay small and dry. Cooking starch mixtures in a double boiler or in a heavy pan over moderate heat will help prevent lumping.

The *time* needed for gelatinization to be completed depends on the kind of starch and the cooking temperature. Once gelatinization occurs, cook the starch mixture for a short time longer to thoroughly cook the starch. This will prevent a raw starch flavor in the finished product.

The amount of *agitation* a starch mixture receives can affect its texture. Gentle stirring during cooking will help keep the starch mixture smooth. If you stir the mixture too rapidly or for too long a time, the starch granules may rupture (break down). As a result, the cooked starch mixture will be thinner.

A recipe will usually tell you which *mixing method* to use when adding starch to a hot liquid. If you add starch directly to a hot liquid, the starch granules usually will lump. To prevent lumping, you must separate the starch granules from one another before you add them to the hot liquid. You can separate starch granules by using one of three techniques

- coating with fat
- combining with sugar
- mixing with a cold liquid to form a paste

Cooking Cereal Products

The relative low cost and high energy value of cereals make them an important part of the diet. Cereals are popular as breakfast foods. However, you can serve a variety of cereal products at meals throughout the day, 14-7.

Food Science Principles of Cooking Cereal Products

Cereal products contain large amounts of starch. Therefore, the principles used in cooking starches also apply to cooking cereal products. Cooking improves both palatability and digestibility of cereal products.

During cooking, the starch granules in cereal products absorb water and swell, causing the products to increase in volume. This swelling causes rice and dried pasta products to soften. It causes cereals to become thicker until they reach a point of maximum thickness (gelatinization).

When cooking cereal products, you must use enough water to permit the starch granules to swell. The amount of water needed will vary depending on the product. You can find correct proportions of cereal products to water along with cooking times on cereal, rice, and pasta packages.

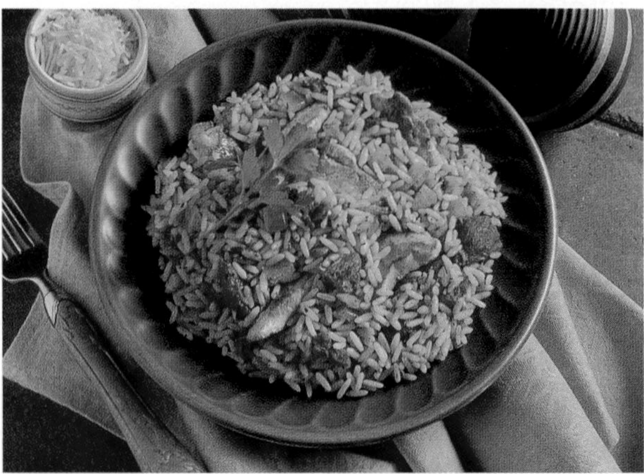

USA Rice Federation

14-7 Rice is a cereal product that serves as the basis for this flavorful dinner entree.

Q: Is it necessary to add salt to the cooking water when preparing cereal products?

A: Adding salt to the cooking water is optional. However, if you wish to add salt, ½ teaspoon (2 mL) of salt per 1 cup (250 mL) of uncooked cereal, rice, or pasta is ample.

Preparing Cooked Breakfast Cereals

To prepare cooked cereal, bring the recommended amount of water to a boil. The size of the cereal particles and whether the bran layer is present determine the amount of cooking water needed. Whole grain cereals will cook more quickly if you first soak them to soften the bran. (If you do not soften the bran, it can block the passage of water into the center of the kernel and delay swelling.) If you soak a whole grain cereal, you should cook it in the soaking liquid, adding more water, if needed.

All the cereal particles must have equal contact with the water and heat so the starch granules can swell uniformly. You may add the cereal to the boiling water in one of two ways to prevent lumping. One way is to slowly add the dry cereal directly to the boiling water. The other way is to wet the cereal with cold water and then add it. (You can mix granular cereals, such as farina, with enough cold water to form a smooth paste. Then you can add the paste to the boiling water.)

Gently stir the cereal with a fork when you are adding it to the boiling water. This preliminary stirring helps separate the cereal particles and prevent lumping. Stirring throughout the remaining cooking time should be gentle and minimal. Too much stirring will break up the cereal particles, and the cooked product will be gummy.

Cook the cereal until it thickens and absorbs all the water. Cooking time will vary depending on the type of cereal and cooking method. Cereals that are finely granulated or precooked will cook faster than cracked or whole grain cereals. Cereal cooked over direct heat will take less time to cook than cereal prepared in a double boiler. Cooking temperature will also affect cooking time. Low to moderate heat is best, as temperatures that are too hot can cause lumping and scorching.

Like starch mixtures, you should cook cereals for a short time after gelatinization is complete to prevent a raw starch flavor. Cooked cereals should be free of lumps. (Flaked cereals should contain separate and distinct flakes.) Cooked cereals should be thick, but they should flow when poured into a serving bowl. See 14-8.

Preparing Rice

When cooking rice, the goal is to obtain tender kernels that hold their shape. Properly cooked rice is tender and fluffy. The rice kernels should not stick together and form a gummy mass.

You may cook rice over direct heat, in a double boiler, or in the oven. The proportion of water to rice varies somewhat. As a rule, white rice requires about twice its volume of water. You can substitute milk, bouillon, or another liquid for all or part of the cooking water. The rice should absorb all the liquid used in cooking.

You can use the same preparation methods for brown rice you use for white rice. However,

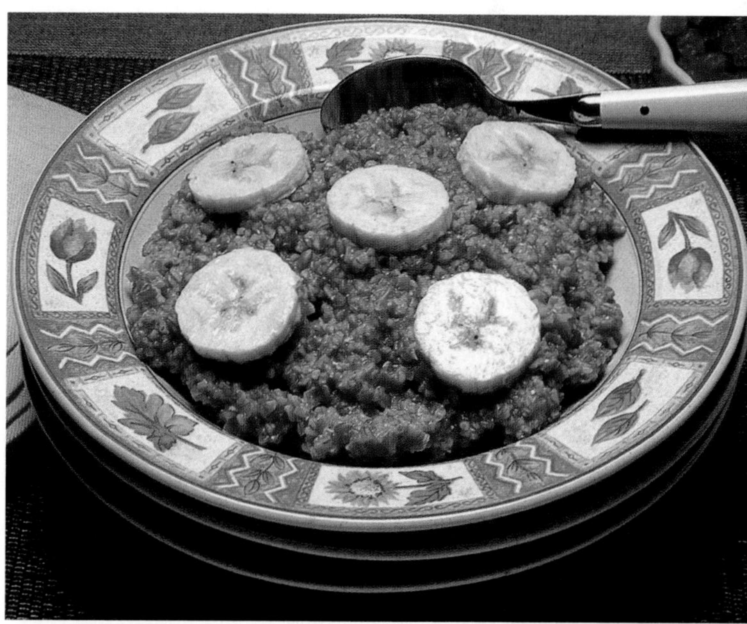

Wheat Foods Council

14-8 Properly prepared cooked cereal should have a thick texture with distinct cereal grains.

Q: How can I keep cooked pasta from sticking together?

A: Adding 1 tablespoon (15 mL) of vegetable oil to the cooking water can help prevent cooked pasta from forming a sticky mass.

brown rice will take about twice as long to cook unless you soak it first. Soaking softens the outer bran layer so the rice will absorb the cooking liquid more quickly. You may also want to soak wild rice before cooking. Follow package directions for soaking and cooking brown and wild rices.

Precooked or instant rice cooks in a very short time. Add the rice to boiling water. Remove the pan from the heat and cover it tightly. When the rice has absorbed all the liquid, it is ready to serve.

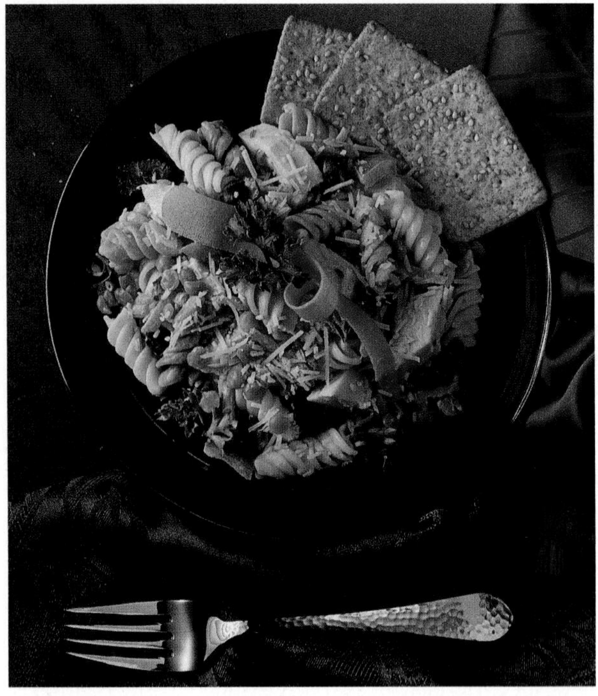

USA Dry Pea & Lentil Council

14-9 These colorful pastas are tender enough to be fully cooked but firm enough to hold their shape.

Preparing Pasta Products

To cook macaroni, spaghetti, and other kinds of pasta, bring water to a boil. Use 2 quarts (2 L) of water for each 8 ounces (225 g) of pasta. Pasta requires more water than other cereal products so it can move freely as it cooks. Add the pasta gradually to the boiling water. The water should not stop boiling. If it does, the pasta may stick together as it cooks. As the starch granules swell, the pasta will double in size. Simmer the pasta just until tender and drain. Do not rinse pasta products after draining. Water-soluble nutrients can be lost by rinsing. Properly cooked pasta is tender, but it holds its shape, 14-9.

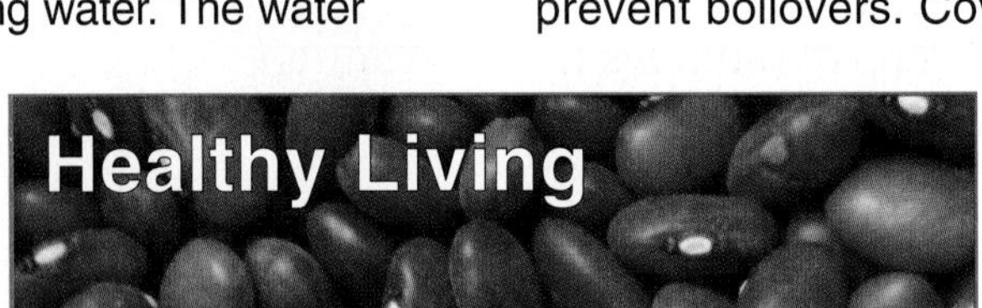

Healthy Living

Seasoned rice mixes can be high in fat and sodium. When preparing them, add only half the amount of fat listed on package directions. Mix some leftover plain rice with the prepared rice mix to reduce the amount of sodium per portion. You can follow these tips to reduce the fat and sodium in seasoned pasta mixes, too.

Microwaving Cereal Products

Cereals, rice, and pasta do not microwave much faster than they cook conventionally. However, these foods are less likely to stick and burn when prepared in a microwave oven. You can also prepare and serve them in the same dish, which saves time on cleanup.

When microwaving cereal products, be sure to use containers that are large enough to prevent boilovers. Cover these foods for microwave cooking. You can serve pasta immediately after microwaving. Allow rice and cereal to stand a few minutes before serving. Cereals, rice, and pasta can be reheated in a microwave oven without stirring or adding water.

You may wish to use quick-cooking rather than conventional cereal products when making casseroles in a microwave oven. If using conventional products, precook them a bit less than if you were going to serve them immediately.

Chapter 14 Review
Grain Foods

Summary

Corn, wheat, rye, oats, rice, and barley are important crops throughout the world. These grains are made into a variety of staple food products, including breakfast foods, flours, and pasta. These products are generally nutritious, inexpensive, and easy to store.

Starches obtained from cereals are used chiefly as thickening agents in gravies, puddings, and sauces. When mixed with liquid and heated, starches absorb water and swell, causing the mixture to thicken. As they cool, most starch mixtures form gels. Temperature, time, agitation, and mixing method used affect the cooking of starch mixtures.

Cooked breakfast cereals, rice, and pasta all contain large amounts of starch. Therefore, you need to keep the principles of cooking starches in mind when preparing these foods. During cooking, cereal products absorb water and increase in volume. The amount of water needed to make the starch granules in cereal products swell varies depending on the product. Cooked breakfast cereals require moderate temperatures and gentle stirring. The water for pasta should boil constantly throughout cooking. Properly cooked cereal products are tender, but they hold their shape and have no raw starch flavor. Microwaving cereal products does not save time, but it may reduce cleanup tasks.

Review What You Have Read

Write your answers on a separate sheet of paper.

1. Describe the three parts of a kernel of grain.
2. How do whole grain cereals differ from refined cereals?
3. List three products, other than breakfast food and flour, that come from grain.
4. True or false. Wild rice is not really rice.
5. Pasta is made from _____.
   A. all-purpose flour
   B. cake flour
   C. self-rising flour
   D. semolina
6. What are two factors that affect the cost of cereal products?
7. The swelling and thickening of starch granules when heated in water is called _____.
8. Describe three ways to separate starch granules to prevent lumping.
9. True or false. Rice should absorb all of its cooking liquid.
10. How can the cooking time of whole grain cereals be shortened?
11. True or false. Cereals should be stirred vigorously throughout the entire cooking time.
12. How can a raw starch flavor be prevented when cooking cereals?
13. How can pasta be kept from sticking together during cooking?
14. True or false. Cereal products can be microwaved in about one-fourth the time needed for conventional cooking.

Build Your Basic Skills

1. **Writing.** Research the types of grains people in different parts of the world use as staple foods. (Use the international foods chapters in this textbook as one of your sources of information.) Summarize your findings in a two-page report.
2. **Math.** Choose one of the following types of cereal products: breakfast foods, flours, pastas, or rice products. Visit a grocery store and make a list of as many products as you can find in the group you chose. Don't forget to list canned and frozen products as well as dried products. Make a poster showing a price graph of all the products you listed.

Build Your Thinking Skills

1. **Compare.** Prepare two white sauces. To prepare the first sauce, make a paste with the fat and flour. Add the milk slowly, stirring constantly, and cook the sauce until thickened. To prepare the second sauce, warm the milk with the fat. Add the flour all at once. Cook until thickened, stirring constantly. Compare the two sauces. Which would you rather serve? Why?
2. **Analyze.** Prepare two recipes of cherry sauce. Thicken one with cornstarch. Thicken the other with flour. Analyze the differences in appearance, texture, and flavor between the two sauces. Which one would you rather serve? Why?
3. **Summarize.** Prepare old-fashioned oatmeal, quick-cooking oatmeal, and instant oatmeal. Taste each type of oatmeal. Summarize how the flavor, texture, and appearance of each product affected your preference.

Apply Technology

1. Research how modified atmosphere packaging (MAP) is used to preserve fresh pasta products.
2. Work in a small group to investigate how and why biotechnologists develop new varieties of grains. Share your findings with the rest of the class through a poster presentation.

Using Workplace Skills

Tom is a miller at the Olde Towne Granary. The granary grinds several varieties of corn and wheat brought in by local farmers. Tom supervises and coordinates the activities of workers who run the cleaning and grinding machines. Whenever the workers have a scheduling problem or a safety concern, Tom has to handle it.

To be an effective worker, Tom needs skill in negotiating. In a small group, answer the following questions about Tom's need for and use of this skill:

A. Why can't the workers handle scheduling problems and safety concerns themselves?
B. How might the workers respond if Tom lacks skill in negotiating?
C. How might Olde Towne Granary be affected if Tom lacks skill in negotiating?
D. What is another skill Tom would need in this job? Briefly explain why this skill would be important.

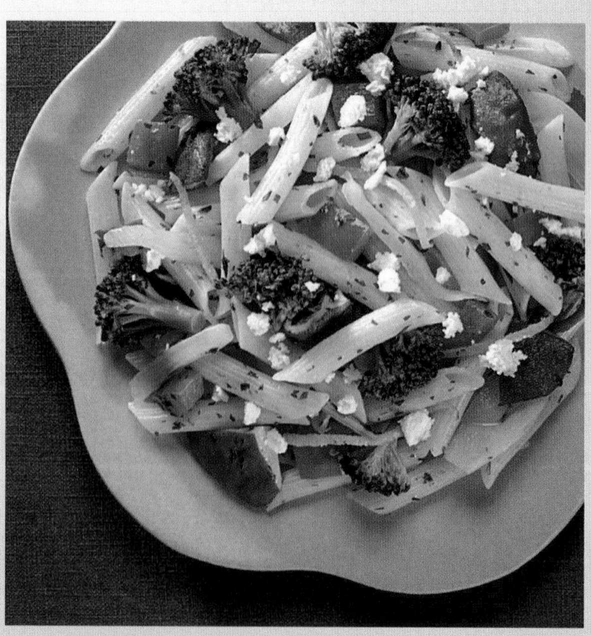

Chapter 15
Vegetables

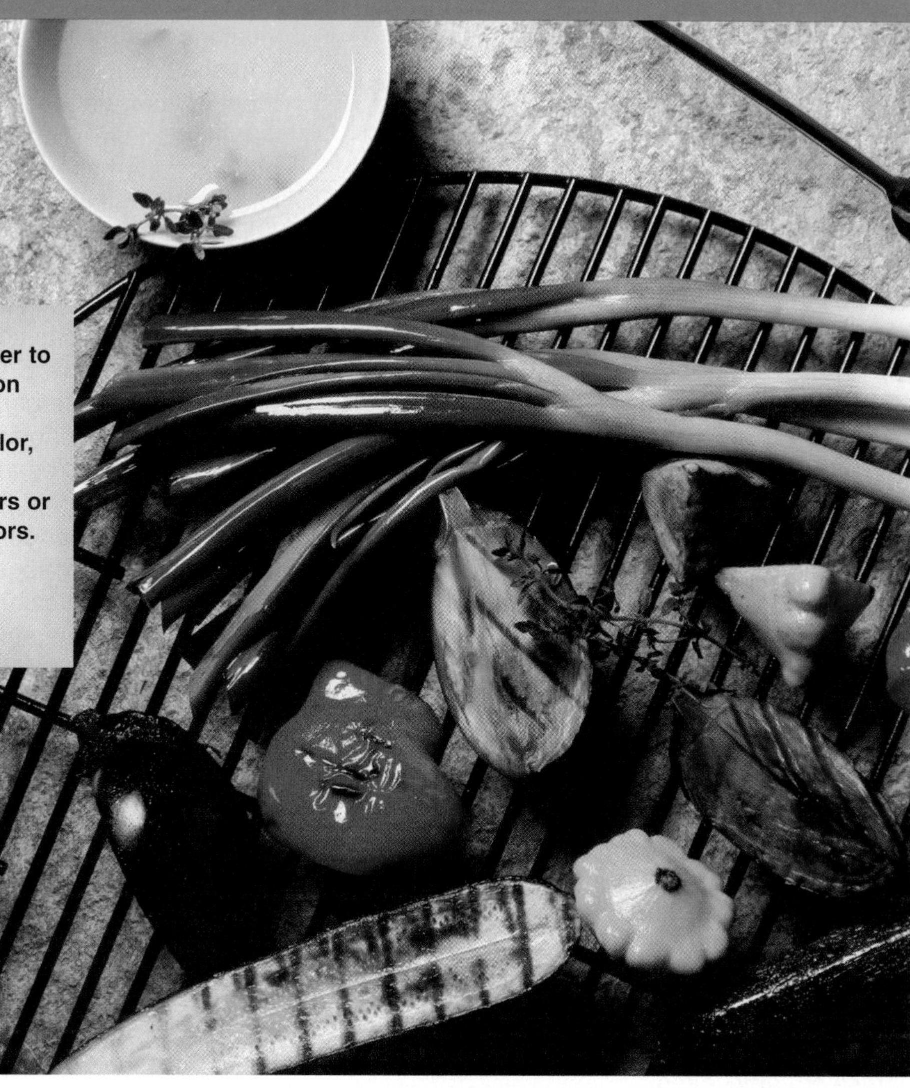

Vegetable Harvest Worker
Harvests vegetables, such as cucumbers, onions, lettuce, and sweet corn, by hand or using a knife, according to the method appropriate for the type of vegetable.

Vegetable Sorter
Works as a crewmember to segregate vegetables on conveyor belt or table according to grade, color, and size and places vegetables in containers or on designated conveyors.

Botanist
Studies development and life processes, physiology, heredity, environment, distribution, anatomy, morphology, and economic value of plants for application in such fields as agronomy, forestry, horticulture, and pharmacology.

Terms to Know

legumes
crisp-tender
chlorophyll
carotene
flavones
anthocyanin
new potatoes

Objectives

After studying this chapter, you will be able to

- explain how to properly select and store vegetables.
- describe food science principles of cooking vegetables.
- identify methods for cooking vegetables.
- prepare vegetables, preserving their colors, textures, flavors, and nutrients.

Most vegetables are fairly low in cost and calories. Vegetables are versatile enough for you to use in any menu. You can serve them raw or cooked to add color, flavor, texture, and nutrients to meals. They are also good choices for between-meal snacks.

Many vegetables are readily available year-round. You can purchase them fresh, frozen, canned, and dried.

Choosing Fresh Vegetables

Methods of growing and shipping vegetables have improved over the years. These improvements have made a greater variety of fresh vegetables available in grocery stores for longer periods. You can purchase many fresh vegetables all year long.

Vegetable Classifications

Vegetables are often grouped according to the part of the plant from which they come. Garlic and onion are *bulbs*. Artichokes, broccoli, and cauliflower are *flowers*. Tomatoes, cucumbers, eggplant, okra, peppers, pumpkins, and squash are *fruits*. Asparagus and celery are *stems*. Brussels sprouts, cabbage, lettuce, and spinach are *leaves*. Peas, corn, and beans are *seeds*. Potatoes and Jerusalem artichokes are *tubers*. Beets, carrots, parsnips, radishes, rutabagas, sweet potatoes, and turnips are *roots*. See 15-1.

Two other ways to classify vegetables are according to flavor or color. For instance, cabbage, Brussels sprouts, turnips, and cauliflower are examples of strong-flavored vegetables. Peas, beans, and potatoes are mild-flavored vegetables. Spinach, Swiss chard, and kale are leafy green vegetables. Carrots, sweet potatoes, and pumpkin are deep yellow vegetables.

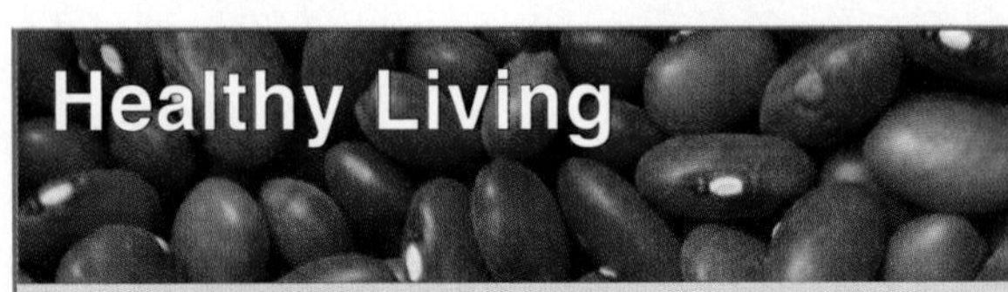

You should eat a diet rich in vegetables and low in fats. Research indicates some of the substances in vegetables may have protective effects against some forms of cancer. Researchers state that eating a lot of vegetables will not guarantee you will never get cancer. However, researchers have concluded that eating vegetables may reduce your cancer risk.

Nutritional Value of Vegetables

Vegetables are excellent sources of many vitamins and minerals needed for good health. You should include three to five servings of them in your diet each day. Remember that a serving equals 1 cup (250 mL) of raw leafy vegetables. One-half cup (125 mL) cooked or chopped vegetables or ¾ cup (175 mL) vegetable juice also equals one serving.

The leafy green and deep yellow vegetables are excellent sources of carotene. This is a substance the body can convert into vitamin A. Tomatoes, broccoli, Brussels sprouts, cabbage, and cauliflower are good sources of vitamin C. Leafy green vegetables are good sources of folate. All vegetables are good sources of fiber. However, fresh vegetables are the best form of vegetables for fiber content. Seeds, roots, and tubers are starchy vegetables. They have more carbohydrate and calories per serving than other types of vegetables.

Selecting Fresh Vegetables

The effects of temperature and handling may reduce the quality of vegetables during shipping. When shopping for fresh vegetables, follow these guidelines

- Look for good color, firmness, and absence of bruises and decay. See 15-2.
- Avoid wilted and misshapen vegetables.
- Handle vegetables carefully to prevent bruising.
- Choose vegetables that are medium in size. Very small vegetables can be immature and lack flavor. Very large vegetables can be overmature and tough.
- Buy only what you will use within a short time. Fresh vegetables lose quality quickly.
- Vegetables that are in season usually are high in quality and low in price.

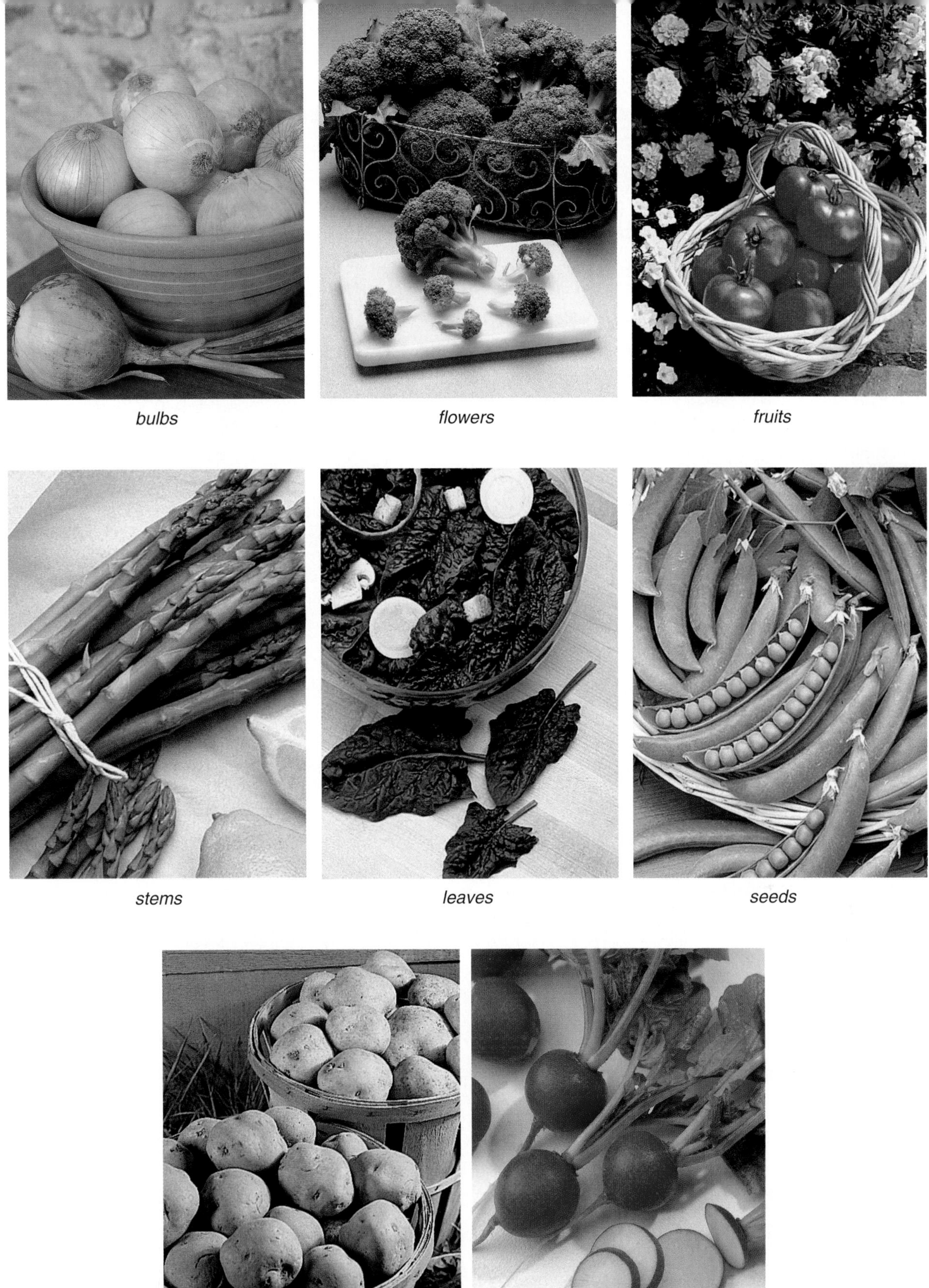

courtesy of W. Atlee Burpee & Co.

15-1 *Vegetables come from various parts of the plant.*

How to Buy Fresh Vegetables		
Vegetables	**Choose**	**Avoid**
Asparagus	Rich, green color; tender stalks; closed, compact tips; round spears	Open, moldy, or decayed tips; ribbed spears; excessive sand
Beans (snap)	Bright color, tender beans, crisp pods	Thick, tough, or wilted pods; serious blemishes
Beets	Slender roots; rich red color; smooth, round bulbs	Wilted, elongated beets; brown, scaly patches
Broccoli	Stems not too thick or tough; firm, compact clusters of small flower buds; deep green color	Open buds; wilted, soft condition; yellow color
Brussels sprouts	Bright green color, tight outer leaves, no blemishes	Yellow or wilted leaves, holes or ragged edges
Cabbage	Firm heads, heavy for size; bright red or green color; fresh; no blemishes	Wilted, decayed, yellow outer leaves; worm holes
Carrots	Bright color; well-rounded, smooth, firm roots	Flabby, decaying roots; patches of green
Cauliflower	Creamy white to white heads; compact, clean, solid florets	Discolored spots, wilting
Celery	Bright color; smooth, rigid stalks; fresh leaves	Discoloration; flabby or pithy stalks; wilting
Corn	Ears with plump, not overly mature kernels; fresh, green husks; silk ends free from damage	Yellow, wilted, or dried husks; kernels that are very small, very large, or dark yellow
Cucumbers	Well-shaped, rounded bodies; bright green color; firm	Signs of wilting, large diameter, yellowing
Lettuce	Bright color, crisp leaves for iceberg and romaine, soft texture for leaf lettuce, no blemishes	Very hard heads of iceberg lettuce, poor color, brown or soft spots, irregular heads
Mushrooms	White, creamy color; small to medium size; caps closed or slightly open around stem; pink or light tan gills	Badly pitted or discolored caps, wide open caps, dark gills
Onions		
Yellow, white, and red	Hard, smooth, and firm with small necks; papery outer covering	Wet or soft necks, woody or sprouting areas
Green	Fresh, green tops; well-formed, white bulbs	Yellow, wilted, or decayed tops
Peppers (bell)	Bright color, glossy sheen, firm walls, heavy for size	Thin, wilted; cut or punctured walls; decayed spots
Potatoes	Firm, well-shaped, free from blemishes and sunburn	Large cuts, bruises, or green spots; soft and decaying areas; signs of sprouting or shriveling
Radishes	Plump, round, and firm; medium size; bright red color	Large or flabby radishes, decaying tops
Squash		
Summer	Tender, well-developed, firm body, glossy skin	Dull appearance; hard, tough skin
Winter	Hard, tough rind; heavy for size	Tender rind; cuts; soft, sunken, or moldy spots
Tomatoes	Well-formed, smooth, free from blemishes, bright red for fully ripe, pink to light red and slightly firmer for ripening	Soft spots, moldy areas, growth cracks, bruises

15-2 Choose vegetables that are brightly colored, firm, and at their peak of ripeness.

Storing Fresh Vegetables

You should use all vegetables as soon as possible for best flavor, appearance, and nutritive value. However, you can keep most vegetables fresh in the refrigerator for at least a few days. Place most vegetables in the crisper or in plastic bags or containers. Store sweet corn in the husks. Allow tomatoes to fully ripen at room temperature before storing in the refrigerator uncovered. Wrap leafy green vegetables in a damp towel and place them in a perforated plastic bag before refrigerating.

Store onions in open containers at room temperature or slightly cooler. Air should circulate freely around them.

Store potatoes, hard-rind squash, eggplant, rutabagas, and sweet potatoes in a cool, dark, dry place. Use potatoes stored at room temperature within a week, as they will sprout and shrivel if kept longer. Potatoes that are exposed to light will turn green and develop a bitter flavor. Cut away green portions before using potatoes.

Cost of Fresh Vegetables

The cost of fresh vegetables depends a great deal on the time of year. Vegetables cost less when purchased during their peak growing season. During other seasons, costs vary due to storage, handling, and shipping charges.

Choosing Canned, Frozen, and Dried Vegetables

Most people prefer fresh vegetables for salads and relish trays. For use in recipes or as hot side dishes, however, canned, frozen, and dried vegetables often work just as well.

Canned Vegetables

Canned vegetables can be whole, sliced, or in pieces. Most are canned in water. A few, like Harvard beets, are canned in sauces.

Most canned vegetables are packed in cans. A few are available in jars. Choose a container size to meet your needs.

Buying and Storing Canned Vegetables

Canned vegetables usually cost less than either frozen or fresh produce. Cost per serving depends on brand, can size, quality, and packing liquid. Choose house brands to save money. Use generic products when making soups and other recipes where appearance is not vital.

Choose cans that are free from dents, bulges, and leaks. Choose the quality that meets your needs and intended use. Store all cans in a cool, dry place. After opening, store unused portions in the refrigerator.

Frozen Vegetables

Frozen vegetables retain the appearance and flavor of fresh vegetables better than canned and dried vegetables. However, freezing may alter their texture somewhat. They are available in paper cartons and plastic bags. Some vegetables are frozen in combinations or in sauces.

Q: Don't fresh vegetables contain more nutrients than canned or frozen vegetables?

A: Canned and frozen vegetables are processed right after they are harvested. Modern processing methods preserve most of the nutrients. Fresh vegetables, on the other hand, can lose nutrients through prolonged storage or incorrect cooking techniques. Therefore, the nutrients in canned and frozen vegetables are likely to match or surpass those in fresh produce.

Buying and Storing Frozen Vegetables

Frozen vegetables usually cost less than fresh. Green beans are one example. During winter months, frozen green beans are less expensive than fresh green beans. (During the summer months when green beans are in season, fresh beans may cost less than frozen.) Prices will vary according to brand, packaging, size of container, and added ingredients such as butter and sauces.

Choose packages that are clean and solidly frozen. A heavy layer of ice on the package may indicate the food thawed and refroze. Store packages in the coldest part of the freezer.

Dried Vegetables

A few vegetables are dried. The dried ***legumes***—peas, beans, and lentils—are the most commonly purchased dried vegetables.

Legumes are high in protein. They are also excellent sources of fiber. They are used as meat substitutes in many dishes. Many people use dried navy beans, lima beans, split peas, and lentils in soups. They use pinto and red beans in chili and many Mexican foods. Black-eyed peas are a popular side dish in the South. Garbanzo beans and kidney beans are tasty in salads. Soybeans are often used in combination with other foods. See 15-3.

Buying and Storing Dried Vegetables

Choose legumes that are uniform in size, free of visible defects, and brightly colored. Store them in covered containers in a cool, dry place.

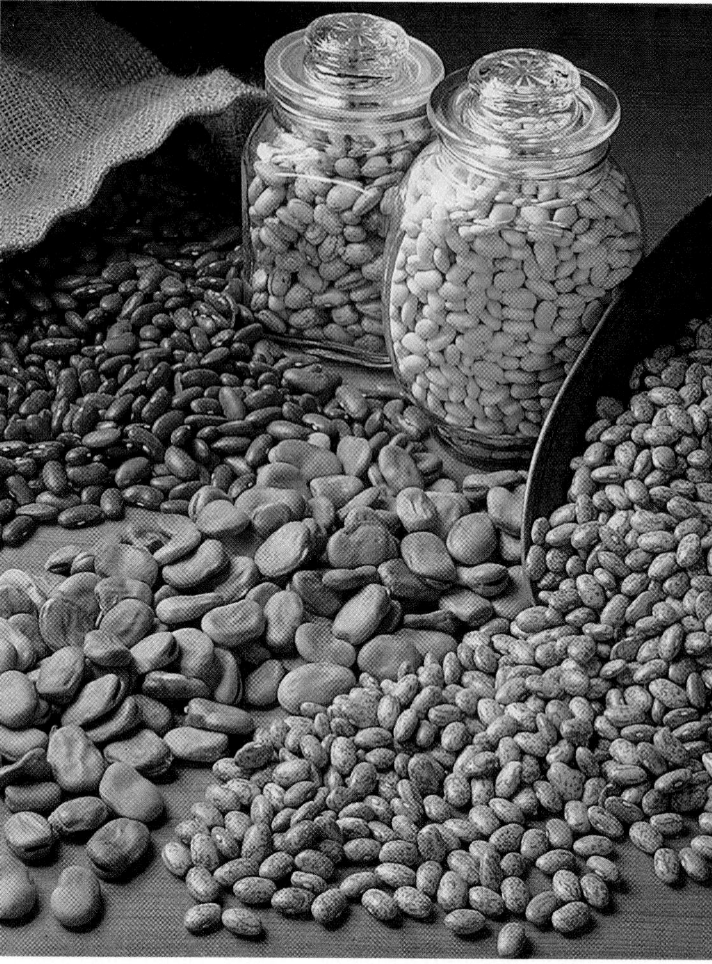

courtesy of W. Atlee Burpee & Co.

15-3 *Dried beans are an excellent source of incomplete protein and an inexpensive meat extender.*

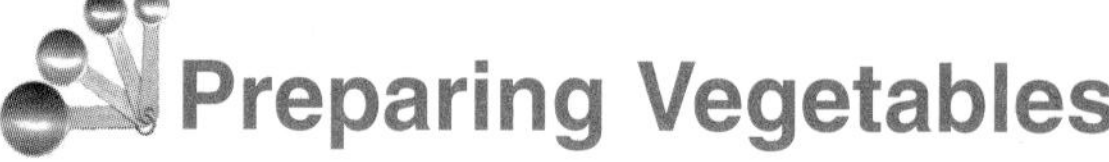

Preparing Vegetables

Vegetables come in a spectrum of colors and a range of flavors. These characteristics, combined with various cooking methods, allow you to use vegetables in countless ways to add interest to meals.

Preparing Raw Vegetables

You can eat many vegetables raw. You probably have eaten raw celery, salad greens, cucumbers, radishes, tomatoes, green peppers, and carrots. You may also have eaten raw cabbage, cauliflower, and broccoli. Raw vegetables are attractive to serve because they are colorful, and their crunchiness adds texture to meals and snacks.

If you have seen a vegetable garden, you know the edible part of most vegetables grows in or near the soil. Soil can carry harmful bacteria, so it is important to wash all vegetables. Careful washing removes dirt, bacteria, and pesticide residues.

Whether you are preparing fresh vegetables to eat raw or cooked, the first step is to wash and trim them. You should even wash vegetables with rinds and peels that you are going to discard, such as winter squash and onions. Wash vegetables in cool running water. A vegetable brush will remove stubborn dirt from crevices. Wash vegetables carefully, but do not let them soak. Water-soluble nutrients can be lost during soaking. Trim any bruised areas, wilted leaves, and thick stems. When peeling vegetables, use a vegetable scraper or floating edge peeler rather than a paring knife. This will help protect as many nutrients as possible. See 15-4.

You can eat raw vegetables out-of-hand. You can use them on relish trays and in salads.

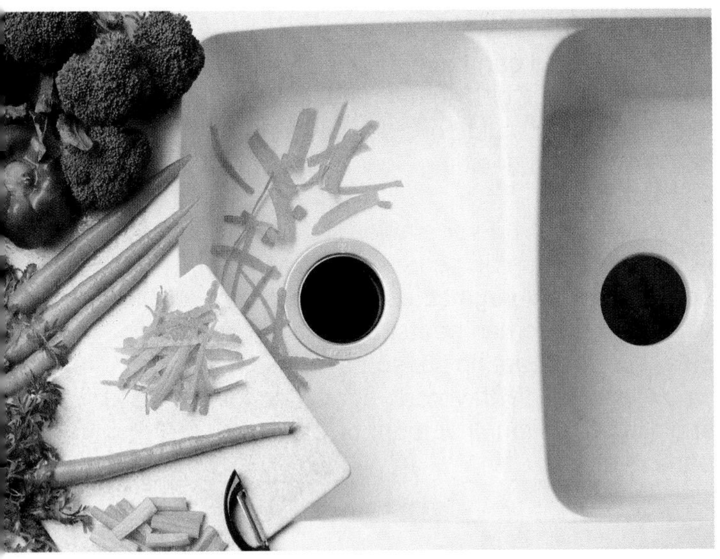

GE Appliances

15-4 Wash and trim fresh vegetables before eating or cooking them.

Cut raw vegetables into pieces that are easy to handle. Sticks, wedges, slices, rings, and florets are good choices. Raw vegetables also make colorful garnishes. Carrot curls, celery fans, and radish roses add nutrients and eye appeal to many dishes.

Raw vegetables taste best when served cold. You can place a relish tray on a bed of ice or arrange vegetables in a bowl lined with ice. Store washed and thoroughly drained vegetables in covered containers in the refrigerator.

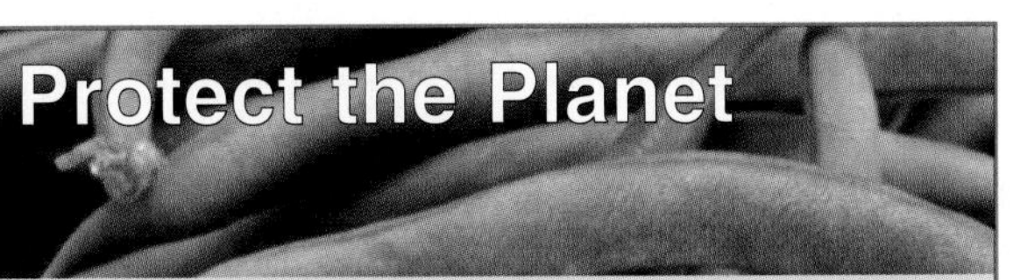

Protect the Planet

Although vegetable scraps are biodegradable, they will not break down rapidly in a landfill. Therefore, do not throw scraps like potato peelings and carrot tops into the garbage when preparing fresh vegetables. Instead, compost your vegetable trimmings.

Find a small area in your yard where you can start a compost pile. A corner of a garden or a spot behind some bushes will work fine. Collect all your organic kitchen waste in a small covered container. Every day or two, empty the scrap container onto your compost pile. Soon, your scraps will decompose into compost.

You can mix your compost into the soil in your garden. This will condition the soil and create a rich medium for planting new vegetables.

Food Science Principles of Cooking Vegetables

When you cook vegetables, several changes take place. The cellulose (fiber) in vegetables softens to make chewing easier. Starch absorbs water, swells, and becomes easier to digest. Flavors and colors undergo changes, and some of the nutrients may be lost.

Properly cooked vegetables are colorful and flavorful. They also have a ***crisp-tender*** texture. This means they are tender, but still slightly firm. You can pierce them with a fork but not too easily.

Overcooked or incorrectly cooked vegetables may suffer undesirable changes in color, texture, and flavor. They also may lose many of their nutrients. The amount of cooking liquid and the cooking time greatly affect nutrient retention and degree of doneness.

Amount of Cooking Liquid

Some nutrients in vegetables, including minerals, vitamin C, and the B vitamins, are water-soluble. They will dissolve in cooking liquid. Vegetables cooked with no added water or in a small amount of water retain more of these water-soluble nutrients.

Cooking Time

Cooking vegetables too long causes several undesirable changes to take place. Heat-sensitive nutrients, such as thiamin, are lost. Unpleasant flavor, texture, and color changes also occur. Vegetables cooked for a short time retain more heat-sensitive nutrients, flavor, texture, and color.

In most cases, you should cook vegetables for a short time in a small amount of water. Serve them when they are crisp-tender.

Effect of Cooking on Vegetable Color

Cooking can affect the color of vegetables. For this reason, cooking times and methods may need adjustment to suit the vegetables you are cooking. See 15-5.

Vegetables can be green, yellow, white, or red. *Green vegetables* contain the green pigment ***chlorophyll.*** Heat affects chlorophyll. Overcooked green vegetables lose their bright green color and look grayish-green.

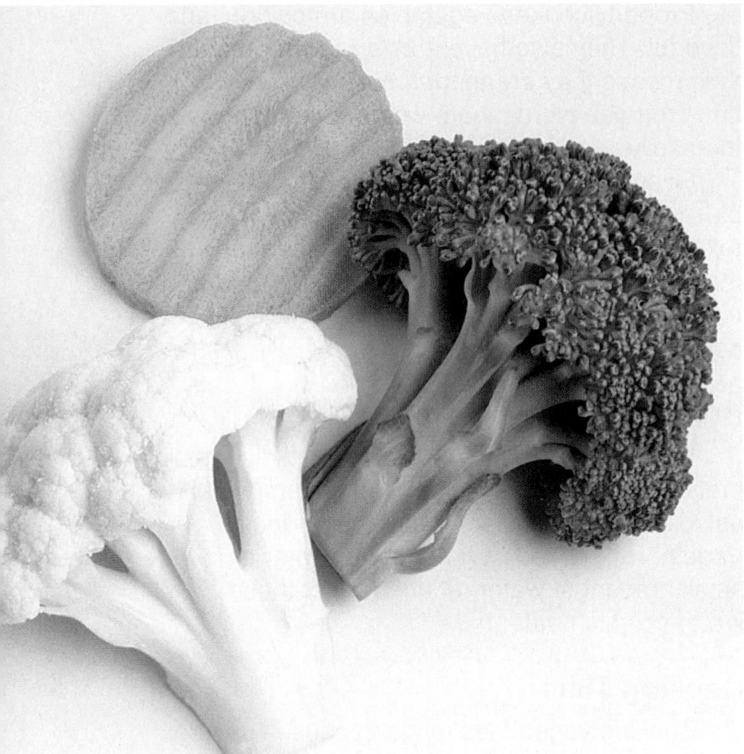

photo courtesy of Mann Packing Co., Inc., Salinas, CA

15-5 The color of vegetables can help you determine the method you should use to cook them.

To keep vegetables green, cook them in a small amount of water. Use a short cooking time and keep the pan lid off for the first few minutes of cooking. Then cover the pan for the remainder of the cooking period.

Yellow vegetables contain ***carotene,*** a source of vitamin A. Carotene gives vegetables a yellow or orange color. Heat does not destroy it. However, if you overcook a yellow vegetable, the cellular structure will break down and release the carotene into the cooking liquid. You should cook most yellow vegetables in a small amount of water with the pan covered.

White vegetables contain pigments called ***flavones.*** Flavones are soluble in water. If you overcook white vegetables, they turn yellow or dark gray. Take care when cooking to avoid these undesirable color changes.

Red vegetables contain a pigment called ***anthocyanin.*** An alkali present in some water can affect this pigment. If the cooking water is alkaline, the red pigment will turn purple. A small amount of vinegar or lemon juice (an acid) added to the water will neutralize the alkali and keep red vegetables red. Cook most red vegetables in a small amount of water, with the pan lid on, just until tender.

Effect of Cooking on Vegetable Flavor

Vegetables can have mild, strong, or very strong flavors. Cooking can affect these flavors. Therefore, you must consider flavors as well as colors when deciding how to prepare a vegetable.

Mildly flavored vegetables include green vegetables, such as peas, green beans, and spinach. Yellow vegetables, such as corn; red vegetables, such as beets; and white vegetables, such as parsnips, also have mild flavors. Cook most mildly flavored vegetables for a short time in a small amount of water with the pan covered.

Q: Won't adding a pinch of baking soda to the cooking water help keep vegetables green?

A: Baking soda is a weak alkali, which will turn chlorophyll a bright green. However, it can also cause a loss of important nutrients. Therefore, adding it to green vegetables is not recommended.

Strongly flavored vegetables, such as cabbage, broccoli, Brussels sprouts, yellow turnips, and rutabagas, are exceptions to general cooking rules. Cover these vegetables with water. Cook them in an uncovered pan for a short time. Following these guidelines will allow some of the strong flavor substances to escape into the water and air.

Very strongly flavored vegetables, such as onions and leeks, should also be covered with water. You should cook them in an uncovered pan for a longer time. As they cook, these vegetables will release strong flavor substances and develop a milder flavor.

Methods of Cooking Vegetables

You can cook vegetables by boiling, steaming, pressure-cooking, baking, frying, stir-frying, broiling, and microwaving. Regardless of the cooking method, vegetables cooked in their skins retain more nutrients. Consider your taste preferences and the other items in your menu when choosing a cooking method. See 15-6.

Cooking Vegetables in Water

Use a pan with a tight-fitting lid when cooking vegetables in water. Add salt to a small amount of water and bring the water to a boil. Add the vegetables, cover, and quickly bring to a boil again. Then reduce the heat and cook the vegetables at a simmering temperature until they are crisp-tender. Drain and serve the vegetables immediately.

After vegetables have cooked, do not throw away the cooking liquid. It contains many valuable nutrients. You can serve a small amount of the cooking liquid with the vegetables in a separate dish. If you do not want to use the liquid right away, freeze it in small amounts. (Ice cube trays work well.) Later, you can add the frozen liquid to sauces, soups, and gravies.

Steaming Vegetables

You can steam young tender vegetables that cook quickly. To steam vegetables, place them in a steaming basket over simmering water. Tightly cover the pan and steam the vegetables until they are tender. You can successfully steam shredded cabbage, broccoli, diced root vegetables, celery, sweet corn, and French-style (thinly sliced) green beans.

Pressure-Cooking Vegetables

To pressure-cook vegetables, follow the directions that accompany the pressure cooker. The pressure in a pressure cooker produces high temperatures, so foods cook quickly. Time vegetables carefully to prevent overcooking.

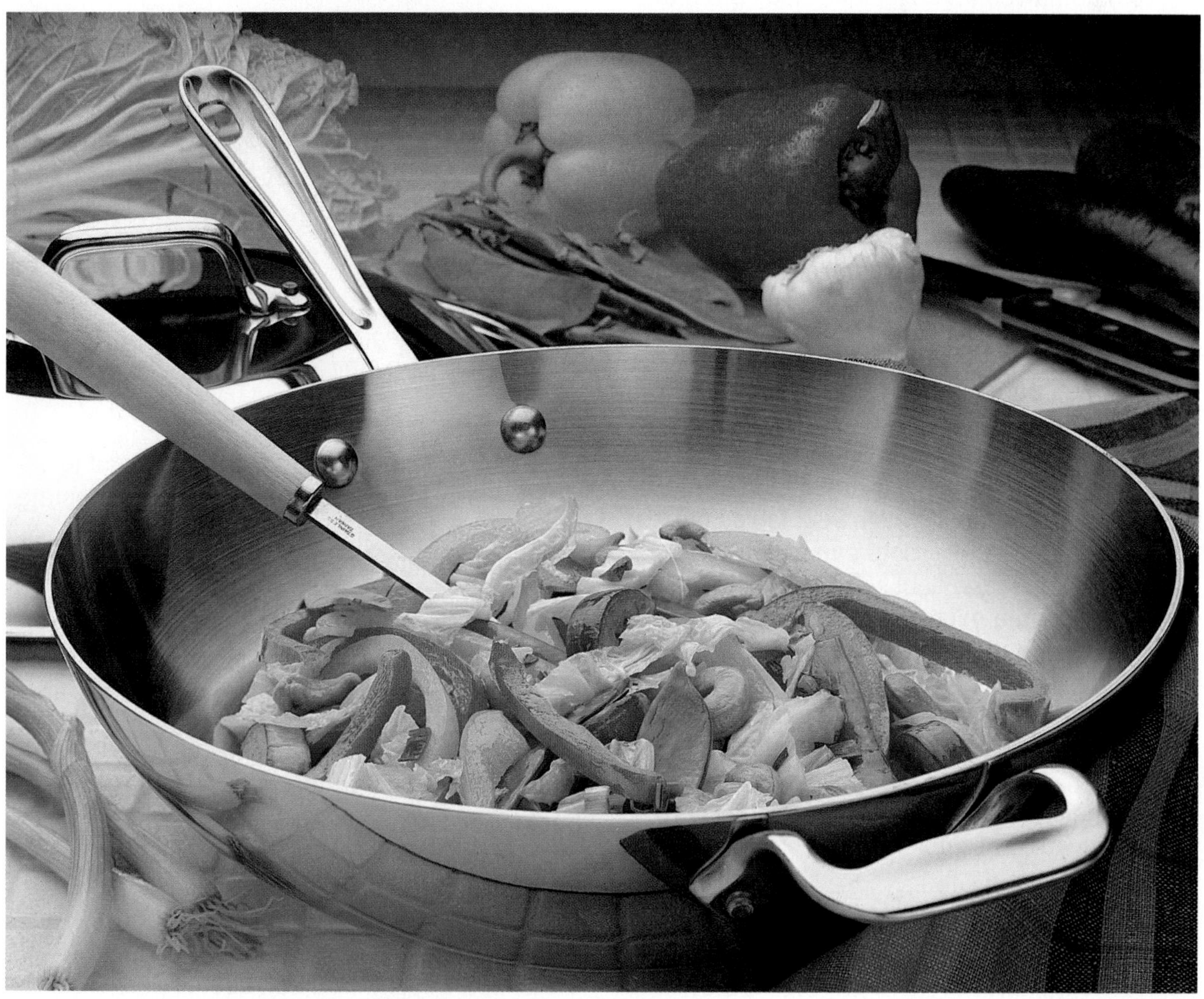

recipe photography courtesy of All-Clad Metalcrafters, Inc.

***15-6** This colorful vegetable stir-fry takes just minutes to cook.*

Baking Vegetables

You can bake vegetables peeled or in their skins. Wrap peeled vegetables in foil or place them in a covered casserole with a small amount of liquid before baking. Potatoes, tomatoes, and onions are popular vegetables for baking. Baking takes longer than other cooking methods.

Frying Vegetables

You can dip vegetables in batter and deep-fry them. You can sauté them in a small amount of fat. Stir-frying works well with vegetables that have a high moisture content.

To stir-fry vegetables, shred them or cut them into small pieces. Place the vegetables in a heavy pan or wok. Use a small amount of oil to help prevent sticking. Place the pan over medium-high heat and stir the vegetables constantly, just until tender.

Broiling Vegetables

Tomato halves and eggplant slices are often broiled. To broil vegetables, brush the cut surfaces with oil or melted fat. Place the vegetables under the broiling unit and broil until tender. Because vegetables cook quickly under the broiler, you must watch them carefully.

Microwaving Vegetables

Vegetables cooked in a microwave oven retain their shapes, colors, flavors, and nutrients. This is due to the short cooking time and the use of little or no cooking liquid. See 15-7.

Use high power to cook vegetables in a microwave oven. Remember to allow standing time for vegetables to finish cooking. Stir vegetable dishes during the cooking period to redistribute heat. Rearrange whole vegetables during the cooking period to ensure even cooking. Vegetables that have tight skins can explode when cooked in a microwave oven. To prevent this, you should pierce their skins in several places before microwaving.

You can prepare frozen vegetables in a microwave oven as easily as fresh vegetables. Slit pouches of vegetables to allow steam to escape. Place vegetables that do not come in pouches in a microwavable casserole for cooking.

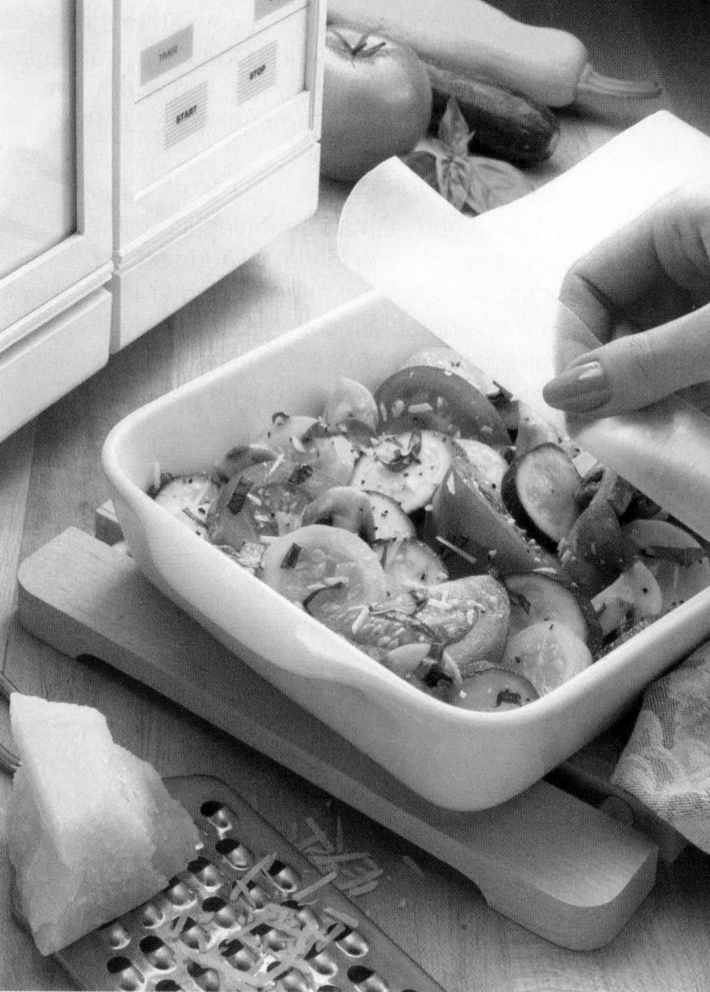

photograph courtesy of The Reynolds Kitchens

15-7 Covering vegetables helps hold in steam and speed cooking in a microwave oven.

Potatoes

Although potatoes are a vegetable, they are treated somewhat differently from other vegetables. The cooking method followed to prepare potatoes depends on the type of potato being used.

Potatoes are classified on the basis of appearance and use. Common varieties are long or round with white skins or round with red skins. They can be all-purpose potatoes, baking potatoes, or new potatoes. (***New potatoes*** are not a variety. They are potatoes that are sent to market immediately after harvesting.)

New potatoes and round red varieties are best for boiling, oven-browning, frying, and making potato salad. This is because these varieties hold their shape when cooked. Baking or russet potatoes are best for baking and mashing. Their mealy texture allows them to break apart easily. You can use all-purpose potatoes for both baking and boiling.

Q: Aren't potatoes fattening?

A: Simply eating potatoes or any other food will not cause you to gain weight. Consuming more total calories than you burn causes weight gain. A medium potato provides only about 100 calories. However, adding high-fat toppings such as butter or mayonnaise can easily double the number of calories potatoes provide. Of course, frying potatoes in fat adds a lot of calories, too.

Preparing Potatoes

Four popular potato preparations are boiling, mashing, frying, and baking. To prepare boiled potatoes, wash, peel, and halve them. Cover the potatoes with lightly salted water and simmer until tender. (You can also cook potatoes in one inch (2.5 cm) of simmering salted water. Check them during cooking to be sure the water has not boiled away. Add more water, if needed.) Drain potatoes and season as desired.

Prepare potatoes for mashing the same as boiled potatoes. Then add butter, milk, and salt and beat the potatoes with an electric mixer or mash them by hand.

French fries, hash browns, and home fries are just a few of the fried potato dishes people enjoy. Some fried potato dishes are made with raw potatoes, and others are made with boiled potatoes. French fries are made by deep-frying raw potato strips. Hash browns are made from shredded cooked potatoes. To prepare home fries, place sliced cooked potatoes in a heavy nonstick skillet with a small amount of melted fat. Season the potatoes with salt and pepper. Cook over low heat until the slices brown on the bottom. Then turn the potatoes to brown the other side.

To prepare baked potatoes, scrub potatoes under cool running water. Pierce potatoes in several places with a fork. This prevents steam from building up inside the skin, which could cause the potato to explode. Bake potatoes in a 400°F (205°C) oven until they are tender, about 40 to 60 minutes. (You can adjust baking time and temperature so potatoes can bake with other foods.) See 15-8.

Preparing Canned, Frozen, and Dried Vegetables

Canned vegetables have already been cooked. Many vegetables suffer changes in color and texture during canning. Therefore, they will look and taste better if you heat them no more than necessary before serving.

To prepare canned vegetables, place the vegetables and the liquid from the can in a saucepan. Cook over low heat until the vegetables are heated through. Add seasonings to taste.

Frozen vegetables have already been blanched (preheated in boiling water or steam for a short time). Blanching reduces the cooking time needed to about half that needed for fresh vegetables.

To prepare frozen vegetables, bring a small amount of salted water to a boil. Add the

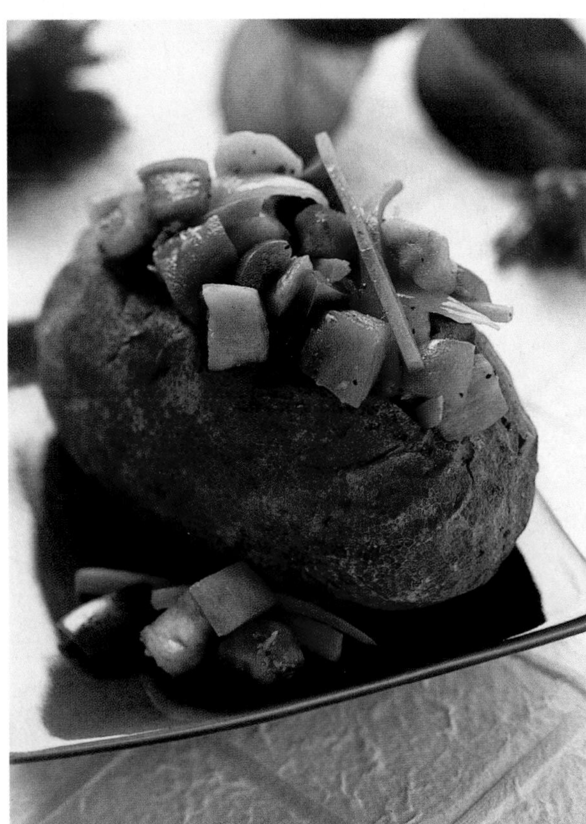

Washington State Potato Commission

***15-8** This colorful vegetable topping turns a plain baked potato side dish into a healthful entree.*

vegetables and cover the saucepan. Quickly bring the water back to a boil. Then reduce the heat and simmer the vegetables until tender. Add seasonings to taste.

Before cooking, rinse and sort dried legumes. Remove any debris that may have been packaged with the vegetables. Dried beans must be soaked before cooking so they will absorb water and cook more evenly. To soak beans, place them in a large pot with plenty of water. Bring the water to a boil for two to three minutes. Cover the pot and remove it from the heat. Allow beans to soak for at least one hour. You should discard the soaking water and use fresh water for cooking. This will help reduce the gas-causing properties of beans. Dried lentils and peas need no soaking. Reconstitute other dried vegetables according to package directions.

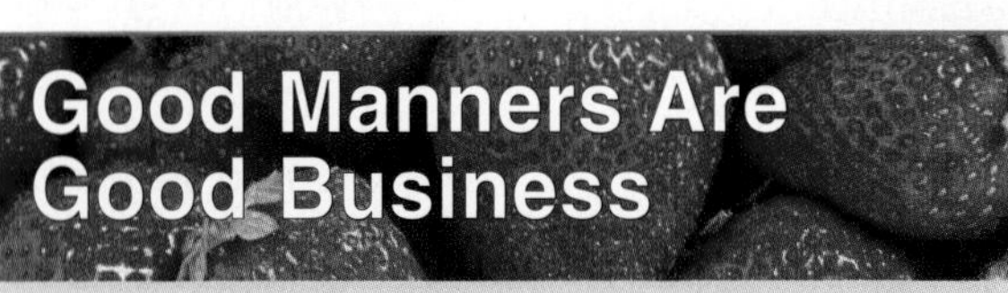

Eating catsup with French fries is acceptable during informal business meals. However, you should not pour catsup over the French fries. Instead, pour a small amount on the side of your plate. Then dip your French fries as you eat them.

This guideline applies to all bottled condiment sauces being used on any food. The exception is that you can pour condiments directly on sandwiches.

Serving Vegetables

You can serve vegetables in many creative and delicious ways. Some people prefer their vegetables served simply, seasoned with herbs or a sprinkling of salt. Others enjoy vegetables topped with crisp onion rings, chopped nuts, crumbled bacon bits, or sliced hard-cooked eggs. With just a little extra effort, you can add variety to a vegetable with a smooth cream sauce or a tasty cheese sauce. Glazes of brown sugar or honey are also popular. See 15-9.

Cottage cheese is a tasty, lowfat alternative to sour cream for topping baked potatoes. Try sprinkling boiled potatoes with chopped parsley. Shape mashed potatoes into patties and brown them in shortening. You can also make them into colcannon by combining them with melted margarine and shredded, cooked cabbage. Brown small whole potatoes around a roast. Serving vegetables in these different ways adds variety to meals.

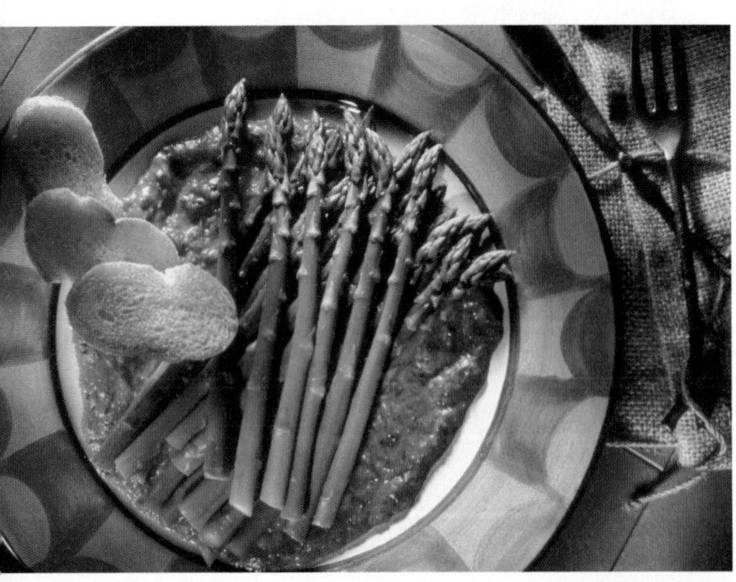

California Asparagus Commission

***15-9** A tangy tomato sauce adds color, flavor, and nutrients to fresh asparagus.*

Chapter 15 Review
Vegetables

Summary

You can group vegetables according to flavor, color, or the part of the plant from which they come. Vegetables are low in fat, high in fiber, and rich in vitamins and minerals. When buying fresh vegetables, choose items that are in their peak growing season to get the best buy. Select medium-sized pieces that have good color and are free from bruises and decay. Store most vegetables in the refrigerator.

Canned, frozen, and dried vegetables can be a good buy when fresh vegetables are not in season. Choose packages that are intact. Store frozen vegetables in the freezer. Keep canned and dried vegetables in a cool, dry place.

To prepare fresh vegetables, begin by washing and trimming them. Cooking affects the pigments in green, yellow, white, and red vegetables. Cook most vegetables for a short time in a small amount of liquid. This will help preserve flavors, textures, colors, and nutrients.

Aside from cooking in liquid, you can steam, pressure-cook, bake, fry, broil, and microwave vegetables. The method you choose will depend on your taste preferences. Canned and frozen vegetables cook more quickly than fresh vegetables. Dried vegetables often require soaking before cooking.

Review What You Have Read

Write your answers on a separate sheet of paper.

1. List the eight parts of plants used as vegetable classifications. Give an example of a vegetable from each group.
2. List three guidelines to follow when shopping for fresh vegetables.
3. What form of vegetables best retains the flavor and appearance of fresh vegetables?
4. What vegetables are most commonly purchased in dried form?
5. Why is it important to wash fresh vegetables? How should you wash them?
6. List three changes that take place in vegetables when you cook them.
7. The pigments in white vegetables are called _____.
   A. anthocyanins
   B. carotenes
   C. chlorophylls
   D. flavones
8. List the three flavor categories of vegetables and give cooking guidelines for each.
9. List four methods for cooking vegetables. Describe two.
10. How can vegetable cooking liquid be used?
11. What type of potato is the best choice when making mashed potatoes?
12. True or false. Canned vegetables have already been cooked.

Build Your Basic Skills

1. **Math.** Compare the unit cost of a vegetable in fresh, frozen, and canned form.
2. **Science.** Cook red cabbage in water made alkaline with baking soda and in water made acidic with vinegar. Compare color.

Build Your Thinking Skills

1. **Evaluate.** Evaluate the flavor, color, and texture of equal amounts of green beans prepared in each of the following ways:
   A. in a small amount of water for a short time with the pan covered
   B. in a small amount of water for a short time with the pan uncovered for the first few minutes of cooking
   C. in a large amount of water for a long time with the pan covered
   D. in a small amount of water for a short time with baking soda added and the pan covered
2. **Compare.** Prepare two portions of small, whole onions. Use a small amount of water and a covered pan for one portion. Use a large amount of water and an uncovered pan for the other portion. Compare flavor and aroma.

Apply Technology

1. Investigate the use of biotechnology in the development of the Flavr Savr tomato.
2. Slice and/or chop vegetables using a food processor. Compare the appliance with a knife in terms of speed and ease of performance.

Using Workplace Skills

Yoshi is a botanist who works for The Green Thumb, a seed catalog company familiar to many home gardeners. Yoshi is working to develop a strain of green beans that has a longer growing season and better keeping quality. He needs to keep detailed records of his procedures and observations. When Yoshi successfully develops the new strain, The Green Thumb will duplicate his work. They will offer seeds for the beans in their catalog.

To be a successful employee, Yoshi needs basic writing skills. Put yourself in Yoshi's place and answer the following questions about your need for and use of these skills:

A. How would having basic writing skills help you when you get to work each day?
B. How would your company's ability to duplicate your results be affected if you do not have adequate writing skills?
C. How would your writing skills affect home gardeners?
D. What is another skill you would need in this job? Briefly explain why this skill would be important.

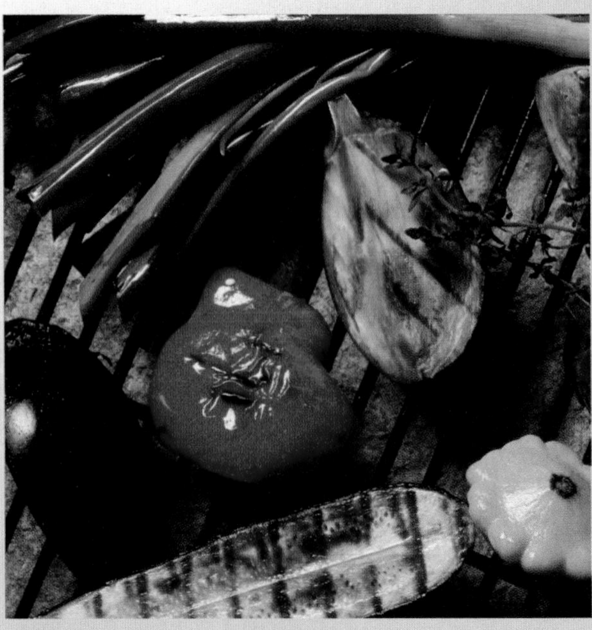

Chapter 16
Fruits

Extractor-Machine Operator
Tends machines that extract juice from citrus fruit.

Produce Broker
Sells bulk shipments of produce to wholesalers and other buyers for growers and shippers on a commission basis.

Grove Supervisor
Supervises and coordinates activities of workers engaged in cultivating, pruning, spraying, thinning, propping, and harvesting tree crops, such as apples, lemons, oranges, and peaches.

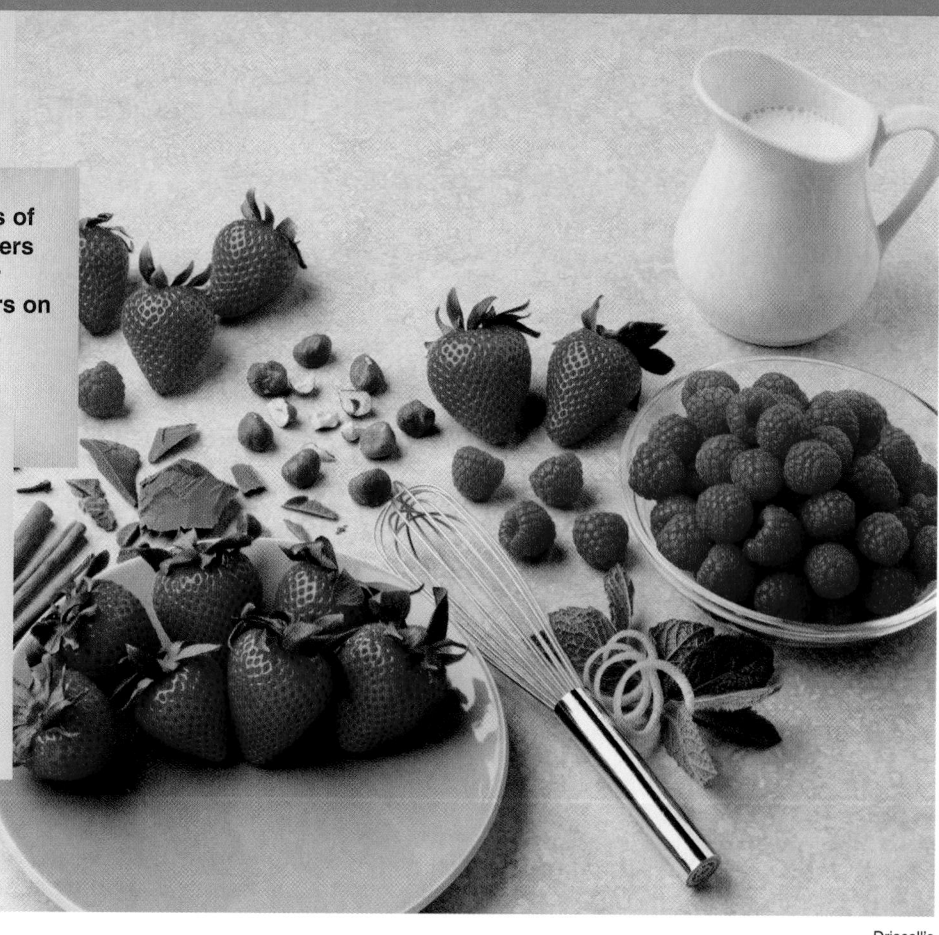

Driscoll's

Terms to Know

berries
drupes
pomes
citrus fruits
melons
tropical fruits
underripe fruit
immature fruit
enzymatic browning
fritters

Objectives

After studying this chapter, you will be able to

- describe how to properly select and store fruits.
- identify the principles and methods of cooking fruit.
- prepare fruits, preserving their colors, textures, flavors, and nutrients.

Fresh, canned, frozen, and dried fruits add flavor, color, and texture contrasts to meals. They are generally nutritious and low in calories, so they are good choices for desserts and snacks.

You can eat fruits raw or cooked. For example, you could pack an apple in a school lunch and eat it plain. You could also use it to make applesauce or a pie. You might toss fresh blueberries into a fruit cup. You could sprinkle them on breakfast cereal or bake them into a cobbler, too.

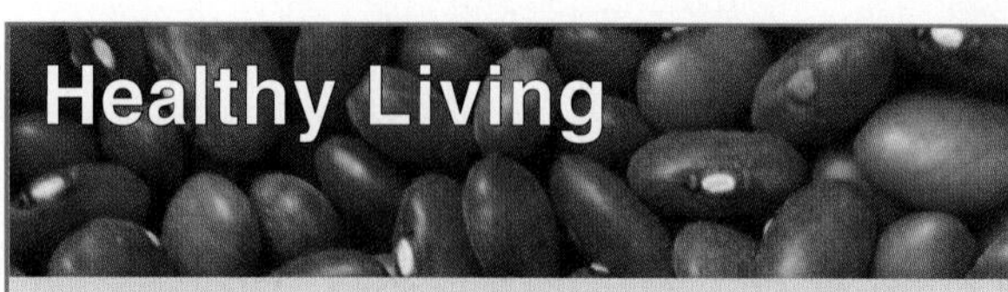

Do not forget tropical fruits for a nutritious change of pace. One-half cup (125 mL) guava has more than twice the vitamin C of a medium orange. A serving of mango beats apricots for vitamin A value.

Choosing Fresh Fruit

Many varieties of fresh fruit are available year-round. Others are available for only a short time. Knowing how to recognize high-quality fresh fruit will help you be a smart consumer.

Fruit Classifications

Fruits can be divided into groups according to physical characteristics. ***Berries*** are small, juicy fruits with thin skins. Blackberries, cranberries, blueberries, red and black raspberries, gooseberries, and strawberries all belong to the berry family. Grapes and currants are also berries. Except for cranberries, all berries are highly perishable.

Drupes have an outer skin covering a soft, fleshy fruit. The fruit surrounds a single, hard seed, which is called a *stone* or *pit.* Cherries, apricots, nectarines, peaches, and plums are all drupes.

Pomes have a central, seed-containing core surrounded by a thick layer of flesh. Apples and pears are pomes.

Citrus fruits have a thick outer rind. A thin membrane separates the flesh into segments. Oranges, tangerines, tangelos, grapefruits, kumquats, lemons, and limes are citrus fruits.

Melons are large, juicy fruits with thick rinds and many seeds. They are in the gourd family and include cantaloupe, casaba, honeydew, crenshaw, Persian, and watermelon.

Tropical fruits are grown in warm climates and are considered to be somewhat exotic. Many species of tropical fruits are available throughout the world. Those most commonly available in the United States are avocados, bananas, figs, dates, guavas, mangoes, papayas, persimmons, pineapples, pomegranates, and kiwifruit. See 16-1.

Nutritional Value of Fruit

According to the Food Guide Pyramid, you should eat two to four servings of fruits each day. A serving is one medium-sized piece of raw fruit. One-half cup (125 mL) chopped, cooked, or canned fruit or ¾ cup (175 mL) fruit juice is also a serving.

Most fruits are high in vitamins and low in fat. (Avocados are a high-fat exception.) Fruits are rich in phytochemicals and provide a good source of fiber.

The citrus fruits are one of the best sources of vitamin C. Oranges usually give the largest amount of vitamin C for the money spent. Cantaloupes and strawberries are also good sources of this important vitamin.

Cantaloupe, apricots, and other deep yellow fruits are good sources of vitamin A because they contain large amounts of carotene. Oranges, strawberries, cantaloupe, and dried fruits are sources of calcium.

Q: Isn't eating grapefruit supposed to help you burn calories?

A: Sorry to say, neither grapefruit nor any other food can speed the burning of calories from the foods you eat. However, grapefruit is a low-calorie, fat free food that is high in vitamin C. It can easily fit into any eating plan.

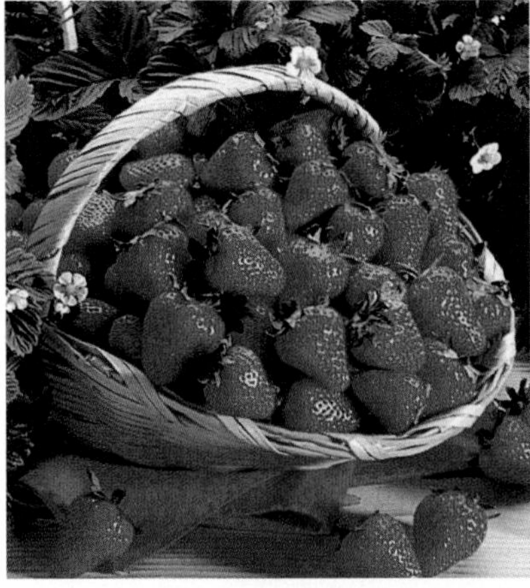
California Strawberry Commission
berries

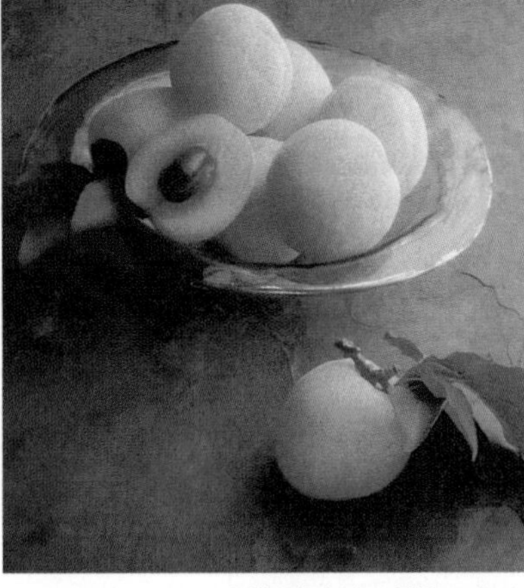
California Apricot Advisory Board
drupes

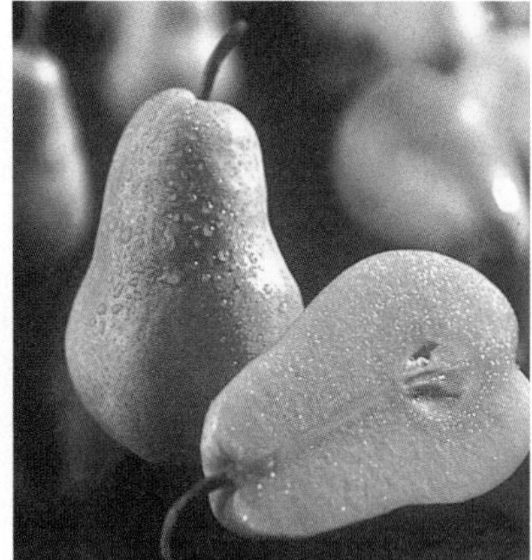
California Tree Fruit Agreement
pomes

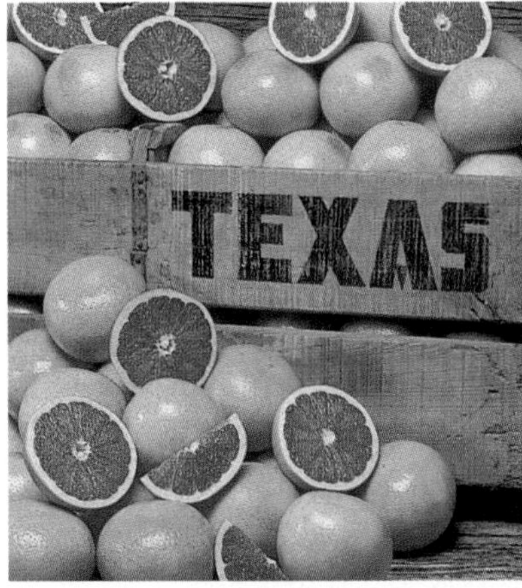

TexaSweet Citrus Marketing, Inc.
citrus fruits

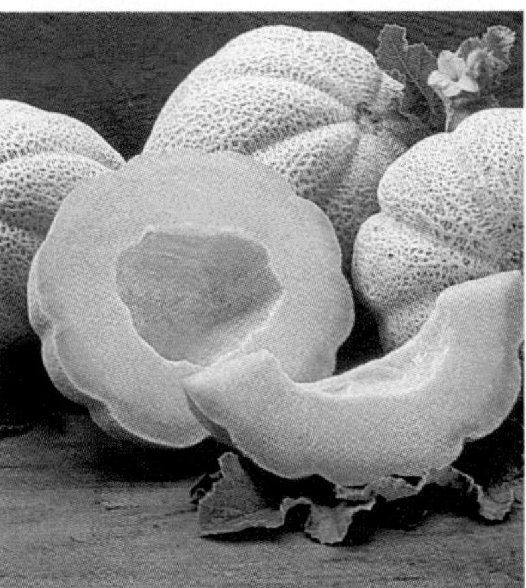
courtesy of W. Atlee Burpee & Co.
melons

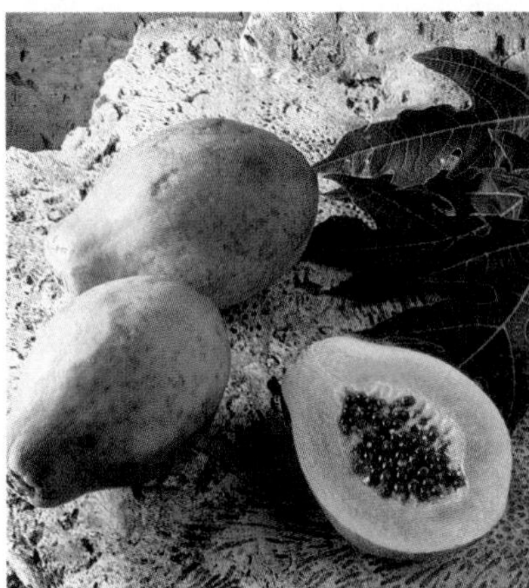
Brooks Tropicals
tropical fruits

***16-1** Fruits are divided into groups by physical characteristics.*

Selecting Fresh Fruit

You can buy some fruits, such as apples, oranges, and grapefruit, in plastic mesh or film bags. You can also buy fruits on cellophane covered trays or loose, as individual pieces.

Ripeness will help you judge the quality of fresh fruits. Ripe fruits are those that have reached top eating quality. Test fruit for ripeness by pressing it gently to see if it gives slightly. ***Underripe fruits*** are fruits that are full-sized but have not yet reached peak eating quality. You can buy some fruits, such as pears and bananas, underripe because they will ripen at room temperature at home.

Color and fragrance are guides to ripeness. Most fruits lose their green color as they ripen. For instance, peaches turn from green to deep yellow. Pineapples and melons have a characteristic fragrance when ripe.

Maturity is another factor that will help you judge the quality of fresh fruits. Do not confuse underripe fruits with immature fruits. ***Immature fruits*** have not reached full size. They are small and have poor color, flavor, and texture. They will not improve in quality when left at room temperature.

When buying fresh fruit

- Buy just what you can use in a short time.
- Look for signs of freshness and ripeness.
- Avoid bruised, soft, damaged, or immature fruits. See 16-2.
- Consider your needs. For instance, use smaller, blemished apples for stewing and pies. Use fancy apples for fruit trays and other dishes in which appearance is important.

How to Buy Fresh Fruits		
Fruit	**Choose**	**Avoid**
Apples	Firm texture, bright color, mature fruit	Immaturity, overripeness, bruises, shriveled skin
Apricots	Uniform color; plump, juicy fruit that yields to slight pressure	Soft, mushy fruit (overripe); pale, greenish-yellow fruit (underripe)
Avocados	Slightly soft fruit that yields to gentle pressure	Dark, sunken spots; cracked or broken surface
Bananas	Firm, bright color	Fruit that is bruised or discolored, dull skin, defects
Blueberries	Dark blue color with silvery bloom, plump fruit, dry skins	Shriveled and discolored skin; brown, soft flesh; defects
Cherries	Bright color; plump, firm fruit	Soft, spongy, shriveled, or discolored fruit
Grapefruit	Well-shaped, firm fruit; heavy for size	Soft, discolored areas
Grapes	Bright color, plump fruit that is firmly attached to stem	Soft, wrinkled, or leaking fruit
Lemons	Bright color, smooth skin, heavy weight for size	Dull color, shriveled skin, soft spots
Limes	Glossy skin, heavy weight for size	Dull, dry skin; soft spots
Melons		
Cantaloupe and Persian	Stemless, thick veining, yellowish rind, pleasant aroma	Soft spots, bright yellow rind
Honeydew	Faint, pleasant aroma; pale yellow to creamy colored rind; slight softening at blossom end	Dead white or greenish colored rind, overly hard fruit, soft areas
Watermelon	Smooth outer surface, rounded ends, bright flesh that is firm and juicy	Pale colored flesh, dry or watery flesh
Oranges	Bright color, heavy weight for size	Light weight for size; dry, dull skin; soft spots
Peaches	Flesh that is still slightly firm or becoming soft, creamy ground color between red areas	Very firm flesh, greenish skin, soft bruised spots
Pears	Firm flesh, characteristic color for variety	Very hard flesh, immature fruit, soft or bruised spots
Pineapples	Pleasant aroma; slight separation of eyes; yellowish-orange color; plump, firm fruit, heavy weight for size	Dry, dull, yellowish-green skin; bruises; soft spots; unpleasant odor
Plums	Fairly firm to slightly soft flesh; good color for variety	Overly hard or soft flesh, brown or shriveled areas
Raspberries and blackberries	Bright, uniform color; plump, tender cells	Hard fruit; irregular color; soft, leaky fruit
Strawberries	Bright red, firm flesh; dry, clean exteriors; attached caps	Pale, soft, or moldy spots; excessive seeds
Tangerines	Deep yellow-orange color, bright luster	Pale, green skin; soft or cut spots

16-2 Each fruit has its own ripeness indicators. Choose fruits that are ripe and high in quality.

Storing Fresh Fruit

Handle all fruits gently to prevent bruising. Let underripe fruits ripen at room temperature and refrigerate ripe fruits. Store strong-smelling fruits in plastic bags or airtight containers. Store other fruits uncovered in a crisper.

You should use berries, melons, grapes, and fruits with pits as soon as possible. You can store apples, pears, and citrus fruits longer, but they too will lose quality after prolonged storage. You can refrigerate bananas for a short time after they have ripened at room temperature. The cold temperature may darken banana skins, but the flavor and texture of the fruit will be unharmed.

Be a Clever Consumer

Fresh fruits are usually least expensive during their peak growing season. They are also at their best quality during this time. Peak season is a good time to buy large quantities of fruit and preserve it for future use.

Choosing Canned, Frozen, and Dried Fruit

You can buy fruit canned, frozen, and dried as well as fresh. Fruits are picked at their peak of quality and then preserved so you can enjoy them all year long.

Canned Fruit

Canned fruits can be whole, halved, sliced, or in pieces. They come packed in juices or in light or heavy syrup. Fruit juices are lower in calories and higher in nutrients than syrups used as packing liquids.

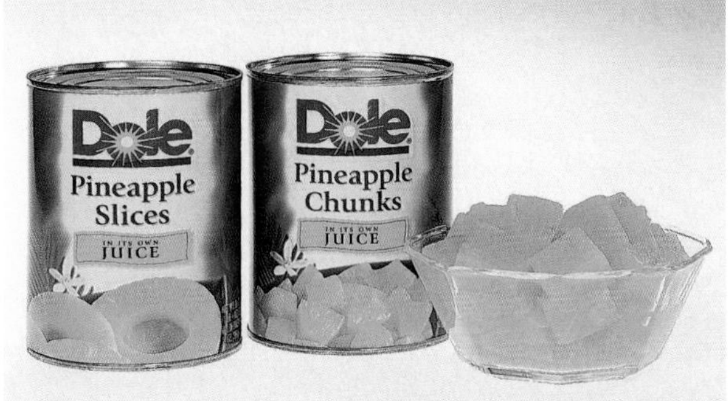

Dole Food Company

16-3 For wholesomeness and quality, avoid dented cans when buying canned fruits.

Canned fruits are packed in cans or jars. You can avoid waste by purchasing the container size that meets your needs.

Buying and Storing Canned Fruits

Canned fruits are usually less expensive than frozen or fresh fruits. Costs vary depending on brand, can size, quality, and packing liquid. To receive the greatest economy from your dollar, choose house brands. Generic products also cost less. They are suitable in fruit dishes where appearance is not important.

Q: Why does fresh fruit have stickers on it in the grocery store?

A: The stickers have numbers on them that help grocery store checkers tell which variety of fruit they are ringing up.

When buying canned fruits, choose cans that are free from dents, bulges, and leaks. Choose jars that are free from cracks and chips. Choose the quality that fits your intended use. Store all cans and jars in a cool, dry place. Cover the fruit after opening and store it in the refrigerator. See 16-3.

Frozen Fruit

Frozen fruits are available sweetened and unsweetened; whole and in pieces. Most frozen fruits come in plastic bags or plastic-coated paper cartons.

Frozen fruits resemble fresh fruits in color and flavor. They may, however, lose some texture qualities during freezing.

Buying and Storing Frozen Fruits

The most common frozen fruits are not available in fresh form year-round. When fresh fruits are out of season, frozen fruits are often less expensive than fresh. However, prices of frozen fruits vary according to brand, packaging, size of container, and added ingredients, such as spices and sweeteners. Be sure to compare prices, especially if the fruit you are buying is in its peak growing season.

When buying frozen fruits, choose packages that are clean, undamaged, and frozen solid. Store in the coldest part of the freezer. After thawing, store the unused portion in a tightly covered container in the refrigerator. Use as soon as possible. Never refreeze.

Dried Fruits

Raisins, prunes, dried plums, and apricots are the most common dried fruits. Dried apples, peaches, pears, figs, pineapple, bananas, and papayas are also available.

Dried fruits usually come in boxes or plastic bags. Sometimes they are loose, so you can buy any quantity you want. Size generally determines the price of dried apples, apricots, and plums. Larger fruits cost more than smaller fruits.

Buying and Storing Dried Fruits

Choose dried fruits that are fairly soft and pliable. Store unopened packages and boxes in a cool, dark, dry place. After opening, store unused portions in tightly covered containers. Some package labels recommend storing opened dried fruits in the refrigerator for best keeping quality.

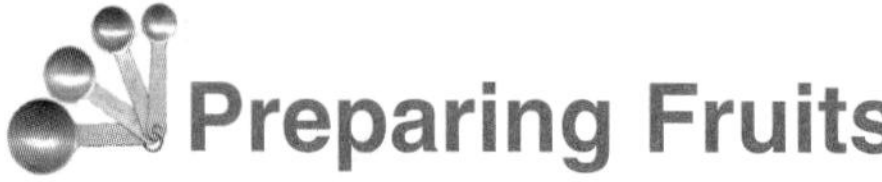

Preparing Fruits

You can serve fruits in a variety of ways to add interest to meals and snacks. You can use them raw or cooked, fresh or preserved. Carefully following preparation techniques will help you maintain fruits' appealing flavors, colors, textures, and shapes.

Preparing Raw Fruits

Raw fruits are delicious when eaten out-of-hand. You can also combine them with other foods in appetizers, salads, and desserts, 16-4.

To prepare raw fruits for eating, wash them carefully under cool running water. You should even wash fruits such as oranges and melons before peeling or removing rinds. Washing removes any soil or sand and many pesticide residues that may be present. Never let fruits soak, as this may cause them to lose flavor and some of their water-soluble nutrients.

Serve raw fruits whole or sliced. Some fruits, such as bananas and peaches, darken when exposed to the air. This is called ***enzymatic browning.*** Dipping these fruits in lemon, orange, grapefruit, or pineapple juice will prevent enzymatic browning and make them look more appealing.

Use a sharp, thin-bladed knife when peeling raw fruit. Peel as thinly as possible to preserve nutrients found just under the skin.

Food Science Principles of Cooking Fruit

People cook some fruits, like rhubarb, to make them more palatable and easier to digest. They cook other fruits, like pears, to give variety to a menu. Cooking allows you to use overripe fruits that are past prime eating quality. For instance, you can use apples that are becoming overripe to make applesauce.

During cooking, several changes take place within fruit. Cellulose softens and makes fruit

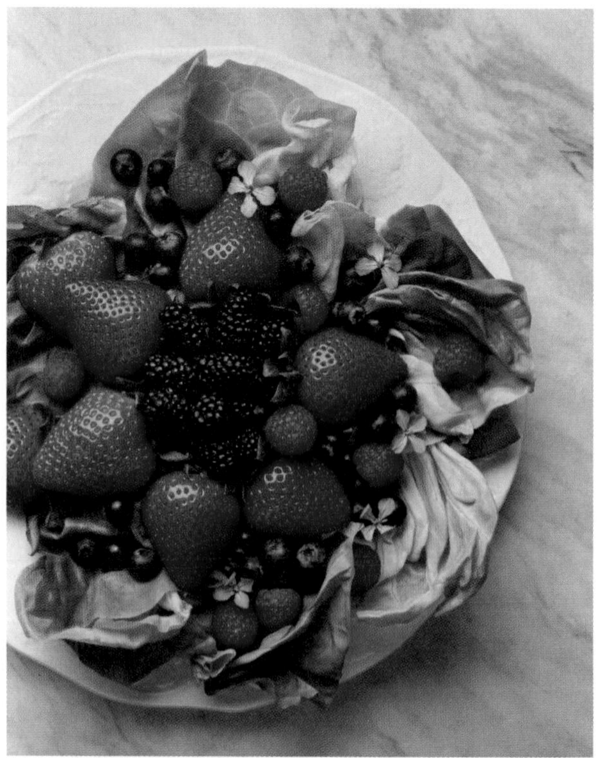

Driscoll's

16-4 *A fresh fruit salad adds color and texture variety to a meal.*

Q: Is it okay to eat fruit and other high-carbohydrate foods at the same meal with meat and other high-protein foods?

A: Yes. The digestive system is wonderfully designed to handle the breakdown of all the nutrients a meal contains.

easier to digest. Colors change. Heat-sensitive and water-soluble nutrients may be lost. Flavors become less acidic and more mellow.

Overcooked fruits become mushy. They lose their colors, nutrients, natural flavors, and shapes. Correctly cooked fruits can retain these characteristics.

Fruits that undergo enzymatic browning will retain their colors if cooked with a small amount of lemon or orange juice. Water-soluble nutrients will be retained if you cook the fruit in a small amount of water just until tender. Natural flavors will be retained if you do not overcook the fruit. Shapes will be retained if you cook the fruit in a sugar syrup instead of plain water.

Sometimes you will want a fruit to retain its shape; other times you will not. For instance, if you are poaching apple slices for a garnish, you will want the slices to retain their shape. If you are making applesauce, however, you will want the apples to lose their shape and form a smooth pulp.

Methods of Cooking Fruit

You can prepare fruits by cooking them in liquid. You might also choose to bake, broil, fry, or microwave fruits.

Cooking Fruit in Liquid

You can use water or sugar syrup when cooking fruits in liquid. Fruits cooked in sugar syrup will retain their shape. Those cooked in water will not. How you intend to use the fruit will determine the cooking method. See 16-5.

When you cook fruits in syrup, use a two-to-one ratio of water to sugar. (Too much sugar will cause the fruit to harden.) Use a low temperature and cook the fruit just until it is tender and translucent. Serve cooked fruit warm or chilled.

When you cook fruits in water, use as little water as possible. Cook the fruit over low heat until tender, then add sugar as your recipe directs. When you add sugar at the end of cooking, it will thin a fruit sauce. Thus, the amount of cooking water used must be small so the sauce will not be too thin. For a smoother sauce, force the cooked fruit through a sieve or run it through a food mill. Serve cooked fruit pulp warm or chilled.

Baking Fruit

You can bake apples, pears, and bananas. Baked fruits should be tender, but they should keep their shape. If you bake a fruit in its skin, the skin will hold in the steam that forms during baking. This steam cooks the interior of the fruit. If you skin the fruit before baking, a covered casserole dish will serve the same purpose as the skin. Bake fruits in a small amount of liquid just until they are tender.

Broiling Fruit

Bananas, grapefruit halves, and pineapple slices often are broiled. Sprinkle these fruits with brown sugar or drizzle them with honey before broiling. Fruits broil quickly, so watch them carefully to prevent overcooking.

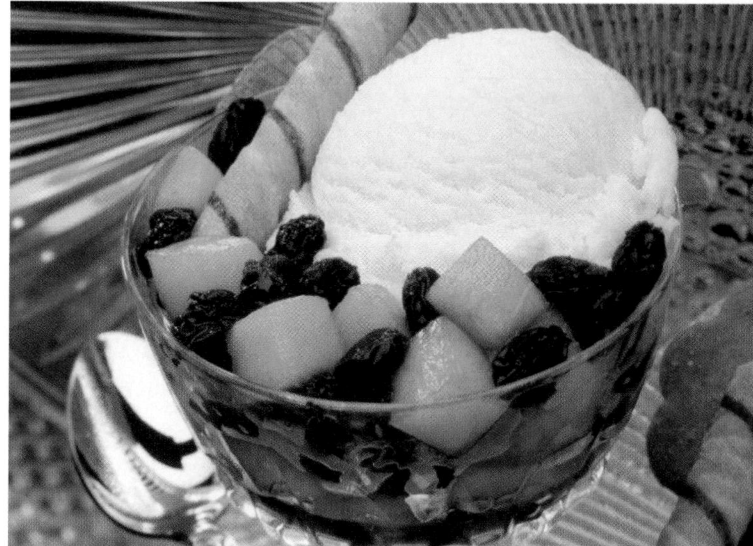

California Raisin Marketing Board

***16-5** The mango chunks in this fruit sauce kept their shape because they were cooked in sugar syrup.*

Frying

You can fry some fruits in a small amount of fat in a skillet. This is called *sauteing.* You can also dip fruits into a batter and deep-fry them. These deep-fried fruits are called ***fritters.*** All fried fruits should be tender, but they should retain their shape.

Good Manners Are Good Business

Business travelers often find themselves entertaining clients in hotel restaurants, where fresh fruits frequently appear on breakfast and lunch buffets. Knowing the proper way to eat fresh fruits will help you make a good impression in business settings. Peel a banana and set the skin aside on your plate. Break off pieces of the banana with your fingers to eat it. You can also cut bananas with a knife and fork. Use your fingers to pick up fresh strawberries by the hulls. Discreetly remove fruit seeds from your mouth between your thumb and forefinger and place them on your plate.

Microwaving Fruit

Fruits cooked in a microwave oven maintain their flavors and nutrients because they cook quickly using little or no water. When microwaving several pieces of fruit, choose pieces of similar size to ensure even cooking. Pierce fruits covered with a tight skin if you are microwaving them whole.

When microwaving fruit, the type of fruit, its size, and its ripeness will affect cooking time. Fruits with a higher moisture content, such as strawberries, will cook more quickly than dense fruits, like rhubarb. Berries and other small pieces of fruit will cook more quickly than larger pieces like apples. Ripe fruit requires less cooking time than firmer, underripe fruit.

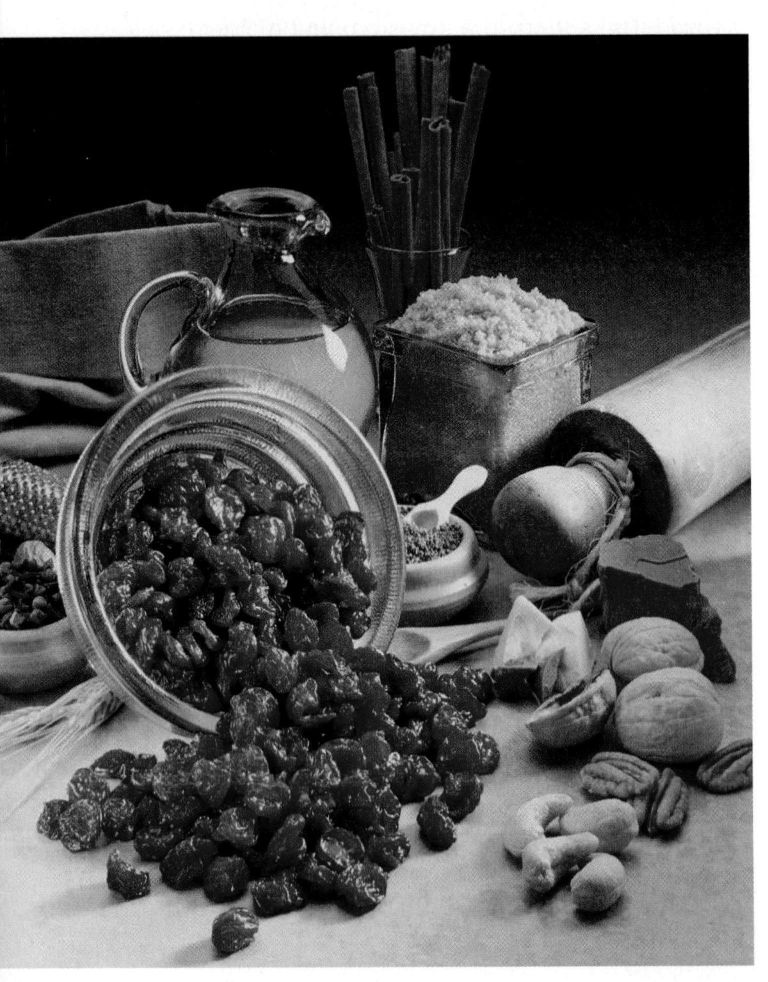

Cherry Marketing Institute

16-6 *Dried tart cherries add a tangy sweetness and a moist, chewy texture to baked goods.*

Preparing Preserved Fruits

You can serve canned fruits right from the can. You may drain them or serve them in the syrup or juice in which they were packed. You can use canned fruits like fresh or frozen fruits. Unless a recipe tells you otherwise, drain canned fruits well before using them in baked products.

Use frozen fruits in the same ways you use fresh and canned fruits. Completely thawing frozen fruits causes them to become soft and mushy. Therefore, serve frozen fruits with a few ice crystals remaining in them.

You can use dried fruits for cooking or baking or eat them right from the package. Before cooking, soak dried fruits in hot water for about an hour. Soaking helps restore the moisture removed during the drying process. Cooking softens the fruit tissues. Because dried fruits vary in moisture content, follow package directions. See 16-6.

Chapter 16 Review
Fruits

Summary

You can group fruits into six basic classifications. No matter what class they are in, however, fruits are high in nutrition. Choose fresh fruits that are mature, ripe, and high in quality. You should store fresh fruits promptly in the refrigerator.

You might choose canned, frozen, and dried fruits when their fresh counterparts are not available. Look for undented cans and solidly frozen packages. Store canned and dried fruits in a cool, dry place. Store frozen fruits in the freezer until you are ready to serve them.

Wash fresh fruits and cut them as desired for serving raw. If necessary, treat cut fruits to prevent enzymatic browning.

Cooking fruits affects their textures, colors, flavors, and nutrients. You can cook fruit in liquid. You can also bake, broil, fry, or microwave it.

You can serve canned fruits right from the can or drain them to use in recipes. Serve frozen fruits with a few ice crystals on them. Eat dried fruits straight from the package or soak them and cook them.

Review What You Have Read

Write your answers on a separate sheet of paper.

1. List the six fruit families and give one example of each.
2. The citrus fruits are one of the best dietary sources of _____.
   A. vitamin A
   B. the B vitamins
   C. vitamin C
   D. calcium
3. Explain the difference between underripe and immature fruit.
4. Give three guidelines for buying fresh fruit.
5. When are fresh fruits usually least expensive?
6. What types of liquids are canned fruits packed in?
7. What should someone look for when buying frozen fruits?
8. How should unused portions of dried fruits be stored?
9. Some fruits darken when they are exposed to air. This is called _____.
10. Describe three changes that take place in fruit during cooking.
11. True or false. Fruits will retain their shape if they are cooked in syrup instead of water.
12. Fruits that are dipped in batter and deep-fried are called _____.
13. List three factors that will affect the microwave cooking time of fruit.
14. What is the general guideline for using canned fruits in baked products?

Build Your Basic Skills

1. **Verbal.** Visit the produce section of a grocery store. Note the different varieties of the same fruit in terms of shape, size, and color. Use visual aids to give a presentation of your findings to the class.
2. **Science.** Slice a banana. Place half the slices on a plate and set aside. Dip the remaining slices in lemon juice, place on a plate, and set aside. Compare slices 30 minutes later.

Build Your Thinking Skills

1. **Design.** Sample and compare one type of fruit in all its available forms. For instance, compare fresh peaches with canned peaches, frozen peaches, and dried peaches. Design a chart describing the differences in flavors, textures, and colors and suggesting ways to serve each form.
2. **Contrast.** Slice an apple into rings. Cook half the slices in sugar syrup and the other half in plain water until tender. Contrast the appearance, texture, and flavor of the two sets of apple rings.

Apply Technology

1. Choose a specific fruit. Then use the Internet to research where and how your selected fruit is grown and harvested. Make printouts from any Web sites that provide worthwhile information.
2. Use a computer and the table function of word processing software to make a table listing 10 popular fruits. Columns of the table should identify how many calories and how much vitamin A, vitamin C, and calcium a serving of each fruit provides. Sort the table in ascending order according to the number of calories per serving and make a printout. Then resort the table in descending order according to the amounts of each of the nutrients and make printouts.

Using Workplace Skills

Margery is a produce broker for citrus growers in Texas. She sells large shipments of oranges and grapefruit to fruit wholesalers throughout the country. Margery is authorized to offer various discounts depending on how much a wholesaler buys. Her computer figures exact discounts when it prints invoices. However, Margery's customers frequently ask her to give them quick estimates of costs when they call to place orders.

To be a successful employee, Margery needs basic math skills. Put yourself in Margery's place and answer the following questions about your need for and use of these skills:

A. What are three specific math skills you would use as a produce broker? Give an example of how you would use each skill.
B. How might wholesalers react if your estimates are too high?
C. How might wholesalers react if your estimates are significantly lower than the amounts shown on their invoices?
D. What is another skill you would need in this job? Briefly explain why this skill would be important.

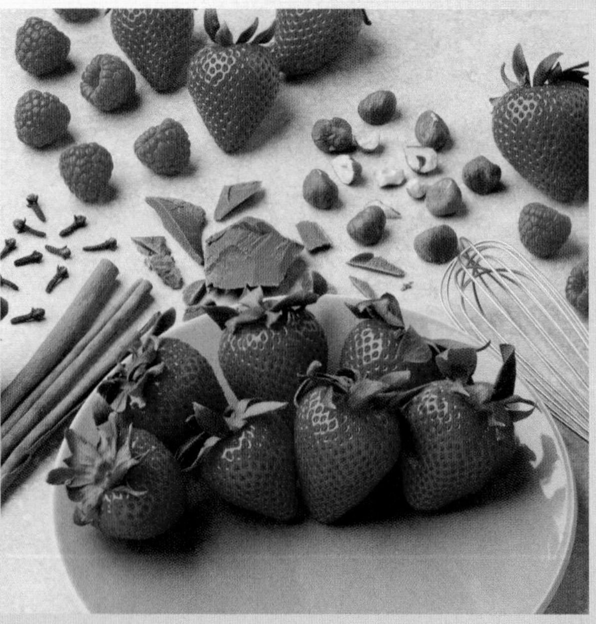

Chapter 17
Dairy Products

Cheese Blender
Prepares charts of quantities, grades, and types of cheese required for blending to make cheese products.

Ice Cream Chef
Mixes, cooks, and freezes ingredients to make frozen desserts, such as sherbets, ice cream, and custards.

Dairy Farm Supervisor
Supervises and coordinates activities of workers engaged in milking, breeding, and caring for cows, and performs lay-veterinary duties on dairy farm.

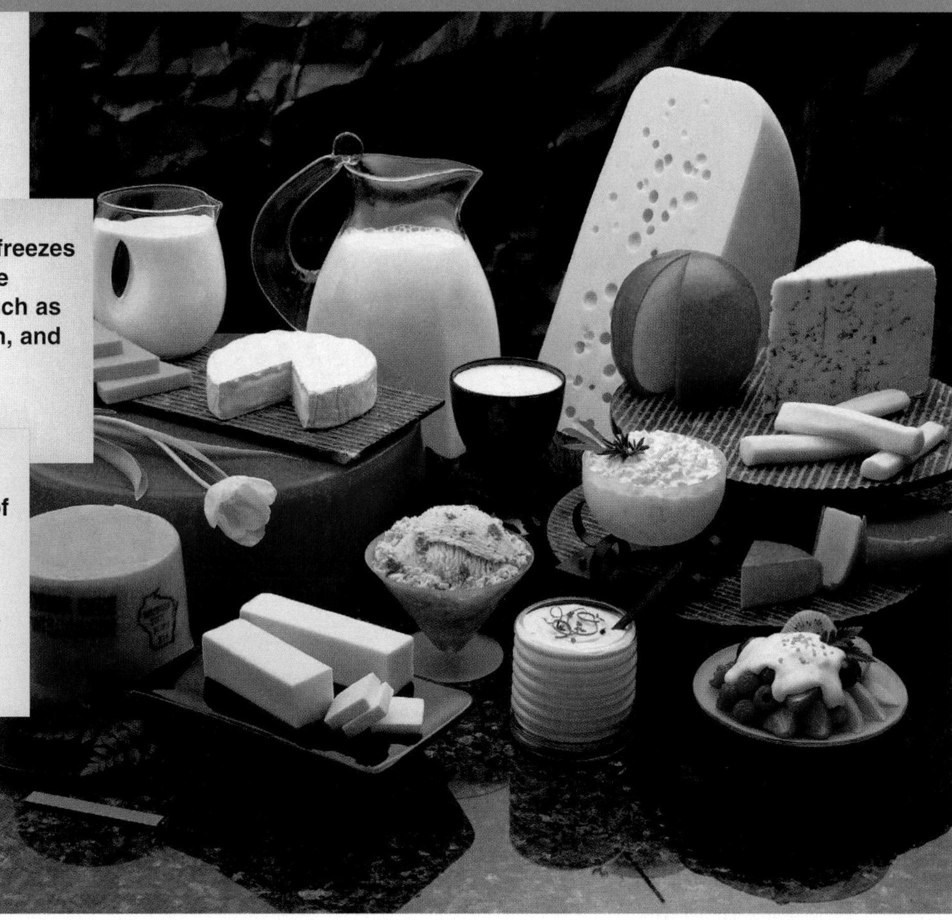

®2002 Wisconsin Milk Marketing Board, Inc.

Terms to Know

pasteurization
ultra-high temperature (UHT) processing
homogenization
milkfat
milk solids
curd
whey
unripened cheese
ripened cheese
process cheese
scum
scorching
curdling
white sauce
roux
slurry
bisque
chowder
gelatin
gelatin cream
hydrate

Objectives

After studying this chapter, you will be able to

- ❑ list factors affecting the selection of dairy products.
- ❑ describe guidelines for preventing adverse reactions when cooking with dairy products.
- ❑ prepare a variety of dishes using milk, cream, cheese, and other dairy products.

Dairy products make up the milk, yogurt, and cheese group of the Food Guide Pyramid. These dairy foods are essential for good health. Teens and older adults should include three servings in their diets each day. People in other age groups should consume two servings daily. Dairy foods are your major source of calcium. They also contain high-quality protein, phosphorous, riboflavin, and vitamins A and D.

Cream, sour cream, ice cream, sherbet, and butter are also dairy products. However, calorie for calorie, they are higher in fat and lower in other nutrients than milk, yogurt, and cheese.

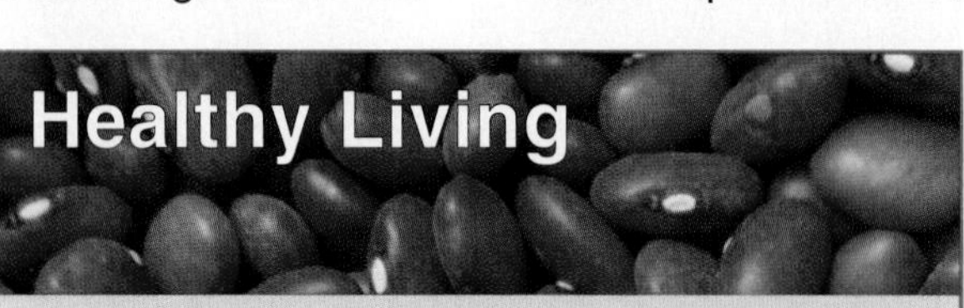

Getting enough calcium in your diet during the teen years is important. You need calcium to support the rapid bone growth that occurs at this stage in your life. A calcium-rich diet during the teen years can also help reduce your risk of osteoporosis (excessive bone tissue loss) later in life.

While all dairy products provide calcium, they do not all provide it in the same amounts. Cottage cheese and ice cream provide about half as much calcium as equal portions of milk or yogurt. Choose three servings of calcium-rich foods and be physically active daily to build strong, healthy bones.

You can enjoy dairy products fresh or use them as ingredients in cooking and baking. Chocolate pudding, pizza, and scalloped potatoes are just a few of the many popular foods that contain dairy ingredients. In addition to contributing important nutrients, dairy products contribute flavor, texture, and richness to many foods. Milk products also help baked goods brown.

Selecting and Storing Dairy Products

You can choose from among a variety of dairy products to meet your drinking and cooking needs. Most dairy products are highly perishable. They require careful storage to maintain their flavors and nutrient qualities.

Milk

Milk, both plain and flavored, is a popular beverage. Milk is also an important ingredient in many foods.

Milk Processing

Milk may go through several processes between the dairy farm and the retail store. Milk and milk products sold in the United States are pasteurized. During ***pasteurization,*** milk is heated to destroy harmful bacteria. Pasteurization improves the keeping quality of the milk. It does not change the nutritional value or the flavor.

Some milk is treated with ***ultra-high temperature (UHT) processing.*** This preservation method uses higher temperatures than regular pasteurization to increase the shelf life of foods like milk. After heating, UHT processed milk is sealed in presterilized boxes. You can store unopened UHT milk products without refrigeration, 17-1.

Fresh whole milk is usually homogenized. ***Homogenization*** is a mechanical process that prevents cream from rising to the surface of milk. This process breaks globules of milkfat into tiny particles and spreads them throughout the milk. Homogenized milk has a richer body and flavor than nonhomogenized milk.

Whole milk is often fortified with vitamin D. Fat free milk may contain added vitamins A and D. Milk fortified with calcium is available for people who are concerned about getting enough calcium in their diets.

Types of Milk

Each type of milk must meet specific standards for its composition. *Whole milk* must contain at least 3.25 percent milkfat and 8.25 percent milk solids. ***Milkfat*** is the fat portion of milk. ***Milk solids*** contain most of the vitamins, minerals, protein, and sugar found in milk.

All types of milk begin as pasteurized whole milk. *Reduced fat milk* has some of the fat removed. *Fat free milk* has nearly all of the fat removed. The less fat the milk has, the fewer calories it provides per serving. Milk with added flavoring becomes flavored milk, such as chocolate milk.

Many people experience gas, cramps, bloating, and diarrhea after drinking and eating regular milk products. They have a condition called *lactose intolerance,* which means their bodies cannot produce enough lactase. Lactase is the enzyme needed to digest lactose—the natural sugar in milk. People with lactose intolerance may choose to buy *lactose-reduced milk,* which has been treated with lactase to break down milk sugar.

Cream

Types of cream are defined according to the amount of milkfat they contain. *Heavy whipping cream* has the most fat, followed by *light whipping cream.* Both hold air when whipped, and they are often used in desserts. *Light cream,* or *coffee cream,* has less fat than light whipping cream. You can use it as a table cream and in cooking. *Half-and-half* is made from half milk and half cream. It has the least amount of fat, so it is the lowest in calories.

Yogurt and Other Cultured Dairy Products

A number of dairy products are made from milk to which helpful bacteria have been added. These bacteria are *cultured,* or specially grown for this purpose. Therefore, dairy products to which they are added are called *cultured dairy products.* The bacteria produce lactic acid, which gives these products a thick texture and tangy flavor.

Yogurt is a cultured dairy product. It may contain added nonfat milk solids and flavorings or fruits. An 8-ounce (227 g) serving of yogurt provides a bit more calcium and protein than a cup (250 mL) of milk. The amount of fat in yogurt depends on whether it was made from whole, reduced fat, or fat free milk. Although yogurt is a nutritious food, fruit-flavored yogurt often contains about 8 teaspoons of added sugar per serving. To limit your sugar intake, try stirring fresh fruit and a drizzle of honey into some plain nonfat yogurt. See 17-2.

Other cultured dairy products include buttermilk and sour cream. People use *cultured buttermilk* for cooking and baking as well as drinking. Regular *sour cream* is made from light cream. *Light* and *reduced fat sour cream* have fewer calories than regular sour cream because they have less fat. These sour cream products can all be used interchangeably in most recipes.

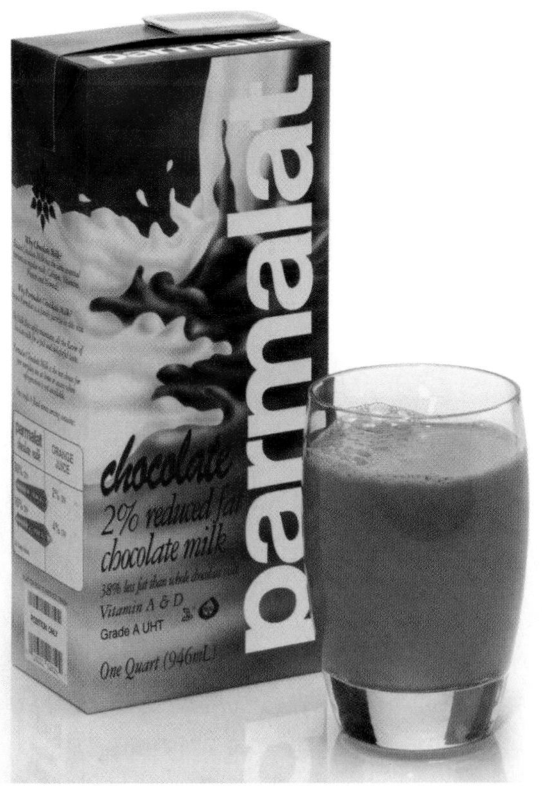

Parmalat

***17-1** UHT processed milk is found in presterilized boxes on the grocer's shelf—not in the dairy case.*

Concentrated Milk Products

Removing water from fluid milk produces concentrated milk products. These products can be canned or dried.

Evaporated milk is sterilized, homogenized whole, reduced fat, or fat free milk that has had some of the water removed. When diluted with an equal amount of water, it matches fresh milk in nutritional value. You can then use it in place of fluid fresh milk for drinking and in recipes. Evaporated milk costs more than fluid whole milk.

Sweetened condensed milk is whole or fat free milk with some of the water removed and a sweetener added. It is used most often in cooking and baking. Sugar affects the flavor and texture of cooked and baked products. Therefore, you should use condensed milk only in recipes that call for it. Sweetened condensed milk cannot be used interchangeably with evaporated milk. You cannot dilute it for use in place of fluid fresh milk, either.

Removing most of the water and fat from whole milk produces nonfat dry milk. You can use nonfat dry milk to add calcium and protein to many foods. You can also reconstitute it and use it like fluid milk. When you add water, it costs one-half to two-thirds less than fluid milk.

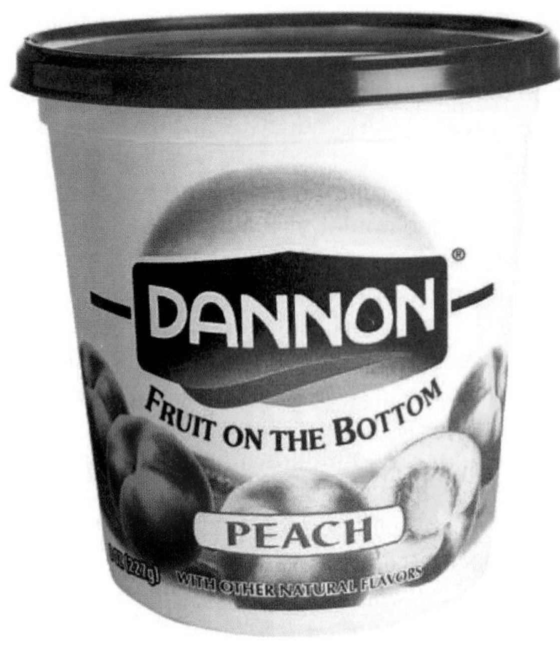

***17-2** Yogurt, like other cultured dairy products, is made by adding cultures of special helpful bacteria to milk. These bacteria cause the milk to thicken and develop a tangy flavor.*

Frozen Dairy Desserts

Ice cream, frozen yogurt, and sherbet are all frozen dairy desserts. The names of these products used on labels indicate fat content. *Reduced fat products* must show at least a 25 percent reduction in fat over regular products. *Lowfat products* must not contain more than 3 grams of fat per serving. *Nonfat products* must contain less than 0.5 grams of fat per serving. See 17-3.

Butter

Churning pasteurized and specially cultured sweet or sour cream produces butter. The churned product is usually salted and artificially colored.

Sweet butter is butter made without salt. Salt acts as a preservative, so sweet butter is more perishable than salted butter. *Whipped butter* is butter that has air whipped into it. It is also more perishable than regular butter.

Nondairy Products

A few products that look and perform like dairy products contain no dairy ingredients. *Nondairy products* include *coffee whiteners, whipped toppings*, and *imitation sour cream.* These products do not contain real cream. They get the body and appearance of dairy products from substances such as soy protein, emulsifiers, and vegetable fats and gums.

Margarine is another nondairy product. Many people use margarine in place of butter. It contains vegetable oil, animal fat, or some of each rather than milkfat like butter.

Cost of Dairy Products

National brand dairy products tend to cost more than local brands. In addition, milk products differ in cost depending on fat content, form, size of container, and place of purchase. Whole milk usually costs more than fat free milk. Fluid fat free milk usually costs more than nonfat dry milk. Ounce for ounce (milliliter for milliliter), milk sold in small containers usually costs more than milk sold in large containers. Home-delivered milk costs more than milk you buy at a store.

The cost of frozen desserts depends on the amount of fat. The kind and amount of extra ingredients, flavorings, and container size also affect cost. Rich ice cream in small containers with many added ingredients costs the most. See 17-4.

The cost of butter depends on form. Sweet butter and whipped butter may cost more than regular butter. Margarine costs less than butter, but prices vary depending on packaging and kind of oil used.

Fat Content of Ice Cream Products

Type of Ice Cream	Typical Percent Milkfat	Fat per 1/2-Cup (125-mL) Serving
Regular ice cream	10.0% or more	6-8 g
Reduced fat ice cream	7.0%	4-5 g
Lowfat ice cream	3.0%	3 g or less
Nonfat ice cream	0.5%	0 g

***17-3** Reading labels can help you determine the fat content of ice cream products.*

Q: Isn't margarine lower in fat and calories than butter?

A: No. Full margarine contains the same amount of fat and calories as butter. Most margarine is lower in cholesterol and saturated fat than butter. However, most stick margarine provides trans-fats. These fats are created when liquid vegetable oils are hydrogenated to make solid margarine. Tub margarines have little or no trans-fat.

Storing Dairy Products

All dairy products are highly perishable. Cover and store them in the coldest part of the refrigerator. Pour out just the amount of milk and cream you intend to use and return the rest to the refrigerator. Keep containers tightly closed to prevent contamination and off flavors.

You can store sealed UHT milk products unrefrigerated for up to six months. Once opened, you should refrigerate them and use them like other milk products.

Cover ice cream and other frozen desserts tightly and store them in the coldest part of the freezer. If frozen desserts become soft, large ice crystals will form when they are refrozen. This damages their textures. For best quality, use these products within a month.

Store dried and canned milk products in a cool, dry place. Reseal opened packages of dried milk carefully. Store reconstituted dry milk like fresh milk. Cover the unused portions of canned milk products and store them in the refrigerator. Use them within a few days.

Refrigerate all butter and margarine. Do not let either product stand at room temperature longer than necessary. Freezing will extend the life of both butter and margarine.

Cheese

Few foods are as versatile as cheese. Its many flavors, textures, and nutrients make it suitable for any meal or snack. See 17-5.

Cheese is a concentrated form of milk, so it is an excellent source of complete protein. A 1-pound (450 g) package of cheese contains the protein and fat of about 1 gallon (4 L) of whole milk. Cheeses are important sources of calcium and phosphorus. They are fair sources of thiamin and niacin. Whole milk cheeses are excellent sources of vitamin A.

Kinds of Cheese

All cheese is made from milk. The milk used can be from cows, goats, or other animals. In simple terms, the milk is coagulated, and the ***curd*** (solid part) is separated from the ***whey*** (liquid part). Cheeses made in this way are sometimes called *natural cheeses*.

Using different kinds of milk and changing the basic steps of production can produce hundreds of different cheeses. All these cheeses may be classified in two main groups: unripened and ripened. ***Unripened cheeses*** are ready for marketing as soon as the whey has been removed. They are not allowed to ripen or age. Cottage cheese, cream cheese, farmer's cheese, and ricotta cheese are examples of unripened cheeses. They are mild in flavor.

Controlled amounts of bacteria, mold, yeast, or enzymes are used to make ***ripened cheeses.*** During ripening, the cheese is stored at a

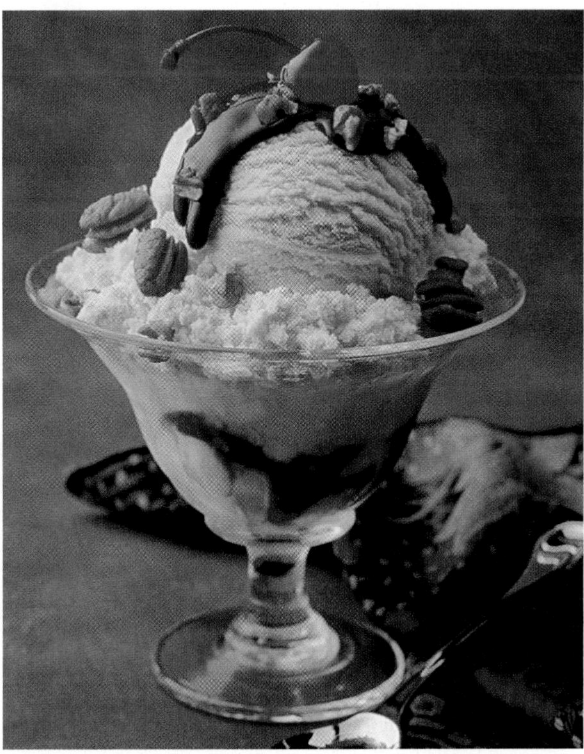

Dairy Management Association

17-4 Premium ice cream with added ingredients costs more than store brands to which you add your own toppings.

specific temperature to develop texture and flavor. Some cheeses become softer and more tender. Others become hard or crumbly. Over 400 varieties of ripened cheeses are produced. Each has a distinctive flavor, ranging from mild to strong. See 17-6.

Some ripened cheeses require further storage to develop flavor. This process is called aging. Cheese is aged anywhere from two weeks to two years, depending on the kind.

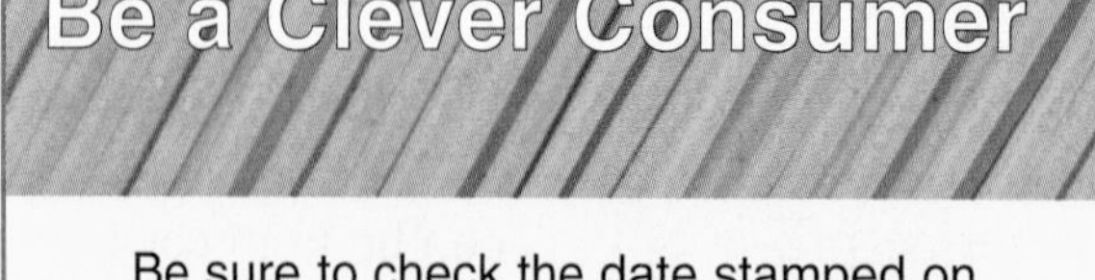

Be sure to check the date stamped on dairy product containers when choosing items at the store. Look for products stamped with the latest date. Keep in mind the date on dairy products is a pull date. This is the last day a store should sell the product. If stored properly, dairy products remain wholesome and can be consumed for a few days past the pull date.

Process Cheese

Natural cheeses can be made into other products called ***process cheeses.*** Several kinds of process cheese products are available in supermarkets and specialty food shops.

Pasteurized process cheese is made from a blend of unripened and ripened cheeses. The cheeses are heated and an emulsifier is added. The finished product is smooth and creamy. *Pasteurized process cheese food* is similar to pasteurized process cheese, but it contains more moisture and less fat. *Pasteurized process cheese spread* has a stabilizer added. It contains less milkfat and more moisture than cheese food.

Coldpack cheese (club cheese) is made from a mixture of unripened and aged ripened cheeses blended without heat. *Coldpack cheese food* is similar to coldpack cheese. It contains additional dairy products like cream, milk, fat free milk, or nonfat dry milk.

Imitation cheese has a large portion of the milkfat replaced by vegetable oils. Imitation cheese may differ in texture and melting

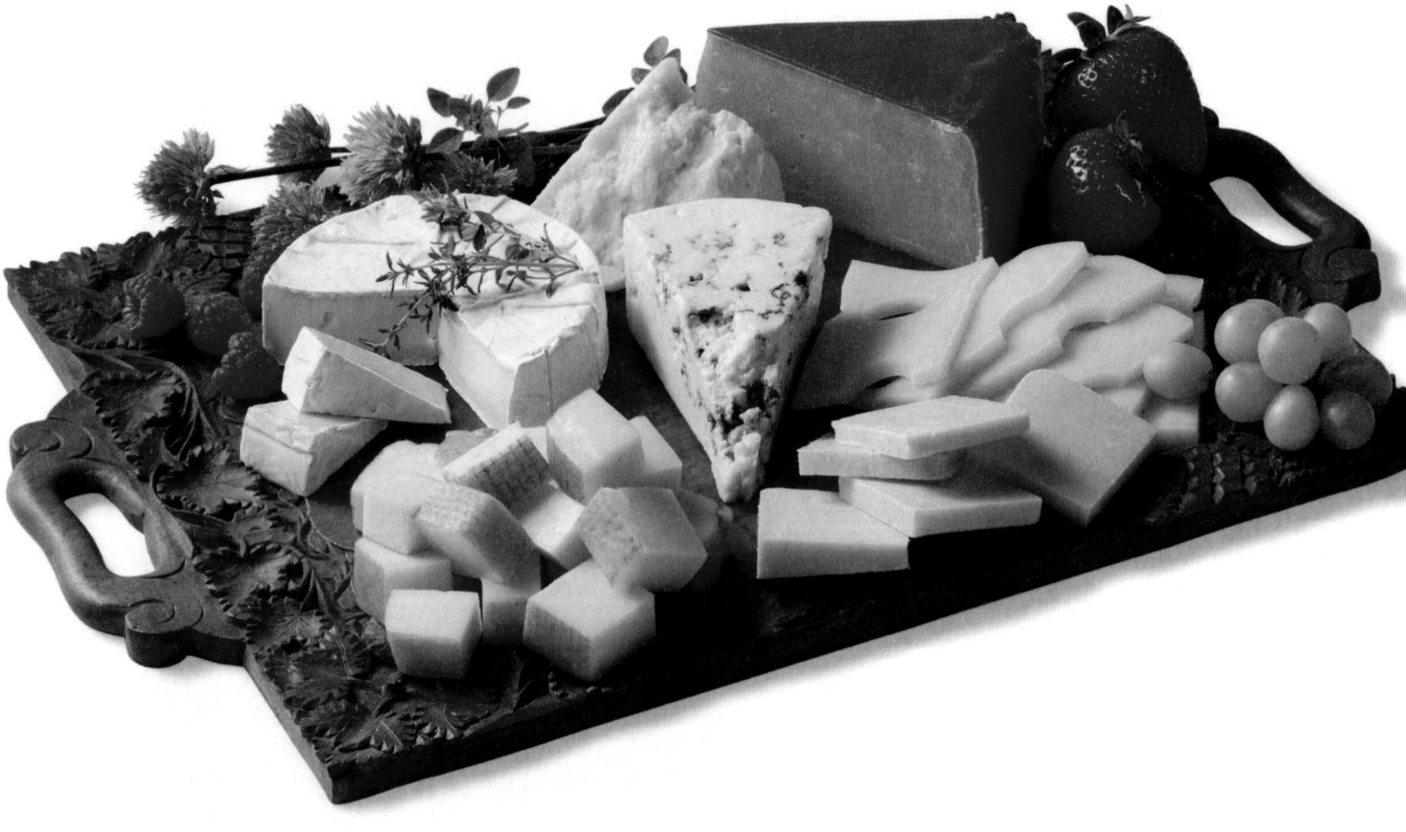

17-5 *Cheese makes a nutritious snack as well as a flavorful ingredient in many recipes.*

Cheese Guide				
Kind	**Color**	**Texture**	**Flavor**	**Use**
Roquefort	White marbled with a blue green mold	Semisoft	Sharp, tangy	Appetizers, snacks, salads, desserts
Blue cheese	Visible veins of blue green mold	Semisoft to crumbly	Spicy, tangy	Appetizers, snacks, salads, desserts
Gorgonzola	Tan surface with creamy interior marbled with blue green mold	Less moist than blue cheese	Tangy, spicy	Snacks, salads, desserts
Cheddar	Light yellow to orange	Hard, smooth	Mild to very sharp	Desserts, snacks, sandwiches, cooking
Colby	Orange	Hard with numerous small holes	Mild	Snacks, sandwiches, cooking
Monterey Jack	Creamy white	Semisoft, smooth	Mild	Snacks, sandwiches
Gouda	Creamy yellow, may have waxy red coating	Hard, open, mealy	Nutlike	Desserts, snacks
Edam	Creamy yellow	Hard, open, mealy	Nutlike	Desserts, snacks
Romano	Yellowish white interior, greenish black surface	Hard, granular	Sharp, tangy	Cooking, seasoning
Parmesan	Light yellow with brown or black coating	Granular, brittle	Sharp, spicy	Cooking, seasoning
Mozzarella	Creamy white	Semisoft, plastic	Mild, delicate	Pizza, sandwiches, cooking
Provolone	Yellowish white	Hard	Mild to sharp or smoky	Salads, cooking
Muenster	Yellow, tan, or white surface with creamy white interior	Semisoft, smooth	Mild to mellow	Sandwiches, snacks
Brick	Light yellow to orange	Semisoft, smooth	Mild	Snacks, sandwiches
Gruyère	Light yellow	Hard with tiny holes	Sweet, nutlike	Snacks, desserts, cooking
Swiss	Light yellow	Hard with large holes	Sweet, nutlike	Sandwiches, snacks, desserts, cooking
Cream cheese	Creamy white	Soft, smooth	Mild	Desserts, snacks, dips
Cottage cheese	White	Soft large or small curds	Delicate	Salads, dips, cooking

17-6 *With a broad range of textures and flavors, cheese is a versatile food.*

characteristics from real cheese. These differences may affect the outcome of cooked foods made with imitation cheese.

Cost of Cheese

You may be able to save money by buying cheese in large pieces rather than sliced, cubed, shredded, or grated. Fully-ripened cheeses often cost more than unripened cheeses or those that ripen for only a short time. Pasteurized process cheese costs less than ripened cheese. Plain cheese costs less than cheese with added ingredients like nuts and herbs.

Q: Isn't cottage cheese a good source of calcium?

A: Actually, cottage cheese has less than half the calcium of an equal portion of milk. An ounce of Cheddar, Swiss, and part skim mozzarella cheeses each provide more calcium than a cup of cottage cheese.

Storing Cheese

You should cover or tightly wrap all cheese and refrigerate it. This will prevent the cheese from becoming dry. It will also prevent the spread of odors and flavors. Strong-flavored cheeses can flavor other foods. Mild-flavored cheeses can pick up flavors from other foods.

Cheese can become moldy if you store it improperly or keep it too long. A small amount of mold on hard cheese is not harmful. Just cut off the moldy section about one-half inch (1.25 cm) into the cheese. Eat the rest of the cheese within a short time. Dispose of hard cheese with large amounts of mold and all moldy soft cheese.

Making the Lowfat Choice

Dairy products contribute a significant amount of fat to the diets of most people in the United States. To meet the Dietary Guideline for a diet moderate in total fat, choose reduced fat or fat free milk products. They can greatly reduce the amount of fat in your diet when used instead of whole milk or cream products. Remember that lower fat means lower calories, too. For every gram of fat you cut from your diet, you save 9 calories.

As an example, you can use plain, nonfat yogurt in place of sour cream in many recipes. Making this simple switch can save 3 grams of fat per tablespoon (15 mL). This may seem like a small difference, but it can really add up. In a recipe calling for a cup (250 mL) of sour cream, you would save 48 grams of fat and 380 calories. (Larger amounts of carbohydrate and protein in yogurt take up some of the calories saved from fat.) Table 17-7 lists some other dairy substitutions that can help reduce fat and calories in your diet.

Cooking with Milk and Cream

White sauce, cream soups, puddings, and frozen desserts are popular milk-based foods. Some of these foods may use cream in place of or in addition to milk.

Fresh milk, sour milk, evaporated milk, dried milk, and condensed milk are used in cooking and baking. Evaporated and dried milks may be used in place of fluid, fresh milk when you mix them with water. You cannot substitute condensed milk for other milk products.

Food Science Principles of Cooking with Milk

When you use milk as an ingredient, you often heat it. Heat affects proteins, and milk is a protein food. Understanding principles for cooking milk will help you avoid undesirable reactions.

The same cooking principles that apply to milk also apply to cream. Because cream is richer than milk (it contains more milkfat), heat and acids affect it more quickly than milk. Therefore, you should take extra care when cooking with cream.

Scum Formation

Scum is a solid layer that often forms on the surface of milk during heating. The scum is made up of milk solids and some fat. Because the scum is rubbery and tough, you should remove it. If you stir the scum into the milk, it will float in small particles throughout the milk.

Scum formation is difficult to prevent. After you remove the scum, another layer will form if heating continues. Stirring the milk during heating or covering the pan will help prevent scum formation. Beating the milk with a whisk or rotary beater to form a foam layer will also help prevent scum from forming.

Boiling Over

Scum formation is the usual cause of milk boiling over. Pressure builds up beneath the layer of scum. The scum prevents the pressure

Lowfat Dairy Substitutions			
Portion	**Whole Milk/ Cream Product**	**Lowfat/Nonfat Product**	**Grams of Fat Saved**
1 cup (250 mL)	whole milk	fat free milk	8
½ cup (125 mL)	regular ice cream	nonfat ice cream	6 or more
1 tablespoon (15 mL)	sour cream	plain, nonfat yogurt	3
1 ounce (28 g)	Cheddar cheese	mozzarella, part skim	4

17-7 *Lowfat or nonfat dairy products can reduce fat in a health-conscious diet.*

from being released as steam. The pressure continues to build until the milk finally boils over. You can prevent milk from boiling over by using low heat and one of the methods suggested for preventing a scum layer.

Curdling

High temperatures, acids, tannins, enzymes, and salts can cause milk proteins to coagulate and form clumps. This is called ***curdling,*** and the clumps are called *curds.* Foods like oranges and tomatoes contain acids. Many fruits and vegetables contain tannins and enzymes. Brown sugar also contains tannins. Cured ham and other meats contain salts. These substances may cause curdling in cream of tomato soup, creamed green beans, scalloped potatoes and ham, and other milk-based foods.

You can prevent curdling by using low temperatures and fresh milk. When you add acid foods to milk, you should thicken either the milk or the acid first. For example, tomato soup made from thickened milk (or tomato juice) is less likely to curdle than tomato soup made from unthickened milk and juice. See 17-8.

Scorching

Scorching is burning that results in a color change. Scorched milk is brown in color and has an off taste.

Milk can scorch because it contains lactose, which is a type of sugar. Like any sugar, lactose can *caramelize,* or change to a brown, bitter substance called *caramel* when it is heated. When you heat milk, the milk proteins coagulate and settle onto the sides and bottom of the pan. If you overheat the milk, the lactose in the coagulated solids caramelizes, thus scorching the milk.

You can prevent scorching by using low heat. Heating milk in the top of a double boiler will also help you avoid scorching.

Q: Shouldn't I avoid high-fat dairy products if I'm trying to watch my weight?

A: Limiting your intake of foods that are high in fat and calories will help you prevent unhealthful weight gain. However, you do not have to completely avoid any food to achieve or maintain a healthy weight. Moreover, many dairy products are low in fat. They serve as excellent sources of protein and calcium that you should include in your diet every day.

Microwaving Milk Products

Use lower settings when microwaving milk and milk products. Higher settings can cause milk to curdle. You should also watch milk carefully, as it can boil over quickly in the microwave oven. Filling containers no more than two-thirds full when microwaving milk products will help avoid this problem. Stirring during the cooking period to prevent scum formation will also help reduce the risk of boiling over.

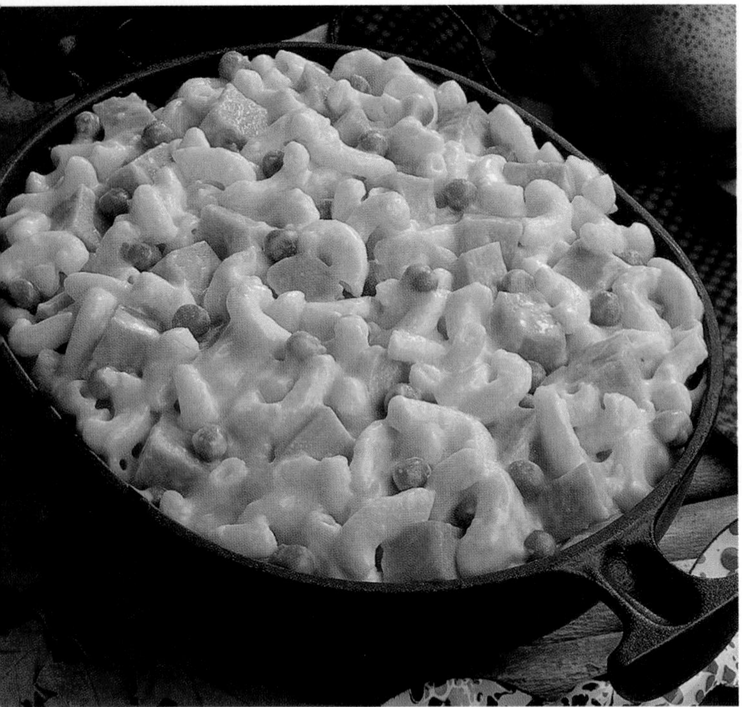

courtesy of National Pork Board

17-8 Thickening the milk before adding the ham to the creamy sauce in this dish will help prevent curdling.

Whipping Properties of Cream

The amount of milkfat affects the volume and stability of whipped cream. Cream must contain at least 25 percent milkfat to whip successfully. However, at least 30 percent milkfat is needed to produce a stable product. More milkfat (up to 40 percent) will produce a product that is still more stable.

When you whip cream, two changes take place. The first is that air bubbles are incorporated in the cream and a foam forms. The second change is that fat particles in the cream clump together. The clumping of the fat particles produces the stiffness in whipped cream. It also is the first step in the churning of butter. For this reason, you must control the amount of beating carefully. When the cream is overbeaten, too much air is incorporated into the cream. The emulsion around the fat particles breaks, the foam collapses, and the cream turns into butter.

Sugar decreases both the volume and stiffness of whipped cream. It also increases beating time if you add it before the cream has begun to stiffen. If you are sweetening the cream, you should add the sugar after the cream has become fairly thick.

Preparing Whipped Cream

For best results when whipping cream, you should thoroughly chill the bowl, beaters, and cream. The bowl to be used for whipping should be large enough to hold the cream after whipping. (Cream doubles or triples in volume during whipping.)

To whip cream, pour the cream into a chilled bowl. Beat it at medium speed until thickening begins. If you are sweetening the cream, gradually start adding sugar at this point. As you add the sugar, increase the beating speed. Continue whipping the cream until it is stiff. Do not overbeat. Serve whipped cream immediately. (If you must hold whipped cream for a short time, refrigerate it promptly.) See 17-9.

Preparing Common Milk-Based Foods

The creamy texture and richness of milk-based foods have made them favorites for generations. Studying basic preparation techniques will allow you to include these popular foods in your menu planning.

White Sauce

A ***white sauce*** is a starch-thickened milk product. It is used as a base for other sauces and as a component in many recipes.

The proportion of starch to milk determines the thickness of white sauce. Use *thin sauce* as the base of cream soups. Use *medium sauce* to cream vegetables and meats and *thick sauce* in soufflés. *Very thick sauce* binds the ingredients in croquettes.

Preparing White Sauce

Classic white sauce is thickened with a ***roux,*** which is a cooked paste of fat and flour. You melt the fat over low heat. Then you stir in flour and seasonings to form a paste. Stir milk into the roux. Stir constantly as you cook the mixture over medium heat until it thickens into a smooth sauce.

You can use a ***slurry*** as the thickening agent in a fat free white sauce. A slurry is a liquid mixture of milk and flour blended together until smooth. Combine fat free milk, flour, and seasonings in a blender container or a small, covered jar. Blend or shake until thoroughly mixed. Cook the slurry in a heavy saucepan

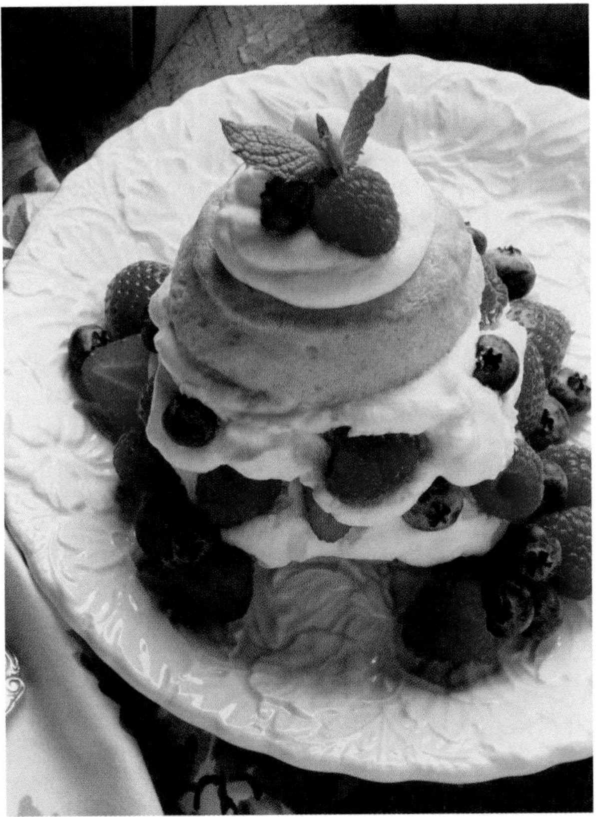

17-9 Whipped cream has the best texture and greatest volume if served right after whipping.

over medium heat, stirring gently, until it reaches a boil. Cook the slurry for one minute longer until the sauce is smooth and thickened. (This cooking will also prevent a raw starch flavor.)

When preparing a white sauce, take care to prevent scorching and lumping. Using moderate heat will prevent scorching. Using cold milk and thorough blending will separate the starch granules in the flour. This, along with gentle stirring during cooking, will prevent lumping and produce a smooth-textured sauce.

The principles of preparing white sauce are also used when preparing gravy. Juices from meat or poultry are used in place of some or all the milk to give gravy flavor. Skim the fat from pan juices remaining after cooking meat or poultry. Stir a slurry into the juices. Cook and stir over medium heat until thickened. To thin or extend gravy, add milk as needed. Season to taste with salt and pepper.

Cream Soups

Milk-based soups, often called cream soups, are popular luncheon and supper dishes. The three basic types of cream soups are thickened cream soups, bisques, and chowders. Use a thin white sauce to make thickened cream soups. They contain vegetables, meat, poultry, or fish that is pureed or cut into small pieces. Cream of mushroom and cream of tomato soups are popular thickened cream soups. See 17-10.

Bisques are rich, thickened cream soups. Light cream often replaces all or part of the milk in a bisque. Bisques usually contain shellfish that is shredded or cut into small pieces. You may have seen lobster bisque listed on a restaurant menu.

Chowders are made from unthickened milk. Chowders can contain vegetables, meat, poultry, or fish. (Most chowders contain potatoes, which help add thickness.) A few chowders use tomatoes and water instead of milk. Tomatoes form the base for Manhattan clam chowder, whereas milk forms the base for New England clam chowder.

Preparing Thickened Cream Soups

The first step in preparing thickened cream soups and bisques is to cook the added ingredients. You must cook the vegetables, meat, poultry, or fish using only a small amount of liquid. This will help preserve as many of the water-soluble nutrients as possible. You may use the cooking liquid later as part of the liquid in the white sauce.

Many cream soup recipes require you to puree the vegetables, meat, poultry, or fish. Use a blender or sieve to make the puree as smooth as possible. You should cut foods that do not require pureeing into small pieces.

The second step in making a cream soup is to add the prepared ingredients to a thin white sauce. Season the soup to taste. You may serve the soup immediately, or refrigerate it and reheat it later. Be sure to use low heat when reheating a cream soup to prevent scorching.

Preparing Unthickened Cream Soups

The cooking method used to prepare chowders differs somewhat from the method used to prepare thickened cream soups. Usually the pieces of vegetables, meat, fish, or poultry are fairly large, and they are cooked in a stock. When they are tender, add the milk to the stock and stir gently until blended. You should add the milk slowly and heat the soup at a low temperature to prevent curdling.

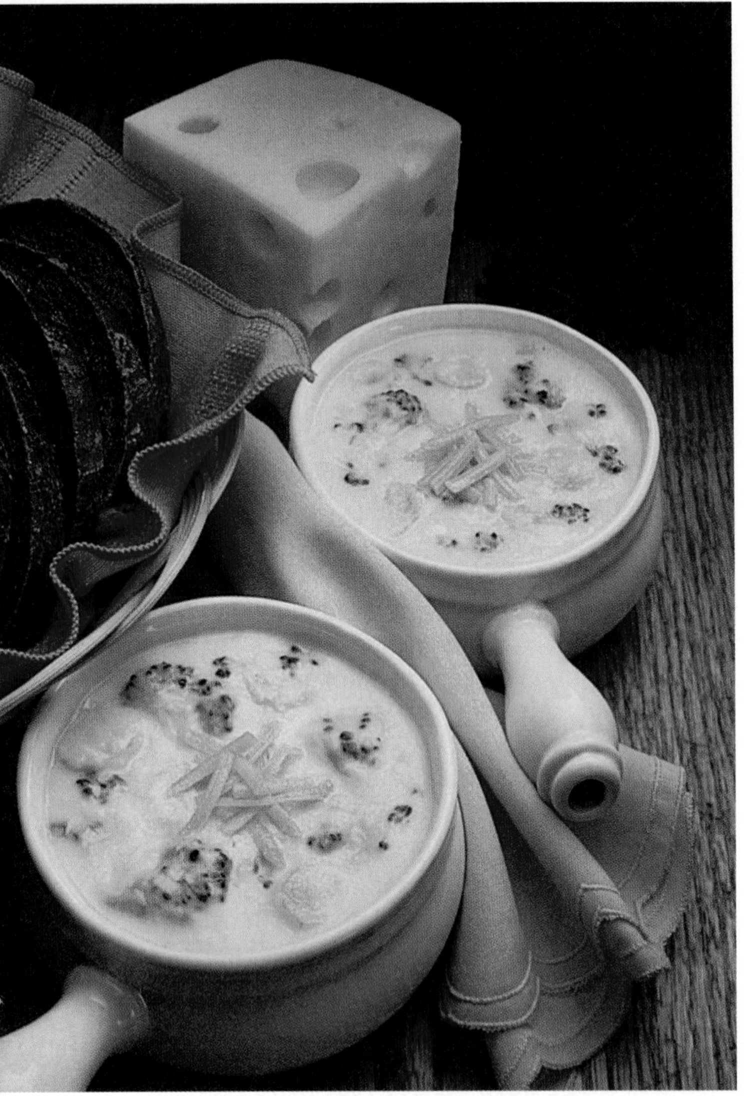

17-10 Creamy cheese soup gets its rich texture from dairy ingredients.

Puddings

Puddings are thickened milk products usually served as desserts. You probably are familiar with cornstarch, tapioca, rice, and bread puddings. You may also have tried Indian pudding. All these puddings contain milk and a thickening agent—cornstarch, tapioca, rice, bread, or cornmeal, respectively. In several types of puddings, eggs contribute additional thickening as well as protein.

Food Science Principles of Cooking Puddings

All puddings require the use of moderate cooking temperatures to prevent scorching and overcoagulation of the egg and milk proteins. You must separate the starch grains before cooking to prevent lumping. You will usually place rice, bread, and Indian puddings in a dish of hot water during baking. This provides further protection against the overcoagulation of proteins.

Some old-fashioned pudding recipes call for *scalded* milk. Scalding means heating to just below the boiling point. In the past, this step was necessary to kill bacteria in unpasteurized milk. Because all milk is now pasteurized, you can skip this step whenever you see it in a recipe.

When you use eggs in pudding, you should first add a small amount of the hot pudding to the beaten eggs. You can then add the diluted egg mixture to the rest of the hot pudding. (Eggs added directly to a hot mixture can coagulate into lumps.) You should cook the pudding a few minutes longer after adding the eggs to completely cook the egg proteins.

Preparing Cornstarch Pudding

Of all the puddings, cornstarch pudding is the most versatile. You can serve it alone or use it to make fillings for other desserts, 17-11.

To prepare a basic cornstarch pudding, combine the sugar, salt, and cornstarch in a heavy saucepan and mix well. Add a small amount of the cold milk and stir to make a smooth paste. (These first steps help separate the starch granules.) Add the remaining milk, stirring constantly.

Cook the pudding over moderate heat, and continue stirring until the pudding boils. Cook for one minute longer to thoroughly cook the starch. Add the flavoring, and pour the pudding into dessert dishes. Chill before serving. A piece of waxed paper placed on the surface of the warm pudding will prevent the formation of a skin.

Gelatin Creams

Gelatin is a gummy substance made from the bones and some connective tissues of animals. In its pure state, it is colorless and tasteless. You will use two types of gelatin in cooking—flavored gelatin and unflavored gelatin. Both types of gelatin are dissolved in a hot liquid. During cooling, the gelatin sets into a jellylike mass.

Gelatin creams are milk-based desserts thickened with unflavored gelatin. They are similar to puddings. Both desserts contain milk products and a thickening agent. However, you thicken puddings with starch instead of gelatin. Three main types of gelatin creams are chiffons, Bavarian creams, and charlottes.

You prepare *chiffons* by adding unflavored gelatin to a stirred custard while the custard is still warm. Chill the mixture until it is almost set. Then fold in cooked, beaten egg whites. Pour the chiffon into a mold and chill until firm.

Good Manners Are Good Business

You can add small oyster crackers to a bowl of soup served at a business meal. However, do not break larger crackers into your soup. Above all else when eating soup, remember to eat it quietly. Slurping soup is one of the quickest ways to make a bad impression at a business meal.

You prepare *Bavarian creams* by folding whipped cream into a chilled soft custard that has been thickened with gelatin. You may wish to add flavorings to the custard. Chill the mixture in a mold until firm and then unmold it for serving.

You prepare *charlottes* by folding whipped cream into a gelatin-thickened custard. Pour the mixture into a mold lined with ladyfingers and chill until set. See 17-12.

Food Science Principles of Preparing Gelatin Creams

When preparing all three types of gelatin creams, you must soak the gelatin in a cold liquid, usually water. This initial soaking ***hydrates*** the gelatin granules, causing them to absorb water. This allows the gelatin to dissolve more easily when you stir it into hot liquid.

Pour a prepared gelatin cream into a mold and chill it until firm. To unmold a gelatin cream, dip the mold quickly in warm water. Run the tip of a paring knife around the edge of the mold. Place the serving dish upside down on top of the mold. Then turn the mold and the dish right side up. Shake the mold gently. The gelatin cream should slip out. If it does not loosen, repeat the previous steps. The gelatin in the mixture helps the dessert hold its shape when you unmold it.

Ice Cream and Sherbet

Ice creams and sherbets are frozen dairy desserts you can make at home. They contain milk, cream, or a combination of both.

Ice cream contains milk, cream, sugar, and flavoring. You can make homemade ice cream that is lower in fat. However, it will be less creamy than regular ice cream. Simply substitute fat free milk for the whole milk and whole milk for the cream found in ice cream recipes.

Sherbet contains fruit juices, sugar, and milk. You may add cooked beaten egg whites, whipped cream, or gelatin to improve the texture of sherbets. The increased sugar in sherbet makes it less creamy than ice cream.

used by permission of Dean Foods

17-11 *Creamy chocolate pudding is a nutritious dessert.*

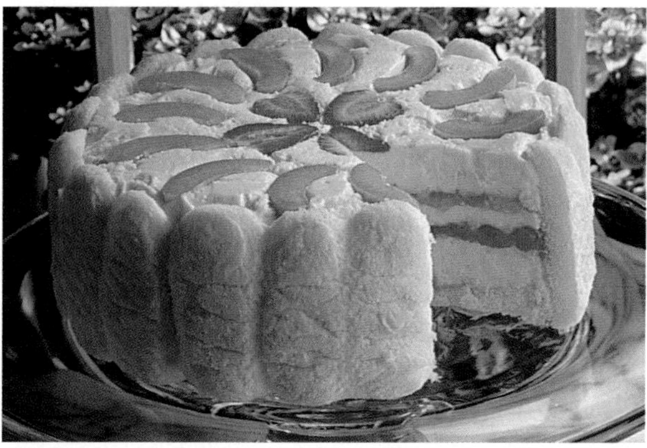

California Apricot Advisory Board

17-12 *A charlotte is a molded gelatin cream surrounded by a ring of ladyfingers.*

Food Science Principles of Preparing Frozen Desserts

You must stir ice cream products and sherbet during freezing to achieve a smooth texture. This is because ice crystals form during freezing. Stirring keeps these ice crystals small. Frozen desserts that have small ice crystals taste creamy. Frozen desserts that have large ice crystals taste grainy. See 17-13.

You can prepare ice cream products and sherbet in an ice cream freezer or in the freezing compartment of the refrigerator. In an ice cream freezer, stirring is continuous, so ice crystals remain small. In the refrigerator freezing compartment, stirring is not continuous. You may add cooked beaten egg whites, whipped cream, whipped evaporated milk, or whipped gelatin to recipes prepared in the refrigerator freezing compartment. These ingredients inhibit the formation of ice crystals.

Preparing Frozen Desserts

Whether prepared in an ice cream freezer or in the freezing compartment of the refrigerator, frozen desserts are frozen by the withdrawal of heat. In an ice cream freezer, ice and salt surround the dessert mixture and withdraw heat. In the refrigerator freezing compartment, cold air surrounds the dessert mixture and withdraws heat from it.

To prepare a frozen dessert in the refrigerator freezing compartment, turn the temperature control to its lowest setting. Pour the dessert mixture into a shallow metal baking pan. Cover it with foil and freeze until mushy. Quickly turn the mixture into a chilled bowl and beat with a whisk or rotary beater. Fold in whipped cream, cooked beaten egg whites, or other ingredients as your recipe instructs. Pour the mixture back into the metal pan. Cover and freeze until firm.

To prepare a frozen dessert in an ice cream freezer, prepare the dessert mixture and chill. Chilling will result in faster freezing.

Rinse the freezer canister first with very hot water and then with cold water. Pour the chilled dessert mixture into the canister, filling it no more than two-thirds full. (The mixture will expand during freezing.) Place the dasher into the canister. Cover the canister and attach the crank handle.

Surround the canister with alternate layers of salt and ice, beginning with ice. Use one part salt to eight parts ice, by weight, for ice cream. Use one part salt to four parts ice for sherbet.

Let the mixture stand four or five minutes and then begin cranking slowly. When the mixture begins to freeze, crank more rapidly. Continue cranking until turning the handle is difficult. (When using an electric ice cream freezer, the motor will stop at this point.)

When cranking is complete, carefully remove the water and salt from the tub. Wipe the top of the canister with a damp cloth. Remove the handle and crank. Then wipe the top again. Remove the lid and push the dessert mixture down with a rubber spatula. Cover the canister tightly. Repack the tub with four parts ice to one part salt. Cover the tub with newspapers, and let the frozen dessert ripen for four hours to develop flavors. Frozen desserts will have more flavor if you allow them to soften slightly before serving.

Cooking with Cheese

You can eat cheeses alone or use them as ingredients in appetizers, sandwiches, casseroles, sauces, salads, and many other dishes. See 17-14. When used as an ingredient, cheese contributes proteins, vitamins, minerals, and flavor to other foods.

Food Science Principles of Cooking with Cheese

Cheese is a concentrated form of milk. Therefore, it is a high-protein food. Like all

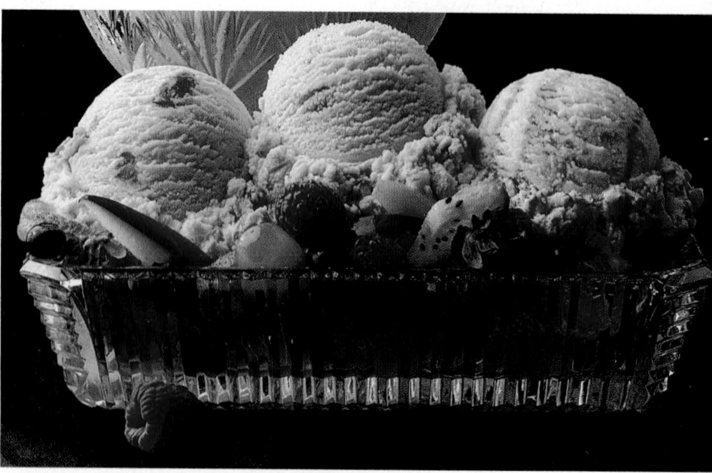

17-13 Keeping the ice crystals small is the key to creamy texture in ice cream.

high-protein foods, heat can adversely affect cheese. If you cook cheese at too high a temperature or for too long a time, its proteins overcoagulate. As a result, the cheese becomes tough and rubbery and the fat in the cheese may separate.

Preparing Cheese Dishes

You combine cheese with liquids in sauces and soups. When combined with liquid, the temperature must be hot enough to melt the fat so the cheese will blend smoothly. However, it must be low enough to prevent toughening of the proteins.

Cheeses that are well ripened blend more easily than less well-ripened cheeses. Well-ripened cheeses also tolerate higher temperatures.

Cheese that is grated, shredded, or cut into small pieces will blend more quickly than cheese cut into large chunks. As a result, you can use a shorter cooking time.

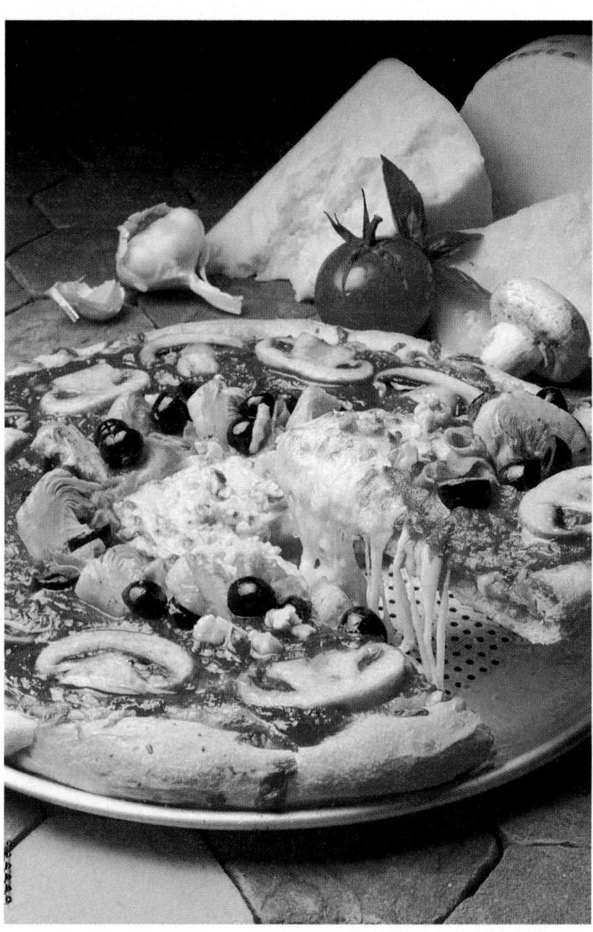

***17-14** Pizza is a favorite among cheese lovers.*

Process cheese blends more easily than natural cheese because of the emulsifiers it contains. A cheese sauce made with process cheese is smooth and less likely to curdle. In comparison, a cheese sauce made with Cheddar cheese has a grainier texture, although the cheese flavor is more pronounced.

When preparing appetizers or cheese sandwiches under the broiler, place the food four to five inches (10 to 12 cm) from the heat. Watch food carefully while broiling. Remove the appetizers or sandwiches when the cheese has melted.

Cheese dishes prepared in the oven, like macaroni and cheese, should bake just until done, 17-15. Cheese dishes cooked on a surface unit should cook over low heat or in the top of a double boiler.

Microwaving Cheese

Cheese requires careful timing and the use of low settings when it is being cooked in a microwave oven. Cooking for too long or at too high a power level can cause cheese to separate and become rubbery. All cheeses microwave well, but some cheeses have better melting qualities than others.

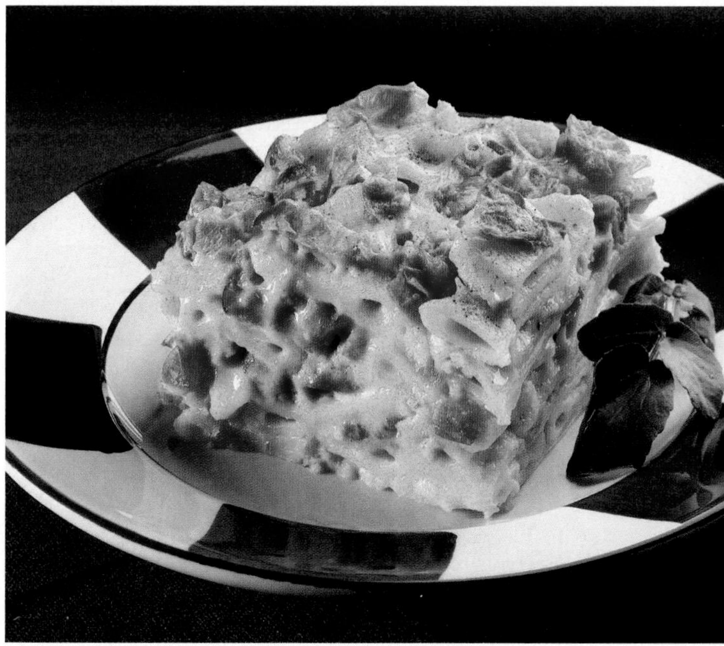

***17-15** Baked dishes containing cheese should stay in the oven just long enough to thoroughly heat the ingredients and melt the cheese.*

Chapter 17 Review

Dairy Products

Summary

Dairy products include a wide range of popular foods, such as milk, cream, yogurt, ice cream, butter, and cheese. Many dairy foods are good sources of protein and calcium as well as a number of vitamins and other minerals. The cost of dairy products varies depending on fat content, container size, brand, and place of purchase. All fresh and frozen dairy products are perishable and require storage in the coldest part of the refrigerator or freezer. Store canned products like fresh products once you have opened them. Store dried products like fresh products after you reconstitute them.

Cream and whole milk dairy products are high in fat. Choosing reduced fat and fat free milk versions of dairy products can help you reduce fat and calories in your diet.

Milk can form a scum layer, boil over, scorch, and curdle during cooking. You can take steps to help prevent these negative reactions.

Many recipes call for dairy products as ingredients. White sauces, cream soups, puddings, gelatin creams, and frozen desserts are just a few of the foods that contain milk. When preparing these foods, you need to remember to use moderate temperatures to prevent scorching and overcoagulating the proteins. You also need to use moderate temperatures when cooking with cheese. This will help keep the cheese from becoming tough and rubbery and prevent the fat from separating.

Review What You Have Read

Write your answers on a separate sheet of paper.

1. The process of heating milk to destroy harmful bacteria is called _____.
2. Which of the following types of cream has the most milkfat?
   A. Coffee cream.
   B. Half-and-half.
   C. Heavy whipping cream.
   D. Light whipping cream.
3. Name three types of cultured dairy products.
4. True or false. Evaporated milk and sweetened condensed milk can be used interchangeably in recipes.
5. True or false. Margarine is a dairy product.
6. Name a cheese that would be suitable for each of the following uses: appetizer, snack, dessert, sandwich, and salad.
7. Describe the difference between ripened and unripened cheeses.
8. True or false. A small amount of mold on hard cheese is not harmful.
9. How can you prevent milk from curdling during cooking?
10. If whipped cream is to be sweetened, when should the sugar be added?
11. List four food products that are made with a white sauce.
12. In what type of cream soup might cream be used in place of milk?
13. How should eggs be added when preparing a cornstarch pudding?
14. Why is it important to stir sherbets and ice creams during freezing?
15. What are two factors that affect how easily cheese blends with other ingredients during cooking?

Build Your Basic Skills

1. **Verbal.** Set up a tasting panel. Compare the tastes of whole milk, reduced fat milk, fat free milk, cultured buttermilk, and reconstituted nonfat dry milk. Discuss how flavors differ.
2. **Writing.** Sample a variety of 10 cheeses. Be sure to choose some you have not tried before. Write a sentence describing the flavor and texture of each. Then write a paragraph describing how you would use one of the cheeses for eating and cooking.

Build Your Thinking Skills

1. **Evaluate.** Whip heavy cream using the following methods:
   A. Chill bowl and beaters. Whip cream and sugar until stiff.
   B. Have bowl and beaters at room temperature. Whip cream until it begins to thicken. Add sugar slowly. Continue beating until stiff.
   C. Chill bowl and beaters. Whip cream until it begins to thicken. Add sugar slowly. Continue beating until stiff.

   Evaluate the beating time, appearance, volume, and stability of each sample.
2. **Compare.** Prepare vanilla ice cream in an ice cream freezer and in a refrigerator freezing compartment. Compare the appearance, texture, and flavor of the products with each other and with commercially made ice cream.

Apply Technology

1. Research how ultra-high temperature pasteurization and aseptic packaging are used to extend the shelf life of milk. Prepare a poster illustrating the pasteurization and packaging processes.
2. Work in a small group to investigate the processes used to produce reduced fat and fat free dairy products. Prepare a visual aid to use in a presentation sharing your findings with the rest of the class.

Using Workplace Skills

Dan is a supervisor at Simons and Son Dairy Farm. He oversees a staff of four farm workers as they attend to the property and a large herd of cows. The workers handle daily chores, like milking and feeding cows. They are also responsible for seasonal and occasional jobs, like planting feed corn and mending fences. Dan needs to be sure the workers do all the critical tasks before the tanker comes for the daily milk pickup.

To be an effective worker, Dan needs skill in making good use of staff. In a small group, answer the following questions about Dan's need for and use of this skill:

A. Why can't Dan simply let the farm workers choose what tasks they want to do each day?
B. How might the farm workers respond if the workdays constantly shift between periods of too little and too much work?
C. How might Simons and Son be affected if Dan lacks skill in making good use of staff?
D. What is another skill Dan would need in this job? Briefly explain why this skill would be important.

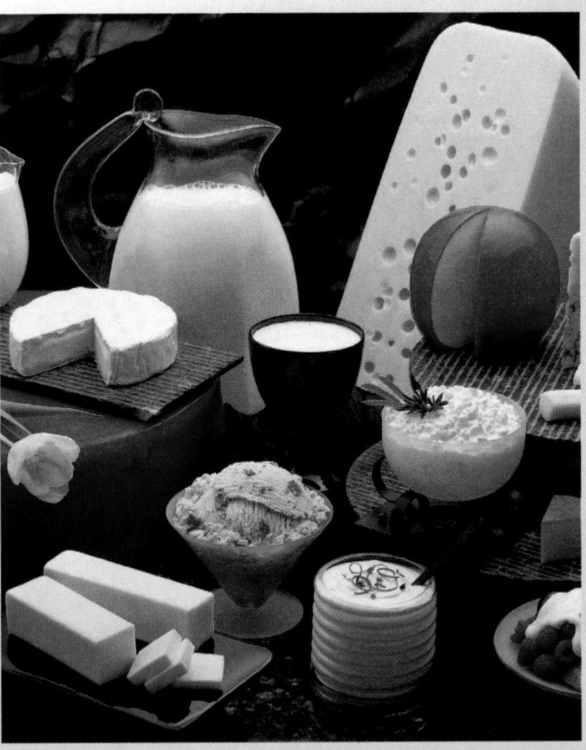

Chapter 18
Eggs

Egg Candler
Inspects eggs to ascertain quality and fitness for consumption or incubation according to prescribed standards.

Egg Pasteurizer
Controls and monitors equipment that pasteurizes liquid egg product.

Egg-Producing Farm Farmworker
Collects eggs from trap nests, releases hens from nests, records number of eggs laid by each hen, and packs eggs in cases or cartons.

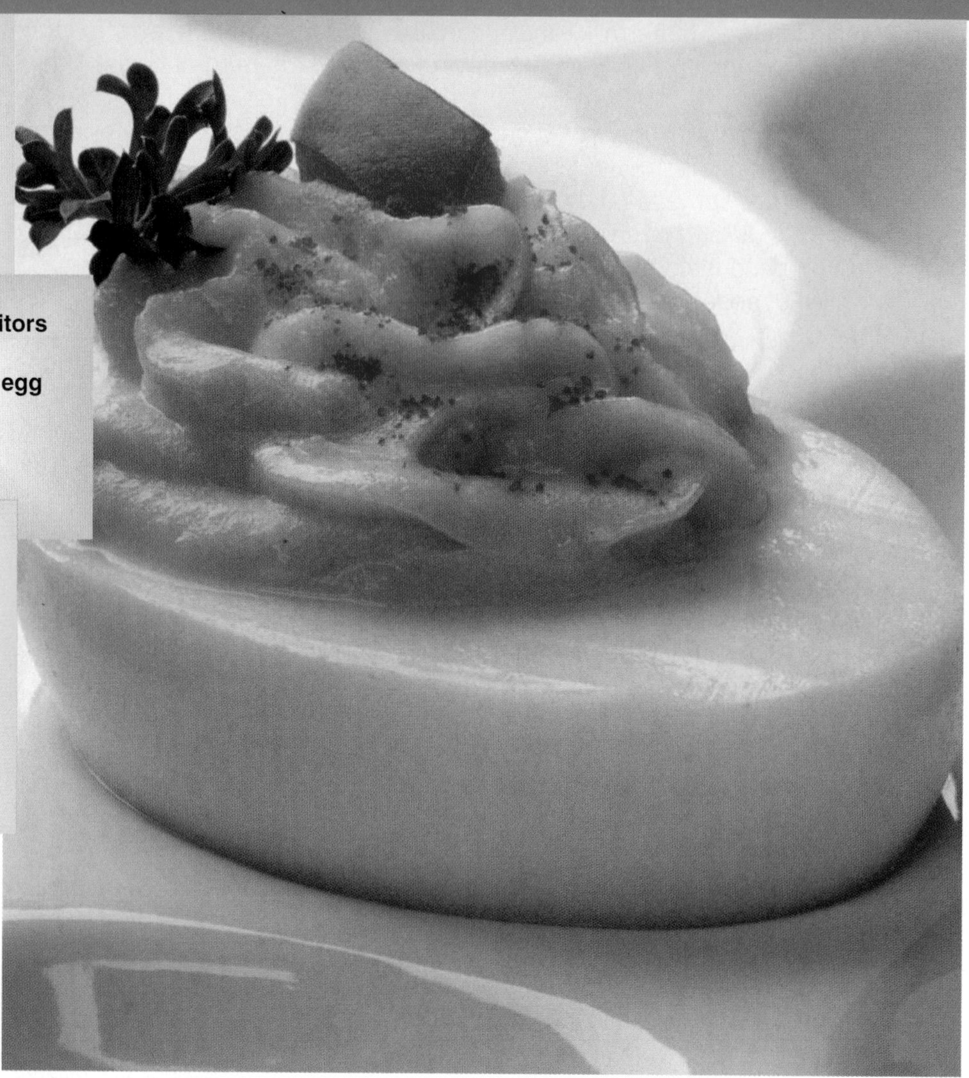

Terms to Know

candling
emulsion
coagulum
omelet
soufflé
meringue
weeping
beading
custard

Objectives

After studying this chapter, you will be able to

- list factors affecting the selection of eggs.
- describe the principles and methods for cooking eggs.
- cook eggs correctly for breakfast menus and use eggs as ingredients in other foods.

Eggs are one of the most versatile and nutritious food sources. You can prepare them in many ways. Because eggs are easy to digest, you can serve them to people at nearly all stages of the life cycle.

Selecting and Storing Eggs

Egg prices vary according to grade and size. Large eggs are the size most shoppers buy, regardless of price.

Nutritional Value of Eggs

Eggs are in the meat and beans group of the Food Guide Pyramid. One egg is equal to 1 ounce of lean, cooked meat. Most people should consume the equivalent of 5 to 7 ounces of lean, cooked meat per day.

Eggs are one of the best sources of complete protein. They also contain a number of vitamins and minerals. Egg yolks are high in cholesterol. Therefore, many health experts recommend using egg yolks and whole eggs with moderation. However, egg whites are cholesterol free, so you can use them freely.

Q: Are eggs a good choice if I'm trying to increase my iron intake?

A: Yes. One egg provides about as much iron as an ounce of lean, cooked meat, fish, or poultry. However, the form of iron in eggs is not as easy for your body to absorb. Having orange juice, or any other food rich in vitamin C, with your eggs will maximize your iron absorption.

Egg Grades

Eggs for retail sale are graded for quality. Grading is done by a system called ***candling.*** The eggs move along rollers over bright lights. The lights illuminate the eggs' structure. Skilled people can then look at the eggs carefully and remove any that do not meet standards.

Look for grade shields on egg cartons or on the tape that seals the cartons. The two grades of eggs available in most supermarkets are U.S. Grade AA and U.S. Grade A. These grades are given to high-quality eggs that have clean, unbroken shells and small air cells. The egg whites are thick and clear, and the yolks are firm and stand high above the whites.

Some eggs are rated Grade B, but you will rarely see these eggs in food stores. They are usually used in other food products.

Egg Size

Eggs are sized on the basis of a medium weight per dozen. Extra large, large, and medium eggs are the most common sizes sold. Size has no relation to quality, however, size does affect price. Eggs of any size can be Grade AA, A, or B. Extra large eggs cost more than large eggs, and large eggs cost more than medium eggs. Most recipes are formulated to use medium or large eggs. See 18-1.

Storing Eggs

Buy eggs only from refrigerated cases. Check to be sure eggs are clean and uncracked before you buy them. Cracked eggs can contain harmful bacteria, which can cause foodborne

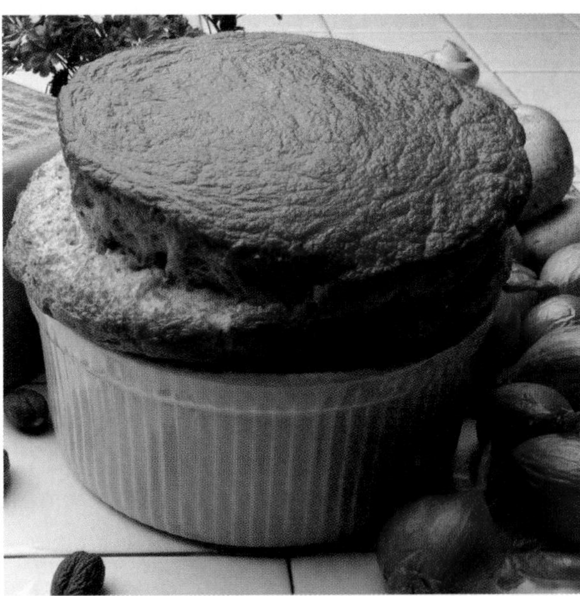

***18-1** Most egg recipes, like the one for this soufflé, are developed to be made with medium or large eggs.*

Q: Are brown-shelled eggs more nutritious than white-shelled eggs?

A: No. The breed of chicken determines egg color. The color of the shell does not affect quality, flavor, or nutritional value.

illness. You should discard any eggs that become cracked or broken during transportation or storage.

Store eggs in your refrigerator as soon as you bring them home from the store. You may safely store fresh eggs in the refrigerator for four to five weeks.

Some recipes call only for egg yolks or egg whites. To store leftover yolks, cover them with cold water and refrigerate in a tightly covered container. Store leftover egg whites in the refrigerator in a tightly covered container, too. Use yolks within one or two days. Use whites within four days.

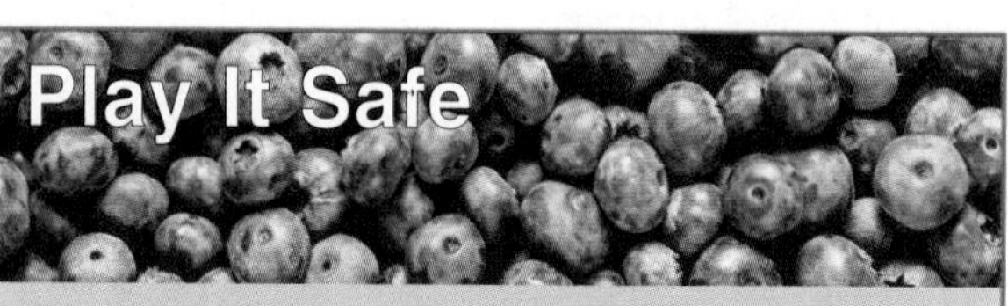

Play It Safe

Some eggs contain illness-causing bacteria. These bacteria can multiply rapidly at warm temperatures. Smell, taste, or appearance will not help you identify a contaminated egg. However, proper storage of eggs can help you control any bacteria that may be present. Store eggs, large end up, in their original carton. Keep them in the main compartment of the refrigerator, not on the refrigerator door, which does not stay as cold.

Eggs as Ingredients

Eggs function as emulsifiers, foaming agents, thickeners, binding agents, and interfering agents. They also add structure, nutrients, flavor, and color to foods.

Emulsifiers

An ***emulsion*** is a mixture that forms when you combine liquids that ordinarily do not mix. (Oil and water or a water-based liquid, such as lemon juice, are commonly combined to form an emulsion.) To keep the two liquids from separating, you need an *emulsifying agent.* Egg yolk is an excellent emulsifying agent. The yolk surrounds the oil droplets in an emulsion. It keeps the droplets suspended in the water-based liquid so the two liquids will not separate. Mayonnaise is an example of this type of emulsion.

Foams

Egg foams are used to add air to foods. When you beat air into egg whites, many air cells form. A thin film of egg white protein surrounds each cell. As beating continues, the cells become smaller and more numerous. The protein film also becomes thinner. As a result, the foam thickens.

Factors Affecting Egg Foams

Temperature, beating time, fat, acid, and sugar affect the formation of egg white foams. When preparing egg foams, two temperatures are needed. Eggs separate most easily when they are cold. However, egg whites reach maximum volume when they are at room temperature. Use an egg separator to separate whites from yolks when you take eggs from the refrigerator. Then let the egg whites stand at room temperature for 30 minutes before beating them. Store leftover yolks.

You must avoid both too little and too much beating time when preparing egg foams. Too little beating time produces underbeaten egg whites, which lose volume quickly and do not hold their shape. Too much beating time produces overbeaten egg whites, which also lose volume quickly. In addition, overbeaten egg whites have little elasticity and will break down into curds.

Fat and fat-containing ingredients, such as egg yolk, inhibit the formation of egg white foam. This is why you must be careful that no fat is present on the beaters or in the bowl when beating egg whites.

Acid makes egg white foams more stable. It also adds whiteness. This is why many recipes that use egg white foams call for a small amount of cream of tartar. See 18-2.

Sugar increases the stability of egg white foam. It also increases beating time. You will usually add sugar to the foam after it has reached most of the volume.

Stages of Egg Foams

Recipes will direct you to beat egg whites to one of three stages: foamy, soft peak, or stiff peak. Each stage requires increased beating time. Egg whites at the *foamy stage* have bubbles and foam on the surface. Egg whites beaten to the *soft peak stage* will form peaks that bend at the tips when you lift the beater. Egg whites beaten to the *stiff peak stage* will form peaks that stand up straight when you lift the beater. If you beat egg whites past the stiff peak stage, you have overbeaten them.

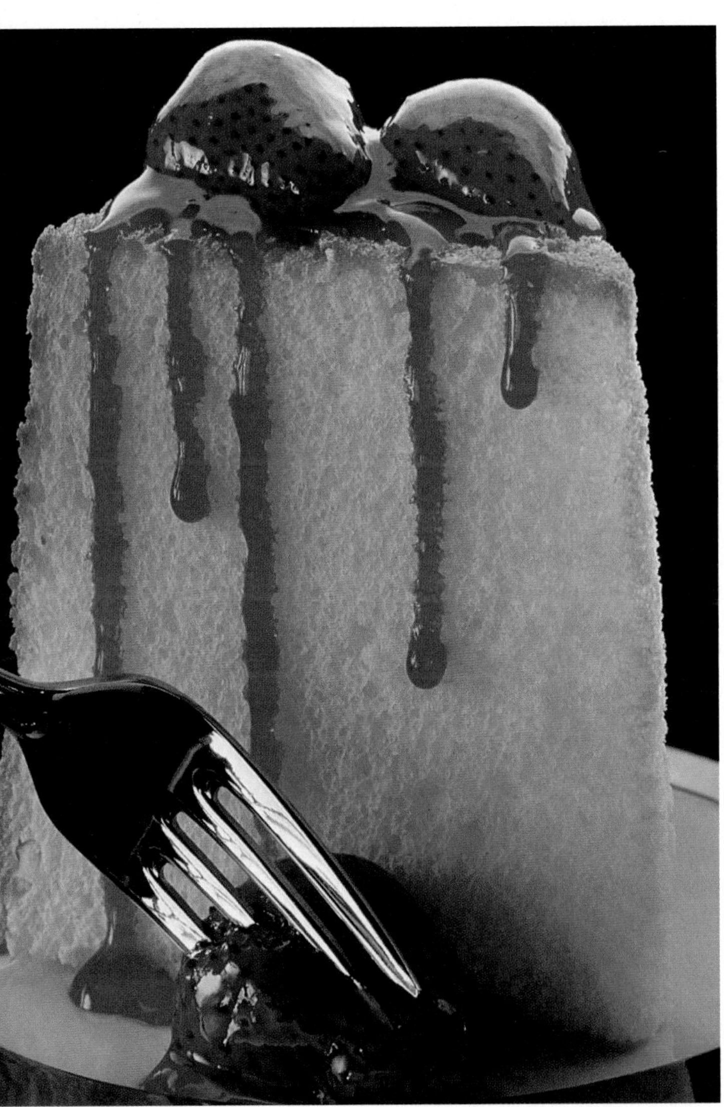

American Egg Board

18-2 *Most recipes for angel food cake call for cream of tartar to create a whiter, more stable egg foam.*

Using Egg Foams

You will use foams to make soft and hard meringues. You will also use them to give structure to angel food and sponge cakes, soufflés, and puffy omelets.

To avoid a loss of air, you must quickly but gently blend other ingredients into egg white foams. This blending process is called *folding.* Wire whisks and rubber spatulas are the best tools for folding. Using either tool, cut down into the mixture, across the bottom, up the opposite side, and across the top. The whisk or spatula should remain in the mixture the entire time you are folding.

Thickeners

Heat causes egg proteins to coagulate (thicken). Because of this property, whole eggs and egg yolks are used as thickening agents in such foods as sauces, custards, and puddings.

When you must add eggs to a hot mixture, you should quickly fold a small amount of the hot mixture into the beaten eggs. Then, you can add the warmed eggs to the rest of the hot mixture. Warming the eggs slightly keeps them from coagulating into lumps.

Binding and Interfering Agents

You can use eggs as binding and interfering agents. Eggs act as binding agents that hold together the ingredients in foods such as meat loaf and croquettes. Frozen desserts like ice cream and sherbet stay creamy because the eggs in them act as interfering agents. The eggs inhibit the formation of large ice crystals, which would ruin the texture of frozen desserts.

Structure

Eggs add structure to baked products, such as muffins and cakes, 18-3. People limiting cholesterol in their diets can still use eggs as ingredients in recipes for baked goods. You can substitute two egg whites for each whole egg. Add 1 teaspoon (5 mL) of oil and decrease liquid in the recipe by 1⅓ tablespoons (20 mL) for each egg being replaced.

Nutrition, Flavor, and Color

Eggs contribute important nutrients to food products. Eggs add flavor and color to foods such as custards and puddings. Eggs also give an appealing color to the interior of baked goods like cakes.

Healthy Living

A small percentage of raw eggs may be tainted with salmonella bacteria, which can cause foodborne illness. Thorough cooking and pasteurization destroy these bacteria. However, they may be present in raw and lightly cooked egg dishes. Children, pregnant women, older adults, and ill people should not eat egg dishes that are not thoroughly cooked. These groups of people are at a greater risk of complications if they contract a foodborne illness.

Using Raw Eggs

The risk of foodborne illness due to contaminated eggs is small, especially for healthy people. However, it is safest not to use raw eggs in any dish that is not thoroughly cooked.

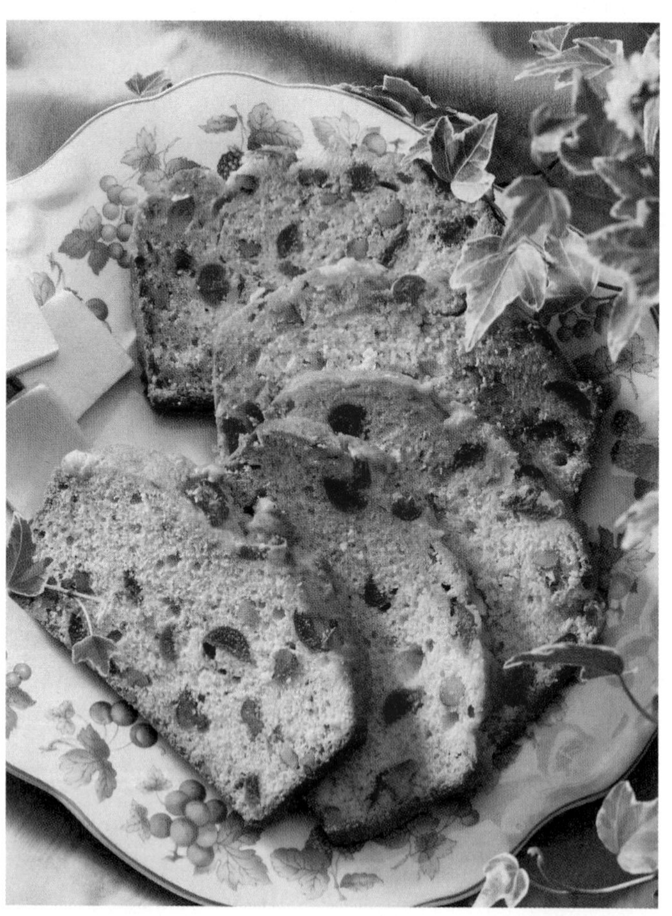

Cherry Marketing Institute

***18-3** Eggs help strengthen the structure of this quick bread.*

If a recipe calls for whole eggs, you can use a pasteurized egg product. A recipe that calls for separated eggs requires some special preparation steps.

Instead of using raw beaten egg whites in an uncooked dish, you can cook the whites. Using a specific technique, you will beat the egg whites into a fluffy frosting before adding them to your recipe. Combine the egg whites with the sugar from the recipe in a heavy saucepan or double boiler. (You will need at least 2 tablespoons [30 mL] of sugar per egg white.) Cook the mixture over low heat while beating it to the soft peak stage with an electric mixer.

Instead of adding raw egg yolks to a recipe, cook them as though you were making stirred custard. Combine the yolks with the liquid from the recipe in a heavy saucepan. (You will need at least 2 tablespoons [30 mL] of liquid per yolk.) Cook the mixture over low heat, stirring constantly until the mixture coats a metal spoon. Cool the mixture quickly and add it to the recipe when you would add the egg yolks.

Another option when preparing uncooked or lightly cooked recipes that call for raw eggs is to use pasteurized shell eggs. These are whole eggs that have been treated using the same heating process used to kill harmful bacteria in milk. This process does not affect the taste or cooking performance of the eggs.

Egg Substitutes

Egg substitutes provide an option for people who want to limit cholesterol and saturated fat from eggs in their diets. Egg substitutes are pasteurized. Therefore, you can use them in place of raw eggs in recipes that will not be cooked.

Egg substitutes are made largely from real egg whites. They contain no egg yolks. Therefore, these products are cholesterol-free, fat-free, and lower in calories than whole eggs. They compare closely to whole eggs in most other nutrient values. However, they may cost over three times as much as fresh eggs.

Egg substitutes are nearly as versatile as whole eggs. You can scramble them or use them to prepare omelets or quiches. You can also use them in most recipes calling for eggs. Typically, you will use ¼ cup (50 mL) of egg substitute in place of each whole egg or egg yolk. You can even use egg substitutes in recipes calling for hard-cooked eggs.

Q: Shouldn't I stop eating eggs if I'm concerned about cholesterol in my diet?

A: Large eggs provide an average of 213 mg of cholesterol each. With balance and moderation, most people can easily include eggs as part of a healthful diet. Also, remember that eggs are only one source of dietary fat and cholesterol. Simply limiting eggs will not lead to a lowfat, low-cholesterol diet. Lowering cholesterol and fat in the diet must become part of a total eating plan.

Food Science Principles of Cooking Eggs

Eggs coagulate when heated during cooking. Temperature, time, and the addition of other ingredients affect coagulation.

Egg white coagulates at a slightly lower temperature than egg yolk. The coagulation temperature of both egg white and egg yolk is below boiling. Temperatures that are too high can cause egg proteins to lose moisture, shrink, and toughen. This is why you should use low to moderate temperatures for cooking eggs. See 18-4.

Cooking time also affects coagulation. Cooking egg proteins too long can cause them to lose moisture and shrink. When both high temperatures and long cooking times are used, moisture loss and shrinkage become even greater.

The addition of other ingredients changes the coagulation temperature of eggs. This is because extra ingredients dilute the proteins found in eggs. As the concentration of egg proteins decreases, the coagulation temperature increases. For instance, eggs scrambled with added milk will coagulate at a higher temperature than eggs scrambled without milk. On the other hand, acid and salt both lower the coagulation temperature of eggs.

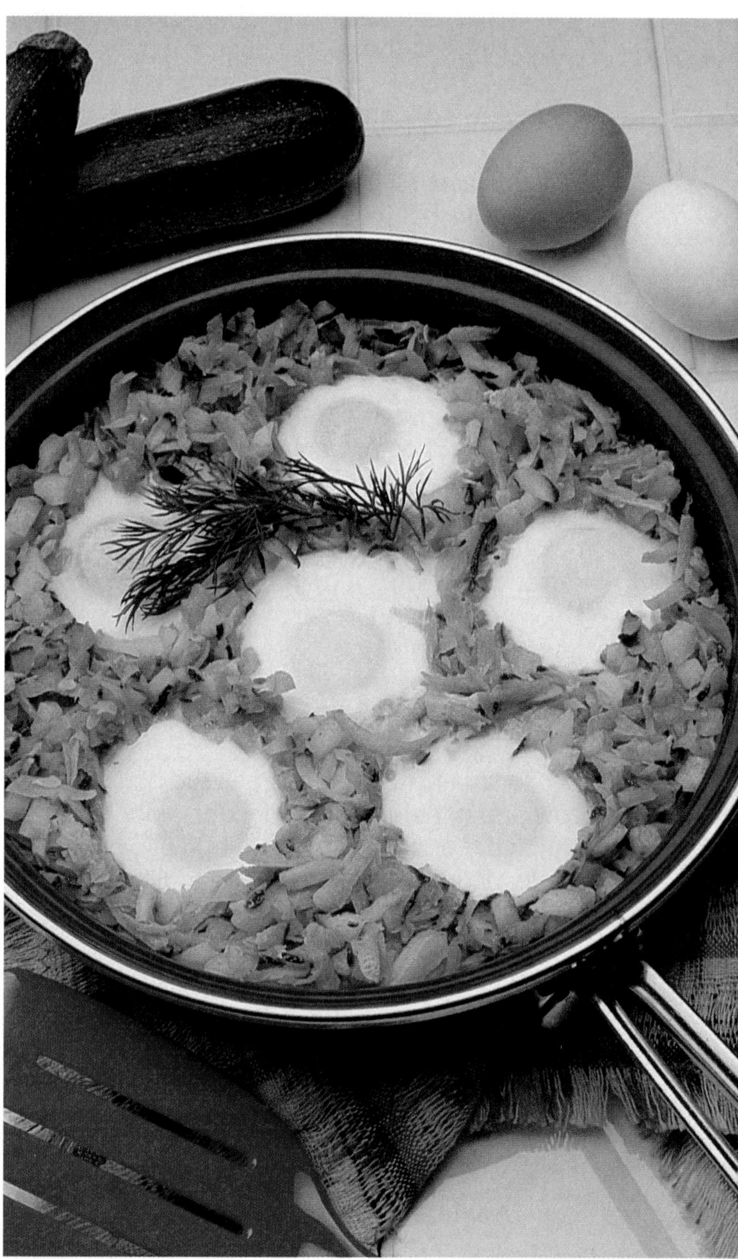

American Egg Board

18-4 Moderate temperatures help egg whites and yolks cook completely without allowing the egg proteins to become tough.

Methods of Cooking Eggs

You can scramble, poach, fry, bake, hard-cook, soft-cook, or microwave eggs. You can use them to prepare plain and puffy omelets, soufflés, soft and hard meringues, and stirred and baked custards, too. In all methods of cooking eggs, low to moderate temperatures and accurate cooking times are important.

Safely cooked eggs have completely set whites and thickened yolks. Yolks do not need to be hard, but they should not be runny. Dishes made with beaten eggs are thoroughly cooked when they no longer contain any visible liquid egg. The most accurate way to test the doneness of casseroles, soufflés, and other egg dishes is with a food thermometer. These dishes should reach the safe internal temperature of 160°F (71°C).

When cooking eggs in a skillet, your pan should be moderately hot before you place the eggs in it. Add any cooking fat you will be using to your skillet before heating it. The skillet is hot enough if a drop of water sizzles when it hits the surface of the pan. Using a pan that is too cool can cause the egg white to spread too far before it sets. As soon as the eggs are in the skillet, you should turn the heat down to low. Cooking temperatures that are too high quickly toughen egg proteins.

Scrambling Eggs

To scramble an egg, break the egg into a bowl. Beat the egg with a fork or whisk until blended. For variety, you can add bits of cooked bacon or finely chopped chives to eggs before scrambling. You can also add milk, tomato juice, or other liquid. However, the amount of liquid cannot exceed the amount of protein available to thicken the mixture. Using too much liquid will cause the eggs to be watery. Use about 1 tablespoon (15 mL) of liquid per egg.

Pour the egg mixture into a lightly greased or nonstick heated skillet. When the egg begins to set, draw a bent-edged spatula across the bottom of the skillet. This will allow more of the liquid egg mixture to come in contact with the hot surface of the skillet. The egg will thicken into large, soft clumps, which are called ***coagulum.*** Gently continue drawing the spatula across the skillet until all the egg mixture has set. However, avoid constant stirring. Too much stirring will cause the coagulum to be small.

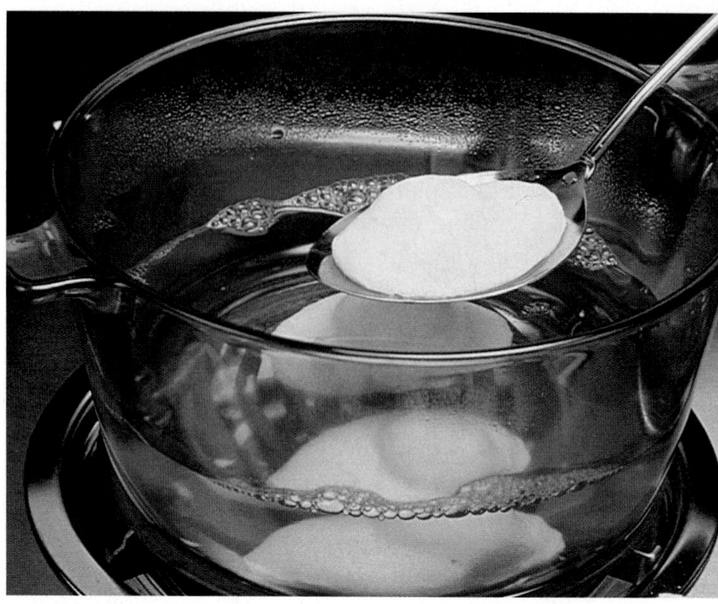

American Egg Board

18-5 *A properly prepared poached egg will have a uniform appearance with a smooth, firm egg white surrounding a thickened yolk.*

Poaching Eggs

You can poach eggs in water, milk, broth, or some other liquid. If using water, you may wish to add a small amount of salt or acid (such as vinegar). This will cause the proteins to coagulate faster and help keep the egg from spreading.

To poach an egg, break the egg into a custard cup. Slip the egg into a saucepan filled with 2 to 3 inches (5 to 7.5 cm) of simmering liquid. Cook the egg until the white is firm and the yolk is thickened. This will take about three to five minutes. Remove the egg from the cooking liquid with a slotted spoon. See 18-5.

Frying Eggs

To fry an egg, add the egg to a moderately hot skillet containing vegetable oil spray or a small amount of fat (1 teaspoon, or 5 mL, per egg). You may add a little water to the skillet, too. Cover the skillet and cook the egg until the white is completely set and the yolk begins to thicken. The steam that forms in the covered skillet will cook the upper surface of the egg. You can also cook the upper surface by gently turning the egg over.

Baking Eggs

Baked eggs are also called *shirred* eggs. To bake an egg, break the egg into an individual, greased baking dish. Then put the baking dish in a shallow casserole filled with 1 inch (2.5 cm) of warm water. Bake the egg in a 350°F (175°C) oven for 12 to 18 minutes, depending on the firmness desired. Try adding variety to baked eggs by sprinkling them with finely chopped green pepper and onion or grated cheese.

Cooking Eggs in the Shell

Eggs cooked in the shell can be soft-cooked or hard-cooked. Time determines the degree of doneness.

To prepare soft-cooked eggs, place the eggs in a deep pan. Add enough cold water to come 1 inch (2.5 cm) above the eggs. Cover the pan and quickly bring the water to a boil. Immediately remove the pan from the heat. Let the eggs remain in the water for four to five minutes, depending on the desired degree of doneness.

To prepare hard-cooked eggs, use the same method used for soft-cooked eggs, but keep the eggs in the water longer. Large eggs will take about 15 minutes. Medium eggs will take only about 12 minutes. Extra large eggs may take about 18 minutes.

Immediately cool soft- and hard-cooked eggs under cold running water or place them in a bowl of ice water. Rapid cooling stops the eggs from cooking and prevents the formation of greenish rings around the yolks. A chemical reaction between iron in egg yolk and hydrogen sulfide in egg white causes this discoloration in overcooked eggs. The discoloration is harmless, but it looks unappetizing.

When soft-cooked eggs are cool enough to handle, they are ready to eat. A popular way to eat them is to place them in eggcups, small end down. Cut off the large end of the egg and eat the egg out of the shell.

When hard-cooked eggs are completely cooled, store them in the refrigerator. You can keep them for up to one week. You should not eat hard-cooked eggs, or any other perishable food, kept at room temperature for over two hours.

Good Manners Are Good Business

Some people like to eat their scrambled eggs with catsup. If you are one of those people, you might want to order something besides scrambled eggs at a business breakfast. Putting anything on any food that was not prepared and served with the food is considered an insult to the chef.

Microwaving Eggs

You can scramble, poach, fry, and hard-cook eggs in a microwave oven. You can also make them into plain omelets or use them to make tasty egg dishes such as quiche, 18-6. However, conventional cooking methods are best for airy egg dishes, such as puffy omelets and soufflés.

Eggs cook rapidly in a microwave oven, and they continue to cook during standing time. Overcooking toughens the protein and produces a rubbery egg. Therefore, start cooking eggs with the minimum time stated in microwave recipes. Remove eggs from the microwave oven just before they are done.

In a microwave oven, steam builds up in foods covered by a tight skin or shell. This buildup could cause these foods to explode. For

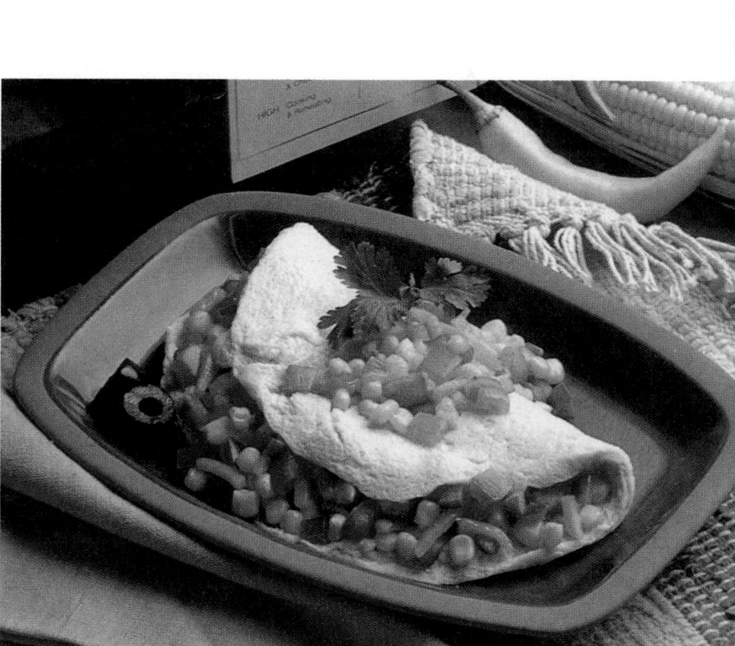

American Egg Board

***18-6** Plain omelets come out moist and delicious when cooked in a microwave oven.*

this reason, you should remove eggs from the shell before cooking them in a microwave oven. In addition, gently puncture egg yolks with a fork or toothpick before microwaving to prevent them from bursting.

Omelets

Omelets are beaten egg mixtures that are cooked without stirring and served folded in half. Omelets can be plain (also called French) or puffy. You make both types of omelets from eggs, a small amount of liquid (usually milk or water), and seasonings. You may serve an omelet with or without a filling.

To make a plain omelet, beat together the eggs, liquid, and seasonings. Pour the mixture into a lightly greased or nonstick heated skillet or omelet pan. The edges of the egg mixture should set immediately. With a wide spatula, gently lift the cooked edges to allow the uncooked egg to run underneath. Tilting the skillet will help. The omelet is ready to fill and serve when the top has set but is still moist.

To make a puffy omelet, beat the egg whites with cream of tartar and water until stiff (but not dry) peaks form. Beat the egg yolks with salt and pepper until they are thick and lemon colored. Gently fold the beaten yolks into the beaten whites. Pour the mixture into a lightly greased ovenproof skillet that is hot enough to sizzle a drop of water. Cook the omelet slowly over medium heat until puffy, about 5 minutes. (The bottom should be lightly brown.) Place the omelet in a preheated 350°F (175°C) oven. Bake it 10 to 12 minutes, or until a knife inserted near the center comes out clean.

Soufflés

Soufflés are fluffy baked preparations made with a starch-thickened sauce that is folded into stiffly beaten egg whites. Like puffy omelets, they use egg whites for structure. You can serve soufflés for dessert or as a main dish.

To prepare a soufflé, add beaten egg yolks to a basic white sauce. The white sauce may contain chocolate, fruit, cheese, or pureed vegetables or seafood. Gently fold the white sauce mixture into the beaten egg whites. Bake the soufflé in a 350°F (175°C) oven until puffy and golden, about 30 to 40 minutes. Serve the soufflé immediately.

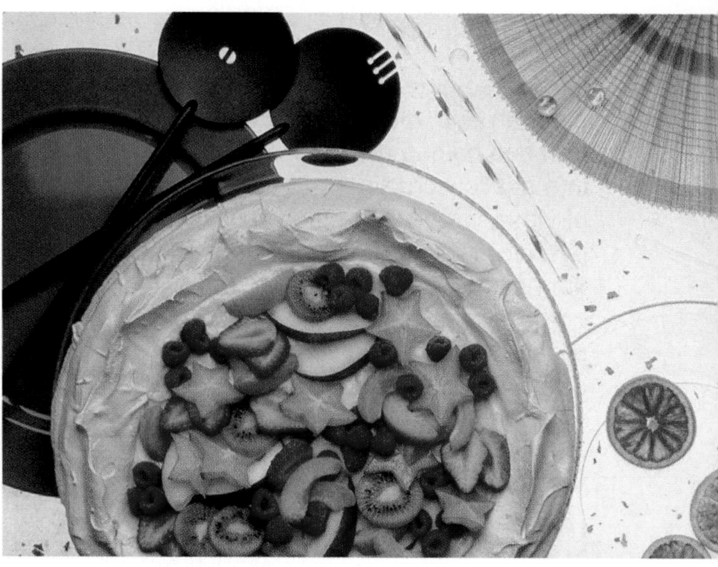

American Egg Board

18-7 *A hard meringue shell filled with fresh fruit makes an elegant dessert.*

Meringues

Meringues are a fluffy, white mixture of beaten egg whites and sugar. Meringues may be soft or hard. Use soft meringues in fruit whips and as toppings on pies and other baked goods like Baked Alaska. Use hard meringues to make meringue shells, which you can fill and serve as desserts, 18-7. You can also use hard meringues to make confections, such as meringue cookies.

Make soft meringues from egg whites, cream of tartar, sugar, and flavoring. Beat the egg whites and cream of tartar to the foamy stage. Add the sugar gradually as you continue beating the egg whites to the upper limit of the soft peak stage. Rub a small amount of meringue between your thumb and forefinger, making sure you do not feel any undissolved sugar. Then beat in the flavoring.

When using a soft meringue on a pie, spread it over hot pie filling. Carefully seal the meringue to the edge of the pastry. These important steps will help minimize weeping and beading. ***Weeping*** is the layer of moisture that sometimes forms between a meringue and a pie filling. ***Beading*** appears as golden droplets on the surface of a meringue. Bake the meringue-topped pie at 350°F (175°C) until lightly browned, about 12 to 15 minutes.

You make hard meringues from the same ingredients as soft meringues. However, they contain a higher proportion of sugar, and you beat them to the stiff peak stage. You will usually shape hard meringues with a spoon and bake them on an oiled or paper-covered baking sheet. Bake hard meringues at 225°F (105°C) for one to one and a half hours. Then turn off the oven and allow the meringues to stand in the oven with the door closed for another hour. This will produce a meringue with a crisp, dry interior.

Custards

Custards are a mixture of milk, eggs, sugar, and a flavoring that is cooked until thickened. Custards can be soft (sometimes called stirred) or baked. You might serve soft custard as a dessert sauce. You can also use it as the base for desserts like English trifle. Serve baked custard plain or with a topping of caramel, fruit, or toasted coconut. You can make bread pudding by pouring custard over bread cubes before baking.

Stir soft custard constantly as it cooks. This breaks up the coagulum as it forms, giving the custard a creamy texture. Be sure to use low heat to prevent *curdling* (the formation of lumps). Soft custard will coat a metal spoon with a thin film when it is fully cooked. Place the pan of cooked custard in a bowl of ice or cold water. Stir the custard for a few minutes to cool it before covering and storing in the refrigerator. See 18-8.

Lack of stirring causes baked custard to become firm enough to hold its shape when removed from the baking dish. Place dishes of custard in a large baking pan. Place the pan in a preheated oven. Then pour very hot water into the pan around the custard dishes. The water should come within ½ inch (1 cm) of the top of the custard. The water helps prevent the custard from overheating, which can result in *syneresis* (the leakage of liquid from a gel). Overbaked custard will have visible bubbles and leakage. To test baked custard for doneness, insert the tip of a knife near the center. If the knife comes out clean, the custard is baked.

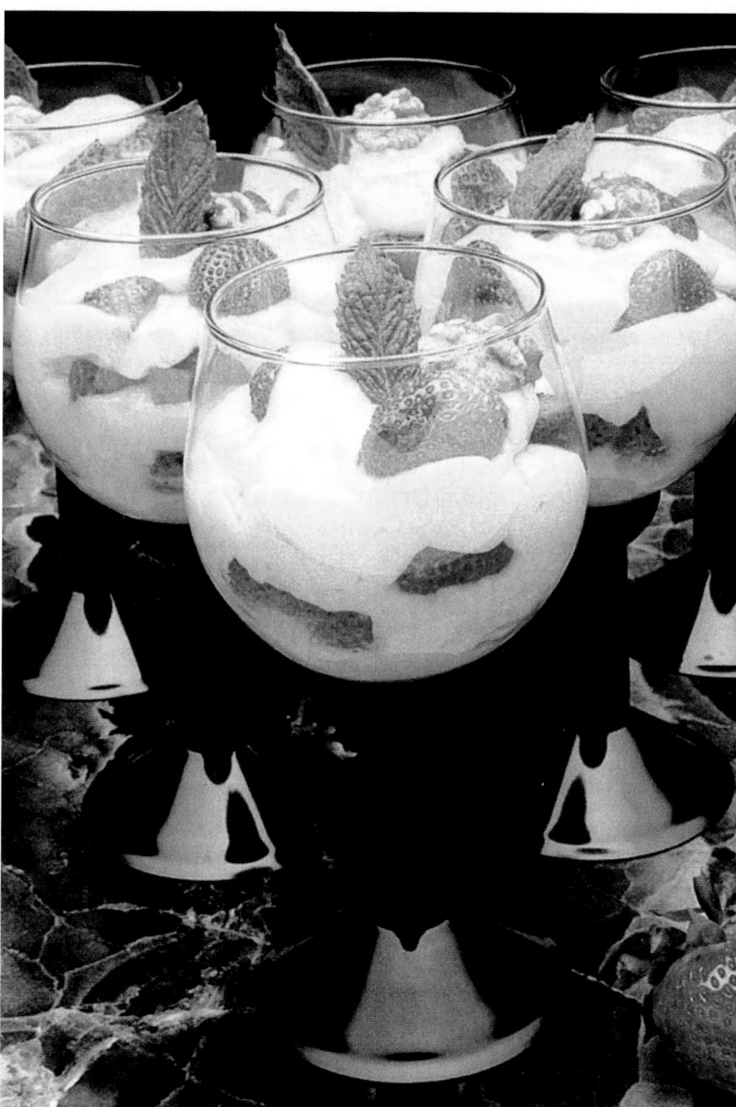

American Egg Board

18-8 *Ripe fruit and creamy custard give this dessert a pleasing combination of textures.*

Chapter 18 Review
Eggs

Summary

Eggs are a nutritious, inexpensive, and versatile food. Grade AA and A are the grades of eggs most commonly sold at retail stores. Extra large, large, and medium are the most common sizes. Fresh eggs keep well in the refrigerator, but require careful handling to prevent cracking.

Eggs serve a number of functions in recipes. They are used as emulsifiers to keep oil suspended in water-based liquids. They are used as foams to add air and give structure to foods like meringues and sponge cakes. They are used to thicken puddings and sauces and to hold ingredients together in foods like meat loaf. They interfere with the formation of ice crystals in frozen desserts. Eggs also add structure, nutrition, flavor, and color to many foods.

Eggs are perishable and require careful handling and thorough cooking to protect against foodborne illness. You can use pasteurized egg substitutes in dishes that call for raw or lightly cooked eggs. These products are also good choices for people trying to limit fat and cholesterol in their diets.

You can use a number of methods to cook eggs. You can also use eggs in a variety of dishes. No matter how you prepare them, eggs require moderate cooking temperatures and carefully monitored cooking times. These factors will prevent egg proteins from shrinking and becoming tough.

Review What You Have Read

Write your answers on a separate sheet of paper.

1. How is candling used in the egg industry?
2. How long can you safely store fresh eggs in the refrigerator?
3. How does egg yolk keep the vinegar and water from separating from the oil in mayonnaise?
4. What are four factors that can affect the formation of egg white foams?
5. How should beaten eggs be added to a hot mixture? Explain why.
6. True or false. To reduce cholesterol, two egg yolks can be substituted for each whole egg in a recipe.
7. How can a recipe for an uncooked dish calling for beaten raw egg whites be prepared safely?
8. True or false. Egg yolk coagulates at a slightly lower temperature than egg white.
9. Describe the appearance of safely cooked whole eggs and beaten egg dishes.
10. Describe two basic egg preparation methods.
11. What precautions should be taken to keep eggs from exploding in a microwave oven?
12. Describe the appearance of a plain omelet that is ready to fill and serve.
13. How are soufflés similar to puffy omelets?
14. Golden droplets of moisture that sometimes appear on the surface of a meringue are called _____.
15. The leakage of liquid from baked custard is called _____.
    A. coagulum
    B. emulsion
    C. syneresis
    D. weeping

Build Your Basic Skills

1. **Science.** In a darkened room, hold an egg directly over the lens of a flashlight. Describe characteristics of the egg that you cannot see in normal room lighting.
2. **Math.** Beat the egg white of a small egg in one bowl. Beat the egg white of an extra large egg in a second bowl. Measure and compare the volume of the two egg white foams.

Build Your Thinking Skills

1. **Compare.** Beat four egg whites to the stiff peak stage. Before beating, add nothing to the first egg white. Add ⅛ teaspoon (0.5 mL) oil to the second egg white. Add ⅛ teaspoon (0.5 mL) cream of tartar to the third egg white. Add ¼ cup (50 mL) sugar to the fourth egg white. Compare volume, appearance, and required beating time of the four samples. Summarize your observations in a brief written report.
2. **Evaluate.** Beat three eggs with milk and seasonings. Divide the mixture into three equal portions. Scramble one portion over high heat. Scramble a second portion over low heat, occasionally drawing a bent-edged spatula across the bottom of the skillet. Scramble the third portion over low heat stirring constantly. Evaluate each product on the basis of appearance, tenderness and size of the coagulum, and flavor.

Apply Technology

1. Research how egg substitutes are made. Summarize your findings in a brief written report.
2. Make a poster illustrating the process used to pasteurize eggs in or out of the shell. Write on the poster why you think pasteurized eggs are of value to consumers.

Using Workplace Skills

Deborah is an egg candler for M-G Farms. She inspects eggs as they move along rollers over bright lights. The lights allow her to see the structure of the eggs and evaluate their quality. She separates the eggs by grade. Grades AA and A are sold to supermarkets. Grade B eggs are sold to food product manufacturers.

To be a successful employee, Deborah needs skill in making decisions. Put yourself in Deborah's place and answer the following questions about your need for and use of this skill:

A. What is a decision you will make every day as an egg candler?
B. How might M-G Farms be affected if you do not have adequate skills in making decisions?
C. How might consumers be affected if you do not have adequate skills in making decisions?
D. What is another skill you would need in this job? Briefly explain why this skill would be important.

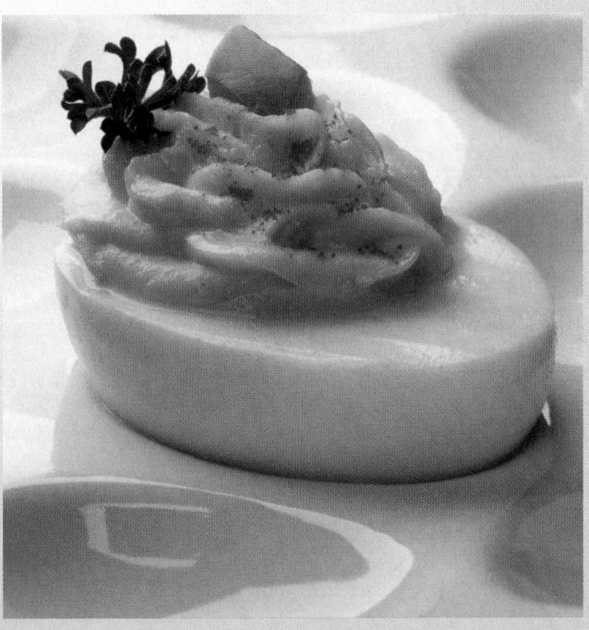

Chapter 19
Meat

Barbecue Cook
Prepares, seasons, and barbecues pork, beef, and other types of meat.

Meat Cutter
Using hand tools and power equipment, such as grinder, cubing machine, and power saw, cuts and trims meat to size for display or as ordered by customer.

Livestock Sales Representative
Sells cattle, hogs, and other livestock to farmers, packinghouses, and other purchasers. Reviews market information and inspects livestock to determine value.

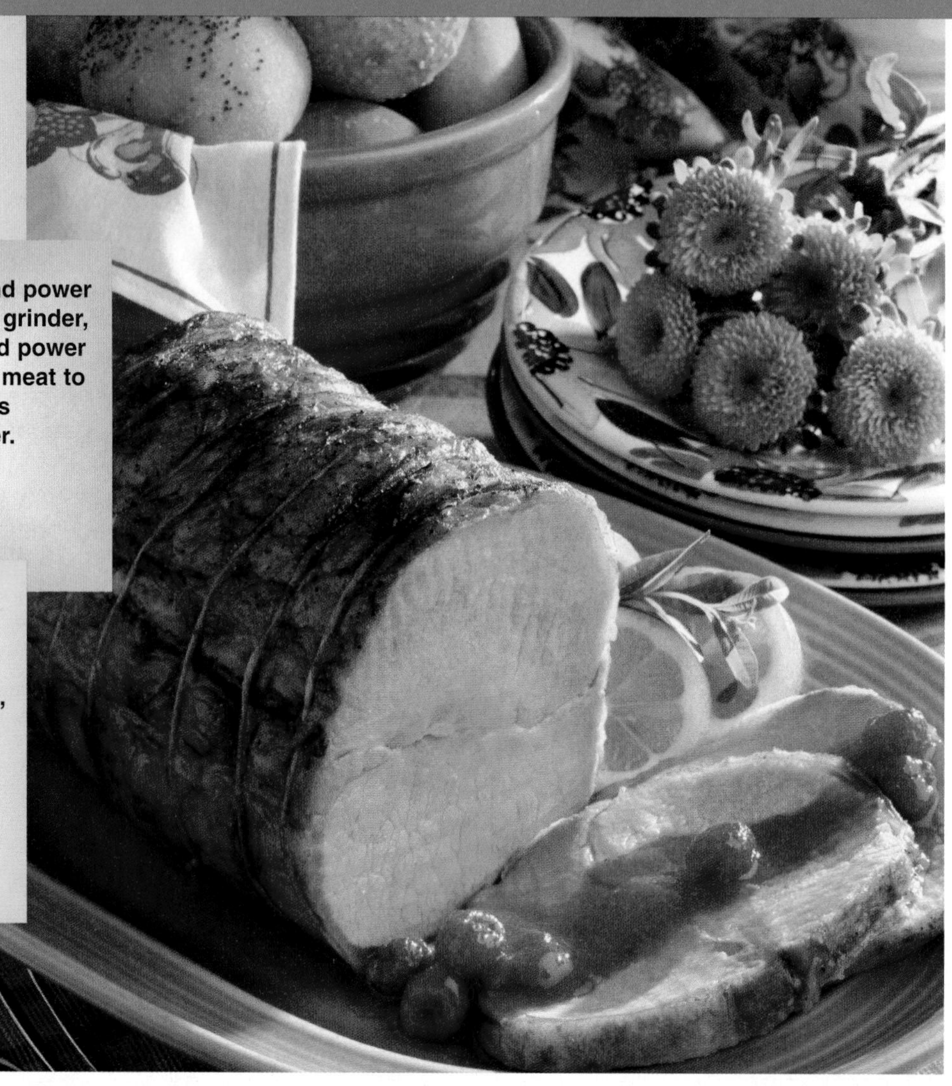

courtesy of National Pork Board

Terms to Know

meat
beef
wholesale cut
retail cut
veal
pork
lamb
variety meats
marbling
elastin
collagen
coagulate
cooking losses

Objectives

After studying this chapter, you will be able to

- ❑ list factors affecting the selection of meats.
- ❑ describe how to properly store meats to maintain their quality.
- ❑ describe the principles and methods of cooking meat.
- ❑ prepare meats by moist and dry cooking methods.

Many meal managers choose the meat course first when planning menus. The meat you prepare should be tender, flavorful, and attractive.

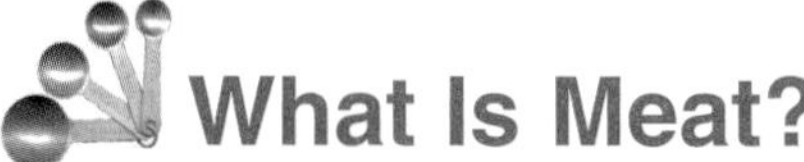

What Is Meat?

Meat is the edible portions of mammals. It contains muscle, fat, bone, connective tissue, and water. The major meat-producing animals in the United States are cattle, swine, and sheep.

Nutritional Value of Meat

You need two to three daily servings from the meat and beans group of the Food Guide Pyramid. These servings should total only the equivalent of 5 to 7 ounces (140 to 190 g) of lean, cooked meat. All meat and meat products contain proteins essential for building and repairing tissue. Meats are also good sources of iron, phosphorus, copper, thiamin, riboflavin, and niacin.

The amount of fat meat contributes to the diet depends on the kind and quality of the meat. Ground meats are generally higher in fat than all other cuts. Fat gives meat flavor and appeal. However, experts recommend that people in the United States limit the percentage of calories they get from fats in their diet. These experts especially stress limiting saturated fats, which occur in larger amounts in meat cuts that are less lean.

Following a few tips can help you limit fat and enjoy meat as part of a healthful diet. Choose lean cuts, such as the round and loin sections of beef and the loin and leg sections of pork. Use cooking methods like broiling and grilling, which allow fat to drip away during cooking. Use nonstick pans when frying and browning meat to eliminate the need for added fat during cooking. Skim the fat from the surface of chilled meat soups and stocks.

Q: Shouldn't people who are trying to limit fat and cholesterol in their diets stop eating red meat?

A: Limiting fats and cholesterol does not mean you have to eliminate meat from your diet. However, you should limit portion sizes to three-ounce (85-g) cooked servings (four ounces, 113 g, of boneless raw meat). A three-ounce (85-g) serving is about the size of a deck of playing cards.

Beef

Beef comes from mature cattle over 12 months of age. It has a distinctive flavor and firm texture. Beef is usually bright, cherry red in color with creamy white fat.

Beef carcasses are classified according to age and sex. Animals sold for meat are most often steers and heifers. *Steers* are young, castrated males. *Heifers* are young females who have never had a calf.

Of all animals used for food, the beef carcass is the largest. The carcass first is cut lengthwise through the backbone into halves. The two halves are called *sides*. The sides are cut into *quarters* and then into smaller pieces, called ***wholesale cuts,*** for easier handling. Meat cutters divide the wholesale cuts into still smaller pieces, called ***retail cuts,*** at the grocery store.

Ground Beef

Some people incorrectly call ground beef, hamburger. *Ground beef* contains only the fat originally attached to the meat before grinding. *Hamburger* can have extra fat added to it during grinding. The fat content of neither ground beef nor hamburger can be more than 30 percent of the total weight. However, you can buy ground beef that is leaner. The label lists the percentage lean.

Veal

Veal is very young beef. It comes from cattle that are less than three months of age. Because the animals are so young, little fat has developed. Thus, most veal is lean. Veal also has quite a bit of connective tissue, but it is still considered to be tender. Veal has a light pink color and a delicate flavor. See 19-1.

A veal carcass is next to beef in size, but it is still much smaller. It does not require splitting for shipment. Because the wholesale cuts are smaller than beef, retail cuts differ somewhat. For example, the loin and rib sections of beef

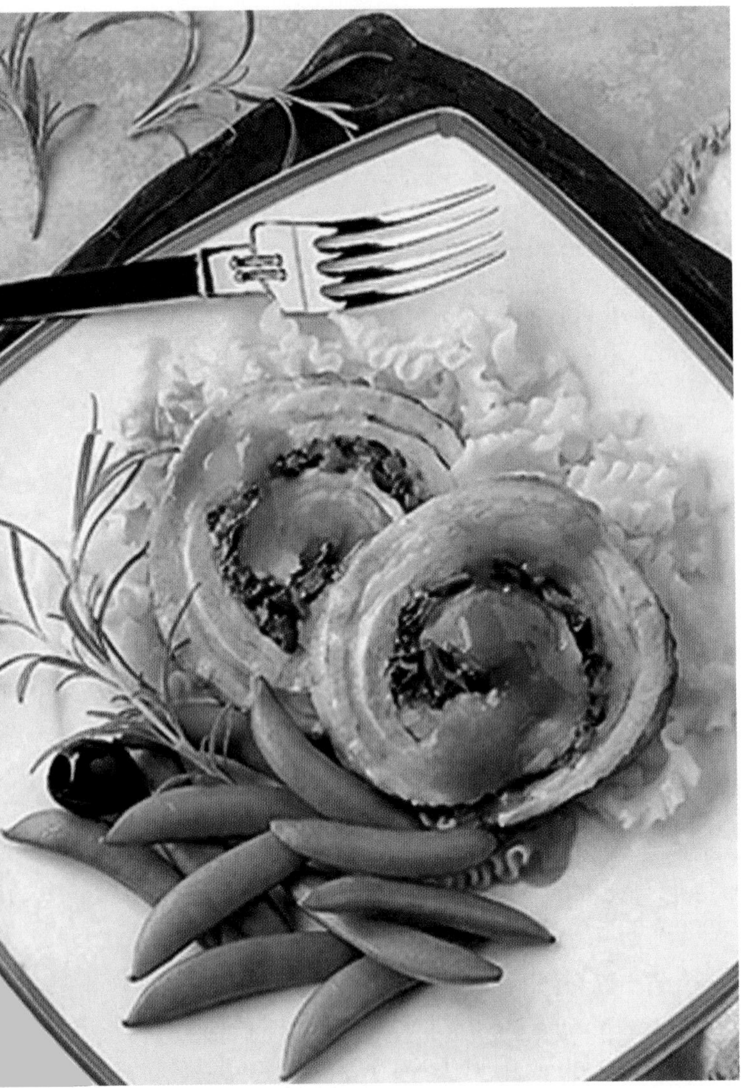

courtesy of National Cattlemen's Beef Association and Cattlemen's Beef Board

19-1 Lean, tender veal has a mild flavor that is enhanced by this olive-mushroom filling.

are used for steaks. Those of veal are used for chops.

Pork

Pork is the meat of swine. Most pork comes from animals that are 7 to 12 months old. Because the animals are so young, most pork is tender. The meat is grayish-pink to light rose in color.

The pork carcass is small enough to be shipped whole, but it is usually split. Pork can be fresh cured or smoked.

Meat packing plants process many pork products. *Ham* comes from the pork leg. It is cured and usually smoked. You can purchase fully cooked canned hams. You can also buy hams that require cooking, which may or may not include the skin and bone. *Bacon* is smoked pork belly meat. You can buy it as a slab, which you slice yourself, or as precut slices. *Canadian bacon* is made from boneless pork loins.

Lamb

Lamb is the meat of sheep less than one year old. It is tender with a delicate flavor. Fresh lamb is pinkish-red in color with white fat. Older animals are marketed as *yearling lamb* (one to two years of age) and *mutton* (over two years of age). Retail outlets do not sell much mutton. It has a stronger flavor than lamb and is less tender.

Lamb is the smallest animal used for meat. Lamb carcasses can be shipped whole. Lamb cuts are similar to veal cuts, but they are smaller in size.

Variety Meats

Variety meats are the edible parts of the animal other than the muscles. Liver, heart, kidney, tongue, and *sweetbreads* (thymus glands) are popular variety meats. Other variety meats include beef *tripe* (stomach lining); brains; *chitterlings* (cleaned intestines); and pork jowls, tail, feet, ears, and snout. Variety meats are usually inexpensive and are rich sources of many vitamins and minerals. For instance, liver is very high in iron.

Inspection and Grading of Meat

Federal inspectors must examine all meat and meat products shipped across state lines. They inspect both the live animal and the carcass. A round purple inspection stamp is placed on all wholesale cuts to indicate the meat is wholesome. This stamp also assures buyers the plant and processing conditions were sanitary. State-supported programs handle the inspection of meat processed and sold within a state.

Animal carcasses may be voluntarily graded for yield and quality. *Yield grades* help wholesalers identify which carcasses will produce the most edible meat per pound. *Quality grades* assure consumers meat has met set standards that predict taste appeal. The USDA oversees the grading program, 19-2.

Quality grades for beef are based on marbling, maturity, texture, and appearance.

Marbling refers to the flecks of fat throughout the lean. Cuts with more marbling are juicy, flavorful, and tender. Higher quality grades go to cuts with more marbling and fine muscle texture. Meat from younger animals that has characteristic color also qualifies for higher quality grades.

The most common grades of beef sold in retail stores are Choice and Select. *Choice meats* are high quality with good marbling. *Select meats* are leaner than Choice meats, and they usually cost less. Restaurants and hotels often offer *Prime meats* on their menus. Prime cuts have received the highest grade.

The standards used for grading veal, pork, and lamb differ somewhat from those used to grade beef. However, the highest grades are given to carcasses that are expected to provide the tastiest meat.

Selecting Meat

Meats are costly food items. Learning how to judge quality factors and identify meat cuts can help you make wise purchases.

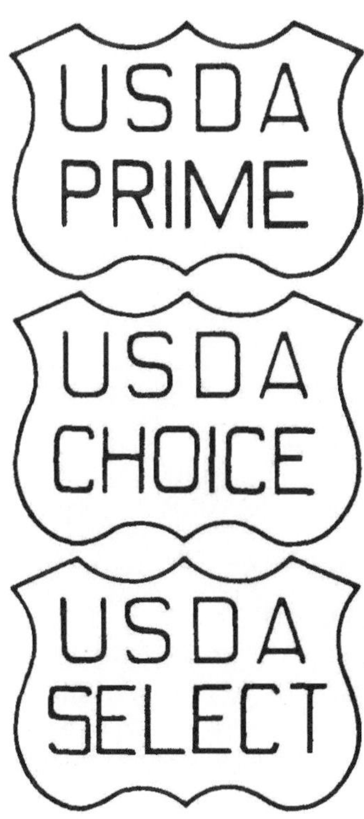

19-2 The USDA grade shield assures consumers meat has met certain standards of quality.

Characteristics of the Fat

Color, firmness, and location of fat affect meat quality. Quality meats will have firm to medium-firm, creamy white fat. Fat that is yellow and coarse is a sign of poor quality.

Marbling indicates tenderness in a cut of meat. Although more marbling means more tenderness, it also means more total fat, saturated fat, cholesterol, and calories. Cooking can tenderize cuts with less marbling. Therefore, to follow the Dietary Guidelines, you should choose leaner cuts most often. Save cuts with more marbling for special occasions.

Location of the Meat in the Animal

Bone shapes can tell you the part of an animal from which meat was cut. Cuts from an animal's short loin, or back, region have T-shaped bones. Flat bones and wedge bones are cross sections of hip bones. Round bones appear in arm and leg cuts. Blade bones come in cuts from the shoulder area of an animal.

The location of muscle tissue in an animal indicates the tenderness of the meat cut the tissue becomes. Rib and loin muscles are quite tender because they lie along the backbone where they receive little exercise. Leg and shoulder muscles are less tender because the animal uses them more. See 19-3.

The tenderness of a meat cut gives you a clue about how to cook it. You can cook tender cuts of meat by dry heat methods, such as broiling or roasting. You can identify these cuts by a T-bone, rib bone, flat bone, or wedge bone. Sirloin and porterhouse steaks, pork and lamb loin chops, and beef and pork rib roasts are examples of tender cuts of meat. Lamb and pork cuts with leg bones are also tender enough to cook with dry heat.

You may prefer to cook less tender cuts of meat by moist heat methods, such as stewing or braising. All cuts containing a blade bone, arm bone, or breast bone are less tender cuts of meat. Beef cuts with a leg bone are also less tender. Examples of these cuts include round steak, rump roast, and shoulder steak.

Meat Labeling

To help consumers with meat selection, most retail stores follow a labeling system. Meat

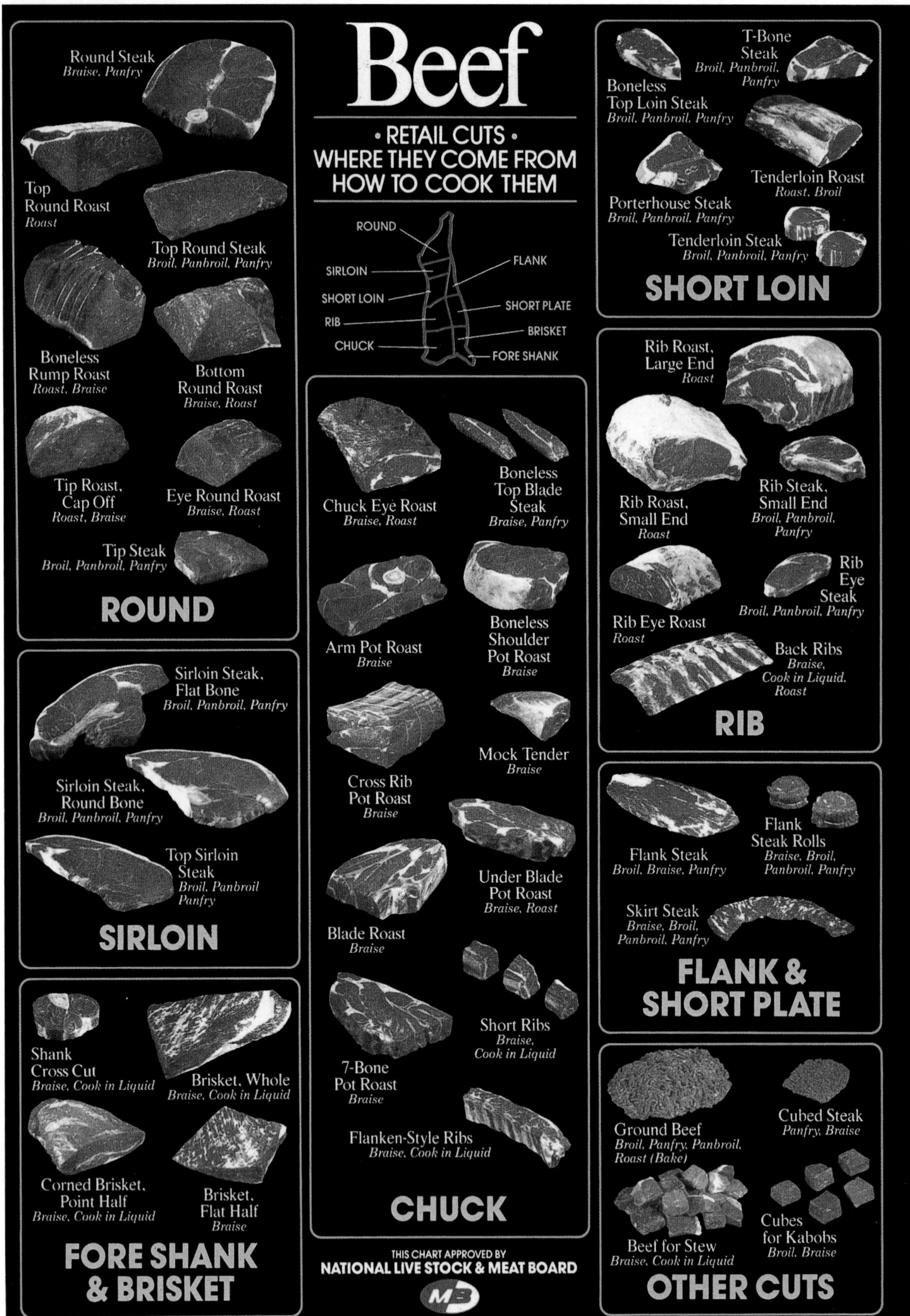

courtesy of National Cattlemen's Beef Association and Cattlemen's Beef Board

19-3 The part of the animal from which meat comes indicates how tender the meat is and how to cook it.

Q: Isn't eating a high-protein diet that includes a lot of meat a good way to build muscle tissue?

A: Amino acids from proteins are needed to build muscle tissue. However, eating more protein will not make your muscles bigger. Eating a diet that contains too much meat may supply excess calories and fat, which could lead to weight gain. Excess protein in the diet can also put a strain on the kidneys and may increase calcium loss from bone tissue.

names on labels follow a three-part format. The kind of meat appears first. This might be *beef.* Next is the name of the wholesale cut. It tells you the part of the animal from which the cut came. *Chuck* is an example of a beef wholesale cut. Third is the name of the retail cut. It tells you from what part of the wholesale cut the meat comes. A *shoulder roast* is an example of a beef retail cut. Using this system, the cut described would be a *Beef Chuck Shoulder Roast.* See 19-4.

The label also lists the net weight of the meat, the price per pound (kilogram), and the price you pay. This information lets you comparison shop more easily.

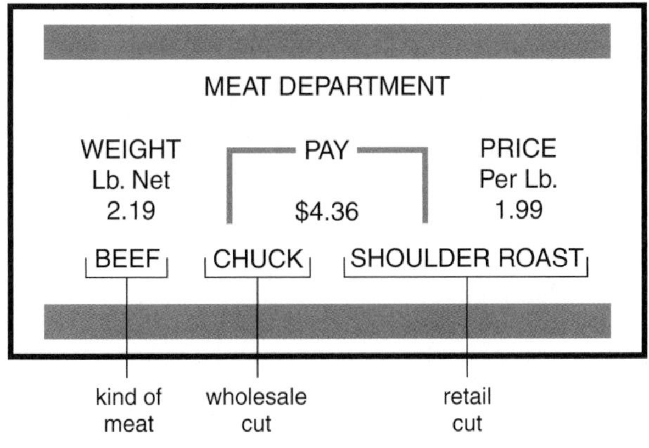

19-4 Standard three-part names on meat labels help consumers identify cuts.

Deciding How Much Meat to Buy

The amount of meat you need to buy depends on several factors. The number of people you will serve and the amount of bone in the meat will affect your purchase. You will also have to keep in mind whether or not you want to have leftovers.

All meat is sold by the pound (kilogram). You need to know how many people 1 pound (0.45 kg) of meat will serve. Boneless meat will serve more people per pound (0.45 kg) than meat with bones. See 19-5.

To determine how much to buy, multiply the amount of meat per serving by the number of people being served. Then add the amount of leftover meat you plan to serve later.

Cost of Meat per Serving

The cost per serving of meat depends partly on the tenderness of the meat. Usually, tender cuts cost more than less tender cuts. That is why sirloin steak costs more than round steak.

The amount of waste in a meat cut also affects the cost per serving. Meat with bones often is priced lower per pound (0.45 kg) than boneless cuts. For example, a bone-in rump roast usually costs less per pound (0.45 kg) than a boneless rump roast.

Meat extenders like dried beans and rice can stretch meat dollars. For instance, ham will go farther when mixed with nutritious navy beans than when served alone.

Storing Meat

Store sausage and fresh, cured and smoked, and ready-to-serve meats (cold cuts) in the refrigerator for use within a few days. You

Meat Purchasing Guide

Amount of Bone	Amount to Buy per Serving
Boneless	1/4 to 1/3 lb (115 to 150 g)
Small bone	1/3 to 1/2 lb (150 to 225 g)
Many bones	1/2 to 3/4 lb (225 to 340 g)

19-5 Use this chart as a rough guide when determining how much meat to buy per serving.

should also refrigerate canned hams until ready for use unless the label says otherwise. Store meats in the meat storage compartment or the coldest part of the refrigerator. The temperature of the refrigerator should be 40°F (5°C) or lower. You can refrigerate prepackaged meats in their original wrappers. After cooking meats, store them in a tightly covered container in the refrigerator.

Freeze meats for longer storage. (You should not freeze canned hams.) The temperature in the freezer should remain at 0°F (-18°C) or colder for maximum keeping quality. To store meats in the freezer, you should rewrap them in moistureproof and vaporproof paper. Label each package with the date and the name and weight of the cut. Be sure to use meats within recommended storage times. See 19-6.

Food Science Principles of Cooking Meat

Cooking meat destroys harmful bacteria that can be present in raw meat. Cooking improves meat's flavor and makes it easier to digest. Cooking also makes some meats more tender.

Remember that meat consists of muscle tissue, connective tissue, fat, and bone. Connective tissue holds together fibers in the muscle tissues. The connective tissue contains two proteins: elastin and collagen. ***Elastin*** is very tough and elastic, and cooking cannot soften it. ***Collagen*** is also tough and elastic, but cooking can soften and tenderize it.

Some meat cuts have more collagen than others. Meat cuts with little collagen are tender. Cuts with a lot of collagen are less tender.

You can use certain food preparation techniques to break down connective tissue in meat before cooking. Elastin can be broken down mechanically or chemically. Pounding, sometimes done to round steak, and grinding, done to ground beef, are two mechanical methods of breaking down elastin. Commercial meat tenderizers can soften collagen chemically. These products contain enzymes that break down the tissue. Marinating meat can also soften collagen chemically. Marinating involves soaking meat in a solution called a *marinade*. The marinade contains an acid, such as vinegar or tomato juice, that helps tenderize the connective tissue. See 19-7.

Storage Times for Meat	
Refrigerated Storage	
Type of Meat	**Time**
Fresh meat cuts	3-4 days
Ground meats	1-2 days
Variety meats	1-2 days
Leftover cooked meats	3 days
Freezer Storage	
Luncheon meats, hot dogs	2 months
Ham	2 months
Ground meats	3 months
Pork cuts	6 months
Lamb	9 months
Beef	12 months

19-6 *Keep fresh meat safe to eat by cooking or freezing it within a few days of purchase. Date frozen meat and use it within recommended storage times for best quality.*

During cooking, heat ***coagulates*** (thickens into a mass) the proteins in the muscle fibers. It also softens the collagen in the connective tissue. You need low temperatures and careful timing when cooking meats. Cooking meats at too high a temperature or for too long a time will make them tough and dry. (Meat cuts cooked in liquid will fall apart.) This is due to overcoagulation of the proteins.

Be a Clever Consumer

Compare meat prices on a cost per serving basis. Sometimes you will find more costly boneless cuts are a better buy. Boneless pork chops may cost $3.99 a pound ($8.78 a kg), while center cut chops cost $3.29 a pound ($7.24 a kg). A pound of boneless chops will give you about four servings at $1.00 a serving. A pound of center cut chops will give you only two and a half servings at $1.32 a serving. Although the center cut chops cost less per pound, much of what you are buying is inedible bone. Therefore, the center cut chops end up costing $.32 a serving more than the boneless chops.

Controlling Temperature When Cooking Meat

Temperature control is a key principle to follow when cooking meat. You need to note the cooking temperature and the internal temperature of the meat.

Using too high a cooking temperature can result in excessive cooking losses. ***Cooking losses*** include fat, water, and other volatile (easily vaporized) substances that evaporate from the surface of the meat. Some of the cooking losses are retained in the pan drippings or cooking liquid. However, loss of these substances causes meat to shrink during cooking, decreasing in size and weight.

Cooking losses are important because they can affect the appearance and eating quality of meat. Meat cooked at too high a temperature can develop a hard crust. This can make carving and eating difficult. Excessive cooking losses can also cause meat to be tough and dry.

Cooking losses can even affect the number of servings meat will provide. For instance, you can expect a 6-pound (2.6 kg) bone-in roast to provide about 15 servings. However, excessive cooking losses could reduce the number of servings by two or more.

Low temperatures will keep cooking losses to a minimum. Meat will be juicier, more flavorful, and easier to carve. Cleanup will be easier because less fat will have spattered on the oven walls or burned onto the pan. Although low cooking temperatures have these pluses, you should not cook meat at temperatures below 325°F (165°C). Temperatures lower than this may allow bacteria to grow before meat has finished cooking.

The second type of temperature you need to be aware of when cooking meat is the internal temperature of the meat. The type of meat and the desired degree of doneness determine the correct internal temperature. Overcooked meat is cooked to an internal temperature that is too high. Such meat has more cooking losses than meat cooked to the correct temperature. See 19-8.

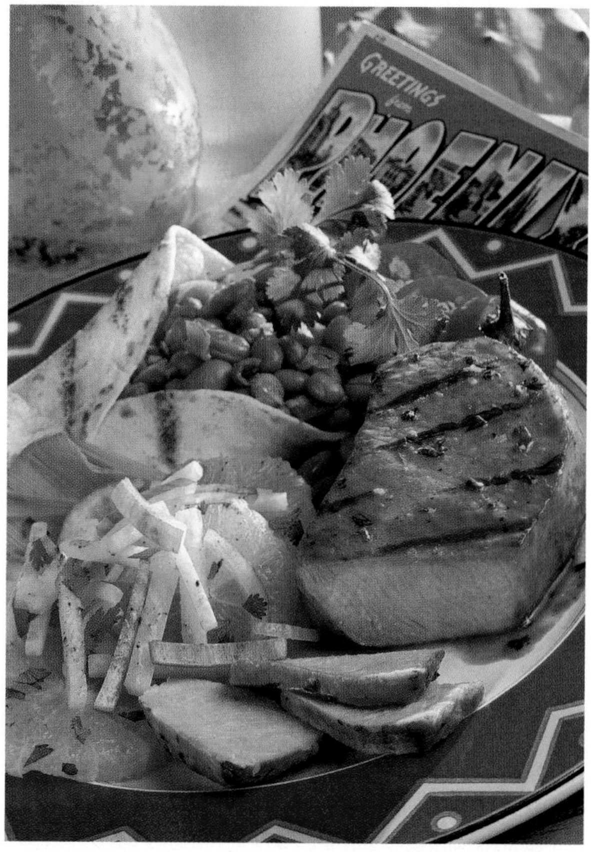

courtesy of National Pork Board

19-7 Besides softening connective tissue, marinades have the advantage of adding flavor to meat dishes.

Recommended Internal Temperatures for Meat	
Medium rare	145°F (65°C)
Medium	160°F (70°C)
Well done	170°F (75°C)

19-8 Meat is moist and flavorful when it has been cooked to the recommended temperature.

The only accurate way to determine the internal temperature of meat is to use a meat thermometer. Insert the thermometer into the thickest part of the muscle. Make sure the probe is not touching bone, fat, or gristle. Check the temperature of uneven cuts in several places. Insert the probe sideways into thin cuts, such as chops and meat patties.

Preventing foodborne illness is also a key reason to be aware of internal temperatures when cooking meat. Thorough cooking kills harmful bacteria. You cannot rely on the color of cooked meat to tell you if the meat has reached a safe internal temperature.

Controlling Time When Cooking Meat

The total time you cook a cut of meat affects its appearance and eating quality just as temperature does. Several factors affect cooking time.

One factor that affects cooking time is cooking temperature. Higher temperatures result in shorter cooking times. Lower temperatures result in longer cooking times. Changing the cooking temperature by just a few degrees can affect cooking time. For instance, suppose you are broiling a steak and open the broiler door every few minutes to check it. Each time you open the door, cool air enters the broiler compartment. This reduces the cooking temperature and will cause the steak to take longer to cook.

The size and shape of the cut of meat are factors that affect cooking time. Large cuts of meat need longer cooking times than small cuts. However, large cuts take fewer minutes *per pound* to cook than small cuts. A rolled rib roast will take longer to cook than a standing rib roast because the meat is more compact.

The desired degree of doneness is another factor that affects cooking time. The cooking time for rare beef is less than for well-done beef. The more well done the meat is to be, the longer it will take to cook.

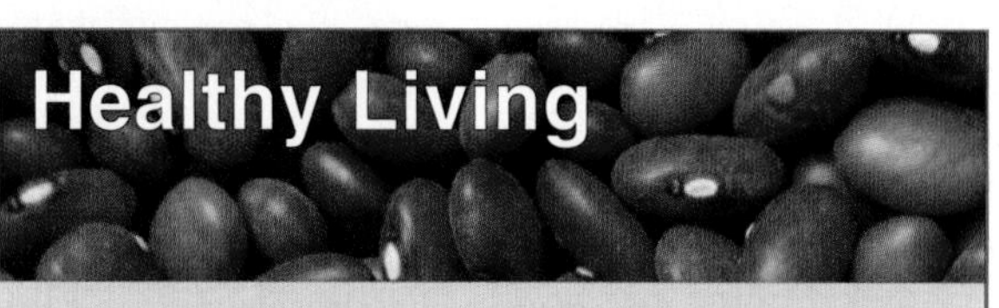

One of the most significant ways you can reduce the fat content of meats is to trim all visible fat. This can reduce the total fat content by about 50 percent. Trimming meat before cooking results in the greatest fat reduction. This prevents fat from melting into the meat during cooking.

Methods of Cooking Meat

You can use variations of six methods for cooking meat: roasting, broiling, panbroiling, frying, braising, and cooking in liquid. Consider the tenderness of the meat and its size and thickness as well as your taste preferences when choosing a cooking method. Roasting, broiling, grilling, panbroiling, and frying are *dry cooking methods*. Use them for tender cuts of meat, such as steaks and rib roasts. Braising and cooking in liquid are *moist cooking methods*. Use them for less tender cuts of meat, such as chuck roasts and corned beef brisket.

Cooking Meat Safely

Meats are often identified as the source of bacteria that cause foodborne illness. Most cases of foodborne illness result from improper food handling. Using care when buying, storing, cooking, serving, and reheating foods will help you avoid illness. Review the food handling precautions outlined in Chapter 6. In addition, be aware of the following guidelines when cooking meat:

- Store meats at or below 40°F (5°C).
- Cook or freeze refrigerated meats within recommended time frames (1 to 2 days for ground meats, 3 to 4 days for nonground products, 3 days for leftovers).
- Wash your hands for 20 seconds with hot, soapy water before you begin cooking. Wash hands again after handling raw meat.
- Thoroughly wash cutting boards and utensils used for raw meat before using them to prepare raw vegetables or cooked meat.

- Marinate meat in the refrigerator, not at room temperature.
- Discard marinade used for raw meat, or bring it to a rolling boil for 1 minute before using it on cooked meat.
- Brush sauces only on cooked surfaces of meat.
- Do not set the oven below 325°F (165°C) when cooking meats.
- Use a thermometer to make sure meat has reached a safe internal temperature. Cook ground meats to an internal temperature of 160°F (70°C) and nonground products to at least 145°F (65°C). See 19-9.
- Reheat leftover meats to an internal temperature of 165°F (75°C).
- Be sure to wash the probe of your meat thermometer in hot, soapy water after each use. Do not reinsert a dirty thermometer into a food or use it to check another food.

Roasting Meat

Roasting is recommended for large, tender cuts of meat. For best results when roasting, place meat with the fat side up on a rack in a large, shallow pan. The fat bastes the meat during cooking, and the rack holds the meat out of the drippings. Season meat with salt and pepper, if desired. Insert a meat thermometer into the thickest part of the muscle, without having the tip touching bone or fat. Roast the meat in a slow oven (325°F to 350°F, 165°C to 180°C), uncovered, until it reaches the desired degree of doneness. (Roast smaller cuts of meat at the higher temperature and larger cuts at the lower temperature.)

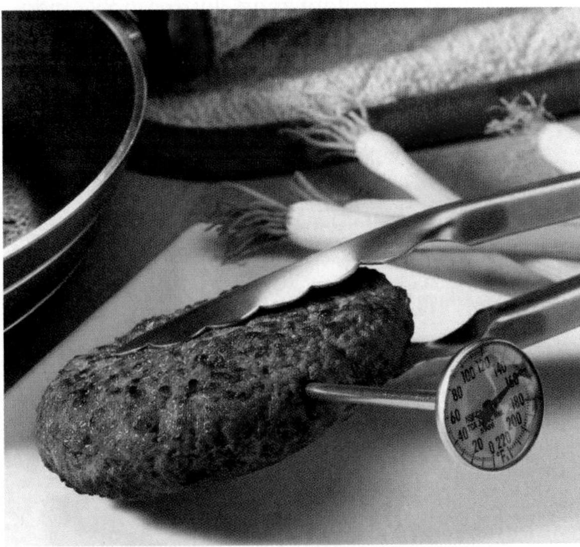

courtesy of National Cattlemen's Beef Association and Cattlemen's Beef Board

***19-9** Insert an instant-read thermometer into the side of a ground meat patty to be sure the meat has reached the safe temperature of 160°F (70°C).*

Allowing a roast to stand for 10 to 15 minutes after taking it from the oven makes it easier to carve. As the roast stands, it will continue to cook. For this reason, you should take the roast from the oven when it is about 5°F (3°C) below the desired internal temperature.

Broiling Meat

You can broil tender beefsteaks, lamb and pork chops, ham slices, ground beef, and ground lamb. Steaks and chops that are too thin will dry out before they are thoroughly cooked. Therefore, these cuts should be at least ¾ inch (2.3 cm) thick for broiling. Ham slices should be at least ½ inch (1.5 cm) thick.

Broiling is done under a direct flame in gas broilers and under the direct heating element in electric broilers. The closer the meat is to the heat source, the shorter the cooking time will be. Place thick cuts of meat farther away from the heat than thin cuts. Place pork far enough away so the meat will not dry out before it is thoroughly cooked. See 19-10.

For best results when broiling meat, place meat on a cold broiler pan. Adjust the broiler rack to the desired distance from the heat source. Broil the top side of the meat until it is brown. (It should be about half cooked at this point.) Turn the meat and season if desired. (You should not salt meats before broiling because salt draws juices from the meat. You should not salt cured meats at all.) Broil the second side until brown.

Time charts can help you determine the correct cooking time when broiling. They are available in basic cookbooks. Use an instant-read thermometer to check the internal temperature of the meat toward the end of the broiling time. This will help you evaluate the degree of doneness. It will also assure you the meat has reached a safe internal temperature. You should cook pork chops and ground meats to the well-done stage.

Grilling Meat

You can successfully grill the same cuts of meat you use for broiling. Indirect grilling is recommended as the most healthful grilling method. For indirect grilling, move hot coals to the sides of the grill. To grill meat indirectly on a gas grill, turn off the central gas burners after preheating the grill. Place seasoned meat in the center of the grill and cover the grill until the meat is done. Because heat surrounds the meat in the covered grill, there is no need to turn the meat. (You will read more about how to set up a grill and prepare coals for cooking in Chapter 25.)

Grill meat for the correct amount of time needed for the particular cut you are cooking. A grilling time chart in a cookbook or the use and care manual for your grill will help you determine cooking times.

To enjoy grilled meats as part of a healthful diet, cut any charred surfaces from meat before eating it. Consider partially precooking meats in a microwave oven immediately before placing them on the grill to reduce grilling time. Also, try wrapping meats in foil for grilling to avoid exposing them to direct flames.

Play It Safe

Many reported cases of foodborne illness caused by E. coli bacteria have been traced to undercooked ground beef. Thorough cooking will kill these bacteria. Therefore, when you broil burgers, or cook them by any other method, check them with a food thermometer. Make sure they have reached an internal temperature of 160°F (70°C).

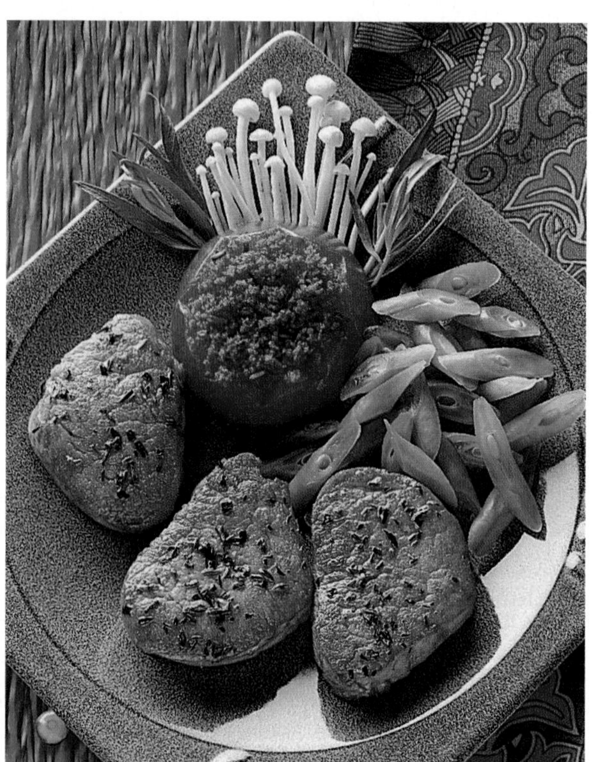

courtesy of National Pork Board

19-10 These ½-inch thick pork tenderloin medallions are cooked just 5 to 6 inches from the direct heat of the broiler.

Panbroiling Meat

Meat cuts that you can broil you can also panbroil if they are 1 inch (2.5 cm) thick or less. Panbroiling is a good method to use when preparing small quantities of meat. It can save energy and cleanup time when cooking just one or two steaks or chops.

For best results when panbroiling, place the meat in a heavy skillet or griddle. Do not cover the pan or add fat. (If the meat is very lean, you might want to lightly brush the skillet with fat to prevent sticking.) Cook the meat slowly, turning it occasionally to ensure even cooking. Pour off any fat that accumulates. Panbroiled meats need only about half the cooking time of broiled meats. Insert an instant-read thermometer sideways into steaks and chops to be sure they have reached the correct internal temperature.

Q: Do grilled meats cause cancer?

A: Research suggests the high heat used in grilling and broiling can allow cancer-causing compounds to form on meat. Meat juices that drip onto hot coals and cause smoke and flare-ups increase the formation of cancer-causing agents. Marinate meat, limit grilling time, and use indirect heat. These steps can greatly help reduce the formation of harmful substances.

Frying Meat

Most fried meats are prepared by panfrying, or sauteing. A few can be deep-fried. Panfry meats in a small amount of fat. You may add this fat before cooking, or it may accumulate during cooking. You can panfry fairly thin pieces of tender meat, tenderized meat, ground meat patties, or cooked meat slices.

For best results when panfrying, brown meat on both sides in a small amount of fat. Season meat after browning or add the seasonings to the breading if you bread the meat. Cook the meat uncovered at a moderate temperature, turning occasionally until done. If the temperature is too high, the fat will smoke, and the meat will burn on the outside before the inside is cooked.

A variation of panfrying is *stir-frying.* Stir-fried meats and vegetables are often served together in Asian dishes. Cook thinly sliced meat in a small amount of oil. Use a wok or frying pan. Cook the meat over high heat and stir it constantly until done.

Braising Meat

Braising is cooking in a small amount of liquid in a tightly covered pan over low heat. You can braise less tender meat cuts and tender cuts of pork and veal. You can braise in the oven or on the surface unit of a range. See 19-11.

For best results when braising, first brown meat slowly on all sides in a small amount of fat. (If the meat has sufficient fat, you will not need additional fat.) Browning adds flavor and color. Season browned meat if desired and add a *small* amount of liquid. You can use water, broth, tomato juice, or a flavorful sauce as the braising liquid. Cover the pan tightly, and cook the meat slowly until tender. (Gently simmer braised meat. The cooking liquid should never boil.) You can thicken the juices that accumulate during cooking and make them into gravy. They contain important vitamins and minerals.

Cooking Meat in Liquid

Unlike braising, when cooking meats in liquid, you cover them with the cooking liquid. Use this method for less tender cuts of meat. When used with whole cuts of meat, this method is called *simmering.* Many people simmer corned beef brisket. When small pieces of meat are cooked in liquid, this method is called *stewing.*

For best results when cooking in liquid, cover the meat entirely with water or stock. This ensures even cooking. Season cooking liquid with salt, pepper, and herbs, if desired. Cover the kettle and simmer until the meat is tender. (Cooking time will vary depending on the meat being cooked. When using this method, you will cook most meat cuts two hours or more.) The cooking liquid should never boil. Boiling can cause meat to shrink and become dry.

If preparing a stew by this method, cut the meat into cubes of uniform size, about 1 to 2 inches (2.5 to 5 cm). Brown the cubes in a small amount of fat, if desired. Cover the meat cubes with liquid and stew until tender. You may add vegetables to the meat later, allowing them to cook just long enough to become tender. Before serving, you can transfer the meat and vegetables to a warm serving platter and thicken the cooking liquid.

Microwaving Meat

Meats cooked in a microwave oven come out flavorful and juicy in a fraction of the time required for conventional cooking. Covering meats in a microwave oven holds in steam. This keeps meats moist and tender and shortens cooking time even further. Remember that microwave cooking time increases as the quantity of food increases. Therefore, large, dense cuts of meat may cook more efficiently in a conventional oven.

You can cook any meat satisfactorily in a microwave oven. However, tender, boneless cuts of uniform shape work best.

Arranging meats will promote even cooking in a microwave oven. Arrange uniformly shaped meat, such as meat patties and sausage links, in a circle. (Remember to pierce the skin on products like sausage to allow steam to escape and prevent bursting.) Overlap sliced meats, such as fully cooked ham or roast beef. Form ground meat into a doughnut-shaped loaf with a hole in the center. Place cuts containing bone with the meatier portions to the outside of the dish. Shield projections and edges on uneven cuts with small pieces of aluminum foil to prevent overcooking. Rotating, turning, and rearranging meats during the cooking period will also help them microwave more evenly.

Large cuts and meat with a high fat content will brown naturally in a microwave oven. However, cuts requiring less time may need the help of a browning agent. You can collect meat drippings by using a rack. You can add these to a gravy mix or browning sauce to cover the meat. Other browning agents include soy, barbecue, and Worcestershire sauces. Sauces have the added advantage of keeping meat moist in the microwave oven. See 19-12.

Cooking Variety Meats

The cooking method used for preparing variety meats depends on the tenderness of each meat. You will cook most variety meats by moist heat. However, you may cook brains, sweetbreads, and the liver and kidneys of veal and calf by dry heat, usually by broiling or frying.

Brains and sweetbreads are very delicate meats. To retain their shape, precook them for

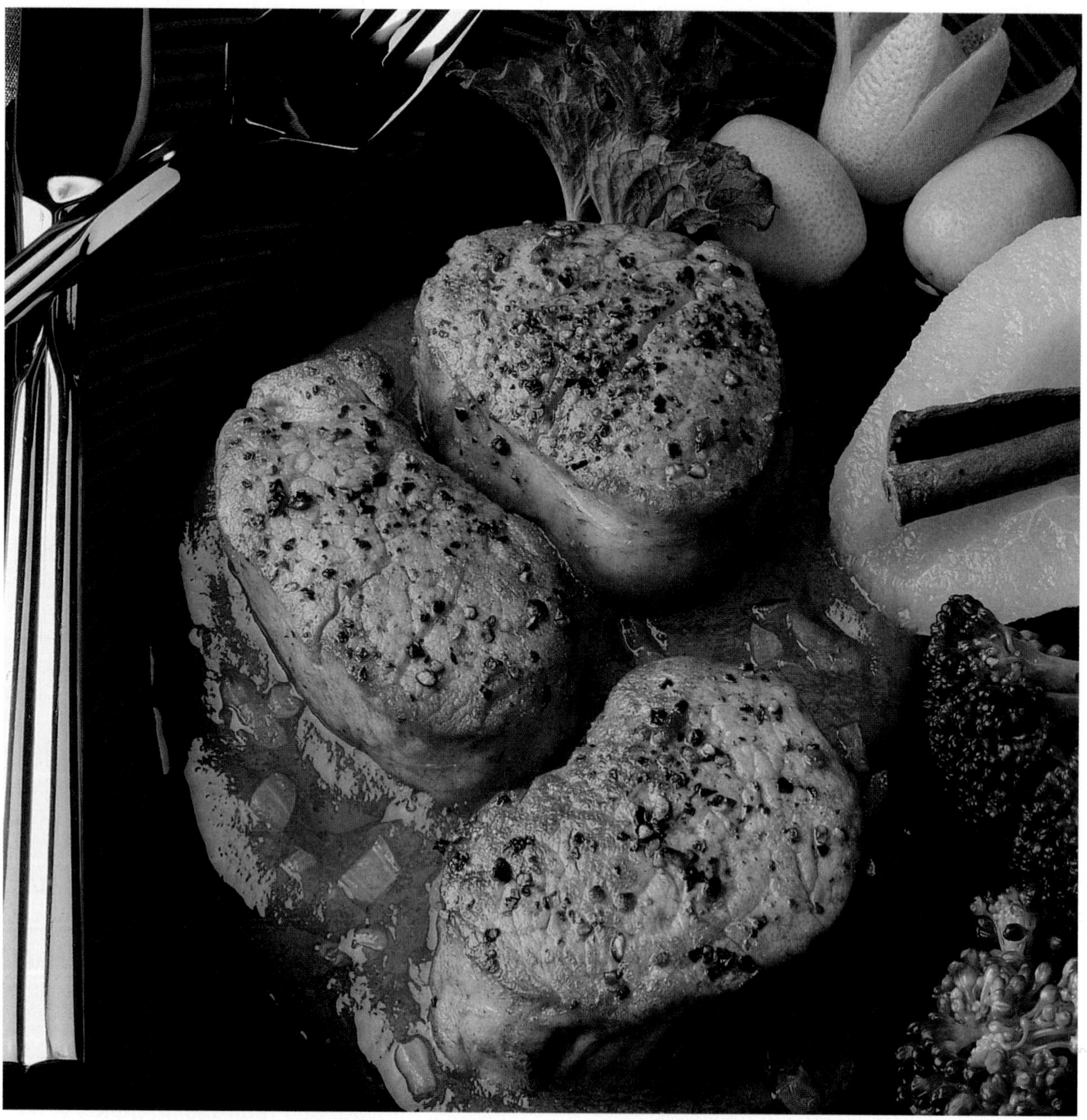

courtesy of National Pork Board

19-11 *These pork medallions braise on top of the range in a matter of minutes.*

about 20 minutes in salted, *acidulated* water (water that contains an acid, such as lemon juice). After precooking, you might choose to fry or broil them.

Cooking Frozen Meat

You can cook frozen meats in the frozen state or defrost them before cooking. Cook prepared frozen meats according to package directions.

For safety, thaw meat in its original wrapper in the refrigerator. Do not thaw meat on the kitchen counter. Harmful microorganisms can grow in meat thawed at room temperature, resulting in foodborne illness.

You must cook frozen meat longer than thawed meat. A frozen roast will need to cook about 50 percent longer than a thawed roast. Cooking time for frozen steaks and chops will vary depending on size and thickness.

When broiling frozen meats, place meat farther away from the heat source. This will prevent the outside from overcooking before the inside is cooked. To panbroil frozen meat, use a hot skillet to brown the meat. Then lower the heat and turn meat occasionally to ensure even cooking.

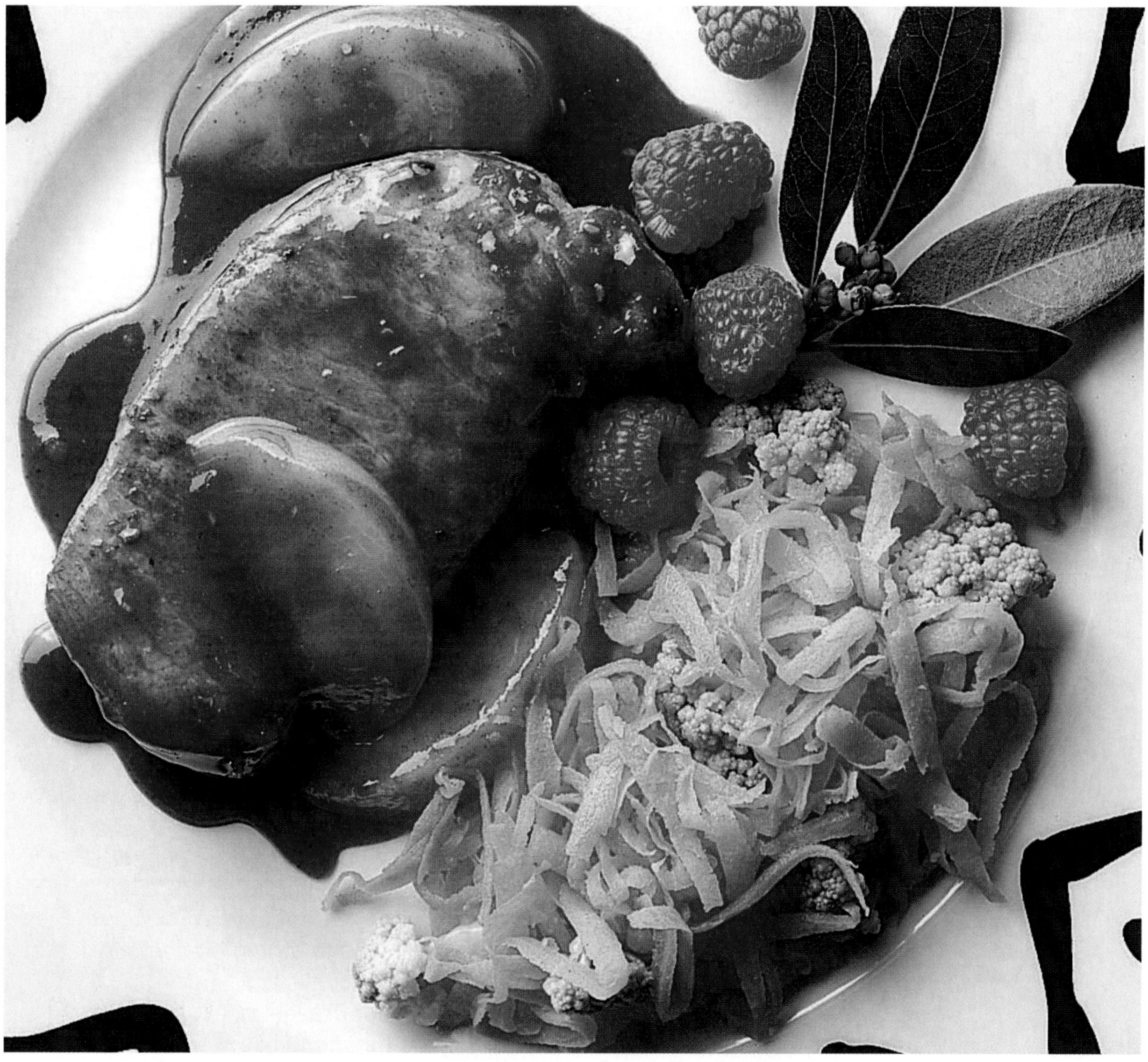

courtesy of National Pork Board

19-12 *Serving a sauce with meat cooked in a microwave will help hide the lack of browning.*

Chapter 19 Review
Meat

Summary

Beef, veal, pork, and lamb are the most commonly eaten types of meat in the United States. They are all high in protein as well as being good sources of several vitamins and minerals.

Meat is inspected for wholesomeness and may be graded for quality. When selecting meat, the appearance of the fat is a sign of quality. Read the label to identify the part of the animal from which the meat comes. This indicates tenderness. When deciding how much meat to buy, remember boneless cuts yield more servings per pound than bone-in cuts. Compare meats in terms of cost per serving rather than cost per pound to get the best buy.

Meats are highly perishable. Store them in the coldest part of the refrigerator and use them within a few days. Wrap them well and put them in the freezer for longer storage.

The connective tissue in meat contains two types of tough, elastic protein. One of these, collagen, can be broken down by mechanical and chemical methods and softened by cooking.

Meats cooked at lower temperatures, large cuts, and well-done meats all require longer cooking times. However, you need to monitor cooking times and temperatures carefully. Temperatures that are too high or cooking times that are too long can make meat tough and dry.

Roasting, broiling, grilling, panbroiling, and frying are dry heat cooking methods. They generally work best for tender cuts of meat. Braising and stewing are moist heat cooking methods. They are recommended for less tender cuts. You can use a microwave oven to defrost and cook meats. You can cook frozen meats in the frozen state or defrost them in the refrigerator before cooking.

Review What You Have Read

Write your answers on a separate sheet of paper.

1. List five nutrients contributed to the diet by meat.
2. Give three tips for selecting and preparing meat to help limit the amount of fat supplied by meat in the diet.
3. Describe the color and fat of high-quality beef.
4. True or false. Hamburger is another name for ground beef.
5. Meat from cattle that are less than three months of age is called _____.
   A. beef
   B. lamb
   C. pork
   D. veal
6. What are the most common grades of beef sold in retail stores?
7. How does the location of the meat in the animal affect the tenderness of a cut?
8. Name two factors that affect the cost per serving of meat.
9. Within what time period should refrigerated fresh meats be used?
10. The tough and elastic meat protein that can be softened and tenderized by cooking is _____.
11. List three characteristics of overcooked meat. List three characteristics of meat cooked to the proper degree of doneness.
12. What are cooking losses and how can they affect the appearance and eating quality of meat?
13. List the seven cooking methods used for meats. After each method, state if it is a moist or dry heat method.
14. Give three tips to promote even cooking of meats in a microwave oven.
15. True or false. Frozen meats must be defrosted before cooking.

Build Your Basic Skills

1. **Writing.** Look at the different cuts of meat in the meat case in a grocery store. Compare the appearance of beef, veal, pork, and lamb. Notice what variety meats are available. Compare the appearance of different grades of meat. Summarize your findings in a brief written report.
2. **Math.** Figure the cost per serving of a boneless cut and a bone-in cut. Which is the better buy?
3. **Verbal.** Discuss different ways to cook less tender cuts to make them more tender and flavorful.

Build Your Thinking Skills

1. **Analyze.** Prepare two identical tender cuts of beef, cooking one with high heat and the other with moderate heat. Compare appearance, flavor, and tenderness to help you analyze the effects of high cooking temperatures on meat.
2. **Describe.** Select one steak labeled *Choice* and one labeled *Select.* Broil both the same length of time. Sample the steaks and describe the tenderness, appearance, and juiciness of each steak.
3. **Compare.** Purchase two cuts of less tender beef. Cook one with dry heat and the other with moist heat. Compare appearance, texture, and flavor.
4. **Evaluate.** Prepare two identical cuts of meat, cooking one in a conventional oven and one in a microwave oven. Compare cooking times, appearance, flavor, tenderness, and juiciness as you evaluate which preparation method you prefer.

Apply Technology

1. Broil a ground beef patty and a patty made of texturized vegetable protein. Compare the two products for appearance, texture, and flavor.
2. Investigate how ultrasound technology is being used to inspect and grade meat.

Using Workplace Skills

Kevin is a meat cutter at DeLong's Grocery Store. The store is known for its hand-trimmed, cut-to-order meats. Kevin always has a steady stream of customers, but the meat department is especially busy just before holidays.

To be an effective worker, Kevin needs competence in serving customers. Imagine you are one of Kevin's customers. Answer the following questions about his need for and use of this skill:

A. What personality characteristics would you expect Kevin to have?
B. How would you respond if you felt Kevin was not providing you with adequate service?
C. How might DeLong's Grocery Store be affected if Kevin lacked competence in serving customers?
D. What is another skill Kevin would need in this job? Briefly explain why this skill would be important.

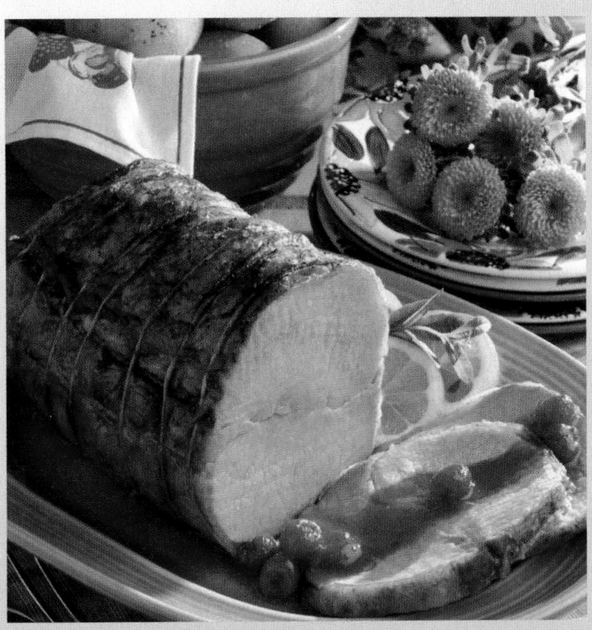

Chapter 20
Poultry

Poultry Farmer
Raises poultry to produce eggs and meat.

Poultry Boner
Cuts, scrapes, and pulls meat from cooked poultry carcasses using fingers and boning knife.

Wholesale Poultry Feed Products Sales Representative
Sells poultry feed products to farmers and retail establishments. Suggests feed changes to improve breeding of fowl.

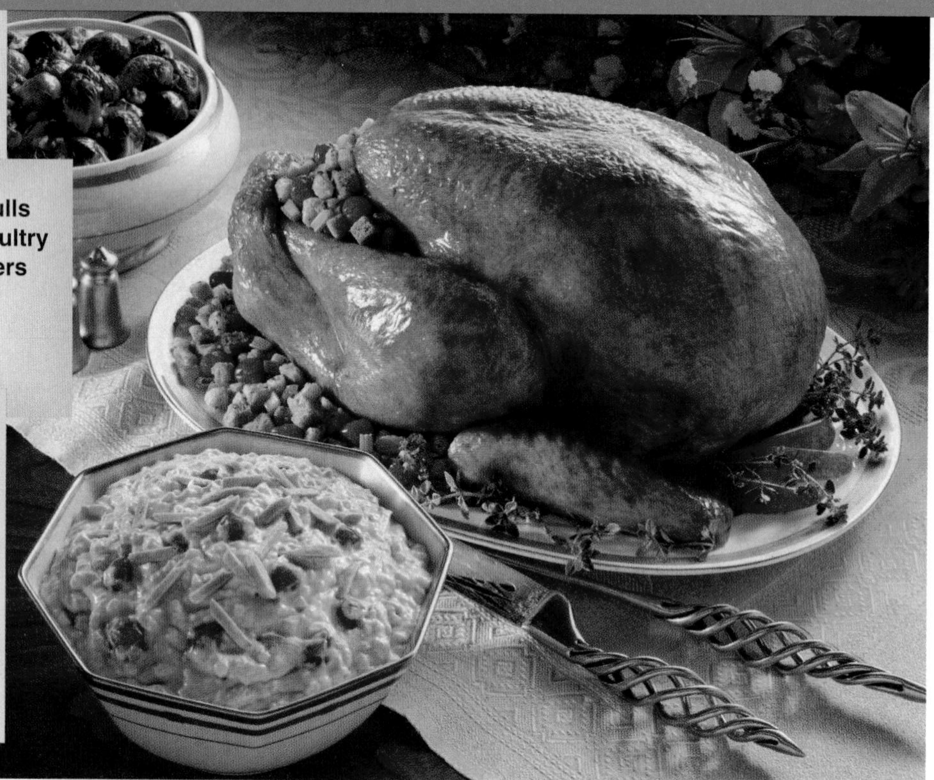

Cherry Marketing Institute

Terms to Know

poultry
giblets

Objectives

After studying this chapter, you will be able to

- list tips for buying poultry.
- describe how to properly store poultry to maintain its quality.
- describe the principles and methods for cooking poultry.
- prepare poultry by moist and dry cooking methods.

The word ***poultry*** describes any domesticated bird. Chicken, turkey, goose, and duck are the types of poultry most commonly eaten in the United States. At one time, chicken and turkey were eaten only on special occasions, but today they are available year-round.

Nutritional Value of Poultry

Poultry is in the meat and beans group of the Food Guide Pyramid. Most people need only the equivalent of 5 to 7 ounces (140 to 190 g) of lean, cooked meat each day. A small chicken breast half is a typical serving size, 20-1

All poultry contains high-quality protein and is a good source of phosphorus, iron, thiamin, riboflavin, and niacin. The amount of fat varies. Older birds have more fat than younger birds. Dark meat is slightly higher in fat than light meat.

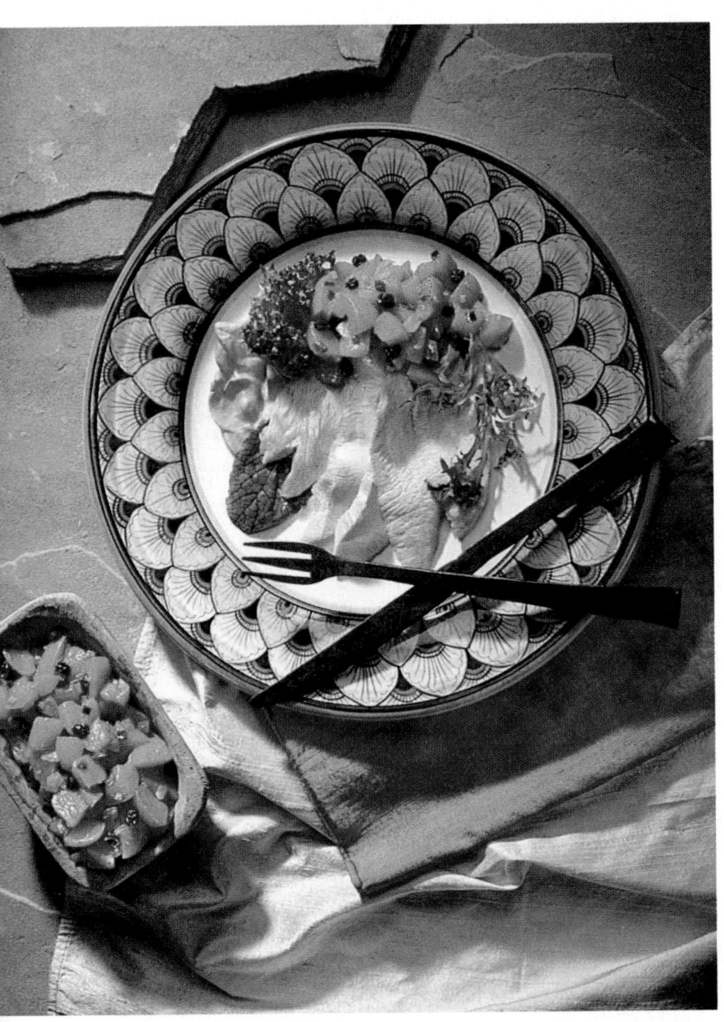

California Apricot Advisory Board

20-1 *A serving of poultry is 3 ounces (85 g) of cooked meat.*

Turkey and chicken are lower in total fat, saturated fat, and calories than many cuts of red meat. This is especially true of the light meat portions of poultry. For this reason, poultry is often included in low-cholesterol and weight reduction diets. Much of the fat in poultry is located just under the skin. Thus, you can reduce the fat content even further simply by removing the skin.

Buying Poultry

Poultry is sold in a variety of forms to meet consumer needs. You can buy poultry fresh, frozen, and in processed poultry products.

Inspection and Grading of Poultry

All poultry sold in interstate commerce must be federally inspected for wholesomeness. Retailers can find a round inspection seal on a tag attached to the wing of approved birds. This seal indicates the bird was healthy, processed under sanitary conditions, and labeled correctly.

Poultry can be voluntarily graded for quality. A grade shield will appear on the wing tag along with the inspection seal. Most poultry sold at the retail level is U.S. Grade A. Grade A birds are full-fleshed and meaty with well-distributed fat. Their skin has few blemishes and pinfeathers. Grade B and C birds are usually used in processed products.

All poultry that is processed and sold as canned poultry is inspected before canning. The quality depends somewhat on the brand.

Buying Fresh and Frozen Poultry

Most fresh and frozen poultry is marketed young. Young birds are tender and suitable for all cooking methods.

You can purchase chickens, turkeys, ducks, and geese fresh-chilled or frozen. Chickens can be purchased whole, cut into halves, or cut into pieces. Breasts, legs, and thighs are meatier

Q: Aren't hot dogs, ham, and luncheon meats made from processed chicken and turkey lower in fat than "regular" meat products?

A: Poultry-based products are generally leaner than other meat products. However, read the Nutrition Facts panels on the products you buy. A large percentage of calories in these poultry products may still come from fat.

than wings and backs. When deciding what type of pieces to buy, compare prices in terms of servings. Chicken, like all poultry, contains more bone in proportion to muscle than does red meat. Therefore, when buying chicken, you need to allow about ½ pound (225 g) of meat per serving. You can allow a little less per serving if you are buying meaty pieces like legs and breasts. You will need to allow a little more per serving if you are buying bony pieces like backs and wings.

Whole turkeys are available in many sizes, making them popular for large gatherings. Turkey parts and ground turkey are also available, 20-2. Allow ⅓ to ½ pound (150 to 225 g) of turkey per serving. Allow more if you want leftovers.

Turkeys as well as chickens have both light and dark meat. Breast meat is light and mildly flavored. The rest of the bird is dark meat, which has a stronger flavor.

Ducks and geese have all dark meat, which is tender and flavorful. Both have more fat than chickens or turkeys. Geese usually have more fat than ducks. Allow ½ pound (225 g) per serving for both duck and goose.

Be a Clever Consumer

Ounce for ounce, skinless chicken breast is lower in fat than ground beef. With this in mind, some consumers will select a chicken sandwich instead of a burger at a fast-food restaurant. They think they are choosing the healthier option. Actually, if the chicken is breaded and deep-fried, it is likely to be higher in fat than the burger. Most fast-food restaurants now make a nutritional analysis of their menu items available to customers. Take the time to review this information so you can be informed about what you order.

When buying poultry

- Choose birds with meaty breasts and legs, well-distributed fat, and blemish-free skin.
- Choose the type and amount of poultry that will suit your intended use.
- Look for frozen birds that are solidly frozen.
- Beware of dirty and torn wrappers and freezer burn (pale, dry, frosty areas).

Buying Processed Poultry Products

Turkey and chicken are available canned. Canned poultry may be whole, cut into pieces, boned, or used in items like chicken chow mein. Generally, canned poultry items are more expensive than fresh-chilled or frozen poultry.

When buying processed poultry products or food items containing poultry, read labels carefully. The ingredient list may include a poultry part, such as *turkey breast* or *chicken leg*. This indicates the fatty skin, as well as the meat, has been used in the product. However, a listing of *breast meat* or *leg meat* indicates the product contains only meat—not skin.

Storing Poultry

All poultry, except canned, is very perishable. Poultry parts are more perishable than whole birds. Poultry needs proper storage to retard spoilage. Proper storage is also important to inhibit the growth of salmonellae, an illness-causing bacteria often found in poultry.

For refrigerator storage, remove store wrapping. Rewrap the bird loosely in waxed paper. Wrap and store giblets separately. Place poultry in the coldest part of the refrigerator and use within two to three days.

For longer storage, rewrap the bird in moistureproof and vaporproof wrapping and store it in the freezer. You should place poultry you buy frozen in the freezer immediately after purchase. You can store poultry in the freezer for six to eight months. Once you thaw poultry, however, you should not refreeze it.

Store all canned poultry products in a cool, dry place. Store all unused portions and cooked poultry in tightly covered containers in the refrigerator. Remove stuffing from cooked poultry and store it separately. Use leftovers within two or three days.

Food Science Principles of Cooking Poultry

Like meat, poultry is a protein food. Cooking principles for poultry are similar to those used for other high-protein foods. Low temperatures and careful timing are important. Cooking poultry for too long or at too high a temperature can make it tough, dry, and flavorless.

A meat thermometer is the only accurate way to test poultry for doneness. When testing a whole bird, insert the probe of the thermometer into the thickest part of the thigh. When testing poultry pieces, insert the probe into the thickest area. The probe should not touch bone. Whole birds, wings, and thighs should reach an internal temperature of 180°F (80°C), 20-3. Breast pieces should reach an internal temperature of 170°F (75°C). Due to the uneven shape of whole poultry and poultry pieces, you should check the temperature in several places.

You must cook poultry to the well-done stage, but you should not overcook it. Pink flesh does not always mean a bird is undercooked. A chemical reaction causes a pink color in cooked poultry. Gases in the oven combine with substances in the poultry and turn the flesh pink. The pink color is not harmful.

Poultry bones will sometimes turn a dark color during cooking. Blood cells in the bone that have broken down during freezing cause this discoloration. When heated, they turn a dark brown. The color has no effect on flavor, and the bird is safe to eat.

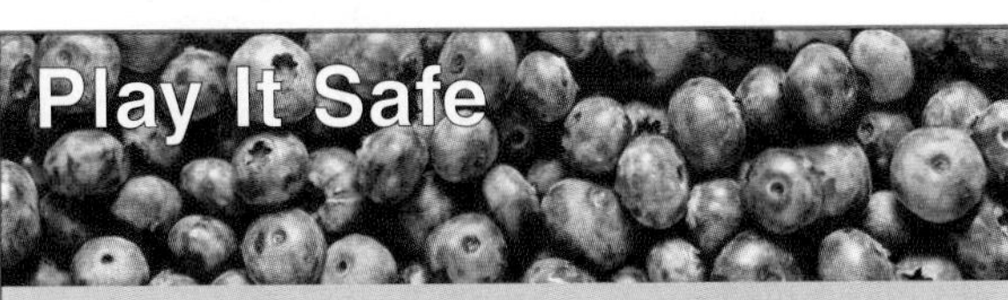

Some fresh poultry carries bacteria that can cause foodborne illness. Therefore, you should put poultry in a separate plastic bag at the store when you take it from the refrigerated poultry case. This will keep poultry drippings from getting on other items in your grocery cart and possibly contaminating them.

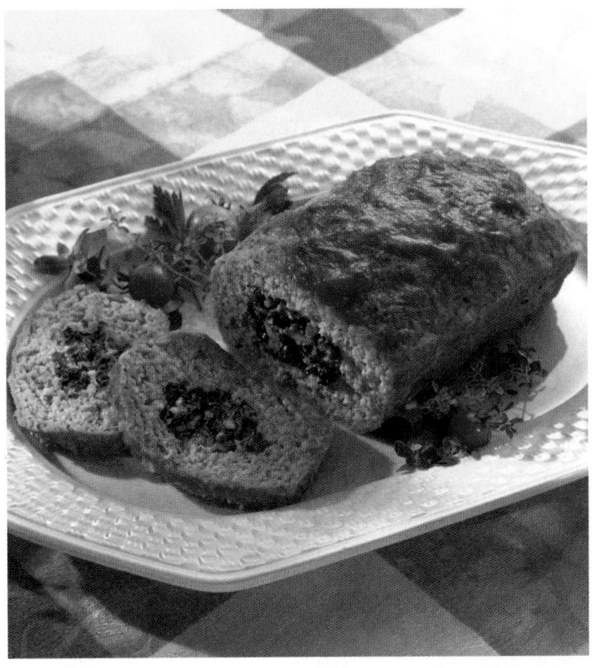

photograph courtesy of The Reynolds Kitchens

20-2 *Ground turkey is a tasty alternative to ground beef for making burgers, meat loaf, and many other dishes.*

Methods of Cooking Poultry

You can roast, broil, grill, fry, braise, or stew poultry. The method you choose will depend mainly on your taste preferences.

Roasting Poultry

Roasting is a popular choice for cooking whole birds. When preparing poultry, be sure to remove the neck and the packet of giblets found inside the cavity of the bird. ***Giblets*** are the edible internal organs, such as the heart and liver. People often use them in appetizers and to flavor soups and gravies.

You should truss large birds before roasting. A *trussed* bird has its wing tips turned back onto the shoulder and the drumsticks tied to the tail. Trussing prevents the wing and leg tips from overbrowning. It also

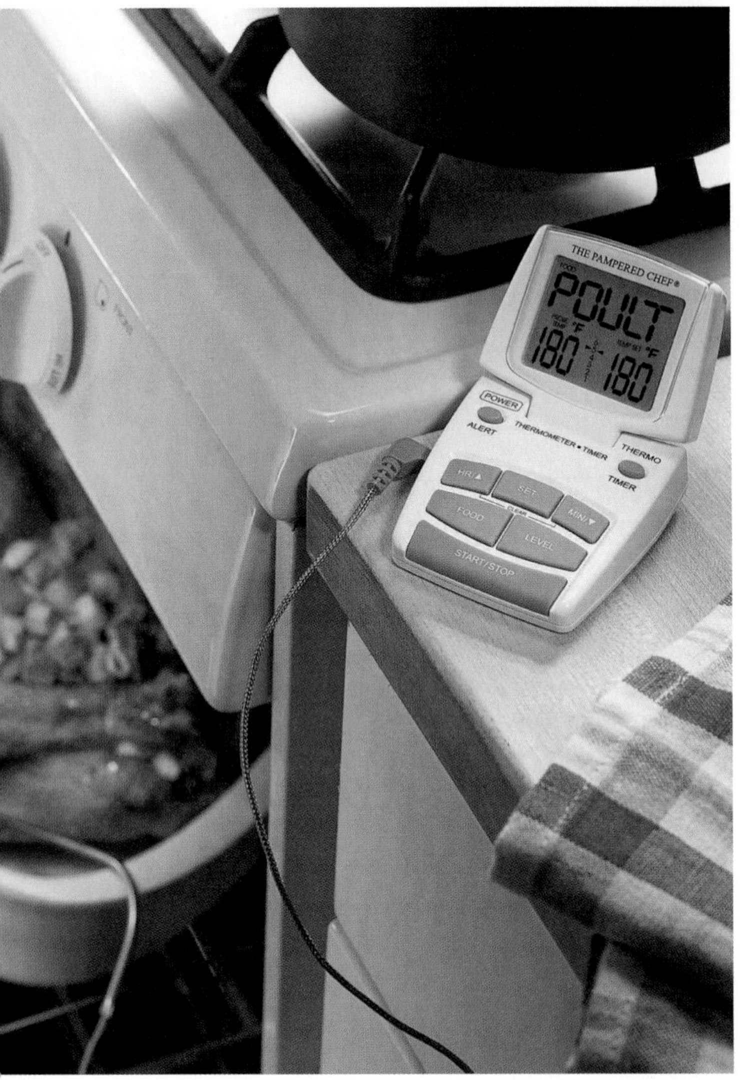

The Pampered Chef®

***20-3** Using a food thermometer to check the internal temperature is the only sure way to be certain poultry is thoroughly cooked.*

makes the bird easier to handle and more attractive to serve.

Place the trussed bird breast side up in a shallow pan. Season the cavity with salt and pepper unless you will be stuffing the bird. Do not add stuffing until you are ready to put the bird in the oven. This will prevent the growth of harmful bacteria, which can cause foodborne illness. Pack the stuffing loosely into the cavity. You can bake any extra stuffing in a greased casserole.

Roast the bird in a 325°F (160°C) oven. Cook the bird until a meat thermometer reads 180°F (80°C). The temperature of the stuffing should reach at least 165°F (75°C). (For faster roasting, you can wrap poultry in aluminum foil and cook it in a 450°F [230°C] oven.) If you allow poultry to stand 10 to 15 minutes after you take it from the oven, it will be easier to carve.

Sometimes the breast of a large bird will brown too quickly during roasting. To prevent overbrowning, you can make a tent out of aluminum foil. Cover the breast with the foil when the bird is about half cooked.

Some people prefer to roast poultry in oven cooking bags. Cooking bags shorten cooking time because they use steam to help cook the bird. Because steam is a form of moist heat, this method is not true roasting. See 20-4.

Broiling Poultry

You can broil turkeys and chickens. To broil poultry, split the bird into halves or quarters. Place pieces on a broiler pan and brush lightly with melted margarine, if desired. Broil 4 to 5 inches (10 to 12 cm) from the heat source until done. Cooking time depends on the size of the bird. Chicken usually will take about 40 minutes. Turkey will take about 80 to 90 minutes. Thinner pieces will cook faster than thicker pieces. Remove pieces from the broiler when they are cooked and keep them warm until ready to serve.

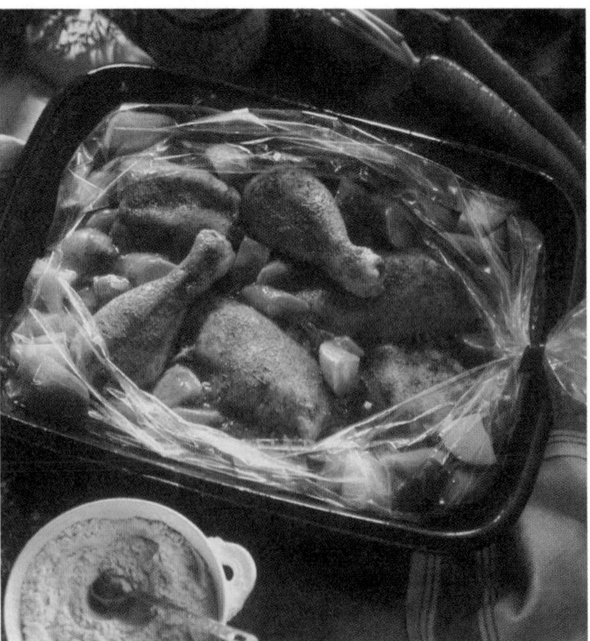

photograph courtesy of The Reynolds Kitchens

***20-4** Cooking bags speed time in the oven and result in poultry that is moist and tender.*

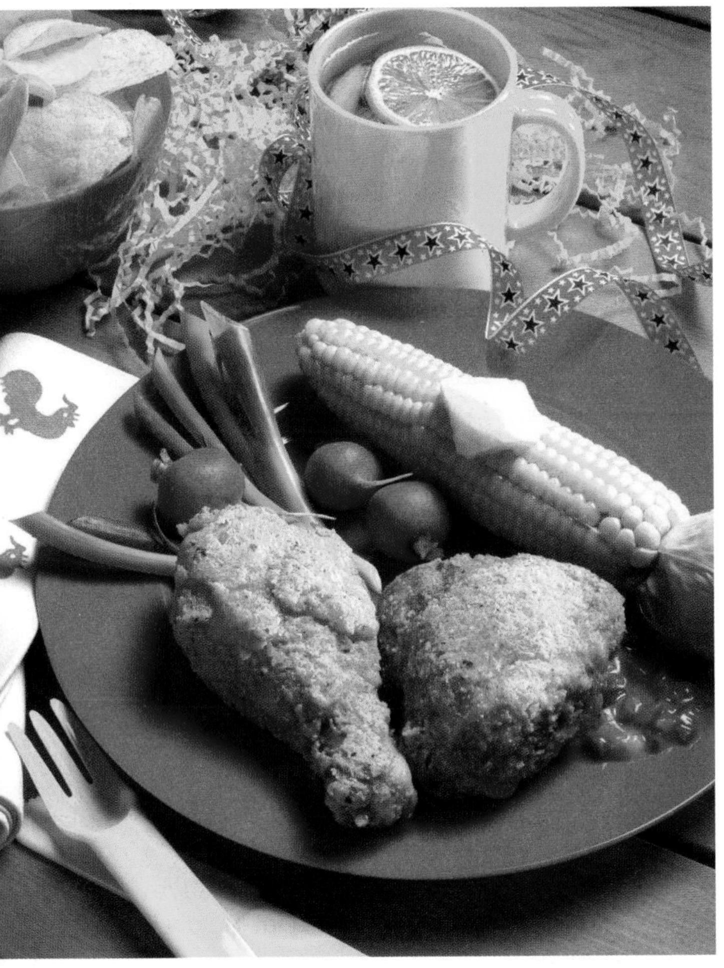

National Chicken Council

***20-5** Fried chicken has a crispy texture and a golden brown color.*

Grilling Poultry

Grilling is a popular way to cook whole birds and poultry pieces, especially during the summer. Grill poultry with bones using indirect heat. Grill boneless poultry pieces over direct heat. Grilling times depend on the size of pieces. Shorten grilling times by partially cooking poultry in a microwave oven immediately before placing it on the grill. Partial cooking also ensures grilled poultry is thoroughly cooked. Use an instant-read thermometer to test the internal temperature of grilled poultry for doneness.

Frying Poultry

You can cut chickens and turkeys into pieces and fry them, 20-5. To fry poultry, first roll the pieces in flour, egg, and bread crumbs or dip them in a batter. Then brown the pieces in about ½ inch (1.5 cm) of hot fat. (The fat should not be so hot that it smokes.) Turn poultry pieces with tongs as they brown. After browning, the bird can finish cooking in the skillet over low heat. You can also complete the cooking in a moderate oven.

Oven-Frying Poultry

Oven-frying is sometimes called baking. You can oven-fry chicken pieces by coating them with seasoned flour. Place them on a baking sheet. Cook in a moderate oven until done. Brushing chicken lightly with melted margarine will produce a crisp golden crust.

Braising Poultry

To braise turkey or chicken, brown individual pieces in a small amount of fat. Add a small amount of water to the skillet and cover tightly. Cook the poultry over low heat until tender, about 45 minutes to 1 hour. You can braise poultry on top of the range or in the oven. For a crisp crust, uncover the pan for the last 10 minutes of cooking.

Stewing Poultry

To stew poultry, put the bird in a big kettle and cover it completely with water. You can add carrots, celery, and seasonings for flavor. Cover the kettle tightly and simmer over low heat until the bird is tender. (You should never allow the

Q: Can eating chicken soup help me feel better when I have a cold or flu?

A: Chicken soup has no medicinal properties to rid you of illness-causing microorganisms. However, steam from the warm liquid may help relieve a stuffed up nose. The warm feeling you get from eating a hot bowl of soup may bring you emotional comfort. Soup will also provide you with nutrients needed to restore your health.

liquid to boil.) If desired, you can easily remove cooled stewed meat from the bone for use in soups and casseroles.

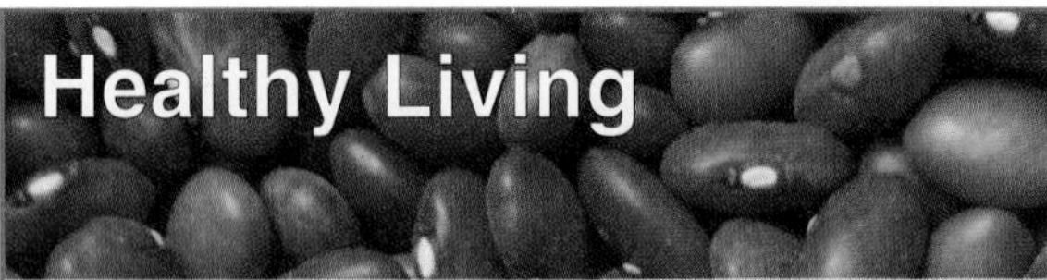

Healthy Living

Choose fried chicken for an occasional treat. For lower fat eating, choose roasted, baked, broiled, and grilled chicken most often. Also, be sure to remove the skin, which is high in fat. When making chicken soup, chill the broth and skim off the fat before serving the heated soup.

Microwaving Poultry

You can use a microwave oven to defrost or partially cook poultry that you are preparing by another method. You can also fully cook chicken and turkey in a microwave oven for poultry that comes out tender and juicy. Poultry generally microwaves in much less time than poultry cooks in a conventional oven. However, when roasting large birds, you may save little or no time by using a microwave oven. In addition, most microwave ovens are not big enough to hold very large birds.

To ensure even cooking in a microwave oven, arrange poultry pieces with the bony portions to the center. Arrange drumsticks like the spokes of a wheel. Place the meaty ends toward the outside of the dish. On whole birds, the breast area and wing and leg tips may cook faster than the rest of the bird. To prevent overcooking, you can cover these areas with foil shields.

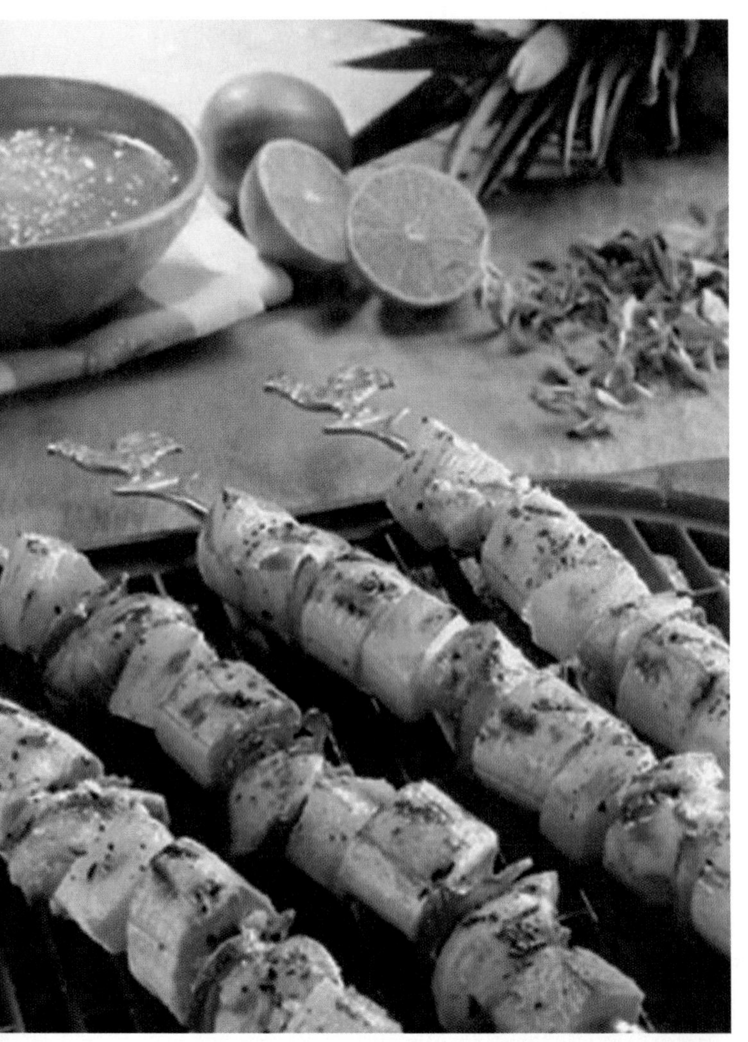

National Chicken Council

***20-6** Use boned chicken to make dishes like these tasty kabobs.*

Frozen Poultry

You should thaw frozen poultry before cooking. (If the bird is commercially stuffed, you should cook it without thawing.) To thaw, leave the bird in its original wrapping and let it thaw in the refrigerator.

For quicker thawing, wrap frozen poultry in a tightly closed plastic bag. Place it in a sink full of cold water. Change the water about every 30 minutes to keep it cold until the bird defrosts.

Boning Chicken

Many recipes call for boneless chicken breasts and thighs, 20-6. Boneless chicken pieces cost more than pieces with bones. You may be able to save money by boning chicken at home. Be sure to thoroughly wash cutting boards, knives, and other utensils after preparing raw poultry. This helps avoid the possibility of transferring harmful bacteria that may be in the poultry to other foods.

Chapter 20 Review
Poultry

Summary

Poultry is a good source of protein and B vitamins. Most poultry is marketed young. When buying poultry, look for meaty birds with well-distributed fat and blemish-free skin.

All poultry is perishable. Store it in the coldest part of the refrigerator and use it within two to three days. You can carefully wrap poultry and place it in the freezer for longer storage.

You should always be sure poultry is thoroughly cooked before you serve it. However, use moderate cooking temperatures and careful timing to avoid overcooking. Overcooking can result in meat that is tough and dry.

Because most poultry is tender, it is suitable for any cooking method. You might choose roasting, broiling, grilling, frying, braising, stewing, or microwaving.

Review What You Have Read

Write your answers on a separate sheet of paper.

1. Name the four kinds of poultry most commonly eaten in the United States.
2. True or false. Most poultry is tender and can be cooked by dry heat methods.
3. Why do you need to allow more weight per serving when buying poultry than when buying red meat?
4. Within what time period should refrigerated poultry be used?
5. True or false. Stuffing should be left inside a poultry carcass for refrigerator storage.
6. What is the recommended internal temperature for cooked poultry?
7. Turning back the wing tips and tying the drumsticks to the tail of the bird before roasting is known as _____.
8. What are two advantages of partially cooking poultry in a microwave oven immediately before placing it on a grill?
9. How should poultry pieces be arranged in a microwave oven to ensure even cooking?
10. Why is it important to thoroughly wash cutting boards and utensils after preparing raw poultry?

Build Your Basic Skills

1. **Writing/verbal.** Write three questions about poultry selection, storage, and preparation. Then contact the U.S. Department of Agriculture's Meat and Poultry Hotline for answers to your questions.
2. **Math.** Compare the price per pound of boneless, skinless chicken breasts with the price per pound of bone-in, skin-on chicken breasts. Calculate the price per ounce of each chicken product. Remove the bone and skin from the bone-in, skin-on breasts. Weigh the bone and skin on a scale. Determine the percentage of waste in the bone-in, skin-on product. Then calculate the cost per ounce of the meat portion of this product. How does this cost compare with the cost of the product sold without bone and skin?

Build Your Thinking Skills

1. **Compare.** Roast chicken, turkey, duck, and goose. Compare the appearance, flavor, and texture of the various meats.
2. **Create.** Find at least three recipes for stuffing. Note what ingredients the recipes have in common and which ingredients are unique to each recipe. Also note the ingredient proportions. Use this analysis to create your own recipe for stuffing. Prepare and sample the recipe. Explain why you would or would not choose to serve it with poultry.

Apply Technology

1. Investigate new techniques being studied to reduce salmonella contamination in poultry. Share your findings in a brief oral report.
2. Research the production procedures used to manufacture poultry-based luncheon meats. Prepare a poster presentation illustrating the procedures.

Using Workplace Skills

Calvin is a sales representative for the Better Bird Feed Company. He sells feed products to poultry farmers all over the Midwest. Each time the company introduces a feed product, someone from the research department gives a presentation to the sales group. The researcher describes the new product's features. Then Calvin receives stacks of detailed handouts about the product. The handouts show lists of ingredients, charts of research results, and graphs comparing Better Bird's feed with other brands.

To be an effective worker, Calvin needs skill in interpreting and communicating information. In a small group, answer the following questions about Calvin's need for and use of these skills:

A. Why wouldn't Calvin simply let his customers read copies of the research handouts to learn about new products?
B. How might Calvin's customers be affected if he does not adequately interpret and communicate information about new products?
C. How might Calvin's company be affected if he does not adequately interpret and communicate information about new products?
D. What is another skill Calvin would need in this job? Briefly explain why this skill would be important.

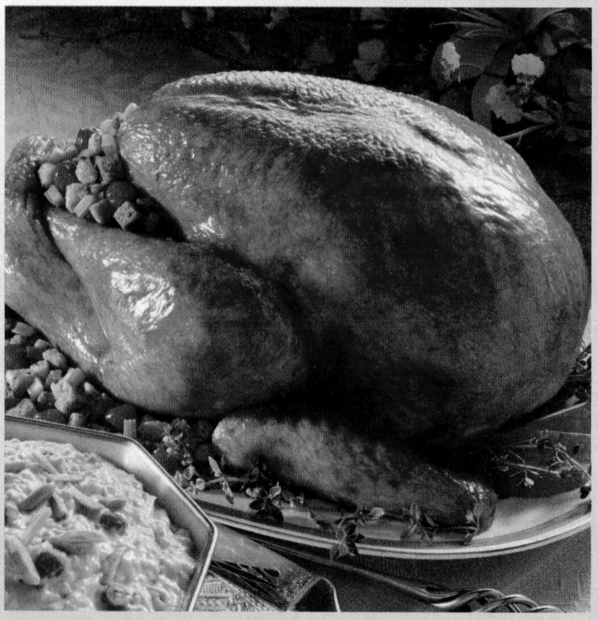

Chapter 21
Fish and Shellfish

Raw Shellfish Preparer
Cleans and prepares shellfish for serving to customers.

Fish Hatchery Attendant
Performs a combination of tasks to trap and spawn game fish, incubate eggs, and rear fry in a fish hatchery.

Net Fisher
Catches finfish, shellfish, and other marine life alone or as a crewmember on shore or aboard fishing vessels using a variety of equipment.

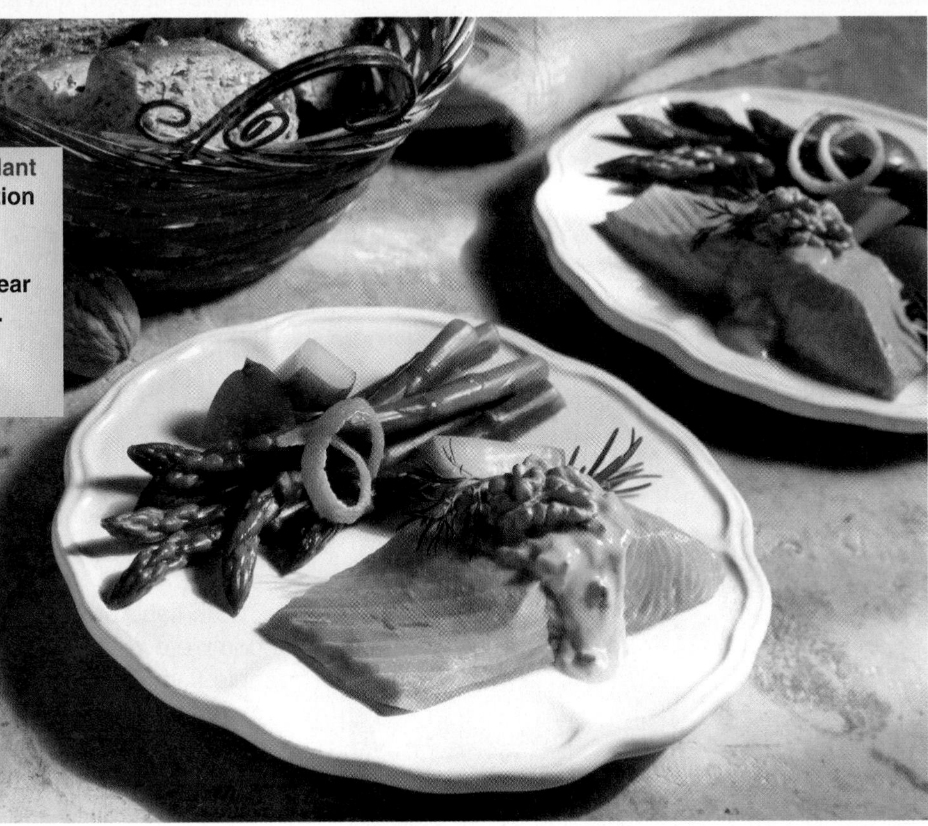

California Asparagus Commission

Terms to Know

finfish
shellfish
lean fish
fat fish
mollusk
crustacean
drawn fish
dressed fish
fish steak
fish fillet

Objectives

After studying this chapter, you will be able to

- list factors affecting the selection of fish and shellfish.
- describe how to properly store fish to maintain its quality.
- describe the principles and methods for cooking fish and shellfish.
- prepare fish by moist and dry cooking methods.

Commercial fishers in the United States catch several billion fish each year for food, 21-1. However, the U.S. is a small consumer of fish and fish products compared with other countries.

Classification of Fish and Shellfish

Two kinds of water animals are eaten as food: finfish (often called *fish*) and shellfish. ***Finfish*** have fins and backbones. ***Shellfish*** have shells instead of backbones. Both finfish and shellfish can be divided into further classes.

Finfish can be lean or fatty. ***Lean fish*** have very little fat in their flesh. Because their flesh is white, they are often called *white fish*. Swordfish, haddock, and cod are lean fish. ***Fat fish*** have flesh that is fattier than that of lean fish. Their flesh is usually pink, yellow, or gray. Mackerel, catfish, and salmon are fat fish.

You can divide shellfish into two groups: mollusks and crustaceans. ***Mollusks*** have soft bodies that are partially or fully covered by hard shells. Oysters, clams, and scallops are mollusks. ***Crustaceans*** are covered by firm shells and have segmented (divided into sections) bodies. Shrimp, lobsters, and crabs are crustaceans.

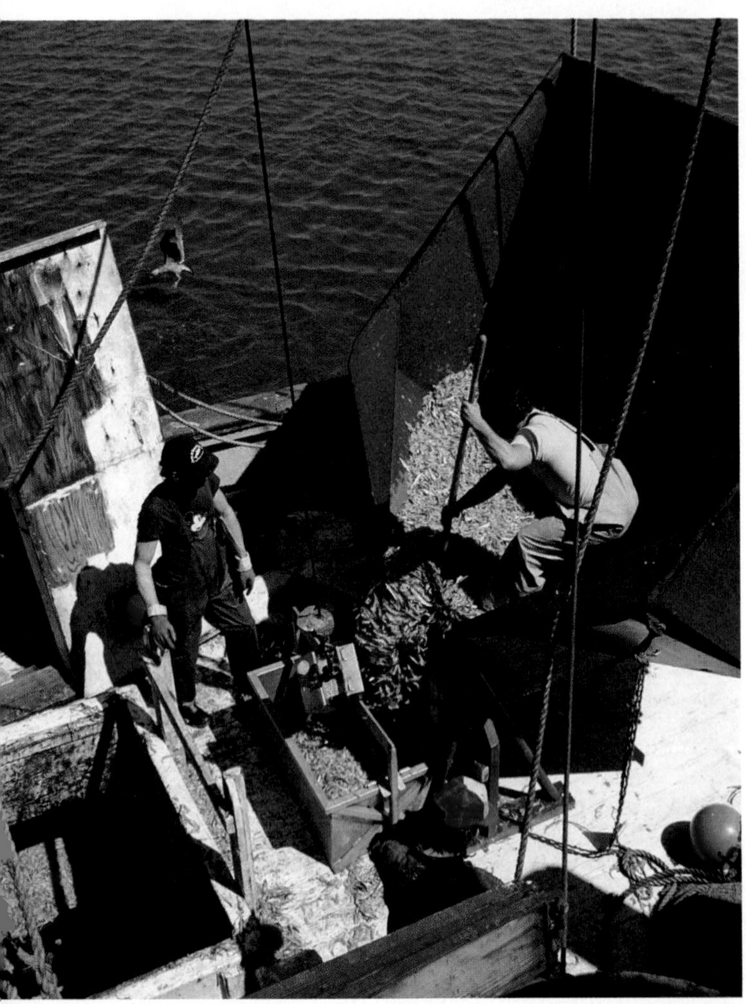

21-1 Commercial fishing is an important industry in coastal regions.

Nutritional Value of Fish and Shellfish

Fish and shellfish are in the meat and beans group of the Food Guide Pyramid. Most people need the equivalent of 5 to 7 ounces (140 to 196 g) of lean, cooked meat, poultry, or fish each day.

Both fish and shellfish are excellent sources of complete protein. In some parts of the world, people use fish flour (concentrated fish protein) to increase the protein level of the diet.

Fat content varies with the kind of fish. Lean fish have fewer calories than fat fish. Most fish have fewer calories and less saturated fat and cholesterol than moderately fat red meat. Including fish in your diet can help you follow the Dietary Guideline about moderating your total fat intake.

Overall, fish is slightly higher in minerals than red meat. Shellfish have even more minerals than finfish. Fish provide fair amounts of iron. Canned salmon and sardines prepared with their bones are especially good sources of calcium. Saltwater fish are one of the most important sources of iodine.

Fish and shellfish contribute the same vitamins as red meat. Fat fish have higher amounts of vitamins A and D.

Selecting and Purchasing Fish and Shellfish

When selecting fish and shellfish, use inspection seals and grade shields to help you determine quality. The appearance and form of fish and shellfish can also guide your purchases.

Inspection and Grading of Fish and Shellfish

The National Marine Fisheries Service provides a voluntary inspection program for the fish industry. All fish products that have passed inspection carry a round inspection seal.

A grade shield appears on fish that have been voluntarily graded. Appearance, odor, flavor, and lack of defects determine quality grades. Most fish at retail markets is U.S. Grade A. These top quality fish are uniform in size and have good flavor and few defects.

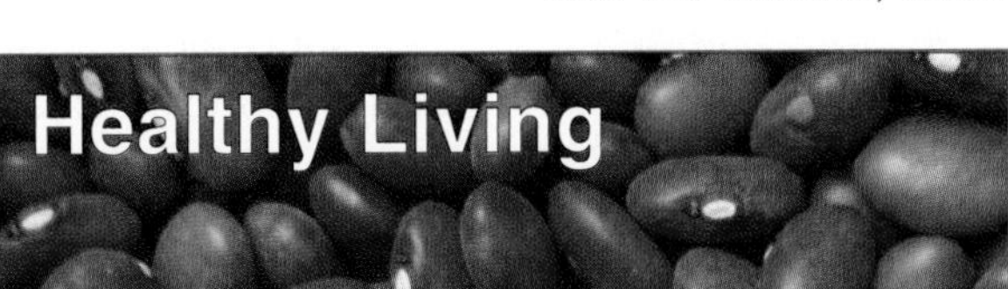

Some nutrition experts suggest including fish in your diet two to three times a week. They believe the omega-3 fatty acids in fish may reduce your risk of heart attack or stroke. Although many experts favor eating fish, most caution against the use of fish oil supplements. These supplements do not contain the other nutrients found in fish. In addition, their use may have some negative side effects.

Forms of Finfish

A fresh fish should have a stiff body, tight scales, and firm flesh. The gills should be red, and the eyes bright and bulging. A finger pushed into the flesh should leave no indentation. The outside should have little or no slime, and the fish should smell fresh.

You can purchase fresh fish whole, drawn, dressed, or as steaks or fillets. A *whole (round) fish* is marketed as it comes from the water. You must clean it before cooking. A ***drawn fish*** has the entrails (insides) removed. A ***dressed fish*** has the entrails, head, fins, and scales removed. It is ready for cooking. ***Fish steaks*** are cross-sectional slices taken from a dressed fish. ***Fish fillets*** are the sides of the fish cut lengthwise away from the backbone. Fillets have few, if any, bones. See 21-2.

Drawn and dressed fish, as well as fish steaks and fillets, can be purchased frozen. Frozen fish should be solidly frozen in moistureproof and vaporproof wrapping. There should be no discoloration and little or no odor.

Q: Can drawn fish be cooked without further trimming?

A: You can cook drawn fish if you shield the fins with foil. However, many people do not care for the presentation of cooked fish with the head still attached.

Types of Shellfish

Shellfish available in most markets include shrimp, oysters, crabs, lobsters, clams, and scallops. See 21-3. Shrimp and oysters are the most important shellfish in the United States in terms of the amount eaten.

Shrimp

You can buy several varieties of shrimp. They differ in color and size when they are raw.

Most shrimp are sold without the head and thorax (middle division of the body). You may have to peel the shell off shrimp. You may also have to remove the intestinal tract before preparing canned or bulk cooked shrimp. The intestinal tract appears as a dark streak that runs along one side of the shrimp. Shrimp sold without the intestinal tract are labeled as *deveined* shrimp.

Shrimp are marketed by sizes such as jumbo, large, medium, and small. Sizes are based on the number needed to weigh 1 pound (0.45 kg). Frozen shrimp may be purchased uncooked, either peeled or unpeeled. Frozen shrimp are also available cooked and peeled or peeled, cleaned, and breaded. When buying fresh shrimp, look for those that are odorless with firmly attached shells.

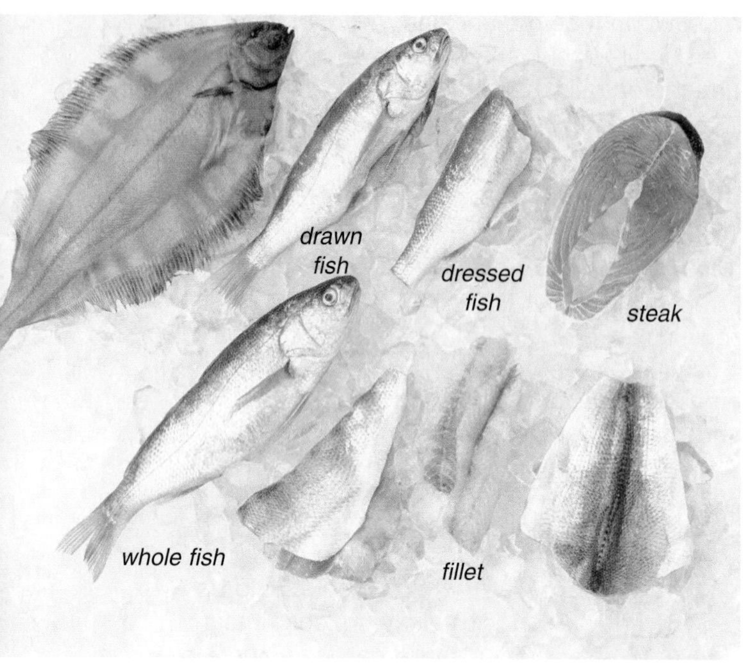

21-2 Fresh fish can be purchased in several forms.

Oysters

You can purchase oysters live in the shell, fresh or frozen shucked (removed from shell), and canned. Like shrimp, they are packed according to size. Live oysters should have tightly closed shells or the shells should close when you touch them. Shucked oysters should be plump, creamy in color, and odorless.

Crabs

The blue crab and Dungeness crab are the two most common species sold in the United States. You can buy them live in the shell, cooked frozen whole, and as frozen or canned cooked meat.

Lobster

Lobster shells are dark blue green when removed from the water. They become red when cooked. You can buy cooked, frozen whole lobsters or lobster tails. You can also purchase lobster as cooked meat taken from the shell and frozen or canned. When buying live lobsters, look for those with tails that snap back quickly after being flattened.

Clams

Several kinds of clams are eaten in the United States. These are available live in the shell, fresh or frozen shucked, and canned. Like shucked oysters, shucked clams should be plump and odorless and have a creamy color. The shells of live clams should be tightly closed or they should close when you touch them.

Scallops

Both tiny bay scallops and the larger deep-sea scallops are available on the market. A fresh bay scallop is creamy white or pink. A fresh deep-sea scallop is white. The whole bodies of these mollusks are edible. However, the large muscle used to close the shell is the only part commonly eaten in the United States. Unlike clams and oysters, you cannot buy scallops in the shell. Scallops are available fresh or frozen.

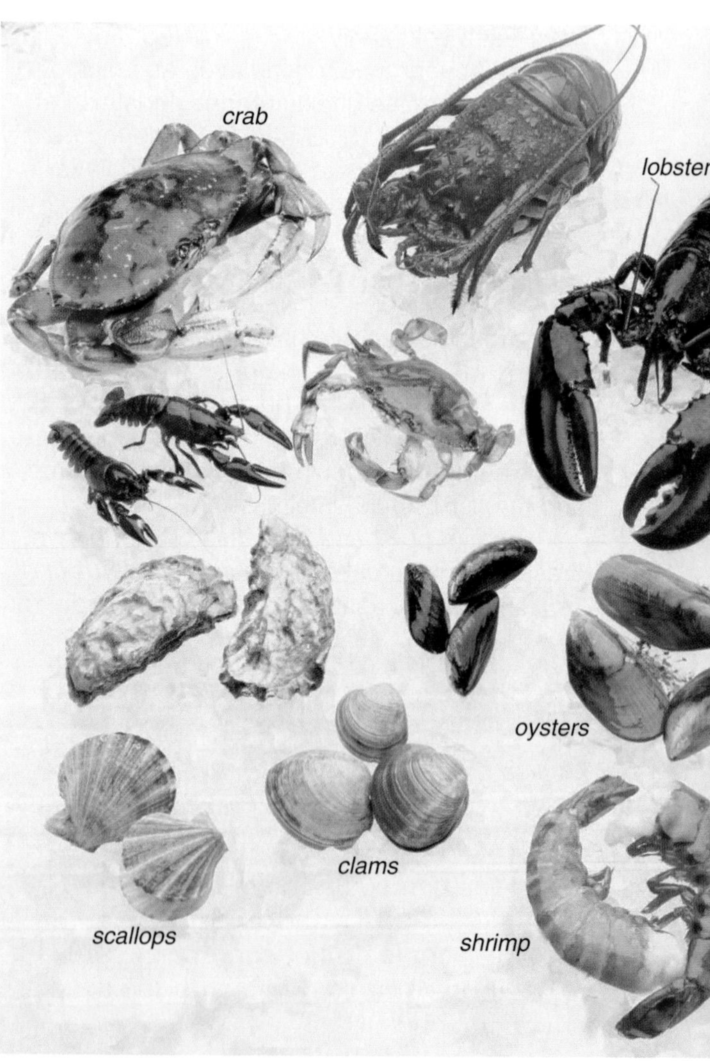

21-3 Both mollusks and crustaceans are available in most markets that sell shellfish.

Canned Fish and Shellfish

Tuna, salmon, sardines, shrimp, crab, lobster, and clams are often canned. Many varieties are available. Read the label carefully to be sure you know what you are buying. To reduce fat in your diet, you should choose tuna packed in water instead of oil. If you are making shrimp cocktail, you might want the large, fancy shrimp rather than the small shrimp.

Play It Safe

Shellfish can carry the hepatitis A virus when the water in which they live is polluted by untreated sewage. The greatest risk comes from raw shellfish. However, cooked shellfish can also carry the virus. To ensure food safety, always buy shellfish gathered from state-approved sources.

Buying Fish and Shellfish

Fresh seafood can be a source of bacteria that cause foodborne illness. To ensure the safety of the fish and shellfish you buy, deal only with reputable sellers. Look for the signs of quality described earlier. Be sure the market is clean and the fish is properly stored on beds of ice, preferably under a cover. The employees should be practicing safe food handling procedures, including wearing disposable gloves when handling your seafood.

The amount of fish you will need to buy depends on the kind and form. Fish, as a rule, have a large amount of waste. Dressed fish have less waste than whole and drawn fish. Fillets and steaks have even less waste, 21-4.

The cost of seafood depends on the form and the region of the country. Fish fillets generally cost more than whole fish because they require more handling. You can often save money by buying dressed fish and filleting it yourself. Fresh fish purchased where it is taken from the water will be less expensive than fish that must be shipped inland. Most shellfish, except for small oysters, is expensive regardless of location.

Storing Fish and Shellfish

Fish is very perishable, so you must store it with care. Wrap fresh fish tightly in waxed paper or foil. Place it in a tightly covered container in the coldest part of the refrigerator. Use stored fish within a day or two. For freezer storage, wrap fish in moistureproof and vaporproof material. Store it in the coldest part of the freezer.

Keep frozen fish in its original package. Place it in the freezer as soon as possible after purchase.

Store canned fish in a cool, dry place. Refrigerate any unused portions in a tightly covered container. Use it within a day or two.

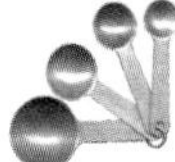

Cooking Finfish

Preparing seafood with care can help you avoid foodborne illness. You need to practice the same precautions when handling seafood that you use when handling meat and poultry. Be sure to wash your hands thoroughly before

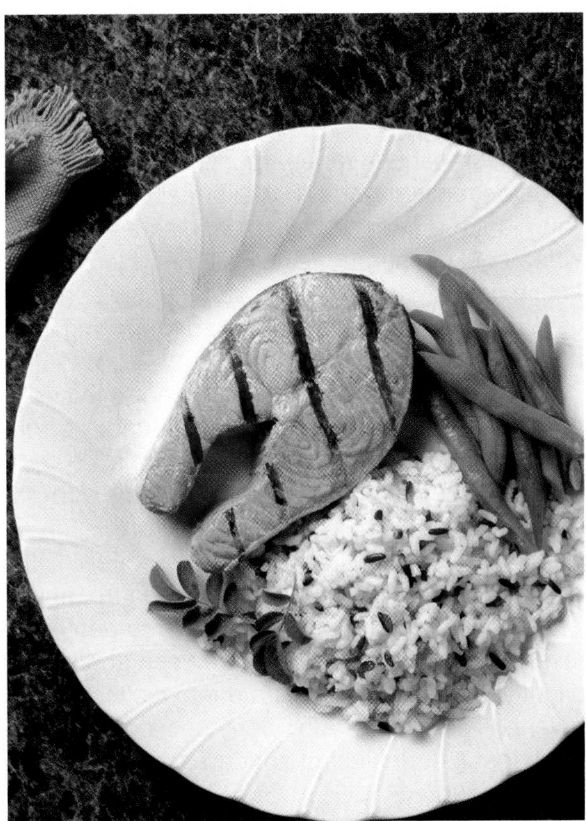

21-4 Fish steaks have less waste than many other forms of fish, so you can get more servings to the pound (450 g).

and after you handle fish and shellfish. Do not thaw frozen products at room temperature. Keep cooked food from touching anything, such as utensils or marinades, that came in contact with raw seafood. Use an instant-read thermometer to be sure the internal temperature of cooked seafood has reached 145°F (63°C). Refrigerate leftover portions promptly.

Q: Is it safe to eat sushi?

A: Sushi contains raw fish. It is safe to eat if purchased from a reputable restaurant where it has been prepared by qualified chefs. However, people in high-risk groups, such as children, pregnant women, and those with immune disorders should avoid eating sushi.

Food Science Principles of Cooking Finfish

Finfish contain tender muscle fibers and little connective tissue. For this reason, tenderizing is not a goal when cooking fish as it is when cooking some meats. You need to cook finfish for only a short time. You must watch them carefully to keep them from becoming dry and overcooked.

You should neither undercook nor overcook fish. Undercooked fish can have an unpleasant flavor and may contain harmful bacteria. Overcooked fish is tough and dry. Some varieties become rubbery; others fall apart.

When you cook a finfish to the proper degree of doneness, the flesh will be firm, and it will flake easily with a fork. (When you gently insert the tines of a fork into the flesh and lift slightly, the flesh will separate into distinct layers.) The flesh of a properly cooked fish will have lost its translucent appearance and will look opaque.

Methods of Cooking Finfish

All finfish are naturally tender, so you can use both dry and moist heat cooking methods. The fat content of the fish usually determines the cooking method. Generally, you should cook fat fish by dry heat and lean fish by moist heat.

Fat fish, such as mackerel, catfish, salmon, and trout, are delicious when broiled, grilled, or baked. Their fat keeps them from drying out during cooking.

Lean fish, like swordfish, halibut, flounder, haddock, and red snapper, are usually fried, poached, or steamed, 21-5. You can cook lean fish by dry heat if you brush them with fat or cook them in a sauce. Likewise, you can poach or steam fat fish if you handle them gently. (Fat fish can fall apart more easily when cooked in liquid.)

Cooking methods used for fish include broiling, grilling, baking, frying, poaching,

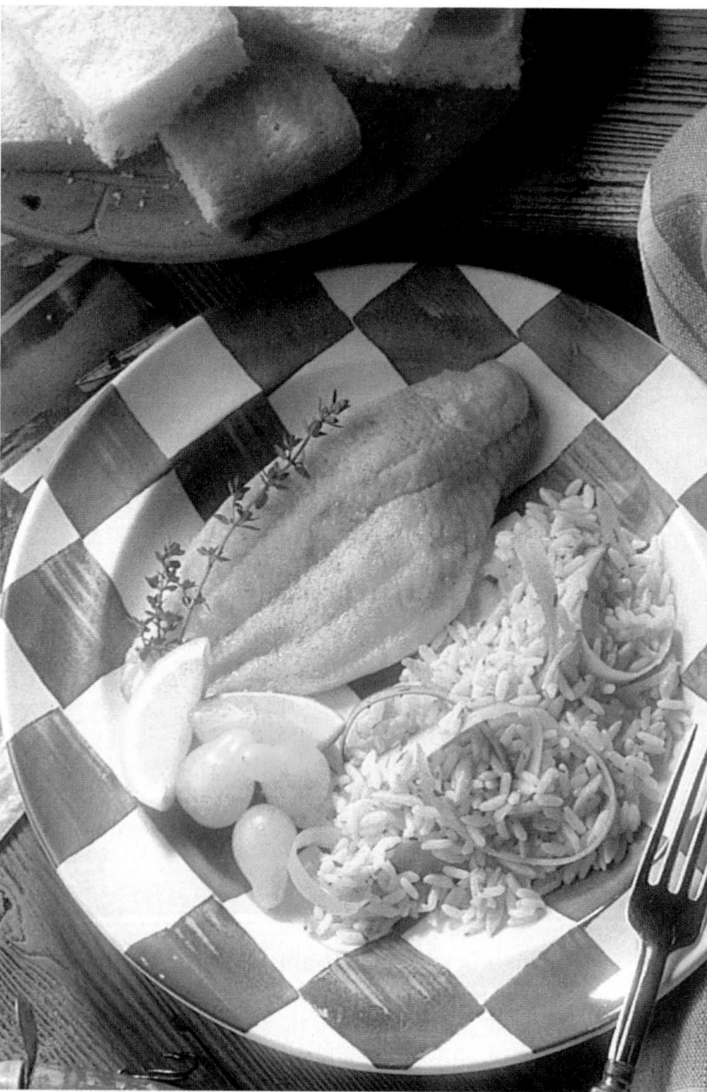

USA Rice Council

***21-5** Steaming is a suitable method for cooking lean varieties of fish.*

steaming, and microwaving. You can use a general guide to time fish cooked by all these methods, except deep-frying and microwaving. Measure fish, including stuffed and rolled fish, at its thickest point. You should cook it about 10 minutes for every inch (2.5 cm) of thickness. Turn thick pieces of fish once during cooking. You do not need to turn fish that is less than ½ inch (1.25 cm) thick. If you wrap fish in foil or cover it with a sauce, you should add 5 extra minutes to the cooking time. Fish cooked from the frozen state will require twice as much time to cook. Test fish for doneness by flaking with a fork.

Broiling Finfish

For broiling, select fish that are at least 1 inch (2.5 cm) thick. You can broil steaks, fillets, and dressed fish. Place the fish on a cold broiler pan and brush the fish with oil if it is lean. Broil until the fish flakes easily with a fork. You can cook thinner fish closer to the heat source than thicker fish. You will need to turn thick pieces once during broiling.

Grilling Finfish

The grilling method used for fish depends on the form of fish you are preparing. Grill steaks and fillets by placing them directly over hot coals. Turn over thick pieces halfway through the grilling time. Use indirect heat to grill dressed fish. Test steaks and fillets with a fork for doneness. Use an instant-read thermometer to check the internal temperature of dressed fish.

Baking Finfish

For baking, select steaks, fillets, and dressed fish. To prevent fish from drying out, brush the pieces with oil or with a sauce. You can stuff dressed fish and fillets just before baking. Bake fish at 400°F to 450°F (200°C to 230°C).

Frying Finfish

You can panfry, oven-fry, or deep-fry fish. You can panfry fillets, steaks, and small dressed fish. Coat fish to be panfried with crumbs or with a batter. Then fry them in a small amount of fat until browned. See 21-6.

Cut fish to be oven-fried into serving-sized pieces and coat them with milk and crumbs. Then drizzle them lightly with oil and place them on a greased baking sheet. To get a crispy texture that resembles fried, bake fish in a 500°F (260°C) oven. At this high temperature, use caution around the oven and watch fish closely as it will cook very quickly. The breading keeps the fish from becoming dry.

Cut fish for deep-frying into serving-sized pieces. Bread them or dip them in batter. Then fry them in 375°F (190°C) fat. If the fat is too hot, the outside of the fish will burn before the inside is cooked. If the fat is too cool, the fish will be soggy and greasy.

Poaching Finfish

Poaching is cooking in simmering liquid. You can use lightly salted water, milk, or water seasoned with spices or herbs as the poaching liquid. You can use any container that is large and deep enough to hold the fish for poaching. It should have a tightly fitting cover.

To poach fish, place the fish in a suitable container. Add enough liquid to barely cover the fish. (If you wrap a dressed fish in cheesecloth or parchment paper or place it on a rack before cooking, it will better retain its shape.) Tightly cover the pan. Poach the fish over low heat until it flakes easily with a fork. After the fish is cooked, you can reduce the volume of the

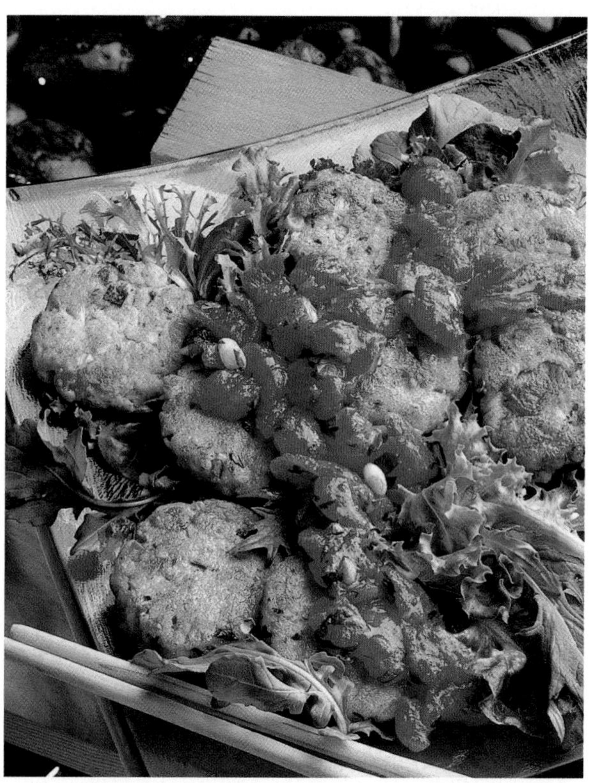

Del Monte Corporation

***21-6** These fish cakes are made with precooked fish and then panfried until golden.*

poaching liquid by simmering it in an uncovered pan. Then you can thicken it and serve it as a sauce.

Steaming Finfish

Steaming differs from poaching only in the amount of liquid used. You can use less liquid because the steam that forms inside the covered cooking utensil will cook the fish. To steam fish, place dressed fish, steaks, or fillets on a rack over simmering liquid. Cover the pan tightly and steam until the fish flakes easily. (You should never allow the water to boil.) You can also steam fish in the oven in a covered pan or wrapped in aluminum foil. The cover or foil holds in the steam that forms so the steam can cook the fish.

Q: Isn't eating fish supposed to make me smart?

A: You need a complete nutritious diet for proper brain development. No single food can improve your intelligence.

Microwaving Finfish

Fish cooked in a microwave oven is tender, moist, and flaky. Fish cooks very quickly in a microwave oven, so you must watch it carefully to avoid overcooking. Do not forget to allow for standing time. Test fish steaks and fillets with a fork. See 21-7.

Remove fish from the microwave oven when it just begins to flake. Rotate dressed fish one-quarter turn several times during the microwave cooking period. This helps to ensure even cooking of the oddly shaped body.

Cooking Frozen Finfish

You can cook frozen fish either frozen or thawed. If you thaw the fish, you can cook it like fresh fish. If you do not thaw it, you must cook it at a lower temperature and for a longer time than fresh fish.

Principles and Methods of Cooking Shellfish

Like finfish, all kinds of shellfish are naturally tender. As a result, you should cook them for a short time at moderate temperatures. Overcooking will cause the proteins to overcoagulate and make the fish tough.

You can simmer, bake, broil, grill, panfry (saute), deep-fry, or microwave shellfish. The cooking method used depends on the kind of shellfish and whether you purchased it live, frozen, or canned.

If you live in an area where fresh shellfish is available, you may purchase your shellfish live. Shellfish purchased in the shell must be alive

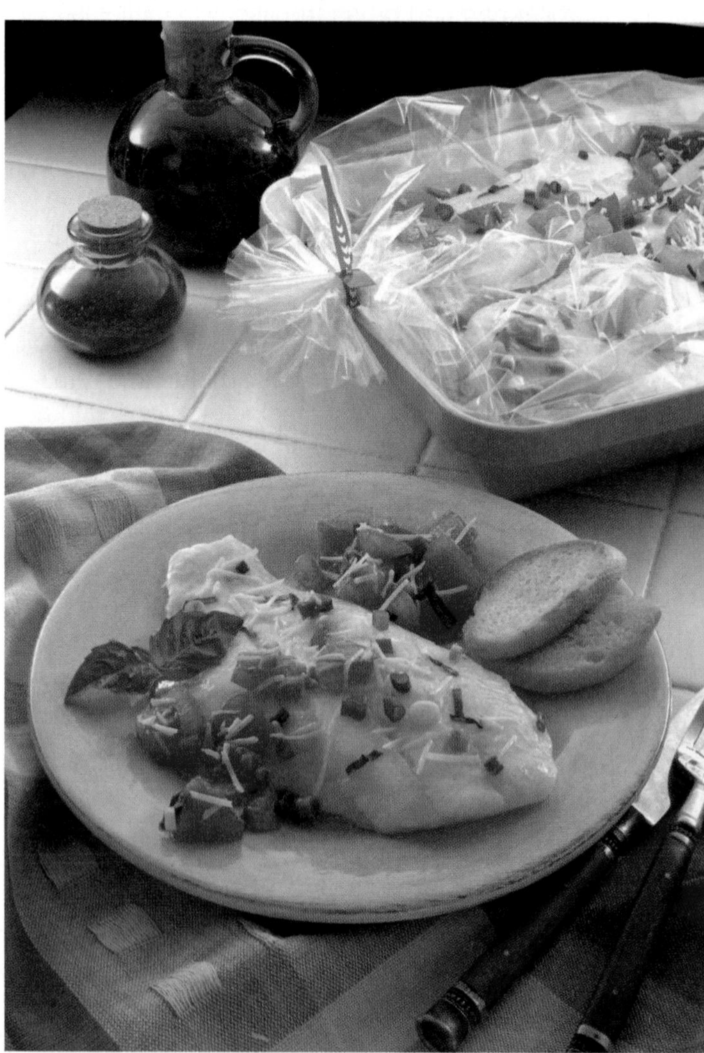

photograph courtesy of The Reynolds Kitchens

21-7 Fish cooked in a microwave oven should be covered to hold in steam, which speeds cooking and keeps fish moist.

when cooked. (Fresh, uncooked shellfish deteriorates very rapidly.)

Parboil live lobster, shrimp, and crab by plunging the shellfish into boiling, salted water until it is partially cooked. (Plunge lobster into the water headfirst.) Shellfish then should be simmered, not boiled. After parboiling, you can broil, grill, bake, panfry, or deep-fry shrimp. You may bake or broil lobster and crab. You may combine all three with other ingredients to make such seafood specialties as Lobster Thermidor, Shrimp Scampi, and Crab Newburg. See 21-8.

The shells of live oysters and clams should be tightly closed. You should discard oysters and clams if their shells are open. When you drop live oysters or clams into simmering water, the shells will open. You can then remove the edible part of the shellfish from the shell. After removal, you can simmer, deep-fry, or saute oysters and clams.

Good Manners Are Good Business

Being served shellfish at a business dinner may make you rather nervous if you are unfamiliar with how to eat them. Clams and oysters often are served in open shells. Use one hand to hold the shell in place on your plate. With your other hand, use a seafood fork to lift the oyster or clam out of the shell. If you wish, dip the shellfish in the accompanying cocktail sauce before eating it in one bite.

Shellfish cooked in a microwave oven require the same timing whether cooked in or out of the shell. Refer to a microwave cookbook for exact cooking times and methods. Remember to place thicker portions of shellfish toward the outside of the dish. This will promote more even microwave cooking.

In inland areas, most of the available shellfish is frozen or canned. Cook uncooked frozen shrimp in salted simmering water until pink. Frozen lobster tails are partially cooked. You may thaw and broil them, or you may cook them in simmering liquid like uncooked frozen shrimp. You may bake, broil, or fry cooked frozen shrimp, crab, or scallops.

You may serve canned shellfish without further cooking. You may also combine them with other foods in salads and main dishes.

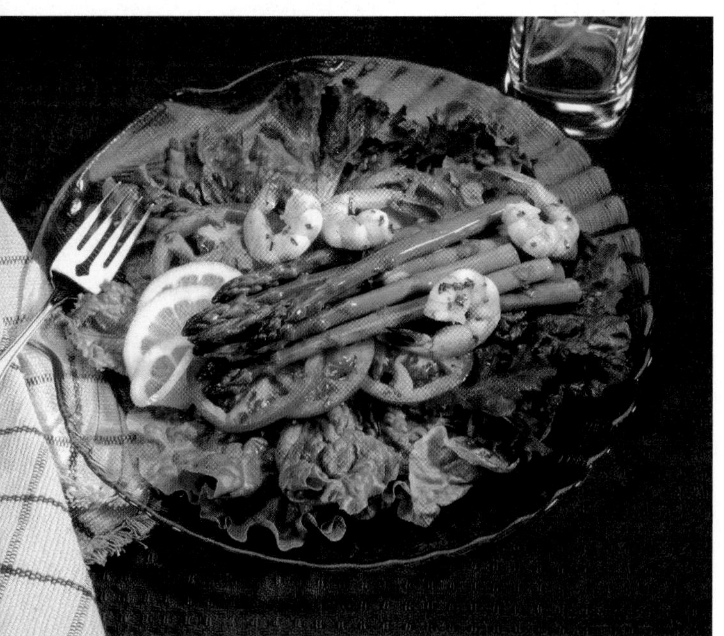

California Asparagus Commission

21-8 Shrimp that have been simmered, chilled, and peeled make a tasty addition to a cool, main dish salad.

Chapter 21 Review
Fish and Shellfish

Summary

Lean fish, fat fish, mollusks, and crustaceans are all good sources of protein, vitamins, and minerals. Finfish are available whole, drawn, dressed, or as steaks or fillets. Shrimp, oysters, crabs, lobsters, clams, and scallops are the most popular types of shellfish in the United States. You can buy both finfish and shellfish fresh, canned, and frozen. Shellfish usually tend to be rather costly. The cost of finfish depends on the form and where you buy it. Both fish and shellfish are quite perishable and should be used soon after purchase.

Both finfish and shellfish require short cooking periods and moderate temperatures. Properly cooked finfish have an opaque appearance and flake easily with a fork. You can use a number of cooking methods to prepare fish. Appropriate methods include broiling, grilling, baking, frying, poaching, steaming, and microwaving. However, fat fish are usually best prepared by dry heat and lean fish are usually best prepared by moist heat. The kind of shellfish, and whether you purchase it live, frozen, or canned, will help you decide how to cook it.

Review What You Have Read

Write your answers on a separate sheet of paper.

1. True or false. Finfish can be lean or fatty.
2. Shrimp, lobster, and crab are examples of _____.
3. Canned salmon and sardines (with bones) are especially good sources of what mineral?
4. List four signs of quality for purchasing fresh fish.
5. A fish that has the entrails removed is called a _____.
   A. drawn fish
   B. dressed fish
   C. fish fillet
   D. fish steak
6. What are deveined shrimp?
7. True or false. Fresh fish is usually less expensive in coastal regions than in inland areas.
8. Describe how to prepare fish for refrigerator storage.
9. What are two characteristics that indicate a finfish has been cooked to the proper degree of doneness?
10. What type of finfish is usually cooked by dry heat?
11. What can you do to prevent baked fish from drying out?
12. How can you help poached fish retain its shape?
13. True or false. Frozen fish is cooked for the same amount of time and at the same temperature as fresh fish.
14. True or false. Shellfish purchased in the shell must be alive when cooked.

Build Your Basic Skills

1. **Math.** Compare the cholesterol and fat content of several varieties of fish and shellfish with those of several cuts of meat. Use Appendix C, "Nutritive Values of Foods," to help you.
2. **Reading.** Find five recipes for broiling lean fish. In each recipe, identify how the fish is prevented from becoming dry.

Build Your Thinking Skills

1. **Predict.** With your foods lab group, examine an unknown type of fish fillet given to you by your teacher. Predict whether the fish would be best prepared by moist or dry heat. Cut the fillet in half. Prepare one half by a moist heat method and the other half by a dry heat method. Compare the flavor and appearance of the two cooked pieces. Write a brief report stating your reasons for your original prediction and an evaluation of whether your prediction was accurate.
2. **Compare.** Panfry, oven-fry, and deep-fry small, dressed fish or fish fillets using both batter and crumb coatings. Prepare a table to compare color, crispness, tenderness, and flavor.

Apply Technology

1. Investigate how commercial fishers use sonar to detect fish in the water.
2. Explore the development of aquaculture and its impact on the supply of fish in consumer retail outlets. Share your findings in an oral report.

Using Workplace Skills

Midori is a raw shellfish preparer at The Barrier Reef, an elegant seafood restaurant. She is responsible for shucking fresh clams, oysters, and scallops; deveining shrimp; cracking crab legs; and splitting lobster tails. The owner of the restaurant prides himself in the presentation of the food. He will not allow the staff to serve anything that looks imperfect. However, he becomes quite angry when food is wasted.

To be an effective worker, Midori needs skill in selecting equipment and tools. In a small group, answer the following questions about Midori's need for and use of this skill:

A. How might the food be affected if Midori does not select the proper tools and equipment for each type of shellfish?
B. How might Midori's customers react if she does not properly prepare each type of shellfish?
C. How might Midori's employer react if she does not properly prepare each type of shellfish?
D. What is another skill Midori would need in this job? Briefly explain why this skill would be important.

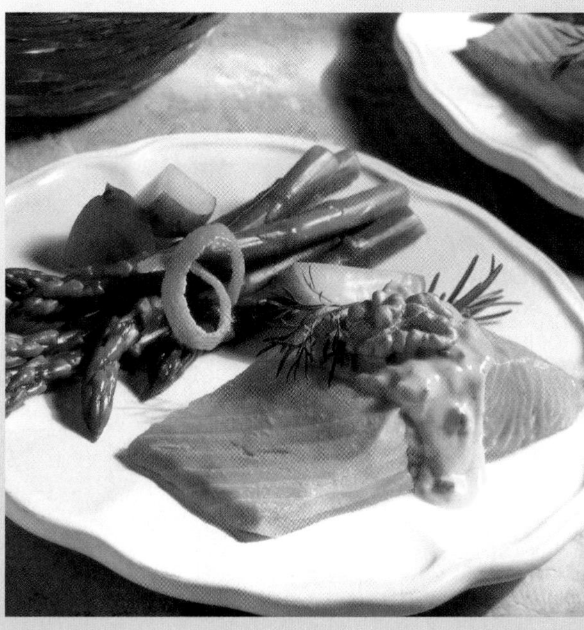

Chapter 22
Salads, Casseroles, and Soups

Salad Maker
Prepares salads, fruits, melons, and gelatin desserts.

Soup Cook
Prepares, seasons, and cooks soups and other foodstuffs for consumption in eating establishments.

Spice Sales Representative
Sells spices to retail food stores, wholesale grocers, restaurants, hotels, or institutions.

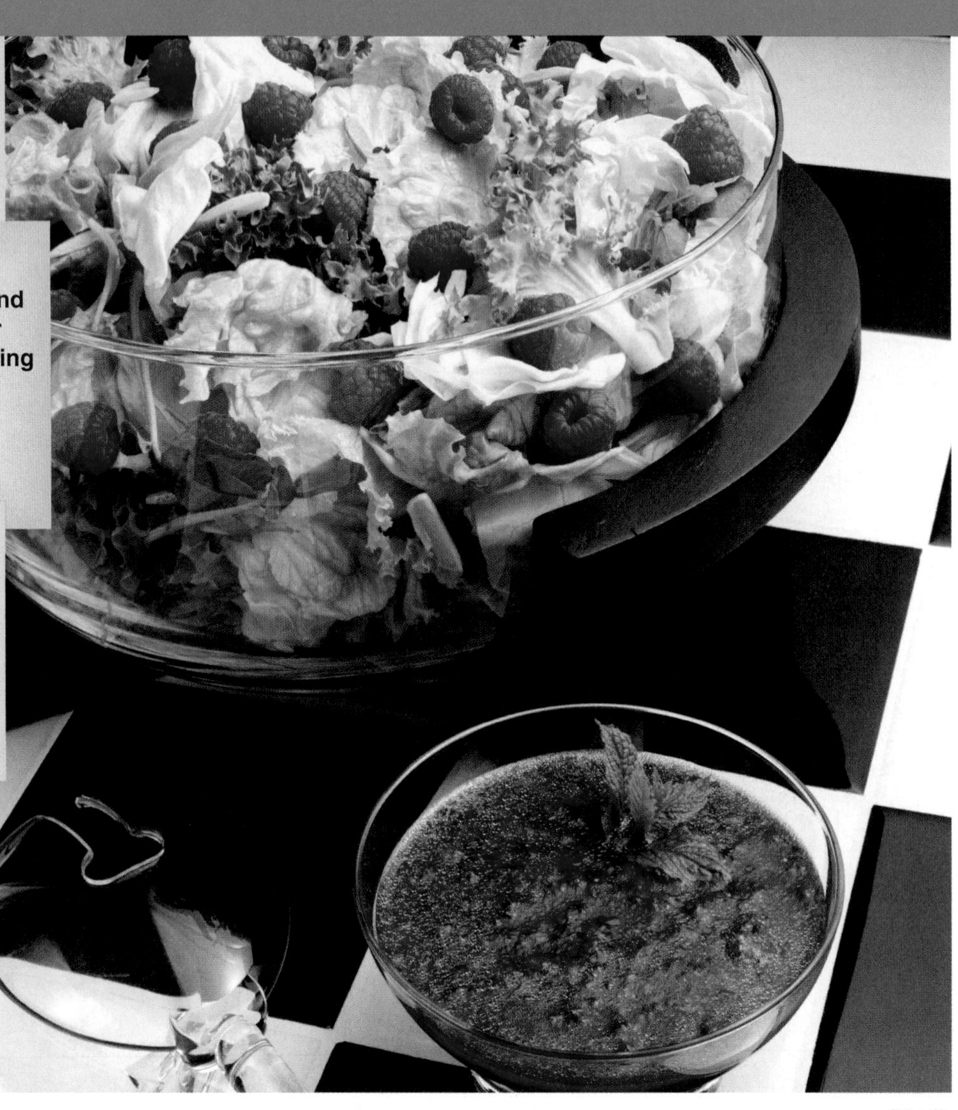

Driscoll's

Terms to Know

salad
temporary emulsion
permanent emulsion
casserole
stock soup
bouillon
consommé
herb
spice
blend
bouquet garni
gourmet

Objectives

After studying this chapter, you will be able to

- explain how to prepare salad ingredients and assemble a salad.
- list the basic ingredients in a casserole.
- prepare nutritious salads, casseroles, and stock-based soups.
- distinguish among herbs, spices, and blends.

Salads, casseroles, and soups add versatility to menus. You may serve them as the main course or as an accompaniment to a meal. These combination dishes are nutritious as well as economical. They include a variety of ingredients, and preparing them can be a way to use leftovers.

Q: Is it true that you can't put pineapple in a gelatin salad?

A: Fresh and frozen pineapple contain an enzyme that will keep gelatin from setting. Fresh and frozen kiwi, gingerroot, papaya, figs, and guava will keep gelatin from setting, too. However, feel free to use cooked and canned forms of these fruits. The heat used in cooking and canning deactivates the enzymes that affect gelatin.

Salads

What is a salad? A ***salad*** is a combination of raw and/or cooked ingredients, usually served cold with a dressing. The vegetables, fruits, and protein foods salads contain contribute important nutrients to the diet. Depending on the ingredients, you can serve salads as any part of a meal—appetizer, main dish, accompaniment, or dessert.

Kinds of Salads

Most salads fit into one of five groups. *Protein salads* make up one group. Some protein salads have small pieces of protein food combined with a dressing. Chicken, ham, crab, and egg salads are examples of this type. Other protein salads have strips or slices of protein food arranged on a plate with cold vegetables or fruits. A chef salad is an example of this type.

Pasta, vegetable, fruit, and gelatin are the other four groups of salads. A *pasta salad* is a combination of cooked pasta, vegetables, possibly a protein food, and a dressing. You can make *vegetable salads* from salad greens; raw vegetables; or cold, cooked vegetables. Tossed salad, coleslaw, and three-bean salad are examples of vegetable salads. Canned, frozen, or fresh fruits served on a bed of greens or in a hollowed fruit shell make a refreshing *fruit salad*. You can use commercial fruit-flavored gelatin or mix fruit and vegetable juices with unflavored gelatin to make a *gelatin salad*. Almost any fruits, vegetables, and/or protein foods can be added to the gelatin for nutrition and variety.

Preparing Salad Ingredients

Most fruits and vegetables used in salads are very perishable. Preserving their freshness is important to keep colors bright, textures crisp, and flavors full. Treating fruits, vegetables, and salad greens carefully will also help protect nutrients.

Trim all bruised and inedible portions on fresh salad ingredients. Discard outer leaves of greens and wash all fresh produce carefully to remove soil and pesticide residues. Avoid soaking fresh ingredients to prevent loss of water-soluble nutrients. Drain fresh salad ingredients well.

To prevent nutrient losses, it is best not to clean fresh salad ingredients too far in advance. Wrap cleaned greens loosely in plastic film or a damp cloth or store them in a vegetable keeper. You can store washed greens for a few hours in the refrigerator. They will be crisp when ready to serve and will still retain important vitamins and minerals. See 22-1.

The size of pieces of food in a salad should be easy to manage. Tear salad greens into bite-sized pieces. Do not cut greens with a knife, as this will cause bruising. Avoid mincing other salad ingredients to keep them from forming a paste when mixed with the dressing.

Treat fresh cut apples, peaches, bananas, and pears with lemon juice. This will prevent enzymatic browning, making your salad look fresher and more attractive.

You may serve canned peaches and pears in large pieces because they are easy to cut with a fork. Be sure to drain liquid from canned fruits and vegetables. Extra liquid will make salads look and taste watery.

Varying the shapes of pieces will add interest to the appearance of a salad. You will

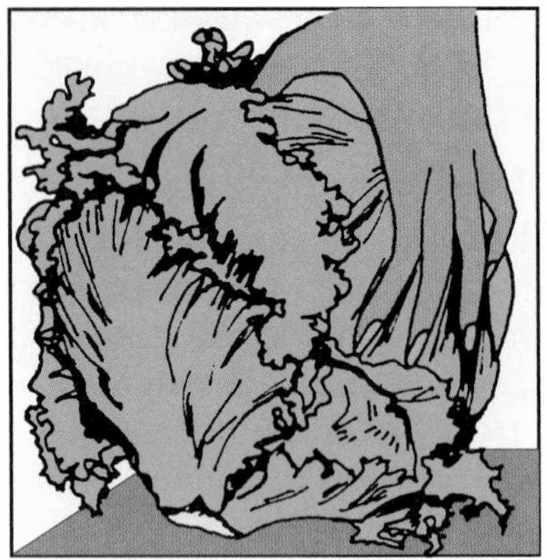
A—Grasp the head firmly. Strike the core end sharply against a counter or wooden cutting board.

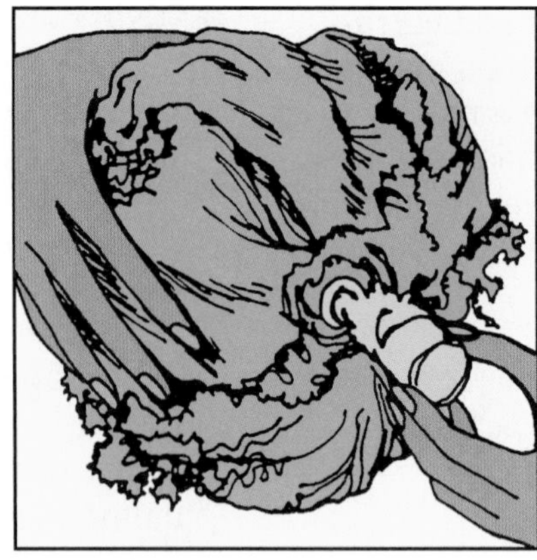
B—Pull the core from the head with a twisting motion.

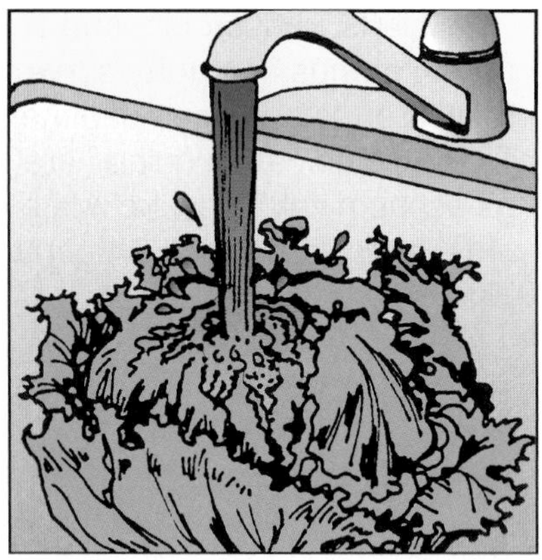
C—Run cold water into the hole left by the core to thoroughly wash the head.

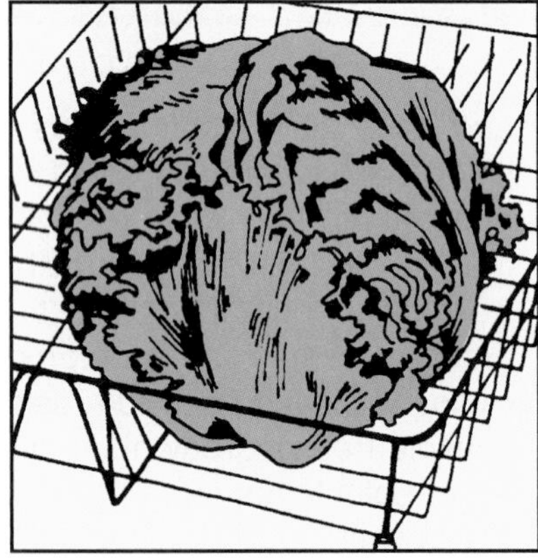
D—Drain lettuce well, using a colander or dish rack.

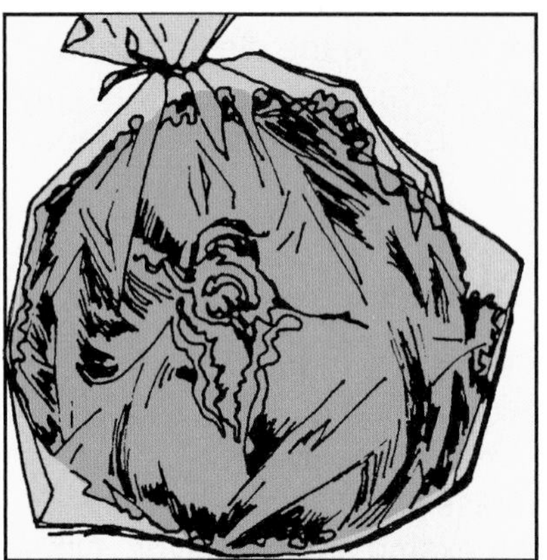
E—Place cleaned and drained lettuce in a loosely closed plastic bag. Store it in the refrigerator.

adapted from Western Iceberg Lettuce

***22-1** When cleaning iceberg lettuce, follow these step-by-step directions.*

usually section citrus fruits. You might cut tomatoes and hard-cooked eggs into wedges. You could slice or shred carrots. You will usually dice meats and poultry. Flake fish with a fork. You might crumble cheese or cut it into strips.

Preparing Salad Dressings

There are three basic types of salad dressings: French, mayonnaise, and cooked. All three types are examples of *emulsions*, which are combinations of two liquids that ordinarily will not stay mixed. In the case of salad dressings, these liquids are usually oil and vinegar, lemon juice, or some other water-based liquid.

You make a true *French dressing* by combining oil, vinegar, and seasonings. When you agitate (shake) the dressing, an emulsion forms. When you stop the agitation and allow the dressing to stand,

Good Manners Are Good Business

Some salad makers do not tear their greens into bite-sized pieces. Do not be unnerved if someone serves you such a salad at a business meal. You should not try to stuff a large piece of lettuce into your mouth. Most salad greens are tender enough to cut with your salad fork. However, if you have trouble, feel free to use your knife to help you cut one bite at a time.

the oil and water-based liquid separate, and the emulsion breaks. Therefore, French dressing is considered a ***temporary emulsion.*** You must shake or stir French dressing to mix it each time you use it.

You make *mayonnaise* from vinegar (or lemon juice), oil, seasonings, and egg yolk. Mayonnaise is an example of a ***permanent emulsion.*** This type of emulsion will not separate on standing. This is because the egg yolk acts as an *emulsifying agent.* This is an ingredient that surrounds the droplets of oil and keeps them suspended in the liquid (vinegar or lemon juice).

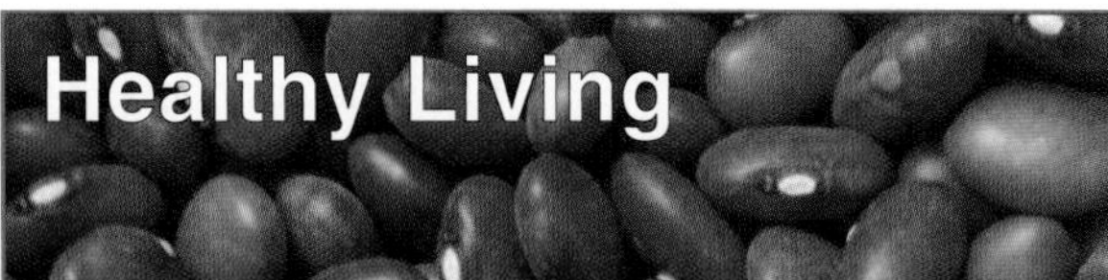

Healthy Living

The dressing can add a lot of fat and calories to a salad. To avoid this, you might try some of the lowfat or fat-free dressings that are available. You can even make your own lowfat dressing. Yogurt can substitute for dressing on many salads. Its texture is similar to mayonnaise, but it is much lower in fat. You can flavor plain yogurt with herbs and use it on vegetable salads. Vanilla and fruit-flavored yogurts make creamy toppings for fruit salads.

A *cooked salad dressing* looks like mayonnaise. However, you thicken it with a food starch, such as cornstarch or flour. It also contains milk or water, an acid ingredient such as lemon juice, and a small amount of oil. Egg and butter are optional ingredients. Cooked salad dressings are permanent emulsions.

You can add other ingredients to mayonnaise or basic cooked dressing. For a fruit salad, you might add whipped cream and crushed pineapple. For Thousand Island dressing, add catsup, pickle relish, and chopped hard-cooked egg.

Assembling a Salad

Assemble salads as close to serving time as possible. Consider flavor, texture, and color when you choose salad ingredients. Avoid too many strongly flavored foods and foods that are all crisp or all soft. Colors should complement each other.

Most salads have three parts: a base, a body, and a dressing. Begin assembling the salad with the *base.* This is the foundation on which you place the main salad ingredients. It provides a contrast in color with the body of the salad. It also keeps the serving dish from looking bare. The base should not extend over the edge of the plate or serving dish.

You will often use salad greens to make the salad base. Many people think of iceberg lettuce when they think of a salad. However, a combination of three or four types of greens can add flavor, color, and texture variety to salads. Romaine, Boston bibb, watercress, spinach, escarole, endive, and leaf lettuce are some of the many salad greens available. See 22-2.

Arrange the salad *body*, or main part of the salad, on top of the base. Be artistic but natural.

If the body of your salad is molded gelatin, you must unmold it before serving. Quickly dip the mold into warm water or cover it with a warm, damp cloth for a few seconds. (Be sure not to keep the mold in the water too long, or the gelatin will lose its shape.) Invert the loosened salad onto a serving plate.

The *dressing* is a sauce served on or with a salad to add flavor. You will usually pour the dressing over the salad just before serving. Avoid using too much dressing. The dressing should not mask the flavors of the other salad

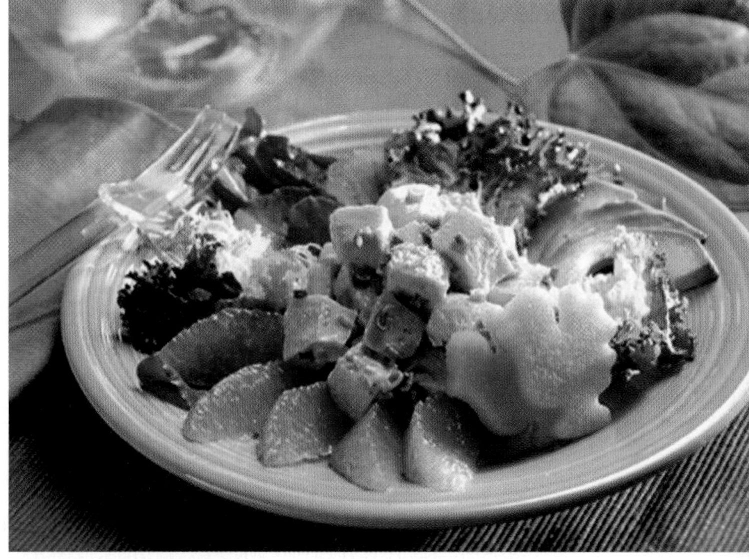

National Chicken Council

22-2 *A combination of red and green lettuce varieties serves as a colorful base for this fruited chicken salad.*

Q: Won't eating spinach salad help build muscles?

A: Thanks to old Popeye cartoons, such myths about spinach are common. Popeye may have been misled by the fact that spinach is a source of iron. Getting enough iron in the diet can help you avoid the fatigue and weakness associated with a lack of iron. However, iron cannot build muscles or make you strong. For that, you need to participate in strength training exercise.

ingredients. Instead, it should complement them. You may also wish to serve dressings separately and allow diners to dress their own salads. For some salads, you will combine the salad ingredients with the dressing several hours before serving to give the flavors a chance to blend.

Some salads have a fourth part—the *garnish.* The main purpose of a garnish is to add eye appeal. It should be simple and should complement the other salad ingredients. Grated hard-cooked egg yolk, pimiento strips, and vegetable curls are popular salad garnishes.

You will serve a few salads, such as German potato salad, hot. Serve most other salads well chilled. Allow a frozen fruit salad to soften slightly before serving. This will give the individual flavors a chance to mellow.

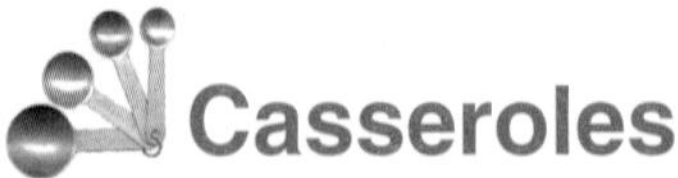

Casseroles

A ***casserole*** is a combination of foods prepared in a single dish. Casseroles are quick and easy to prepare. A simple salad and dessert are all you need to accompany them. Most casseroles freeze well, so you can prepare them ahead of time for emergency meals.

Casseroles are a great way to emphasize plant foods in your diet. Casseroles often include a variety of vegetables and grains and only small amounts of meat. Many hearty casseroles can be made without any meat at all. Tasty combinations of rice and legumes or vegetables and pasta can become nutritious entrees. See 22-3.

Casserole Ingredients

Most casseroles are a combination of a protein food, a vegetable, a starch, and a sauce. Many have a topping made of crumbs, cheese, or chopped nuts.

One or several foods high in protein can form the basis of a casserole. Turkey, chicken, ground beef, ham, luncheon meat, cheese, hard-cooked eggs, and seafood make good casserole bases.

You can use any canned, frozen, or cooked fresh vegetable in a casserole. Try peas, green beans, carrots, spinach, or a combination of vegetables.

You can combine starchy foods, such as potatoes, rice, and pasta, with a variety of protein foods and vegetables. Starchy ingredients help make casseroles filling.

A casserole sauce can be as simple as a can of condensed soup or as fancy as a homemade cheese sauce. Experiment with cream of tomato, shrimp, mushroom, or asparagus soups. As an alternative, try adding grated Swiss cheese and a sprinkle of nutmeg to a basic white sauce.

Extras can add crunch, color, and flavor to a casserole. Bean sprouts, Chinese noodles, celery, almonds, and French-fried onion rings

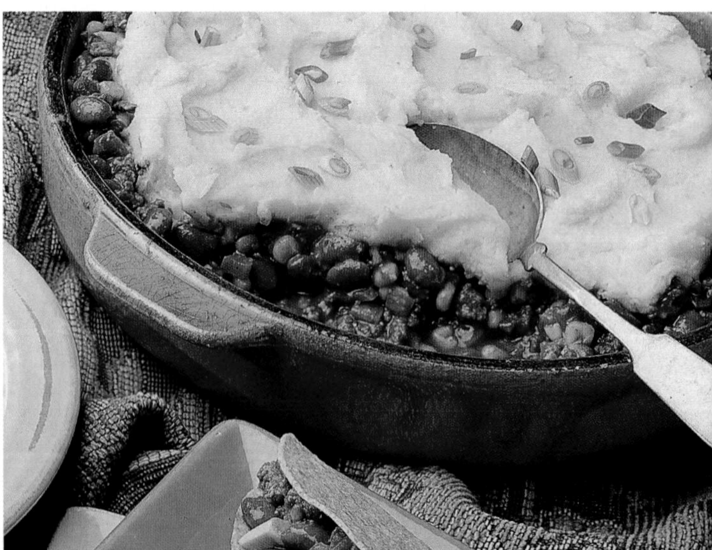

Bush's Chili Magic Chili Starter

***22-3** Onions, tomatoes, corn, beans, and mashed potatoes help a little ground beef go a long way in this tasty, nutritious casserole.*

add crunch. Tomato wedges, green pepper rings, chopped parsley, and pimiento add color. Horseradish, chili sauce, and chopped onions add flavor.

Toppings help keep a casserole from becoming dry. They also add color, flavor, and texture. Buttered bread crumbs are one popular topping. You might want to try crushed cereals, potato chips, or corn chips mixed with a little melted margarine. Dumplings, biscuits, and cornbread squares also make good toppings.

As you prepare casseroles, be aware of the fat and sodium content of sauces and other ingredients. You can adapt many casserole recipes to make them more healthful. For instance, you can easily use reduced-fat mayonnaise or low-sodium condensed soup in place of traditional ingredients. Such changes will make casseroles more nutritious without having much effect on flavor.

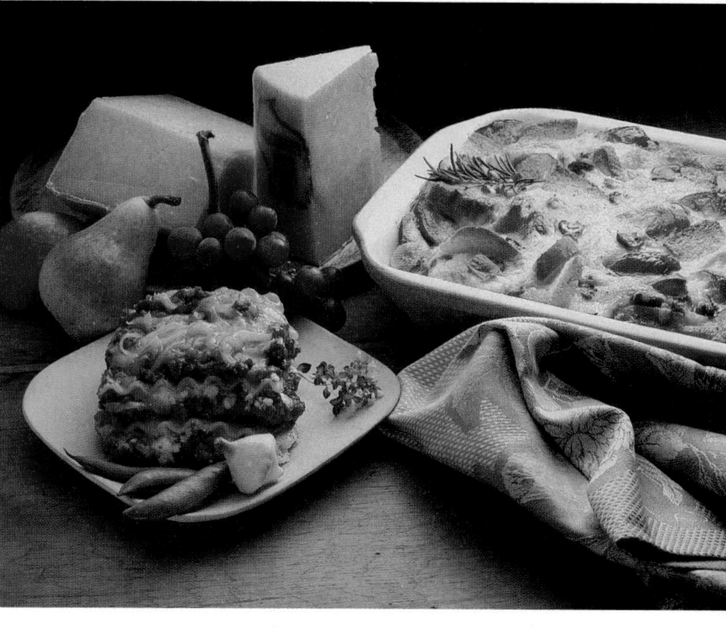

22-4 *Greasing the baking dish before layering in the ingredients will make casseroles easier to serve and clean up.*

Putting It Together

The key to putting a casserole together is combining ingredients that complement each other. Personal likes and dislikes will guide you. Experience will also help.

Until you have become experienced in making casseroles, you probably will want to choose just one item out of each group. Use seasonings sparingly at first. Also avoid using too many highly seasoned foods at one time.

Cleanup of baked casseroles will be easier if you put the casserole in a greased dish, 22-4. You can bake most casseroles in a moderate oven until they are brown and bubbly. Cooking time will depend on the size of the dish and the starting temperature of the casserole. The topping may begin to brown before the casserole heats through. A piece of aluminum foil placed loosely over the top will keep it from getting too dark.

You can prepare some casseroles on top of the range. They are just as quick and easy as oven casseroles. However, they may require some stirring and a bit more attention during the cooking period.

Unlike soufflés and rare roast beef, most casseroles can wait for latecomers. Some casseroles even improve when they are held for a while. This is because their flavors have a chance to blend. When you will not be serving a casserole right away, cover it tightly and keep it warm in a low oven.

Be a Clever Consumer

Making casseroles can help you stretch your food dollars. Starchy foods and vegetables help extend more costly protein ingredients. Because you need to precook casserole ingredients, casseroles can also help you make use of leftovers. Most casseroles are easy to prepare, so they save time as well as money. They are an economical choice when serving a crowd, too.

Microwaving Casseroles

Dinners can be ready in minutes when you assemble casseroles from leftovers and heat them in a microwave oven. The microwave oven is also excellent for reheating and defrosting casseroles.

Make casseroles for the microwave with precooked ingredients. You can prepare and serve most of them in the same dish. This saves time and effort in cleanup.

Stock Soups

People throughout the world serve soup in many forms. It can be hot or cold, hearty or light. It can be an appetizer or a main dish. You can eat it alone or serve it with other foods. Soup is most popular in the United States as an appetizer or luncheon dish.

You can make soup in two ways. You make ***stock soups*** with rich-flavored broth in which meat, poultry, or fish; vegetables; and seasonings have been cooked. You make *cream soups* with milk instead of broth. This chapter discusses stock-based soups. Chapter 17 discussed milk-based or cream soups.

Make stocks from less tender meat cuts, poultry, and fish. You might want to add vegetables such as celery and carrots for flavor.

Preparing Stocks

Stocks obtain their flavor from the flavors of their ingredients. Meats, poultry, fish, and vegetables release their flavors slowly. To make stocks rich and flavorful, cook them over low heat for a long time.

To make a stock more flavorful, you will want to increase the amount of surface area exposed to the cooking liquid. To do this, cut the meat, poultry, fish, and vegetables for a stock into small pieces. Also, crack any large bones that you put into a stockpot.

If you are making a *brown stock,* begin by browning the meat. If you are making a *light stock,* use poultry, fish, or unbrowned meat, 22-5.

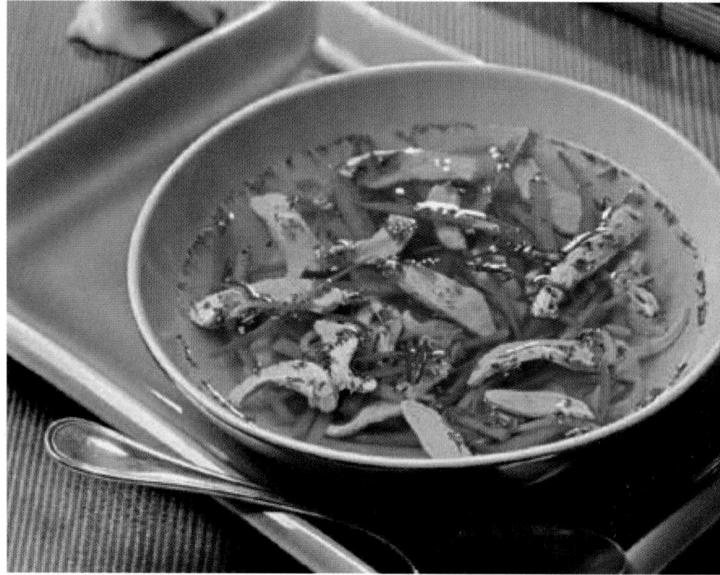

National Chicken Council

22-5 Chicken soup is made with a light stock.

To prepare a stock, place all the ingredients in a large pan with a tightly fitted lid. Cover them with cold water, and cook them slowly for several hours at a simmering temperature. The liquid should never boil.

During the first stage of cooking, foam will rise to the surface. Skim it from the stock. You can use a wooden spoon or paddle for skimming.

During the final stages of cooking, fat will rise to the surface of the stock if you have used fatty meats. You can remove the fat with a baster while the stock is hot. You can also remove fat after it congeals on chilled stock.

After cooking, strain the stock. *Straining* separates the broth from the solid materials. You can serve the meat, poultry, or fish separately or add it back to the stock to make soup. You can also add vegetables, rice, noodles or other pasta, and seasonings, if desired.

Preparing Bouillon and Consommé

Clear broth made from stock is called ***bouillon.*** Bouillon is most often made from beef stock. Clear, rich-flavored soup made from stock is called ***consommé.*** Both bouillon and consommé are low in calories. They make excellent appetizers and snacks for all age groups.

For both bouillon and consommé, you must first *clarify* the stock. You can clarify strained stock by adding a slightly beaten egg white and a few pieces of eggshell to the boiling broth. As the egg protein coagulates, it traps any solid materials. Strain the clarified stock to remove the egg, solid materials, and eggshell.

To prepare bouillon, reduce the strained and clarified stock in volume by further cooking. This additional cooking concentrates the stock, making it richer and more flavorful.

Prepare consommé by simmering the strained and clarified stock still longer. It has a richer flavor than bouillon.

Microwaving Soups

Stocks are best when prepared on a conventional rangetop. Long, slow cooking allows flavors to blend. Once you have made stocks

Q: Because herbs are natural products, wouldn't herbal supplements be safe?

A: Natural and safe are not synonyms. (Remember, poison ivy is a natural product!) Herbal supplements are not regulated, and the concentrations of herbs used in supplements vary. Much research is still needed to fully evaluate the safety and effectiveness of these products. If you choose to use herbal supplements, do so with caution. Also, be sure to tell your doctor about any herbal supplements you are taking. Some can interact with medications.

into soups, however, you can heat them in a microwave oven in a matter of minutes. You can also prepare convenience soups in a microwave oven.

Microwave most stock soups on high power. Refer to a microwave cookbook for specific instructions. You may want to heat some soups on a lower power to allow ingredients to simmer.

Choose containers of ample size when microwaving soups to avoid boilovers. Cover soups and stir them during the microwaving period to promote more even cooking.

Herbs and Spices

Herbs, spices, and blends can greatly enhance the flavors of salads, casseroles, soups, and all other foods. ***Herbs*** are the leaves of plants usually grown in temperate climates. Basil, bay leaf, and mint are examples of herbs, 22-6. You can purchase some herbs fresh, but most are sold dried.

Spices are the dried roots, stems, and seeds of plants grown mainly in the tropics. Cinnamon, allspice, pepper, and ginger are examples of spices. Sometimes people use the word spice to mean "hot" or pungent. Not all spices are hot, however. Most just give flavor. Spices are sold in whole or ground forms.

Blends are combinations of ground herbs and spices. Poultry seasoning and pumpkin pie spice are examples of blends.

Using Herbs and Spices

You can use herbs fresh or dried. Fresh herbs such as dill sprigs and basil leaves make attractive garnishes. Fresh herbs are not as concentrated as dried herbs. You need to use about three times more to get the same flavor. Unless the recipe tells you otherwise, use dried herbs when you cook.

You can use a microwave oven to dry fresh herbs for use in recipes. Simply microwave ½ cup (125 mL) fresh herbs on high power for two minutes.

Ground spices release their flavor immediately when added to food. Add them toward the end of cooking. Whole spices release their flavor more slowly, so you can add them at the beginning of cooking.

You might want to place whole spices and herbs in a cheesecloth bag before adding them to food. This is called a ***bouquet garni.*** After the herbs and spices have released their flavors, you can easily remove them from the food.

Gourmet Cooking

Gourmets are people who enjoy being able to distinguish the complex combinations of flavors that make up foods. Some people think gourmet cooking requires hours of work and ingredients that are hard to find. However, this is not necessarily the case. Gourmet food is simply food that is expertly seasoned. Creative use of herbs and spices can make gourmet dishes out of some of the simplest foods.

Becoming familiar with a range of herbs and spices can help you prepare foods with a gourmet touch. As you work with seasonings, you will learn that some herbs and spices go especially well with certain foods. For instance, many recipes for custard call for nutmeg. Rosemary and mint complement the flavor of lamb. People often add cinnamon to apple dishes. See 22-7.

Using herbs and spices well requires practice and skill. When learning to use seasonings, start with small amounts. Ideally, herbs and spices should enhance food, not overpower it.

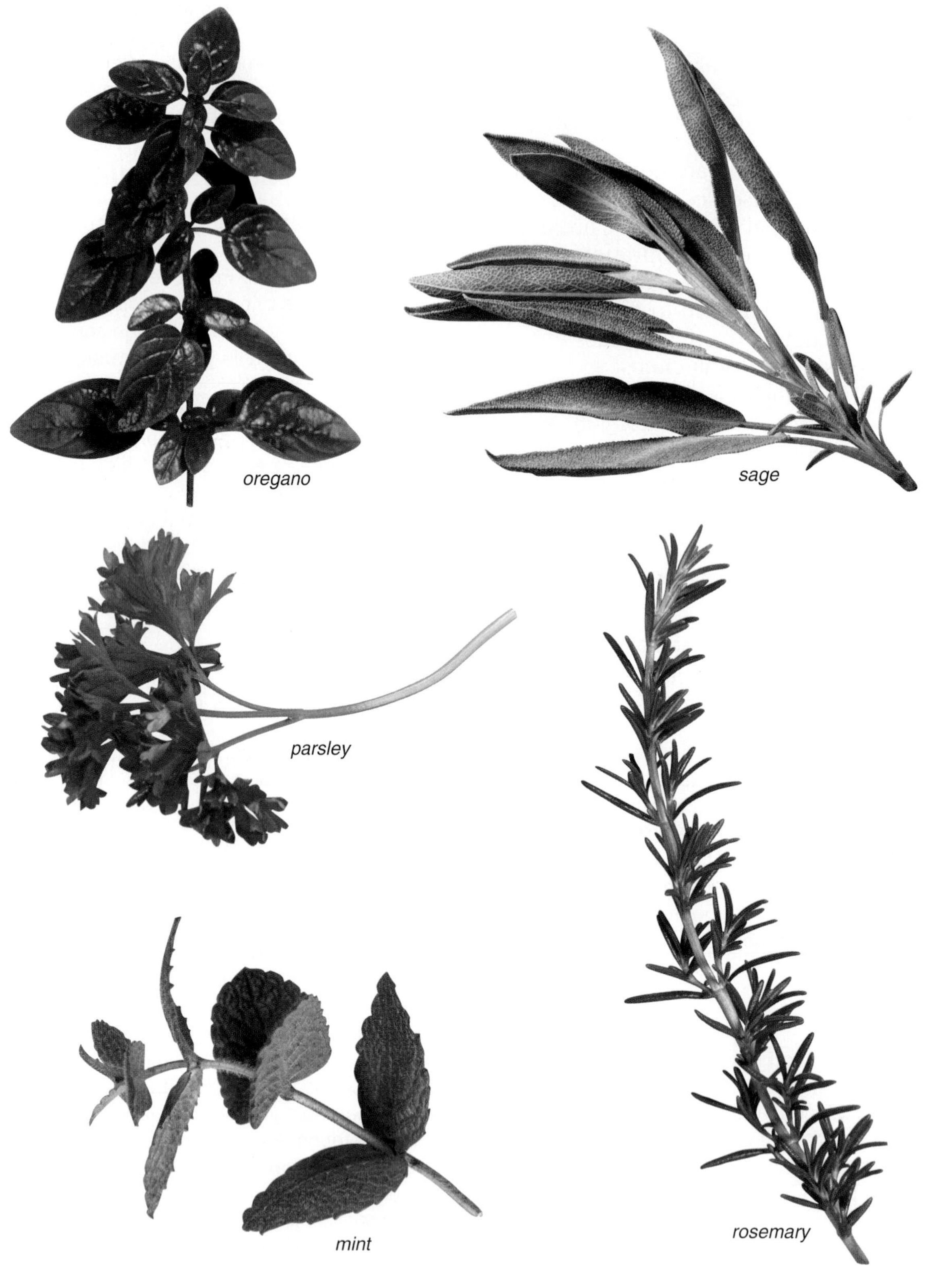

22-6 *Leaves of plants used to flavor foods are called herbs.*

Seasoning Success	
Food Item	**Herbs and Spices**
Beef	*Basil, bay leaves, cayenne, cloves, garlic, ginger, oregano, pepper, sage, tarragon, thyme*
Fish	*Allspice, cayenne, dill weed, garlic, ginger, mint, paprika, rosemary, sage, thyme*
Lamb	*Mint, rosemary*
Pork	*Cloves, cumin, garlic, ginger, sage*
Poultry	*Rosemary, sage, tarragon, thyme*
Eggs	*Basil, cayenne, chives, oregano, paprika, tarragon*
Vegetables	*Allspice, basil, bay leaves, cayenne, cloves, dill weed, garlic, ginger, nutmeg, oregano, paprika, rosemary, tarragon, thyme*
Fruits	*Allspice, cinnamon, cloves, ginger, nutmeg*
Breads and stuffings	*Cayenne, cinnamon, dill weed, rosemary, sage, thyme*
Desserts	*Allspice, cinnamon, cloves, ginger, mint, nutmeg*

22-7 *Learning which seasonings complement various food items can give you the confidence to be creative when combining ingredients and cooking new dishes.*

Storing Herbs and Spices

Always store herbs and spices in a cool, dry place away from light. Keep the containers tightly closed.

Buy herbs and spices in small amounts for ordinary cooking. Most spices and herbs will keep their flavor and aroma for about a year when properly stored. However, they lose their strength as they age, so date all containers. Whole spices will last longer than ground spices. You can tell if a spice or herb has lost its strength. Simply rub a little of it between your hands and smell it. If it has little or no odor, you have stored it too long.

Chapter 22 Review

Salads, Casseroles, and Soups

Summary

You can serve a salad as almost any part of a meal, from appetizer to dessert. There are five main types of salads—protein, pasta, vegetable, fruit, and gelatin. To prepare most salads, you will begin with a base of washed and trimmed salad greens. Cut ingredients for the body of the salad into bite-sized pieces. Salad dressings may be temporary or permanent emulsions. When assembling a salad, keep flavor, texture, and color in mind.

Casseroles are both easy and economical to prepare. They generally contain a protein food, vegetable, starch, sauce, and topping. Although you cook some casseroles on the rangetop, you cook most casseroles in a conventional or microwave oven.

You make stocks by covering meat, poultry, or fish with water and simmering it for a long time. You may also add vegetables for extra flavor. After cooking, you can strain a stock and add ingredients to make a hearty soup. You can also clarify stock and then reduce it through further cooking to prepare bouillon or consommé.

Herbs, spices, and seasoning blends are important ingredients in many foods. With practice, you will learn to use them to enhance the flavor of almost any dish.

Review What You Have Read

Write your answers on a separate sheet of paper.

1. Give an example of each of the five main types of salads.
2. Give two tips for preventing nutrient losses when preparing salad ingredients.
3. What are the three basic types of salad dressings?
4. What are the three main parts of a salad?
5. List five components of a casserole and give an example of each.
6. Give three guidelines you can follow when preparing casseroles.
7. What is a soup stock and how is one made?
8. How does bouillon differ from consommé?
9. List three common herbs and three common spices.
10. When should ground spices be added to food? When should whole spices be added?

Build Your Basic Skills

1. **Math.** Calculate and compare the cost per serving for instant, canned, and homemade bouillon. Taste samples of each and discuss when you might choose to use each product in cooking.
2. **Writing.** Write a paragraph about a real or fictional family and the activities in which each member is involved. In a second paragraph, describe a time during the week when all the family members share a meal. Write two dinner menus featuring meat, fish, or poultry entrees the meal manager might prepare for this meal. Write a third paragraph describing another time during the week when the meal manager has little time to prepare a meal. Then write two more menus featuring casseroles the meal manager could make with the leftovers from the first two menus.

Build Your Thinking Skills

1. **Plan.** Plan and prepare a class salad buffet. Each lab group should prepare one type of salad greens and one type of dressing. Each lab group should also choose a different type of salad to prepare. Coordinate recipe choices with other lab groups to plan for a variety of flavors, textures, colors, sizes, shapes, and temperatures.
2. **Propose.** Smell samples of three herbs and three spices. Use the aromas to propose a food item whose flavor would be enhanced by each herb or spice. Sample your proposed flavor combinations and summarize your conclusions in writing.

Apply Technology

1. Prepare two versions of a soup recipe—one made with salt and the other made with a salt substitute. Compare and evaluate the two products.
2. Investigate how and why spices are irradiated.

Using Workplace Skills

Sandy is the soup cook at The Country Hearth restaurant. The restaurant is known throughout the area for its delicious homemade soups and European-style, hearth-baked breads. Sandy's employer expects her to prepare three soup recipes each day of the week.

To be a successful employee, Sandy needs basic reading skills. Put yourself in Sandy's place and answer the following questions about your need for and use of these skills:

A. How will you use your reading skills as a soup cook?
B. How might customers of the restaurant be affected if you do not have adequate reading skills?
C. How might other people who work at the restaurant be affected if you do not have adequate reading skills?
D. What is another skill you would need in this job? Briefly explain why this skill would be important.

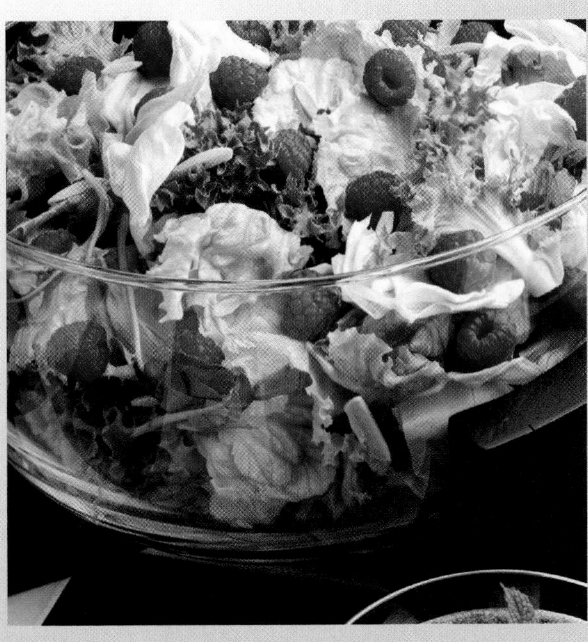

Chapter 23
Breads

Oven Tender
Tends stationary or rotary hearth oven that bakes breads, pastries, and other bakery products.

Baker
Mixes and bakes ingredients according to recipes to produce breads, pastries, and other baked goods.

Dividing-Machine Operator
Tends machines that automatically divide, round, proof, and shape dough into units of specified size and weight, according to work order, preparatory to baking.

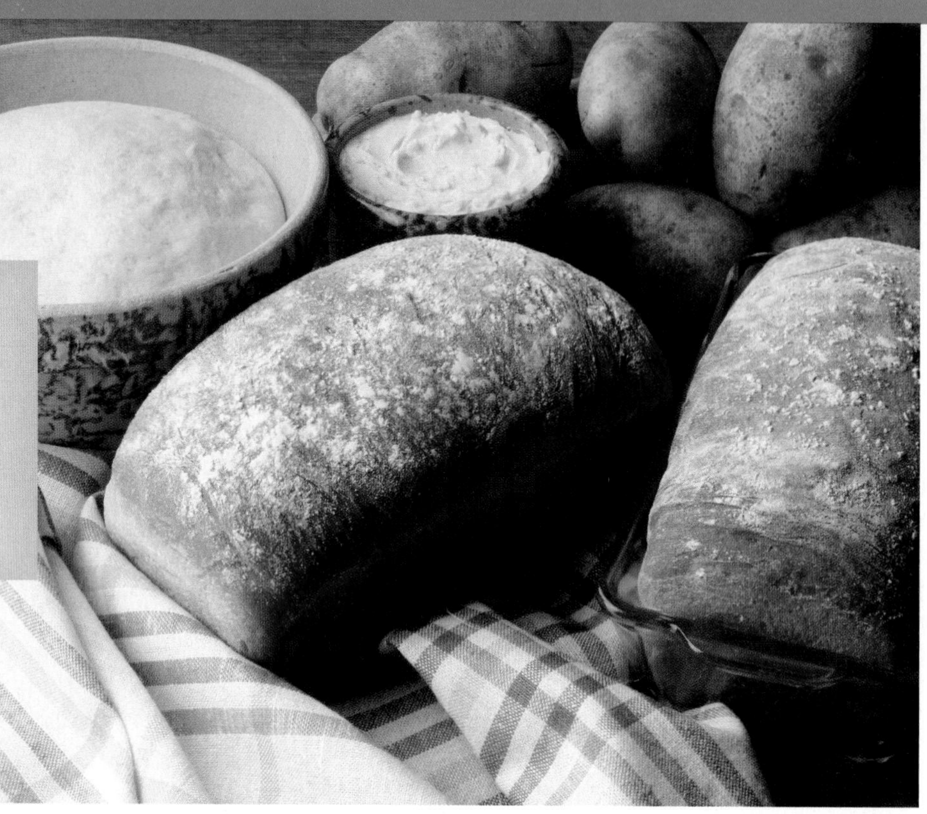

Terms to Know

batter
dough
leavening agent
gluten
fermentation

Objectives

After studying this chapter, you will be able to
- ❑ describe how to select and store baked goods.
- ❑ identify the functions of ingredients in baked products.
- ❑ prepare quick breads and yeast breads.

You can prepare *quick breads* in a short amount of time. Quick breads include biscuits, muffins, popovers, cream puffs, pancakes, and waffles. They also include coffee cakes and breads leavened with baking powder.

Yeast breads require more time to prepare than quick breads. Yeast breads include breads, rolls, English muffins, raised doughnuts, crullers, and many other yeast-raised products.

Selecting and Storing Baked Products

Quick breads and yeast breads are *baked products*. Cakes, cookies, and pies are baked products, too. Some of the following information applies to *all* baked products. However, preparation of cakes, cookies, and pies differs from preparation of breads. Therefore, cakes, cookies, and pies will be discussed further in the next chapter.

You can purchase baked products freshly baked, partially baked, refrigerated, and frozen. *Freshly baked items* are sold in bakeries, in bakery sections of supermarkets, and on supermarket shelves. They are ready to serve. *Brown-and-serve baked goods* are partially baked. They need a final browning in the oven before serving. *Refrigerated doughs* are ready to bake. They are handy for quickly preparing items like biscuits, turnovers, cookies, and rolls. *Frozen doughs and baked goods* require thawing and/or baking. Yeast doughs and cookie doughs are available frozen. You can buy frozen pies, cakes, coffee cakes, and doughnuts, too.

Cost of Baked Products

The cost of rolls, cakes, and other bakery products depends a lot on the amount of convenience. Ready-to-serve items usually cost more than items that require some preparation. Bakery yeast rolls, for instance, usually cost more than frozen yeast rolls.

Bread costs depend on size of loaf, extra ingredients, and brand. Large loaves usually cost less per serving than small loaves. Breads with fruit and nuts cost more than plain white or wheat bread. Store brands generally cost less than national brands.

Storing Baked Products

You can store freshly baked items at room temperature or in the freezer, tightly wrapped, 23-1. Freezing bread in hot, humid weather prevents mold growth. You can take slices of bread from the freezer as needed to thaw and eat. Refrigerate any baked products with cream, custard, or other perishable fillings or frosting.

Keep refrigerated doughs refrigerated until you plan to bake them. Likewise, store frozen doughs and baked products in the freezer until you are ready to use them.

Quick Breads

Quick breads may be made from batters or doughs. Both batters and doughs are mixtures of flour and liquid. ***Batters*** range in consistency

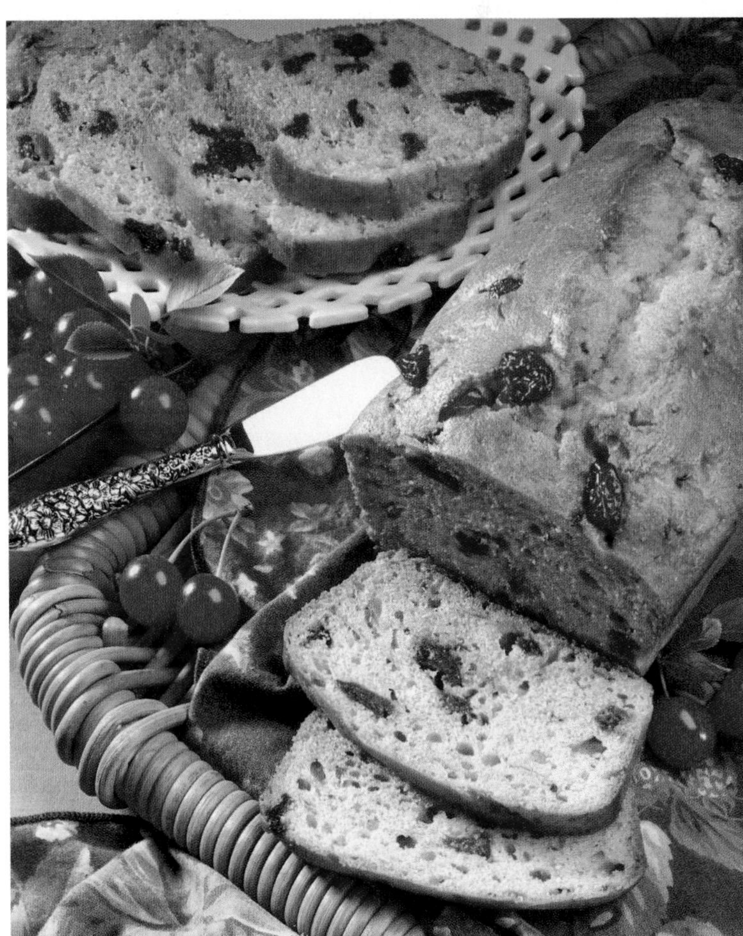

Cherry Marketing Institute

23-1 *This freshly baked bread can be wrapped and stored at room temperature.*

from thin liquids to stiff liquids. Thin batters are called *pour batters.* They have a large amount of liquid and a small amount of flour. You make a pour batter to prepare pancakes and popovers. Stiff batters are called *drop batters.* They have a high proportion of flour, and you can drop them from a spoon. You make a drop batter to prepare drop biscuits and some muffin recipes. ***Doughs*** have an even higher proportion of flour. They are stiff enough to shape by hand. You use soft dough to prepare shortcake and rolled biscuits. You use stiff dough to make rolled cookies and pastry.

Healthy Living

Breads, which are part of the grains group of the Food Guide Pyramid, are an excellent source of complex carbohydrates. You should be eating 6 to 11 servings of bread and cereal products every day to meet your body's energy needs. A typical serving of bread is one slice; one dinner roll; or half of a bagel, sandwich bun, or pita. When buying bread products, choose whole grain items often. They are low in fat and rich in vitamins and minerals. They are also higher in fiber than refined bread products.

Quick Bread Ingredients

Flour is a basic ingredient in all quick breads. However, the kinds of ingredients added to the flour distinguish one product from another. Leavening agents, liquid, fat, eggs, sugar, and salt are among the other ingredients that may be part of quick breads. Each ingredient serves a specific purpose.

Q: Doesn't a slice of toast have fewer calories than a slice of bread?

A: No. The heat of toasting removes water from bread but not calories.

Flour

Flour gives structure to baked products. White wheat flours are most often used for baking. Most quick breads are made with *all-purpose flour.* Some recipes call for *self-rising flour.* This is all-purpose flour with added leavening agents and salt.

Leavening Agents

Leavening agents are ingredients that produce gases in batters and doughs. These gases make baked products rise and become light and porous. Two leavening agents used in quick breads are baking soda and baking powder. Chemical reactions during baking cause these ingredients to release *carbon dioxide* gas.

Baking soda is sodium bicarbonate, which is an alkaline ingredient. It is used in quick bread recipes that contain food acid ingredients, which neutralize the alkali. This prevents a bitter, alkaline taste from forming in the bread. Food acid ingredients include buttermilk, molasses, brown sugar, vinegar, honey, applesauce or other fruit, and citrus juices. See 23-2.

Baking powders contain a dry acid or acid salt, baking soda, and starch or flour. Be sure to follow guidelines for using the recommended amount of baking powder. Too much baking powder will produce too much carbon dioxide, and the baked product will collapse. Too little baking powder will not produce enough carbon dioxide, and the product will be small and compact.

Two gases other than carbon dioxide that make baked products rise are steam and air. *Steam* is produced when liquid ingredients reach high temperatures during baking. Popovers and cream puffs are leavened almost entirely by steam. *Air* is incorporated into baked products by beating eggs, creaming fat and sugar together, folding doughs, and beating batters. All baked products contain some air.

Liquids

Water, milk, and fruit juices are liquids commonly used in baked products. Eggs and fats are also considered to be liquid ingredients.

Liquids serve several functions. They *hydrate* (cause to absorb water) the protein and starch in flour. Proteins must absorb water to later form gluten. Starches must absorb water to gelatinize during baking. Another function of liquids is to moisten or dissolve ingredients such as baking powder, salt, and sugar. Liquids also serve as leavening agents when they are converted to steam during baking.

Be a Clever Consumer

Compare carefully when shopping for baked products. Although added convenience usually means added cost, there are exceptions. For instance, a devil's food cake made from a mix is often less expensive than one made from scratch. Also, keep in mind that convenience can be worth the extra cost when you are in a hurry.

Fat

Fat serves primarily as a tenderizing agent in baked products. The fat coats the flour particles and causes the dough structure to separate into layers. Fat also aids leavening. When you beat fat, air bubbles form. The fat traps these air bubbles and holds them.

Eggs

Eggs help incorporate air into baked products when you beat them. They also add color and flavor and contribute to structure. During baking, the egg proteins coagulate. The coagulated proteins give the batter or dough elasticity and structure.

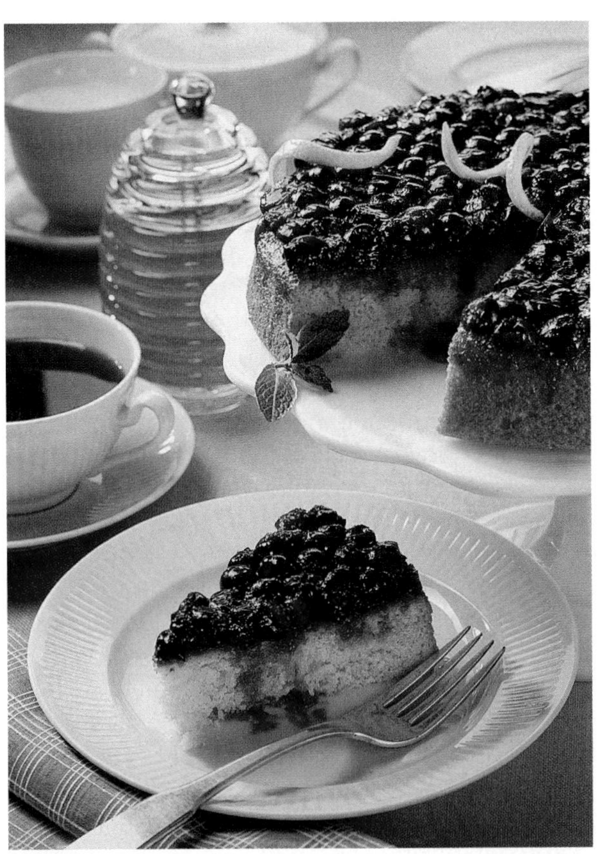

National Honey Board

***23-2** The alkaline baking soda in this coffee cake is neutralized by honey and lemon juice.*

Sugar

Sugar gives sweetness to baked products. It also has a tenderizing effect and helps crusts brown. In yeast breads, sugar serves as food for the yeast. Brown sugar gives a distinctive flavor to baked products. It also produces baked products that are moister than products made with granulated sugar.

Salt

Salt adds flavor to many baked products. In yeast breads, salt also regulates the action of the yeast and inhibits the action of certain enzymes. If yeast dough contains no salt, the yeast will produce carbon dioxide too quickly. The bread dough will be difficult to handle, and the baked product will have a poor appearance.

Adjusting Ingredients

As you have read, baking powder, fat, eggs, sugar, and salt each perform certain functions in baked goods. However, some recipes call for more of these ingredients than is really necessary. You can follow some simple guidelines to adjust quick bread and yeast bread recipes to reduce excess ingredients. Cutting down on unneeded ingredients will result in breads that are lower in calories, fat, and sodium. Such changes are in line with the Dietary Guidelines for Americans.

Table 23-3 shows minimum proportions of fat, eggs, sugar, salt, and baking powder for basic bread recipes. Ingredients are listed in the amounts needed for each cup of flour in the recipe. Many bread recipes call for cornmeal, oatmeal, and bran along with flour to give structure to products. You should count these ingredients as flour when figuring proportions of ingredients. However, these ingredients are heavier and may require a little extra baking powder for proper leavening.

Minimum Ingredient Proportions per 1 Cup (250 mL) of Flour					
Product	Fat	Eggs	Sugar	Salt	Baking Powder
Biscuits	2 tablespoons (30 mL)	—	—	1/4 teaspoon (1 mL)	1 1/4 teaspoons (6 mL)
Muffins	2 tablespoons (30 mL)	1/2	1 tablespoon (15 mL)	1/4 teaspoon (1 mL)	1 1/4 teaspoons (6 mL)
Popovers	1 tablespoon (15 mL)	2	—	1/4 teaspoon (1 mL)	—
Cream puffs	1/2 cup (125 mL)	4	—	1/4 teaspoon (1 mL)	—
Traditional yeast breads	1 tablespoon* (15 mL)	1/2*	1 teaspoon* (5 mL)	1/4 teaspoon (1 mL)	—
Bread machine yeast breads	2 teaspoons (10 mL)	*	1 tablespoon (15 mL)	1/2 teaspoon (2 mL)	—

*Many traditional yeast breads can be made without any fat or eggs. When recipes for richer breads call for these ingredients, the minimums shown here will produce a suitably rich dough. Sugar is not an essential ingredient in traditional unsweetened yeast breads. However, most recipes call for a small amount to serve as food for the yeast. Fat and sugar are not optional ingredients in yeast breads prepared in bread machines. Adding an egg and decreasing other liquids by 1/4 cup (50 mL) will improve structure and volume of whole grain bread machine recipes.

23-3 *Following these proportions will reduce the sugar, fat, and sodium in many quick bread and yeast bread recipes.*

You can make another simple adjustment by substituting fat free milk for whole milk in bread recipes. This change will reduce the fat in each serving of bread products. A recipe for corn muffins has been modified in 23-4.

Food Science Principles of Preparing Quick Breads

You can see food science principles at work in quick breads in the development of gluten. ***Gluten*** is a protein that gives strength and elasticity to batters and doughs and structure to baked products. It also holds the leavening gases, which are what make quick breads rise. Gluten is created by the proteins *gliadin* and *glutenin,* which are found in wheat flour. When you combine wheat flour with liquid and stir or knead the mixture, the glutenin and gliadin form gluten.

To understand gluten, think of a piece of bubble gum. When you first put the gum in your mouth, it is soft and easy to chew. As you chew the gum, it becomes more elastic, and you can blow bubbles. As you continue to chew the gum for a long time, it becomes so elastic it makes your jaws hurt.

Gluten behaves in a similar way. If you mix or handle a batter or dough too much, the gluten will overdevelop. This can cause a quick bread to be compact and tough. To keep quick breads light and tender, mix them for only a short time and handle them carefully.

The different kinds of white wheat flour contain different amounts of gliadin and glutenin. Therefore, the strength of the gluten produced by each of the flours differs. In baking, you must use the type of flour listed in your recipe. This will result in the correct amount of gluten for the particular product you are preparing. Yeast breads require a strong gluten structure. Cakes should have a delicate gluten structure. Most quick breads fall somewhere between.

Another way food science principles are at work in quick breads is in chemical reactions that produce leavening gases. Baking soda is an alkali. When combined with a food acid ingredient, baking soda releases carbon dioxide. Acid ingredients also help neutralize the batter, which would otherwise have a bitter flavor and disagreeable color.

Recipe Comparison	
Traditional Corn Muffins (Makes 12 muffins)	**Light Corn Muffins** (Makes 12 muffins)
1 cup flour	1 cup flour
1 cup cornmeal	1 cup cornmeal
1/4 cup sugar	2 tablespoons sugar
1 teaspoon salt	1/2 teaspoon salt
4 teaspoons baking powder	1 tablespoon baking powder
1 egg	1 egg
1 cup milk	1 cup fat free milk
1/3 cup shortening	1/4 cup shortening

***23-4** Adjusting ingredient proportions in this traditional recipe can save 25 calories, 2 grams of fat, and 115 mg of sodium per muffin.*

Most baking powders are *double-acting baking powders*. They release some of their carbon dioxide when they are moistened. However, they release most of their carbon dioxide when they are heated.

Preparing Biscuits

The method used to mix baked products is another factor that distinguishes one baked product from another. When preparing biscuits, combine the ingredients using the *biscuit method*. This method involves sifting dry ingredients together into a mixing bowl. Use a pastry blender or two knives to cut the fat into the dry mixture. Continue cutting in until the particles are the size of coarse cornmeal. Then add the liquid all at once and stir until the dough forms a ball. This is the same mixing method you will use when making pastry.

The dry ingredients in biscuits are flour, baking powder, and salt. You can also use self-rising flour, which is a mixture of these three ingredients. The liquid in biscuits is milk or buttermilk. Drop biscuits contain a higher proportion of liquid than rolled biscuits. You drop the batter for *drop biscuits* from a spoon onto a greased baking sheet. You gently knead the dough for *rolled biscuits* 8 to 10 times and roll or pat it into a circle. Cut the dough with a biscuit cutter and place the biscuits on an ungreased baking sheet. Bake both types of biscuits in a hot oven until they are golden brown.

Characteristics of Biscuits

A high-quality rolled biscuit has an even shape with a smooth, level top and straight sides. The crust is an even brown. When you break it open, the *crumb,* or soft interior, is white to creamy white. It is moist and fluffy and peels off in layers. See 23-5.

Biscuits require gentle handling. An undermixed biscuit has a low volume and a rounded top with a slightly rough crust. The crumb is tender. An overmixed biscuit also has a low volume and a rounded top, but the top is smooth. The crumb is tough and compact.

Preparing Muffins

When preparing muffins, combine ingredients using the *muffin method*. For this method, measure the dry ingredients into a mixing bowl. Make a well in the center of the dry ingredients. In a separate bowl, combine beaten eggs with milk and oil or melted fat. Pour all the liquid mixture into the well in the dry ingredients. For muffins, stir the batter just until the dry ingredients are moistened. You will also use this mixing method when preparing waffles, pancakes, popovers, and some coffee cakes. Batter for some of these baked products may require more stirring than the batter for muffins.

The dry ingredients in muffins are flour, baking powder, salt, and sugar. Fruits, nuts, cheese, and other ingredients may be added to muffin batter for variety. After combining ingredients, drop muffin batter into a greased muffin pan and bake.

Characteristics of Muffins

A high-quality muffin has a thin, evenly browned crust. The top is symmetrical, but it looks rough. When broken apart, the texture is uniform, and the crumb is tender and light.

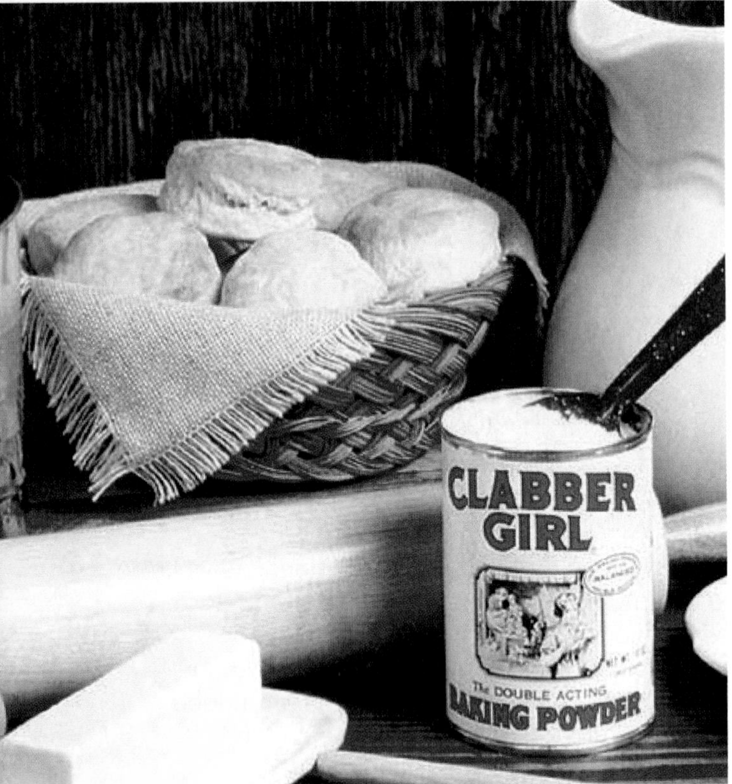

Clabber Girl Corporation

23-5 Light, golden rolled biscuits should have a uniform appearance.

An undermixed muffin has a low volume and a flat top. The crumb is coarse. An overmixed muffin has a peaked top and a pale, slick crust. When broken apart, narrow, open areas called *tunnels* are visible.

Preparing Popovers

Popovers look like golden brown balloons. You can eat them with jam or fill their hollow centers with mixtures of meat, poultry, seafood, and/or vegetables. A variety of sweet fillings, such as ice cream, pudding, fruit, and custard, are also popular in popovers.

Popovers contain flour, salt, eggs, milk, and a small amount of fat. Use the muffin method to combine these ingredients. Then place popovers in a hot oven for the first part of the baking period. This allows steam to expand the walls of the popovers. Following this expansion, lower the temperature to prevent overbrowning before the interior has set. Do not open the oven door to check popovers during baking. If you do and they have not set, the steam can condense and cause the popovers to collapse.

Characteristics of Popovers

A high-quality popover has good volume. The shell is golden brown and crisp, and the interior contains slightly moist (but not raw) strands of dough. See 23-6.

Insufficient baking is one of the biggest causes of popover failures. If you have not baked a popover long enough, it will collapse when you take it from the oven. The exterior will be soft instead of crisp, and the interior will be doughy.

Preparing Cream Puffs

A cream puff is a golden brown, hollow shell with crisp walls. You can fill cream puffs with pudding, custard, ice cream, fruit, or whipped cream and serve them as a dessert. You can fill them with creamed meat, poultry, or fish and serve them as a main dish. You can also fill small cream puffs with cream cheese, shrimp salad, or another light filling and serve them as appetizers. Elongated cream puffs filled with custard are called *eclairs*.

Cream puffs are made from water, fat, flour, and eggs. They require a special mixing method. Begin by bringing the water and fat to a boil. Then add the flour and stir vigorously over low heat until the mixture forms a ball. After removing the mixture from the heat, stir in the eggs until the mixture is smooth. The resulting dough is called *puff paste*.

Drop the puff paste onto an ungreased baking sheet. Begin baking the cream puffs in a hot oven so the steam will cause them to puff (rise). Then reduce the temperature. This will prevent the exteriors of the cream puffs from overbrowning before the interiors have set. Do not open the oven door to check the cream puffs during baking. If you do and the cream puffs have not set, the steam can condense and cause them to collapse.

Characteristics of Cream Puffs

A properly prepared cream puff has a good volume and a brown, tender crust. When broken apart, the interior of the cream puff is hollow. A few strands of moist, tender dough may be visible.

Cream puff failures usually are the result of underbaking. When you take an underbaked cream puff from the oven, it will collapse. The interior is moist and filled with strands of dough.

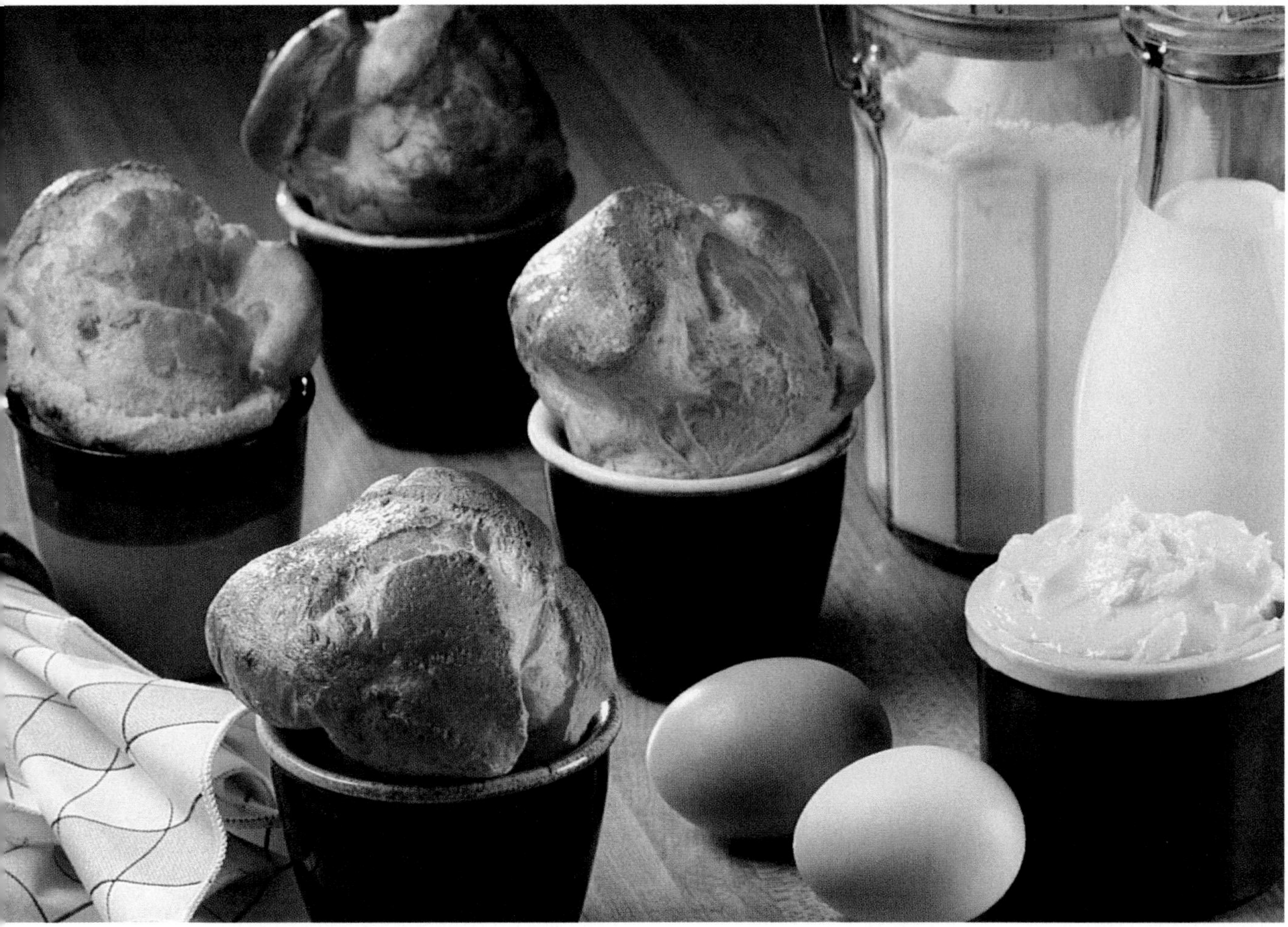

American Egg Board

23-6 High-quality popovers look like golden brown balloons on the outside.

Occasionally, cream puffs will ooze fat during baking. The evaporation of too much liquid can cause this. Evaporation may take place when the water and fat are heated together or when the puff paste is cooked.

Microwaving Quick Breads

You can use the microwave oven to prepare a variety of tasty quick breads in a matter of minutes. Nut breads, muffins, coffee cakes, corn bread, and biscuits all microwave beautifully. You can reheat frozen waffles and pancakes in a microwave oven, too. However, popovers and cream puffs do not microwave well due to the lack of dry heat needed for crust formation.

Many microwave quick bread recipes use baking mixes and refrigerated biscuits for added speed and convenience. You can use a variety of tasty toppings to disguise the lack of browning on these products.

Quick breads will microwave more evenly in ring-shaped pans or muffin rings. A round casserole with a juice glass placed in the center will serve as a ring-shaped pan. Custard cups arranged in a circle can take the place of a muffin ring. You can also use loaf pans, but you should place foil shields on the ends to prevent overcooking in the corners.

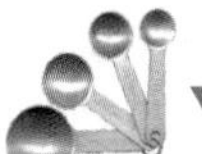

Yeast Breads

Homemade yeast bread is decidedly different from commercially prepared sandwich breads. It has a distinctively appealing sweet smell and delicious taste that cannot be matched, 23-7.

Many meal managers rely on the ease of bread machines to make homemade bread an option in their menu plans. All a meal manager

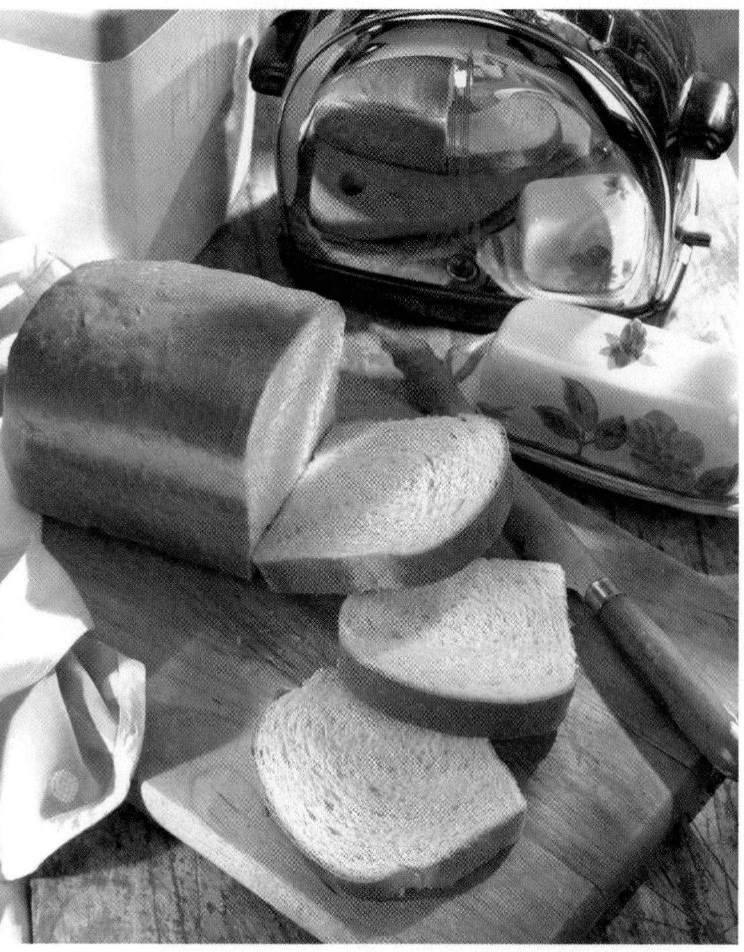

photo courtesy of Fleischmann's Yeast

23-7 *The flavor, texture, and aroma of homemade yeast bread create a feast for the senses.*

has to do is measure the ingredients, and the bread machine does the rest. Even without the convenience of this appliance, however, you can serve homemade breads. Try recipes for brown-and-serve breads and cool-rise and frozen doughs. These recipes allow you to take advantage of time you have available to prepare products you can bake later.

Yeast Bread Ingredients

All yeast breads must contain flour, liquid, salt, and yeast. Most recipes call for a small amount of sugar, and some include fat and eggs. Proportions of ingredients vary somewhat between traditional yeast breads and those prepared in bread machines.

Flour

You can use all-purpose flour for making traditional yeast breads. When mixed with liquid and kneaded, the flour develops gluten to support the carbon dioxide produced by the yeast.

Bread flour contains larger amounts of gliadin and glutenin than all-purpose flour. It produces the strongest and most elastic gluten of all the white wheat flours. Bread flour is recommended when preparing breads in a bread machine. This is because the actions of a bread machine require stronger gluten.

Whole wheat and nonwheat flours, such as rye, soy, corn, and oat, have a lower protein content than all-purpose flour. They will produce a denser loaf than all-purpose or bread flour. Many recipes calling for whole grain flours also call for some all-purpose or bread flour. Such a combination is essential when preparing products in a bread machine. The combination of flours will produce more gluten and help bread rise. Traditional recipes may suggest equal parts of all-purpose and whole grain flours. A ratio of two parts bread flour to one part whole grain flour is recommended for bread machines.

Liquid

You can use plain water, potato water, or milk as the liquid in yeast breads. Milk produces a softer crust and helps breads stay fresh longer than water. Other options for liquid ingredients in yeast breads include buttermilk, fruit juices, yogurt, applesauce, and cottage cheese. These options add nutrients and distinctive flavors.

The temperature of the liquids affects yeast cells. You need to warm liquids used in traditional yeast breads. Your recipe will tell you the temperature to which liquids should be heated. Temperatures that are too high kill the yeast cells. Temperatures that are too low can slow or stop yeast activity. When preparing breads in a bread machine, liquids should be near room temperature, 75°F to 85°F (24°C to 29°C). Using liquids that are too warm may keep yeast breads prepared in a bread machine from rising.

Salt

Salt regulates the action of the yeast and inhibits the action of certain enzymes in the flour. Bread machine recipes require a higher proportion of salt than traditional recipes. Without salt, a traditional yeast dough is sticky and hard to handle. When baked, the bread may look moth-eaten. Omitting salt from a bread machine recipe may cause the top of the loaf to collapse.

Yeast

Yeast is a microscopic, single-celled plant used as a leavening agent in yeast breads. It is available in three forms. *Compressed yeast* is made from fresh, moist yeast cells that are pressed into cakes. You must refrigerate compressed yeast because it is very perishable. *Active dry yeast* is made from an active yeast strain that has been dried and made into granules. *Fast-rising yeast* products are highly active yeast strains. The granules of these products are smaller than those of active dry yeast, which allows them to act more quickly. Active dry and fast-rising yeast are both available in small foil packets and glass jars. Store these yeast products in a cool, dry place and refrigerate jars after opening. For fastest action, buy yeast in small quantities and use it promptly. See 23-8.

For best results, use the amount of yeast specified in your recipe. A general guideline is 3/4 teaspoon (3 mL) active dry yeast or 1/2 teaspoon (2 mL) fast-rising yeast per cup of flour. Using too much yeast will cause the dough to rise too quickly. Excess yeast will also give the bread an undesirable flavor, texture, and appearance. Using too little yeast will lengthen the rising time.

Good Manners Are Good Business

You can use a piece of bread to help you push a bite of food onto your fork at a business meal. However, avoid using your bread to wipe your plate clean.

Sugar

Sugar, brown sugar, honey, and molasses can all be used in yeast bread recipes. These ingredients influence browning, flavor, and texture. They also provide extra food for the yeast so the dough will rise faster. If you use too much sugar, however, the yeast will work more slowly.

Bread machine recipes require a higher proportion of sugar than traditional recipes. In a bread machine, too much sugar can keep bread from rising. Even the sugar contributed by dried fruits can have this effect. Some bread machines have a special cycle for sweet breads. This cycle is designed to produce high-quality products when using recipes with a high sugar content.

Fat

Fat increases tenderness of yeast breads. Fat is optional in some traditional recipes, but it is required in bread machine recipes. Most recipes call for solid fat, but some call for oil.

Eggs

Eggs add flavor and richness to yeast breads. They also add color and improve the structure.

You may wish to add an egg to a bread machine recipe calling for whole grain flour. This will help improve the structure and volume of the finished product. Eggs are considered part of the liquid in yeast bread recipes. Therefore,

Q:If I want more fiber in my diet, shouldn't I eat brown bread instead of white bread?

A: Use the Nutrition Facts panel and the ingredients list rather than color to find bread that is higher in fiber. In some bread, brown coloring comes from food dyes not high-fiber, whole grain ingredients.

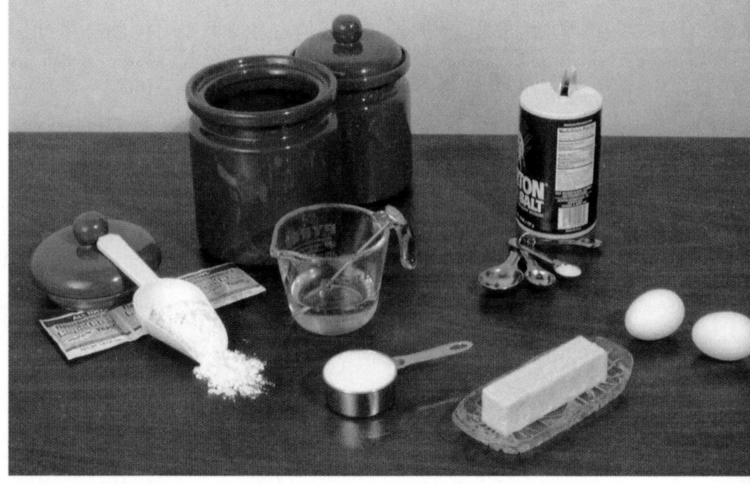

Jack Klasey

23-8 *In addition to yeast, basic yeast bread ingredients include flour, liquid, salt, sugar, fat, and eggs.*

when adding an egg not listed in the recipe, decrease the amount of other liquid ingredients by 1/4 cup (50 mL).

Other Ingredients

You may add other ingredients, such as raisins, nuts, cheese, herbs, and spices, to bread dough. They add flavor and variety. However, these ingredients tend to lengthen the rising time.

Mixing Methods for Yeast Breads

You will use the traditional, one-rise, mixer, or batter method when mixing yeast dough. Your recipe will tell you which method to use.

Traditional Method

For the *traditional method*, dissolve the yeast in a small amount of warm water. The water should be 105°F to 115°F (41°C to 46°C). Then add remaining liquid, sugar, fat, salt, and some of the flour. Like the water used to dissolve the yeast, remaining liquid should be 105°F to 115°F (41°C to 46°C). Cold liquid will slow the rising action when added to activated yeast. If the recipe calls for eggs, stir them in before adding the remaining flour to form a soft dough.

Doughs prepared by the traditional method are allowed to rise twice. The first rising takes place after you mix the ingredients. Then you shape the dough and allow it to rise a second time. See 23-9.

One-Rise Method

The *one-rise method* requires the use of fast-rising yeast. Mix the yeast with some of the flour and all the other dry ingredients. Heat the liquid and fat together to a temperature of 120°F to 130°F (49°C to 54°C). Add the warmed liquids to the dry ingredients. If eggs are required, add them before adding the remaining flour to form a soft dough.

After combining the ingredients, you may knead the dough. Then cover it and allow it to rest for 10 minutes. This resting period replaces

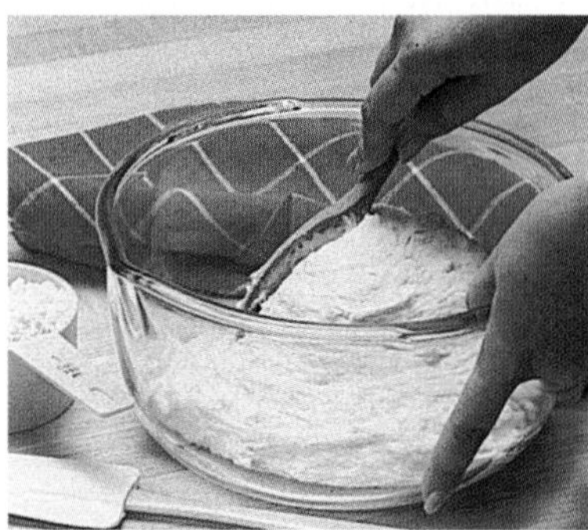

A—Combine ingredients and beat until smooth. Stir in enough additional flour to make a moderately stiff dough.

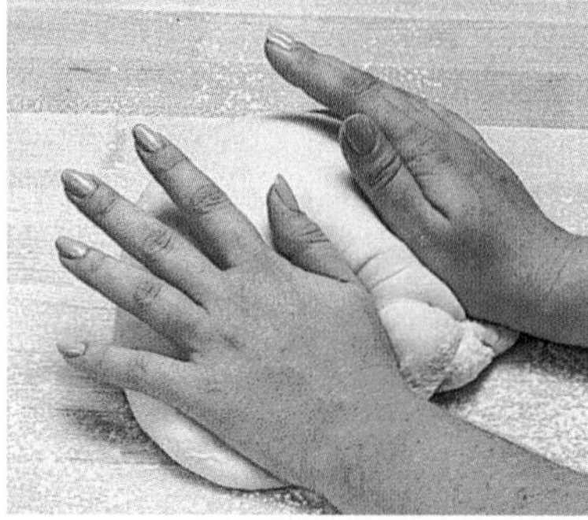

B—On a lightly floured pastry board or cloth, knead dough until smooth and elastic.

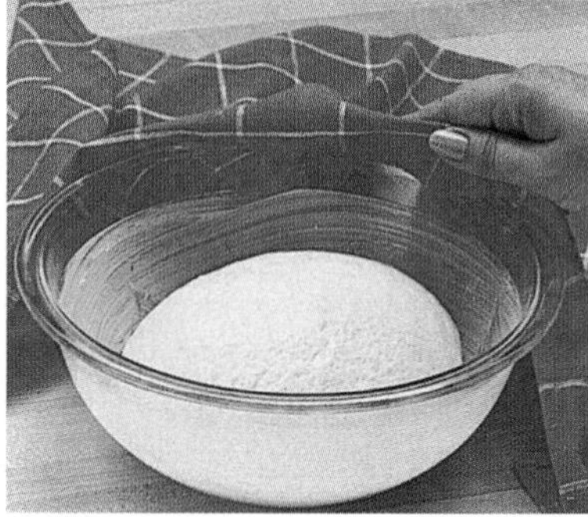

C—Place dough in a lightly greased bowl; turn once to grease top.

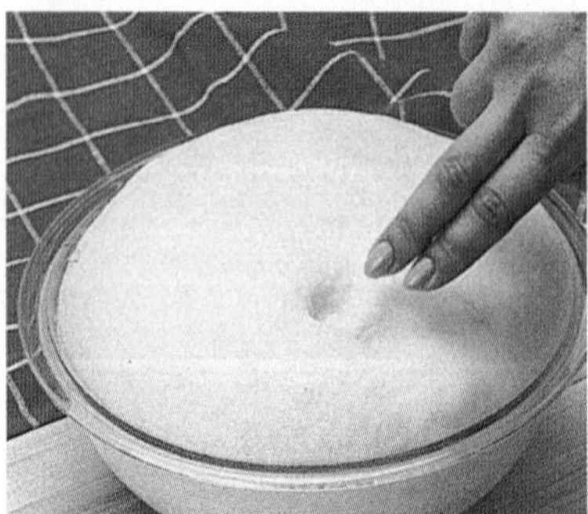

D—Let dough rise in a warm place until double in bulk. Test dough for lightness with two fingers.

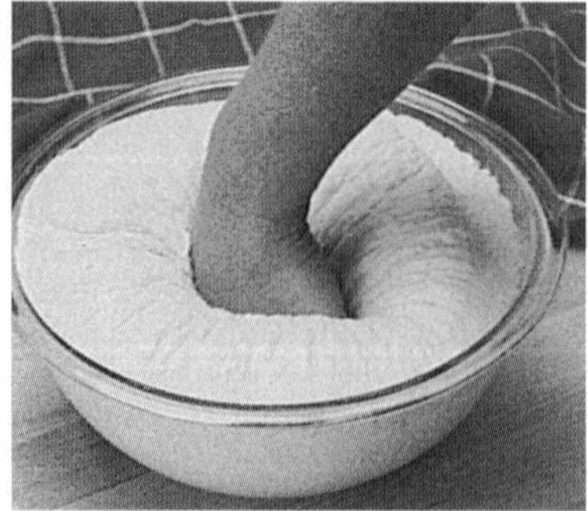

E—When dough is light, punch down.

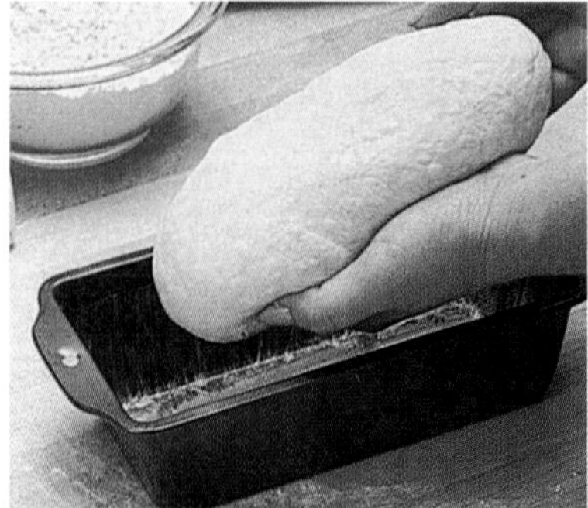

F—Shape dough into loaves or rolls. Allow the dough to rise a second time, then bake as directed.

photo courtesy of Fleischmann's Yeast

***23-9** To prepare yeast bread by the traditional method, follow these easy steps.*

the first rising required in the traditional method. After resting, shape the dough and allow it to rise before baking.

Mixer Method

The *mixer method* works well with active dry or fast-rising yeast. Like the one-rise method, begin by mixing the yeast with some of the flour and all the other dry ingredients. Heat the liquid and fat together to a temperature of 120°F to 130°F (49°C to 54°C). Using an electric mixer, add the warmed liquids to the dry ingredients. Add eggs if required. Then stir in the remaining flour with a spoon to form a soft dough. This method allows ingredients to blend easily. Using the mixer helps develop gluten and, therefore, shortens the kneading time.

Batter Method

Some recipes use the *batter* or *no-knead method*. These recipes use less flour, so the yeast mixture is thinner than dough. Vigorous stirring, rather than kneading, helps develop the gluten. Batter recipes that require two risings rise first in the mixing bowl. Then you spread the batter in a pan for the second rising before baking.

Food Science Principles of Preparing Yeast Breads

Like preparing quick breads, preparing yeast breads requires the development of gluten and the formation of carbon dioxide. During mixing and kneading, the gluten develops. The gluten will form the framework of the bread. It will trap the carbon dioxide produced by the yeast as the dough rises. As the amount of carbon dioxide increases, the dough will rise, giving volume to the bread. The preparation of successful yeast bread depends on careful measuring, sufficient kneading, and controlled fermentation temperatures. Correct pan size and baking temperature are also important.

Kneading

After forming yeast dough by the traditional, one-rise, or mixer method, you must knead it. Although some of the gluten develops during initial beating, kneading develops most of the gluten. To knead, press the dough with the heels of the hands, fold it, and turn it. You must rhythmically repeat this motion until the dough is smooth and elastic. See 23-10.

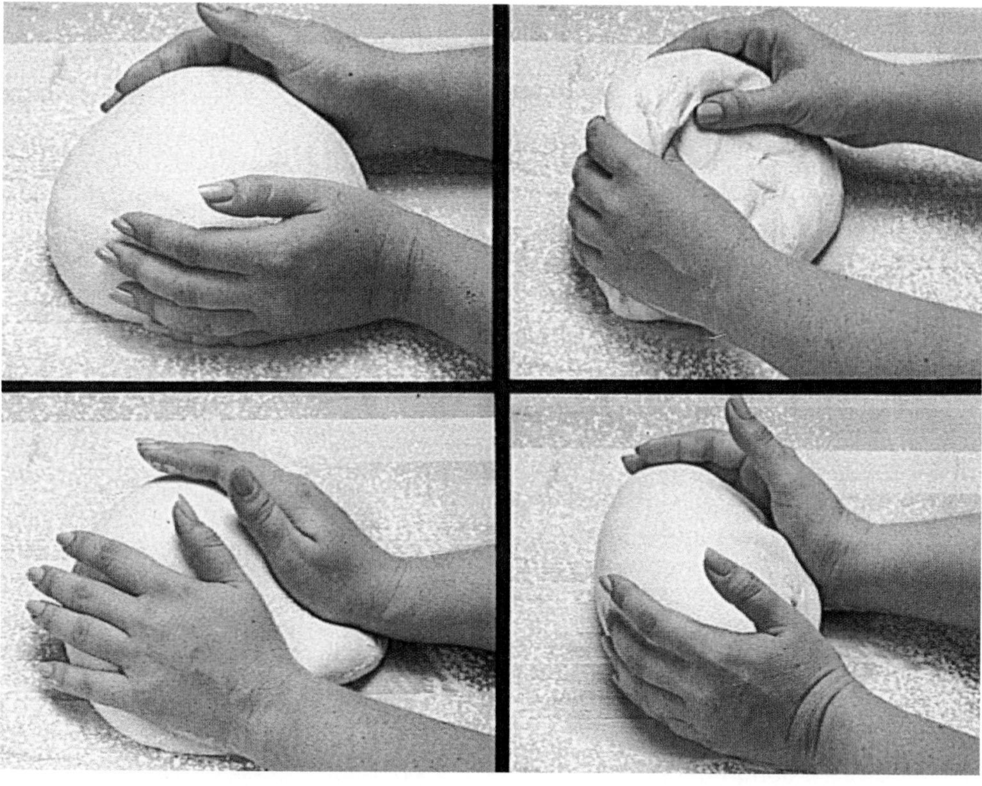

photo courtesy of Fleischmann's Yeast

23-10 *To knead dough, use your fingers to fold it in half toward your body. With the heels of your hands, push against the dough and turn it one-quarter turn.*

Avoid adding too much extra flour when kneading the dough. Too much flour will make the dough stiff. It is also important not to be too rough with the dough. Too much pressure at the beginning of kneading can keep the dough sticky and hard to handle. Too much pressure toward the end of kneading can tear or mat the gluten strands that have already developed.

Fermentation

After kneading yeast dough, you must allow it to rest in a warm place. During this resting time, the yeast acts on the sugars in the bread dough to form alcohol and carbon dioxide. This process is called ***fermentation***. The alcohol evaporates during baking. The carbon dioxide causes the bread to rise.

The dough should at least double in volume during fermentation. To see if dough has doubled in size, gently push two fingers into the dough. If an indentation remains, the dough has risen enough.

Fermentation time varies depending on the kind and amount of yeast, the temperature of the room, and the kind of flour. Breads made with fast-rising yeast rise up to 50 percent faster than products made with regular yeast. The dough should be kept in a warm place for optimal fermentation. The temperature range of 80°F to 85°F (27°C to 29°C) is ideal for the production of carbon dioxide by the yeast. You can create such a warm environment by placing the bowl of dough over a pan of steaming water. Avoid temperatures that are too warm, which will cause the yeast to work too quickly, causing the dough to rise too fast.

Punching the Dough

When the dough is light (has completed the first rising), you must punch it down to release some of the carbon dioxide. Punch dough down by firmly pushing a fist into the dough. Then fold the edges of the dough toward the center, and turn the dough over so the smooth side is on top. At this point, some doughs require a second rising time. (Doughs made with bread flour need a second rising.)

Shaping

After punching the dough down, use a sharp knife to divide it into portions as the recipe directs. Allow the divided dough to rest about 10 minutes. After resting, the dough will be easier to handle and shape as desired.

To shape yeast dough, first flatten the dough into a rectangle. The width of the dough should be about the length of the bread pan. Using a rolling pin will help you to work out any large air bubbles. Fold the ends of the rectangle to the center, overlapping them a little. This should give you a smaller rectangle. Use your rolling pin to flatten the rectangle into a square. Roll the dough into a cylinder. Pinch the edge of the dough into the roll to seal it. Seal each end of the roll by pressing down on it with the side of your hand. Fold the ends under. Place the shaped dough, seam side down, in a greased loaf pan. Brush the top with melted shortening, if desired. Cover the loaf with a clean towel, and shape the remaining dough. Let the loaves rise in a warm, draft-free place until they have doubled in bulk.

Baking

Baking times and temperatures vary somewhat depending on the kind of dough and size of the loaf. Place most yeast breads in a moderately hot oven. During baking, the gas cells formed during fermentation expand. The walls of dough around these cells set and become rigid. During the first few minutes of baking, the dough will rise dramatically. This rapid rising is called *oven spring.*

After baking, immediately remove bread from the pans and place it on cooling racks. Cool the bread thoroughly before you slice and store it, 23-11.

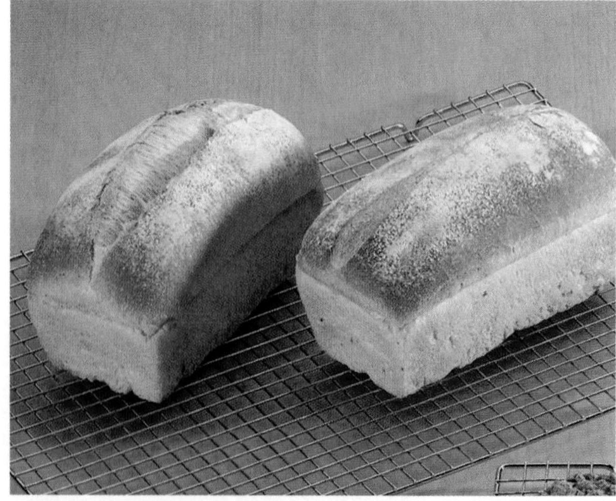

Baker's Secret

23-11 *Using a cooling rack will keep the bottom of yeast bread from getting soggy due to trapped steam.*

Characteristics of Yeast Bread

A high-quality loaf of yeast bread has a large volume and a smooth, rounded top. The surface is golden brown. When sliced, the texture is fine and uniform. The crumb is tender and elastic, and it springs back when touched.

If yeast dough has been under- or overworked, the finished product will have a low volume. This is because carbon dioxide has leaked out of the dough.

If you allow bread to rise for too long a time before baking, it may have large, overexpanded cells. The top of the loaf may be sunken with overhanging sides, much like a mushroom. The texture is coarse, and it may be crumbly.

If you have not allowed bread to rise long enough before baking, it may have large cracks on the sides of the loaf. Its texture is compact.

Timesaving Yeast Bread Techniques

Bread making no longer has to be the all-day task it once was. Fast-rising yeast can cut rising time in half. Using the one-rise mixing method saves rising time. The mixer method speeds the blending of ingredients and shortens kneading time. The batter method eliminates kneading entirely.

Besides timesaving ingredients and mixing methods, some recipes allow you to fit bread making conveniently into your schedule. These include recipes for cool-rise, refrigerator, and freezer doughs. Of course, a bread machine is the ultimate time-saver.

Cool-Rise Doughs

Cool-rise doughs are prepared from recipes that are specially designed to rise slowly in the refrigerator. You mix ingredients and knead the dough. Then after a brief rest, you shape the dough and place it in a pan. You cover the dough and place it in the refrigerator. The dough will rise and be ready to bake at your convenience any time from 2 to 24 hours later.

Refrigerator Doughs

Like cool-rise doughs, *refrigerator doughs* are prepared from recipes that are specially designed to rise slowly in the refrigerator. The batter method is often used to prepare these doughs. Therefore, they are not kneaded like cool-rise doughs. Refrigerator doughs are also shaped after, rather than before refrigeration. Refrigerator doughs can usually remain in the refrigerator for 2 to 24 hours. Then you shape the dough, let it rise, and bake it.

Freezer Doughs

Another type of specially formulated yeast bread recipe is for *freezer doughs*. These recipes allow you to mix and knead dough. Then you can freeze the dough before or after shaping. Store dough in the freezer for up to one month. When you are ready to eat it, simply thaw, shape if necessary, let rise, and bake.

Q: Isn't bread fattening?

A: Bread provides mostly complex carbohydrates, which supply 4 calories per gram, or about 70 calories for the average slice. If you're worried about calories, go easy on high-fat spreads, such as butter and margarine.

Bread Machines

Few people would argue that bread machines are the fastest, easiest way to produce homemade bread. However, these marvelous appliances are not foolproof. Each machine model behaves a bit differently. The best way to ensure success when using your machine is to carefully follow the manufacturer's directions. See 23-12.

The consistency of the dough in a bread machine indicates the quality of the bread that will result. You can check the texture of the dough by opening the machine's lid partway through the first knead cycle. The dough should form a soft ball that is somewhat sticky to the touch. If the dough is too moist, the loaf will collapse during baking. To correct this, add bread flour 1 tablespoon (15 mL) at a time. If the dough is not moist enough, it may produce a small, compact loaf. To correct this, add liquid 1 tablespoon (15 mL) at a time.

Weather conditions can have an effect on dough prepared in a bread machine. Therefore,

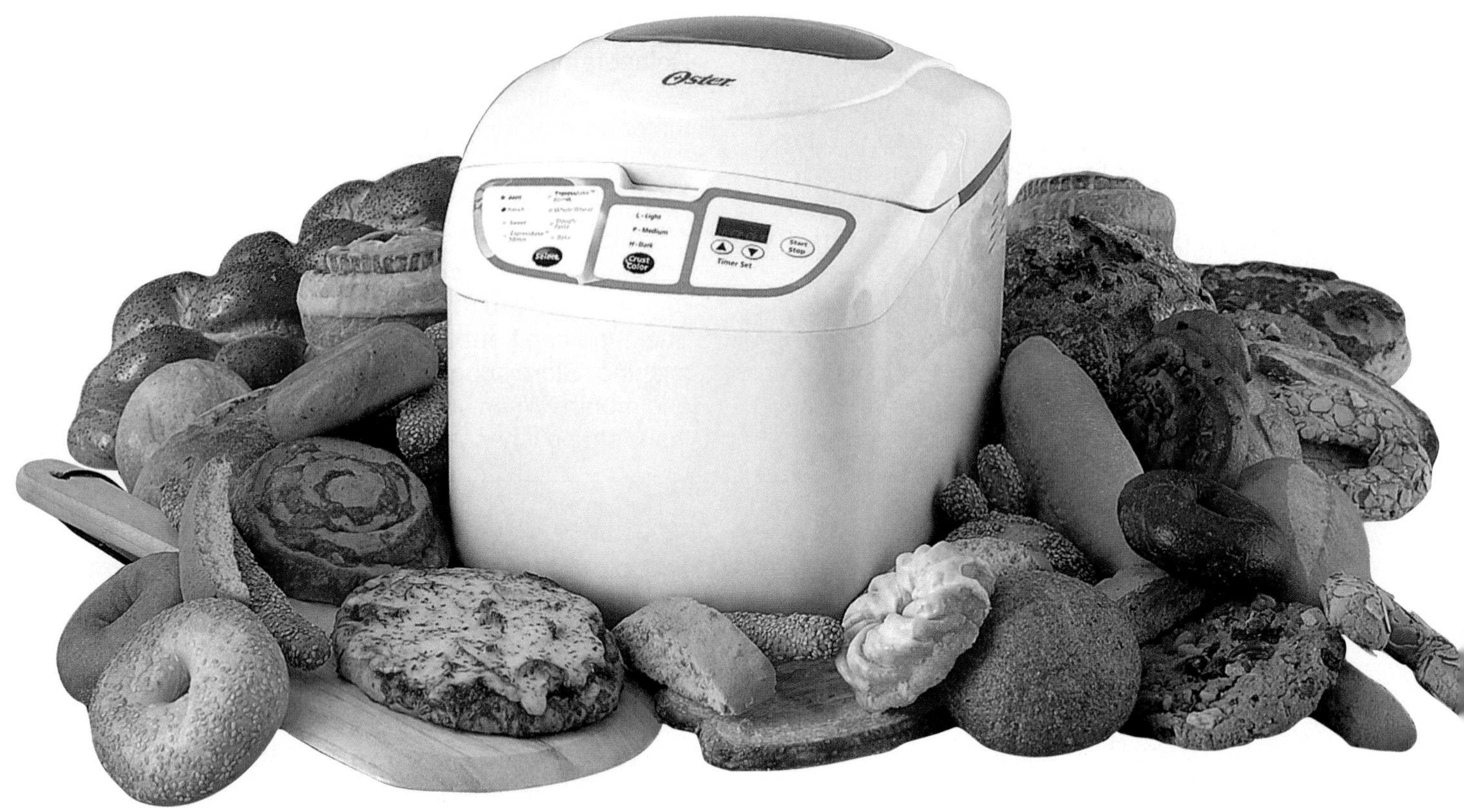

Oster

23-12 A bread machine simplifies the process of making yeast bread at home.

a recipe may produce satisfactory results one time and unsatisfactory results another time. For advice on specific problems with your bread machine, use the toll-free consumer information number provided by the manufacturer. Your county extension agent may also be able to offer suggestions related to your specific situation.

Microwaving Yeast Breads

You may be able to use a microwave oven to help you with some steps in yeast bread preparation. For instance, you can defrost frozen bread dough in a microwave oven. Start by microwaving 1 cup (250 mL) of water for 3 to 5 minutes on high power until boiling. This creates a warm, moist atmosphere for the dough. Then place the frozen dough in a greased, microwavable loaf pan. Microwave on the defrost setting for 3 minutes. Turn dough over and rotate the pan. Microwave on defrost for another 3 minutes until the dough is soft to the touch. Allow the dough to stand for 5 minutes to become pliable.

You can raise dough in a microwave oven by placing the dough in a greased bowl. Turn the dough to grease all sides. Cover the bowl with waxed paper and place it in a dish of warm water. Microwave on low power for 1 minute. Let the dough stand in the oven for 15 minutes. Rotate the dish one-quarter turn. Repeat the microwaving, standing, and rotating process as needed until the dough is doubled in size.

Some recipes are even designed to be baked in a microwave. However, the resulting loaves will lack the crisp, brown crusts of conventionally baked breads. Batter breads work especially well in a microwave oven because they do not have crusts. Raised coffee rings with toppings and dark breads also microwave well because they do not show the lack of browning.

Bread baked in a microwave oven is microwaved on medium power until it is almost done. Complete the last few minutes of microwaving on high power until bread is no longer doughy. You may place bread in a preheated conventional oven for a final few minutes to brown the crust.

Yeast Bread Variations

Add variety to yeast bread by combining white flour with whole wheat flour, rye flour, or cornmeal. Try adding dried fruits, nuts, herbs, or cheese to the basic dough. Brush the tops of the loaves with butter and sprinkle them with poppy, sesame, or caraway seeds.

You can shape basic bread dough into rolls. After punching the dough down, allow it to rest for a short time. Then divide it into portions and shape it into rolls. Crescent rolls, cloverleaf rolls, Parker House rolls, fan tans, and bows are popular roll shapes. You can find directions for shaping rolls in many cookbooks. See 23-13.

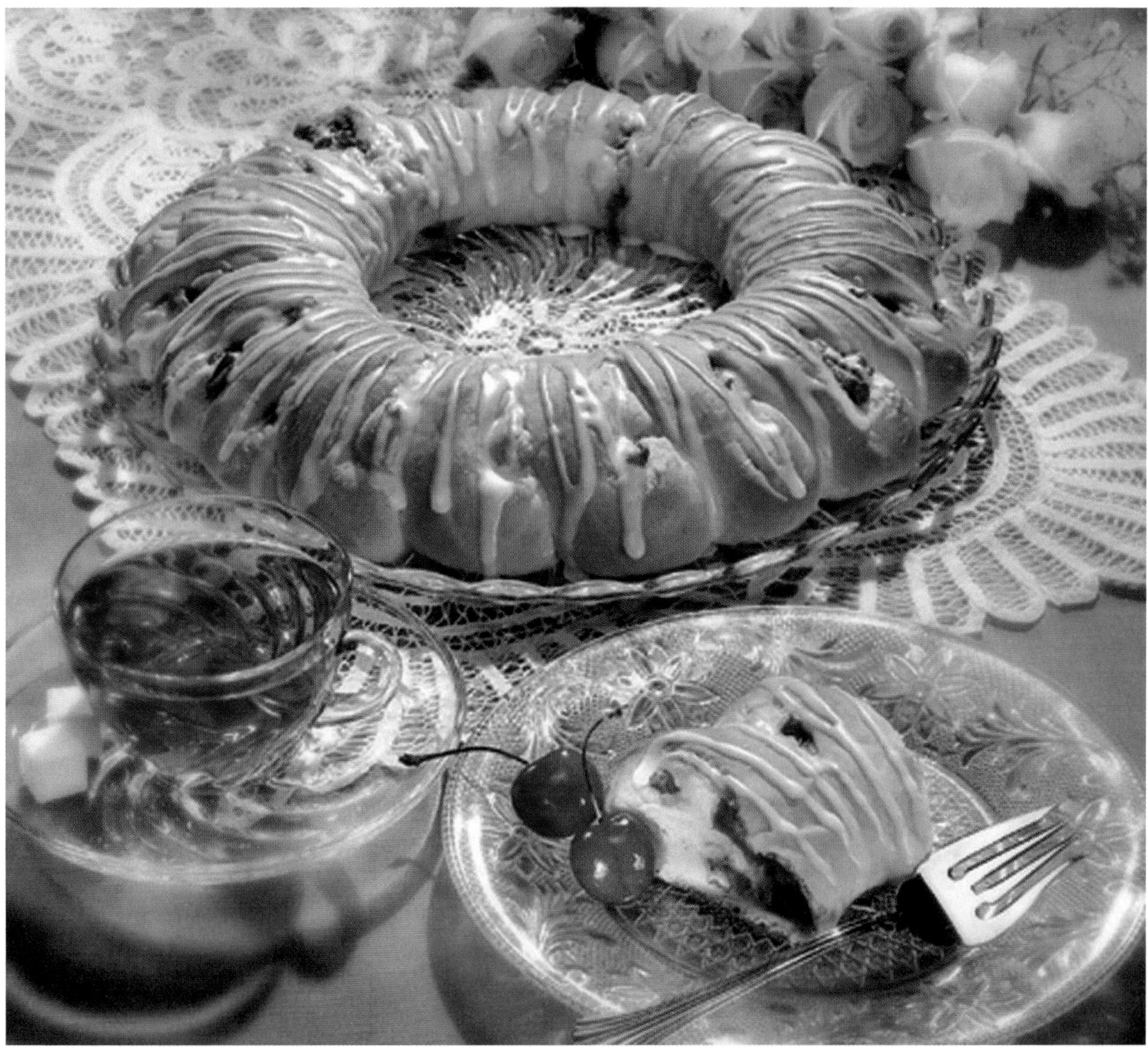

photo courtesy of Fleischmann's Yeast

***23-13** Fruit filling and a fancy shape turn ordinary yeast dough into a festive coffee cake.*

Chapter 23 Review
Breads

Summary

Quick breads and yeast breads are baked products. All baked products are available in various forms. Convenience tends to affect the cost of these products. Unless they contain perishable fillings or frostings, you can keep most baked products at room temperature. Use the freezer for longer storage.

Biscuits, muffins, popovers, and cream puffs are four popular types of quick breads. Flour, leavening agents, liquids, fat, eggs, sugar, and salt each serve specific functions in these baked products. Varying ingredient proportions and mixing methods results in the distinctive differences among these baked products.

The mixing methods used to prepare yeast breads are different from those used to prepare quick breads. Most yeast breads require kneading to develop the gluten needed to form the structure of the bread. Yeast breads also need time for fermentation to occur. This is the time during which yeast acts on sugars, causing the dough to rise. You must punch the dough down and shape it before baking. Adding different ingredients to the dough and changing the shaping can produce a variety of yeast breads.

Review What You Have Read

Write your answers on a separate sheet of paper.

1. Explain the difference between quick breads and yeast breads. Give three examples of each.
2. What is the advantage of freezing bread in hot, humid weather?
3. What is the difference between a batter and a dough?
4. What are the three gases that make baked products rise?
5. What is the minimum amount of fat, sugar, and salt needed per cup of flour when preparing muffins?
6. Why is it important to use the type of flour listed in a recipe?
7. Match the following quick breads with their descriptions:
   _____ May be rolled or dropped.
   _____ Has a peaked top and tunnels when overmixed.
   _____ Leavened almost entirely by steam; baked in muffin pans or custard cups.
   _____ Made with a dough called puff paste.
   A. biscuit
   B. cream puff
   C. muffin
   D. pancake
   E. popover
8. What two quick breads do not microwave well?
9. What is a main difference between liquids used in traditional yeast breads and liquids used in bread machine yeast breads?
10. Which mixing method for yeast breads eliminates the need for kneading?
    A. The traditional method.
    B. The one-rise method.
    C. The mixer method.
    D. The batter method.
11. What is the function of kneading yeast dough?
12. List three factors that affect the length of fermentation for yeast doughs.
13. What is the proper consistency of dough in a bread machine and how can it be checked?
14. True or false. Yeast breads can be baked in a microwave oven.

Build Your Basic Skills

1. **Math.** Visit the bread aisle in a local grocery store. List 25 bread products in order according to cost, beginning with the least expensive. Share your findings in a class discussion on factors that affect bread costs.
2. **Science.** Use a microscope to watch yeast grow. Explain how yeast differs from other leavening agents.

Build Your Thinking Skills

1. **Compare.** Prepare biscuits from scratch, from a refrigerated biscuit product, and from biscuit mix. Taste and compare. Which would you rather eat and why?
2. **Analyze.** Prepare a plain muffin batter. Drop half of the batter from a large spoon into a muffin pan. Place it in the oven and bake it as the recipe directs. Continue beating the remaining batter for two more minutes. Drop it into another muffin pan and bake as the recipe directs. Analyze the differences in appearance, flavor, and texture of the two products.
3. **Evaluate.** Bake a traditional loaf of white bread and a loaf in a bread machine. Evaluate the two loaves along with a loaf of purchased white bread. Rate each product in terms of appearance, texture, flavor, and cost.

Apply Technology

1. Research the mass production processes used to manufacture bread.
2. Compare convenience features available on various models of bread machines to identify the model you would prefer to own.

Using Workplace Skills

Darnell is a baker at The Village Bakeshop, a popular spot among commuters who ride the morning train. Darnell arrives at work at 3 o'clock every morning to begin making a variety of breads and pastries. Using cool-rise dough prepared the day before, Darnell shapes, bakes, fills, and frosts loaves, rolls, and coffee cakes. When the bakeshop opens at 6:00 a.m., Darnell must have a variety of baked goods ready to sell.

To be a successful employee, Darnell needs skill in making good use of time. Put yourself in Darnell's place and answer the following questions about your need for and use of this skill:

A. How will having skill in making good use of time help you as a baker?
B. How might commuters respond if you lack skill in making good use of time?
C. How might The Village Bakeshop be affected if you lack skill in making good use of time?
D. What is another skill you would need in this job? Briefly explain why this skill would be important.

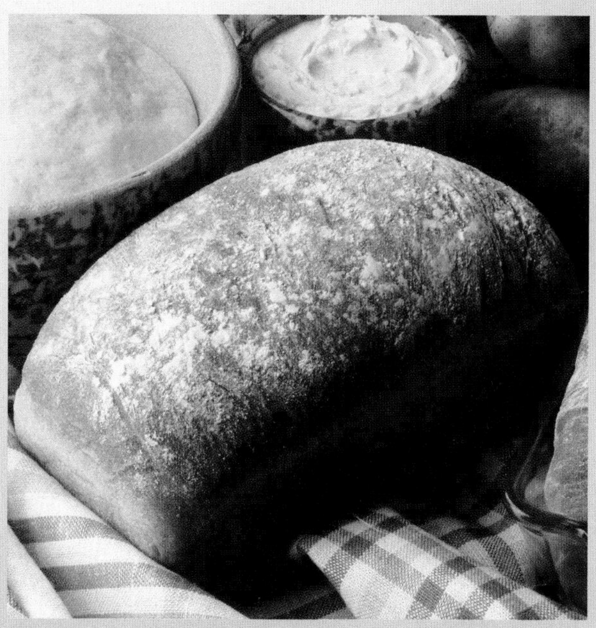

Chapter 24

Cakes, Cookies, Pies, and Candies

Cake Decorator
Decorates cakes and pastries with designs using icing bag or handmade paper cone.

Pastry Chef
Supervises and coordinates activities of cooks engaged in preparing desserts, pastries, confections, and ice cream.

Candy Maker
Mixes and cooks candy ingredients by following, modifying, or formulating recipes to produce product of specified flavor, texture, and color.

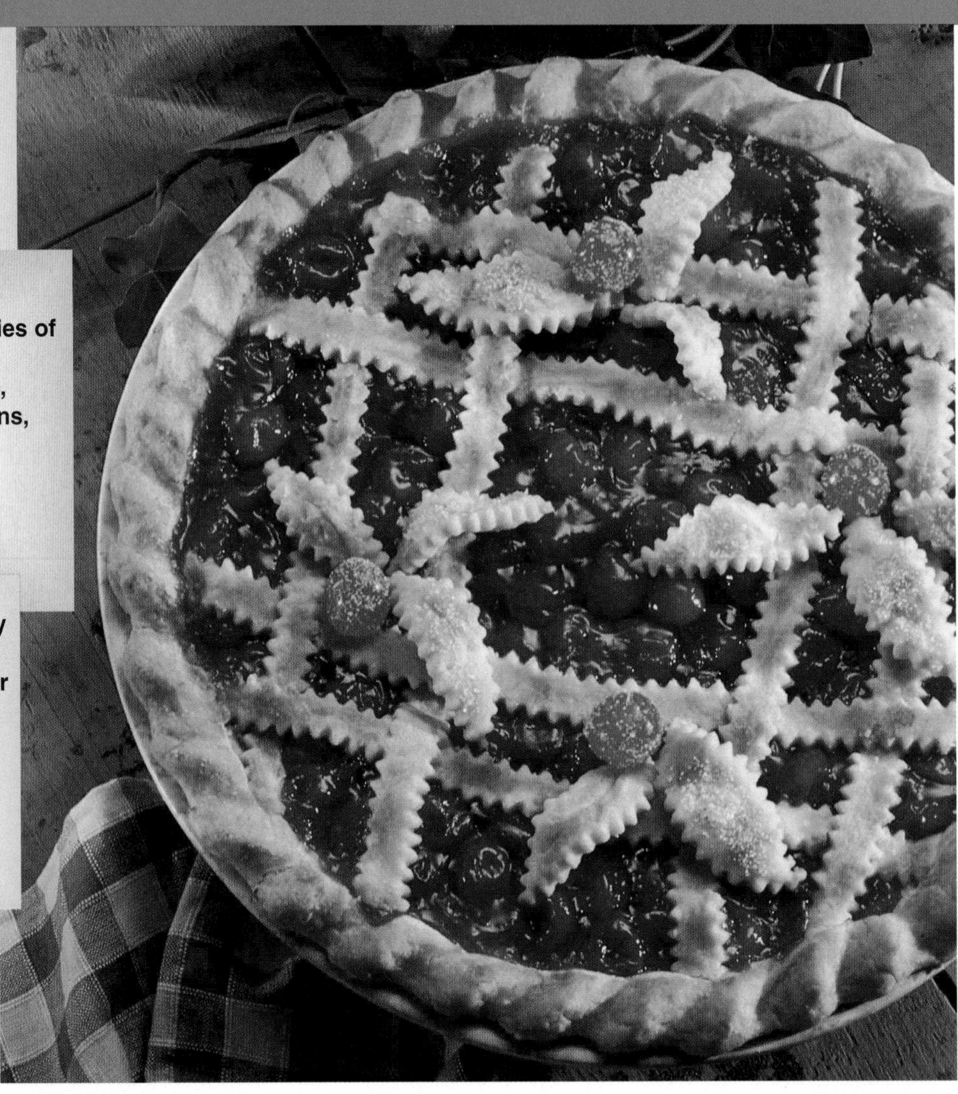

Cherry Marketing Institute

Terms to Know

shortened cake
unshortened cake
chiffon cake
pastry
crystalline candy
noncrystalline candy
sugar syrup

Objectives

After studying this chapter, you will be able to

- ❏ describe the functions of basic ingredients used in cakes.
- ❏ identify six types of cookies.
- ❏ explain principles of pastry preparation.
- ❏ compare characteristics of crystalline and noncrystalline candies.
- ❏ prepare cakes, cookies, pies, and candies.

For many people, a meal is not complete without something sweet. Restaurants are famous for the richness of their cheesecakes. Bakeries pride themselves on their pastries. Candy stores guard their recipes for fudge, peanut brittle, and English toffee.

Cakes, cookies, and pies are three of the most popular desserts. Candies are not really desserts, but because they are sweet, many people serve them at the end of a meal.

Most desserts are high in calories because they contain large amounts of sugar and fat. Desserts should never replace grain foods, fruits, vegetables, dairy products, or protein foods in the diet. However, they can add variety to meals and provide extra energy for people who are active.

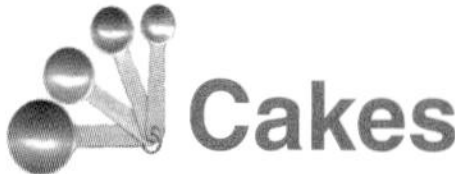

Cakes

Cakes are a favorite dessert of many people. They add festivity to many special occasions. They also add variety to lunch boxes and make a plain meal something special.

Q: Doesn't eating too much sugar make children hyperactive?

A: Research has not proven this to be true. Children often seem excited after eating sweets at a party. However, they are more likely responding to the active games and party atmosphere than the sweets.

Kinds of Cakes

Cakes are classified into two groups: shortened and unshortened. ***Shortened cakes*** contain fat. This is why some people call shortened cakes *butter cakes.* Most shortened cakes contain leavening agents. Shortened cakes are tender, moist, and velvety.

Unshortened cakes, sometimes called *foam cakes,* contain no fat. They are leavened by air and steam rather than chemical leavening agents. Angel food and sponge cakes are unshortened cakes. The main difference between these two cakes is the egg content. Angel food cakes contain just egg whites. Sponge cakes contain whole eggs. Unshortened cakes are light and fluffy. See 24-1.

Chiffon cakes are a cross between shortened and unshortened cakes. They contain fat like shortened cakes and beaten egg whites like unshortened cakes. They have large volumes, but they are not as light as unshortened cakes.

Cake Ingredients

Cakes contain flour, sugar, eggs, liquid, and salt. All shortened cakes also contain fat, and most cakes contain a leavening agent. Unshortened cakes contain cream of tartar, too.

Flour gives structure to a cake. The gluten that develops when flour is moistened and

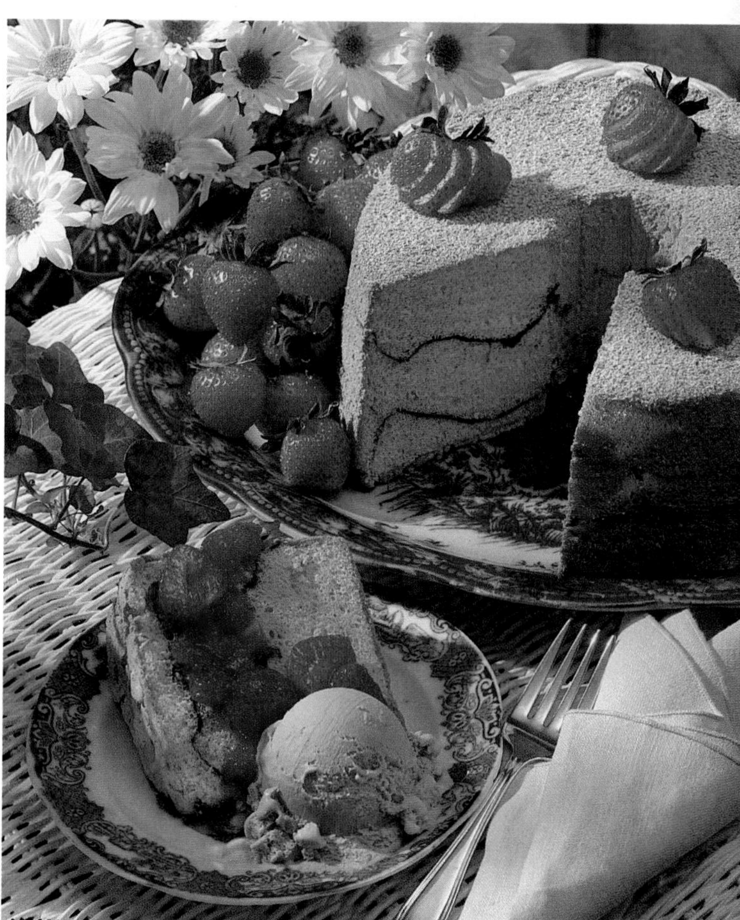

Wilton Industries

24-1 *Angel food cake is leavened by air beaten into egg whites.*

mixed holds the leavening gases that form as cakes bake. You can make cakes with cake flour or all-purpose flour. Cakes made with cake flour are more delicate and tender. This is because cake flour has lower protein content, so it yields less gluten. It is also more finely ground than all-purpose flour.

Sugar gives sweetness to cakes. It also tenderizes the gluten and improves the texture of cakes. Recipes may call for either granulated or brown sugar. Both should be free of lumps.

Eggs improve both the flavor and color of cakes. The coagulated egg proteins also add structure to cakes. In angel food and sponge cakes, eggs are important for leavening. Eggs hold the air that is beaten into them, and the evaporation of liquid from the egg whites creates steam.

Liquid provides moisture and helps blend ingredients. Most cake recipes call for fluid fresh milk. However, some call for buttermilk, sour milk, fruit juices, or water instead. In angel food cakes, egg whites are the only source of liquid needed.

Salt provides flavoring. Cakes require a smaller amount of salt than quick breads and yeast breads.

Fat tenderizes the gluten. Shortened cakes may contain butter, margarine, or hydrogenated vegetable shortening. Chiffon cakes contain oil instead.

Leavening agents are added to most shortened cakes to make the cakes rise and become porous and light. Most recipes call for baking powder or baking soda and sour milk.

Angel food and sponge cake recipes call for *cream of tartar*. Cream of tartar is an acid that makes egg whites whiter and makes the cake grain finer. Cream of tartar also stabilizes the egg white proteins, which increases the volume of the baked cake.

Flavorings are not essential ingredients in cakes, but they help make cakes special. You can add spices, extracts (concentrated flavors), fruits, nuts, poppy seeds, and coconut to cake batters for variety.

Like bread recipes, many dessert recipes call for more of some ingredients than are needed to perform their specific functions. Table 24-2 shows minimum proportions of fat, eggs, sugar, salt, and baking powder for some desserts. Try using these proportions to adjust cake, cookie, and pastry recipes. Your results will be products that are lower in fat, sugar, and sodium.

Food Science Principles of Preparing Cakes

Successfully preparing a cake depends on measuring, mixing, and baking. You must measure ingredients accurately and mix them correctly. You must bake the cake batter in the correct pans at the correct temperature. You also need to watch baking time carefully.

Measuring Ingredients

Flour, fat, sugar, liquid, and eggs affect the development of gluten. The correct proportions of each ingredient will produce a cake that is light and tender. Too much or too little of one or more ingredients may affect the finished product.

The optimum amount of flour provides the correct amount of gluten needed for structure. A cake made with too much flour is compact and dry. A cake made with too little flour is coarse, and it may fall.

Optimum amounts of fat and sugar tenderize gluten. Too much fat or sugar overtenderizes the gluten and weakens it. A cake made with too much of either ingredient will be heavy

Minimum Dessert Recipe Proportions per 1 Cup (250 mL) of Flour

Product	Fat	Eggs	Sugar	Salt	Baking Powder
Shortened cakes and dropped cookies	2 tablespoons (30 mL)	1/2	1/2 cup (125 mL)	1/8 teaspoon (0.5 mL)	1 teaspoon (5 mL)
Pastry	1/4 cup (50 mL)	—	—	1/2 teaspoon (2 mL)	—

24-2 *Using these proportions can help you cut the calories, fat, and sodium from some dessert recipes.*

and coarse, and it may fall. A cake made with too little of either ingredient will be tough.

The optimum amount of liquid provides the moisture needed for gluten to develop. Too much liquid will make a cake soggy and heavy. Too little liquid will make a cake dry and heavy.

The optimum number of eggs contributes proteins that strengthen the gluten framework. Too many eggs will make a cake rubbery and tough.

Mixing Cakes

You must mix the correct proportions of ingredients according to the method your recipe directs. Cake batters should be neither overmixed nor undermixed. Overmixing will cause the gluten to overdevelop. As a result, the cake will be tough. Overmixing angel food and sponge cakes will cause air to be lost from the beaten egg whites. As a result, the volume of the cake will be smaller.

Baking Cakes

Bake cake batter in pans that are neither too large nor too small. If the pans are too small, the batter will overflow. If the pans are too large, the cake will be too flat and may be dry. The correct pan size will produce a cake with a gently rounded top.

You should grease the pans for most shortened cakes and flour them lightly. You may grease and flour both the bottoms and sides of the pans or just the bottoms. You should not grease the pans for unshortened cakes. This is because angel food and sponge cake batters must cling to the sides of the pan during baking.

Place cakes in a preheated oven set at the correct temperature and bake them just until they test done. Cakes baked at too high a temperature may burn. Cakes baked too long may be dry. See 24-3.

Preparing a Shortened Cake

You can mix shortened cakes by the conventional method or the quick mix method. For the *conventional method,* cream the fat and sugar together until light and fluffy. Beat the eggs into the creamed fat and sugar. Then add the dry ingredients alternately with the liquid.

The *quick mix method,* also called the *one-bowl method,* takes less time than the conventional method. Measure the dry ingredients into the mixing bowl. Beat the fat and part of the liquid with the dry ingredients. Add the remaining liquid and unbeaten eggs last.

Pour cake batter into prepared pans. Then arrange the pans in the oven so the heat circulates freely around the cake. The pans should not touch each other or any part of the oven. If they do, hot spots may form, and the cake may bake unevenly.

To test a cake for doneness, lightly touch the center with your fingertip. If the cake springs back, it is baked. You can also insert a toothpick into the center of the cake. If the toothpick comes out clean, the cake is baked.

Most recipes will tell you to let cakes cool in the pans for about 10 minutes after

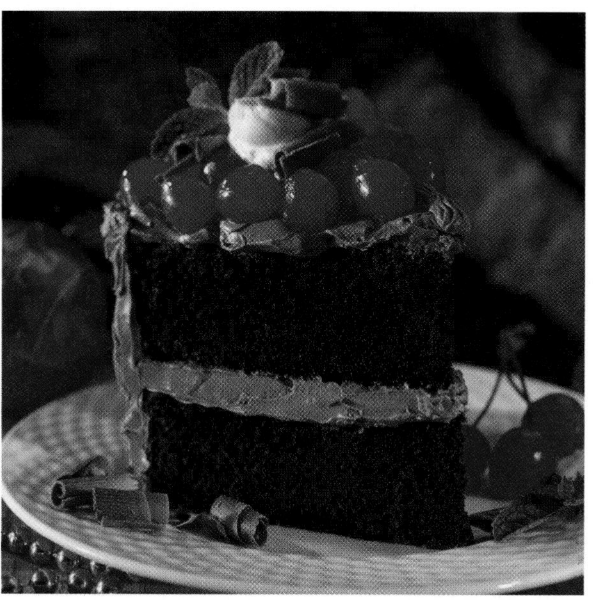

Cherry Marketing Institute

24-3 A cake that is baked at the correct temperature for the right amount of time is light with a velvety interior.

Be a Clever Consumer

Many consumers who want to cut fat and calories in their diets are buying reduced fat margarines. In order to achieve the reduction in fat and calories, manufacturers replace some of the fat in these products with water. These products may be fine for spreading on toast. However, they cannot perform the function of fat in cooking and baking. Read labels carefully. For best results in cooking and baking, margarines need to contain at least 80 percent oil.

removing the pans from the oven. This cooling period makes it easier to remove the cakes from the pans. To remove a cake from the pan, run the tip of a spatula around the sides of the cake to loosen it. Invert a cooling rack over the top of the pan and gently flip the cooling rack and the pan. The cake should slide out of the pan. Carefully remove the pan and place a second cooling rack on top of the cake. Flip the cake and the cooling racks so the cake is right side up. Let cake layers cool thoroughly before frosting them.

Characteristics of a Shortened Cake

A high-quality shortened cake is velvety and light. The interior has small, fine cells with thin walls. The crusts are thin and evenly browned. The top crust is smooth or slightly pebbly and gently rounded. The flavor is mild and pleasing.

Pound Cakes

Pound cakes are shortened cakes that contain no chemical leavening agents. Pound cakes rely on air and steam for leavening. You must thoroughly cream the fat and sugar when making pound cake. Beat the eggs into the creamed mixture until fluffy to incorporate enough air. Add the dry ingredients and the liquid to the creamed mixture. Pound cakes are more compact than other shortened cakes, and they have a closer grain, 24-4.

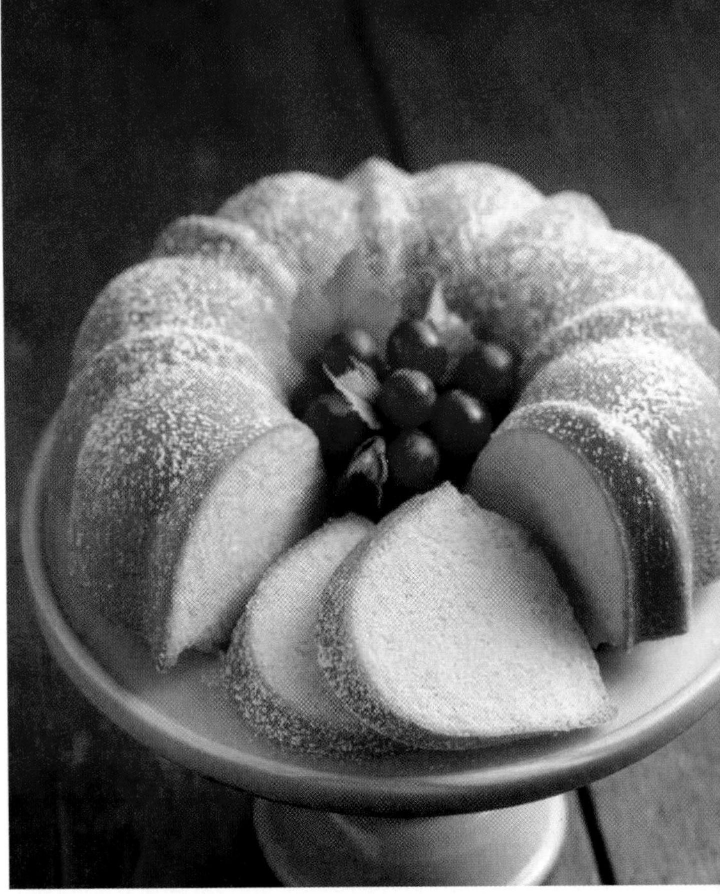

photo courtesy of Land O'Lakes, Inc.

24-4 Pound cake is so moist and rich, it needs no frosting.

Preparing an Unshortened Cake

Angel food cake is the most frequently prepared unshortened cake. When preparing an angel food cake, the ingredients should be at room temperature. Egg whites that are cold will not achieve maximum volume when beaten.

Angel food and sponge cakes are mixed by a different method from those used for shortened cakes. For an angel food cake, beat the egg whites with some of the sugar until stiff. Carefully fold the flour and remaining sugar into the beaten egg whites. For a sponge cake, beat the dry ingredients into the egg yolks. Then fold the beaten egg whites into the egg yolk mixture.

Carefully pour the batter for an unshortened cake into an ungreased tube pan. Run a spatula through the batter to release large air bubbles and seal the batter against the sides of the pan. Bake the cake in a preheated oven for the recommended time. Test the cake for doneness by gently touching the cracks. They should feel dry and no imprint should remain.

When you remove an unshortened cake from the oven, immediately suspend the pan upside down over the neck of a bottle. Hanging the cake upside down prevents a loss of volume during cooling. Cool the cake completely before removing it from the pan.

Characteristics of an Unshortened Cake

A high-quality angel food cake has a large volume. The interior is spongy and porous and has thin cell walls. The cake is tender and moist, but it is not gummy.

Sponge Cakes

Sponge cakes contain whole eggs rather than just egg whites. To make a sponge cake, you will use a variation of the mixing method used for angel food cakes. Beat the egg yolks until they are thick and lemon colored. Add the liquid, sugar, and salt to the yolks. Continue beating until the mixture is thick. Gently fold the flour into the yolk mixture. Then fold the stiffly beaten egg whites into the flour-yolk mixture.

Preparing a Chiffon Cake

Mix a chiffon cake by combining the egg yolks, oil, liquid, and flavoring with the dry ingredients. Beat the mixture until smooth. Beat the egg whites with the sugar and cream of tartar. Then fold the egg white mixture into the other mixture.

Characteristics of a Chiffon Cake

A high-quality chiffon cake has a large volume, although not quite as large as that of an angel food cake. The interior is moist and has cells with thin walls. The cake is tender and has a pleasing flavor, 24-5.

Microwaving Cakes

Shortened cakes prepared in a microwave oven come out moist and tasty. Unshortened cakes require a long cooking period and do not microwave well. For best results, prepare unshortened cakes and chiffon cakes in a conventional oven.

Microwaved cakes will not have the characteristic browning of conventionally prepared cakes. Lack of browning is less noticeable on chocolate, spice, and other dark cakes. Frosting will hide the lack of browning on white and yellow cakes.

Microwave cakes one layer at a time. Use microwavable round or ring-shaped pans for the most even cooking. Begin cooking at a medium power level. Then rotate the cake and complete the last few minutes of cooking on high power. Test cakes for doneness with a toothpick, as in conventional baking.

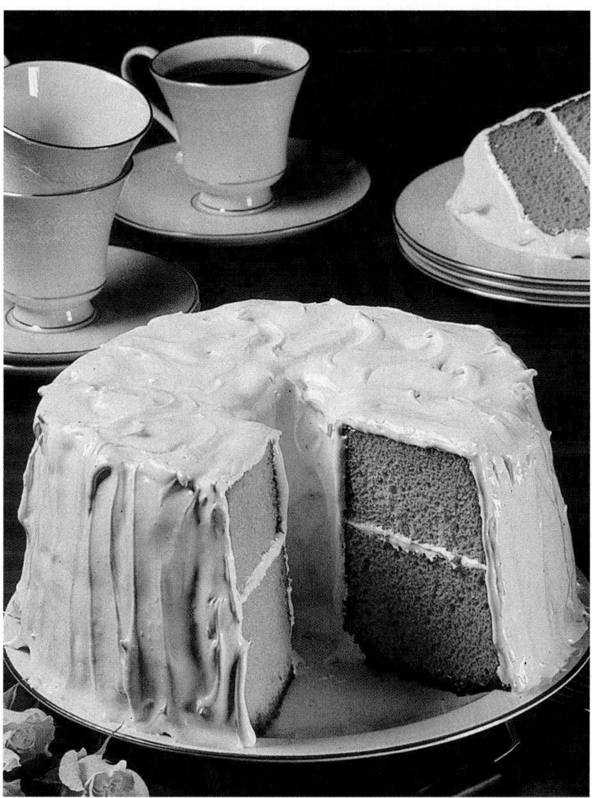

American Egg Board

24-5 Chiffon cake has a large volume and a light, but moist texture.

Filling and Frosting Cakes

Fillings and frostings can make a simple cake into a really special dessert. Fillings and frostings come in as wide a variety as the cakes they enhance.

Fluffy whipped cream, creamy puddings, and sweet fruits are among the popular fillings for cakes. You can spread fillings between layers of cake or roll them into the center of a jelly roll. You can also spoon them into a cavity dug into the middle of a cake.

Canned frostings and frosting mixes are available, but you can easily make frostings from scratch. Frostings may be cooked or uncooked. Cooked frostings use the principles of candy making. They include ingredients that interfere with the formation of crystals in a heated sugar syrup. Then you beat them until fluffy.

Uncooked frostings are popular for their creamy texture. You can easily make them by beating the ingredients together until they reach a smooth, spreadable consistency. Cream cheese frosting and butter cream are well-liked uncooked frostings.

Frostings not only enhance the flavor of cakes, they also enhance the appearance. You can cut cake layers into pieces and reassemble them to form the shapes of animals and objects. Use frosting as the "glue" to hold the pieces together.

Use decorators' frosting to personalize cakes and trim them with pretty flowers and fancy borders. A few simple tools are all you need. A *decorators' tube* is a cloth, plastic, or paper bag you fill with frosting. A *coupler* holds various plastic or metal *decorating tips* onto the tube. Squeeze the frosting through these tips to create various designs. See 24-6.

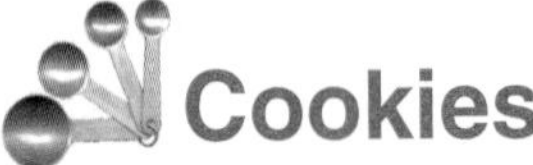

Cookies

Children and adults find it hard to resist a cookie jar filled with fresh homemade cookies. People enjoy chocolate chip, peanut butter, oatmeal, and sugar cookies year-round. At holiday time, many families make special cookies like Swedish pepparkakor, Norwegian krumkakke, and Scottish shortbread.

Kinds of Cookies

All cookies belong to one of six basic groups: rolled, drop, bar, refrigerator, pressed, or molded. The ingredients used to make different kinds of cookies are similar. However, the doughs differ in consistency, and you shape them differently.

You use stiff dough to make *rolled cookies*. Roll the dough on a pastry cloth or board to a thickness of ⅛ to ¼ inch (3 to 6mm). Cut the cookies from the dough with a cookie cutter and transfer them to a cookie sheet. Cookie cutters are available in many shapes and sizes. Sugar cookies are popular rolled cookies.

You use soft dough to make *drop cookies*. Drop or push the dough from a spoon onto cookie sheets. Leave about 2 inches (5 cm) of space between cookies. Drop cookies will spread more than rolled cookies. Chocolate chip cookies are popular drop cookies.

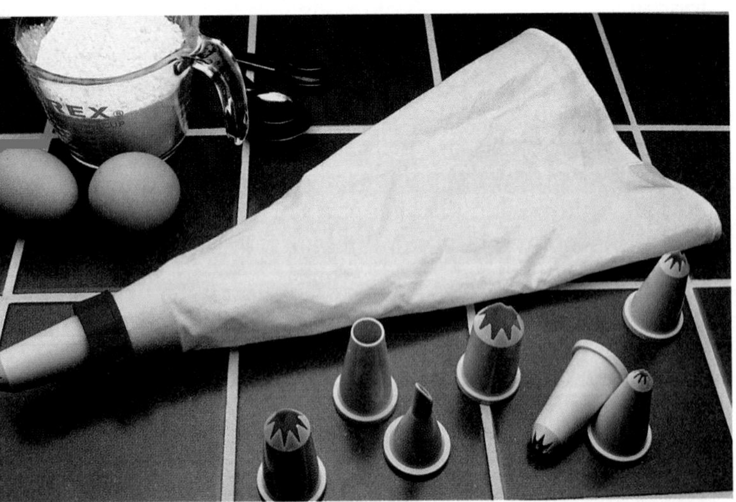

Progressive International Corp.

***24-6** These accessories can be used to give any cake a festive trim. They are available at cake and candy supply stores.*

You also use soft dough to make *bar cookies*. Spread the dough evenly in a jelly roll pan or square cake pan and bake it. Depending on the thickness of the dough, bar cookies may be chewy or cakelike. You can cut bar cookies into different shapes after baking. Brownies are popular bar cookies.

Refrigerator cookies contain a high proportion of fat. Form the stiff dough into a long roll, about two inches (5 cm) in diameter. Wrap the roll in foil or plastic wrap and refrigerate it until firm. When the dough has hardened, cut it into thin slices. Place the cookies on lightly greased cookie sheets and bake them. Pinwheel cookies are popular refrigerator cookies.

You use very rich, stiff dough to make *pressed cookies*. Pack the dough into a *cookie press*. This utensil has perforated disks through which you push the dough onto cookie sheets. The cookies vary in shape and size, depending on the disk used. Swedish spritz cookies are pressed cookies.

You also use stiff dough to make *molded cookies*. Break off small pieces of dough and shape them with your fingers. Crescents and small balls are popular shapes, 24-7.

Cookie Ingredients

Cookies contain the same basic ingredients you use to make cakes. They contain flour, sugar, liquid, fat, salt, egg, and leavening agents. Most cookies contain more fat and sugar and less liquid than cakes. Rolled cookies often contain no liquid. The proportion of ingredients, as well as the way you shape the cookies, determines if cookies are soft or crisp.

Many cookie recipes call for ingredients such as spices, nuts, coconut, chocolate chips, and dried fruits. Some recipes tell you to add these ingredients to the dough during mixing. Other recipes say to sprinkle cookies or roll them in colored sugars, coconut, or nuts after baking.

Mixing Methods for Cookies

You will make many cookies using the conventional mixing method you use for shortened cakes. Blend the sugar and fat until smooth. Add the eggs, liquid, and flavorings, followed by

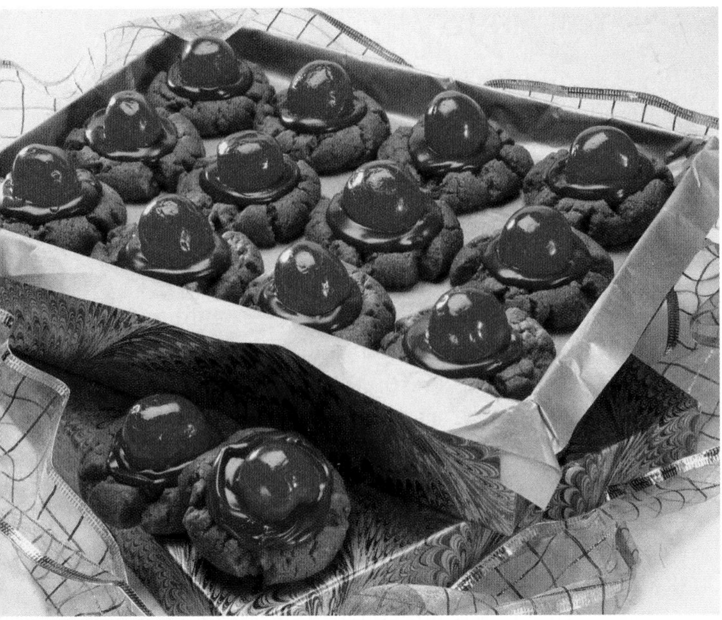

Cherry Marketing Institute

24-7 The indentations in these molded thumbprint cookies are filled with chocolate and topped with delicious, colorful cherries.

the dry ingredients. Cookies are crisp or chewy rather than light and delicate. Therefore, you do not need to cream the fat and sugar as thoroughly as you do for a cake. Also, you can add the flour all at once rather than in parts.

Macaroons, meringues, and kisses contain beaten egg whites. You mix them like angel food and sponge cakes. You mix a few cookies, like Scottish shortbread, using the biscuit method. (Chapter 23 describes the biscuit method.) Your recipe will tell you which method to use.

Pans for Baking Cookies

Bake drop, rolled, refrigerator, pressed, and molded cookies on flat baking pans or cookie sheets. Cookie sheets should not have high sides, or cookies will bake unevenly. Bake bar cookies in pans with sides.

Baking pans made of bright, shiny aluminum reflect heat. Cookies baked on bright, shiny cookie sheets will have light, delicate brown crusts. Dark pans absorb heat. Cookies baked on dark cookie sheets will have dark bottoms. See 24-8.

Cookie sheets should be cool when you place cookies on them for baking. Warm sheets will cause cookies to spread and lose their shape.

If you bake two sheets of cookies at one time, you may have to rotate the pans during baking. This will help the cookies brown evenly. Baking pans should never touch each other or the sides of the oven.

Healthy Living

Modifying cake, cookie, and pastry recipes will help these foods fit more easily into a nutritious diet. However, they will still be higher in calories and lower in nutrients than many other food choices. Therefore, you will still need to eat them in moderation.

Microwaving Cookies

Most microwave ovens are not large enough to efficiently cook dozens of individual cookies. However, bar cookies work well in a microwave oven because the whole pan cooks at once. If using a square or oblong pan, use foil shields to keep the corners from overcooking. Like cakes, bar cookies are often microwaved on medium power and tested with a toothpick for doneness.

Storing Cookies

Store crisp cookies in a container with a loose-fitting cover. To retain their crispness, crisp cookies need to remain dry. Store soft cookies in a container with a tight-fitting cover. Exposure to the air will dry out soft cookies. (Never store crisp and soft cookies together. The soft cookies will soften the crisp cookies.) You can store bar cookies in their baking pan if you cover them, and if you will be eating them in a short time.

For longer storage, you can freeze cookies. Many cookies freeze well both in dough form and after baking.

To freeze refrigerator cookie dough, wrap the shaped rolls tightly in plastic wrap and then in aluminum foil. Label the package and freeze. You can shape molded, rolled, and drop cookie doughs into large balls. Then wrap and label them for freezer storage. You will need to thaw the dough before molding, rolling, or dropping it. You can freeze bar cookie dough in the baking pan. You can press dough for pressed cookies or drop dough

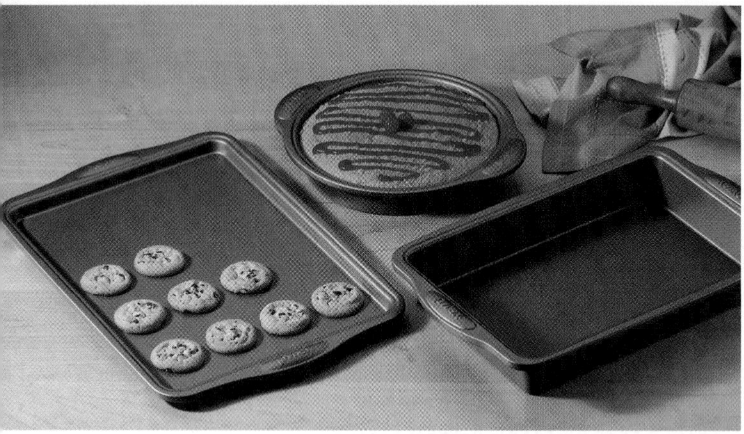

Pyrex

24-8 The dark coating on this cookie sheet will help give the bottoms of these cookies a darker brown crust.

for drop cookies onto cookie sheets and quickly freeze it. You can then remove the frozen dough from the cookie sheet with a spatula. Place the unbaked cookies in airtight containers or plastic bags. Before baking, thaw the cookies at room temperature on a cookie sheet. To freeze baked cookies, pack them in a sturdy container with a tight-fitting cover. Separate layers of cookies with waxed paper or plastic wrap. Cover the container tightly and label.

Freshening Stale Cookies

You can freshen cookies that have lost their characteristic texture. If crisp cookies have become soft or begun to stale, you can make them crisp again. Place cookies on a cookie sheet in a 300°F (150°C) oven for a few minutes. If soft cookies have become hard, you can make them soft again. Place a piece of bread, an apple slice, or an orange section in the cookie container. Replace bread or fruit every other day.

Pies

Apple pie is a favorite dessert in the United States. Who can resist the flavor, aroma, and eye appeal of golden flaky pastry filled with warm, spicy apples? Apple pie begins with pastry. ***Pastry*** is the dough used to make piecrusts. Pastry making is not difficult. However, it does require practice and patience.

Uses for Pastry

You can use pastry in many ways. You may mainly use it when making dessert pies. However, you can use pastry when making main dish pies, such as meat pies and quiche, 24-9. You can fill small pastry shells with foods such as creamed tuna or chicken a la king to make potpies. You can use small pastry shells to make tarts filled with pudding or ice cream. You can fold pastry squares in half over fruit filling to make turnovers. You also use pastry to make appetizers such as cheese sticks.

Kinds of Pies

The four basic kinds of pies are fruit, cream, custard, and chiffon. *Fruit pies* usually are two crust pies. They may have a solid top crust, or they may have a lattice or other decorative top. You may use commercially prepared pie filling or make filling from canned, frozen, dried, or fresh fruit.

Q: Is there anything wrong with eating some of the dough when I'm making cookies?

A: Most homemade cookie dough contains raw eggs, which can be a source of illness-causing bacteria. If you enjoy eating unbaked cookie dough, choose refrigerated dough that you buy at a grocery store. It is made with eggs that have been pasteurized to kill harmful bacteria. You could also use pasteurized eggs in your homemade cookie recipes

Cream pies usually are one-crust pies. Use a cornstarch-thickened pudding mixture to make a cream filling. Cream pies often have a meringue topping.

Custard pies are one-crust pies filled with custard made from milk, eggs, and sugar. The custard may or may not contain other ingredients. Pumpkin pie is a popular custard pie.

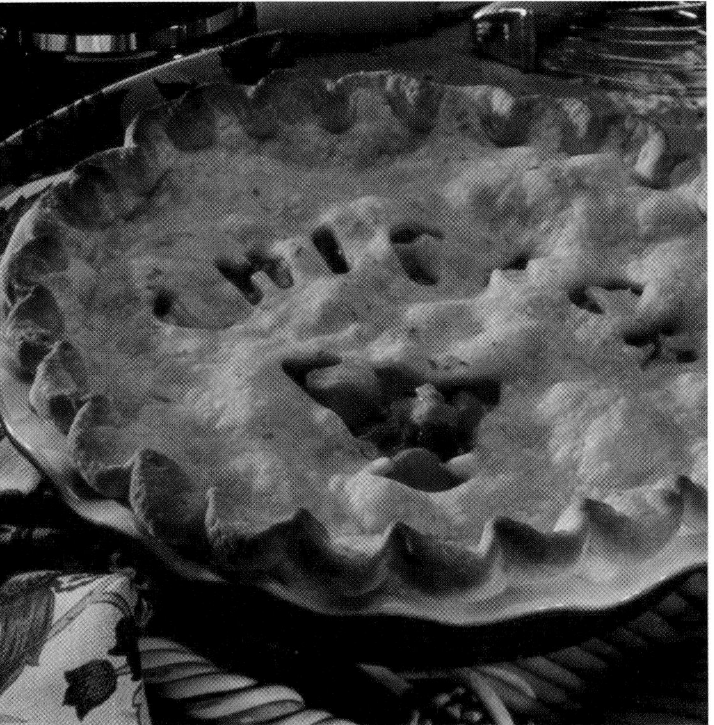

National Chicken Council

***24-9** Tender, flaky pastry can be used to make hearty main dishes, such as chicken potpie.*

Chiffon pies are light and airy. They are one-crust pies filled with a mixture containing gelatin and cooked beaten egg whites. Some chiffon pie fillings also contain whipped cream. Chill all chiffon pies until the filling sets.

Ingredients for Pastry

You will use four basic ingredients to make pastry—flour, fat, water, and salt. When combined correctly, the four ingredients will produce pastry that is tender and flaky.

Flour gives structure to pastry. Most home bakers use all-purpose flour to make pastry.

Fat makes pastry tender by inhibiting the development of gluten. It contributes to flakiness by separating the layers of gluten. Most bakers use lard or hydrogenated vegetable shortening. These fats produce tender and flaky pastry. Some pastry recipes call for oil. Oil-based pastry will be tender, but it will be mealy rather than flaky.

Water provides the moisture needed for the development of the gluten and the production of steam. You need only a small amount of water. For each 1 cup (250 mL) of flour, 2 tablespoons (30 mL) of water is ample.

Salt contributes flavor to pastry. If you eliminate the salt, it will not affect the pastry in any other way.

Food Science Principles of Preparing Pastry

To make pastry that is both tender and flaky, you must use the correct ingredients. You must measure them accurately. You must also handle the dough gently and as little as possible. See 24-10.

Measuring the Ingredients

Flour, fat, and liquid all affect the tenderness and flakiness of pastry. If you do not measure these ingredients accurately, a poor-quality pastry will result.

Gluten develops when you moisten and stir the flour. The gluten creates a framework that traps air and holds steam formed during baking. This trapped air and steam is what causes pastry to be tender and flaky. Too much flour will make pastry tough.

The fat forms a waterproof coating around the flour particles. This prevents too much water from coming in contact with the proteins of the flour. It also prevents the subsequent development of too

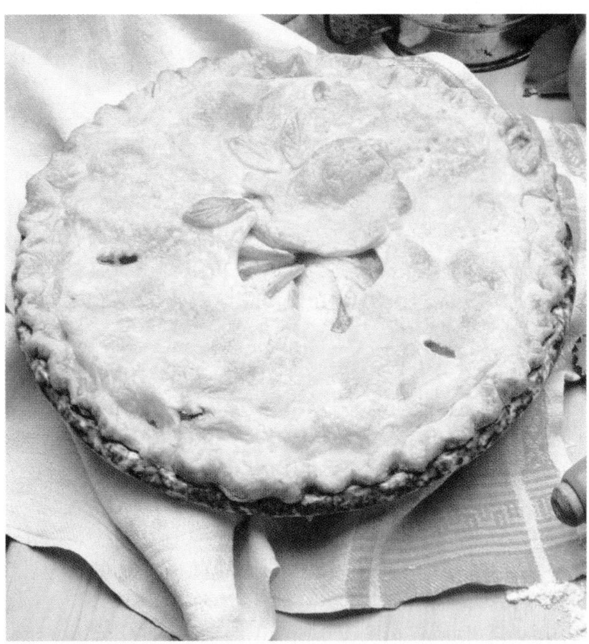

***24-10** The texture of pastry is affected by the proportions of the ingredients and the handling of the dough.*

much gluten. Layers of fat physically separate the layers of gluten that form. As a result, the pastry is both tender and flaky. Too little fat will make pastry tough; too much fat will make pastry crumbly.

Water hydrates the flour so the gluten will develop. It also produces the steam needed for flakiness. The right amount of liquid will moisten the flour just enough to develop the optimum amount of gluten. Too much liquid will make the pastry tough. Too little liquid will make it crumbly and difficult to roll.

Handling the Dough

Too much flour, too much liquid, and too little fat can make pastry tough. Too much handling can also make pastry tough. Handling causes gluten to develop. The more the gluten develops, the tougher the pastry will be.

You should handle pastry gently at all times. You should also handle it as little as possible to prevent overdeveloping the gluten. It is especially important not to

- overmix the dough when adding the liquid
- use the rolling pin too vigorously when rolling the pastry
- stretch the pastry when fitting it into the pie plate

Preparing Pastry

You can use several methods to mix pastry, but the biscuit method (sometimes called the pastry method) is most popular. This method produces pastry that is both tender and flaky. See 24-11.

When making a one-crust pie you will fill after baking, flute the edges. Prick the bottom and sides of the piecrust with a fork to prevent blistering during baking. Do not prick the bottom or sides of a crust you will fill before baking.

Characteristics of Pastry

High-quality pastry is both tender and flaky. The amount and distribution of gluten determines tenderness. Flakiness is due to layers of gluten (with embedded starch grains) separated by layers of fat and expanded (puffed up) by steam.

If pastry is tender, it will cut easily with a fork and "melt in the mouth" when eaten. If pastry is flaky, you will be able to see thin layers of dough separated by empty spaces when you cut into the pastry with a fork.

Aside from having pastry that is tender, flaky, and crisp, a pie should be lightly and evenly browned. The filling should have a pleasing flavor and be neither too runny nor too firm.

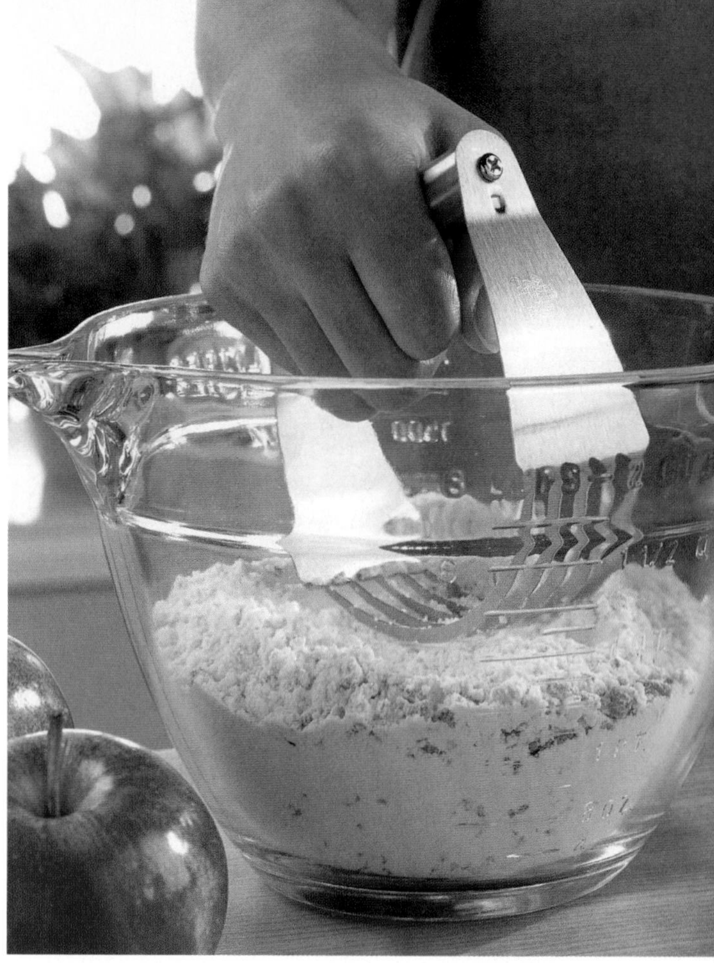

The Pampered Chef®

***24-11** Using a pastry blender to cut shortening into flour is a basic step of preparing pastry by the biscuit method.*

Microwaving Pie

You can prepare both pastry crusts and pies successfully in a microwave oven. You should prepare both in glass pie plates to allow the microwaves to penetrate.

Pastry crusts can be microwaved in six to seven minutes. As with many foods, however, pastry will not brown in a microwave oven. You can add cocoa or instant coffee to the flour when making pastry. You also could brush the pastry with a mixture of molasses and egg yolk before baking. Either technique will produce a crust that appears more traditionally brown.

Microwave times for pies vary according to the filling. Fruit pies are best when you place them in a preheated conventional oven for 10 to 15 minutes after microwaving.

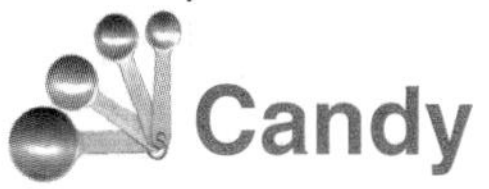

Candy

People enjoy candy throughout the year. At holiday time, however, candy making becomes an important activity in many homes. Homemade fudge, divinity, peanut brittle, toffee, and caramels are fun to make and give as gifts.

To make good candy, you must follow directions exactly. You must mix candies correctly and cook them to the exact temperature specified in the recipe. Otherwise, they are likely to fail.

Kinds of Candy

You can make many kinds of candy at home. A few kinds of candies do not need to be cooked, but these require special recipes. You will cook most candies. Cooked candies are either crystalline or noncrystalline candies.

Crystalline candies contain fine sugar crystals. They taste smooth and creamy. Fudge, fondant, and divinity are crystalline candies.

Noncrystalline candies do not contain sugar crystals. They can be chewy or brittle. Caramels, peanut brittle, and toffee are noncrystalline candies, 24-12.

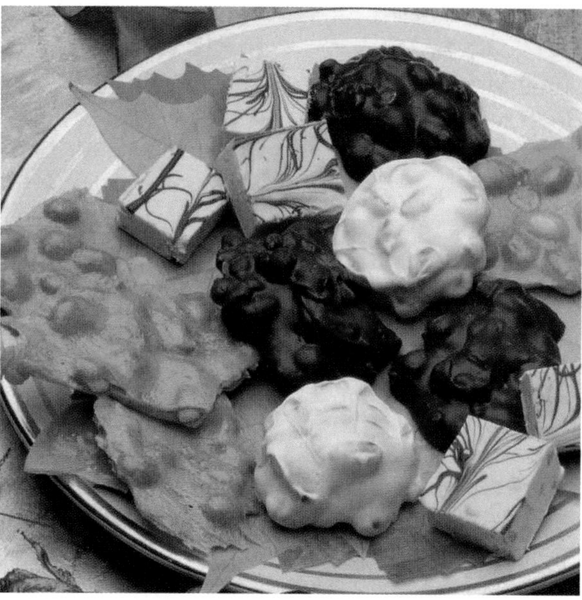

National Peanut Board

24-12 *Golden peanut brittle is a well-liked noncrystalline candy that many people enjoy making at home.*

Food Science Principles of Candy Making

All cooked candies begin with ***sugar syrup.*** This is a mixture of sugar and liquid that is cooked to a thick consistency. Successful candy making depends on how you treat this sugar syrup.

When making crystalline candies, you want the sugar syrup to form crystals. However, you want these crystals to be very small and fine. To produce small sugar crystals, you must heat the sugar syrup to a specific temperature. You must then cool it to a specific temperature and beat it vigorously.

Fudge is one of the most popular crystalline candies. High-quality fudge tastes smooth and creamy because it contains small sugar crystals. It has a deep brown color and a satiny sheen. Poor-quality fudge tastes grainy because it contains large sugar crystals.

When making noncrystalline candies, you do not want the sugar syrup to form crystals. You can prevent crystal formation by heating the syrup to a very high temperature. You can add substances like corn syrup, milk, cream, or butter, which interfere with crystallization. You can also use a combination of high temperatures and interfering substances to prevent crystals from forming.

Peanut brittle is a popular noncrystalline candy. High-quality peanut brittle has a golden color and looks foamy. Cooking the candy to a very high temperature and using interfering substances prevent crystal formation.

Whether you are making crystalline or noncrystalline candies, temperature is very important. A candy thermometer is the most accurate method of testing the temperature of sugar syrups. Each type of candy requires a specific temperature. The candy thermometer will accurately tell you when sugar syrup reaches the correct temperature.

You will also want to use a heavy saucepan to cook candy. Mixtures that contain large amounts of sugar burn easily. A heavy saucepan will help prevent scorching.

Microwaving Candy

A microwave oven works well for melting chocolate, caramels, and marshmallows for use in recipes. These candies are less likely to stick and burn in a microwave oven than on a conventional range.

In addition to melting prepared candies, you can make fresh candy in a microwave oven. You can successfully prepare both crystalline and noncrystalline candies. Cooking procedures for candies vary. Refer to a microwave cookbook for specific directions.

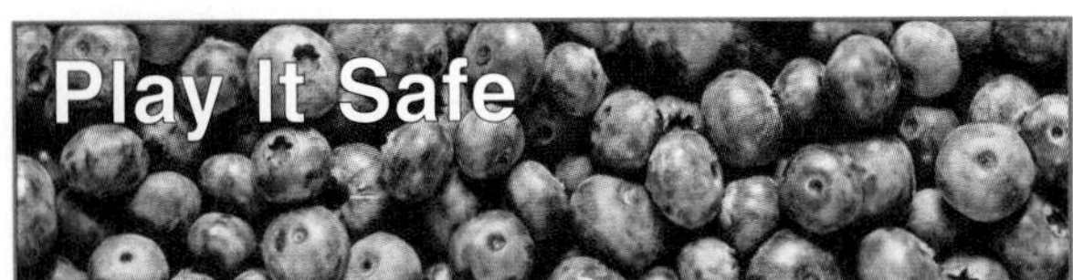

Sugar syrups are extremely hot and can cause severe burns if they come in contact with the skin. Use caution when handling sugar syrups. Never leave children unattended while making candy.

Chocolate

In the minds of some sweet lovers, no candy can match chocolate. The most exquisite chocolates may be best left to professional candy makers. However, even novices can melt chocolate at home. You can pour melted chocolate into molds. You can use it to make clusters of raisins, nuts, or coconut. You can also dip fondant or caramels in a coating of melted chocolate, 24-13.

Chocolate is made from the beans of the cacao tree. The beans are first roasted. Then they are shelled, pressed, and heated until they form a liquid, which is called *chocolate liquor*. At this point, some of the fat, or *cocoa butter*, may be removed. However, a high cocoa butter content is a sign of quality in chocolate.

Baking and eating chocolate is made from chocolate liquor. It comes in various degrees of sweetness. *Unsweetened chocolate* contains no sugar. *Bittersweet, semisweet,* and *milk chocolate* each contain progressively more sugar. Sweetened chocolates also contain vanilla, and milk chocolate contains milk solids.

Other products related to chocolate include cocoa, white chocolate, and imitation chocolate. Cocoa is made from dried chocolate liquor that has been ground to a fine powder. *White chocolate* is made from cocoa butter, sugar, milk solids, and flavorings. Because it contains no chocolate liquor, it is not truly chocolate. *Imitation chocolate* or chocolate-flavored products are made with vegetable oil instead of cocoa butter. Imitation chocolate is less expensive than real chocolate. However, it lacks the creamy smoothness and delicious flavor characteristic of true chocolate.

To melt chocolate, chop bars into small pieces or use chocolate chips. Place chocolate in the top of a double boiler over hot water and stir constantly. Remove chocolate from heat as soon as it is melted to prevent scorching. You can also melt chocolate in a microwave oven. Place the chocolate in a glass bowl. Microwave on high power for 30 seconds at a time until chocolate is melted. Be sure to stir the chocolate after each microwaving period.

Q: Isn't chocolate high in caffeine?

A: Chocolate supplies only a small amount of caffeine. A cup of coffee has more than 20 times the caffeine found in a serving of chocolate milk or an ounce of milk chocolate.

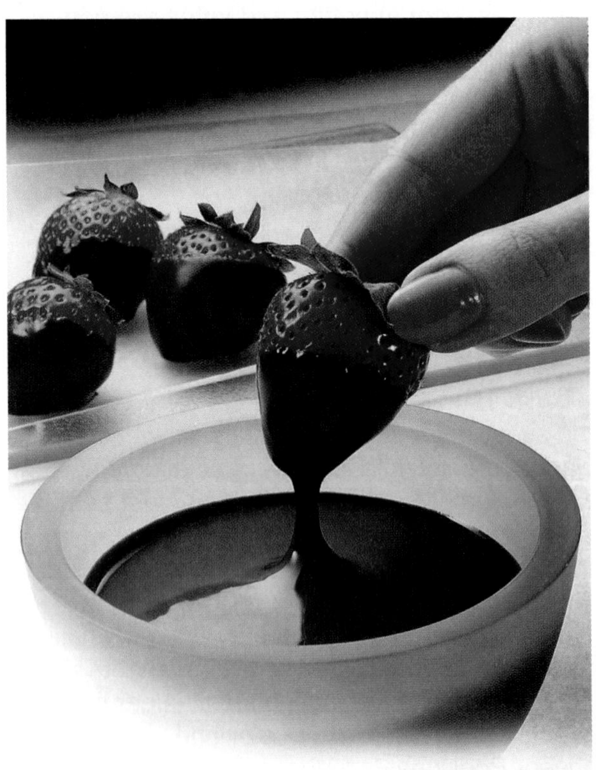

photograph courtesy of The Reynolds Kitchens

***24-13** Creamy melted chocolate makes a delicious coating for fresh strawberries.*

Chapter 24 Review

Cakes, Cookies, Pies, and Candies

Summary

The two basic types of cakes are shortened, which contain fat, and unshortened, which do not contain fat. Chiffon cakes are a cross between shortened and unshortened cakes. All cakes contain the same essential set of ingredients, each of which performs a specific function. You must measure ingredients carefully and then mix them using the method described in your recipe. You also must use correct pan sizes, oven temperatures, and baking times to make sure cakes bake properly. After baking, you can fill and/or frost a cake to enhance its flavor and appearance.

Rolled, drop, bar, refrigerator, pressed, and molded cookies all contain ingredients similar to cakes. You will mix most cookies by the conventional mixing method and bake them on a cookie sheet. You should store crisp cookies in containers with loose-fitting lids and soft cookies in containers with tight-fitting lids.

Pastry is the primary component of fruit, cream, custard, and chiffon pies. Flour, fat, water, and salt are the basic ingredients in pastry. Carefully measuring these ingredients and gently handling the dough will help you produce tender, flaky pastry.

You can make both crystalline and noncrystalline candies at home. Both types begin with sugar syrup. You will heat, cool, and then beat sugar syrups for crystalline candies to produce fine sugar crystals. You will heat sugar syrups for noncrystalline candies to high temperatures and/or add interfering substances to keep crystals from forming.

Review What You Have Read

Write your answers on a separate sheet of paper.

1. True or false. Both shortened and unshortened cakes contain chemical leavening agents.
2. List the seven basic ingredients of a shortened cake (other than pound cake) and briefly describe a major function of each.
3. What are two functions of cream of tartar in angel food cake?
4. What would happen if a cake were made with too much fat?
5. Why do baking pans need to be the correct size when baking a cake?
6. What are the two most common mixing methods for making shortened cakes?
7. True or false. An angel food cake should be removed from the pan as soon as it comes out of the oven.
8. True or false. Both shortened and unshortened cakes can be microwaved successfully.
9. How do proportions of cookie ingredients differ from proportions of cake ingredients?
10. Describe the appearance of cookies baked on a shiny aluminum cookie sheet and cookies baked on a dark cookie sheet.
11. How will pastry be affected if salt is omitted from the recipe?
12. List three reasons pastry might be tough.
13. What two characteristics are used to describe high-quality pastry?
14. Describe two techniques that can be used to give a brown appearance to a pastry crust prepared in a microwave oven.
15. How does a crystalline candy differ in texture from a noncrystalline candy?

Build Your Basic Skills

1. **Science.** Prepare two angel food cakes. In one cake, add cream of tartar to egg whites during beating. Do not add cream of tartar to the egg whites used in the other cake. Discuss the appearance, texture, and volume of the two cakes.
2. **Math.** Choose a favorite cookie recipe. Write down the amount of each ingredient you would need to prepare a double batch. Also note the yield for the double batch.
3. **Writing.** Prepare enough pastry for a two-crust pie. Divide the dough in half. Roll half the dough and cut it into 1-inch (2.5-cm) strips. Place the strips on a cookie sheet. Knead the other half of the dough for several minutes. Roll and cut the dough into 1-inch (2.5-cm) strips and place them on a second cookie sheet. Bake the pastry strips. After comparing the appearance and texture of the two samples, write a paragraph explaining why overhandling pastry should be avoided.

Build Your Thinking Skills

1. **Compare.** Prepare two batches of a shortened cake recipe—one with granulated sugar and the other with brown sugar. Store the cakes in covered containers for several days. Compare the flavor and texture.
2. **Analyze.** Prepare two batches of fudge. Follow directions exactly for the first batch. For the second batch, stir fudge occasionally during cooling. After the fudge has set, rate the texture, flavor, and appearance of both samples. Analyze the impact of stirring fudge during cooling.

Apply Technology

1. Find out how the automatic measuring feature available on some of the newest electric mixer models works. Predict how you think this feature would affect the preparation of cake and cookie recipes.
2. Prepare a cake or cookie recipe. Then prepare a second version of the recipe using an artificial sweetener in place of the sugar. Compare and evaluate the two products.

Using Workplace Skills

Judi is the pastry chef on the Caribbean Empress, which is a cruise ship noted for its world-class meals. Judi supervises three dessert cooks. Each day they prepare pastries, confections, and ice cream to coordinate with the executive chef's elaborate menus. Once a week, they also put together an expansive dessert buffet, which becomes a highlight of every cruise. Judi makes sure the cooks correctly prepare and attractively plate each of 1,800 servings of dessert daily.

To be an effective worker, Judi needs leadership skills. In a small group, answer the following questions about Judi's need for and use of these skills:

A. How might Judi's leadership skills help the dessert cooks do their work?
B. How might the ship's guests be affected if Judi lacks leadership skills?
C. How might the Caribbean Empress be affected if Judi lacks leadership skills?
D. What is another skill Judi would need in this job? Briefly explain why this skill would be important.

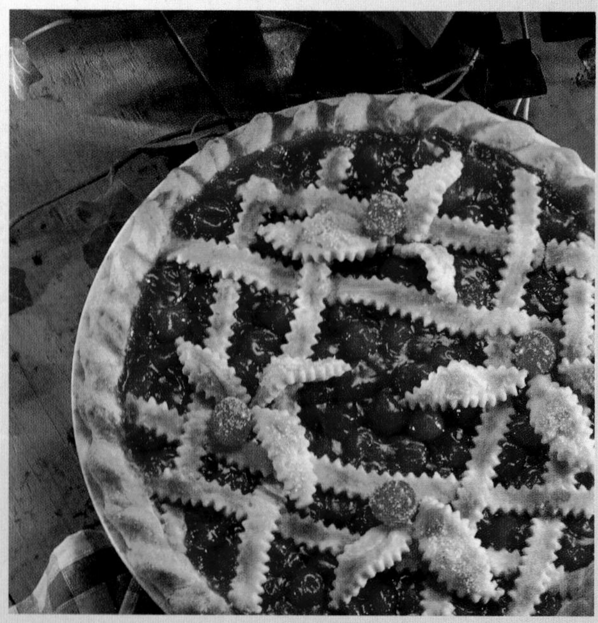

Chapter 25
Food and Entertaining

Social Director
Plans and organizes recreational activities and creates friendly atmosphere for guests in hotels and resorts or for passengers on board ships.

Formal Waiter
Serves meals to patrons according to established rules of etiquette, working in a formal setting.

Food and Beverage Analyst
Examines food samples and food-service records to determine sales appeal and cost of preparing and serving foods in establishments such as restaurants.

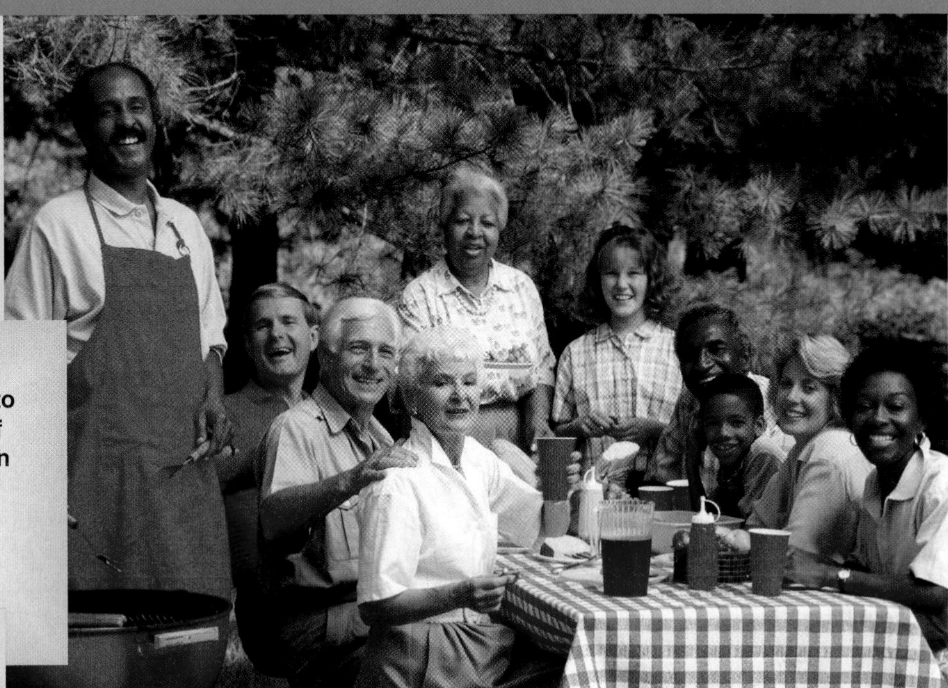

Terms to Know

RSVP
American (family style) service
Russian (continental) service
English service
compromise service
blue plate service
buffet service
manners
etiquette
appetizer
reservation
entree
table d'hôte
a la carte
Dutch treat
gratuity
tip

Objectives

After studying this chapter, you will be able to

- plan a social gathering.
- wait on a table correctly.
- prepare appetizers.
- describe guidelines for safely preparing, transporting, and serving food for outdoor entertaining.
- use appropriate behavior when dining out.

Eating food is more enjoyable when others eat it with you. Entertaining and dining out give people chances to renew longstanding relationships and meet new friends.

Planning for Entertaining

Most people enjoy getting together with friends and family members. You might host a formal dinner party, a special birthday celebration, or an impromptu get-together. No matter what the event is, a little planning will help it go more smoothly.

Social gatherings should allow both guests and hosts to enjoy themselves. Guests may find it hard to relax if their host is running around tending to last minute details. Hosts may find it hard to have a good time if they have not completed preparations before their guests arrive. Careful planning helps prevent these problems and set a festive mood for a party.

Planning a gathering involves money, time, and energy. The kind of gathering you have and the number of guests you invite depend on these and other important factors.

The Theme

Social gatherings often have themes. You can turn almost any idea into a party theme. Sports events and holidays are popular themes. You could plan a gathering with an international theme using information from the last part of this text.

The theme helps determine what people should wear and what foods you might serve. The theme can give you ideas for decorations and activities, too. For instance, guests could wear sombreros to go with a Mexican theme. You could serve tacos and enchiladas, 25-1. You might hang a piñata for a decoration. Later, you could invite guests to help break it as one of the activities.

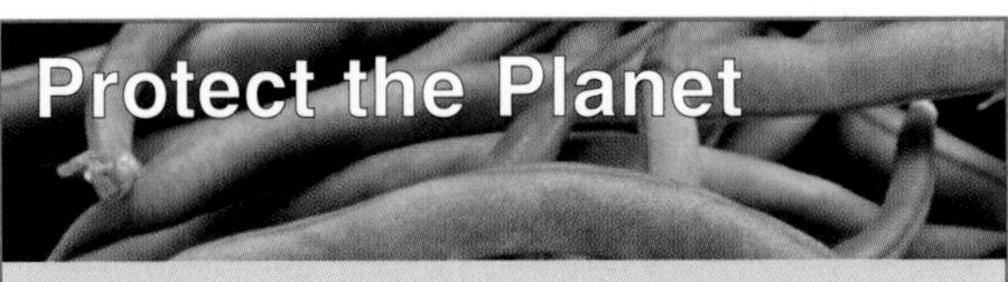

Paper plates and cups and plastic flatware can be convenient for informal entertaining. However, natural resources are required to make these items. After one use, they end up in a landfill. Washing dishes or loading a dishwasher takes only a few minutes when cleaning up from a party. To help give the environment a break, plan to use nondisposable dinnerware at your next social gathering.

The Guest List

When putting together your guest list, keep people's interests and personalities in mind. Common interests will help your guests get to know one another. Compatible personalities will help create a setting in which everyone gets along and has a good time.

The number of people invited to a party should fit comfortably in the amount of space available. Your guest list should also fit your cooking skills and available equipment. Unless you have extra help or a large freezer, very large parties might not be practical.

The Invitations

Most parties have no rules for invitations. You might invite friends for a spur-of-the-moment party or casual gathering in person or over the phone. For large parties, handwritten notes or printed invitations are more convenient. A formal event always requires a written invitation.

All invitations should include the date, the time, and the place of the party. Invitations should specify if a party is to honor a special event, such as a birthday. They should also indicate any need for special clothing, such as swimsuits for a pool party.

You may wish to include the letters ***RSVP*** on your invitations. This is the abbreviation for a French phrase that means "please respond." Also include your phone number so your guests can let you know if they are coming.

Keep a list of all replies as you receive them. You will need this list for later planning.

The Menu

Almost any foods can be party foods. Sometimes the kind of gathering you are giving helps you plan the menu. You might serve cookies and hot chocolate at a sledding party. You might choose heartier foods, such as sandwiches and pizza, for an after-the-game get-together.

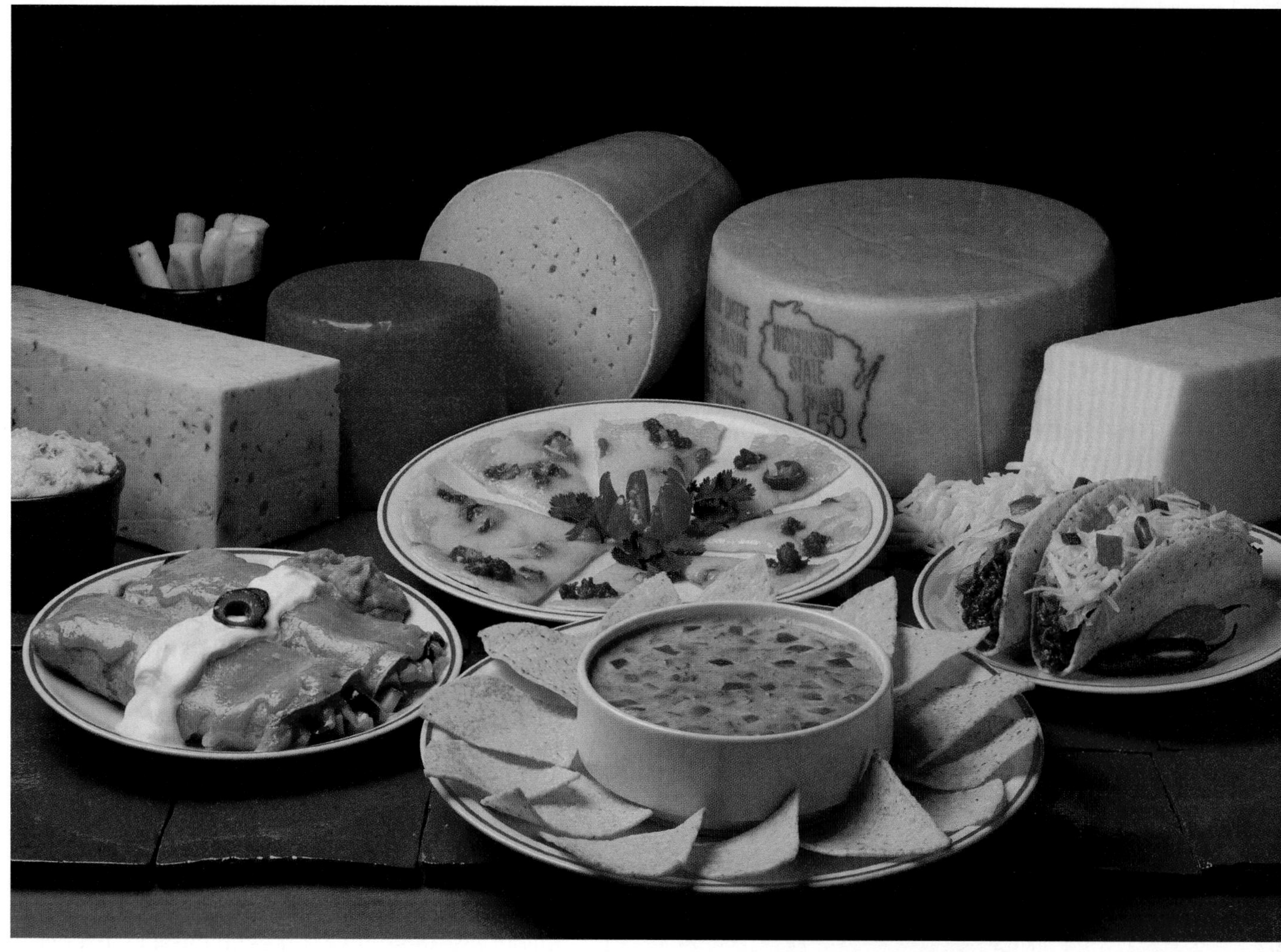

25-1 *Tacos, enchiladas, and other Mexican dishes might make up the menu at a party with a Mexican theme.*

Of course, a key consideration when planning a menu is your guests' food preferences. You want to choose foods you think your guests will like. If any of your guests has special dietary needs, try to serve some foods and drinks that meet those needs. For instance, offer meatless items for guests who are vegetarians. Also, avoid serving foods to which you know a guest is allergic.

Other factors to consider when planning a party menu include your budget, cooking skills, time schedule, and equipment. Party food can be costly. Preparing food yourself is likely to be less expensive than buying ready-made snacks. You may wish to give a party with friends who can help share the costs. For a casual gathering, you might ask your friends to bring some of the food.

When you are having guests, choose familiar recipes you know you can prepare successfully. Save new recipes for a trial run later with your family or close friends. Limit the number of dishes that will require your last minute attention. Choose one or more dishes you can prepare in advance. This gives you more time to enjoy your guests.

Do not finalize the menu until you check your equipment. See if you have all the cookware and serving utensils you will need. For instance, if you do not have a deep, straight-sided dish, do not plan to make a soufflé. Also check to see when you will need to use certain appliances. You may not have enough room to microwave two dishes at the same time. (You may be able to borrow or rent equipment, but check first.)

Appetizers

Appetizers are small, light foods served to stimulate the appetite. They are often served at the beginning of a meal. Appetizers are also popular as party foods, 25-2.

You can prepare many appetizers in advance, so they require little last minute attention. You can conveniently serve appetizers to a large group because guests can eat them while standing. You are also likely to spend less money for party food when serving appetizers than when serving a full meal.

Instead of serving chips and pretzels at your next party, be creative and try making your own appetizers. Choose appetizers that guests will find easy to nibble while they mingle. Remember to select both hot and cold appetizers, using ingredients with a variety of flavors, colors, and textures.

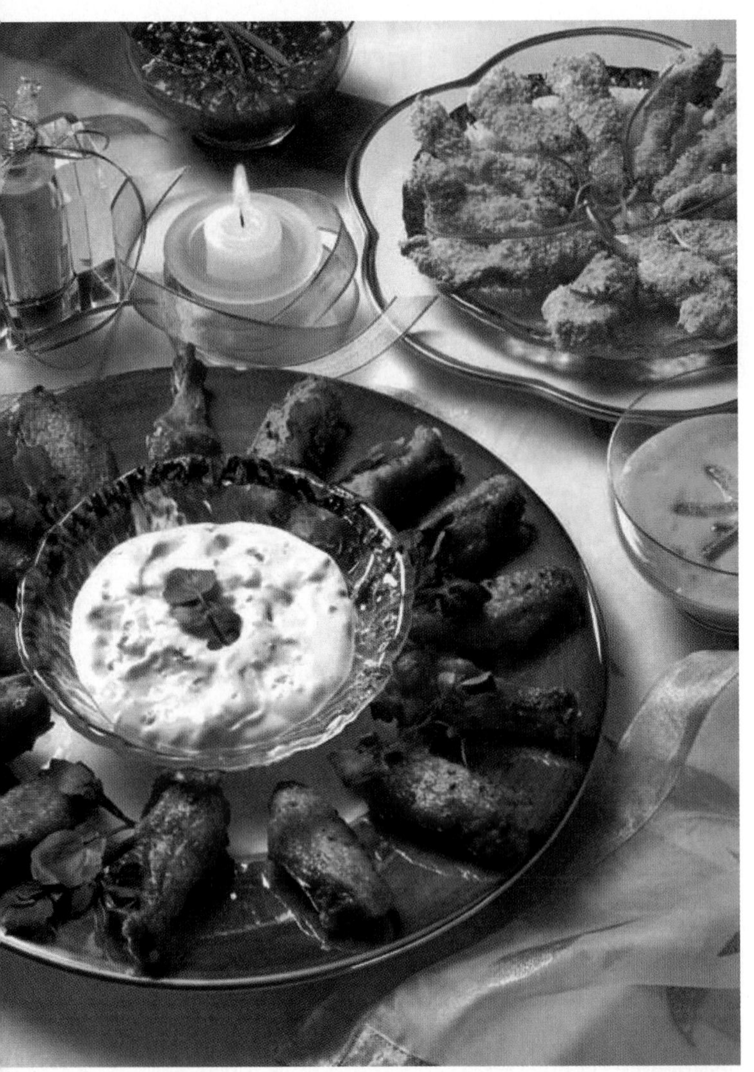

National Chicken Council

***25-2** A variety of tasty appetizers may be served in place of a meal at a social gathering.*

You might use a microwave oven to save time when preparing hot appetizers. Mini pizzas, toasted nuts, cocktail sausages, chicken wings, and hot dips are just a few of the tasty appetizers that can be microwaved. You can prepare many of these foods ahead of time and then microwave them at the last minute.

You can adapt many conventional appetizer recipes for the microwave oven. Appetizers containing delicate ingredients, such as sour cream, cheese, eggs, milk, and mayonnaise, should be microwaved at lower settings. Stir dips and sauces halfway through the cooking period to promote even heating. Spread toppings on crackers or toast points just before microwaving to prevent them from getting soggy. Place egg rolls and foods with cracker bases on paper towels to help absorb excess moisture.

Serving Party Foods

You should always try to make food look appetizing when you serve it. This is especially important when serving foods to guests. Arrange food attractively on platters and trays and in serving bowls. Use garnishes to add color and give guests a hint of what is in foods. For example, you might use jalapeño peppers to garnish a spicy hot Mexican cheese dip. You might use fresh raspberries to garnish a chocolate raspberry torte.

Be sure an appropriate serving utensil accompanies each dish. Use serving spoons for soft foods and serving forks for meats. Tongs work well for serving individual items, such as shrimp and fresh vegetables. When guests will be approaching a buffet table from both sides, place two serving utensils with each dish.

The Meal Service

If you are serving a meal at your gathering, you will need to decide how to serve it. You might want to serve appetizers in the living room before the meal. This will help eliminate clutter at the table. Likewise, you can serve dessert in the living room after the meal. This will give you a chance to clear the table and start to clean up the kitchen. Trays or a serving cart can help you serve both of these courses away from the table more easily.

You can serve meals in several ways. The style of service you select will depend on the formality of the meal, the menu, and the availability of help.

The six major styles of meal service are American or family, Russian or continental, English, compromise, blue plate, and buffet. They differ in the way the guests are served and in the number of courses.

American or ***family style*** service is the style most often used in homes in the United States. In this style of service, the host fills serving dishes in the kitchen and takes them to the table. Diners serve themselves as they pass the serving dishes around the table. After clearing the table, the host may serve dessert at the table or from the kitchen.

Russian or ***continental service*** is the most formal style of meal service. In Russian service, serving dishes are never placed on the table. Instead, waiters serve guests filled plates of food, one course at a time. Plate replaces plate as one course is removed and another is served. This type of service is often used in fine restaurants and at state dinners.

In ***English service,*** one of the hosts fills plates at the table and passes them from guest to guest until everyone is served. Because English service requires a lot of passing, it is best for use with small groups.

Compromise service is a compromise between Russian service and English service. The salad or dessert course is often served from the kitchen. For the other courses, one of the hosts fills the plates and passes them around the table. One person acts as waiter to clear one course and bring in the next.

Blue plate service is used at home when serving small groups of people. It is also used at banquets where waiters are able to serve a crowd quickly, 25-3. In blue plate service, the host fills plates in the kitchen and carries them to the dining room. The host may offer second helpings at the table or refill plates in the kitchen. One person clears the main course and then brings in the dessert course.

Buffet service is often used for serving large numbers of people. A dining table, a buffet, or another surface may hold the serving dishes and utensils, dinnerware, flatware, and napkins. The guests serve themselves from the buffet.

Depending on the amount of space available, guests may eat at one large table, at several smaller tables, or from lap trays. If space is limited, they may eat from plates held in their hands while sitting or standing. If guests will be seated at a table, the host may place napkins, flatware, and beverageware on the table ahead of time.

Buffet service requires careful menu planning. Equipment may be needed to keep hot foods hot and cold foods cold. Precutting foods into individual servings and pouring beverages ahead of time will make serving easier.

The Host's Responsibilities

As the host, you have certain responsibilities to your guests. Before your guests arrive, be sure the house is clean and tidy. Put fresh soap

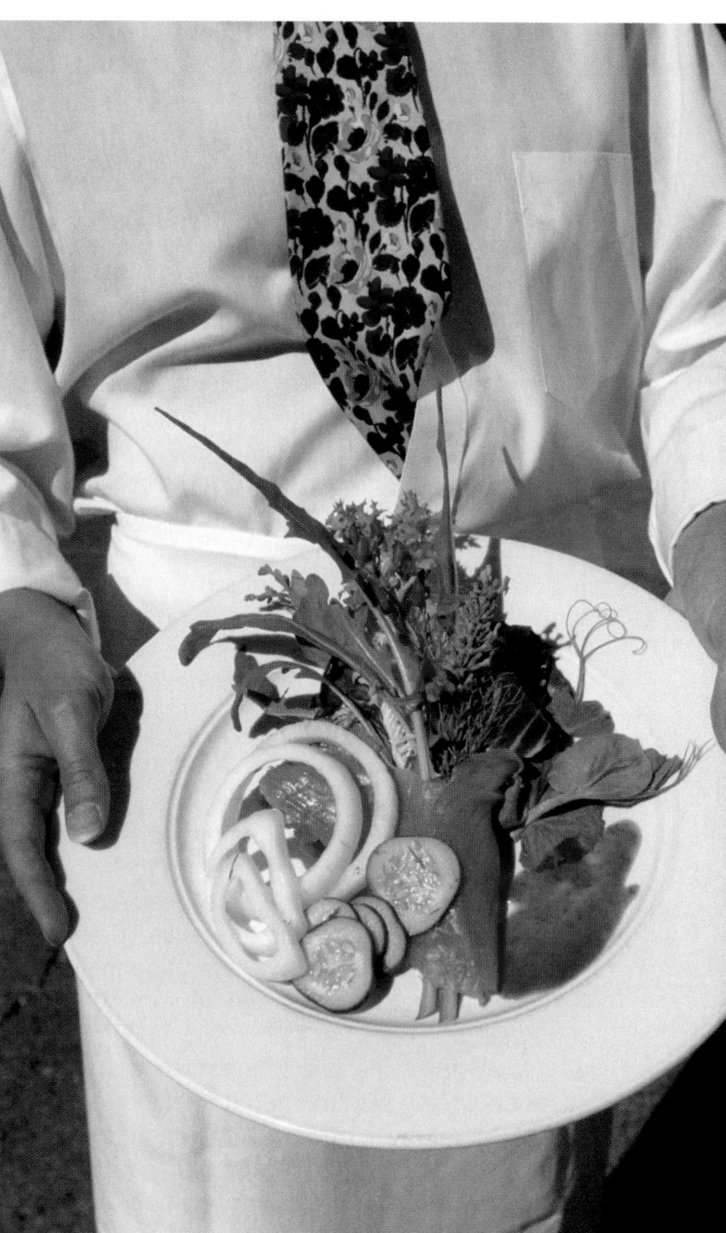

25-3 *A waiter bringing a filled plate to a banquet guest is using blue plate service.*

Q: How can I keep food safe on a buffet table for several hours during a social gathering?

A: Put food in small serving dishes so foods will heat and chill quickly. Refill or replace serving dishes as needed. Place hot foods in slow cookers or on warming trays to keep them at a safe, hot temperature. Place containers of cold food in deep trays filled with ice.

and clean towels in the bathroom. Be sure to have a specific place for your guests' coats.

As your guests begin to arrive, make introductions. Introduce a younger person to an older person by giving the older person's name first. Try to say something interesting about each person for a conversation starter. You might say, "Mary Lewis, I would like you to meet LaVarre Johnson. LaVarre worked as a camp counselor last summer."

A planned activity helps people get to know one another. Games, music, and dancing are good ways to break the ice.

Try to participate in your party as much as possible. Circulate from guest to guest instead of spending the evening with just one or two close friends. It is up to you to make all your guests feel welcome.

Waiting on the Table

If your gathering includes a meal, one of your responsibilities as host will be to wait on the table. Rules for waiting on the table are as flexible as rules for setting the table. The style of service and the menu help determine the way in which you clear the table and serve new courses.

Clear the table in a counterclockwise direction, beginning with the person seated to your right. Serve a new course in the same manner. You will use both hands when serving and clearing, but usually at different times. When serving or clearing plates, you should stand at the guest's left and place or remove the plate with your left hand. This avoids a possible collision with the water glass on the right.

Remove beverageware and unused knives and spoons from the guest's right side with your right hand. Place dessert flatware in the same manner, and pour water from the right with the right hand.

When clearing or serving, a cart or large tray can save time and steps. The order for removing and serving a course is listed in 25-4.

The Guest's Responsibilities

A good guest also has responsibilities. These begin with the invitation. Always answer an invitation as soon as possible. You may be able to give an immediate response to a telephoned invitation. If not, you should answer within a day or two. Formal events require a written response. When responding to an invitation, repeat the time and the date to avoid any misunderstandings.

Arrive at a party at the designated time. Guests who arrive too early can disrupt last minute preparations. Guests who arrive late can be the cause of a ruined meal.

Greet any members of your host's family who happen to be present. Follow house rules and always be courteous.

Table Manners

When dining in a friend's home, you should use your best table manners. ***Manners*** refer to social behavior. Society sets rules of ***etiquette,*** which guide manners. Knowing proper etiquette will help you relax in unfamiliar settings because you will know how to behave. Those around you will also feel more at ease because your behavior will not be offensive to them. The table manners below will help you feel more comfortable and show your consideration for others when eating.

- A man should help seat women who are sitting near him.
- Shortly after sitting down, open your napkin to a comfortable size and place it in your lap.
- When passing dishes at the table, always pass them in one direction.
- Wait for the host to begin eating.
- Try to eat at least a small portion of each food served. If you cannot eat something, leave it without comment.

Waiting on the Table	
Removing a Course	
1.	Remove all serving dishes and utensils from the table and take them to the kitchen.
2.	Beginning with the appropriate person, remove the dinner plate from each cover with your left hand. Transfer the first plate to your right hand. Place the second plate on top of the first plate. Then remove the third plate with your left hand. Take cleared plates to a serving cart or the kitchen. Continue this process around the table in a counterclockwise direction until you have cleared all covers.
3.	Use a small tray to remove flatware and other items not needed for the next course.
4.	If necessary, refill water glasses from each guest's right, using your right hand. Use a clean napkin to catch drips.
Serving a Course	
1.	Place needed flatware, such as cake forks or dessertspoons, at each cover.
2.	Place cream, sugar, and other needed items on the table.
3.	Place needed dinnerware at each cover.
4.	Place food and/or beverages.

***25-4** Following a standard order for clearing and serving courses makes meal service more efficient.*

- Use eating utensils in the order in which they have been placed on the table—from the outside toward the plate.
- Never set a used eating utensil on the table. Place dirty utensils on the plates with which you used them. For instance, leave your salad fork on your salad plate.
- If you drop an eating utensil, do not use it anymore. Your host should give you another one.
- Do not place your elbows on the table while eating.
- Keep one hand in your lap while eating.
- Do not reach in front of another diner for food. Ask someone to pass the food to you. Take helpings of average size.
- Corn on the cob, pizza, and hot dogs are generally considered to be finger foods. At informal events, you can also pick up fried chicken, French fries, and whole fresh fruits with your fingers, 25-5. However, you should use utensils when eating these foods at formal gatherings. Even at formal events, you may use your fingers when eating many appetizers.
- Do not put foods into a bowl of dip after you have had them in your mouth. Use a serving spoon to put a small amount of dip on your plate for dipping chips and vegetables.
- Do not take a bite from a whole slice of bread. Tear bread into quarters; tear biscuits and rolls in half. Put butter on your bread and butter plate with the knife that accompanies the butter. Then use your table knife to spread butter on one piece of bread, biscuit, or roll at a time.
- Remove seeds, pits, or fish bones from your mouth with your fingers as inconspicuously as possible. Place them on the side of your plate.
- If you cough or sneeze at the table, use your handkerchief and quietly excuse yourself. If you have a coughing or sneezing spell, quietly excuse yourself and leave the table.
- When you have finished eating, place your knife on the rim of the plate with the sharp edge pointing toward the center. Place the fork parallel to the knife. Lay your napkin casually to the left of the plate. Wait for your host to invite you to leave the table.

Offer to assist with last minute details or cleanup tasks if you see the host needs help. Most hosts will appreciate your help

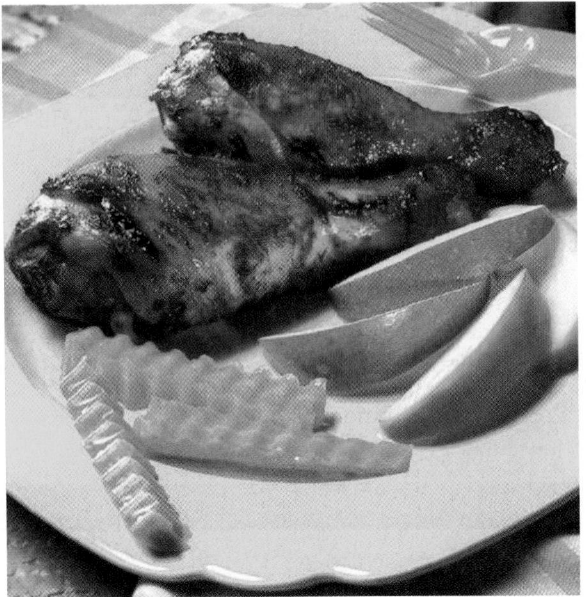

National Chicken Council

25-5 You can use your fingers to eat fried chicken and cut fresh fruits and vegetables at an informal gathering.

filling serving dishes or picking up used glasses and plates. If the host refuses help, do not insist.

Outdoor Entertaining

Outdoor meals are an important part of warm weather entertaining. An outdoor meal can be as simple as fresh fruit, cheese, and a loaf of bread shared on a park bench. A neighborhood clambake on the beach is a more elaborate type of outdoor entertaining.

You can prepare picnic foods at home or cook them at the picnic site. Besides traditional hot dogs and hamburgers, consider expanding your picnic menus to include casseroles, soups, and ethnic dishes, 25-6.

The food you serve for a picnic and how you carry it depend somewhat on transportation and available facilities. If you plan to bicycle or hike to your picnic site, you will need foods that are compact and easy to carry. Finger foods, such as sandwiches, vegetable relishes, fresh fruits, and bar cookies, would be good choices.

Picnics on the water usually have some space limitations, though not as many as bicycle picnics. On small boats, serve foods prepared in advance. On larger boats with cooking facilities, you can finish last minute preparations on the boat. Drinking water is often limited on board boats. For this reason, you might want to carry some high-moisture foods and avoid salty foods when picnicking on the water.

Grilling

Picnics that include grilled foods are called cookouts or barbecues. You can cook food over an open fire or on a grill.

Tools

The grill is the major barbecuing tool. Except for gas and electric grills, all grills use charcoal briquettes for fuel. You place charcoal in the grill's *fire box*, and cook the food on the *grate*.

In addition to a grill, you might want to invest in tongs, a long-handled fork, and a broad turner. A basting brush, fireproof mitts, and heavy-duty foil also come in handy when grilling. If your grill is not gas or electric, you will need charcoal briquettes and an electric starter or lighter fluid.

Cooking

Light the charcoal in a grill about 30 minutes before you want to begin cooking. The time will

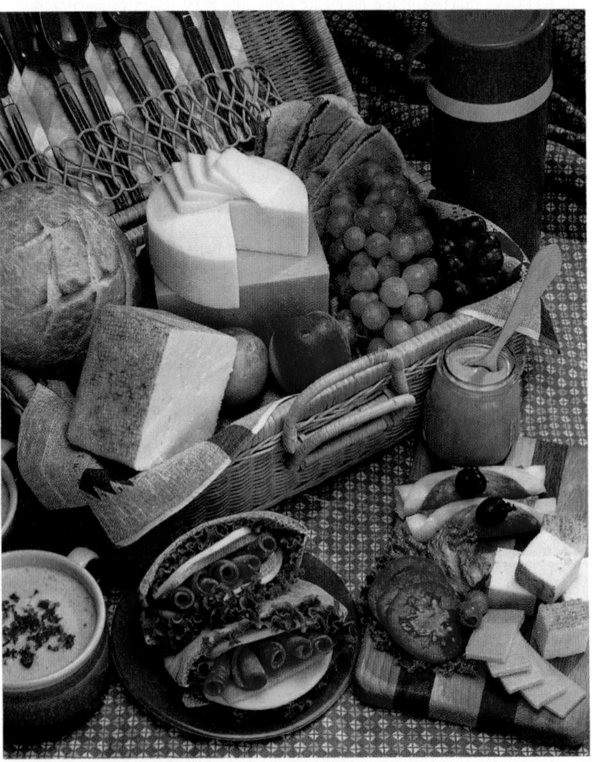

©2002 Wisconsin Milk Marketing Board, Inc.

25-6 Picnic food can include almost anything you can pack into a basket or cooler.

vary somewhat depending on the wind, the location of the grill, and the kind of charcoal. Coals covered with a gray ash are ready for good heat distribution.

You can cook many foods outdoors. Meats, fish, and poultry are probably the most commonly grilled foods. You can put fruits and vegetables on skewers and cook them as kabobs. You might also try wrapping them in heavy-duty foil and cooking them over the coals. You can wrap breads and biscuits in foil and warm them on a grill, too.

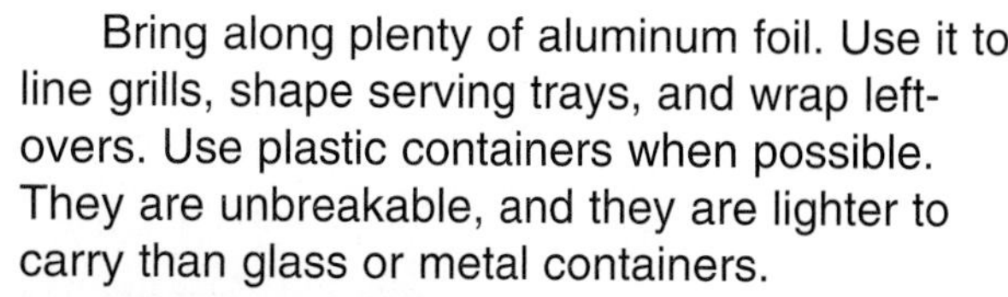

Play It Safe

Safety precautions are important when cooking outdoors. You need to protect yourself, other people, and the environment.

Always place the grill in the open, away from trees, shrubbery, furniture, and buildings. Keep all flammable materials, such as lighter fluid, away from the fire.

Wear tight-fitting clothes and a heavy-duty apron. If you have long hair, tie it back away from your face.

Never use gasoline or kerosene to start the fire. Never pour lighter fluid over the coals once the fire has started. Keep a container of water and a baster handy. Use them to extinguish flare-ups, which can occur when fat drips onto hot coals.

Transporting and Serving Food Outdoors

You must keep hot foods hot and cold foods cold when transporting and serving foods for outdoor meals. (See Chapter 6.) Vacuum containers and insulated picnic coolers can keep foods at proper temperatures during transport. Keep foods for grilling in the cooler until the coals are ready. See 25-7.

Remove food from coolers in small amounts. You can always serve second helpings. Return all perishable foods to the insulated cooler as soon as possible.

Bring along plenty of aluminum foil. Use it to line grills, shape serving trays, and wrap leftovers. Use plastic containers when possible. They are unbreakable, and they are lighter to carry than glass or metal containers.

Keep a supply list inside your picnic basket. Frequently forgotten items include can openers, paring knives, salt and pepper, paper towels, eating utensils, and matches.

Cleaning Up

Litter is unsightly and often illegal. It attracts insects and animals, and it can cause fires. Most parks, forest preserves, and camping grounds have refuse containers available. Be sure to use them to properly dispose of all refuse.

Also, pack a couple of large plastic bags with your picnic supplies. They will come in handy if you find yourself picnicking in an area that does not have refuse containers. Use one of the bags to hold trash until you find a suitable container. Use the other bag to collect cans and bottles to take home with you for recycling.

Be sure to extinguish all fires, whether in a grill or on the ground. Use plenty of water and stir the coals. Be sure all the embers have stopped smoldering before you leave. Place your hand above the ashes. If they still feel warm, add more water.

Q: How long can food be safely left out at a picnic?

A: The general guideline is to leave food at room temperature for no more than two hours. However, if temperatures are 90°F (32°C) or higher, food should not be left out for more than one hour.

Dining Out

When you want to socialize without going to a lot of trouble, dining out is an option for entertaining. However, eating in restaurants is not just for social occasions. With today's busy lifestyles, many people eat out often. Meal managers use eating out as an alternative to food preparation time.

The cost of eating out varies according to where you go and what you order. However, eating out almost always costs more than eating

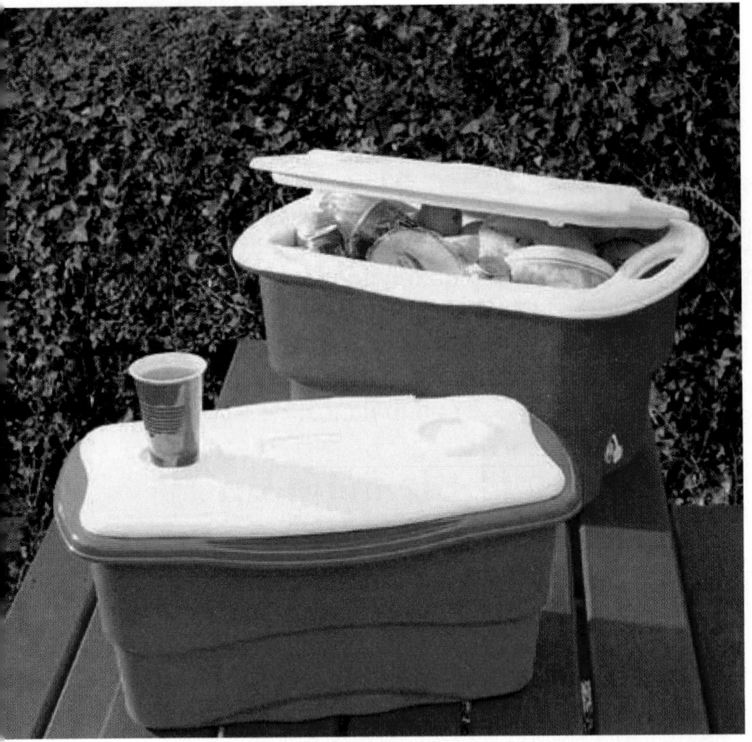

Rubbermaid

25-7 Having a separate cooler for drinks helps avoid the need to repeatedly open a cooler containing perishable foods.

at home, even when you consider the cost of labor. The cost difference may be small when you look at the price of a single meal. The difference increases when you figure the price of feeding a family.

Eating out requires time as well as money. You save shopping, preparation, and cleanup time. However, you tend to spend more time at the table when dining out. You must allow time to be seated, place your order, receive your food, eat, and pay your check.

Restaurant Basics

Regardless of the time and cost factors, dining out is an enjoyable experience. Following some basic guidelines will help you feel comfortable in any restaurant setting.

Being Seated

A ***reservation*** is a request for a restaurant to hold a table for a guest. Some small or formal restaurants require reservations. In busy restaurants, reservations can ensure you will get a table when you arrive. To make a reservation, call the restaurant and request a table for the number of people in your group. Give your name and state the day and time you would like the table.

In some casual restaurants, diners seat themselves. Most restaurants, however, have a host. The host will greet you at the door and ask how many people are in your group. If you have made a reservation, give the host your name. The host will often ask if you prefer sitting in the smoking or nonsmoking section. The host will then show you to a table when one is available.

Ordering from a Menu

As you are seated, you will receive a printed menu listing the food items that are available. Items will generally be grouped under headings, such *Appetizers, Salads, Entrees*, and *Desserts*. (***Entrees*** are main courses.) Being familiar with terms used on menus will help you know how foods are prepared. This will allow you to choose items that suit your tastes. See 25-8.

Pricing of menu items may be table d'hôte or a la carte. ***Table d'hôte*** pricing means there is one price for an entire meal. Usually, this price includes salad, bread, a main course, and

Menu Terms

a la. In the style of. For instance, *a la Suisse* means Swiss style.
a la Kiev. Containing butter, garlic, and chives.
a la king. Served with a cream sauce that contains mushrooms, green peppers, and pimientos.
a la mode. Served with ice cream.
almondine. Made or garnished with almonds.
au gratin. Served with cheese.
au jus. Served with natural juices.
du jour. Of the day. For instance, *soup du jour* means soup of the day.
en brochette. Broiled and served on a skewer.
en coquille. Served in a shell.
en croquette. Breaded and deep-fried.
en papillote. Cooked in parchment paper to seal in juices.
Florentine. Prepared with spinach.
lyonnaise. Sliced and sauteed with onion.
marengo. Sauteed with mushrooms, tomatoes, and olives.
picata. Prepared with lemon.
piquant. Highly seasoned.
Provençale. Prepared with garlic and olive oil.

25-8 Becoming familiar with these terms will help you when ordering from restaurant menus.

side dishes. It may also include an appetizer, soup, dessert, and beverage. ***A la carte*** pricing means there is a separate price for each menu item.

You will have a few minutes to decide what you want to eat. Then your waiter will come to your table and ask what you wish to order. If you would like an appetizer, order it first. Then tell the waiter what entree you would like. State your preferences for optional items, such as side dishes and salad dressings. On some menus, items are numbered. You can simply order the number of the meal or food item you want.

Restaurants generally serve food in courses. Your waiter will usually bring out beverages right after you place your order. If you have ordered appetizers, your waiter will serve them first. He or she will then serve soups and salads followed by entrees and side dishes. Your waiter will serve dessert last. You may order dessert with the rest of the meal or after you have finished eating your entree.

Dining in Public

When dining in public, you are a guest of the restaurants to which you go. Your behavior should be that of a well-mannered visitor. You should dress appropriately for the setting of the restaurant. Even in casual restaurants, it is important to look neat and clean and use good table manners. Follow the same guidelines you would use when eating in a friend's home.

Occasionally, you may have a problem with the food or service in a restaurant. Perhaps your food seems unwholesome or is not prepared as you ordered it. Maybe the service is slow or the waiter forgot part of your order. Whatever the problem is, quietly call it to your waiter's attention. Avoid making a scene and disturbing other diners. If the waiter is unwilling or unable to correct the problem, ask to speak to the manager.

Your satisfaction can affect the success of a restaurant. In most cases, restaurant staff members will do their best to make your dining experience a pleasant one.

Paying the Bill

At the end of your meal, the waiter will bring a bill showing how much money you owe. When dining with others, you should know in advance who is going to pay the bill. When someone invites a person to go out for a meal, the person extending the invitation generally pays. When a group of friends goes out to eat, they often go ***Dutch treat***. This means each person pays for his or her meal.

Sometimes it may be easiest to simply split the bill equally among everyone in the group. Other times, each person will pay just for the foods he or she ordered. If you intend to pay this way, ask the waiter when ordering if you can have separate checks. This will make it easy for each person to know how much he or she owes.

Sometimes the bill will be in a folder or on a plate or small tray. Place either cash or a credit card in the folder or on the plate or tray. The waiter will take the payment and bring you your change. (If you are paying with a credit card, your waiter will bring you a receipt to sign.) In casual restaurants, you may pay a cashier on the way out the door. See 25-9.

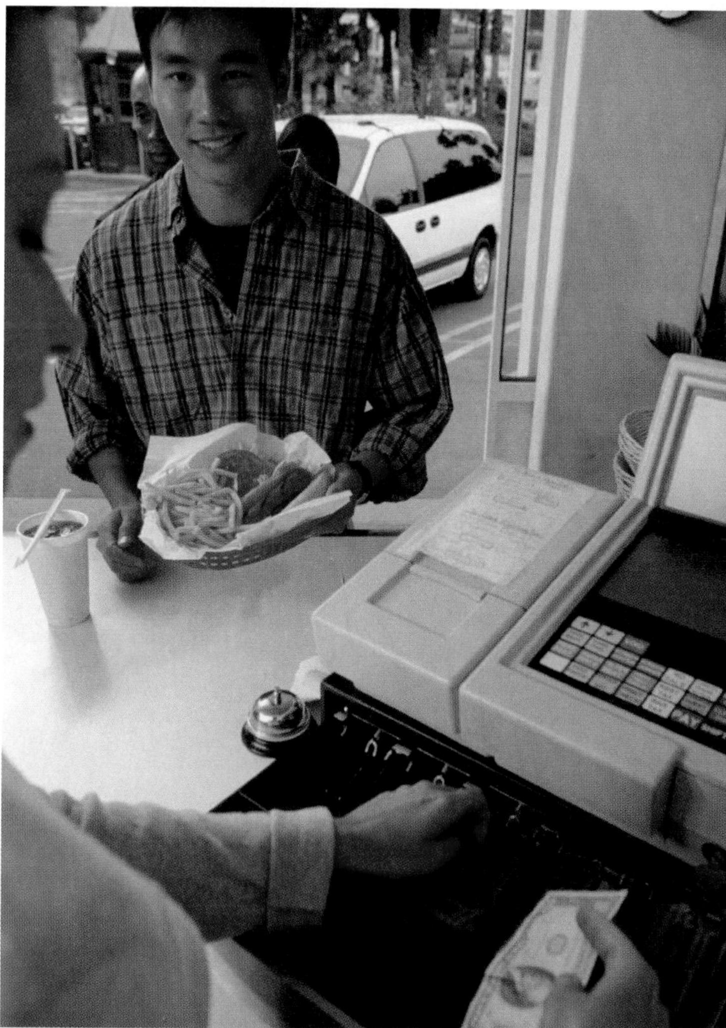

25-9 *At fast-food restaurants, you pay at the counter when you place your order.*

Whether you pay the waiter or a cashier, it is customary to leave a ***gratuity,*** or ***tip,*** for service received. Some restaurants automatically include a gratuity on the bill, especially for larger groups. If no gratuity is indicated, leave whatever you feel is proper. For average service, about 15 percent of the total bill is usually appropriate. If a waiter has given you special service, you may want to leave a larger tip.

If the waiter collects payment, you can leave the tip in the folder or on the plate or tray. If you pay the cashier, leave the tip inconspicuously on the table. If you pay with a credit card, you can write the amount of your tip on the receipt. Then add the cost of the meal and the tip. Write the total on the receipt before signing your name.

Good Manners Are Good Business

If you invite someone to a business lunch, that person considers you to be hosting the meal. This is especially true when you are asking the other person for his or her opinions or advice. When you are the host, the other person will expect you to pay the check.

If you are the guest at a business meal, show consideration for your host. He or she is not likely to have an unlimited expense account. Therefore, follow the lead of your host when ordering from the menu. If your host does not order the most expensive item on the menu, you shouldn't either.

Q: If I'm trying to watch my weight when eating out, isn't a salad a good choice?

A: The fresh vegetables used in many salads are low in fat and calories and high in fiber. However, dressings, meats, and cheeses added to salads can add a lot of fat and calories. To keep your salads light, order these items on the side. Use them to subtly flavor rather than cover your salad.

Types of Restaurants

The variety of restaurants is almost limitless. Restaurants offer all cuisines and a range of prices and formality.

Fast-Food Restaurants

Fast-food restaurants specialize in speedy service. They cater to people who are looking for quick, inexpensive meals.

Most fast-food restaurants have rather limited menus. The menu is usually posted above the counter near the restaurant entrance. All the foods on the menu can be prepared quickly. Many items are fried because frying allows foods to cook rapidly.

Food at fast-food restaurants is relatively inexpensive. The high sales volume and limited service help keep prices down. Because customers do not receive service from waiters, they do not have to leave tips in fast-food restaurants. This also saves customers money.

Cafeterias and Buffets

Cafeterias have a variety of prepared foods placed along a serving line. Customers carry a tray along the line and select the foods they want. Foods are served in individual portions and each item is priced separately. Customers pay for the items on their tray when they reach the end of the line.

Buffets are similar to cafeterias as far as the way the food is served. However, at buffets, customers generally pay a fixed price for the meal. They can serve themselves as much of each food on the buffet line as they like. They can also return to the serving line for more food as many times as they wish.

Neither cafeterias nor buffets have waiters to take customers' food orders at the table. However, servers may take beverage orders, refill coffee, and clear dirty dishes. For these services, leaving a tip of about 10 percent of the food bill is appropriate.

Family Restaurants

Family restaurants offer casual, comfortable dining. These restaurants appeal to people dining out with children. Prices are reasonable, so meals can fit into a family food budget. Family restaurants offer a variety of popular menu items. This allows each family member to order a different favorite food.

Formal Restaurants

Formal restaurants offer an elegant dining atmosphere, 25-10. Customers dine on fine foods and receive excellent service. In keeping with the atmosphere, guests in formal restaurants should dress formally.

Skilled chefs usually prepare the foods served at formal restaurants. They use only the freshest ingredients. Menus may list daily specials created by the chef.

The high-quality food and service at formal restaurants often cause them to be rather expensive. Some people also tend to tip a bit more in these restaurants than they would elsewhere. Be prepared for these expenses before you go to a formal restaurant.

Specialty Restaurants

Specialty restaurants focus on a specific type of food. Pizza parlors, steak houses, and ethnic restaurants are all specialty restaurants.

Specialty restaurants come in all price ranges. Some fast-food, family, and formal restaurants are also specialty restaurants.

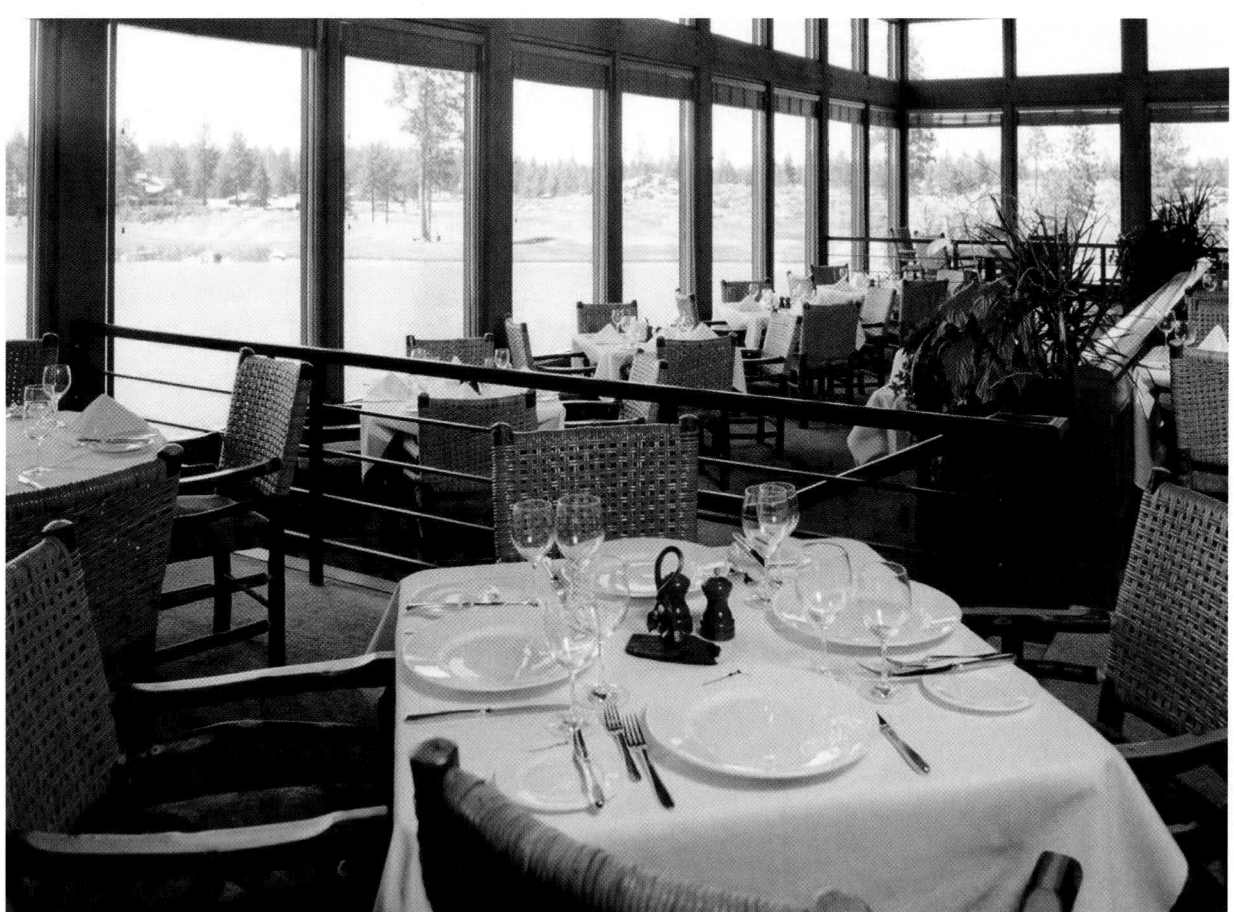

***25-10** Attractive surroundings help set the mood in a formal restaurant.*

Chapter 25 Review
Food and Entertaining

Summary

Planning a gathering begins with choosing a theme. Then you need to make up a guest list and extend invitations. You need to choose a menu and determine how you will serve it. As a host, you have the responsibility of making your guests feel comfortable in your home. In return, your guests have the responsibility of using their best manners and respecting your property.

Almost everyone enjoys picnics and barbecues when the weather is nice. No matter what type of outdoor entertaining you do, you need to transport and serve food carefully to keep it safe. You also need to be sure the outdoor area is clean when your party leaves.

Dining out can be an everyday experience or a special treat. Knowing how to make reservations, order, and tip in a restaurant will help you feel more comfortable when dining out. Your choice of restaurants includes fast-food, cafeteria, buffet, family, formal, and specialty establishments. You should be able to find a menu and a price range to suit any taste.

Review What You Have Read

Write your answers on a separate sheet of paper.

1. What information should be included on all invitations?
2. List four factors that should be considered when planning a party menu.
3. True or false. Appetizers containing sour cream, cheese, eggs, milk, and mayonnaise should be microwaved at lower settings.
4. What type of meal service is used most often in homes in the United States?
5. Give three responsibilities of a host.
6. List five examples of table manners.
7. List four important safety precautions you should follow when cooking outdoors.
8. True or false. Picnic foods should sit out so picnickers can enjoy them all afternoon.
9. On what type of restaurant menu are food items priced individually?
10. What would be an appropriate tip for average service on a restaurant bill totaling $13.35?
11. What terms might be used on a menu to describe foods prepared in the following ways?
    A. Garnished with almonds.
    B. Sauteed with mushrooms, tomatoes, and olives.
    C. Served with ice cream.
    D. Prepared with spinach.
12. What type of restaurant offers a variety of individually priced food items along a serving line?
    A. Buffet.
    B. Cafeteria.
    C. Family restaurant.
    D. Specialty restaurant.

Build Your Basic Skills

1. **Verbal.** Investigate where and when one of the styles of meal service developed. Share your findings in a brief oral report.
2. **Writing.** Investigate foodborne illnesses that can result from improperly handling food. Write a two-page report about how to safely transport and serve picnic and barbecue food in order to avoid illness.

Build Your Thinking Skills

1. **Plan.** Working in a small group plan a social gathering. Begin by choosing a theme. Then create an invitation and write a menu.
2. **Analyze.** Analyze menus from several restaurants ranging from casual to formal. Identify each menu as table d'hôte or a la carte. Find terms from Chart 25-8 used in the menus.

Apply Technology

1. Use a computer and card-making software to create party invitations. Use the computer's printer to print addresses on the envelopes or make address labels in an attractive font before sending the invitations.
2. Use the Yellow Pages to identify local carryout restaurants that accept food orders by fax machine.

Using Workplace Skills

Rashid is a formal waiter at Emerald Palms Restaurant. This elegant restaurant is known for its wonderful Caribbean cuisine and impeccable service. Each day, the chef plans a unique menu of exotically named dishes prepared with the freshest ingredients available. Like other waiters at Emerald Palms, Rashid is not permitted to write down patrons' food orders. If he gets an order wrong, however, he may be suspended from his job.

To be a successful employee, Rashid needs basic listening skills. Put yourself in Rashid's place and answer the following questions about your need for and use of these skills:

A. How will you use your listening skills as a formal waiter?

B. How might customers of the restaurant be affected if you do not have adequate listening skills?

C. How might other people who work at the restaurant be affected if you do not have adequate listening skills?

D. What is another skill you would need in this job? Briefly explain why this skill would be important.

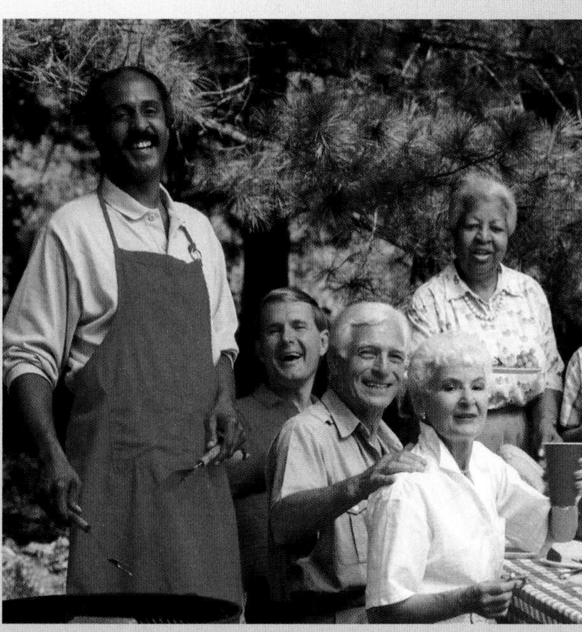

Chapter 26
Preserving Foods

Pickler
Pickles prepared food products in preservative or flavoring solutions.

Freezer Tunnel Operator
Tends freeze tunnel to quick-freeze food products.

Dehydrator Tender
Tends sulfur and drying chambers to bleach and dehydrate fruit.

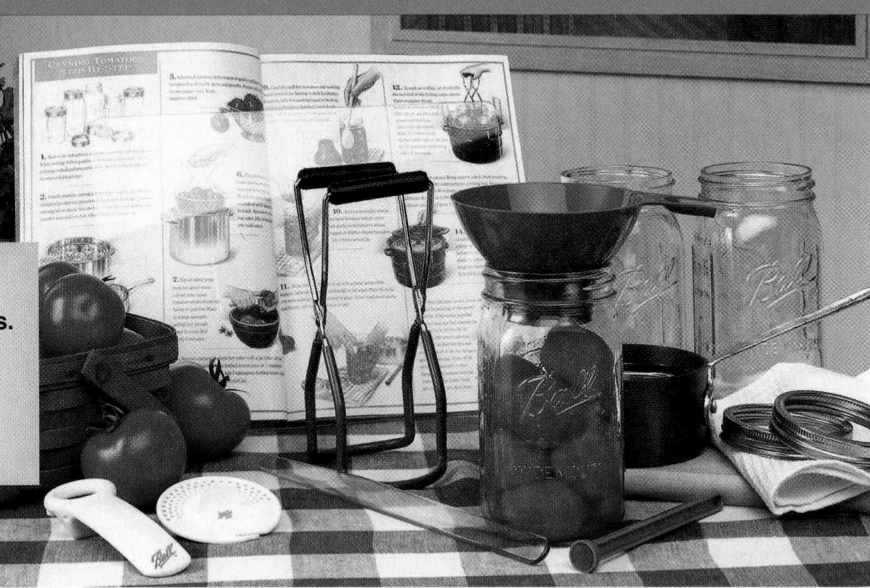

Alltrisia Consumer Products Company, marketers of Ball brand home canning products

Terms to Know

mold
yeast
enzyme
canning
raw pack
hot pack
headspace
processing time
botulism
pectin
quick-freezing
freezer burn
ascorbic acid
sulfuring
freeze-drying
aseptic packaging
retort packaging
irradiation
shelf life

Objectives

After studying this chapter, you will be able to

- ❑ generalize about factors that cause food spoilage.
- ❑ describe techniques for home canning and making jellied products.
- ❑ explain procedures for freezing and drying foods.
- ❑ identify methods of commercial food preservation.

Even primitive people realized food was perishable (subject to spoilage). They understood they needed some form of preservation to keep food from decaying. They learned to preserve food when it was bountiful for times of scarcity.

Today's homemakers can buy foods in all seasons, but many people still like to preserve food. This is especially true of people who have fruit and vegetable gardens. Three popular methods of food preservation are canning, freezing, and drying.

Food Spoilage

Bacteria, mold, and yeast are all microorganisms related to food preservation. Chapter 6 discussed how bacteria can cause foodborne illnesses. Bacteria can also cause chemical reactions in food, some of which lead to spoilage. ***Mold*** is a growth produced on damp or decaying organic matter or on living organisms. ***Yeast*** is a microscopic fungus that can cause fermentation in preserved foods, resulting in spoilage.

These microorganisms, along with enzymes, have both good and bad effects on food. (***Enzymes*** are complex proteins produced by living cells that cause specific chemical reactions.) Some bacteria are used to make buttermilk and sauerkraut. Certain molds are used in curing some cheeses such as Roquefort and Camembert. Yeast makes breads rise. Enzymes ripen foods and tenderize meats.

The bad effect of microorganisms is food spoilage. Enzymes can cause foods to deteriorate. They can soften the texture, change the color, and impair the flavor of foods. To preserve food, you must inactivate or destroy bacteria, mold, yeast, and enzymes.

Microorganisms need food, moisture, and favorable temperatures to grow. By removing one of these conditions, you can stop the spoiling action of microorganisms and preserve foods. Freezing temperatures prevent microorganisms from growing and retard the action of enzymes. High temperatures, as those used in canning, destroy both microorganisms and enzymes. Drying preserves food by removing moisture needed for the growth of microorganisms. To control enzyme activity, fruits and vegetables are treated before drying.

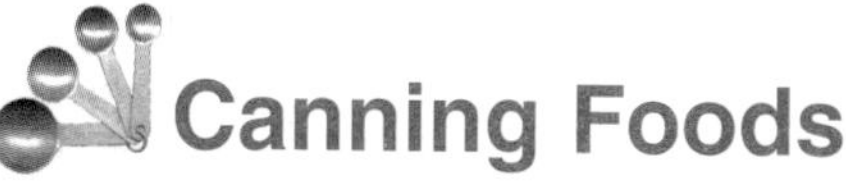

Canning Foods

Canning is a food preservation process that involves sealing food in airtight containers. The food is heated and held at a high temperature for a period long enough to kill harmful microorganisms. See 26-1.

People can foods at home for many reasons. Many home canners enjoy preserving their own special recipes of items like barbecue or spaghetti sauces. Some people can to avoid wasting an overabundance of seasonal fruits and vegetables. Others want to avoid the preservatives added to commercially canned foods.

Still another reason for home canning is the low cost. Home canning can reduce food costs if you do it frequently. The equipment is expensive, so buy it only if you plan to can for several years. You can save more money if you grow the food yourself.

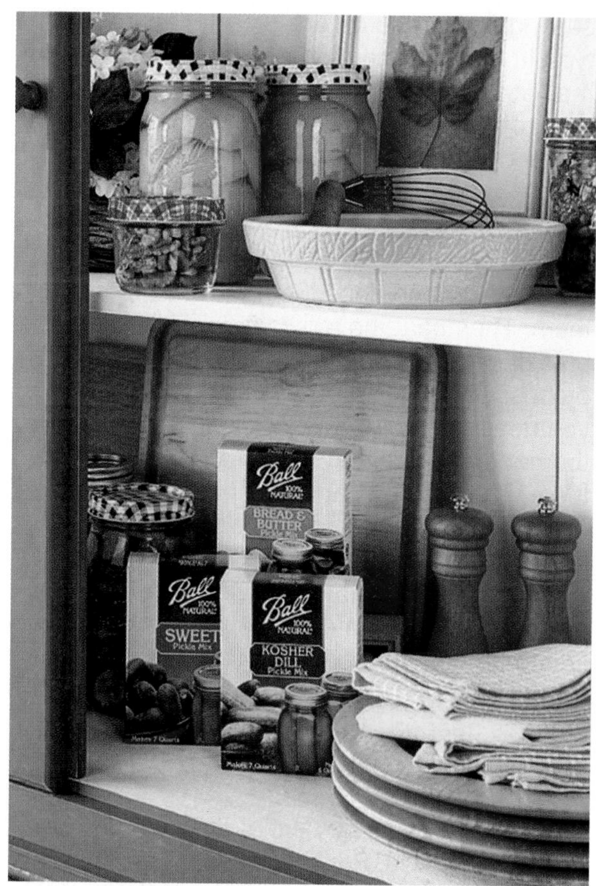

Alltrista Consumer Products Company, marketers of Ball brand home canning products

26-1 *Properly sealed home-canned foods can be safely stored for up to a year.*

You must follow canning procedures carefully to ensure proper preservation of food. You can obtain step-by-step directions on home canning from manufacturers of canning products and county extension agents.

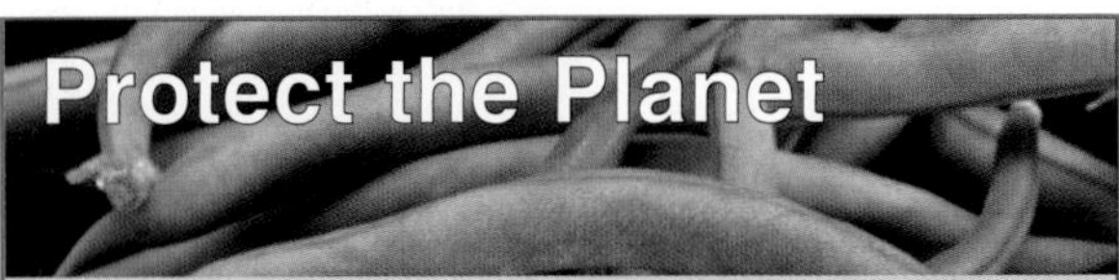

You should use a flat metal lid with sealing compound only once. However, you can reuse canning jars and screw bands as long as they are in good condition. Be sure all jars are perfect. Discard jars that have cracks or chips, as these defects prevent airtight seals. Discard metal bands that are dented or rusty.

Canning Jars and Closures

Most foods that are canned at home are put into *glass* jars. Use only jars especially made for home canning. Do not use jars from commercially canned foods, such as peanut butter or mayonnaise. These will not seal tightly.

The most popular canning jar closures are two-piece vacuum caps. The pieces are a metal screw band and a flat metal lid that has a sealing compound on one side. When using this type of closure, wipe the rim of the filled jar. Put the flat lid on the jar with the sealing compound next to the glass. Then screw the band down tightly over the lid.

Preparing Jars and Closures

You should wash all canning jars in hot, soapy water and rinse them well before using them. Then heat the jars to help keep them from breaking. When canning foods that are processed less than 10 minutes, such as jellies, you need to sterilize the jars. Leave the jars in the hot environment until you are ready to use them. Then remove and fill them one at a time.

Like the jars, you need to wash the lids and screw bands before using them. After washing in hot, soapy water, dry the screw bands and set them aside. Allow the flat metal lids to heat in very hot, but not boiling, water for at least 10 minutes. Remove them one at a time, as needed.

Filling Canning Jars

You may fill jars by either the raw pack or hot pack method. For ***raw pack,*** pack raw fruits or vegetables into containers. Cover with boiling water, juice, or syrup. For ***hot pack,*** heat food in water, steam, syrup, or juices. Pack loosely in jars and cover with cooking liquid or boiling water.

When you fill the jars, leave some headspace. ***Headspace*** is space between the food and the closure of a food storage container. Follow your canning recipe to determine the correct amount of headspace. Leaving too much or too little headspace may prevent jars from sealing properly. See 26-2.

Liquid in the canning jars should fill all spaces between food and cover all the food. Food that is not covered tends to darken. Remove air bubbles trapped in the food with a nonmetal spatula to prevent food from darkening.

Pressure Canning

The high temperatures used in canning destroy microorganisms and enzymes. The temperatures obtained vary with the canning method. Since some microorganisms are more heat-resistant than others, the canning method used depends on the type of food being canned.

Use *pressure canning* for green beans and other low-acid vegetables. Use it for meats, poultry, and fish, too. These foods need a higher temperature than that of boiling water to destroy food-spoiling microorganisms and enzymes.

You do this type of canning in a *pressure canner*. This type of canner can reach 240°F to 250°F (115°C to 120°C) by building up steam under pressure. Pack low-acid foods into

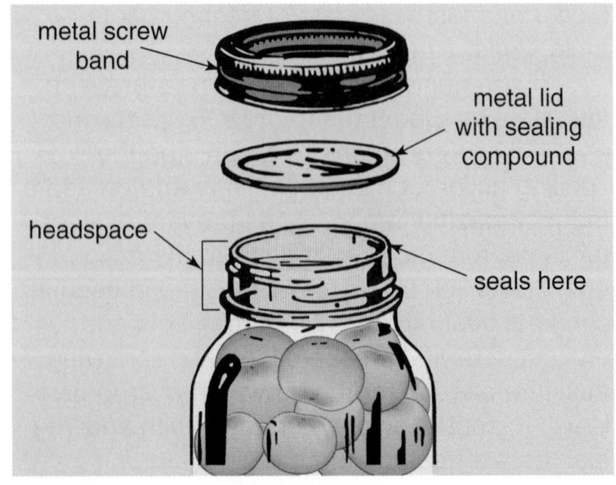

26-2 *The amount of headspace left between food and the two-piece vacuum cap sealing a canning jar depends on the food being canned.*

sterilized canning jars. Cover the food with liquid, and cap the jars. Put water in the bottom of the canner, and place the filled jars in the canner on a rack. Lock down the lid of the pressure canner to make the canner steam-tight. After sealing the canner, place it on the range.

A vent in the lid, called a *petcock,* allows air to be exhausted and steam to be released as needed. When the petcock is closed, the temperature and pressure inside the canner rise. A *pressure gauge* measures steam pressure inside the canner. A *safety valve* in the lid prevents explosions. It works only if pressure or temperature inside the canner becomes dangerously high. See 26-3.

Processing Time

When the proper pressure has been reached inside the canner, processing time begins. ***Processing time*** is the amount of time canned goods remain under heat (or under heat and pressure) in a canner. Processing time varies according to the food being processed.

When processing time is complete, remove the canner from the heat and allow pressure to return to zero. Lift the cover of the canner away from your body to prevent steam burns. Then remove the jars from the canner and allow them to cool.

Boiling Water Canning

Use boiling water canning for high-acid foods, such as acidified tomatoes, fruits, and pickled vegetables. You do this method of canning in a *boiling water canner.* The temperature of boiling water is enough to destroy the microorganisms and enzymes that cause food spoilage in these foods.

For this method of canning, pack food into clean canning jars, cover it with liquid, and cap the jars. For raw-pack jars, heat water in the canner until it is hot. For hot-pack jars, heat the water to boiling. Set the filled jars on the rack in the canner so water surrounds each one. Add boiling water to bring the water level above the tops of the jars. Cover the canner and allow the water to come to a rolling boil.

When the water comes to a rolling boil, the processing time begins. As with pressure canning, processing time varies with the type of food being canned. The water boils steadily throughout the processing time. When processing time is up, quickly remove the jars from the canner and allow them to cool.

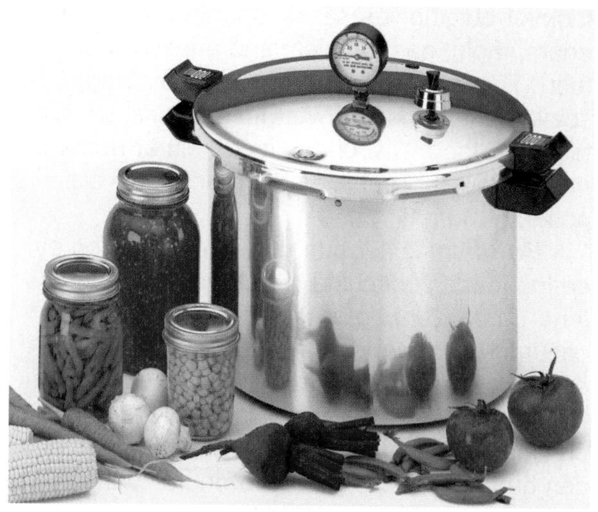

photo courtesy of National Presto Industries, Inc.

26-3 *The buildup of pressure in a pressure canner allows canned foods to be processed at temperatures above the boiling point.*

After Canning

Test the seals the day after canning. To do this, press the center of each lid. Make sure it is concave and does not flex up and down. Then remove the screw band and make sure you cannot lift the lid off with your fingertips. If the jars pass this inspection, they have formed a good vacuum seal.

If you find a leaky jar, use the food right away. You could also can the food again, treating it as if it were fresh. Check jars and lids carefully for defects before using them again.

When jars are completely cool, carefully remove screw bands. Wash bands and store them in a dry place for future use.

Wipe jars clean with a soapy cloth, rinse them well, and dry them thoroughly. Label each jar, listing the type of food and the date. If you canned more than one lot on the same day, list the lot number, too.

Properly canned foods stored in a cool, dry, dark place will last as long as a year. A cool temperature helps foods maintain appearance, flavor, and nutrients. Do not allow canned foods to freeze, as this will cause a loss of texture and appeal. Dampness may corrode metal lids and cause leakage. This makes the foods spoil. Heat and light may cause food to lose some of its eating quality after only a few weeks.

Checking for Spoilage

Before eating home-canned foods, take certain safety precautions. When you open jars, look for bulging lids, leaks, spurting liquid, off odors, mold, gas bubbles, and unusually soft food. These are signs of broken seals and spoilage. If you see any of these signs, do *not* taste the food. Dispose of it so neither humans nor animals will eat it. Use a food waste disposer, or burn it.

Botulism is a foodborne illness caused by eating foods containing the spore-forming bacteria *Clostridium botulinum*. These bacteria can occur in home-canned foods that were improperly processed. Botulism is the most dangerous type of foodborne illness. Even a taste of food containing the toxin produced by these bacteria can be fatal. This is why following only the latest, researched recommendations for canning methods and processing times is so important. Using proper canning methods is especially important for low-acid foods.

The texture of foods spoiled by botulism may be very soft and mushy. The foods may smell like rancid cheese. However, some spoiled foods look and smell normal. If you have any question about the safety of a home-canned food, you should not take any chances. Boil the food for 10 to 15 minutes in an uncovered saucepan before eating it. This will destroy any toxins and microorganisms. If the food looks spoiled, foams, or has an off odor during heating, *destroy it!*

Q: If I'm watching calories, would all-fruit spread be a better choice than jam on my toast?

A: Check Nutrition Facts panels to compare calories per serving. Some all-fruit spreads replace sugar with fruit juice concentrates that provide about the same number of calories.

Making Jellied Products

Canning principles are used in making jellied products, 26-4. Jellied products include jelly, jam, marmalade, preserves, and conserves. *Jelly* is a firm, clear product made from fruit juice. *Jam* is a less firm product made from crushed fruit that is cooked to a fairly even consistency. *Marmalade* is a tender jelly containing small pieces of fruit and fruit rind. It is often made from citrus fruit and it may contain a mixture of fruits. *Preserves* are slightly jellied products that contain whole fruits or large pieces of fruit in thick syrup. *Conserves* are jams made from a mixture of fruits, usually including citrus fruits and sometimes raisins and nuts. *Fruit butters* are not jellied products. They are spreads made from cooked, pureed fruit.

Ingredients

You need four basic ingredients to make good jellied products. The first of these is fruit. Fruit gives jellied products their flavors and colors. You can use almost any flavorful fruit. Fruit also contributes some or all of two other basic ingredients—pectin and acid.

Pectin is a carbohydrate found in all fruits. It makes fruit juices jell. Some fruits have more pectin than others. If the fruit you are using is low in pectin, you can buy pectin in powdered or liquid form. You can use either kind with any fruit. However, they are not interchangeable. Follow your recipe. Use the form and amount of pectin it suggests.

Acid is the third basic ingredient in jellied products. It works with pectin to make the products jell. It also adds flavor. All fruits contain varying amounts of acids. You can add lemon juice or citric acid to fruits that are low in acid.

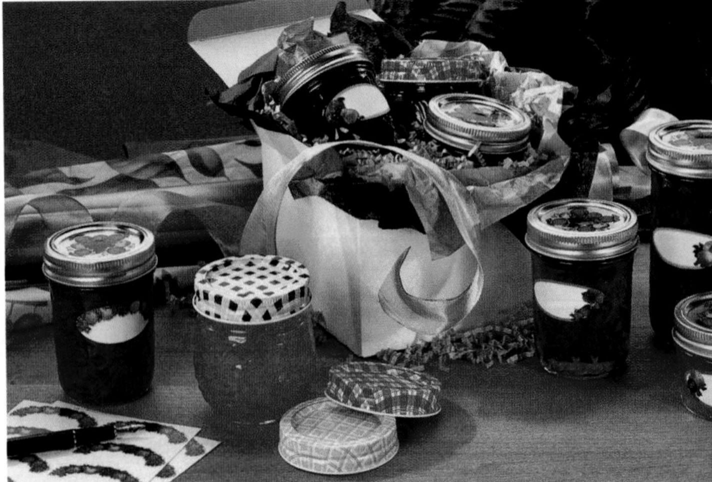

Alltrista Consumer Products Company, marketers of Ball brand home canning products

***26-4** The flavors of fresh fruits can be captured and enjoyed for months in home-canned jellied products.*

Sugar is the fourth basic ingredient. It helps jellied products become firm. It also adds flavor and helps preserve the products. Leaving some of the sugar out of a recipe will cause the jellied product to be runny. However, recipes are available for making jellied products with artificial sweeteners for people who want to avoid sugar.

Good Manners Are Good Business

Homemade jam or preserves would be a special treat to offer your guests when hosting a business meal. However, you should not put the canning jar on your table. Instead, put the jellied product into a small dish with a spoon. If you wish to enjoy some of the jellied product on your food, spoon some onto your bread plate. Then use your knife to spread it on your food.

Processing Jellied Products

You must process jellied products by the boiling water method. After you combine and boil the ingredients, pour the mixtures into hot, sterilized canning jars. Then seal and process the jars. After cooling, label the products and store them in a dark, dry, cool place.

Uncooked jam is a jellied product that is easy to make and does not require boiling water processing. You can prepare it by adding sugar and commercial pectin to crushed, fully-ripe fruit. Uncooked jams keep up to three weeks in the refrigerator or up to a year in the freezer. However, they spoil quickly at room temperature.

Freezing Foods

One of the best ways to preserve the fresh flavor of food is to freeze it. Frozen foods are popular because they offer consumers many advantages. Frozen foods have the appearance, taste, and nutritive value of fresh foods. They are available at any time of year, and they are easy to prepare. Frozen foods can also help you save money. You can buy them when prices are low and store them for later use. See 26-5.

Many frozen foods that you buy at the grocery store are preserved by ***quick-freezing.*** Quick-frozen foods are subjected to temperatures between -25°F and -40°F (-32°C and -40°C) for a short time. These extremely low temperatures produce very small ice crystals in foods. When foods are frozen more slowly, larger ice crystals may form. These large crystals damage the cell structure of foods and change their textures. After quick-freezing, foods are maintained at a normal freezing temperature of 0°F (-18°C).

Foods frozen at home have the same advantages as commercially frozen foods. Using the right equipment and following recommended procedures will ensure the highest quality in home-frozen foods.

Equipment

You need to have a properly operating freezer and suitable containers to freeze foods at home. Chapter 9 described the styles and features of home freezers you might consider.

Containers used in freezing must be moisture- and vapor-resistant. This protects foods from exposure to air and loss of moisture during frozen storage. Foods that you have not wrapped securely may develop off flavors and lose nutrients, texture, and color. Some foods may develop ***freezer burn,*** or dry, tough areas. Freezer burn occurs where dry air from the freezer has come in contact with food surfaces, causing dehydration.

Properly sealed aluminum, glass, plastic-coated paper, and plastic containers are all suitable for freezer storage. You can also use aluminum foil and plastic-coated or transparent

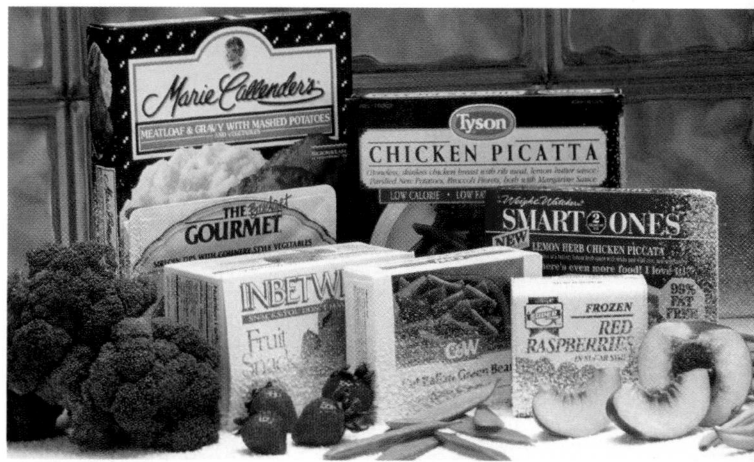

Agricultural Research Service, USDA

26-5 *Frozen foods retain much of the flavor and nutrition of fresh foods.*

freezer wraps. These flat packaging materials work especially well when freezing bulky items, such as roasts and cakes.

Freezing Fruits and Vegetables

When selecting fresh produce for freezing, choose ripe, top-quality fruits and young, tender vegetables. Work with small batches. Carefully sort and wash each piece but do not allow them to soak. Pit, trim, and slice fruits and vegetables as desired.

Preparing Fruits and Vegetables for Freezing

Some fruits need treatment with ascorbic acid to prevent darkening. ***Ascorbic acid*** is a food additive that prevents color and flavor loss. It also adds nutritive value. (Ascorbic acid is another name for vitamin C.) Ascorbic acid is available in crystalline form or in a mixture with sugar and perhaps citric acid. Follow manufacturer's instructions for use.

You must blanch most vegetables in boiling water or steam before freezing. This inactivates the enzymes. When blanching is complete, cool vegetables quickly and drain well. Quick cooling prevents vitamin loss and spoilage.

Packing Fruits and Vegetables for Freezing

Pack most vegetables and some fruits using the *dry pack* method. Carefully pour prepared produce into freezer containers. Gently tap containers to pack food closely without crushing. Do not add liquid.

Frozen sweetened fruits, usually have a better texture than unsweetened fruits. Therefore, you may wish to use the sugar pack or syrup pack method when freezing fruits. For the *sugar pack* method, place prepared fruit in a shallow pan. Add sugar. Turn pieces of fruit gently until the sugar dissolves and forms a syrup. Carefully pack fruit into freezer containers. Gently tap each container to exclude air. For the *syrup pack* method, prepare syrup and chill. Place prepared fruit directly into container. Pour chilled syrup over fruit.

For all packing methods, leave 1 inch (2.5 cm) headspace to allow for expansion. Wipe top of container with a clean, damp cloth. Seal tightly and label with the name of the food and the date. See 26-6.

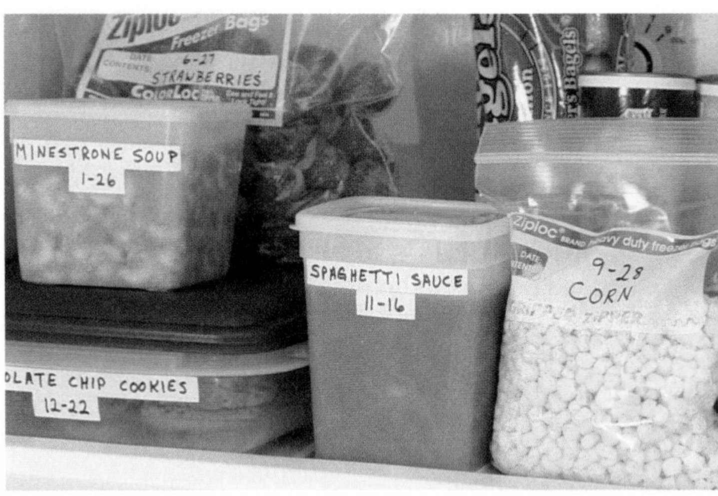

Jack Klasey

26-6 *Label foods clearly for freezer storage.*

Freeze all foods at 0°F (-18°C) or lower immediately after packing. When food freezes too slowly, a loss in quality or food spoilage may occur. Freeze food in batches, giving each batch a chance to freeze before adding the next batch. This will keep freezer temperature constant. Leave a little space between items in the freezer to allow room for cold air to circulate. Follow your freezer manufacturer's instructions concerning quantity and placement of foods.

Freezing Meat, Poultry, and Fish

Meats require no special preparation before freezing. You may, however, wish to trim large cuts and package them in serving-sized pieces. Choose only top quality meat cuts for freezing.

Examine poultry for hairs and feathers. Wash and dry thoroughly. You may freeze poultry whole or in pieces.

Purchased fish also require washing and drying before freezing. You must scale and eviscerate (remove entrails) game fish before freezing. You should also remove their heads and fins.

Do not freeze meat, poultry, or fish in their original wrappers. Rewrap them in moisture-proof and vaporproof paper, excluding as much air as possible. Seal and label with product name, weight, and date.

Freeze meat, poultry, and fish as soon as possible after purchasing them. Turn the freezer control to its lowest possible setting for the first 24 to 48 hours. Then maintain the temperature at 0°F (-18°C) as for fruits and vegetables.

Q: Is it safe to refreeze meat once it has thawed?

A: If meat is partially thawed but still firm, you can refreeze it. The meat will suffer a loss in quality, but it will still be safe to eat. Refreeze it and use it as soon as possible. If the meat is fully thawed but still very cold, refrigerate it and use it immediately. Do not refreeze.

Freezing Prepared Foods

Baked pastry, cookies, breads, and cakes all freeze well. Wrap these items carefully in moistureproof and vaporproof wrapping.

You can freeze casseroles and stews in their baking dishes. To save space, line the baking dish with foil. Fill the dish with food, wrap well, and freeze. When frozen, remove the food from the dish. Wrap it well, label it, and return it to the freezer. You can then use the casserole dish for other foods.

Be sure to label all prepared foods with the name of the product and the date. Freeze promptly and use within the recommended time.

Some foods do not freeze well. These include salad greens, custards, gelatin products, meringues, sour cream, and hard-cooked egg whites. Sandwiches containing salad dressing or mayonnaise do not freeze well, either.

You can store some foods longer than others. Beef, cheese, whole turkeys, and vegetables, for example, can be stored for a year. You can store cookies and soups for six months and unbaked pies for three months.

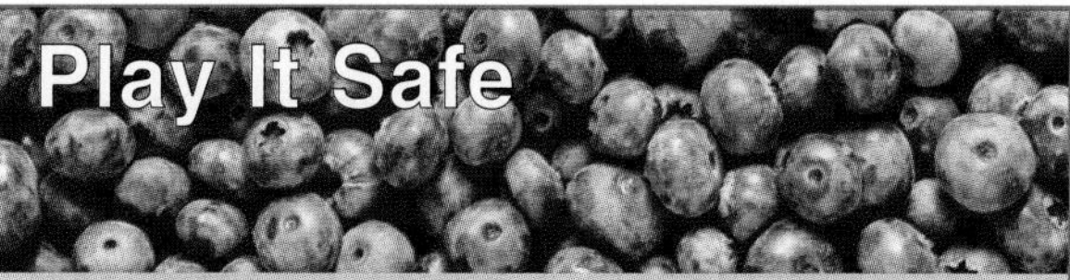

Organisms that cause foodborne illnesses multiply quickly at room temperature. Therefore you should never thaw foods, especially meat, poultry, and fish, at room temperature. Allow them to thaw overnight in a refrigerator. Use the defrost setting on a microwave oven to thaw foods quickly right before cooking. You can also allow them to thaw during the cooking process.

Thawing Frozen Foods

You should cook some frozen foods, such as vegetables, without thawing. Thaw prepared and baked products in their original wrappers to prevent dehydration. Thaw fruits in their original covered containers to prevent *enzymatic browning* (discoloration caused by exposure to air). Fruits have the best flavor if served with a few ice crystals remaining.

You can cook meats, poultry, and fish either frozen or thawed. Cooking frozen food, however, takes longer than cooking fresh or thawed foods. You must consider the extra cooking time when planning meals.

Drying Foods

Food drying is one of the oldest and simplest methods of food preservation. Microorganisms that cause food spoilage need moisture to grow. Drying removes moisture, thus stopping the growth of microorganisms. When drying foods, speed is important. Using a temperature that will dry food without cooking it is important, too.

The many advantages of dried foods make them especially popular with campers, cyclists, and backpackers. Dried foods are lightweight. They take up less space than fresh foods, and they taste good. See 26-7.

Campers are not the only ones who use dried foods. In the home, many people add dried vegetables to soups. A variety of dried mixes are popular convenience products. People enjoy jerky and dried meat sticks as snacks. You can add dried fruits to salads, desserts, and a variety of other foods.

Fruit leathers are pliable sheets of dried fruit puree. You can make them from almost any fruit. Fruit leathers are nutritious and lightweight for packing in school lunches or taking on camping trips.

Preparing Fruits and Vegetables for Drying

You must dry vegetables completely to prevent spoilage. Fruits, because of their high sugar content, may retain more moisture than vegetables.

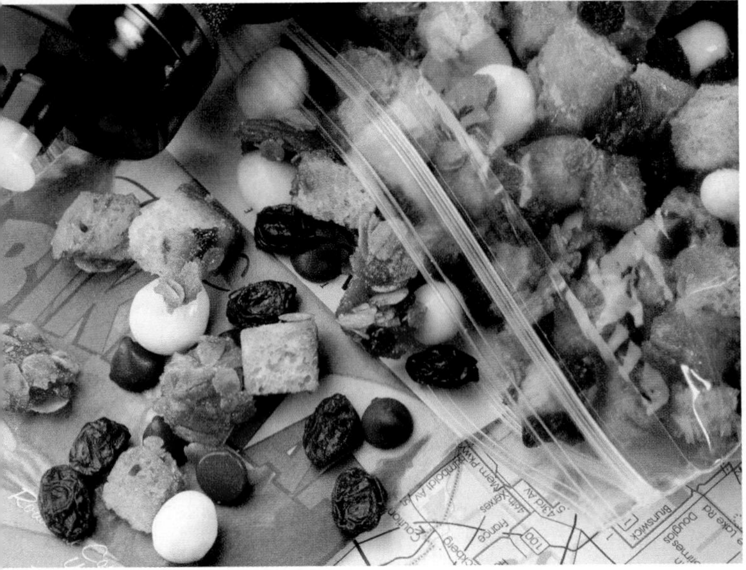

California Raisin Marketing Board

26-7 Snack mixes made with dried fruits such as raisins are well-liked by cyclists because they are lightweight and packed with energy.

Choose fruits at optimum maturity. Wash, sort, and discard bruised, overripe fruit. Peel and core fruits, if necessary. You can dry berries and other smaller fruits whole. Larger fruits will dry more evenly and quickly if cut into halves, quarters, or 1/4-inch (6 mm) slices.

You can also use a salt solution to keep fruit from darkening. You can also use ***sulfuring*** as an antidarkening treatment for some fruits. Prepare a sulfuring solution using sodium metabisulfite purchased from a drugstore. Soak fruits for 15 minutes. Drain. Spread fruit to dry.

Select young, tender vegetables in prime condition. Wash vegetables thoroughly and drain. Trim and cut them into small pieces. Smaller pieces dry more quickly and evenly. Blanch prepared vegetables using steam or boiling water. Drain well and dry with a towel.

Procedure for Drying

Two popular methods of drying fruits and vegetables at home are sun drying and oven drying. Sun drying is less costly, but it relies on the weather.

Drying in the oven does not depend on the weather, so you can do it at any time. You can do oven drying in a food dehydrator following manufacturer's instructions, 26-8. You can also do oven drying in a conventional oven.

To dry food in a conventional oven, spread food evenly in a single layer on trays. Make trays of wire screening tacked to a wooden frame or stretch and secure cheesecloth around oven racks. Preheat oven to 150°F (64°C) or as low as the oven thermostat will allow. Place lower oven rack about 3 inches (7.5 cm) from oven bottom. Stack trays evenly.

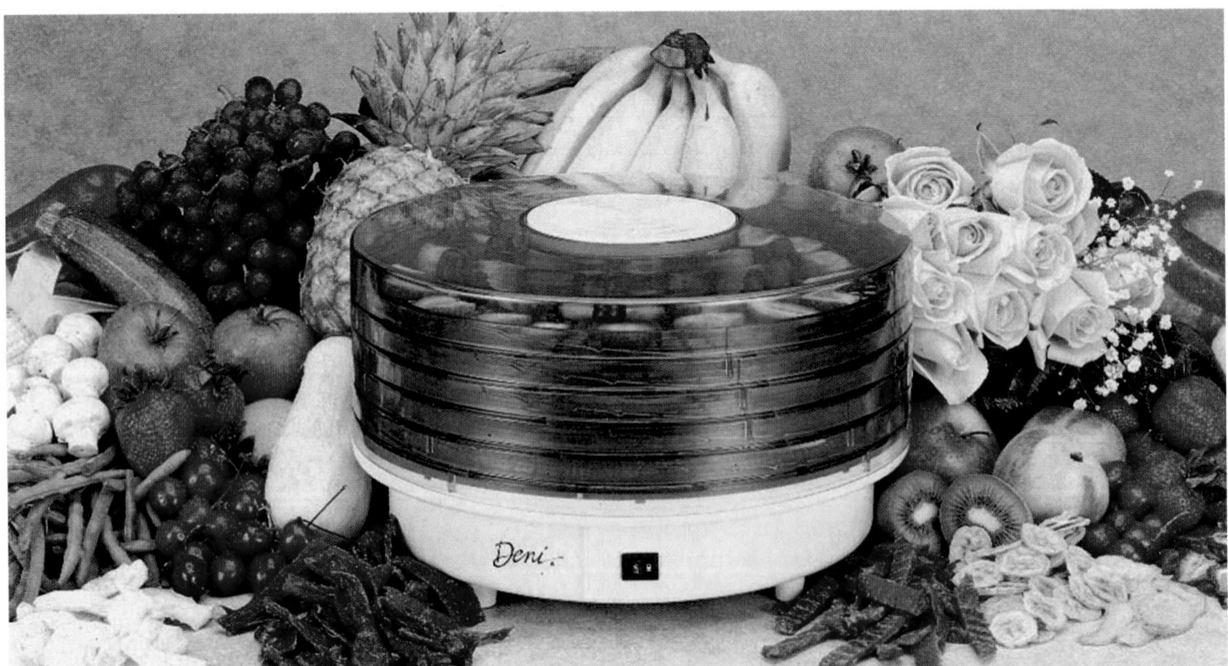

Deni/Keystone Manufacturing Company, Inc.

***26-8** A food dehydrator maintains the proper temperature for drying foods. It allows air to circulate around several trays so a number of foods can be dried at once.*

Rotate trays periodically because food on trays near the bottom of the oven will dry more quickly. Occasional stirring ensures even drying.

Drying time depends on the food being dried. When dry, vegetables will feel hard and brittle. Fruits will feel leathery but pliable. Cool thoroughly.

Storing and Using Dried Foods

Package dried foods in insectproof and moistureproof containers. Plastic containers, glass jars, and waxed cartons are all suitable. Seal, label, and store them in a cool, dark place.

You may eat dried fruits in their dry state, or you can rehydrate them. You will rehydrate most dried vegetables. To rehydrate, soak foods for an hour or two. Simmer in the same liquid used for soaking until foods are tender. Do not overcook.

Commercial Food Preservation

Of course, canning, freezing, and drying are not just home preservation methods. They are common commercial food preservation methods as well. Technical advances in food processing have improved the quality of preserved foods in recent years. Commercially preserved foods keep more nutrients than foods preserved at home. Commercial processing is done quickly and very soon after foods are harvested. This allows preserved foods to have nutritional values that are close to fresh foods.

The principles used in commercial food preservation are the same as those used at home. Moisture and temperature conditions are controlled to stop the spoiling action of microorganisms and enzymes.

Freeze-Drying

Food manufacturers preserve foods in a number of ways besides canning, freezing, and drying. One of these ways is freeze-drying. ***Freeze-drying*** involves the removal of water vapor from frozen foods. This process produces high-quality food products. It also saves transportation and refrigeration costs. Freeze-drying is used to preserve a variety of foods, including instant coffee.

Aseptic Packaging

With ***aseptic packaging,*** a food and its packaging material are sterilized separately. Then the food is packed in the container in a sterile chamber. Aseptic packaging allows you to store some perishable foods without refrigeration. Foil-lined paper boxes used for milk products and juices are examples of aseptic packaging, 26-9.

Retort Packaging

Retort packaging is similar to aseptic packaging. In ***retort packaging,*** food is sealed in a foil pouch. Then it is sterilized in a steam-pressure vessel known as a retort. This type of packaging is often used for shelf-stable entrees.

The advantages of aseptic and retort packaging include improved flavor and nutrition. The packages use minimal storage space and require no refrigeration. You can easily prepare the foods inside these packages in minutes.

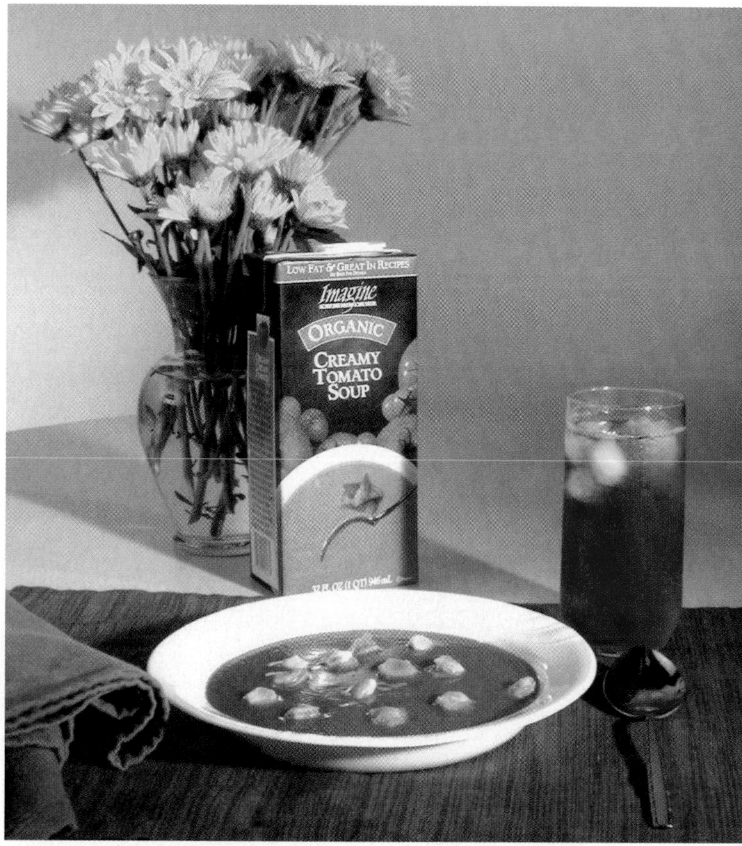

Jack Klasey

26-9 *Aseptic packaging allows perishable foods to be stored for months without refrigeration.*

Q: Doesn't irradiation destroy the nutrients in food products?

A: Irradiation causes very little nutrient loss in foods. Irradiated foods have nutrient values that are close to fresh foods.

Irradiation

Irradiation exposes food to controlled doses of gamma rays, electron beams, or X rays. Irradiation can limit sprouting in potatoes. It can slow the ripening of fruits and vegetables. It can control insects and microorganisms in seasonings and wheat. It can also control disease-causing trichinae in pork and salmonella in chicken. The FDA has approved all of these uses of irradiation. Even so, irradiation has not caught on as a trend in the food industry. Currently, irradiation in the United States is mainly being used to preserve spices, 26-10. Use of irradiation may increase in the future if it becomes more economical for food processors. It must also gain a wider degree of acceptance among consumers.

Irradiated food products are labeled with the statement "treated with radiation" or "treated by irradiation." A special logo also appears on the label of irradiated foods.

Preservation techniques increase a food's ***shelf life.*** This is the amount of time a food can be stored and remain wholesome. However, you cannot keep preserved foods forever. Table 26-11 shows how long you can store various foods in a refrigerator, freezer, or pantry.

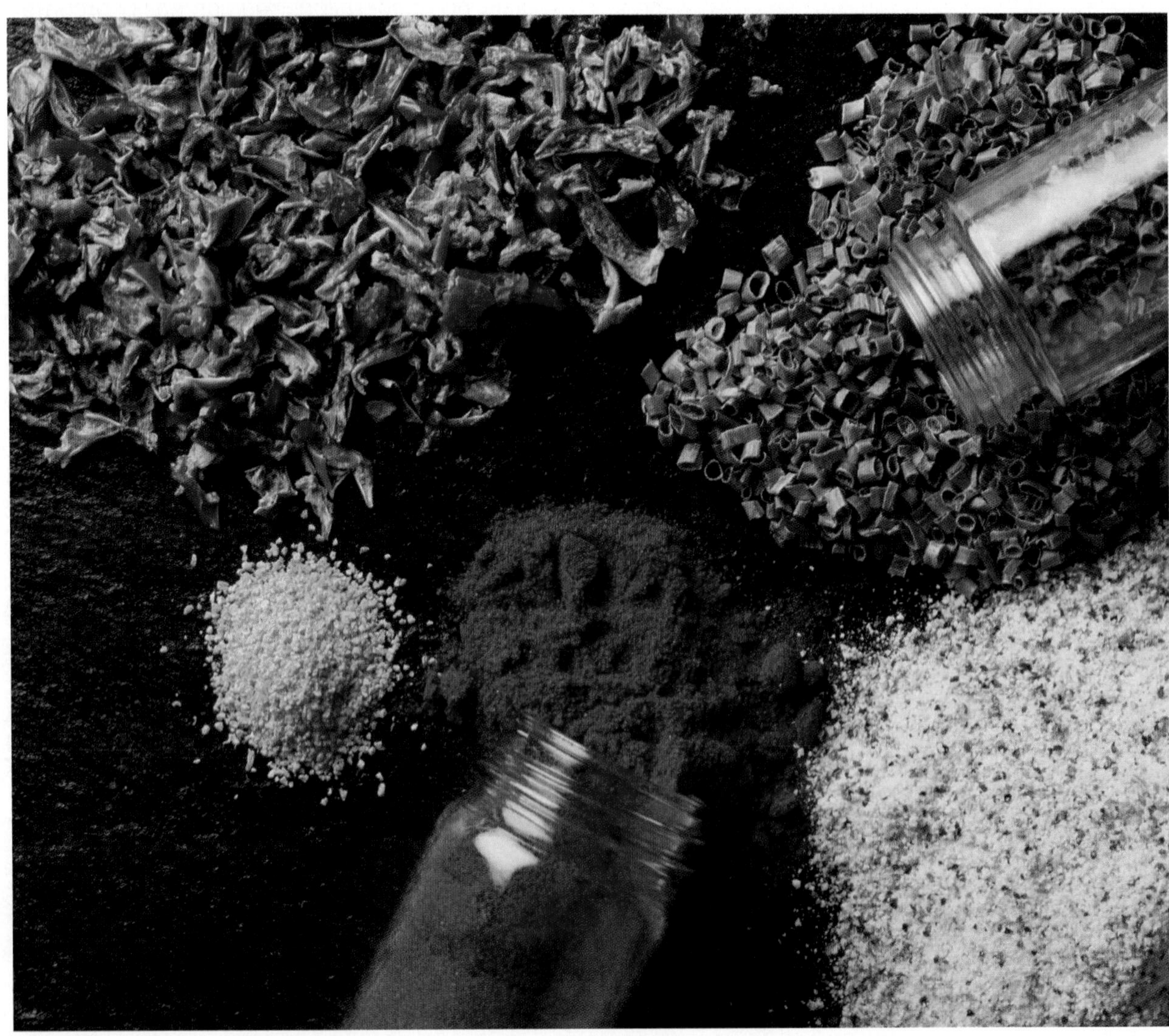

26-10 *Spices are the most commonly irradiated food product.*

Shelf Life of Foods	
Foods Stored in a Refrigerator	
beef, pork, lamb	2 to 4 days
poultry, fish	1 to 2 days
bacon, ham	5 to 7 days
milk	1 week
butter	2 weeks
natural, process cheeses	4 to 8 weeks
fruits and vegetables	varies according to type
Foods Stored in a Freezer	
beef	6 to 12 months
pork	3 to 6 months
lamb	6 to 9 months
ground beef, pork, lamb	3 months
ham, hot dogs	2 months
poultry	6 to 8 months
fish	3 to 4 months
fruits and vegetables	9 to 12 months
bread	2 to 3 months
ice cream	2 months
Foods Stored at Room Temperature	
dried fruits and vegetables	1 year
staple items (cereal, flour, sugar)	1 year
home-canned foods	1 year
onions and potatoes	4 weeks
commercially packaged foods in unopened cans and jars	1 year
aseptically packaged products (milk products, juices, soups)	6 months
freeze-dried foods	1 year
shelf-stable entrees	6 months

26-11 *Even preserved foods have a limited storage life.*

Chapter 26 Review
Preserving Foods

Summary

Enzymes and microorganisms cause food spoilage. Food, moisture, and favorable temperatures need to be present for spoilage to occur. Removing any one of these items will help preserve food.

Canning uses high temperatures to preserve foods. Home-canned foods are stored in jars with two-piece vacuum caps used as closures. You need to process low-acid foods in a pressure canner. You can process high-acid foods in a boiling water bath. After canning, you need to check the lids on canning jars to be sure they have formed good seals. Label canned foods clearly and store them in a cool, dry, dark place. Always check for signs of spoilage before using home-canned foods.

Jellied products are popular home-canned foods. The four basic ingredients in jellied products are fruit, pectin, acid, and sugar. Besides jelly, you can make marmalade, jams, preserves, conserves, and fruit butters.

Freezing uses low temperatures to preserve foods. A freezer and food storage containers are all you need to keep foods on hand for months. Some fruits need an antidarkening treatment before freezing. Most vegetables need blanching before freezing. You must thaw some frozen foods before preparing them. You can cook others in their frozen state.

Drying removes moisture to preserve foods. You need to blanch vegetables and sulfur some fruits before drying. You can dry foods in the sun or in a conventional oven. You should store dried foods in tightly sealed containers to prevent moisture from affecting them.

Commercial food preservation follows the same principles as home preservation. Freeze-drying, aseptic packaging, retort packaging, and irradiation are all commercial preservation techniques.

Review What You Have Read

Write your answers on a separate sheet of paper.

1. True or false. Bacteria, mold, and yeast can have good effects on food.
2. What are three reasons people can foods at home?
3. Space between the food and the closure of a food-storage container is called _____.
4. What are two foods that must be processed by pressure canning? Explain why.
5. List three factors that can cause home-canned foods to lose eating quality during storage.
6. What are five signs of spoilage in home-canned foods?
7. A tender jelly containing small pieces of fruit and fruit rind is _____.
8. What is the function of each of the four basic ingredients needed to make jellied products?
9. True or false. Because acid and sugar act as natural preservatives, jellied products do not require further preservation methods.
10. Describe the advantage quick-frozen foods have over foods frozen more slowly.
11. What are the three packing methods that may be used when freezing fruits?
12. List five foods that do not freeze well.
13. What are two methods for drying fruits and vegetables at home?
14. What type of commercial food preservation involves separate sterilization of a food and its packaging material?
    A. Aseptic packaging.
    B. Commercial canning.
    C. Freeze-drying.
    D. Retort packaging.

Build Your Basic Skills

1. **Writing.** Design a brochure about the safe use of home-canned foods. The brochure should describe how to check for spoilage. Also list types of spoilage of which people should be aware. Explain what to do with spoiled food. Finally, discuss how to prepare foods that appear to be wholesome.
2. **Verbal.** Prepare an oral report explaining how the food industry prevents food spoilage by microorganisms and enzymes.

Build Your Thinking Skills

1. **Analyze.** Make two batches of a jellied product. Add commercial pectin to one batch. Do not add pectin to the other batch. Analyze the effects of added pectin on the flavor, consistency, cooking time, yield, and appearance of the jellied product.
2. **Evaluate.** Make a batch of cookies. Sample and evaluate for quality. Package and freeze half of the remaining cookies in a loosely rolled paper bag. Package and freeze the other half of the cookies in a tightly sealed plastic container. After one month, thaw, sample, and evaluate the cookies. Which type of container best preserved the flavor, texture, and appearance of fresh cookies?
3. **Compare.** Compare the flavor, texture, appearance, and drying time of oven-dried and sun-dried apples.

Apply Technology

1. Identify five food products sold in aseptic or retort packaging.
2. Prepare a poster illustrating the procedure used to irradiate foods.

Using Workplace Skills

Henry is a dehydrator tender for the Nature Made company. Nature Made produces a variety of dried fruits. Henry spends his entire shift spreading fresh fruit onto trays for drying and emptying dried fruit into totes for packaging. The drying tunnel requires only one person to tend it, so Henry does his routine work alone.

To be a successful employee, Henry needs skills in self-management. In a small group, answer the following questions about Henry's need for and use of these skills:

A. What characteristics of Henry's job make having good self-management skills so important?
B. How will having self-management skills help Henry as a dehydrator tender?
C. How might the quantity and quality of Nature Made's dried fruit products be affected if Henry lacks self-management skills?
D. What is another skill Henry would need in this job? Briefly explain why this skill would be important

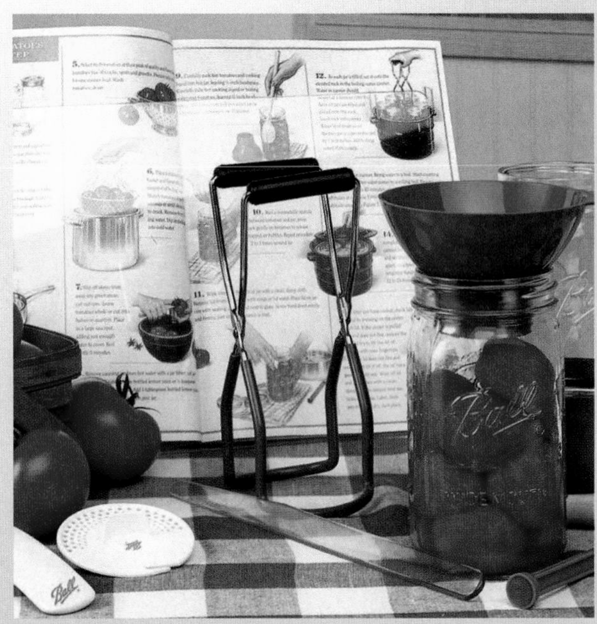

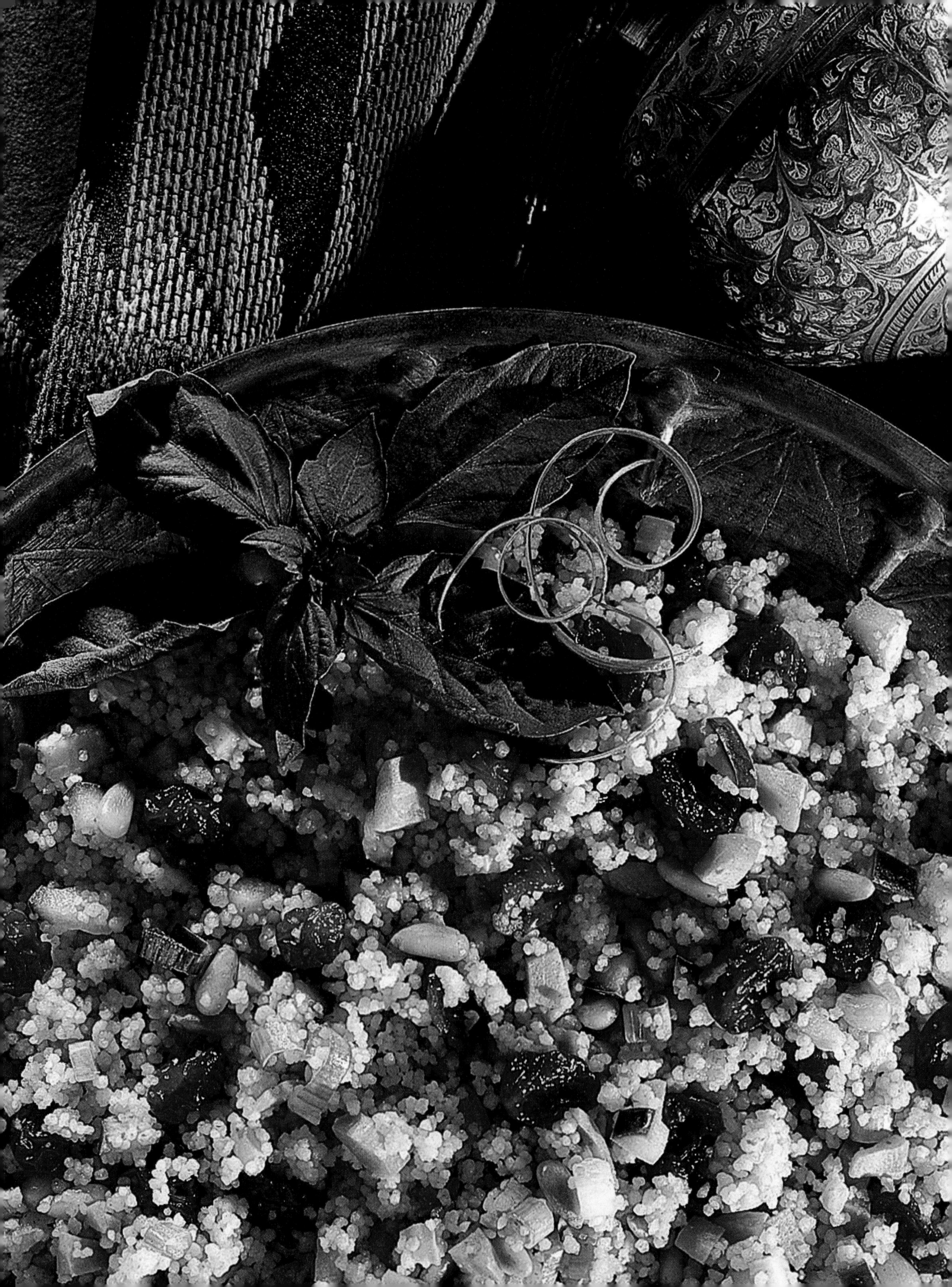

Part 4
Foods of the World

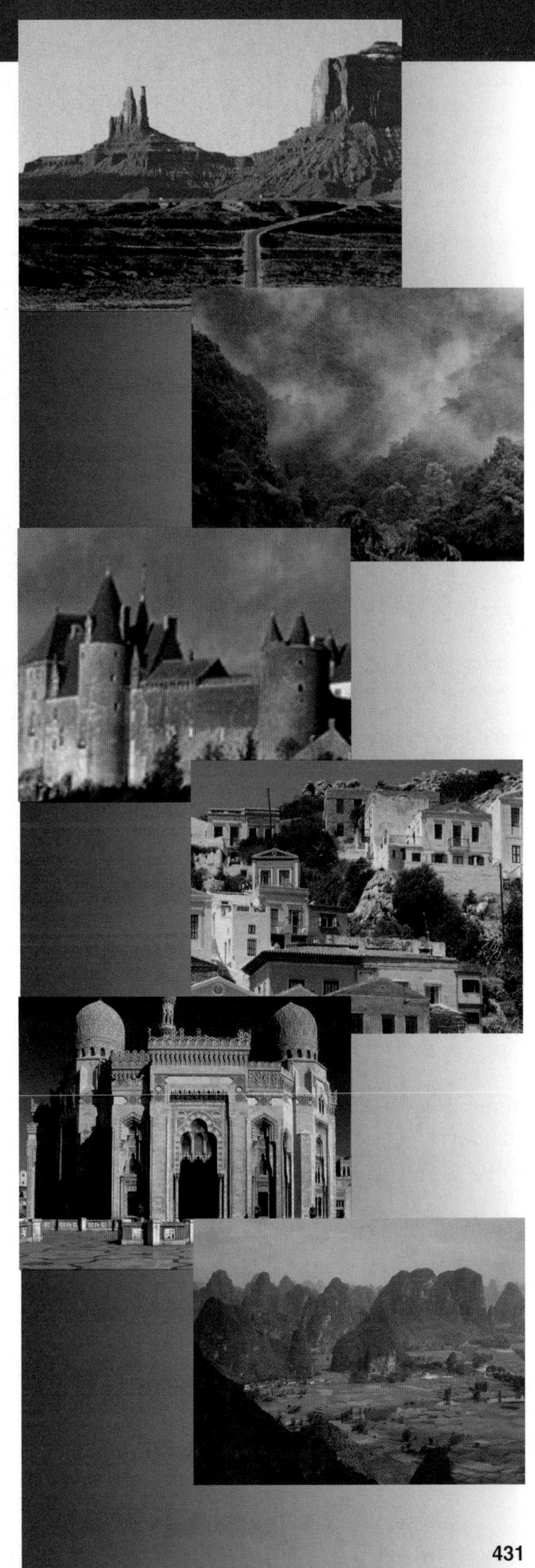

◄ Cherry Marketing Institute

Chapter 27
The United States and Canada

Restaurant Critic
Writes critical reviews of restaurants for broadcast and publication.

Tourist-Information Assistant
Provides travel information and other services to tourists at State Information Centers.

Travel Writer
Travels to various locations to gather information in order to write articles about rates and amenities of lodging and dining facilities and local points of interest.

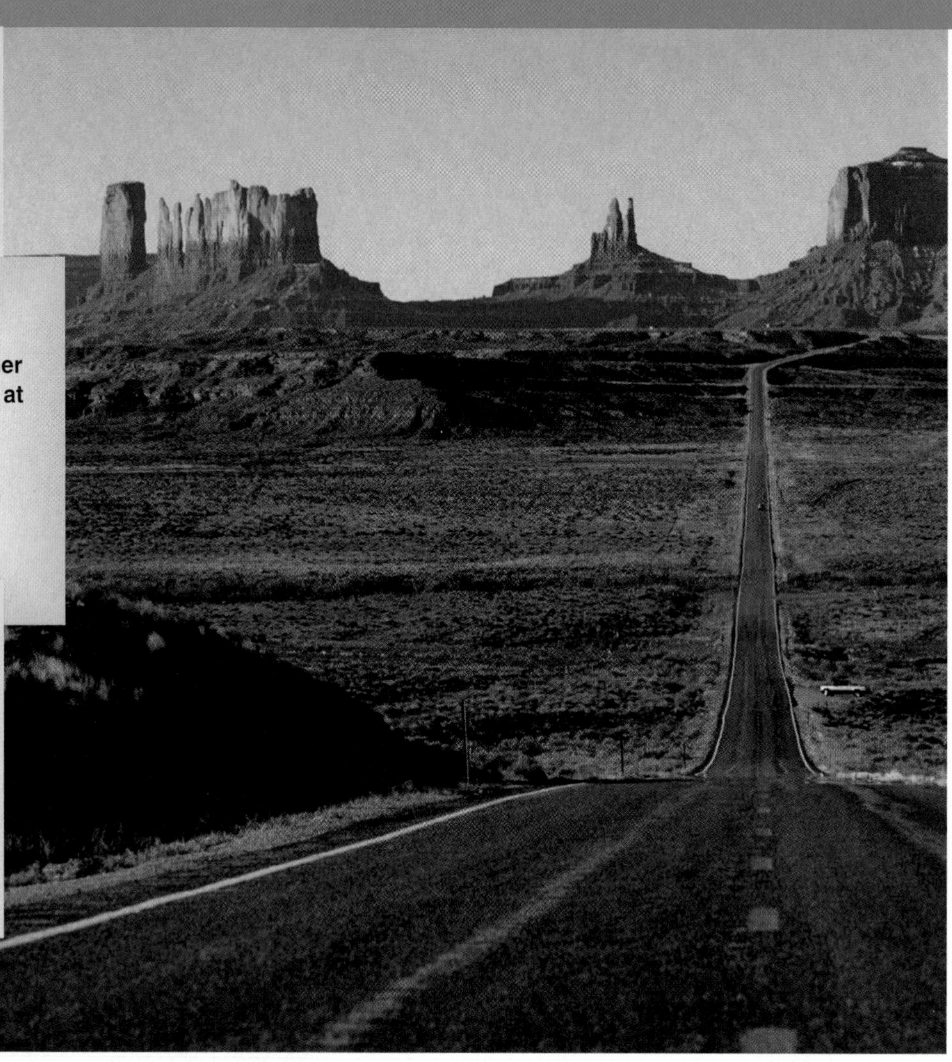

Terms to Know

Pennsylvania Dutch
soul food
okra
yam
Creole cuisine
filé
gumbo
jambalaya
Cajun cuisine
potluck
sourdough
luau
imu
Aboriginal

Objectives

After studying this chapter, you will be able to

- identify the origins of foods of the seven main regions of the United States.
- explain how geography, climate, and culture affected the development of Canadian cuisine.
- prepare foods that are representative of the United States and Canada.

The food customs of the United States and Canada are as diverse as the inhabitants of these nations. People who live in these two countries have roots that stretch around the world.

A Historical Overview of the United States

Since shortly after Columbus' arrival in North America in 1492, people began leaving their homelands to move to the New World. They had many reasons for making this major life change. Some moved to escape debtor's prison. Others sought religious freedom. Many fled famine and disease. Some came as forced laborers, whereas others came in search of fame and fortune.

The First Inhabitants and Early Settlers

Food customs of the United States began with the *Native Americans*. The Native Americans were excellent farmers. Although they cultivated many fruits and vegetables, beans, corn, and squash supplied the basis of their diets. They hunted wild game, gathered nuts and berries, and fished to supplement these staple foods. The high nutritional quality of their diets made the Native Americans healthier than the Europeans of that time.

The British and Spanish were the first permanent colonists in the United States. They established the early settlements of Jamestown and Plymouth (British) and St. Augustine (Spanish). The French who settled in the United States established provinces in Louisiana. A little later, the Dutch arrived and established the New Netherland Colony, which later became New York.

Good Manners Are Good Business

Regional foods, perhaps arranged in an attractive basket, make a thoughtful business gift. International business associates or those living in other regions will especially enjoy foods from your region.

Business people often send gifts to celebrate successes, such as mergers and promotions. They also send them to thank people for their help. For instance, you might send a gift to someone who helps you get a job or increase business.

Each group of settlers had to adjust to the climate and geography of the area in which they settled. However, they were able to adapt many of their food customs to take advantage of New World ingredients.

The life of the first colonists was a struggle for survival. The Native Americans contributed to the success of the first colonial settlements in the New World. They taught colonists how to hunt, fish, and plant crops. Within a few years, the colonists had cleared land, built small groups of homes, and planted simple gardens. The colonists grew new varieties of vegetables and fruits. They learned to eat animals and fish that had been unfamiliar to them.

As the colonists' knowledge grew, they added many new dishes to their diets. They used local lobster, crab, and other fish in seafood chowders. They salted pork and preserved beef for use in a variety of meat dishes throughout the winter. They used pumpkin and wild berries to make pies, puddings, and cakes.

The Immigrants

As more and more people came to the New World, communities sprang up along the east coast. People also began to settle on more fertile lands farther inland. Many immigrants stayed together in groups and settled in particular regions. Many British, Dutch, German, and French people settled in the Northeast. British, French, and Spanish immigrants settled in the Deep South. Other Spanish settlers chose to live in the Southwest. As the South was settled, the slave trade became established. Africans were brought to the United States to work on Southern plantations.

During the 1800s, many people came to the United States in search of economic opportunities, land, and freedom. Most of these immigrants tended to settle in areas with climates similar to those of their homelands. Chicago, New York, and other large industrial cities attracted large groups of Poles, Irish, French, and Italians. Many of these immigrants worked as unskilled laborers. Scandinavians and Germans traveled to Wisconsin and Minnesota to farm. Chinese, Japanese, and other South Asians settled along the Pacific Coast where they mined and worked on the railroads.

The new immigrants brought their native food customs with them to North America. They adapted their recipes to the foods that were readily available. Italian immigrants made rich pasta sauces from tomatoes, basil, and onions sold by street vendors in New York. The Chinese used chicken, bamboo shoots, and water chestnuts to make their chow mein. The Poles stuffed cabbage leaves with ground beef and tomato sauce to make their traditional cabbage rolls. These citizens of the New World helped create the cuisine eaten in the United States today.

Holidays in the United States

Immigrants brought their holiday traditions to the United States along with their food customs. Many holidays are ethnic celebrations. Therefore, some holidays are celebrated only in regions of the country where certain ethnic groups are found.

One regional holiday in the United States is *Mardi Gras.* It is celebrated in some parts of the South, where French settlers introduced it. Mardi Gras is French for fat Tuesday. It falls on the day before Ash Wednesday, which marks the beginning of Lent in the Christian church. Lent is a 40-day period of prayer and fasting. Mardi Gras began as a last celebration before entering into this solemn time. Festivities often begin the week before the actual holiday. They include colorful parades with floats and marching bands. People wear ornate costumes and masks and attend gala balls and parties.

Cajun favorites featuring locally caught seafood are served at many Mardi Gras parties. A typical menu might include shrimp mold appetizer, crab bisque, and crawfish stew. The classic Mardi Gras dessert is king cake. This is a ring of cinnamon-filled dough decorated with purple, green, and gold sugar. A tiny plastic baby doll is baked inside the cake. Whoever gets the piece of cake containing the doll is supposed to throw the next Mardi Gras party. See 27-1.

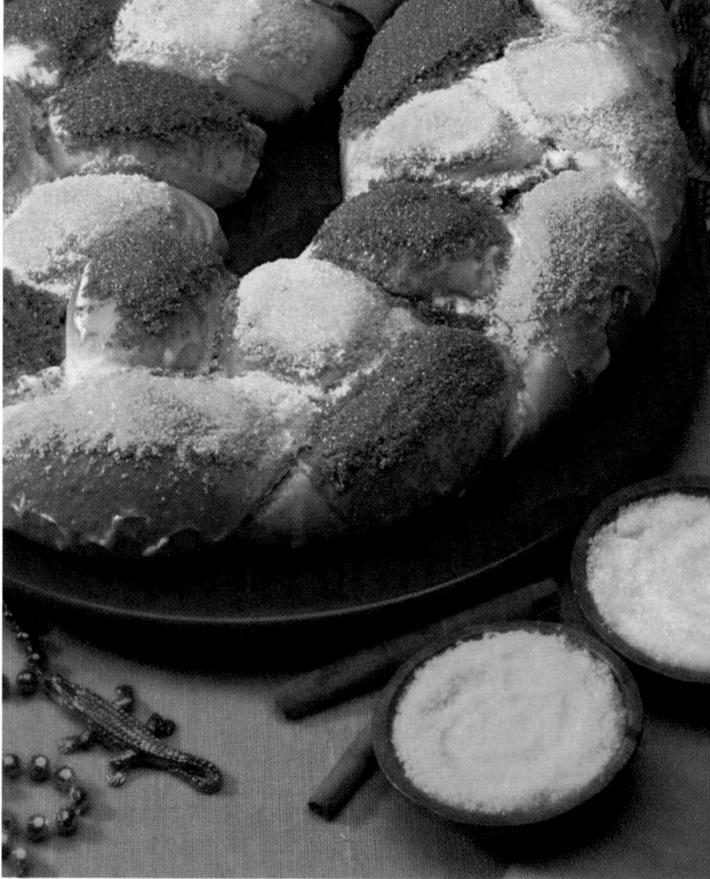

photo courtesy of Fleischmann's Yeast

***27-1** The purple, green, and gold colors used to decorate Mardi Gras king cake symbolize justice, faith, and power, respectively.*

Only people of a certain culture observe some holidays. *Cinco de Mayo* is a cultural holiday observed by Mexican Americans. The name is Spanish for Fifth of May, which is the day of celebration. It marks the victory of severely outnumbered Mexican troops over French troops at the Battle of Puebla in 1862. Parades, music, dancing, and carnivals are all part of the celebration. The day may conclude with Mexican foods, including sweet breads and coffee or hot chocolate flavored with cinnamon.

A newer cultural holiday is *Kwanzaa.* This is a family-centered observance of cultural unity among people of African heritage. The name comes from a Swahili word for first fruits. This weeklong celebration occurs between Christmas and New Year's Day. People use this time to think about their ancestry, family, and community. On the next to the last night of Kwanzaa, families hold the *karamu,* which is a ritual feast. Kwanzaa was developed in the United States. However, this celebration is becoming popular among people of African descent all over the world.

New England

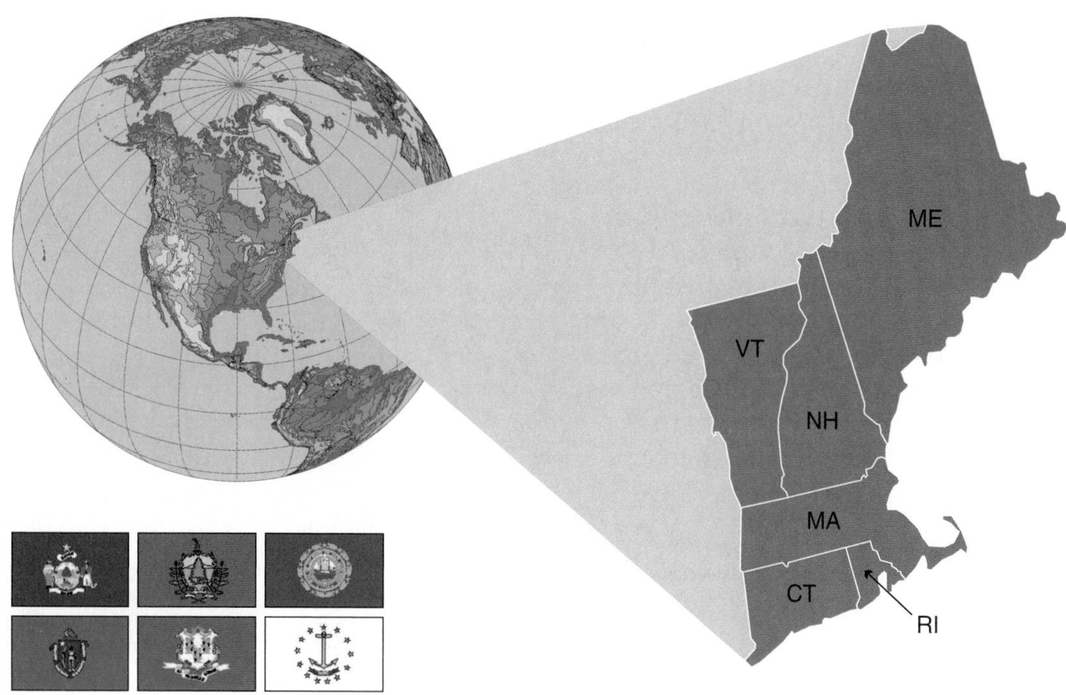

The British were the first people to settle in the area now called New England. Much of the land was rocky, mountainous, or forested, and winters were long and severe. The early colonists had to work hard to survive.

The character of the people and the land they inhabited shaped the character of New England cooking. Most of the farms that sprang up were isolated and self-sufficient. Seafood and wild game supplemented the foods New Englanders could grow at home. The waters provided lobsters, crabs, clams, and other shellfish, which later became New England specialties. The forests provided wild turkeys, geese, ducks, and pheasants.

Each home had a large fireplace the family used for cooking. New Englanders prepared most foods in iron pots that hung over the fire. They made baked goods in covered Dutch ovens over the coals of the fireplace or in beehive ovens. These baked goods included Indian bread, Sally Lunn, and johnnycakes.

New England cooks used foods that were readily available to create hearty, substantial meals. For instance, they used corn to make corn sticks, Indian pudding, and cornmeal mush. They also used it for succotash (a combination of corn and lima beans).

To survive the long, cold winters, the early New Englanders learned to dry and salt foods to preserve them. They commonly dried beans, corn, and apples. Later, they soaked these foods in water and cooked them until tender. Early New Englanders made baked beans in this way. The Native Americans taught the early settlers how to soak the dried beans overnight. Then cooks would flavor the beans with

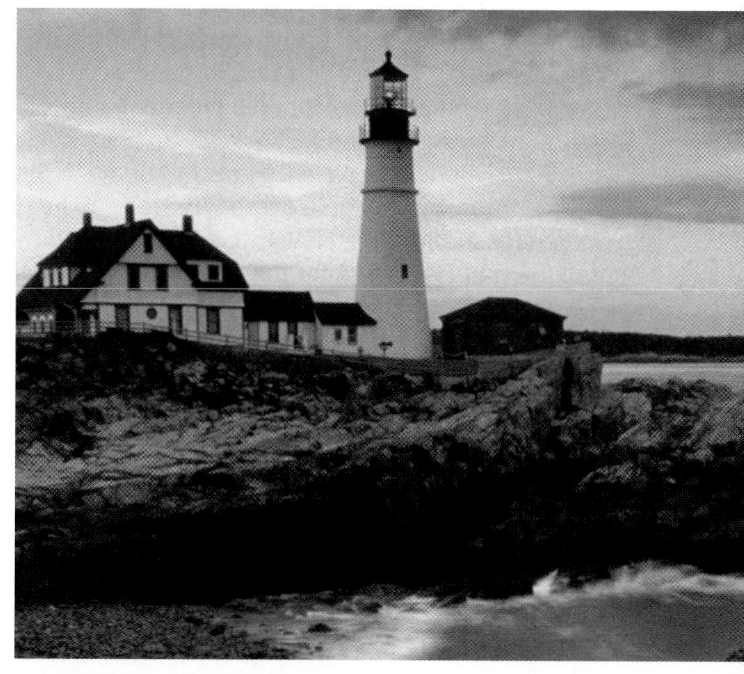

A lighthouse on a rocky Maine coast helps guide ships safely in the Atlantic Ocean.

Q: What is the difference between pure maple syrup and maple-flavored syrup?

A: Pure maple syrup is made from the sap of sugar maple trees. Maple-flavored syrup, also known as pancake syrup, is made with corn syrup that may contain natural or artificial maple flavoring. Although maple-flavored syrup is less costly, true syrup lovers believe pure maple syrup is worth the higher price.

molasses and salt pork and cook them slowly in big pots.

One-dish meals were popular in New England because they gave the cooks more time to do other tasks. One of the most common one-dish meals of that time, the *New England boiled dinner*, is still popular today. It is a combination of meat (usually corned beef), potatoes, onions, carrots, beets, cabbage, and other available vegetables. The ingredients cook together slowly until they are tender.

The colonists used a variety of meats, seafood, and vegetables to make stews and chowders. Clam chowder was one of the most popular. Many people continue to associate New England cooking with this creamy soup made with potatoes and clams, 27-2.

From the sap of New England's sugar maple trees came maple syrup. Native Americans taught the New Englanders how to tap the maple trees. After the colonists boiled down the sap, they used the syrup to make cakes, candies, sauces, and puddings. They also used it to flavor baked beans, squash, and other vegetables.

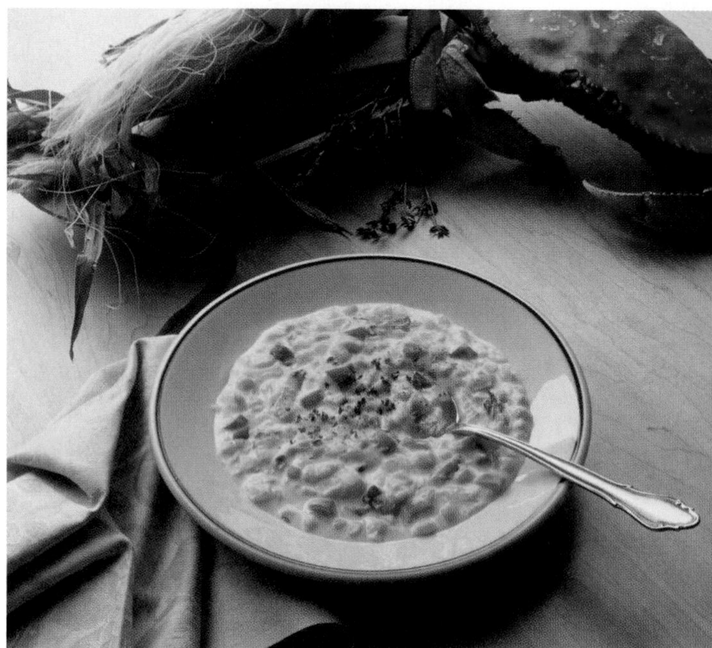

27-2 *Creamy seafood chowders have been part of New England cuisine since colonial days.*

Blueberries, cranberries, blackberries, and other fruits were another important food source. New England cooks gathered the berries and used them to make a variety of nourishing desserts. Two examples are *blueberry mush* (a steamed pudding) and *blueberry grunt* (berries simmered in a thickened sauce and topped with fluffy dumplings).

New Englanders used leftovers in creative ways. For instance, they would grind the leftovers from a boiled dinner and fry them in a large iron skillet. Beets give this dish a red color, which reminded the New Englanders of red flannel underwear worn during the cold winters. Thus, the dish earned the name *red-flannel hash.*

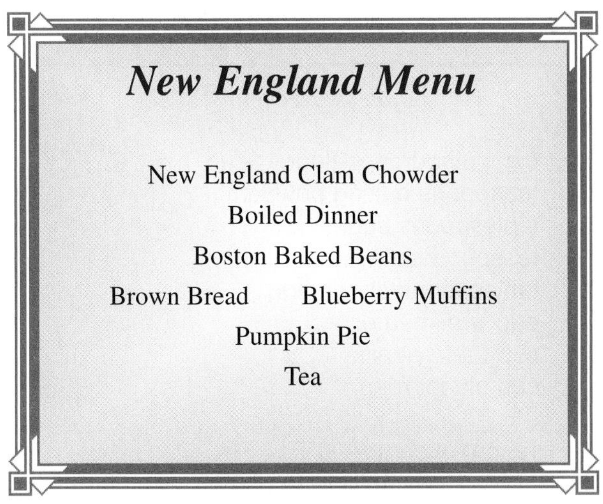

New England Menu

New England Clam Chowder
Boiled Dinner
Boston Baked Beans
Brown Bread Blueberry Muffins
Pumpkin Pie
Tea

New England Clam Chowder

Serves 6

3 slices bacon
2 cans minced clams, 8 ounces each
1 large potato, peeled and cubed
1 medium stalk celery, chopped
1/2 cup finely chopped onion
1/4 teaspoon pepper
1/8 teaspoon thyme
2 cups fat free milk
1 1/2 cups evaporated fat free milk

1. In large, heavy saucepan, cook bacon until crisp.
2. Remove bacon to a piece of absorbent paper to drain. Pour excess fat from pan.
3. Drain clams, reserving liquid. Set clams aside.
4. In saucepan used to cook bacon, add potato, celery, onion, pepper, and thyme to liquid from clams. Bring to a boil; simmer covered until vegetables are tender (about 10 minutes).
5. Add milk, evaporated milk, and clams and heat almost to the boiling point. Taste to see if additional seasonings are needed. Serve immediately.

Per serving: 268 cal. (13% from fat), 28 g protein, 30 g carbohydrate, 4 g fat, 54 mg cholesterol, 1 g fiber, 261 mg sodium.

Boiled Dinner

Serves 8

2 pounds corned beef
8 medium-sized beets*
2 pounds green cabbage, cored and quartered
4 medium-sized red potatoes, scrubbed, peeled, and cut in half
8 small carrots, scraped
16 small white onions, peeled and trimmed
parsley, chopped

1. Place corned beef in a large kettle of cold water (water should rise at least 2 inches above meat). Bring to a boil and skim off any scum that rises to surface.
2. Cover kettle and reduce heat to slow simmer; cook corned beef 3 to 4 hours or until tender. (Check water level during cooking.)
3. Scrub beets, cut off tops leaving 1 inch and cover with water. Simmer until tender. Cool slightly and slip off skins.
4. Cook cabbage, potatoes, carrots, and onions in salted, simmering water until tender.
5. To serve the dinner, slice the meat and arrange on serving platter. Surround meat with vegetables and top with chopped parsley. Serve with horseradish sauce or mustard.

*One medium can whole beets can be substituted for fresh.

Note: Vegetables (with the exception of the beets) can be added to the corned beef about 30 to 40 minutes before serving as is done in New England. However, some people object to the salty flavor the corned beef gives the vegetables.

Per serving: 417 cal. (39% from fat), 23 g protein, 45 g carbohydrate, 18 g fat, 61 mg cholesterol, 8 g fiber, 229 mg sodium.

Boston Baked Beans

Serves 8

2 cups dried great northern or navy beans*
8 cups water
1/2 cup molasses
1/2 cup brown sugar
1/3 cup onions, coarsely chopped
2 teaspoons dry mustard
1/2 teaspoon pepper
2 slices Canadian bacon

1. Place beans in large saucepan and cover with cold water (water should be at least 2 inches higher than the beans). Bring beans to a boil and let boil 2 minutes.
2. Remove pan from heat and let beans soak about 1 hour.
3. Return pan to heat, bring water to a boil. Reduce heat and slowly simmer beans until

almost tender (about 1 to 1½ hours); drain and reserve liquid.
4. Preheat oven to 300°F.
5. Place beans in 2-quart bean pot or heavy casserole.
6. Add enough water to bean liquid to make 2 cups.
7. Combine bean liquid, molasses, brown sugar, onions, dry mustard, and pepper; pour over beans.
8. Cut Canadian bacon into bite-sized pieces and add to beans.
9. Cover pot tightly; bake beans 1½ to 2 hours, stirring occasionally and adding water if needed.
10. Remove cover and bake beans an additional 30 minutes without stirring.

*Three 16-ounce cans beans can be substituted for dried. Begin recipe preparation with step 4.

Per serving: 266 cal. (4% from fat), 12 g protein, 54 g carbohydrate, 1 g fat, 3 mg cholesterol, 5 g fiber, 142 mg sodium.

Brown Bread

Makes 3 small loaves

1 cup whole wheat flour
1 cup rye flour
1 cup cornmeal
1½ teaspoons baking soda
½ teaspoon salt
¾ cup raisins
2 cups buttermilk
¾ cup dark molasses
2 tablespoons melted shortening

1. Preheat oven to 350°F.
2. Grease three 1-pound coffee cans.
3. In large mixing bowl, combine flours, cornmeal, soda, salt, and raisins; mix well.
4. Combine buttermilk, molasses, and melted shortening; add to dry ingredients mixing well.
5. Pour batter into greased cans filling ⅔ full; cover with foil.
6. Place cans on rack in shallow pan. Place pan in oven. Pour boiling water around cans to depth of 2½ inches.
7. Steam breads 3 hours until toothpick inserted in center comes out clean.
8. Cool 15 minutes and remove from cans. Serve warm.

Per slice: 85 cal. (13% from fat), 2 g protein, 17 g carbohydrate, 1 g fat, 1 mg cholesterol, 2 g fiber, 103 mg sodium.

Blueberry Muffins

Makes 12 muffins

2 cups all-purpose flour
2½ teaspoons baking powder
3 tablespoons sugar
½ teaspoon salt
3 tablespoons shortening
1 egg, well beaten
1 cup fat free milk
1 cup blueberries

1. Preheat oven to 400°F.
2. Stir flour, baking powder, sugar, and salt together in mixing bowl.
3. Melt shortening; cool.
4. Combine egg and milk; add cooled shortening.
5. Add liquid ingredients to dry ingredients all at once. Stir only until blended. (Batter will be lumpy.)
6. Gently fold in blueberries.
7. Fill greased muffin pans ⅔ full of batter.
8. Bake muffins 20 to 25 minutes or until brown.

Per muffin: 173 cal. (26% from fat), 3 g protein, 22 g carbohydrate, 4 g fat, 23 mg cholesterol, 1 g fiber, 167 mg sodium.

Pumpkin Pie

Makes one 9-inch pie

2 eggs
¾ cup light brown sugar, packed
2 cups canned pumpkin
1½ cups evaporated fat free milk
1 teaspoon cinnamon
½ teaspoon ground cloves
½ teaspoon ginger
½ teaspoon nutmeg
1 unbaked pastry shell, 9-inch

1. Preheat oven to 450°F.
2. In large mixing bowl, beat eggs slightly; add pumpkin, milk, and spices and mix well.
3. Pour mixture into pastry shell.
4. Bake 10 minutes.
5. Reduce temperature to 300°F and continue baking until knife inserted in center comes out clean, about 40 to 50 minutes.
6. Cool. Serve with whipped cream.

⅙ of pie: 394 cal. (28% from fat), 10 g protein, 63 g carbohydrate, 13 g fat, 94 mg cholesterol, 2 g fiber, 284 mg sodium.

Mid-Atlantic

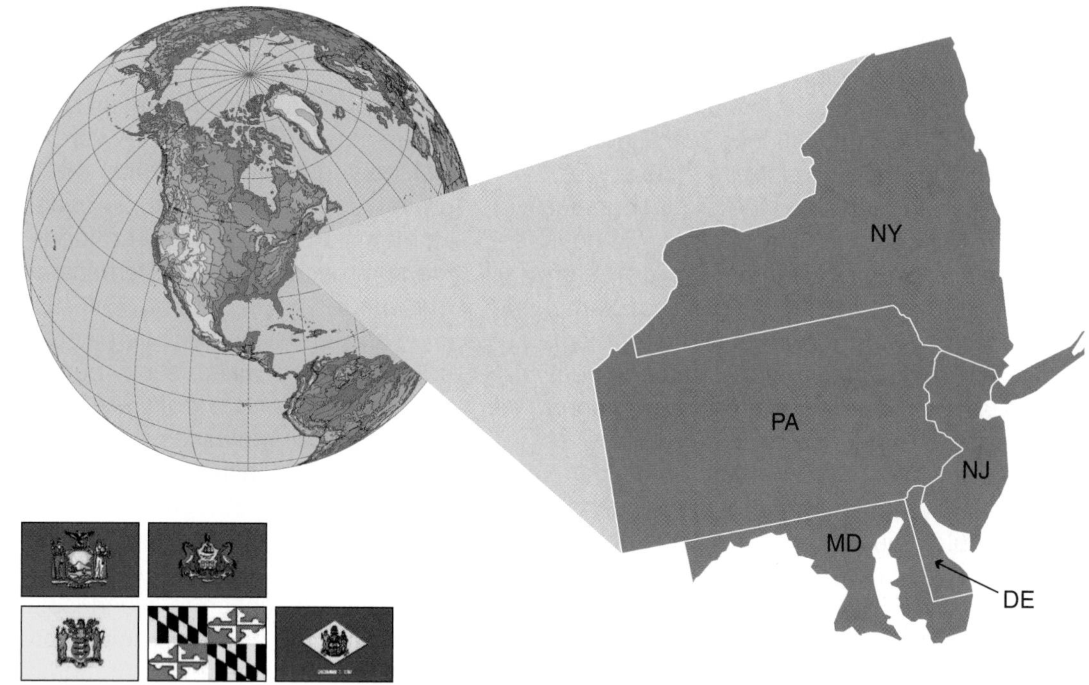

South of New England, the climate is milder. The land in the mid-Atlantic region is rich and fertile, and farming is profitable. New Jersey is a major center of fresh fruit and vegetable production. New Jersey ships apples, peaches, beans, cranberries, tomatoes, onions, asparagus, cucumbers, peas, and melons to many parts of the country.

The mid-Atlantic region was settled by Dutch, German, Swedish, and British immigrants. The Dutch were excellent farmers. They had large vegetable gardens and kept their root cellars well stocked. Many had their own orchards, too.

The Dutch were also excellent bakers. Cookies (koekjes), doughnuts (olykoeks), molasses cake, and gingerbread figures all have Dutch origins. The Dutch also introduced waffles, coleslaw, cottage cheese, and griddle cakes.

The Pennsylvania Dutch

One group of mid-Atlantic settlers, the Pennsylvania Dutch, deserves special mention. The ***Pennsylvania Dutch*** were a group of German immigrants who settled in the southeast section of Pennsylvania. (The word *Dutch* comes from the word *Deutsch,* which means German.) These immigrants came from the Rhine Valley, where they were farmers. When they came to the United States, they were successful in adapting their farming techniques to the soil in Pennsylvania.

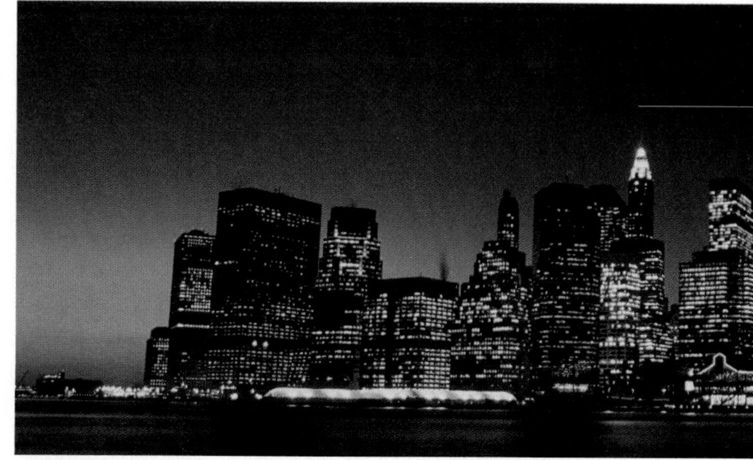

From Amish farms in Pennsylvania to the bustle of New York City, the Mid-Atlantic region encompasses a full range of lifestyles.

The food customs of the Pennsylvania Dutch were very different from those of their neighbors. They developed a style of cooking that was rural, hearty, and inventive. They based it on cooking techniques practiced in the Old World. The thrifty *hausfraus* (housewife) canned, pickled, and dried the produce, meat, and poultry raised on the farm. They did not waste anything. They used their thriftiness and ingenuity to create many new dishes. Examples are pickled pigs' feet, blood pudding, *scrapple* (pork combined with cornmeal), smoked beef tongue, stuffed heart, sausages, and bologna.

Soup was one of the most popular dishes. The Pennsylvania Dutch made it from whatever foods were available. Since they were especially skillful in the production of vegetables and poultry, they served vegetable and chicken soups often. *Chicken corn soup* remains a traditional favorite.

Hearty German foods, such as sauerbraten, sauerkraut, liverwurst, and pork, were mainstays of the Pennsylvania Dutch diet. Noodles, dumplings, potato pancakes, and other filling foods were served as accompaniments. See 27-3.

Each meal included seven sweets and seven sours. These usually were in the form of pickled vegetables and fruits, relishes, jams, preserves, salads, and apple butter. Homemakers made all these foods during the summer and stored them in cellars for the winter.

The Pennsylvania Dutch were excellent bakers. Coffee cakes, sticky buns, funnel cakes, crumb cakes, and *shoofly pie* (pastry with a filling made of molasses and brown sugar) are some of their specialties.

Several religious groups, including the Amish and the Mennonites, shared a German heritage with the Pennsylvania Dutch. However, these peoples chose to live in isolated groups. Their isolation, however, helped preserve their hearty homestyle cooking and native crafts. Some small colonies of these peoples still exist throughout the country.

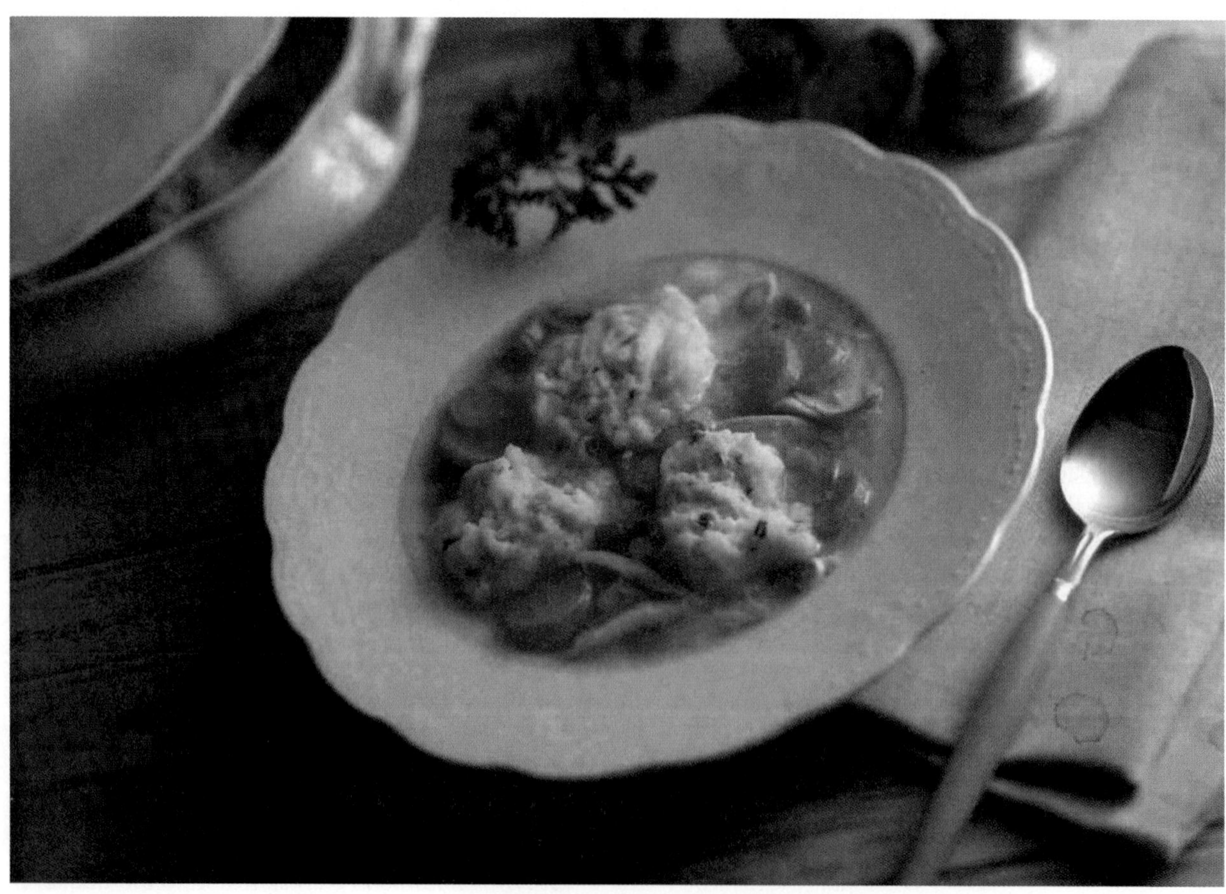

photo courtesy of Land O'Lakes, Inc.

***27-3** A hearty bowl of chicken soup with dumplings might be the focus of a satisfying Pennsylvania Dutch meal.*

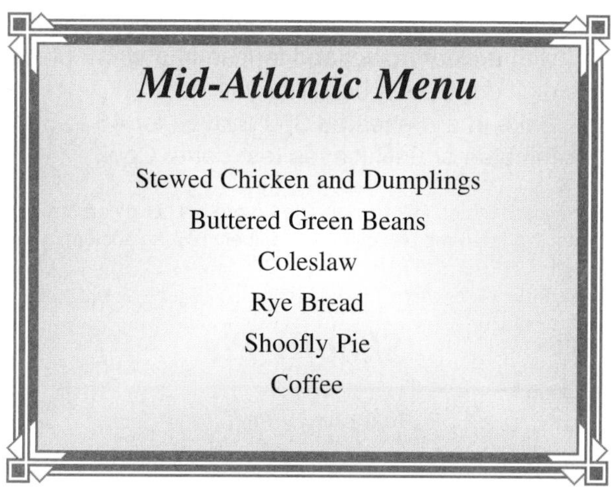

Mid-Atlantic Menu

Stewed Chicken and Dumplings
Buttered Green Beans
Coleslaw
Rye Bread
Shoofly Pie
Coffee

Stewed Chicken and Dumplings

Serves 8

- 4 skinless chicken breast halves
- 4 skinless chicken legs and thighs
- 1 onion, quartered
- 3 stalks celery, cut in 1/2-inch slices
- 3 carrots, diced
- 1/2 teaspoon sage
- salt and pepper
- cold water
- 1/4 cup all-purpose flour
- 1 cup cold fat free milk

Dumplings:

- 1 1/4 cups all-purpose flour
- 1/4 teaspoon salt
- 2 1/2 teaspoons baking powder
- 1/4 cup shortening
- 1/2 cup fat free milk

1. Wash chicken and place in a large kettle with onion, celery, carrots, sage, and salt and pepper to taste. Add enough cold water to barely cover chicken and vegetables.
2. Cover kettle and bring to a boil over high heat.
3. Reduce heat and simmer 1 hour, until chicken is tender.
4. About 45 minutes after the chicken begins to simmer, start to mix the dumplings. Begin by stirring the flour, salt, and baking powder together into a medium mixing bowl.
5. Cut in shortening with pastry blender or two knives until particles are the size of coarse cornmeal.
6. Add milk, stir with a fork to make a sticky dough.
7. Divide the dough into eighths and drop by spoonfuls onto the chicken (not into the liquid). Allow space between dumplings for them to double in size.
8. Cover pan and continue to simmer chicken for 15 more minutes without lifting the lid.
9. Lift out the dumplings onto a plate.
10. Place chicken on a serving platter.
11. Shake 1/4 cup flour with 1 cup cold milk in a small covered container until thoroughly blended.
12. Stir flour mixture into the chicken stock.
13. Heat and stir until stock thickens.
14. Pour thickened stock and vegetables over chicken. Arrange dumplings on top.

Per serving: 331 cal. (24% from fat), 31 g protein, 26 g carbohydrate, 9 g fat, 74 mg cholesterol, 2 g fiber, 298 mg sodium.

Buttered Green Beans

Serves 6

- 2 pounds fresh green beans*
- 3/4 cup water
- salt
- margarine
- pepper

1. Wash beans under cool running water. Snap off ends; then snap beans in half.
2. Place water and salt in medium saucepan; bring to a boil.
3. Add beans. Return to a boil, then reduce heat and simmer beans gently just until crisp-tender, about 10 to 15 minutes.
4. Drain beans, top with margarine, and season with salt and pepper to taste. Serve immediately.

* Two 10-ounce packages of frozen green beans may be substituted for fresh. Follow package directions for cooking.

Per serving: 47 cal. (36% from fat), 1 g protein, 7 g carbohydrate, 2 g fat, 0 mg cholesterol, 3 g fiber, 202 mg sodium.

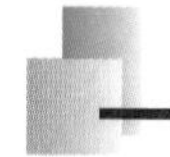

Coleslaw

Serves 6 to 8

- 1 large white cabbage, shredded
- 2 large carrots, shredded
- 1 medium green pepper, diced

- 1/2 cup evaporated fat free milk
- 3/4 cup plain nonfat yogurt
- 1 teaspoon prepared mustard
- 3 tablespoons lemon juice
- 1 tablespoon sugar
- 1 teaspoon celery seed
- salt and pepper

1. Combine vegetables in large mixing bowl.
2. In small bowl, beat together the evaporated milk, yogurt, mustard, lemon juice, sugar, celery seed, and salt and pepper.
3. Pour over vegetables, tossing well.
4. Refrigerate 1 hour before serving.

Per serving: 68 cal. (6% from fat), 4 g protein, 13 g carbohydrate, 1 g fat, 1 mg cholesterol, 2 g fiber, 76 mg sodium.

Rye Bread

Makes 2 loaves

- 2 cups all-purpose flour
- 3 tablespoons brown sugar, firmly packed
- 1 1/2 teaspoons salt
- 1 teaspoon caraway seeds
- 1/2 teaspoon baking soda
- 2 packages active dry yeast
- 1 cup buttermilk
- 1/4 cup dark molasses
- 1/4 cup shortening
- 1 cup water
- 4 to 4 1/4 cups rye flour

1. In large mixing bowl, combine all-purpose flour, brown sugar, salt, caraway seeds, baking soda, and dry yeast. Mix well.
2. In small saucepan, heat buttermilk, molasses, shortening, and water until very warm (120°F to 130°F).
3. Add milk mixture to dry ingredients blending at lowest speed of electric mixer until moistened.
4. Beat at medium speed 3 minutes.
5. By hand, stir in enough rye flour to make a stiff dough.
6. Turn out onto lightly floured board or pastry cloth. Knead until smooth and elastic, about 5 minutes.
7. Place in greased bowl, turning once to grease top. Cover with a clean towel; and let rise in warm place until doubled in bulk, 1 to 1½ hours.
8. Punch down.
9. Shape into two round loaves.
10. Place on lightly greased baking sheet. Cover with a clean towel and let rise in a warm place until doubled in bulk, about 1 hour.
11. Bake in a preheated 350°F oven for 45 to 50 minutes or until loaves test done. Cool.

Per slice: 114 cal. (16% from fat), 4 g protein, 21 g carbohydrate, 2 g fat, 0 mg cholesterol, 3 g fiber, 125 mg sodium.

Shoofly Pie

Makes one 9-inch pie

- 1 unbaked pastry shell, 9-inch
- 1 1/2 cups all-purpose flour
- 1/2 cup margarine
- 1 cup light brown sugar, packed
- 1 teaspoon baking soda
- 1 cup boiling water
- 1/2 cup molasses
- 1/2 cup honey

1. Preheat oven to 375°F.
2. In large mixing bowl, cut margarine into flour with pastry blender or two knives until mixture resembles small peas.
3. Stir in brown sugar and set aside.
4. Dissolve soda in boiling water. Then add molasses and honey.
5. Pour molasses mixture into pastry-lined pie plate with fluted edge.
6. Sprinkle the flour mixture over the top.
7. Bake pie at 375°F for 10 minutes.
8. Reduce heat to 350°F and continue baking another 25 to 30 minutes or until the filling has set.
9. Cool completely before serving.

1/8 of pie: 507 cal. (33% from fat), 4 g protein, 83 g carbohydrate, 19 g fat, 0 mg cholesterol, 1 g fiber, 407 mg sodium.

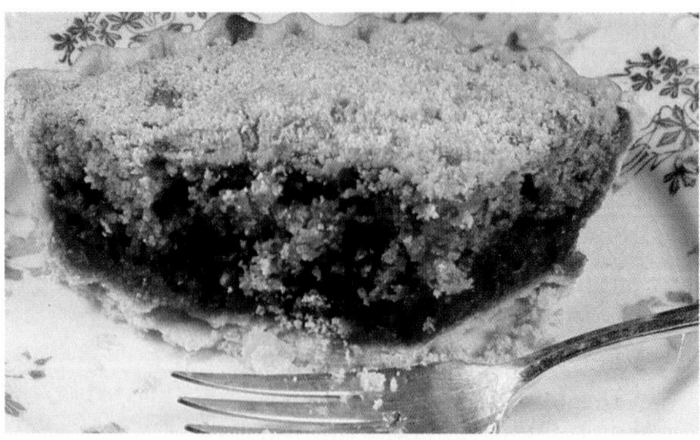

Pennsylvania Dutch Convention & Visitors Bureau, Lancaster, PA

Molasses and brown sugar are used to make the rich filling of shoofly pie.

South

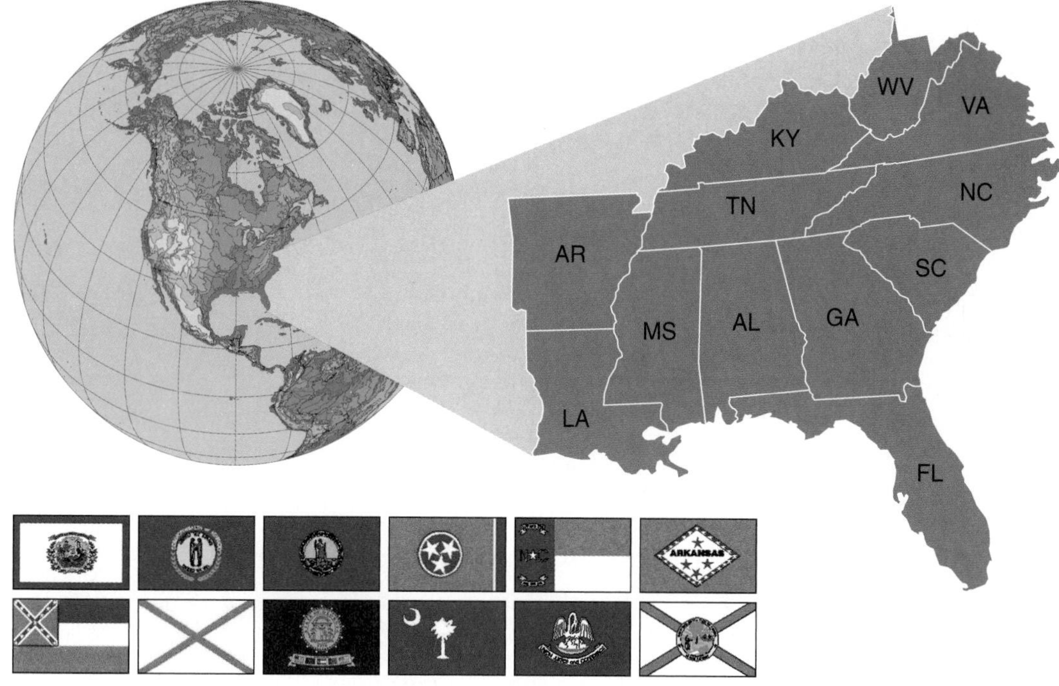

Immigrants from France, England, Ireland, Scotland, and Spain settled in the South. Once they were established, they brought African slaves to the United States. The slaves worked on the large plantations and served in the huge mansions.

The mild climate of the South made year-round production of many crops possible. Sugarcane, rice, and peanuts were the most economically important food crops. Southern farmers also grew fruits and vegetables, but on a smaller scale.

The waters and forests of the South were important sources of food. Southerners found catfish, bass, trout, and terrapin (turtle) in rivers and streams. They found crabs, crayfish, oysters, and shrimp in the Gulf waters. Wild game was abundant. Squirrel, goose, and turkey were especially well liked. From these foods evolved the popular *Brunswick stew* (vegetables and game, poultry, or beef cooked together slowly until tender).

Corn is a staple food in the South. Southerners serve it in many ways. At breakfast, they serve corn as hominy or hominy grits. They use cornmeal to make delicious hot breads, such as corn bread and spoon bread. *Spoon bread* is baked in a casserole like a pudding until it is crispy on the outside but still soft in the center, 27-4.

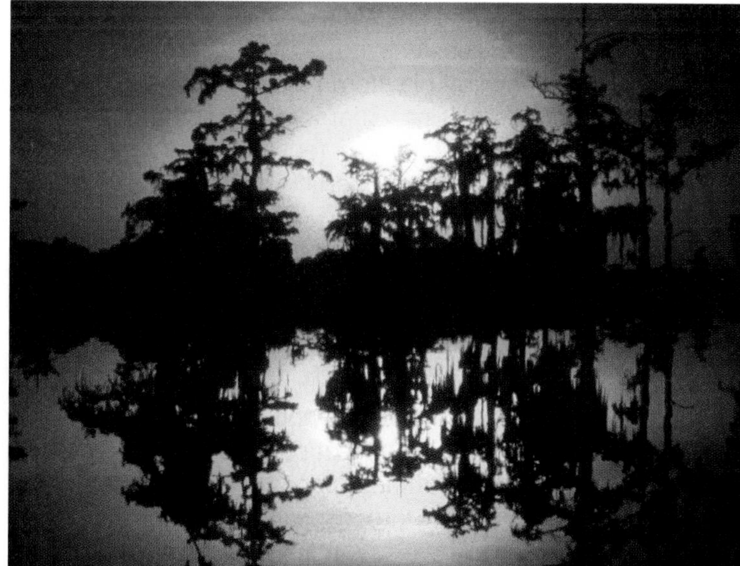

Louisiana Office of Tourism

The Black Bayou in Louisiana serves as a refuge for a variety of birds and wetland animals.

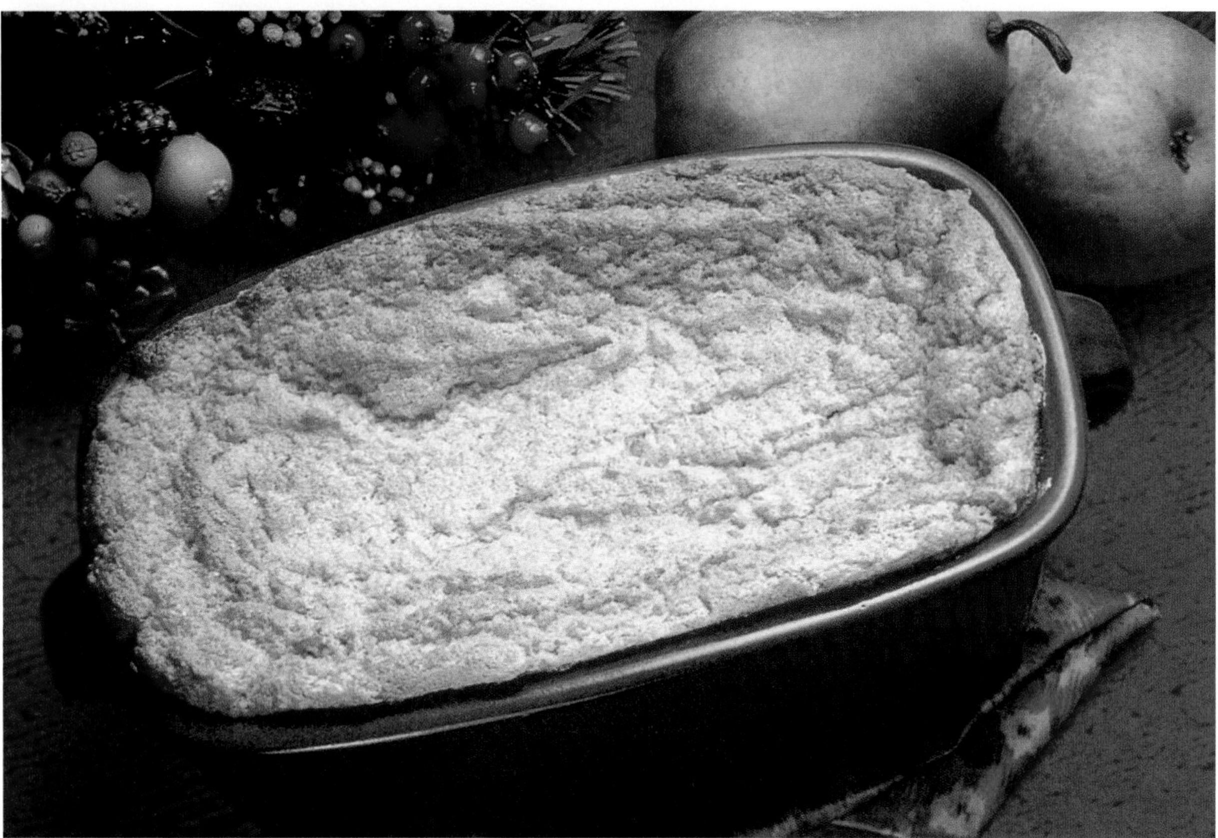

American Egg Board

27-4 Spoon bread is so soft that it is baked in a casserole rather than being shaped into a loaf.

Two other hot breads, buttermilk biscuits and shortnin' bread, are also Southern specialties. Today, Southern cooks still pride themselves on the tenderness and lightness of their biscuits.

Pigs and chickens were the most common types of livestock in the South. As a result, pork and chicken played an important part in the region's cuisine. Spareribs, cured ham, fat back, chitterlings, and pigs' feet often appeared on Southern tables. Fried chicken became a Southern specialty.

Rice grew abundantly in the Carolinas. Southern cooks used it in many of their dishes. They often combined rice with beans, meat, or seafood to make economical and nutritious dishes.

Aside from corn, popular vegetables included beans, sweet potatoes, and a variety of greens. Southern cooks often prepared turnip and dandelion greens with pork fat for flavor. Black-eyed peas, yams, and nuts were other staple foods used in Southern cooking. *Hoppin' John* (a combination of black-eyed peas and rice) and pecan pie are two popular dishes made from these staple foods.

Soul Food

Soul food is a distinct cuisine that developed in the South. ***Soul food*** combines the food customs of African slaves with the food customs of Native Americans and European sharecroppers. It developed around those few foods that were readily available to all three groups of people.

Some plantation owners allowed their slaves to have small gardens. Some slave families were also able to keep a few chickens, but no other domestic animals were allowed. Fishing, however, was allowed, and the slaves could eat all the catfish they were able to catch. Those slaves who worked in the fields received a small amount of meat at harvest time. They also received the less desirable parts of the hogs and cattle. Poor sharecroppers and Native Americans had small gardens and they hunted game animals, such as squirrel, deer, and opossum.

Slaves used the few foods available to them in many creative ways. They mixed leftovers from the plantation house with rice or beans for nutritious and tasty main dishes. The cooks used the cornmeal portions allotted to each family member to make a variety of hot breads and puddings. Batter bread, hush puppies, corn bread, hoecake, and cracklin' corn bread were a few of the most popular ones.

The slaves used all the parts of hogs and cattle discarded by the plantation owners. They cleaned *chitterlings* (the intestines of the hog) and boiled them with spices or dipped them in batter for deep-frying. They even used the hogs' feet, tails, snouts, and ears. Slaves often pickled these parts or boiled them to add to stews, soups, beans, or rice.

Vegetables used in soul food dishes included corn, squash, black-eyed peas, okra, and greens. Corn and squash had been grown in the South by Native Americans for many years. ***Okra*** is a green, pod-shaped vegetable that was brought to the United States from Africa. Slaves breaded and fried it or added it to soups and stews.

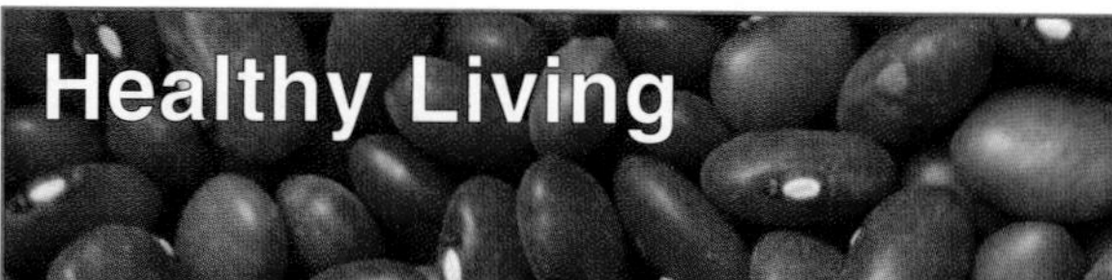

Many traditional Southern recipes are high in fat. Try revising some old favorites to reduce the fat. For instance, instead of deep-frying chicken with the skin on, try oven-frying skinless chicken. You will end up with a similar taste and texture, but only a fraction of the fat.

Greens, such as spinach, mustard, sorrel, beet tops, collards, turnip, kale, dock, and dandelion, grew wild and in gardens. When cooked with salt pork, bacon, pork shank, pork jowl, or ham bone, they were nutritious and flavorful.

Yams are sweet potatoes that have moist, orange flesh. Slaves added them to stews, fried them as fritters, and made them into a pudding called *pone*. They also used yams to make the popular *sweet potato pie,* 27-5.

Creole Cuisine

New Orleans is the home of Creole cuisine. However, people throughout the South enjoy Creole dishes.

Creole cuisine combines the cooking techniques of the French with ingredients of the Africans, Caribbeans, Spanish, and Native

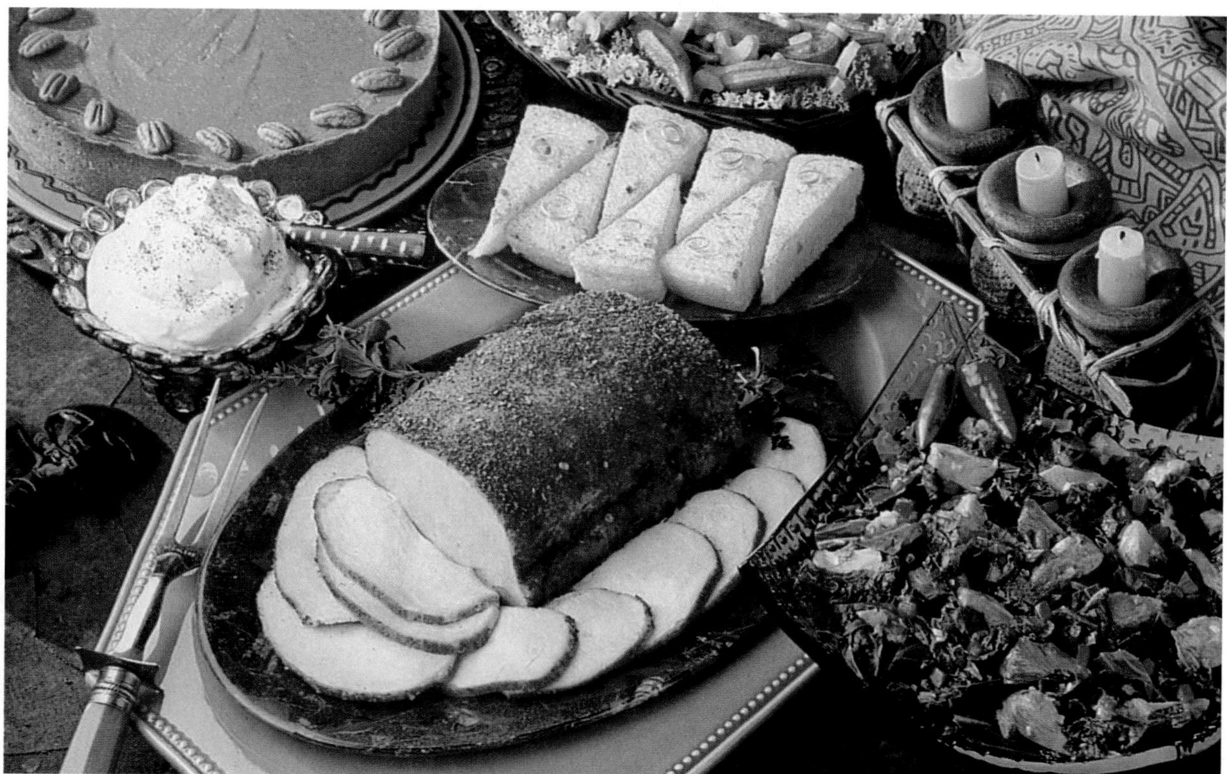

courtesy of National Pork Board

27-5 *Traditional soul foods include okra, grits, greens, pork, and sweet potato pie—foods that were available to African slaves in the South.*

Americans. The contributions of each group have come together to give Creole foods a character all their own. For instance, the French contributed *bouillabaisse* (a highly seasoned fish stew), court bouillon, and pastries. The Africans contributed okra, which is used as both a vegetable and a thickening agent in soups and stews. The Spanish contributed tomatoes, red and green peppers, and mixtures of rice, seafood, poultry, and meat. The Choctaw Indians were the first to use filé. (***Filé*** is a flavoring and thickening agent made from sassafras leaves, which are dried and ground into a powder.) The addition of red beans, rice, and a variety of fish and seafood native to Louisiana resulted in many unusual and delicious dishes.

Gumbo is a soup that reflects the various cultures of Southern Louisiana. Although recipes vary, meats, poultry, seafood, okra, and other vegetables are common ingredients. Cooks may thicken gumbo with roux, okra, or filé. Families often hand their gumbo recipes down from generation to generation.

Jambalaya is a traditional Creole rice dish. It contains rice; seasonings; and shellfish, poultry, and/or sausage. Some cooks also add tomatoes. Creole cooks use a hot pepper sauce to season both gumbo and jambalaya.

Gumbo, jambalaya, and red beans and rice (a main dish made from red beans simmered with a small amount of meat) are economical. Creole cooks often made these dishes from leftovers. See 27-6.

Other Creole specialties include beignets, café au lait, café brulot, and pralines. *Beignets* are deep-fried squares of bread dough. Small cafés scattered throughout New Orleans serve them hot with a dusting of powdered sugar. Strong coffee flavored with chicory usually is served with them. *Café au lait* is a beverage made from equal portions of this chicory-flavored coffee and hot milk. *Café brulot* is strong coffee flavored with spices, sugar, citrus peel, and brandy. It often is flamed. *Pralines* are a sweet, rich candy made with sugar, pecans, and sometimes milk or buttermilk. They are sold in candy shops all over the South.

Cajun Cuisine

Cajun cuisine is the hearty fare of rural Southern Louisiana. It reflects the foods and cooking methods of the Acadians, French, Native Americans, Africans, and Spanish. (Acadians are French-speaking immigrants from a part of Nova Scotia called Acadia.) Like Creole cuisine, jambalayas and gumbos characterize Cajun cuisine. These dishes are seasoned heavily with hot peppers and other spicy seasonings. Cajun dishes are generally prepared from foods that are commonly available in Southern Louisiana. Crawfish, okra, rice, pecans, beans, and *andouille* (smoked pork sausage) frequently appear in Cajun recipes. Many dishes center around locally available game and seafood. They are creative combinations of whatever happens to be on hand and are often prepared from leftovers.

Traditional Cajun dishes include chaudin, rice dressing, and tartes douces. *Chaudin* is braised pig stomach stuffed with ground pork, onions, bell peppers, garlic, and diced yams. *Rice dressing* is rice cooked with bits of chicken liver, chicken gizzard, and/or ground pork and seasoned with parsley and onion tops. *Tartes douces* are pies made with a soft, sweet crust and fillings like custard, blackberry, coconut, or sweet potato.

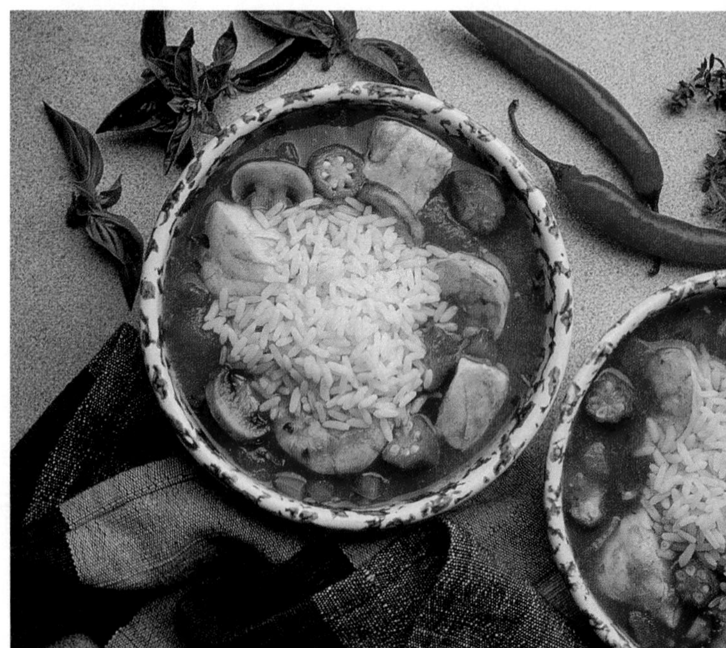

USA Rice Federation

27-6 *Gumbo recipes vary throughout the South. This one contains seafood and vegetables thickened with okra.*

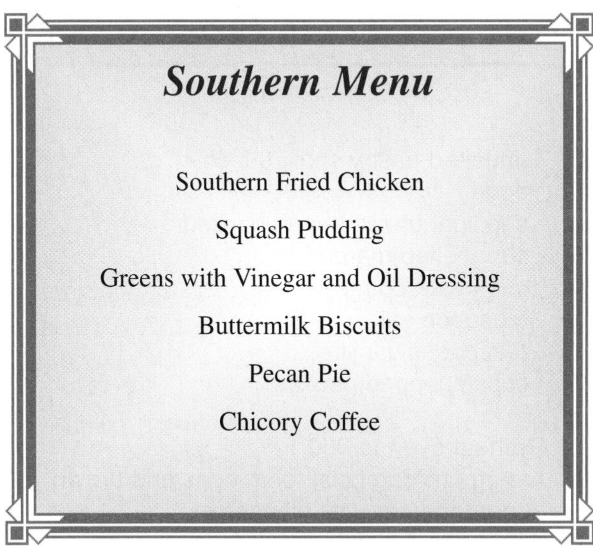

Southern Menu

Southern Fried Chicken

Squash Pudding

Greens with Vinegar and Oil Dressing

Buttermilk Biscuits

Pecan Pie

Chicory Coffee

Southern Fried Chicken

Serves 5

1 3-pound fryer, cut into pieces
1/2 cup all-purpose flour
1 teaspoon salt
1/4 teaspoon pepper
1/2 cup evaporated fat free milk
1 egg
shortening or oil for frying

1. Wash chicken pieces and pat dry with a paper towel.
2. Combine flour, salt, and pepper in a shallow pan.
3. Beat milk and egg together in a pie plate.
4. Dip chicken pieces in seasoned flour, then in milk mixture, then in flour. Set aside until all pieces are coated.
5. In large, heavy skillet, heat shortening or oil until hot but not smoking.
6. Add chicken pieces, a few at a time. Brown all sides, turning occasionally.
7. When all pieces have been browned, return them to the skillet. Reduce heat, cover tightly, and cook chicken until tender, about 30 minutes. Remove cover the last 10 minutes to crisp chicken.

Per serving: 349 cal. (59% from fat), 29 g protein, 6 g carbohydrate, 23 g fat, 135 mg cholesterol, 0 g fiber, 330 mg sodium.

Squash Pudding

Serves 6 to 8

2 cups hot butternut squash, mashed
1 1/2 tablespoons margarine
1/2 cup sugar
1/3 cup fat free milk
1/2 teaspoon salt
1 teaspoon cinnamon
1 teaspoon nutmeg
3 eggs

1. Preheat oven to 325°F.
2. Add margarine to squash; stir until melted.
3. Add sugar, milk, salt, cinnamon, and nutmeg.
4. Beat with an electric or rotary beater until blended.
5. Beat eggs; blend in squash mixture.
6. Pour into a greased 1 1/2-quart casserole.
7. Bake until internal temperature reads 160°F on a thermometer, about 30 minutes.

Per serving: 163 cal. (33% from fat), 4 g protein, 24 g carbohydrate, 6 g fat, 137 mg cholesterol, 2 g fiber, 253 mg sodium.

Greens with Vinegar and Oil Dressing

Serves 8

1 bunch beet tops
1 bunch kale
1 bunch spinach
1 bunch collards
1/4 cup water
6 slices bacon, cooked and cut into pieces
1 clove garlic, chopped

1. Clean greens. Trim tough ends and bruised spots. Tear into pieces.
2. Place greens in large saucepan with water, bacon, and garlic.
3. Cover and simmer slowly until tender, about 15 minutes.
4. Drain and serve with vinegar and oil.

Per serving: 77 cal. (65% from fat), 3 g protein, 4 g carbohydrate, 6 g fat, 4 mg cholesterol, 0 g fiber, 143 mg sodium.

Buttermilk Biscuits

Makes about 15 biscuits

2 cups all-purpose flour
1 tablespoon baking powder
1/2 teaspoon salt
1/4 cup shortening
2/3 to 3/4 cup buttermilk

1. Preheat oven to 425°F.
2. In large mixing bowl, combine flour, baking powder, and salt.
3. Using a pastry blender or two knives, cut in shortening until mixture resembles small peas.
4. Add buttermilk, stirring gently with fork until soft dough forms.
5. Turn dough out onto lightly floured board. Knead 8 to 10 times.
6. Roll to 1/2-inch thickness. Cut into rounds with 2-inch biscuit cutter.
7. Place biscuits close together on an ungreased baking sheet.
8. Bake 10 to 12 minutes or until golden brown. Serve hot.

Per biscuit: 97 cal. (34% from fat), 2 g protein, 14 g carbohydrate, 4 g fat, 0 mg cholesterol, 1 g fiber, 147 mg sodium.

Pecan Pie

Makes one 9-inch pie

1 unbaked pastry shell, 9-inch
4 eggs
1/3 cup light brown sugar, packed
1/4 cup melted margarine
1 1/4 cups dark corn syrup
1/2 teaspoon salt
1 1/2 teaspoons vanilla
1 1/4 cups chopped pecans

1. Preheat oven to 350°F.
2. In large mixing bowl, beat eggs and brown sugar together until blended.
3. Add melted margarine, corn syrup, salt, vanilla, and chopped pecans and mix thoroughly; pour into unbaked pie shell.
4. Bake until filling is puffed and golden brown, about 35 to 40 minutes.
5. Serve pie slightly warm or cool and top with whipped cream.

1/8 of pie: 426 cal. (56% from fat), 6 g protein, 42 g carbohydrate, 28 g fat, 137 mg cholesterol, 2 g fiber, 388 mg sodium.

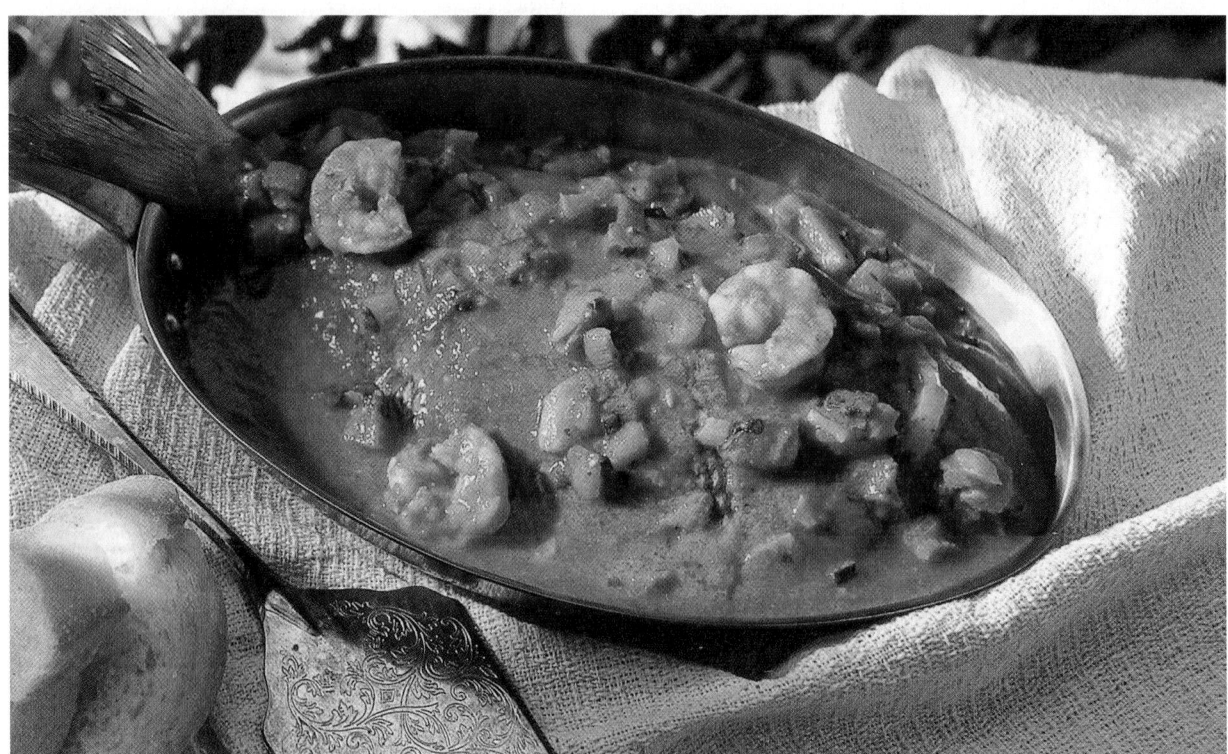

Louisiana Office of Tourism

Shrimp Creole is a highly seasoned dish made with tomatoes, peppers, okra, and rice.

Midwest

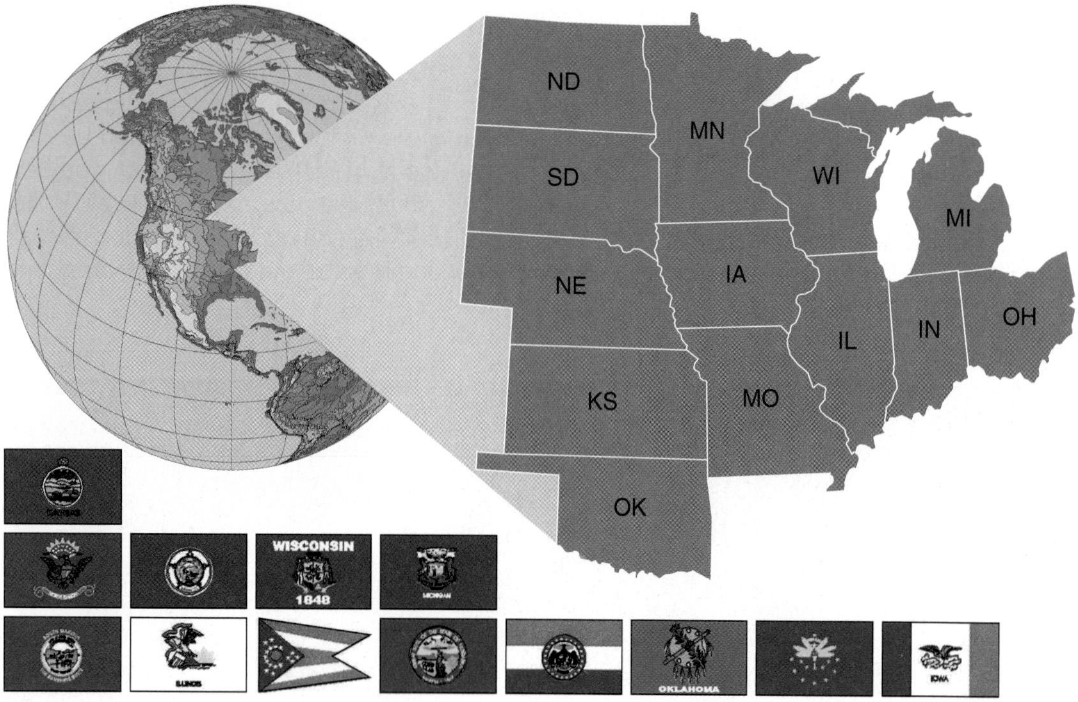

People often call the Midwest the "breadbasket" of the nation. Rich soil, good climate, and advanced farming techniques have made the Midwest one of the world's most agriculturally productive regions. Corn, wheat, and soybeans grow in large enough quantities to be exported to many parts of the world.

Beef, pork, lamb, and poultry are produced in large quantities in the Midwest. Lakes and streams in this region provide a variety of fish. People throughout the United States recognize Wisconsin and Minnesota for their dairy products. Small farms throughout the Midwest grow many kinds of fruits and vegetables.

Fairs, festivals, and picnics are popular in the Midwest. Food plays an important part at these gatherings, 27-7. Homemade breads, cakes, pies, cookies, jams, and jellies are judged at county and state fairs. Cities and towns in many parts of the Midwest hold festivals centered on apples, pumpkins, strawberries, and other fruits and vegetables.

Buffet dinners and potlucks are traditional gatherings in the Midwest. For a buffet dinner, cooks fill a large table with meat dishes, potatoes, other vegetables, fruits, and baked goods. A ***potluck*** is a shared meal to which each person or family brings food for the whole group to eat. These meals get their name from a tradition of hospitality in which a prepared meal would be shared with an unexpected guest. Since the cook did not know the guest was coming, the guest

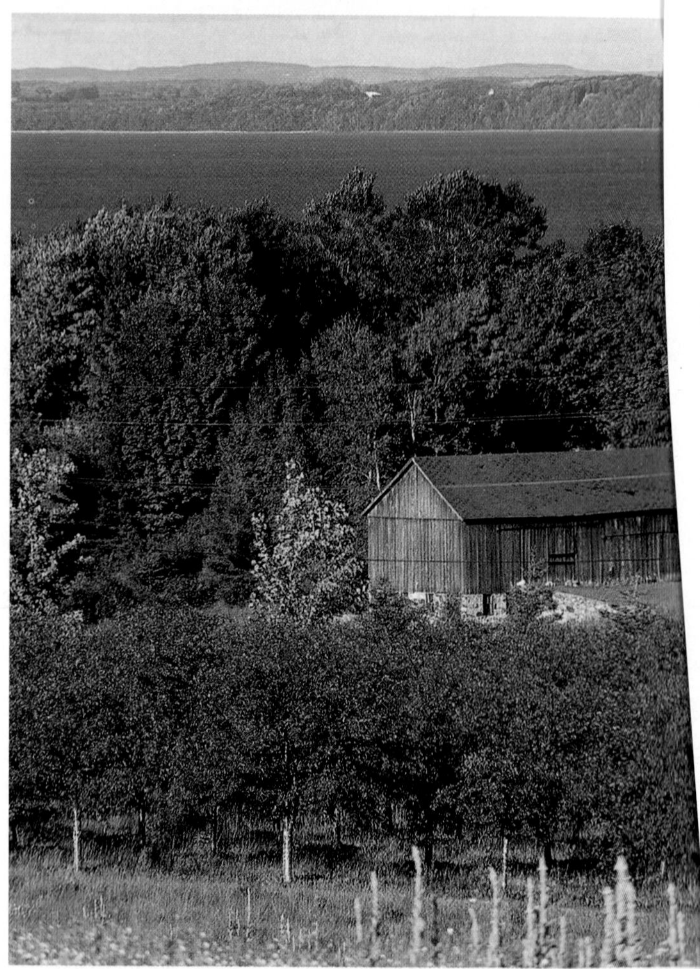

Cherry Marketing Institute

The Midwest is home to many fruit orchards as well as grain fields.

would have to take "the luck of the pot." Potlucks are popular social gatherings with churches, clubs, and family groups.

Midwestern cooking, as a whole, is hearty and uncomplicated. Broiled steak, roast beef, baked and hash brown potatoes, and corn on the cob are staples of the Midwestern diet. Coleslaw, fresh tomatoes from the garden, home baked rolls, apple pie, and brownies also belong to the Midwest. Fruit, hot cereal or cornmeal mush, pancakes, bacon, eggs, toast, and coffee might be served at a filling Midwestern breakfast.

Ethnic foods from immigrants who settled in large Midwestern cities have been added to the foods of the farm. Swedish meatballs, Greek moussaka, German bratwurst, Polish sausage, and Italian lasagna have become almost as common as steak and potatoes.

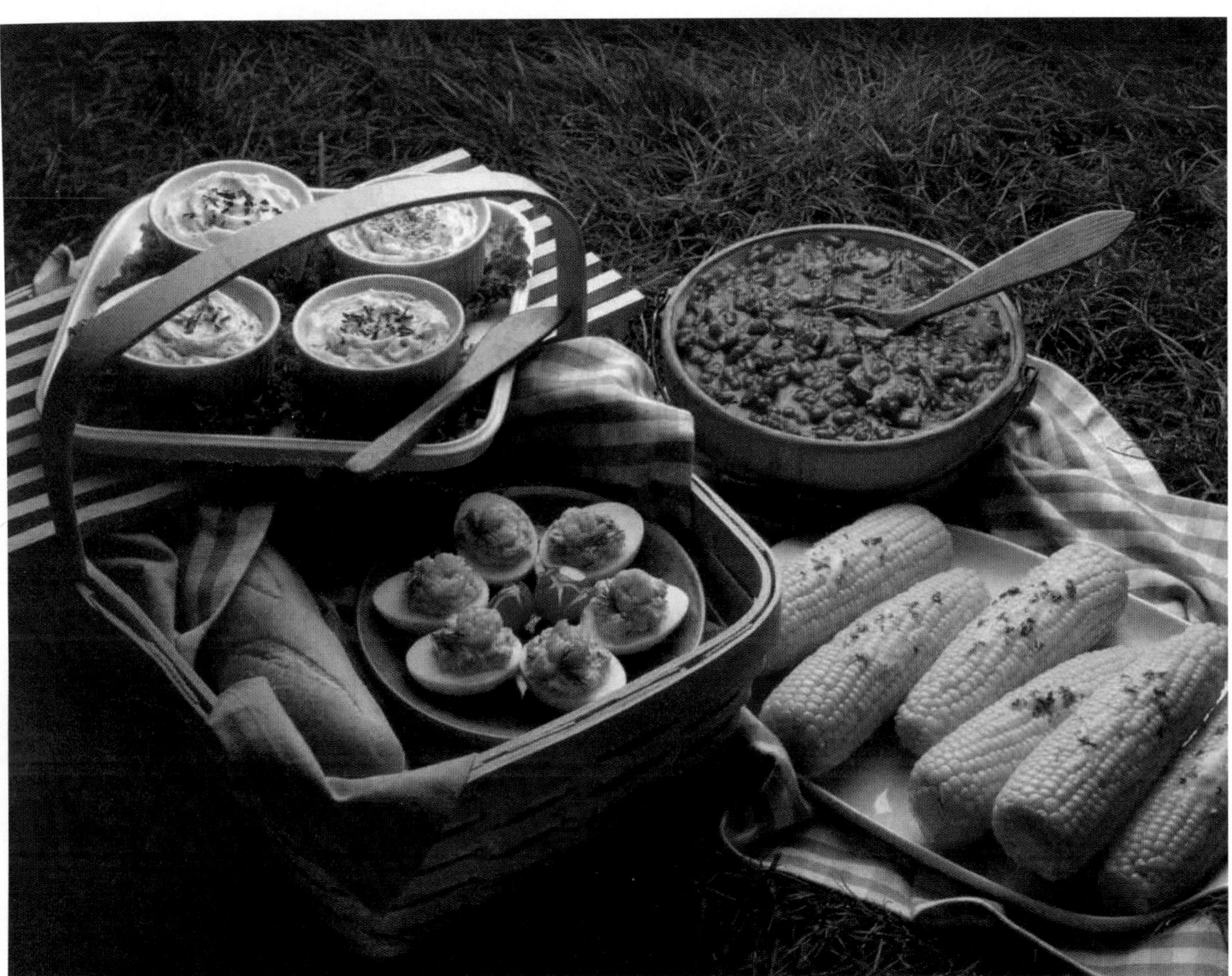

photo courtesy of Land O'Lakes, Inc.

27-7 Baked beans, deviled eggs, and corn on the cob are among the tasty foods that are likely to be served at a Midwestern picnic.

Midwestern Menu
Broiled Steak
Baked Potatoes
Sauteed Zucchini
Sliced Tomatoes
Warm Whole Wheat Bread
Deep Dish Apple Pie
Milk Coffee

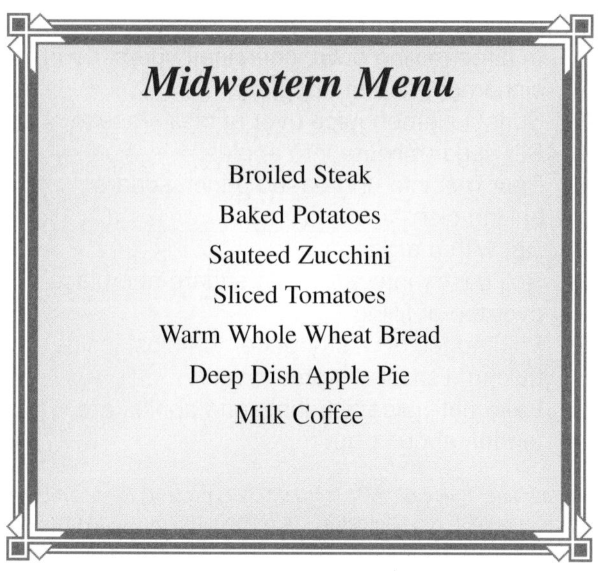

Broiled Steak

Serves 8

2 sirloin steaks, each about 1-inch thick and weighing 1 pound, 10 ounces
salt
pepper
garlic powder

1. Preheat broiler.
2. Trim fat from edges of steaks with a sharp knife.
3. Wipe steaks with damp paper towels; place on broiler pan.
4. Broil steaks 2 to 3 inches from the heat until brown.
5. Season with salt, pepper, and garlic powder and turn; finish broiling. Test doneness with a meat thermometer. Medium rare steaks should reach an internal temperature of 145°F in about 18 to 22 minutes. Medium steaks should reach an internal temperature of 160°F in about 20 to 25 minutes.

Per serving: 196 cal. (38% from fat), 29 g protein, 0 g carbohydrate, 8 g fat, 83 mg cholesterol, 0 g fiber, 240 mg sodium.

Baked Potatoes

Serves 6

6 medium baking potatoes
margarine
salt
pepper

1. Preheat oven to 350°F.
2. Scrub potatoes under cold running water.
3. Pierce skins in several places with the tines of a fork.
4. Place potatoes in oven and bake until fork pierces potato easily, about 45 minutes to 1 hour.
5. Remove from oven.
6. Using pot holders, roll potatoes gently between hands for a minute or two.
7. Make a slit in the top of each potato and push gently.
8. Top with margarine, salt, and pepper. If desired, serve potatoes with shredded reduced fat cheese or plain nonfat yogurt and chives.

Per potato: 180 cal. (19% from fat), 3 g protein, 34 g carbohydrate, 4 g fat, 0 mg cholesterol, 3 g fiber, 410 mg sodium.

Sauteed Zucchini

Serves 6

6 small zucchini
2 tablespoons margarine
3/4 teaspoon dried dill weed

1. Wash zucchini. Trim and discard ends. Cut into 1/4-inch slices.
2. Melt margarine in a skillet. Add zucchini and saute until crisp-tender (about 5 to 8 minutes), stirring occasionally.
3. Sprinkle with dill weed. Serve immediately.

Per serving: 61 cal. (59% from fat), 2 g protein, 6 g carbohydrate, 4 g fat, 0 mg cholesterol, 2 g fiber, 51 mg sodium.

Whole Wheat Bread

Makes 2 loaves

5 1/2 to 6 cups all-purpose flour
2 cups whole wheat flour
3 tablespoons sugar
2 teaspoons salt
2 packages active dry yeast
2 cups fat free milk
3/4 cup water
1/4 cup softened margarine

1. On a large sheet of waxed paper, combine all-purpose and whole wheat flours.
2. In large mixing bowl, combine 2½ cups flour mixture, sugar, salt, and dry yeast.
3. In small saucepan, combine milk, water, and margarine. Heat over low until very warm (120°F to 130°F). Margarine does not need to completely melt.
4. Gradually add warm liquids to dry ingredients; beat at medium speed of electric mixer two minutes.
5. Add 1 cup flour mixture and beat on high speed another 2 minutes, scraping bowl occasionally.
6. Stir in enough additional flour mixture to make a stiff dough.
7. Turn dough out onto lightly floured board or pastry cloth. Knead until smooth and elastic, about 8 to 10 minutes.
8. Cover with plastic wrap and then a towel. Let rest 20 minutes.
9. Divide dough in half. Roll each half into a rectangle.
10. Shape into loaves and place in two greased 9 × 5-inch loaf pans.
11. Brush tops with oil.
12. Cover with plastic wrap and refrigerate 2 to 24 hours.
13. When ready to bake, remove dough from refrigerator; let stand 10 minutes.
14. Using a greased toothpick, prick any bubbles that may have formed.
15. Bake bread at 400°F about 40 minutes or until loaves are golden and sound hollow when tapped with knuckles.
16. Remove bread from pans and cool thoroughly before storing.

Per slice: 134 cal. (12% from fat), 4 g protein, 25 g carbohydrate, 2 g fat, 0 mg cholesterol, 2 g fiber, 159 mg sodium.

Deep Dish Apple Pie

Serves 9

1 cup sugar
½ cup light brown sugar, packed
½ cup all-purpose flour
1 teaspoon cinnamon
¾ teaspoon nutmeg
2 tablespoons lemon juice
12 cups sliced, pared tart apples
2 tablespoons margarine, cut into chunks
pastry for a single-crust, 9-inch pie

1. Preheat oven to 425°F.
2. In large mixing bowl, combine sugars, flour, cinnamon, and nutmeg; mix well.
3. Sprinkle lemon juice over apples. Toss to coat.
4. Stir sugar mixture into apples.
5. Pour fruit into ungreased 9-inch square baking dish.
6. Dot with margarine.
7. Roll pastry into a 10-inch square and place over top of filling.
8. Fold edges of pastry under to fit just inside baking dish. Make steam vents.
9. Bake until juice is bubbly and apples are tender, about 1 hour.

Per serving: 366 cal. (22% from fat), 2 g protein, 72 g carbohydrate, 9 g fat, 0 mg cholesterol, 4 g fiber, 165 mg sodium.

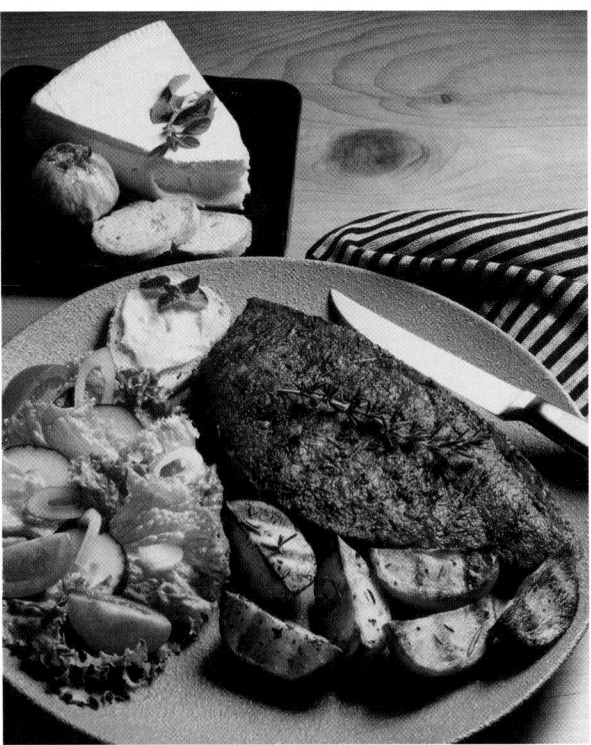

A classic Midwestern menu might include steak, potatoes, and a salad.

West and Southwest

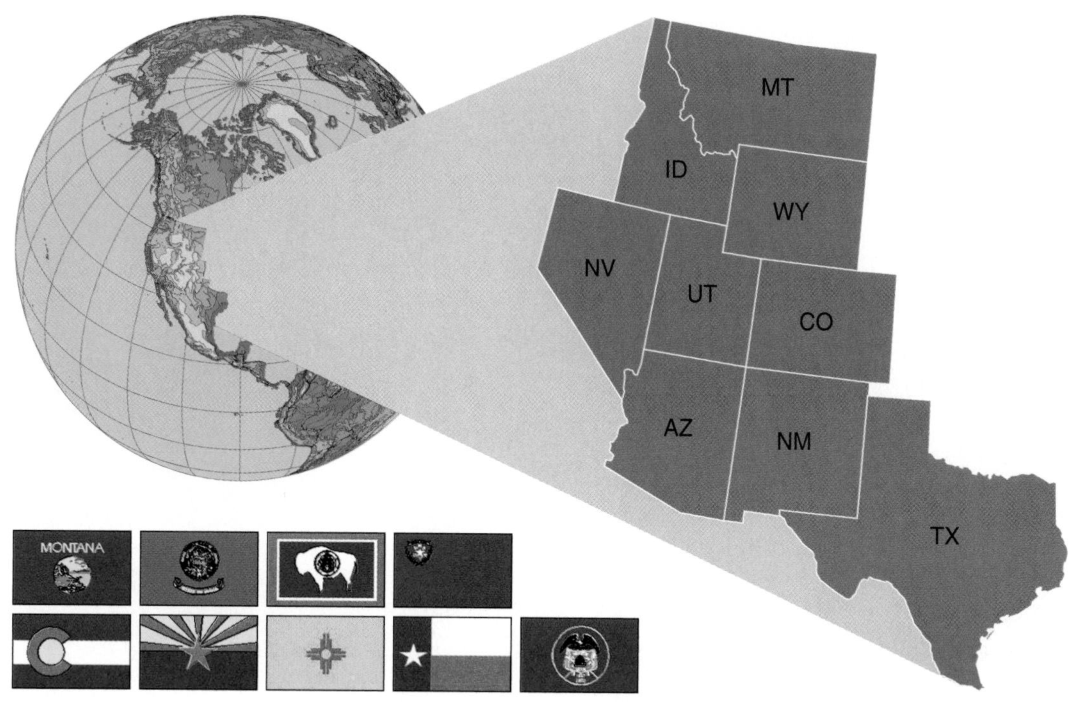

The western part of the United States is a land of contrasts. Abandoned mining towns, desolate deserts, sprawling ranches, mountains, plateaus, and oil fields make up much of the landscape.

Westerners tend to eat simply. They enjoy meat and game, homemade breads and biscuits, and locally grown fruits and vegetables.

Beef plays an important part in Western cooking. Western cooks grill, spit barbecue, and pit barbecue. Depending on the occasion, they might roast a whole steer at one time.

Lamb is also quite popular in some parts of the West. It usually is roasted or stewed. In remote areas, wild game accounts for quite a bit of the meat in the diet. Antelope, rabbit, deer, and pheasant are among the game animals used for meat.

Many people associate chuck wagons and cowboys with the Southwest. However, Native Americans, Spaniards, and Mexicans also influenced the development of Southwestern cuisine. The foods of Native Americans in this region included corn, squash, and beans. To these, the Spanish added cattle, sheep, saffron, olive oil, and anise. The Aztecs of Mexico introduced red and green peppers.

The cattle introduced by the Spanish eventually developed into the longhorn breed. They

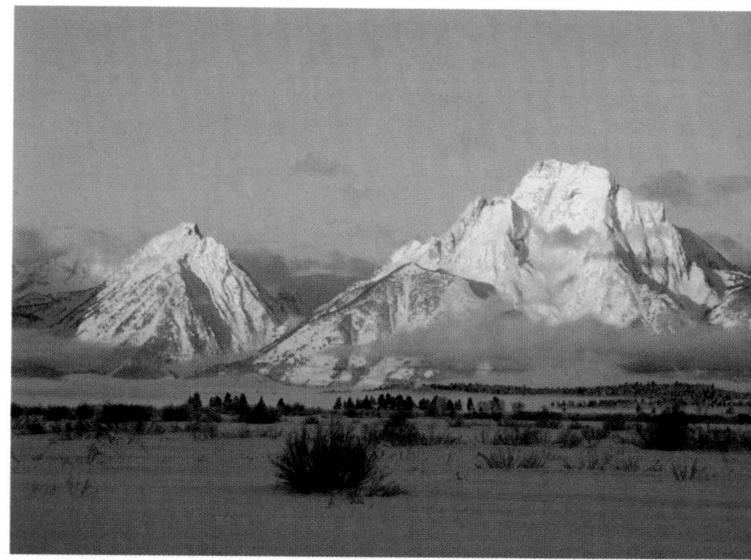

The peaks of the majestic Teton Range rise more than a mile above the valley floor below.

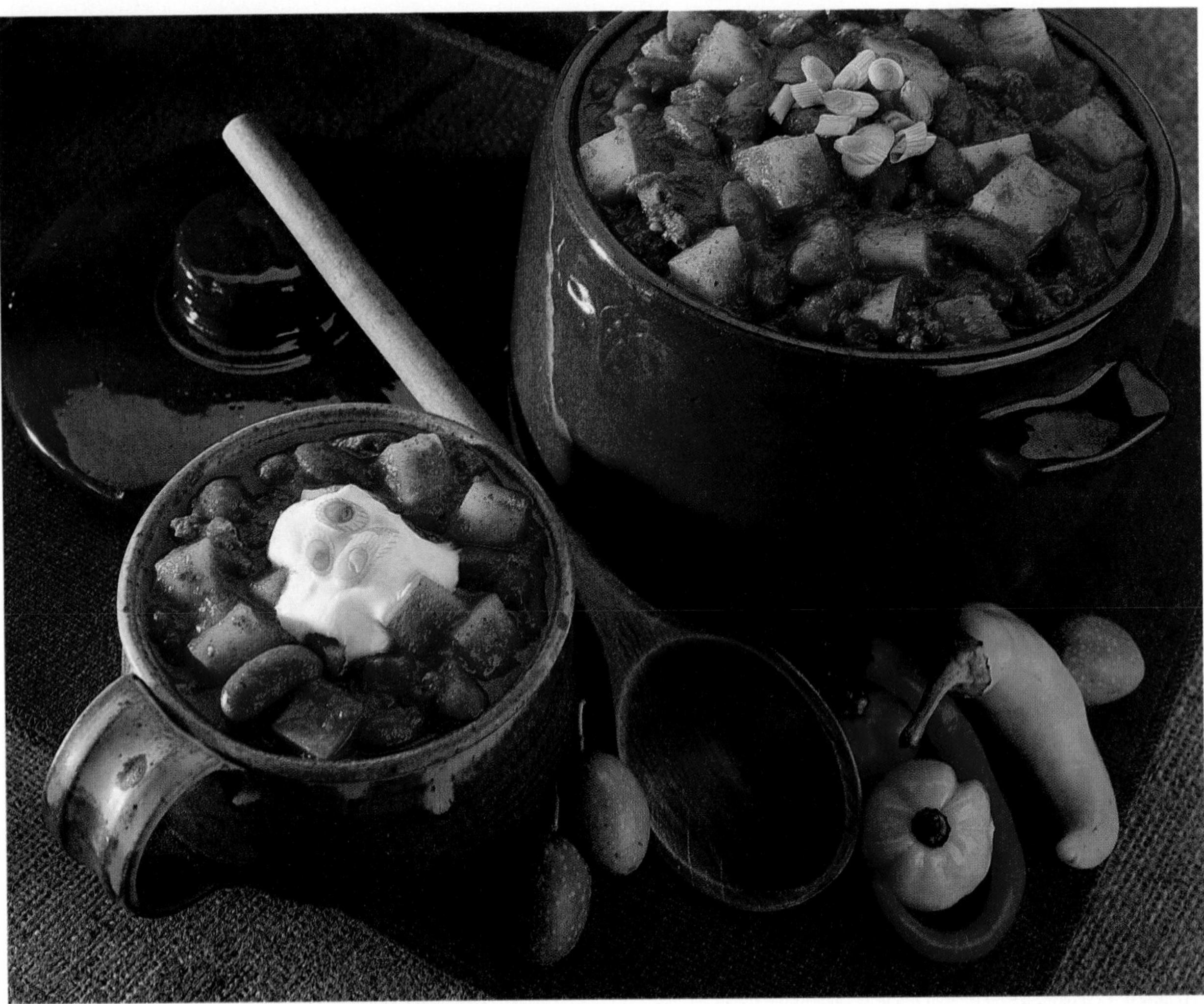

Idaho Potato Commission

27-8 Many variations of chili have evolved since the first spicy version developed by the Texans.

roamed the plains from Texas to California and north into the Dakotas. Long cattle drives ended at the railroad yards where the cattle were shipped east. Here, stories of the cowboy and the chuck wagon originated.

Beef has always been an important staple food in the Southwest. Trail cooks used the tongue, liver, sweetbreads, and heart of a freshly slaughtered steer to make *son-of-a-gun* stew, a favorite of the cowboys. They often served beans and homemade biscuits with the spicy stew. They used chunks of beef in chili, chuck wagon beans, and many other filling dishes. Although some people think of chili as a Mexican dish, Texans claim to have originated it. They made the first chili with cubes of beef, peppers, and seasonings. It did not include beans, 27-8.

From across the Rio Grande came the spicy Mexican foods, which the Southwesterners quickly adopted. Beans, corn, and dishes like tortillas, tostadas, and tacos all have Mexican origins. Other popular Southwestern foods that originated in Mexico are *tamales* (a mixture of cornmeal and peppered ground meat that is wrapped in corn husks and steamed) and *sopapillas* (sweet fried pastries).

Barbecues continue to be an important part of Southwestern cooking. People in this region often baste their meat with a spicy tomato-based sauce during grilling.

The climate of the Southwest is hot and sunny, so many fruits and vegetables grow year-round. Texas produces large quantities of grapefruit, oranges, and strawberries. Farmers in the Rio Grande valley grow early season melons, lettuce, and other fruits and vegetables. Refrigerated trucks transport these fruits and vegetables to all parts of the United States.

Southwestern Menu
Nachos
Barbecued Beef Short Ribs
Three Bean Salad
Tossed Greens with Ranch Dressing
Mexican Cornbread
Sopapillas
Coffee

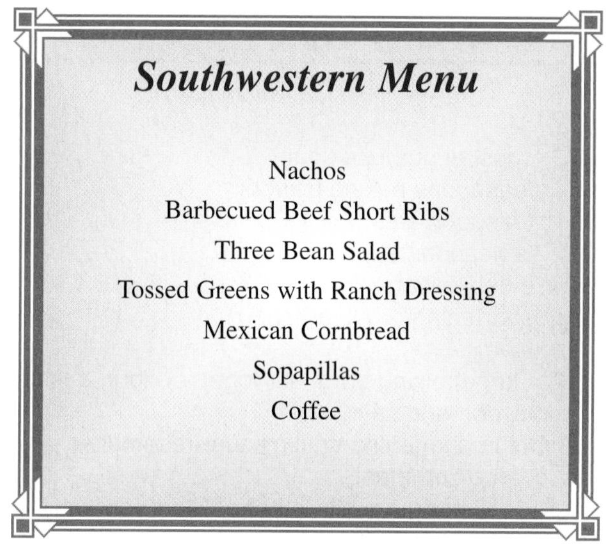

Nachos

Makes 24 appetizers

- cooking spray
- 6 corn tortillas
- 1/4 pound sharp Cheddar cheese, grated
- 3 jalapeno peppers, sliced
- 1/2 cup light sour cream

1. Coat a baking sheet with cooking spray.
2. Cut tortillas into quarters and spread on prepared baking sheet.
3. Bake at 350°F for 10 minutes, or until golden and crispy.
4. Remove baking sheet from oven. Sprinkle tortilla wedges with grated cheese and top each with a jalapeno slice.
5. Place pan under broiler and broil just until cheese melts.
6. Top each nacho with a teaspoon of sour cream. Serve immediately.

Per nacho: 36 cal. (50% from fat), 2 g protein, 3 g carbohydrate, 2 g fat, 6 mg cholesterol, 0 g fiber, 33 mg sodium.

Barbecued Beef Short Ribs

Serves 6

- 3 pounds beef short ribs, cut into serving-sized pieces
- 1 1/2 cups tomato sauce
- 1 teaspoon beef bouillon granules
- 1/3 cup red wine vinegar
- 1/4 cup brown sugar, firmly packed
- 2 tablespoons Worcestershire sauce
- 1 1/2 teaspoons garlic salt
- 1 1/2 teaspoons prepared mustard
- 2 lemons, sliced thinly
- 1 medium onion, sliced thinly

1. Preheat oven to 350°F.
2. Place short ribs in a deep roasting pan.
3. In a small bowl, combine tomato sauce, bouillon granules, red wine vinegar, brown sugar, Worcestershire sauce, garlic salt, and prepared mustard.
4. Pour sauce over ribs; place lemon and onion slices over sauce.
5. Bake ribs, covered, until tender, 1 1/2 to 2 hours.
6. Serve ribs with sauce.

Per serving: 304 cal. (41% from fat), 27 g protein, 19 g carbohydrate, 14 g fat, 75 mg cholesterol, 2 g fiber, 456 mg sodium.

Three Bean Salad

Serves 6 to 8

- 1 1/2 cups canned red kidney beans, drained
- 1 cup canned green beans, drained
- 1 cup canned chickpeas, drained
- 1/2 cup finely chopped onion
- 1/4 teaspoon garlic powder
- 1 1/2 tablespoons chopped parsley
- 2 small green peppers, seeded and chopped
- 1/2 teaspoon salt
- dash pepper
- 1/3 cup red wine vinegar
- 1 teaspoon sugar
- 1/3 cup vegetable oil

1. Using a strainer or colander, rinse drained beans and chickpeas under cold running water; drain and rinse beans again. Pat beans dry with paper towels.
2. In a large bowl, combine beans, chickpeas, onion, garlic powder, parsley, green pepper, salt, and pepper; mix well.
3. In small bowl, combine vinegar, sugar, and oil.
4. Pour dressing over beans and toss.
5. Let salad stand in refrigerator for an hour before serving.

Per serving: 171 cal. (50% from fat), 5 g protein, 17 g carbohydrate, 10 g fat, 0 mg cholesterol, 5 g fiber, 318 mg sodium.

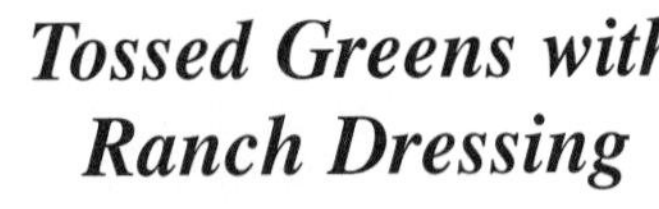

Tossed Greens with Ranch Dressing

Serves 6

- 3/4 cup plain nonfat yogurt
- 1 1/2 teaspoons prepared mustard
- 1 1/2 teaspoons lemon juice
- 1 tablespoon chopped green onion (tops and bottoms)
- 1 tablespoon chives
- 5 to 6 cups assorted salad greens

1. In small bowl, combine yogurt, mustard, lemon juice, onion, and chives.
2. Cover and refrigerate dressing until well chilled.
3. Clean salad greens and tear into bite-sized pieces.
4. When ready to serve, place greens in large salad bowl. Toss with dressing and serve immediately.

Per serving: 33 cal. (17% from fat), 3 g protein, 5 g carbohydrate, 1 g fat, 2 mg cholesterol, 1 g fiber, 60 mg sodium.

Mexican Corn Bread

Serves 8

- 1 cup cornmeal
- 1 cup all-purpose flour
- 1 cup buttermilk
- 3/4 teaspoon baking soda
- 1/4 teaspoon salt
- 1/2 cup onion, chopped
- 2 eggs, beaten
- 2 tablespoons cooking oil
- 1 can cream-style corn, low sodium
- 1/2 cup green pepper, chopped
- 1/4 pound Cheddar cheese, grated

1. Preheat oven to 350°F.
2. In medium bowl, combine all ingredients except cheese.
3. Pour half the batter in a 2 1/2-quart casserole.
4. Cover with half the grated Cheddar cheese.
5. Add the other half of the batter and cover with the remaining cheese.
6. Bake until corn bread is golden brown and tests done, about 40 minutes.

Per serving: 219 cal. (41% from fat), 9 g protein, 26 g carbohydrate, 10 g fat, 69 mg cholesterol, 4 g fiber, 334 mg sodium.

Sopapillas

Makes about four dozen pastries

- 2 cups all-purpose flour
- 2 1/2 teaspoons baking powder
- 1/2 teaspoon salt
- 1 tablespoon shortening
- 1/2 cup lukewarm water
- shortening or oil for frying

1. In large mixing bowl, stir together flour, baking powder, and salt.
2. Cut in shortening until mixture resembles coarse cornmeal.
3. Add water gradually, stirring with a fork until dough clings together.
4. Turn dough out onto lightly floured board or pastry cloth. Knead until smooth.
5. Divide dough in half. Let rest for 10 minutes.
6. Roll each half into a 10 × 12-inch rectangle about 1/8-inch thick.
7. Cut into 2-inch squares.
8. In deep fryer or large saucepan, heat shortening or oil until it reaches 375°F.
9. Add sopapillas, a few at a time. Fry about 1/2 minute on each side.
10. Serve warm with butter and honey or sprinkle with confectioner's sugar.

Per sopapilla: 31 cal. (41% from fat), 1 g protein, 4 g carbohydrate, 1 g fat, 0 mg cholesterol, 0 g fiber, 39 mg sodium.

Pacific Coast

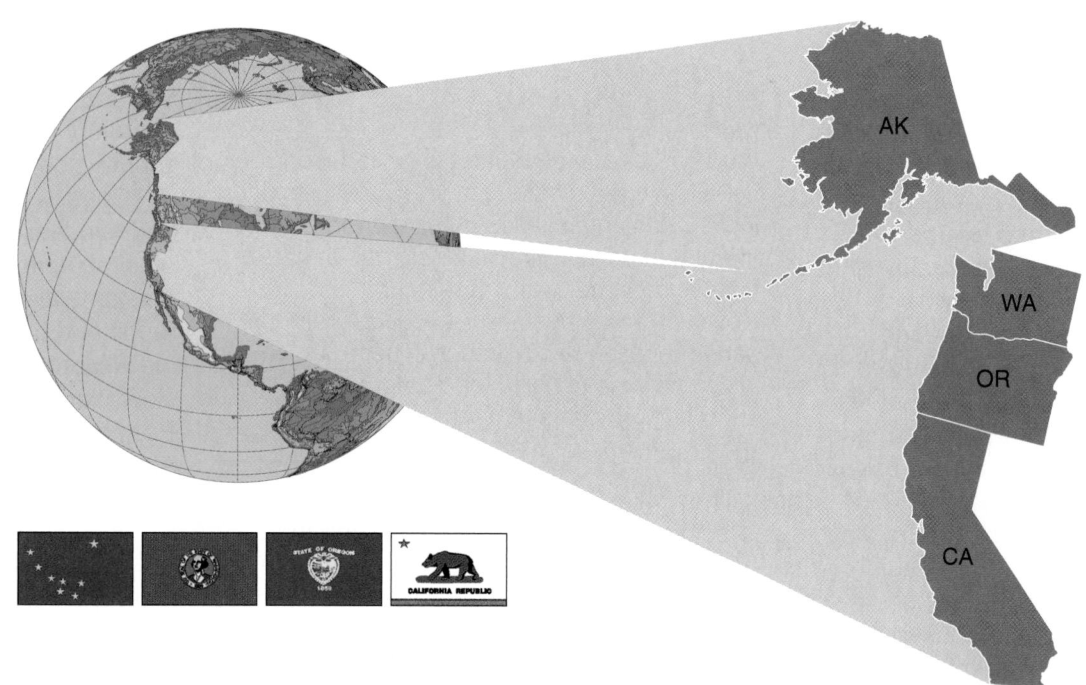

The Pacific Coast includes the states of California, Oregon, Washington, and Alaska. These diverse states vary widely in geography, climate, culture, and food customs.

Most parts of California have rich, fertile soil; a warm, sunny climate; and adequate rainfall. Fruits and vegetables of all kinds grow in abundance. Avocados, papayas, pomegranates, dates, Chinese cabbage, kale, and okra are common, as are oranges, grapefruit, lettuce, and tomatoes.

The ocean and inland lakes provide a bounty of fish and shellfish. Shad, tuna, salmon, abalone, lobsters, crabs, shrimp, and oysters are especially popular.

Few rules or traditions hamper California-style cuisine. They might simply broil salmon steaks and top them with a fresh dill sauce. However, more unusual combinations, such as crab and artichoke hearts or chicken and anchovies, are also popular.

Many of the foods that are part of California's cuisine are also available in Oregon and Washington. Many fruits, including peaches, apples, apricots, strawberries, raspberries, blackberries, blueberries, and boysenberries, grow in Washington and Oregon. Other fruits and vegetables are shipped there from California.

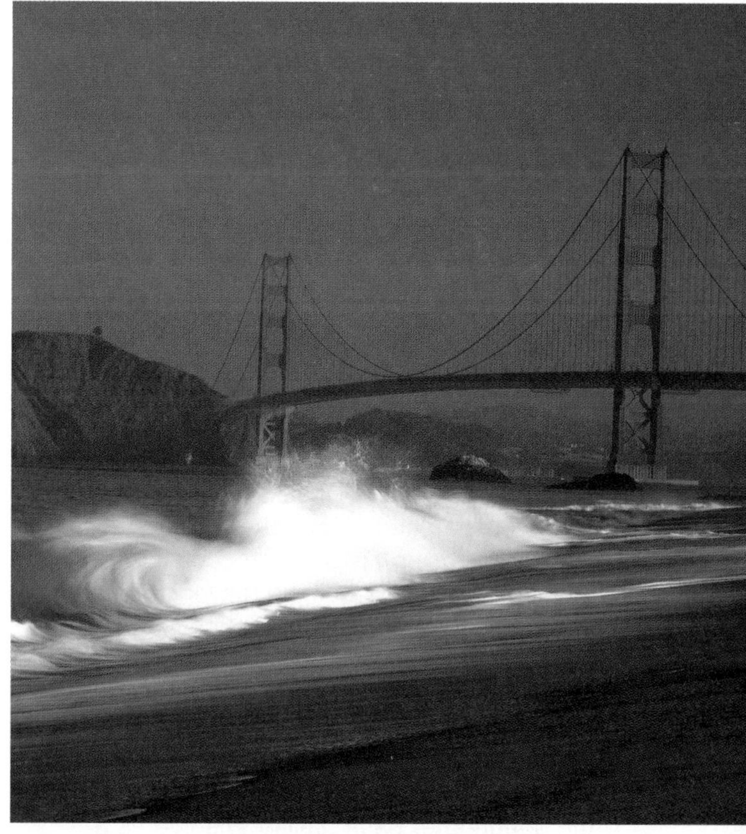

The Golden Gate Bridge in San Francisco is a triumph of twentieth century construction technology.

Steaks, chops, and other standard fare of the United States make up much of the diet of the Pacific Northwest. These foods are supplemented by wild game, fish, and seafood. Dungeness crabs, butter clams, Columbia River salmon, and Olympia oysters are especially popular.

Be a Clever Consumer

If your vacation budget is limited, consider traveling in the off-season. Many facilities offer lower rates at this time. Off-season travel has the added benefit of smaller crowds at attractions and shorter waits at restaurants. However, some businesses reduce their operating hours in the off-season. Therefore, you would be wise to call ahead before going to shop, eat, or sightsee.

Cooking techniques of all the Pacific states are, for the most part, simple. They take advantage of the natural flavors and colors of the foods. Cooks usually bake or broil fresh fish and shellfish. They serve vegetables raw in large salads or cooked just until crisp-tender. They often serve fresh fruits for dessert.

The people who settled the Pacific Coast influenced California's cuisine (and to a lesser extent that of Oregon and Washington). From the Far East came Chinese, Japanese, and Koreans, and from the South Pacific came Polynesians. Many of these immigrants worked as cooks, thus contributing native foods and dishes. Chop suey, for example, was supposedly invented in California by a Chinese cook. He named the dish chop suey, which means everything chopped up.

The Mexicans who settled in Southern California brought native dishes with them. Tacos, tamales, enchiladas, guacamole, chili, and refried beans are all popular in this area of the state. The Spanish brought a type of stew called *cocido* (a mixture of vegetables, beef, lamb, ham, fowl, and a sausage called chorizo).

The prospectors who flocked to the Pacific states in search of gold brought sourdough with them. ***Sourdough*** is a dough containing active yeast plants. It is used as a leavening agent. The prospectors made sourdough by mixing together flour, water, and salt. They exposed the mixture to the air to absorb yeast plants. Then they added the dough to flour, water, and other available ingredients to make a variety of baked products. They always kept a small amount of the dough after each baking to serve as a starter for the next batch. They replenished the starter by adding more flour and water.

Only that part of Alaska that lies within the Arctic region has the long, frigid winters many people associate with the state. Farther south, the climate is more mild, and vegetable, grain, and dairy farms dot the countryside.

Caribou sausage and reindeer steak are Alaskan specialties. Alaskans also enjoy rabbit and bear hunted in the wilderness. The icy, clear waters of the Pacific Ocean provide Alaskan king crab. Glacier-fed lakes and streams provide delicious salmon and trout, 27-9.

Alaskan cooks use the blueberries, huckleberries, and cranberries that grow wild to make pies and sauces. Other Alaskan specialties include fiddlehead ferns (young leaves of certain ferns eaten as greens), raw rose hips (the ripened false fruit of the rosebush), and cranberry catsup.

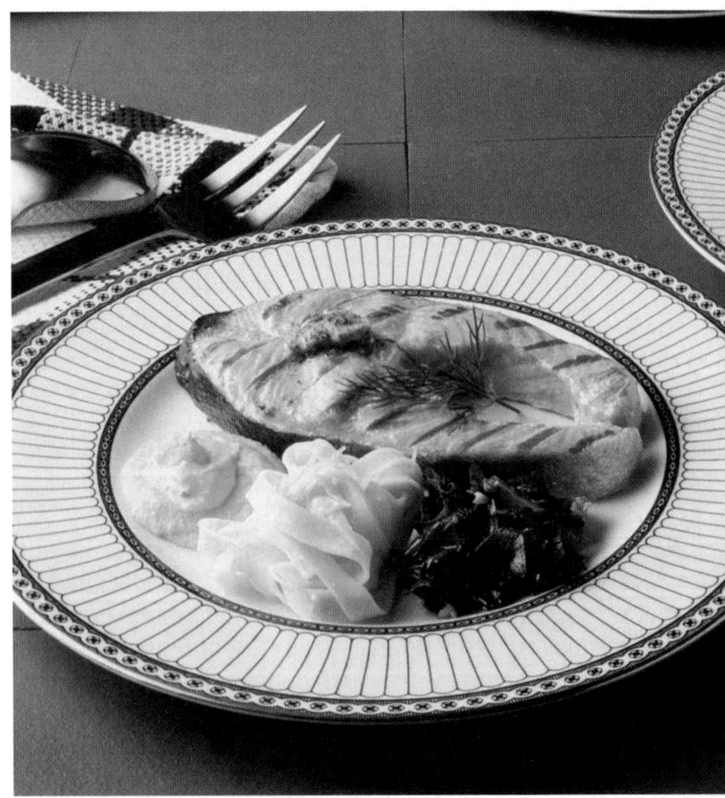

27-9 Alaskan salmon is a popular entree throughout the United States.

Pacific Coast Menu
Salmon Steaks with Dill Sauce
New Potatoes and Peas
Avocado Salad
Sourdough Bread
Blackberry Buckle
Iced Tea

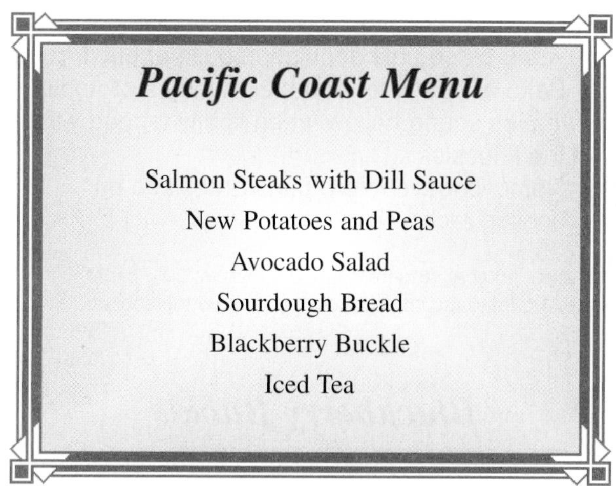

Salmon Steaks with Dill Sauce

Serves 6

1 teaspoon dehydrated minced onion
1 teaspoon chicken bouillon granules
1/2 tablespoon lemon juice
1 teaspoon dill weed
2 cups water
3 salmon steaks (about ½ pound each)
2 tablespoons all-purpose flour
3/4 cup evaporated fat free milk
1/4 cup plain nonfat yogurt
2 teaspoons dill

1. In large skillet, combine onion, bouillon granules, lemon juice, dill weed, and water. Bring to a boil.
2. Add salmon steaks. Reduce heat and cover pan tightly. Simmer steaks over low heat about 8 to 10 minutes or until fish flakes easily with a fork.
3. Remove salmon to a heated platter and keep warm. Reserve ¼ cup poaching liquid.
4. Shake flour and evaporated milk in a small covered container until thoroughly blended.
5. Pour flour mixture into the skillet; add reserved poaching liquid.
6. Cook sauce over low heat, stirring constantly, until smooth and bubbly.
7. Remove from heat and quickly stir in yogurt and dill.
8. Pour sauce over salmon steaks and serve immediately.

Per serving: 306 cal. (44% from fat), 33 g protein, 7 g carbohydrate, 15 g fat, 98 mg cholesterol, 0 g fiber, 299 mg sodium.

New Potatoes and Peas

Serves 5 to 6

1 1/2 pounds new potatoes (or small red skinned potatoes)
1 3/4 cups fresh or frozen peas
margarine
salt and pepper

1. Carefully scrub potatoes.
2. With vegetable peeler or paring knife, remove one thin strip of peel from around the center of each potato.
3. Place potatoes in large saucepan.
4. Cover with cold, lightly salted water. Bring to a boil.
5. Reduce heat and simmer potatoes until tender, about 20 to 25 minutes.
6. About 15 to 20 minutes before you are ready to serve (a little less if frozen peas will be used), shell and wash peas.
7. Bring a small amount of salted water to a boil.
8. Add peas and return water to a boil.
9. Reduce heat and simmer peas, covered, 15 to 20 minutes or until tender. (Check package directions for cooking time for frozen peas.)
10. Drain both potatoes and peas.
11. Toss together with margarine and sprinkle with salt and pepper. Serve immediately.

Per serving: 179 cal. (12% from fat), 5 g protein, 35 g carbohydrate, 2 g fat, 0 mg cholesterol, 5 g fiber, 82 mg sodium.

Avocado Salad

Serves 8

1 large pink grapefruit (or 1 cup canned grapefruit sections)
2 large navel oranges
1 cup green grapes
1/2 cup pomegranate seeds (optional)
4 cups mixed salad greens
2 avocados
1/3 cup walnuts, chopped
3/4 cup lowfat French dressing

1. Section grapefruit and oranges; set aside.
2. Wash grapes and drain well.
3. Remove seeds from pomegranate; set aside.
4. In large salad bowl or on individual salad plates, arrange salad greens. Top with orange and grapefruit sections.

5. Peel and slice avocados. Arrange avocado slices over citrus fruits.
6. Sprinkle with grapes, pomegranate seeds, and walnuts.
7. Serve with French dressing.

Per serving: 167 cal. (54% from fat), 5 g protein, 16 g carbohydrate, 11 g fat, 1 mg cholesterol, 3 g fiber, 27 mg sodium.

Sourdough Bread

Makes 3 loaves

Sourdough starter:
3 1/2 cups bread flour
1 tablespoon sugar
1 package active dry yeast
2 cups warm water
Sourdough bread:
5 to 6 cups all-purpose flour
1 package active dry yeast
3 tablespoons sugar
1 1/4 teaspoons salt
3/4 cup fat free milk
1/4 cup water
2 tablespoons margarine
1 1/2 cups sourdough starter

1. In large bowl or crock, prepare starter by combining flour, sugar, and yeast.
2. Gradually add warm water, beating until smooth.
3. Cover starter tightly and let stand in a warm place for 2 days.
4. When ready to prepare bread, combine 2 1/2 cups flour, yeast, sugar, and salt in a large mixing bowl.
5. Heat milk, water, and margarine until very warm (120°F to 130°F). Margarine does not need to completely melt.
6. Gradually add milk mixture and sourdough starter to dry ingredients. Beat 2 minutes at medium speed, scraping bowl occasionally. Then beat 2 more minutes at high speed.
7. Add enough additional flour to form a stiff dough.
8. Turn out onto a lightly floured board or pastry cloth and knead dough until smooth and elastic, about 8 to 10 minutes.
9. Cover dough with a clean towel and let rise in a warm place until doubled in bulk, about 1 hour.
10. Punch down and divide dough into three equal parts.
11. Shape each into a round loaf.
12. Place loaves on lightly greased baking sheet and slash tops with sharp knife.
13. Cover with a clean towel and let rise in a warm place until doubled in bulk, about 1 hour.
14. Bake at 400°F for about 25 minutes or until loaves sound hollow when lightly tapped with the knuckles.
15. Remove loaves from pans and place on cooling racks.

Per slice: 100 cal. (8% from fat), 3 g protein, 20 g carbohydrate, 1 g fat, 0 mg cholesterol, 1 g fiber, 85 mg sodium.

Blackberry Buckle

Serves 9

1/4 cup margarine
1/2 cup sugar
1 egg, well beaten
1 cup all-purpose flour
1 1/2 teaspoons baking powder
1/8 teaspoon salt
1/3 cup fat free milk
1 teaspoon vanilla
2 cups blackberries
Topping:
1/4 cup sugar
2 tablespoons margarine
2 tablespoons all-purpose flour
1/4 teaspoon cinnamon

1. Preheat oven to 375°F.
2. In medium mixing bowl, cream margarine and sugar until light and fluffy.
3. Add egg and beat well.
4. Sift together flour, baking powder, and salt. Add vanilla to milk.
5. Add liquid and dry ingredients alternately to creamed mixture, beginning and ending with dry ingredients.
6. Pour batter into a greased and floured 9 x 9-inch pan. Cover with blackberries.
7. In small bowl, combine sugar, margarine, flour, and cinnamon.
8. Sprinkle topping over blackberries.
9. Bake buckle for 40 minutes or until cake tests done.
10. Serve warm with whipped cream or ice cream.

Per serving: 221 cal. (36% from fat), 3 g protein, 33 g carbohydrate, 9 g fat, 32 mg cholesterol, 2 g fiber, 183 mg sodium.

Hawaiian Islands

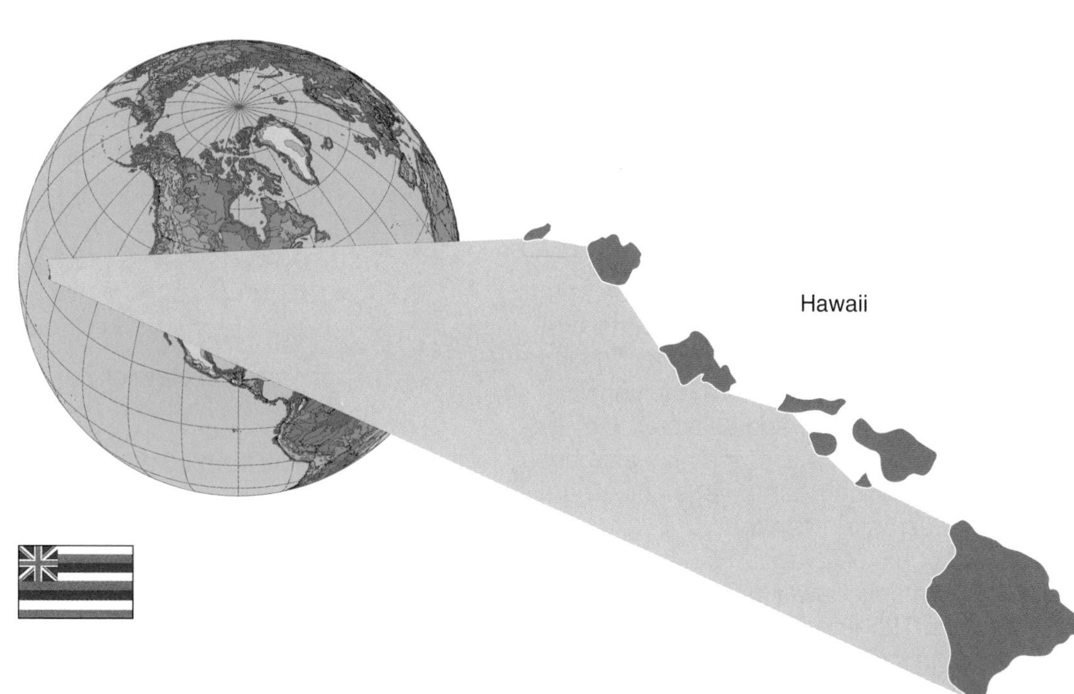

The Hawaiian Islands are much more than a tourist's paradise. They have a rich history and colorful culture. They also have beautiful scenery and delicious food.

Historians believe Hawaii's first settlers were Polynesians from other Pacific islands. After their arrival, Hawaii was isolated from the rest of the world for many years. Although no written records exist, the Hawaiians have a rich heritage of songs and stories.

One of the outstanding figures in Hawaiian history is Kamehameha. Kamehameha eventually captured all of the islands and became king. He was able to establish order and peace throughout the islands.

Christian missionaries and European traders came to Hawaii in the 1800s. Some enterprising foreigners began large sugar plantations. The increasing numbers of Europeans slowly weakened the traditional monarchy. It finally ended with the death of Kamehameha V. Then, in 1898, the United States annexed Hawaii. Hawaii became a state in 1959.

During the last century, Hawaii has grown rapidly. Today, pineapple, sugarcane, and tourism are Hawaii's three largest industries.

The traditional Hawaiian diet was not highly varied. It consisted mainly of *poi,* a smooth paste made from the starchy root of the taro plant. The Hawaiians also ate *limu,* or seaweed, as a relish. Their main sources of protein were

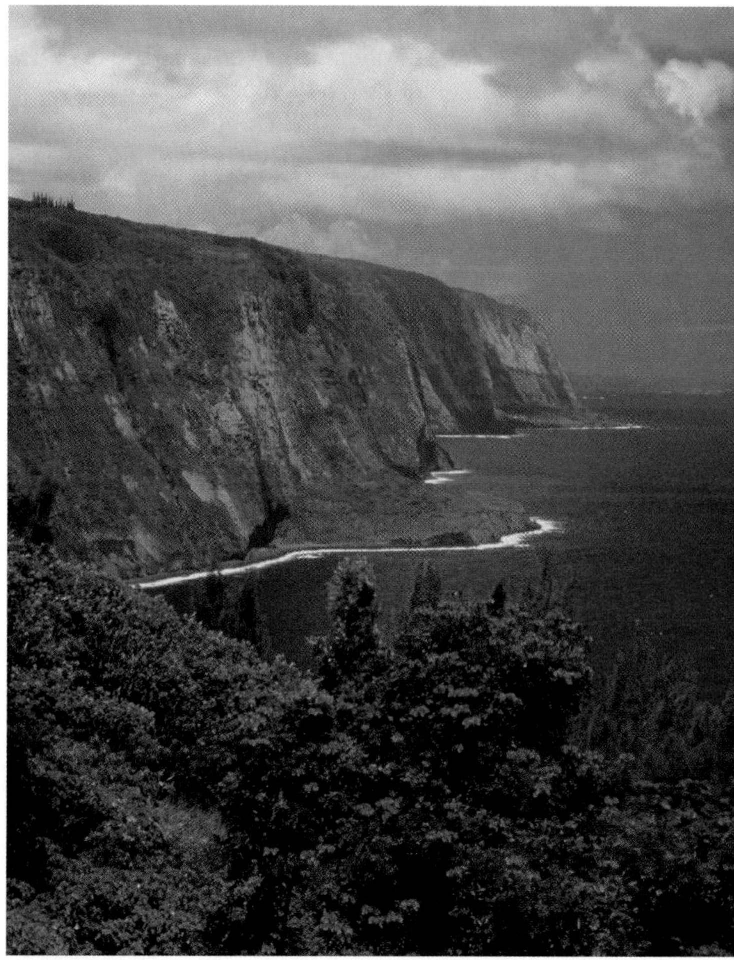

This lush landscape of steep cliffs plunging to the ocean is exemplary of Hawaii's natural beauty.

the numerous varieties of fish they harvested from the waters surrounding the Islands.

The early Hawaiians had some interesting food customs. Unlike many cultures, in the Hawaiian culture men typically prepared the food. Men and women were not permitted to eat at the same table. Their foods were not allowed to be prepared in the same oven, either.

Today, most Hawaiians eat three meals a day. Many Hawaiians have adopted food customs of the mainland. Breakfast may consist of fruit, cereal, eggs, and coffee. However, lunch and dinner may incorporate more traditional Hawaiian foods. Poi, fish, and seaweed may be a typical noon meal. These foods may also be served for dinner, along with a vegetable and a dessert, such as baked bananas.

Throughout history, various groups of people who came to Hawaii each contributed different foods. The first Polynesians are thought to have brought coconuts and *breadfruit* (a round, starchy fruit). European traders are believed to have introduced chicken and pork. The missionaries brought the stews, chowders, and corn dishes of their native New England. Curries reflect Indian influence.

Sugar plantation owners imported large groups of Chinese workers to labor in the fields. The Chinese brought rice, bean sprouts, Chinese cabbage, soybeans, snow peas, and bamboo shoots. They also introduced the stir-fry technique for cooking foods quickly over high heat.

A number of Japanese immigrated to the Hawaiian Islands. They brought with them a variety of rice and fish dishes and pickled foods.

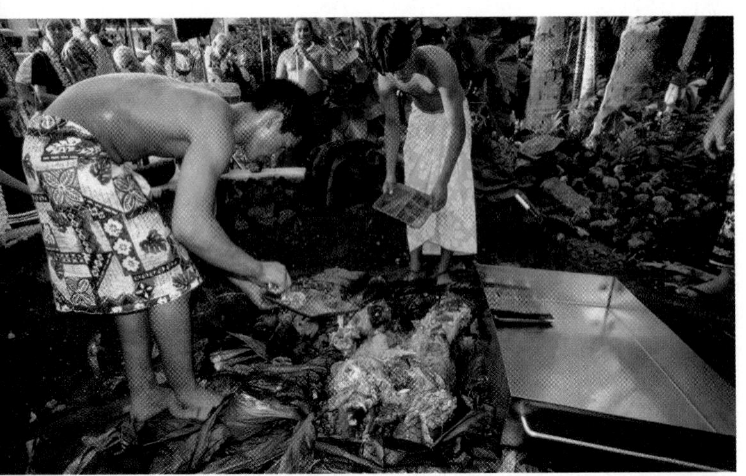

HVCB/Kirk Lee Aeder

27-10 *Foods at a traditional Hawaiian luau are cooked in a pit in the ground called an imu.*

Q: What food group would poi be in?

A: Poi is made from the starchy taro root, which is high in complex carbohydrates. Its nutritional profile is most like that of foods in the breads, cereals, rice, and pasta group.

Contributions from all these groups led to the amazing variety visitors find in Hawaiian markets today. Water chestnuts, watercress, squash, and lotus root are just a few of the many vegetables sold. Papayas, mangoes, and pineapples are among the many locally grown fruits. Lobsters, crabs, opihi (a clamlike mollusk), oysters, shrimp, tuna, snapper, and salmon come from the bounty of the surrounding waters. Other popular items are fresh *tofu* (bean curd), soybean cakes, Japanese fish cake, Korean kim chee, and persimmon tea.

The native Hawaiians held lavish feasts on special occasions. ***Luaus*** are elaborate outdoor feasts that are still popular in the islands today. At these feasts, *kalua puaa* is often served as a main course. This is a whole, young pig that is dressed, stuffed, and cooked in a pit called an ***imu.*** The imu is lined with hot rocks covered with banana leaves. The dressed pig is stuffed with hot rocks and placed on a wire rack. More leaves are placed over the top of the imu followed by more hot rocks and earth. Bananas, sweet potatoes, and meat or seafood dishes wrapped in leaves may be roasted with the pig. After several hours, the pig and other foods are dug from the pit and are ready to serve. See 27-10.

No traditional Hawaiian meal would be complete without poi. Other Hawaiian foods that may be served at a luau include *kamano lomi.* This is salted salmon that is mashed with tomatoes and green onions. *Haupia* is a pudding made of milk, sugar, cornstarch, and grated fresh coconut. A variety of fresh fruits, macadamia nuts, and kukui nuts may be served along with the haupia for dessert.

Musical entertainment, singing, and dancing usually accompany a luau. Guests often join in the festivities.

Hawaiian Menu
Shrimp Curry
Rice
Spinach with Evaporated Milk
Banana Biscuits
Tropical Fruit Medley
Coffee

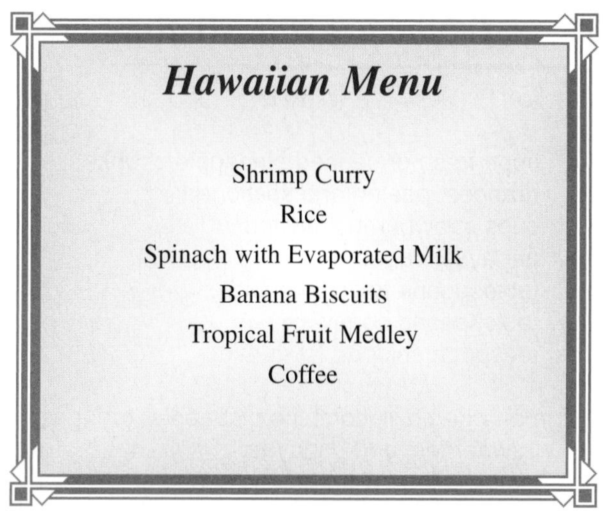

Shrimp Curry

Serves 8

- 1 1/2 pounds fresh shrimp*
- 1 tablespoon margarine
- 2 finely chopped green onions
- 1 teaspoon grated fresh ginger root*
- 3 tablespoons flour
- 1 cup cold fat free milk
- 1 1/2 cups coconut milk*
- 1/2 teaspoon salt
- 2 to 3 teaspoons curry powder
- 6 cups cooked brown rice

1. Clean, peel, and devein the shrimp. Set aside.
2. Melt margarine in a skillet over medium-high heat.
3. Add onion and ginger root. Saute 2 to 3 minutes until onion is tender.
4. Shake flour and milk in a small, tightly covered container until thoroughly blended.
5. Reduce heat to low. Add flour mixture to skillet. Cook sauce, stirring constantly, until smooth and bubbly.
6. When sauce begins to thicken, stir in coconut milk, salt, and curry powder.
7. Cover and allow mixture to simmer over low heat for 10 minutes.
8. Add shrimp. Continue simmering just until shrimp are cooked through, about 5 minutes.
9. Serve over rice. Pass small dishes of several of the following accompaniments: shredded coconut, finely chopped green pepper, finely chopped green onion, pineapple chutney, and/or orange marmalade.

*You can substitute 1 1/2 pounds cooked boneless, skinless chicken breast cut into bite-sized pieces for the shrimp. You can use 1 1/2 teaspoons ground ginger in place of the fresh ginger root. If canned coconut milk is not available, combine 1 1/2 cups shredded packaged coconut with 1 1/2 cups fat free milk in a small saucepan. Allow coconut to soak for 20 minutes. Then simmer over low heat for 10 minutes. Allow mixture to cool. Then strain through two thicknesses of cheesecloth, squeezing out as much milk as possible.

Per serving: 369 cal. (32% from fat), 24 g protein, 39 g carbohydrate, 13 g fat, 167 mg cholesterol, 3 g fiber, 383 mg sodium.

Spinach with Evaporated Milk

Serves 8

- 2 pounds fresh spinach
- 1/2 teaspoon salt
- 1 tablespoon margarine
- 1/4 cup water
- 1/4 cup fat free evaporated milk

1. Wash spinach thoroughly and remove stems.
2. Place spinach, salt, margarine, water, and evaporated milk in a large nonstick saucepan. Cover and cook over medium heat until the spinach begins to wilt.
3. Uncover and cook until spinach is tender, stirring frequently. Serve immediately.

Per serving: 43 cal. (42% from fat), 4 g protein, 5 g carbohydrate, 2 g fat, 0 mg cholesterol, 3 g fiber, 255 mg sodium.

Banana Biscuits

Makes about 15 biscuits

- 1 1/2 cups all-purpose flour
- 2 teaspoons baking powder
- 2 teaspoons sugar
- 1/2 teaspoon salt
- 1 cup mashed bananas
- 3 tablespoons shortening
- 1/4 cup fat free milk
- 1 egg, beaten

1. Preheat oven to 425°F.
2. In a large mixing bowl, combine flour, baking powder, sugar, and salt.

3. In a smaller bowl, thoroughly combine mashed bananas with shortening.
4. Add banana mixture to flour mixture. Using a pastry blender or two knives, cut in bananas until mixture resembles small peas.
5. Combine milk with beaten egg. Gently stir liquids into flour mixture with a fork until a soft dough forms.
6. Turn dough out onto lightly floured board. Knead 8 to 10 times.
7. Roll to 1/2-inch thickness. Cut into rounds with a 2-inch biscuit cutter.
8. Place biscuits close together on an ungreased baking sheet.
9. Bake 12 to 15 minutes or until golden brown. Serve hot.

Per biscuit: 86 cal (31% from fat), 2 g protein, 13 g carbohydrate, 3 g fat, 14 mg cholesterol, 1 g fiber, 114 mg sodium.

Tropical Fruit Medley

Serves 8

2 cups fresh or canned pineapple chunks
2 oranges, peeled and sectioned
3 cups strawberries, halved
2 papayas, cubed
3 tablespoons fresh lime juice
3 tablespoons honey
1 teaspoon snipped fresh mint

1. In a large bowl, combine pineapple, oranges, strawberries, and papayas.
2. Combine lime juice, honey, and mint.
3. Pour dressing over fruit and toss gently to blend. Serve chilled.

Per serving: 106 cal. (8% from fat), 1 g protein, 27 g carbohydrate, 1 g fat, 0 mg cholesterol, 4 g fiber, 3 mg sodium.

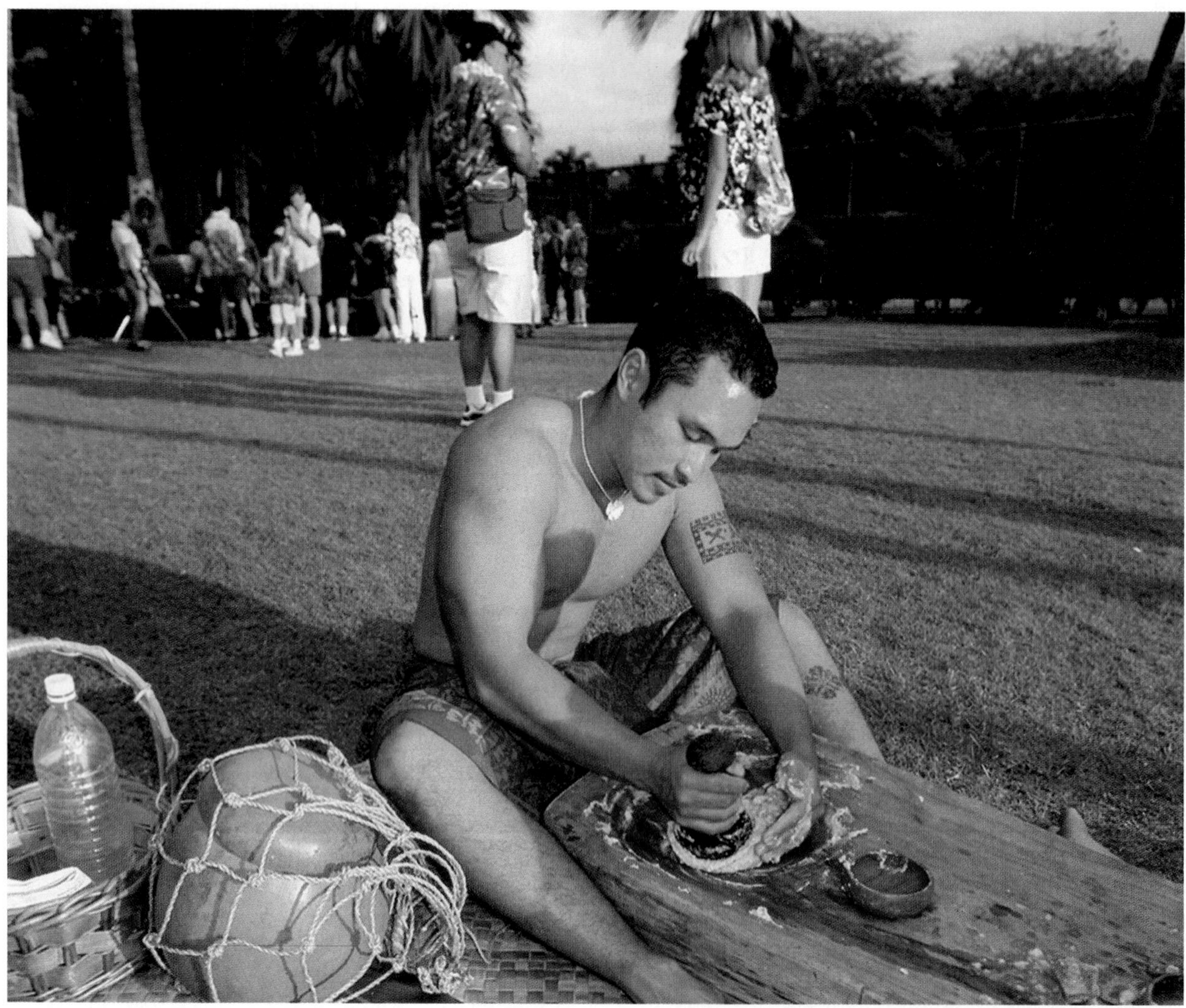

HVCB/Kirk Lee Aeder

Hawaiians orginally made poi by pounding steamed taro root in a wooden trough until it formed a thick, smooth paste.

Canada

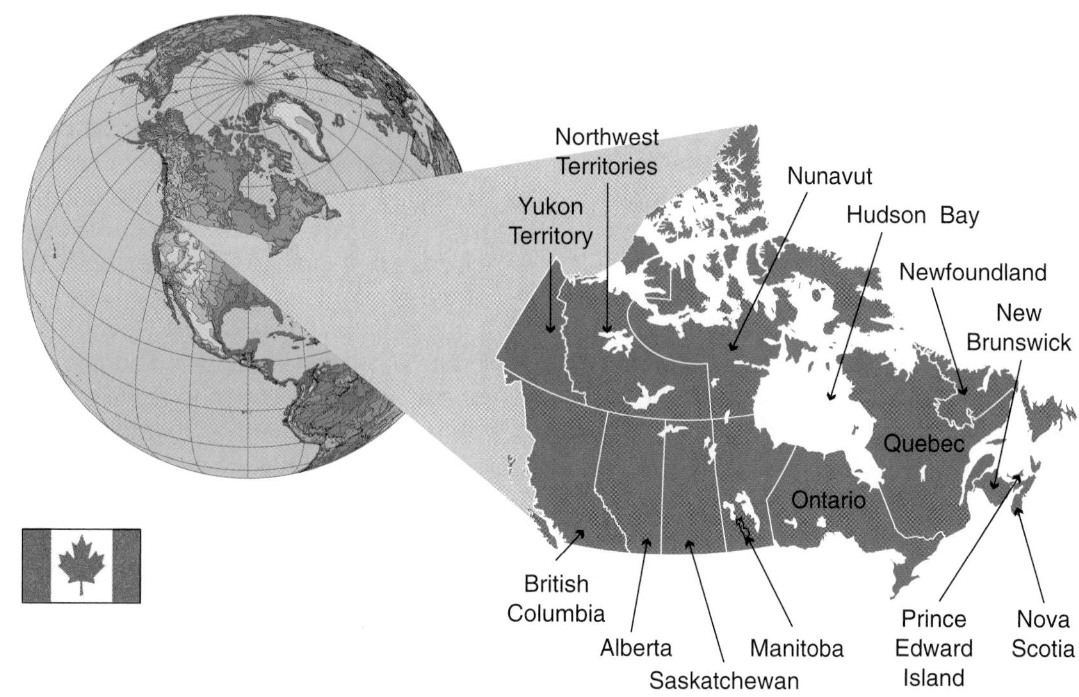

In terms of land mass, Canada is the second largest country in the world. However, it has a population smaller than the state of California. The majority of Canadians live within a few hundred miles of the country's southern border. Over half the people live in the area around the Great Lakes and the St. Lawrence River.

Like the United States, Canada is a land that was settled by immigrants from many nations. These settlers combined their cultures with those of native peoples. Their food customs were major influences on Canadian cuisine.

Geography and Climate of Canada

Canada is divided into 10 provinces and 3 territories. Diverse geography partly accounts for the country's varied climate. Canada boasts the world's longest coastline. On the Atlantic side, air currents from over the ocean bring high annual levels of rain and snow. Along the Pacific coast, ocean airstreams give British Columbia the warmest average temperatures throughout the year. Just off the mainland, Vancouver Island's tremendous annual rainfall combines with the warm air to create a rain forest climate. The Arctic Ocean to the north surrounds many islands. It borders a region with long, dark winters. Temperatures here stay below freezing all but a few weeks a year.

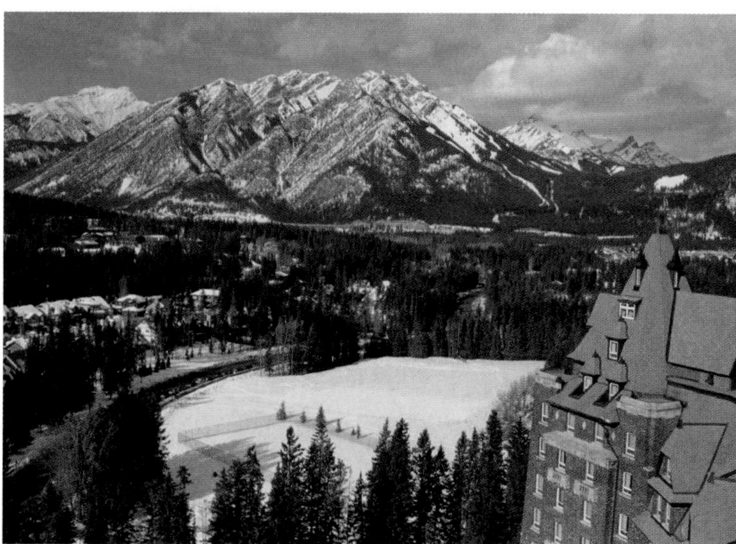

The beauty of Banff National Park in the Canadian Rockies attracts millions of visitors every year.

Several mountain ranges break up the landscape and shape the climate of Canada's interior regions. Rain and snow are common in the mountain areas. The valleys, by contrast, are often described as desertlike.

The key geographical feature of central and eastern Canada is a rocky, U-shaped region called the Canadian Shield. This area, which encircles Hudson Bay, is made up mostly of low hills and lakes. The soil in this region is not very suitable for farming.

Between the Rocky Mountains and the Canadian Shield lie the vast Interior Plains. The southern part of this region is home to some of the most productive grain fields in the world. This region reports some of the lowest levels of annual rainfall in Canada. However, much of the rain that falls comes in the spring, preparing the fields for planting. The summers in this area are hot, but the winters bring some of the lowest temperatures south of the Arctic.

Canadian Culture

By European standards, Canada is a young country. Despite its youth, Canada has developed into one of the world's leading nations. It is strengthened by a rich history and a diversity of cultures.

Influences on Canadian Culture

The ***Aboriginals,*** or first inhabitants of the land, influenced Canadian culture and food customs. Canadian Aboriginals form two groups—*First Nations* and *Inuit.* First Nations lived throughout Canada. Some were farmers; others were fishers or nomadic hunters. Inuit (once known as Eskimo) lived in the far northern regions where the land was not suitable for cultivation. Therefore, Inuit hunted inland game animals or marine mammals.

In the early 1600s, British and French fur trappers and traders began establishing settlements in Canada. The British settled primarily along the Atlantic coast and in the Hudson Bay area. The French explorers claimed a vast territory along the St. Lawrence River and the Great Lakes. This territory became known as New France. The Inuit had little contact with these early settlers. However, the First Nations helped the settlers learn how to hunt, fish, and plant crops.

A series of wars between the French and English colonists in Canada took place between 1689 and 1763. As a result, most of New France came under British rule and was renamed Quebec. Through the Quebec Act in 1774, Britain granted the French-speaking citizens in this area political, religious, and linguistic rights.

The following year, the Revolutionary War broke out in the American colonies. Thousands of colonists who chose to remain loyal to the British crown moved north into Canada. This led Britain to split Quebec into two colonies. They were later reunited as the Province of Canada. In 1867, this colony was joined with Nova Scotia and New Brunswick to form a new country—the Dominion of Canada. Each of the former colonies became a province in the new country.

Exploration and settlement of western Canada had been increasing since the first half of the early 1800s. Within four years of the formation of the Dominion of Canada, two more provinces were added. By 1949, a total of 10 provinces had joined the Dominion.

Modern Canadian Culture

Today, Canada is a federal state with a democratic parliament. The Parliament is modeled after the British government system. It is made up of a Senate and a House of Commons.

Canada has a multicultural society. Most of Canada's people have a British or French background. However, many Canadians claim ties to other European countries. Others have an Asian heritage. In addition, three to four percent of Canada's people are of native descent. See 27-11.

Canada has two national languages. English is the primary language of the majority of Canadians. However, French is the main language of a sizable percentage of the people. The largest segment of the French-speaking population lives in the province of Quebec.

Canadian Agriculture

Food products play a large role in the Canadian economy. Much of Canada's land is well suited for agriculture. Wheat, barley, apples, berries, and potatoes are among the economically important crops grown by Canadian farmers. Dairy products and livestock are significant, too. Fishing is an important industry in coastal regions. Cod, flounder, lobster, and salmon are among the most valuable catches brought in by Canadian fishers.

Canadian Holidays

As in all countries, holidays are an important part of the lifestyle in Canada. Many of these events involve the sharing of traditional foods.

Spring and summer holidays include Easter and Canada Day. Spring vegetables, such as asparagus and fiddlehead ferns, are often served with ham for Easter dinner. Canada Day, which is observed on July 1, honors Canada's freedom from British rule. Strawberry festivals are often held at the time of this holiday. Picnics, fireworks, parades, and concerts are also part of the festivities.

The fall and winter months bring a number of holidays in Canada. Thanksgiving is observed on the second Monday in October. A turkey dinner ended with hot pumpkin pie is the typical feast. A traditional Christmas dinner reflects the British heritage of many Canadians. This meal is likely to include roast goose with plum pudding. Shortbread and fruitcake are also common holiday treats.

Canadian Cuisine

Good nutrition for the Canadian people is a top goal of health experts. In fact, Canadian scientists have been working with the Food and Nutrition Board in the United States. Together they are developing the new Dietary Reference Intakes (DRIs). These are recommended levels of nutrient intake for people in the United States and Canada.

The typical Canadian diet is nutritious. It includes a variety of foods. It features a bounty of fruits, vegetables, and grain products. Meat and dairy products have traditionally played a key role in Canadian cuisine. If portions are moderate, however, lean meats and lowfat dairy products can be part of a healthful diet. See 27-12.

Canada's diverse climate and geography have caused available foods to vary from one part of the country to another. Different native and immigrant influences also affected each area. Like the United States, therefore, Canada has a regional cuisine.

Traditional Canadian foods were based largely on native ingredients. Canadian cooks could not obtain these ingredients all year long. Therefore, classic Canadian cuisine was seasonal in nature. The distinctive qualities of what was once standard Canadian fare have become less striking in recent years. Food products are made by large manufacturers instead of small-scale entrepreneurs. Busy lifestyles have led to widespread use of processed foods. Modern transportation has brought cooks a broad range of foods that are not produced in Canada. It has also allowed year-round availability of foods that were once seasonal. These factors have worked together to remove some of the unique character from everyday menus in Canada. However, traditional dishes still appear at holidays and other special occasions.

In the past, food was central to many Canadian social events, such as teas, church suppers, and quilting bees. It was the main focus of parties celebrating the harvest of such foods as strawberries, smelts, apples, and maple sugar. Food also played a key role at weddings, funerals, picnics, and other family gatherings. At these functions, cooks proudly displayed their pickles, preserves, and baked goods for all to enjoy.

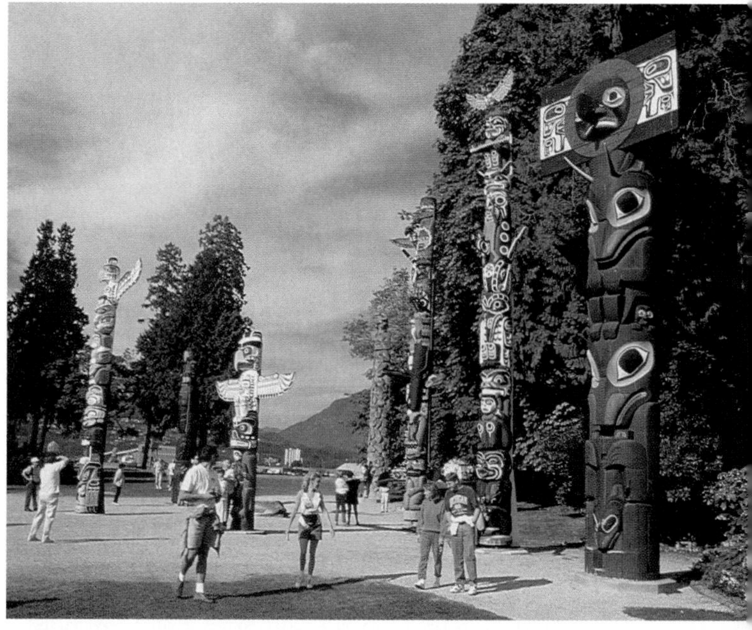

Tourism Vancouver

27-11 Canada's Aboriginal people are an important part of the country's multicultural society.

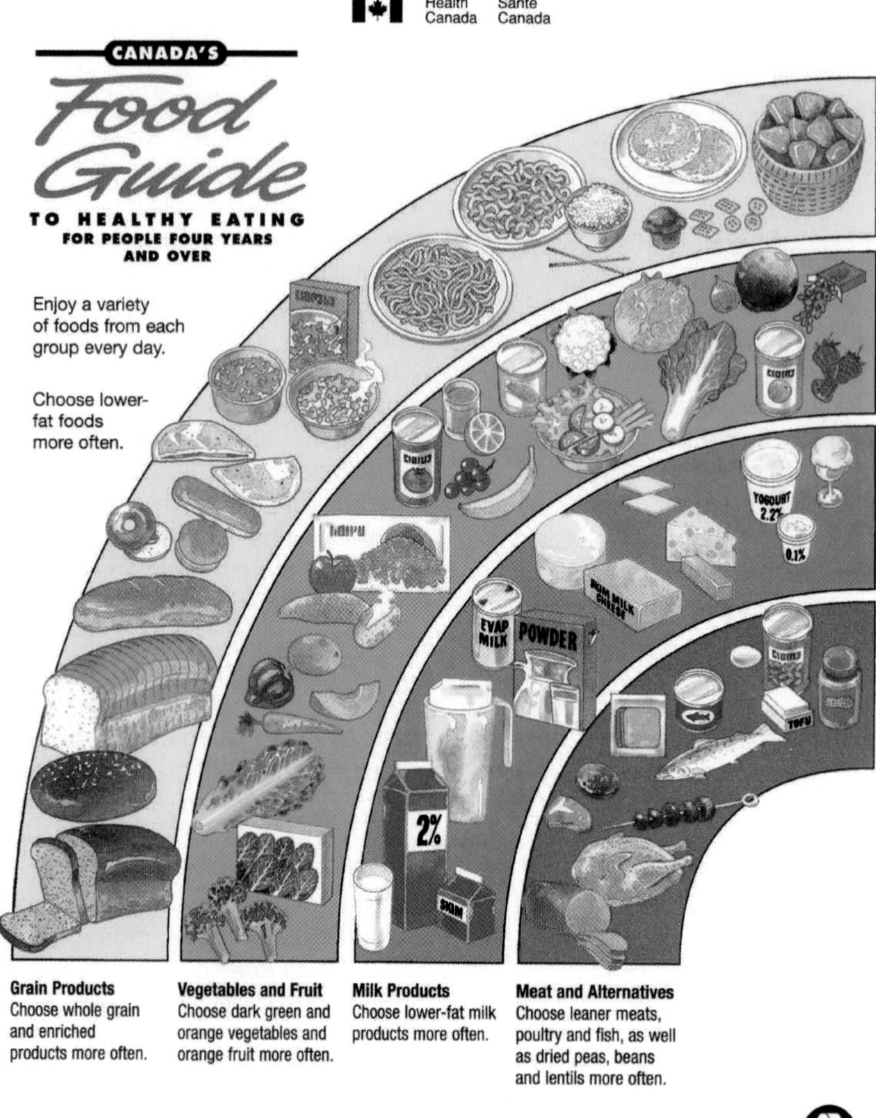

Health Canada

27-12 Canada's Food Guide to Healthy Eating groups foods similarly to the Food Guide Pyramid used in the United States.

Immigrant Influence on Canadian Cuisine

British, Scottish, Irish, French, and German settlers all had an effect on the development of Canadian cuisine. British influence can be seen in the popularity of such dishes as steak and kidney pie. *Yorkshire pudding* is a British food that appears in some Canadian cookbooks. It is a quick bread flavored with drippings from beef roast. Tea (both the drink and the light afternoon meal) are also signs of British influence on Canadian cuisine. Scones, custards, and baked and steamed puddings are other British favorites that have become part of Canadian fare. (You will read more about many of these foods in Chapter 29, "Europe.")

Two traditional entrees served in Canada for Christmas and New Year's dinners are Irish in origin. Spiced beef and stuffed pork tenderloins are often the center of winter holiday meals.

Provincial French influence is most prominent in the cuisine of Quebec. It also plays a role in the foods of the East Coast provinces. Hollandaise sauce and oil and vinegar salad dressings flavored with garlic are examples of French influence.

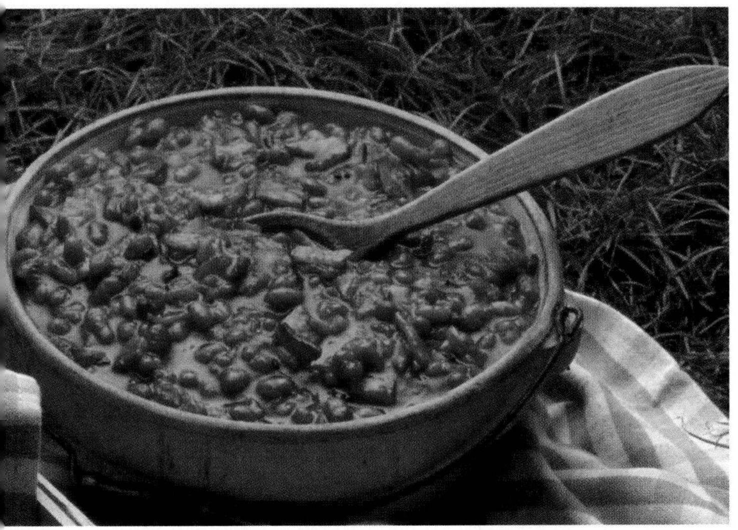

photo courtesy of Land O'Lakes, Inc.

***27-13** Baked beans are among the dishes that were brought to Canada by immigrating New Englanders.*

German influence is seen in foods brought to Canada by groups of Mennonite and Amish settlers. One example is dandelion salad with bacon and sour cream dressing. German influence is also seen in the quality baked goods that are popular in areas with large Amish and Mennonite populations.

Even the United States influenced the cuisine of Canada. Many people from New England moved north and settled along the east coast of Canada. Their effect is seen in such dishes as seafood chowders, baked beans, and steamed brown bread, 27-13. People from the mid-Atlantic states settled in Ontario. Pancakes, gingersnap cookies, and hearty soups may be among the Canadian foods that reflect their influence. Another example of U.S. influence is in the traditional foods served for Thanksgiving in Canada—turkey, cranberries, and pumpkin pie.

Canadian Main Dishes

Main dishes in Canada generally include meat, poultry, or fish. Not surprisingly, menus in the coastal provinces often feature seafood. The East Coast is known for cod, flounder, lobster, crab, and oysters. In this part of Canada, seafood chowders, boiled lobster, oyster dressing, and fish salads are popular dishes. Salmon is the primary catch in the West Coast province of British Columbia. Canadians enjoy salmon poached, smoked, broiled, and grilled. Inland lakes and streams, especially in the northern provinces, provide freshwater fish including trout, pickerel, and whitefish. Commercial ice fishing makes these fish widely available during the winter months. Pan-frying and baking with stuffing are two popular preparation methods.

Canadian people eat more beef than any other meat. Throughout Canada, people enjoy grilled steaks, roast prime rib, and beef sandwiches. Spiced beef, which is preserved with a mixture of salt, cloves, nutmeg, and allspice, is a Canadian Christmas specialty.

Pork was once the most commonly eaten meat in some parts of Canada, and it is still quite popular. In Canada's early days, hogs were raised on almost every farm. Butchering and sausage making were annual fall events. Most pork cuts were salted to preserve them for use throughout the winter. Better cuts, such as the hams, were cured in brine and smoked. This extra processing inspired many people to save hams for special occasions, such as Easter dinner.

Poultry is also common as a Canadian main dish. Chicken is most popular, and it is served in a variety of ways. Roasted chicken, grilled chicken, and chicken salads are favorite entrees. Canadians enjoy other types of poultry, too, especially at holiday times. Turkey is the traditional entree for Thanksgiving in Canada. Goose is often the bird of choice for Christmas dinner.

Game meats are not unusual on the menus of people living in rural northern regions. Bear, caribou, and moose are abundant in these wilderness areas. In other parts of Canada, rabbit is a more likely game entree. Stewing and roasting are two favorite cooking methods.

Q: What are gooseberries and how did they get their name?

A: Gooseberries are a round, tart fruit that may be used in pies and other desserts. Their name may come from the fact that English people centuries ago enjoyed serving them with roast goose.

Canadian Fruits and Vegetables

The soil and climate in Southern Canada are suitable for growing a wide variety of fruits and vegetables. Apples are probably the most popular fruit in Canada. Different species are available from midsummer to late fall. Canadians use apples to make cider, apple butter, and a number of desserts and condiments.

Gooseberries, strawberries, and rhubarb are available in Canada in the spring. Blueberries, raspberries, and blackberries are part of the harvest of summer fruits. Plums, peaches, and cherries are among the tree fruits grown in this region. With this range of fruits, few would wonder why fruit pies are such popular desserts in Canada. Canadians also have a long tradition of putting up their bounty of native fruits in jams, jellies, and other preserves.

Canadian vegetables are just as varied as the fruits. Asparagus and watercress are often the first vegetables ready for picking in the spring. Peas, leaf lettuce, radishes, tomatoes, cucumbers, and corn follow in the summer. Canadians enjoy vegetables in soups, salads, and side dishes.

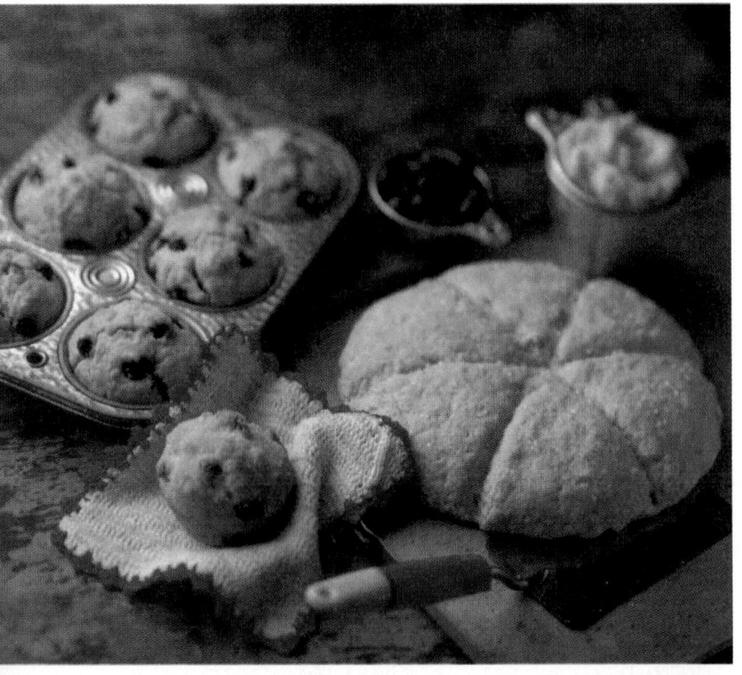

photo courtesy of Land O'Lakes, Inc.

***27-14** Blueberry gems, or muffins, would be a welcome sight on a Canadian breakfast table.*

Canadian Grain Products

Canada has an abundant wheat crop, and bread products are part of most meals. Breakfasts may include buckwheat pancakes or muffins, which are sometimes called *gems*, 27-14. Lunches and teas are likely to feature sandwiches on hearty yeast breads. Yeast rolls or quick breads flavored with fruits are popular accompaniments to dinner entrees.

Baked goods such as cakes, cookies, and pies are also Canadian standards. Early Canadian cookbooks included a wealth of recipes for these treats, which were the pride of many cooks. Many of these traditional recipes were sweetened with maple sugar or maple syrup, which was made locally every spring.

Classic Canadian menus seldom include pasta products. However, wild rice may appear as a side dish or in a stuffing. Wild rice grows in shallow Canadian lakes and streams. It must be harvested by hand from canoes and then dried. The labor-intensive harvesting process causes wild rice to be fairly costly.

Canadian Dairy Products

Large herds of dairy cows make dairy products popular in Canada. A variety of flavorful cheeses are produced throughout the country. Cheddar may be the most commonly produced cheese, but Oka, Ermite blue, and St. Benoit are uniquely Canadian.

The use of dairy products is prominent throughout traditional Canadian recipes. Oysters may be poached in milk. Cream is added to various soups, which are a filling first course in many winter menus. In the summer, homemade ice cream is a classic dessert.

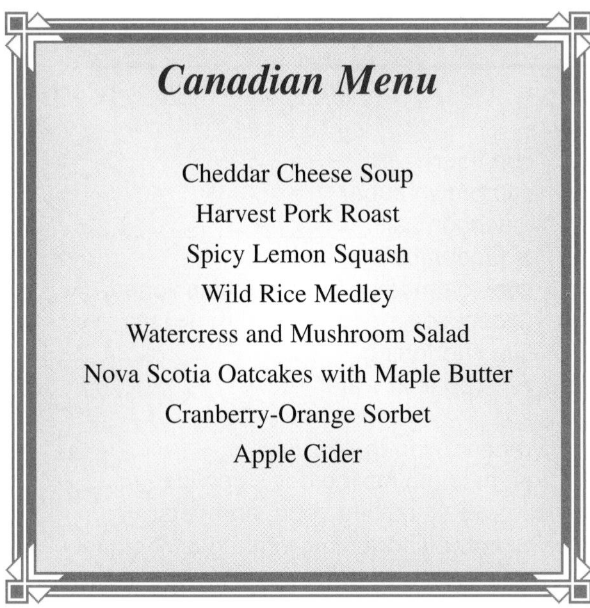

Canadian Menu

Cheddar Cheese Soup
Harvest Pork Roast
Spicy Lemon Squash
Wild Rice Medley
Watercress and Mushroom Salad
Nova Scotia Oatcakes with Maple Butter
Cranberry-Orange Sorbet
Apple Cider

Cheddar Cheese Soup

Serves 6

1/3 cup minced onion
1 tablespoon butter
2 1/2 cups low-sodium chicken broth
1/2 cup fat free milk
2 tablespoons flour
1 1/2 cups evaporated fat free milk
1 1/2 cups shredded Cheddar cheese
1/2 teaspoon dry mustard
1/8 teaspoon cayenne pepper

1. In a large nonstick saucepan, saute onion in butter over medium heat until tender.
2. Stir in chicken broth, reduce heat to low, and simmer for 15 minutes.
3. Combine milk and flour in a small, tightly covered container. Shake vigorously to mix thoroughly.
4. Slowly pour flour mixture into broth, stirring constantly. Continue stirring gently until soup begins to thicken.
5. Add evaporated milk, cheese, dry mustard, and cayenne pepper.
6. Continue stirring gently until cheese is melted and soup is heated through. Do not allow soup to boil.

Per serving: 211 cal. (51% from fat), 14 g protein, 12 g carbohydrate, 12 g fat, 37 mg cholesterol, 0 g fiber, 347 mg sodium.

Harvest Pork Roast

Serves 6

1 2-pound boneless pork loin roast
1 tablespoon oil
1/2 cup apple cider
1/2 teaspoon dried thyme
1/4 teaspoon dried marjoram
1 tablespoon dried parsley

1. Trim exterior fat from pork loin.
2. Combine oil and apple cider in blender. Blend for 15 seconds.
3. Generously brush cider mixture over the pork loin. Sprinkle moist surface with thyme, marjoram, and parsley.
4. Place pork loin on a rack in a shallow roasting pan.
5. Place roasting pan in 350°F oven and roast for 45 minutes to an hour, until internal temperature measures 155°F to 160°F on a meat thermometer.
6. Remove pork loin from oven. Let it stand for 10 minutes before slicing.

Per serving: 176 cal. (41% from fat), 24 g protein, 2 g carbohydrate, 8 g fat, 67 mg cholesterol, 0 g fiber, 58 mg sodium.

Spicy Lemon Squash

Serves 6

1 teaspoon grated lemon peel
1/4 cup brown sugar
1/2 teaspoon ground ginger
1/2 teaspoon ground cinnamon
1/4 teaspoon ground nutmeg
3 tablespoons butter, melted
1 teaspoon rum extract
3 acorn squash

1. In a small bowl, combine lemon peel, brown sugar, ginger, cinnamon, and nutmeg.
2. Stir in butter and rum extract.
3. Wash squash. Cut in half and remove seeds.
4. Sprinkle the insides of the squash with the spice mixture.
5. Place squash halves, cut sides up, in a shallow baking dish. Add 1/4 inch of water to the dish.
6. Cover the dish with aluminum foil and bake at 400°F for 30 minutes, or until tender.

Per serving: 128 cal. (42% from fat), 1 g protein, 18 g carbohydrate, 6 g fat, 16 mg cholesterol, 3 g fiber, 63 mg sodium.

Wild Rice Medley

Serves 6

1/4 cup chopped onion
1/4 cup minced celery
1 tablespoon butter
1/2 cup wild rice
2 3/4 cups low-sodium chicken broth
1/4 teaspoon salt
1/2 cup brown rice
1 tablespoon chopped fresh parsley

1. In medium saucepan, saute onion and celery in butter over medium heat until tender.
2. Add wild rice, chicken broth, and salt. Increase heat to high and bring to a boil.
3. Cover, reduce heat to low, and simmer for 15 minutes.
4. Add brown rice, cover, and simmer an additional 30 minutes.
5. Remove from heat. Drain any unabsorbed liquid. Sprinkle with parsley.

Per serving: 133 cal. (20% from fat), 5 g protein, 23 g carbohydrate, 3 g fat, 5 mg cholesterol, 2 g fiber, 197 mg sodium.

Watercress and Mushroom Salad

Serves 6

1/4 pound mushrooms, sliced
1 tablespoon chopped fresh parsley
1 tablespoon chopped fresh chives
1/4 cup vegetable oil
1 tablespoon lemon juice
1/2 teaspoon dry mustard
1/4 teaspoon pepper
1/4 teaspoon salt
2 bunches watercress

1. Place mushrooms, parsley, and chives in a large bowl.
2. Combine the oil, lemon juice, dry mustard, pepper, and salt and pour over mushroom mixture. Stir gently, cover, and refrigerate for 15 minutes.
3. Meanwhile, wash the watercress and pat dry with paper towels.
4. Add the watercress to the mushrooms. Toss well to blend. Serve immediately.

Per serving: 75 cal. (84% from fat), 1 g protein, 2 g carbohydrate, 7 g fat, 0 mg cholesterol, 1 g fiber, 108 mg sodium.

Nova Scotia Oatcakes

Makes 36

1 cup flour
1/3 cup brown sugar
3/4 teaspoon salt
1/2 teaspoon baking soda
3 cups oatmeal, quick or old fashioned, uncooked
1/2 cup shortening
1/3 to 1/2 cup cold water

1. Preheat oven to 425°F.
2. In a medium mixing bowl, combine flour, sugar, salt, baking soda, and oats.
3. Cut in the shortening with a pastry blender or two knives until the mixture resembles coarse crumbs.
4. With a fork, add water a tablespoon at a time until dough will hold together but is not sticky.
5. Press dough into a greased 10 x 15-inch jelly roll pan.
6. Cut dough into 36 squares (divide 10-inch side into fourths and 15-inch side into ninths); do not separate.
7. Bake in preheated oven for 15 minutes, or until browned.
8. Separate squares into a napkin-lined basket. Serve warm with maple butter.

Per oatcake: 71 cal. (38% from fat), 1 g protein, 9 g carbohydrate, 3 g fat, 0 mg cholesterol, 1 g fiber, 67 mg sodium.

Maple Butter

Makes 3/4 cup

1/3 cup butter, softened
3 tablespoons brown sugar
1/4 cup maple syrup
1/8 teaspoon cinnamon

1. In a small mixer bowl, beat butter until light and fluffy.
2. Beat in brown sugar, maple syrup, and cinnamon.

Per teaspoon: 25 cal. (72% from fat), 0 g protein, 3 g carbohydrate, 2 g fat, 5 mg cholesterol, 0 g fiber, 18 mg sodium.

Cranberry-Orange Sorbet

Serves 6

2 cups fresh or frozen cranberries
3/4 cup water
3/4 cup sugar
1 cup water
1/2 cup orange juice concentrate

1. In a small saucepan, combine the cranberries and 3/4 cup water. Cook over medium heat until cranberries are tender, about 10 minutes.
2. Remove from heat and set aside to cool.
3. In a separate saucepan, bring sugar and 1 cup water to a boil, stirring to dissolve sugar.
4. Boil for 5 minutes. Set aside to cool slightly.
5. Press cooled cranberry mixture through a large strainer into a mixing bowl.
6. Stir in orange juice concentrate and cooled sugar syrup.
7. Cover mixture and chill.
8. Pour the mixture into the canister of a 1-quart ice cream freezer and freeze according to the manufacturer's directions.

Per serving: 150 cal. (0% from fat), 1 g protein, 38 g carbohydrate, 0 g fat, 0 mg cholesterol, 2 g fiber, 4 mg sodium.

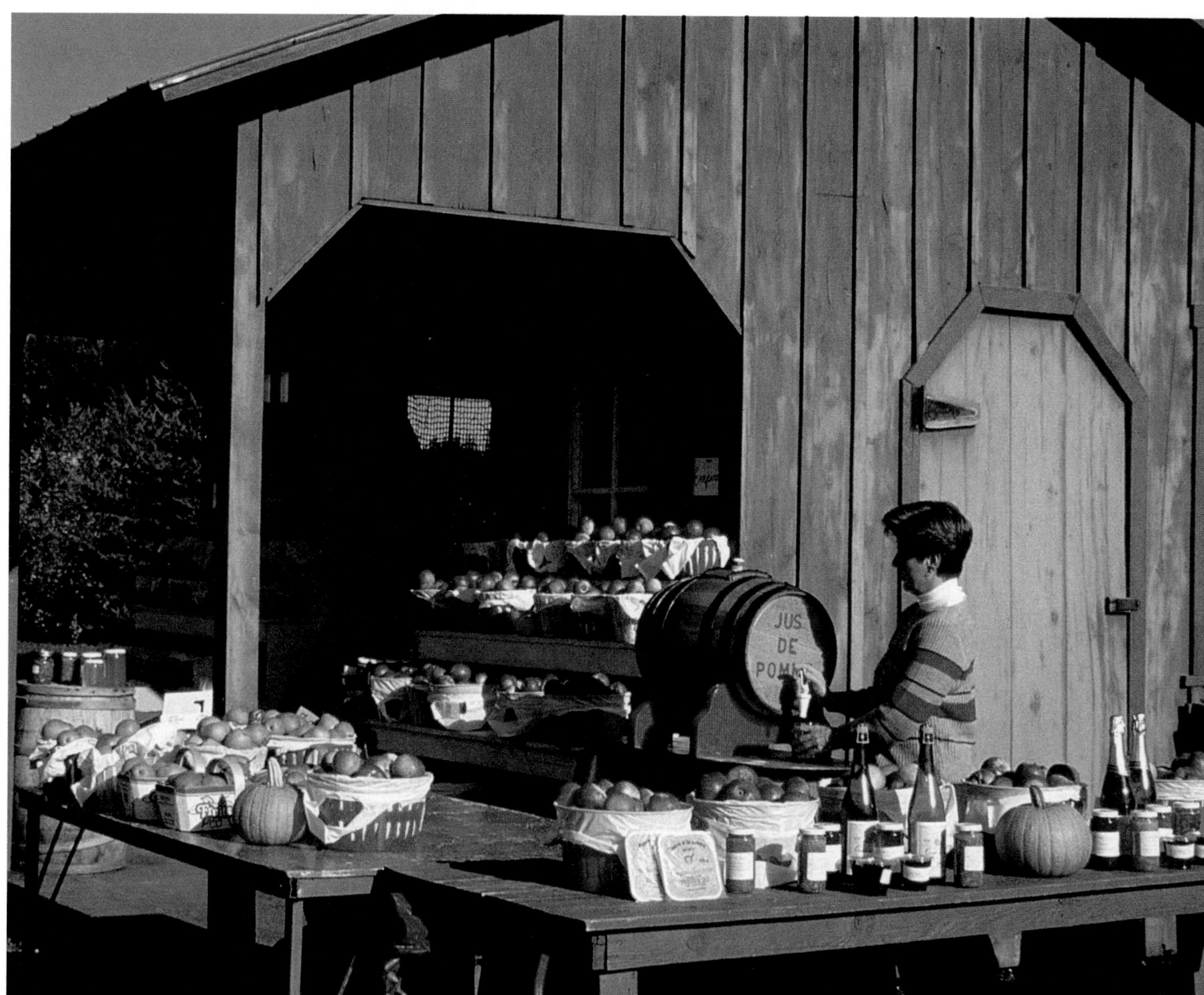

Tourisme Québec, Giles Rivest

Apples harvested from Canadian orchards are often available at roadside markets.

Chapter 27 Review

The United States and Canada

Summary

The Aboriginals and the first explorers laid the foundations of cuisine in the United States and Canada. As immigrants came from many parts of the globe, they added foods and cooking techniques from their homelands. This blend of cultures and traditions has evolved into the cuisines found in the United States and Canada today.

Immigrants from certain countries tended to settle together. Therefore, the cuisine of the United States has some regional characteristics. For instance, hearty one-dish meals and foods made with locally produced maple syrup are popular in New England. German foods of the Pennsylvania Dutch can be found in the mid-Atlantic region. The South is known for fried chicken and buttermilk biscuits. Soul food and Creole cuisine also originated in the South. In the Midwest, where much of the nation's grain is grown, meat and potatoes are standard fare. Native Americans, Mexicans, and Spaniards influenced the foods of the West and Southwest. Chili and barbecued meats are favorites in this region. Sourdough bread, Alaskan seafood, and fresh fruits and vegetables are typical of the Pacific Coast. Tropical fruits and vegetables, often prepared with an Asian flair, are common in Hawaii.

Classic Canadian dishes were created with ingredients that were locally produced. Canada's climate and geography caused available foods to vary from area to area. Seasonal and regional distinctions are less apparent in Canadian cuisine today. In coastal regions, main dishes often feature seafood. Beef and pork are more standard in inland areas. Apples and potatoes are common. However, Canadian meals feature a broad range of fruits and vegetables. Baked goods made from wheat grown in the prairie provinces are staples of the Canadian diet. Dairy products, including cheeses, cream soups, and frozen desserts, are also well liked.

Review What You Have Read

Write your answers on a separate sheet of paper.

1. Name three reasons immigrants came to the New World.
2. How did New Englanders preserve foods for winter?
3. Name three culinary contributions of the Pennsylvania Dutch.
4. Name two distinct forms of cooking that developed in the South.
5. Name six agricultural products of the Midwest.
6. What four groups of people had the most influence on cooking in the Southwest?
7. How did the prospectors make and use sourdough?
8. Identify three groups that influenced Hawaiian cuisine and give an example of a food contributed by each group.
9. Match the following foods to the regions of the United States with which they are associated:

    _____ poi
    _____ baked beans
    _____ salmon
    _____ tamales
    _____ gumbo
    _____ shoofly pie

    A. New England
    B. mid-Atlantic
    C. South
    D. Midwest
    E. West and Southwest
    F. Pacific Coast
    G. Hawaii
10. Identify foods that are typically associated with two Canadian holidays.
11. How did people in the United States influence the cuisine of Canada?
12. True or false. Pasta is a common side dish on Canadian menus.

Build Your Basic Skills

1. **Writing.** Research the first Thanksgiving in the United States or Canada. Write a report about the foods that were served. Note how many of these foods are still served today.
2. **Reading.** Visit a local butcher to learn more about the parts of the hog used in the preparation of soul food. Then find some interesting recipes using chitterlings or jowls and prepare them.
3. **History.** Prepare a time line illustrating important dates in Canada's history.

Build Your Thinking Skills

1. **Develop.** Divide into seven groups, one group for each major region of the United States. Research the history and foods of your region. Then develop a menu for a typical meal and prepare it for the other class members.
2. **Plan.** Work with your school's music and athletic departments to plan a fund-raising luau. Your class can prepare the food, while the other groups furnish the entertainment.

Apply Technology

1. Use a computer and word processing software to prepare a template for a travel journal. If you have access to a laptop computer, take the computer with you on a trip and use your template files to create documents for each day's journal entries.
2. Use map-making software or visit a map-making Web site on the Internet. Use these resources to plan a travel route from your school to the U.S. or Canadian destination of your choice. You should also investigate tourist attractions along your route and identify restaurants, gas stations, and lodging facilities at which you would stop.

Using Workplace Skills

Zaleeka is a tourist-information assistant at a state information center in the South. She provides travel information to tourists, helping them map routes to places of interest around the state.

To be an effective worker, Zaleeka needs skill in organizing and processing symbols, pictures, graphs, and other information. In a small group, answer the following questions about Zaleeka's need for and use of this skill:

A. What types of symbols, pictures, and graphs might Zaleeka be required to interpret in her job?
B. How would the clients Zaleeka serves be affected if she lacked skill in organizing and processing symbols, pictures, graphs, and other information?
C. How might the tourism industry in Zaleeka's state be affected if she lacked skill in organizing and processing symbols, pictures, graphs, and other information?
D. What is another skill Zaleeka would need in this job? Briefly explain why this skill would be important.

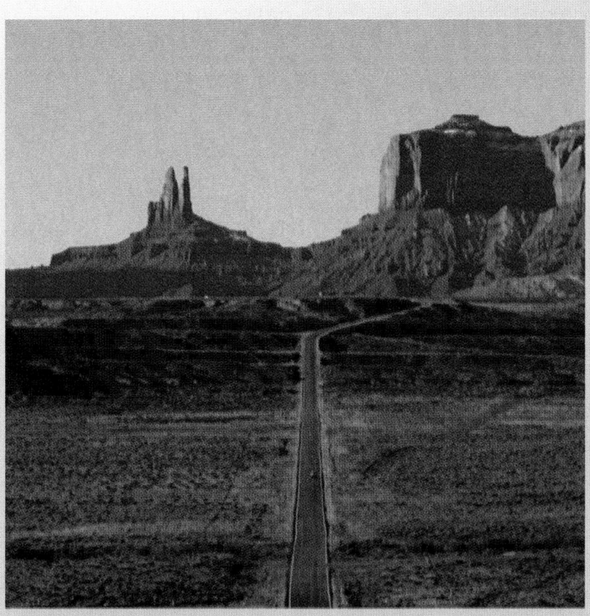

Chapter 28
Latin America

Spanish Interpreter
Translates spoken passages from Spanish into one or more other languages.

Mexican-Food-Machine Tender
Tends machine that automatically dispenses cheese onto tortillas to form enchiladas or ground meat onto taco shells to form tacos.

Mexican Food Cook
Supervises and coordinates activities of workers engaged in preparing, cooking, portioning, and packaging ready-to-serve Mexican food specialties, such as chili, tamales, enchiladas, and tacos.

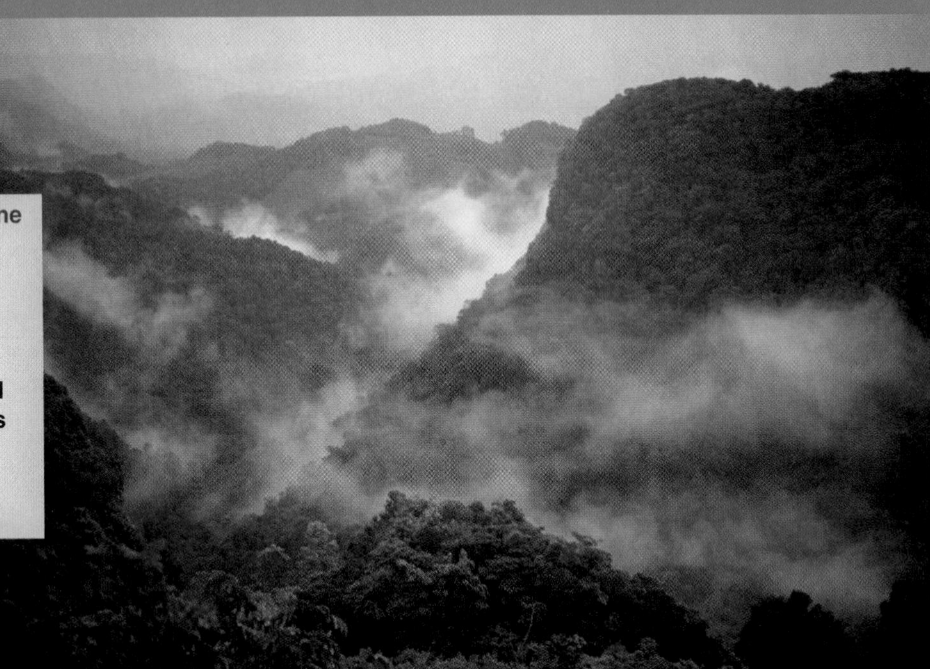

Terms to Know

Latin America
Aztecs
conquistador
tortilla
frijoles refritos
chilies
guacamole
mole
plantain
comida
siesta
Inca
manioc
cassava
arepa
ají
ceviche
gaucho
empanada
dendé oil
feijoada completa

Objectives

After studying this chapter, you will be able to

- ❑ identify geographic and climatic factors that have influenced the characteristic foods of Mexico and the South American countries.
- ❑ describe cultural factors that have affected the food customs of Mexico and South America.
- ❑ prepare foods native to Latin America.

The landmass that stretches southward from the Rio Grande to the tip of South America is known as ***Latin America.*** It is called Latin America because the official language of most of the countries is either Spanish or Portuguese, both of which are based on Latin.

Latin America was first explored and settled by the Spanish. Later, other Europeans established settlements. A large number of Portuguese settled along the eastern shores of South America in what today is Brazil.

Extremes are the rule rather than the exception in Latin America. Dense, tropical rain forests are as common as snow-capped mountains. Large, modern cities may not be far away from wild jungles.

The food customs of Latin America are rich and varied. They reflect the culture, climate, and geography of each country. The ancient Aztecs and the Spanish conquistadores influenced Mexico. The foods of Peru reflect the ancient Inca civilization. The foods of Argentina are an unusual mixture of European influences and native foods grown in the rich soil. The foods of Brazil reflect strong African and Portuguese heritage.

For the most part, the cuisines of Latin America are healthful. They include large amounts of fruits and vegetables and daily portions of grains and beans. In many regions, meat and poultry are costly, so people use them in limited amounts. Experts believe this plant-based diet is partly the reason for the low cancer rates in many Latin American countries. One aspect of Latin American cuisine that is a health concern is the frequent use of animal fats in cooking. The popularity of pickled, smoked, and salted foods in some regions is a nutritional concern, too. These factors have been linked with increased cancer risk.

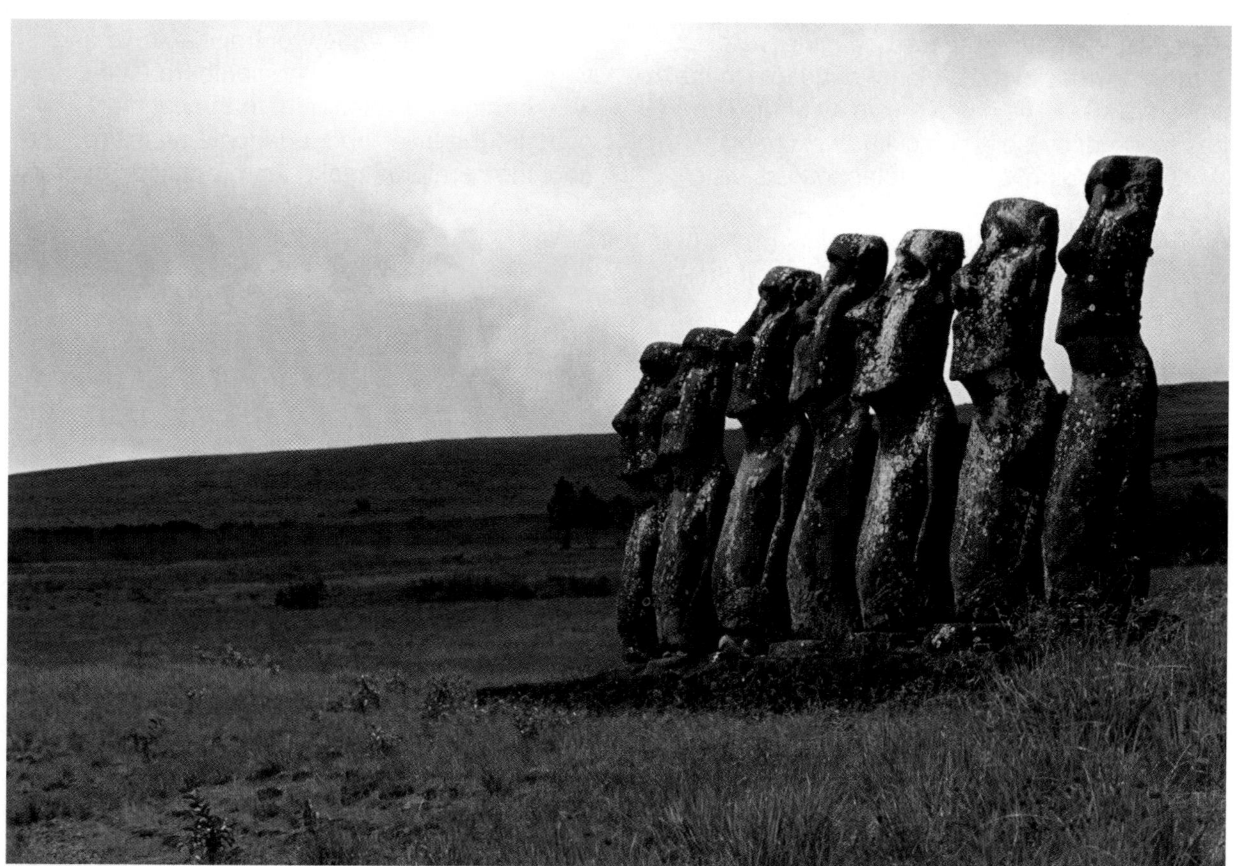

Easter Island, which is off the coast of Chile, is known for these mysterious statues carved by tribespeople centuries ago.

Mexico

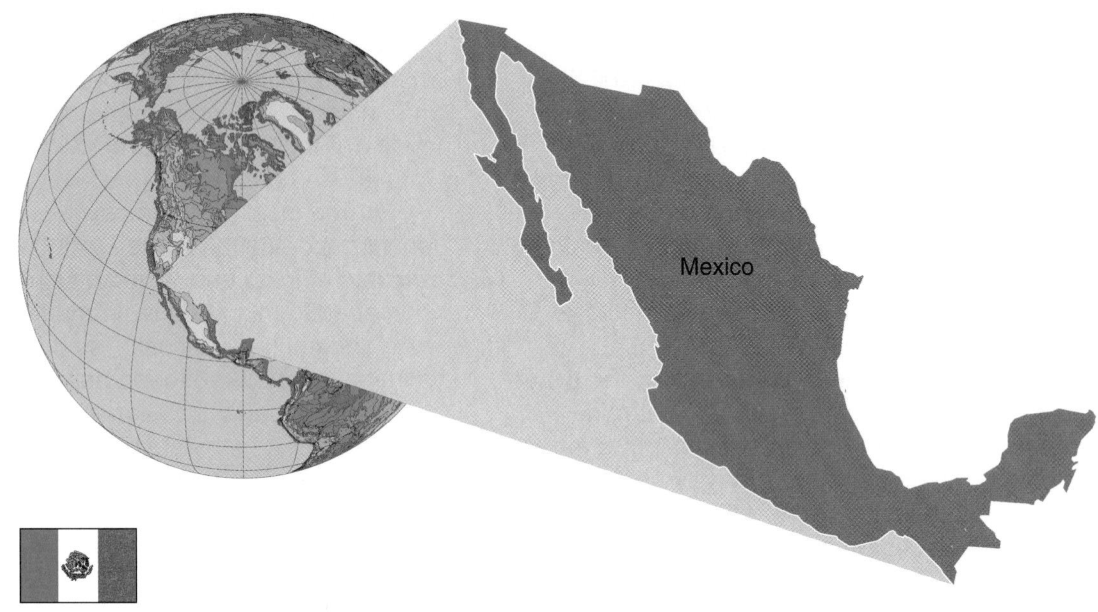

Of all the Latin American countries, Mexico is most familiar to the majority of people in the United States. The close proximity of Mexico has made possible a rich cultural exchange.

Thousands of United States tourists visit Mexico each year. Mexican foods, such as tacos, enchiladas, and refried beans, are popular in the Southwest and throughout the United States.

Geography and Climate of Mexico

Mexico is a land of deserts, mountains, grasslands, woodlands, and tropical rain forests. The Rio Grande separates Mexico from Texas. The Pacific Ocean, Gulf of California, Caribbean Sea, and Gulf of Mexico form its coastline. Much of Mexico is mountainous, with valleys separating the different ranges. Although the climate in a few regions is wet and humid, nearly half of Mexico is arid or semiarid.

Both geography and climate have affected food customs in Mexico. In those sections of the country bordered by water, fish is an important part of the cuisine. The areas that border the United States have land that is too dry for large scale crop production. However, it is suitable for raising cattle. As a result, beef is a staple food in these areas. A variety of tropical fruits and vegetables grow along the southern Gulf Coast where rainfall is adequate. In the central plateau, the level land, adequate moisture, and cool temperatures make the production of crops like corn and beans profitable.

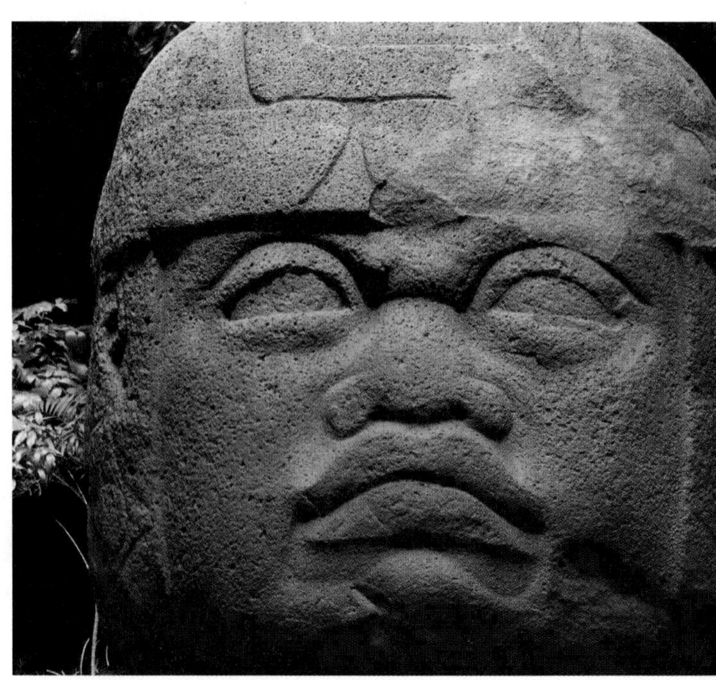

The Olmec Head is representative of the artwork left in Mexico by the ancient Mayan people.

Mexican Culture

The ***Aztecs*** were the original inhabitants of Mexico. They had a very advanced civilization for their time in history. In 1520, Hernando Cortes and the Spanish ***conquistadores*** (conquerors) explored Mexico and plundered villages for gold that decorated Aztec palaces and temples.

The Spanish controlled Mexico, except for a few years, until the middle of the nineteenth century. Their influence greatly affected the development of Mexican culture, especially architecture, language, and food customs.

Good Manners Are Good Business

You will make a better impression when dealing with business associates in other countries if you demonstrate sensitivity to cultural differences. Do not expect everyone to speak English and conduct business as it is conducted in the United States.

In Mexico, for instance, executives often take a rather relaxed view of scheduling. Just because you have an appointment and are waiting outside, a manager is not likely to rush through an earlier meeting. Rather than getting upset, you would be wise to schedule your appointments for early in the day. This will help you avoid being kept waiting.

Mexican Lifestyle

Living quarters in all but the wealthiest Mexican homes are simple. Beds, tables, and chairs are often hand-carved. Many dishes and cooking utensils are handmade.

Traditionally, Mexican families are close-knit. Children learn to help their parents at an early age. The children of rural families work in the fields, help with housework, and take care of their younger brothers and sisters. Many city children must work to supplement the family income.

Mexican Holidays

Most Mexicans are Roman Catholic. Many holidays throughout the year center around religious celebrations.

Food plays a role in some Mexican holidays. The Feast of Epiphany on January 6 falls at the end of a 22-day Christmas celebration. This day celebrates the coming of three kings to see the infant Jesus. People get together and share a special supper, which includes a ring-shaped cake with a tiny plastic baby baked inside. The person who gets the piece of cake with the baby hosts a tamales party for all who are present. This party is held on February 2, which is Candlemas Day. Mexicans celebrate this as the day Jesus' parents took him to the temple in Jerusalem.

The observance of the Days of the Dead also involves a food tradition. Mexicans believe dead souls return to visit the living between October 31 and November 2. During this time, many families set up altars in the corners of their homes. They set these altars with candles, photos, and favorite foods and drinks of dead loved ones.

Mexican Agriculture

A little more than half of Mexico's people are farmers. Because good, rich soil is scarce, farming is difficult. Many farmers cannot afford modern machinery or fertilizers. As a result, crop yields are poor. In recent years, government irrigation projects and credit to farmers have helped farmers improve yields.

Corn is Mexico's major crop. Bean production is second. Other important crops include sugarcane, coffee, tomatoes, green peppers, peas, melons, citrus fruits, strawberries, and cacao beans. Wheat is grown in the North as are smaller amounts of barley, rice, and oats. Cattle graze on northern pastures.

Coastal waters provide a variety of seafood. Large quantities of shrimp are caught and exported, 28-1. Sardines, tuna, turtles, and mackerel are also important.

Mexican Cuisine

Both the Aztecs and the Spaniards made many contributions to Mexican cuisine. The Aztecs contributed chocolate, vanilla, corn, peppers, peanuts, tomatoes, avocados, squash, beans, sweet potatoes, pineapples, and papayas. The Aztecs boiled, broiled, or steamed their food or ate it raw. Their more elaborate dishes were similar to modern stews.

The Spanish added oil, wine, cinnamon, cloves, rice, wheat, peaches, apricots, beef, and chicken. With the introduction of oil, many of the early Aztec foods could be fried. Today, frying is an important part of Mexican cooking. Mexican cooks fry foods in deep fat or on lightly greased griddles.

Another contribution to Mexican cuisine was made in the mid 1860s by emperor Maximilian. Maximilian was from Austria. He introduced dishes from his homeland as well as sophisticated French and Italian dishes to Mexico.

Characteristic Foods of Mexico

Corn, beans, and peppers are staple ingredients in Mexican cuisine. Mexican cooks use a variety of other locally grown vegetables and fruits, too. Flavorful sauces and stews, as well as some distinctive desserts and beverages, are also typical foods of Mexico.

Corn

Corn has formed the basis of Mexican cuisine since the days of the Aztec civilization. Mexican cooks use corn in many ways, but its most important use is in the production of tortillas. A ***tortilla*** is a flat, unleavened bread made from cornmeal and water. The dough is shaped into a thin pancake in a tortilla press. Then it is cooked on a lightly greased griddle called a *comal.*

Mexican cooks make many popular dishes from tortillas, 28-2. They fill tortillas with a mixture of shredded meat or sliced chicken, onions, garlic, and chilies to make *enchiladas.* Then they bake and serve the enchiladas with cheese and a red or green tomato sauce. Mexicans fry tortillas until crisp and garnish them with chopped onion, chilies, beans, shredded lettuce, meat, and cheese to make *tostadas. Quesadillas* are deep-fried turnovers made of tortillas filled with meat, sauce, cheese, beans, or vegetables. Tortillas wrapped around a meat or bean filling are called *burritos.* Crisp, fried tortillas filled with meat, beans, shredded lettuce, and cheese and seasoned with chili are called *tacos.*

Mexican cooks never waste corn. They do not even discard the husks. They use the husks to make *tamales.* The cooks stuff small amounts of corn dough with meat and beans and tuck it into the corn husks. They fold the husks into small parcels and steam them or roast them over an open fire.

Beans

Like corn, beans are a staple food in Mexico. Local farmers grow many varieties of beans. Sometimes people boil the beans and eat them from the pot as was done during Aztec

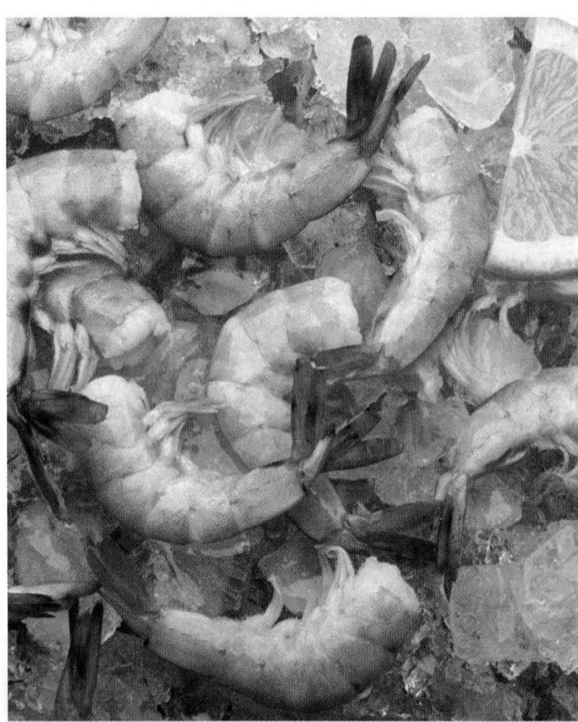

28-1 *Shrimp are an important product in the economy of Mexican people living near coastal waters.*

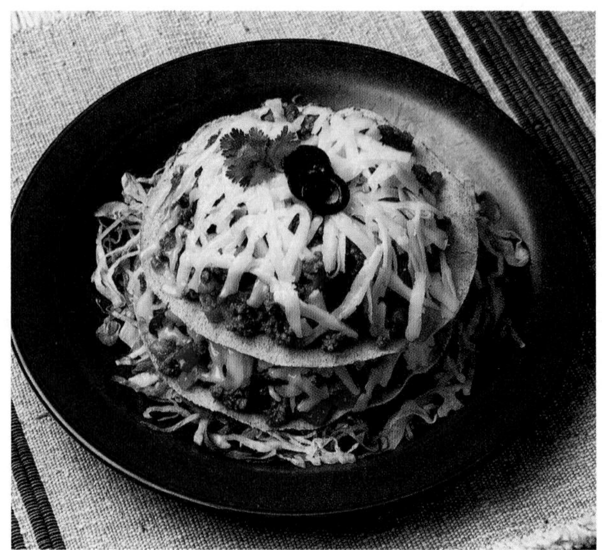

28-2 *Flat, unleavened corn cakes called tortillas form the basis of many Mexican dishes.*

times. Often they cook the beans until they are soft, then they mash the beans and fry them slowly. The Mexicans call this dish ***frijoles refritos*** (refried beans) and frequently serve the beans with grated cheese.

Peppers

People throughout Latin America use peppers, but they are especially important in Mexico. Strings of peppers hang outside many Mexican homes to dry.

Mexican cooks use over 30 varieties of peppers. The peppers range in size and color. They can be sweet, pungent, or burning hot. Generally, the mild peppers are called *sweet peppers,* and the hot ones are called ***chilies.***

The peppers used most often in cooking can be divided into two groups according to color—red and green. Mexican cooks use red peppers dried, except for ripe red bell peppers and pimientos. They use green peppers fresh. See 28-3.

Mexican Vegetables and Fruits

Mexican farmers grow a variety of vegetables. Mexicans usually do not eat vegetables plain. Instead, they add them to casseroles and use them as garnishes for other dishes.

Mexican vegetables that are common in the United States include zucchini, artichokes, white potatoes, spinach, chard, lettuce, beets, cauliflower, and carrots. Less common are *huazontle* (wild broccoli), *jicama* (a large, gray root), *nopole* (tender cactus leaves), and *chayotes* (a tropical squash).

Many fruits grow in Mexico. Avocados have a bland flavor and are often added to other foods. ***Guacamole,*** for example, is a spread made from mashed avocado, tomato, and onion. It may be served with tortillas or crisp

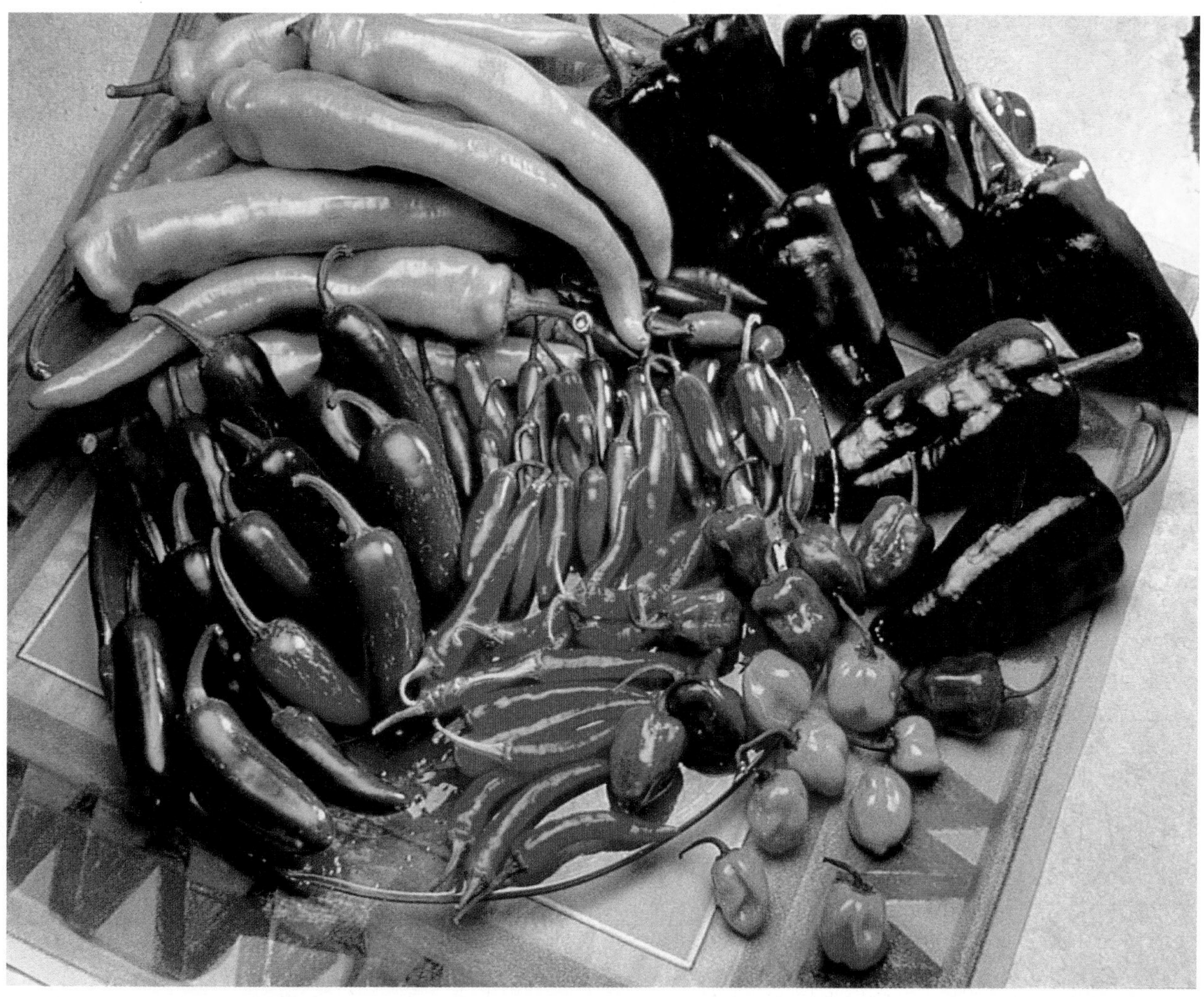

courtesy of W. Atlee Burpee & Co.

28-3 Mexican cooking is flavored with a variety of chilies.

Q: Is it true that hot peppers can actually burn your skin?

A: Yes. That's why chefs recommend you wear rubber or plastic gloves when working with raw peppers. Also, be careful not to touch your eyes or face after handling fresh peppers until you have thoroughly washed your hands.

corn chips. Bananas, pineapples, guavas, papayas, and prickly pears are other tropical fruits that are popular in Mexico. The fruits are often served alone or in a syrup as a light, refreshing dessert.

Sauces and Stews

Mexican cooks often use thick sauces. They pour some sauces over other foods. Other sauces contain pieces of meat, vegetables, tortillas, or beans and are served as main dishes.

Very simple sauces are made from chilies and/or sweet peppers mixed with finely chopped onions and tomatoes. More complex sauces are called ***moles.*** The word mole is derived from the Aztec word *molli,* which means a chili-flavored sauce. Cooks make one type of mole from a variety of chilies, almonds, raisins, garlic, sesame seeds, onions, tomatoes, cinnamon, cloves, coriander seeds, and anise seeds. They finely chop these ingredients and add them to chicken stock. They add the final ingredient, unsweetened chocolate, just before serving. This type of mole is part of turkey mole, which is a traditional dish.

Mexican stews are as unique as moles. Stews begin with a sauce. Cooks grind dried peppers and mix them with ground spices and vegetables. They add some meat or poultry stock to the ground mixture to make a thick paste. Then they fry the paste, thin it, and add it to cooked meat or poultry. See 28-4.

Long, slow cooking gives Mexican stews their characteristic flavors. Because of the high altitude, the boiling point in many parts of Mexico is lower. As a result, stews can be simmered for many hours to develop flavor without becoming overcooked.

Mexican Desserts

Other than fresh fruits and sweet tamales, the Aztecs had few desserts. Catholic convents begun by the Spaniards developed many of the desserts and sweets eaten in Mexico today. Early Spanish and Portuguese cooks influenced those desserts that use large amounts of egg and sugar, such as *flan* (a caramel custard).

Mexican Beverages

Chocolate drinks and coffee are popular Mexican beverages. The cacao bean, known since the days of the Aztecs, is toasted and ground into cocoa or made into chocolate. Mexican chocolate is similar to the hot chocolate drink served in the United States. However, it has a different texture and is lighter than the chocolate served in other Latin American and European countries. A tool called a *molinillo* is used to beat the chocolate into a foam before

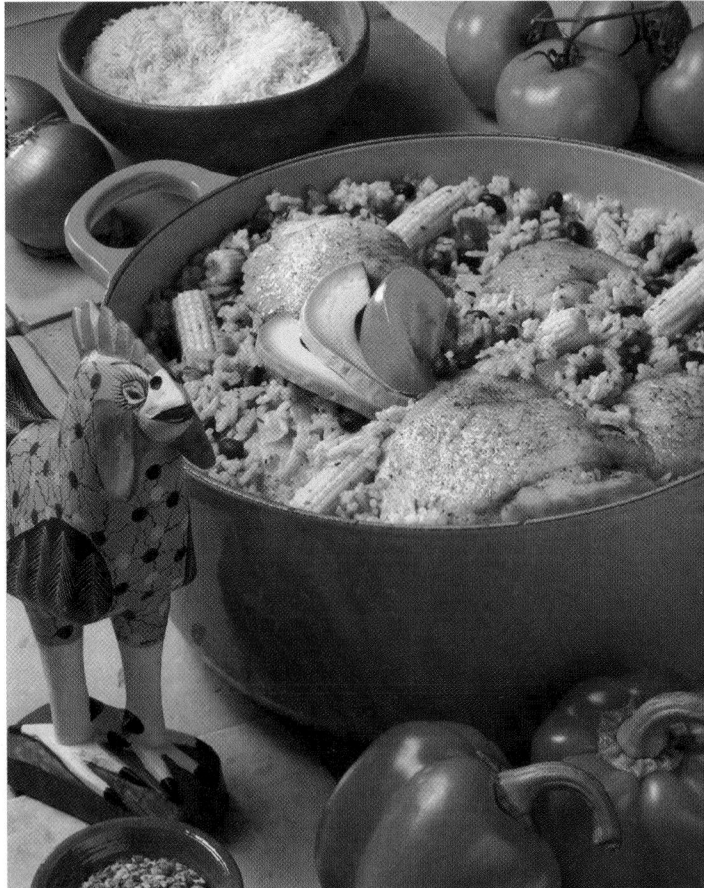

National Chicken Council

28-4 *Arroz con pollo—rice with chicken—is a stewed Mexican dish that is flavored with chilies, cumin, and cilantro.*

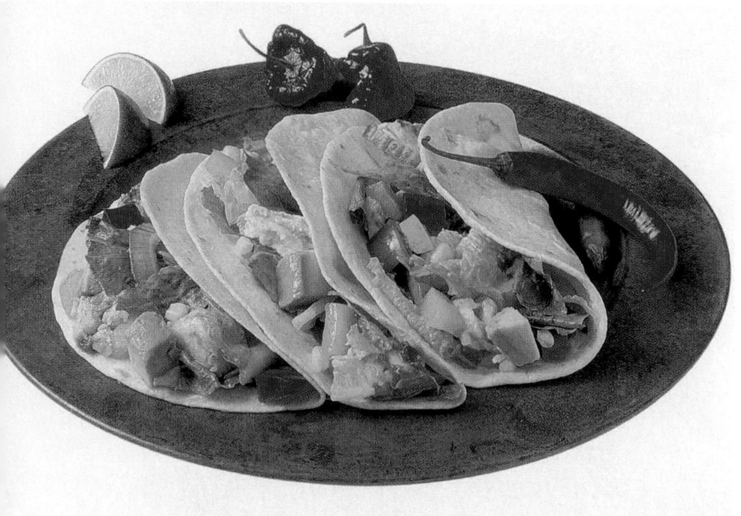

Dole Food Company

28-5 In coastal regions of Mexico, fish becomes a common filling for tortillas.

serving. Coffee often is served with milk and called *café con leche.* It also can be boiled to a thick syrup and served black or with sugar.

Mexican Regional Cuisine

Although many foods are common throughout Mexico, regional differences exist. These occur mainly as a result of geographic and climatic conditions.

In the climate of northern Mexico, farmers can grow wheat and raise cattle. Therefore, tortillas in this area are made from wheat rather than corn. People commonly eat beef, which they may dry or cook with onions, peppers, and tomatoes and serve with beans. Cheese is also popular in several northern states. In Chihuahua, for example, people fry beans in lard and then carefully heat them with cheese. In Senora, cooks cover a potato soup with a thick layer of melted cheese.

Finfish and shellfish are important protein sources for people living in coastal areas. People in these regions use seafood in appetizers, soups, and main dishes, 28-5. Cooks near the Gulf coast make a popular dish from plantains. ***Plantains*** are green, starchy fruits that have a bland flavor and look much like large bananas. The cooks fry the plantains with onions and tomatoes and serve the mixture with shrimp (or other seafood) and chili sauce. *Paella,* derived from the Spanish dish with the same name, contains seafood, chicken, and peas cooked in chicken broth and served with rice.

Wild duck is popular in eastern Mexico. Turkey is one of the most important foods of the Yucatan (peninsula that forms Mexico's southern tip).

Squash blossoms and sea chestnuts (a type of crustacean) are popular in southern Mexico. Because banana trees are abundant, tamales in this region are wrapped in fresh banana leaves rather than corn husks.

Q: Which are more nutritious, corn tortillas or flour tortillas?

A: Corn tortillas are generally made with whole grain, so they are higher in fiber than most flour tortillas. Corn tortillas also tend to be lower in fat than flour tortillas.

Mexican Meals

Mexican meal patterns differ somewhat from those of the United States. Families with ample incomes often eat four meals a day.

The first meal of the day, *desayuno*, is a substantial breakfast. Fruit, tortillas, bread or sweet rolls, eggs or meat, and coffee or chocolate are served. *Huevos rancheros* (eggs prepared with chilies and served on tortillas) are a popular breakfast dish.

The main meal of the day, ***comida,*** is served in the middle of the day between one and three o'clock. Six courses are not unusual. These may consist of an appetizer, a soup, a small dish of stew, a main course, beans, dessert, and coffee. Tortillas are traditionally served, but bread sometimes is substituted. A ***siesta*** (rest period) usually follows comida.

A light snack, *merienda,* is served around five or six o'clock. It includes chocolate or coffee, fruit, and *pan dulce* (sweet breads), 28-6.

Mexicans may eat *cena,* supper, between eight and ten o'clock. Cena is similar to comida, but smaller and lighter. (Many Mexican families combine merienda and cena and eat one meal in the early evening.)

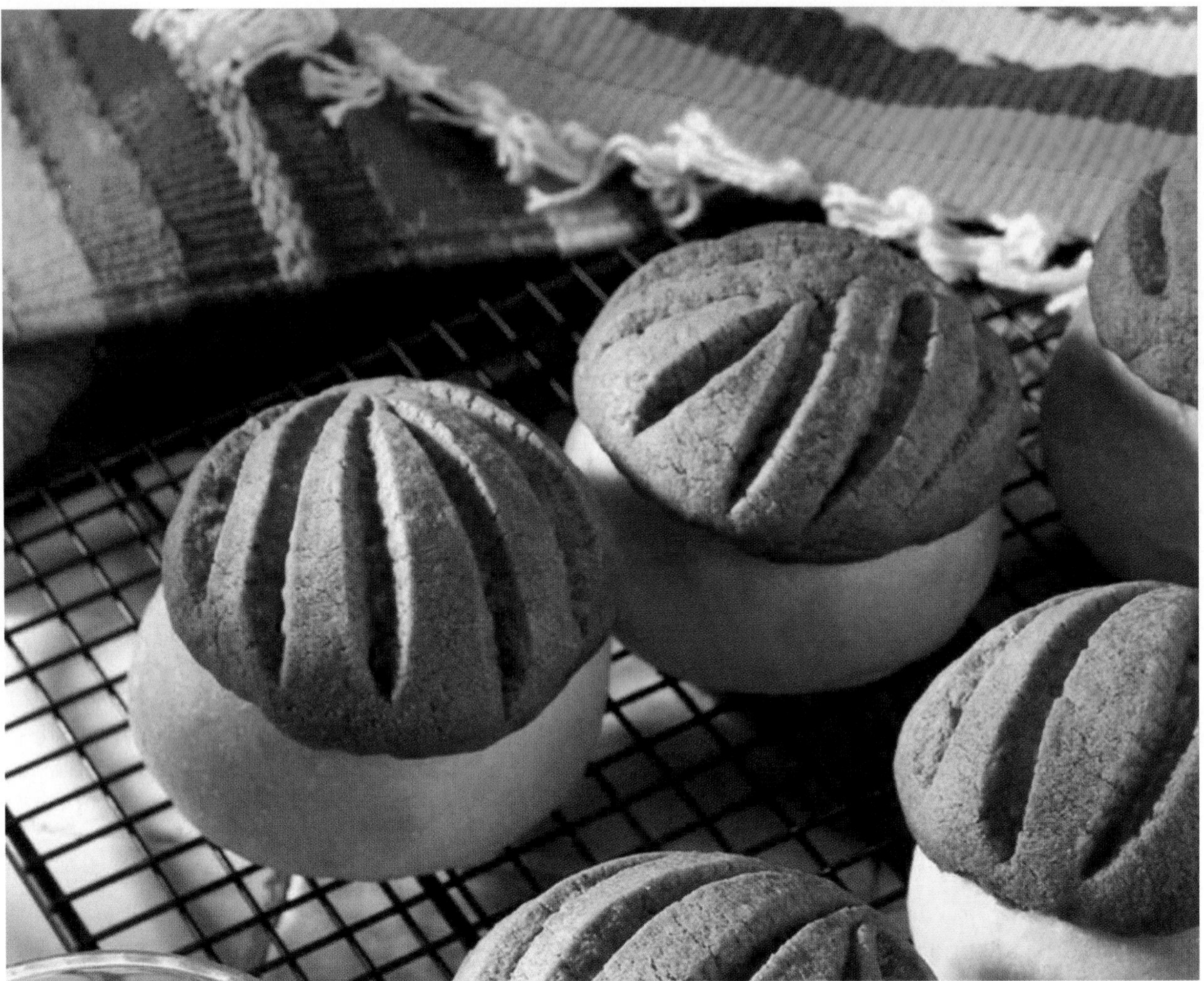

photo courtesy of Fleischmann's Yeast

28-6 *Cocoa and cinnamon give pan dulce their brown, "mushroomlike" tops.*

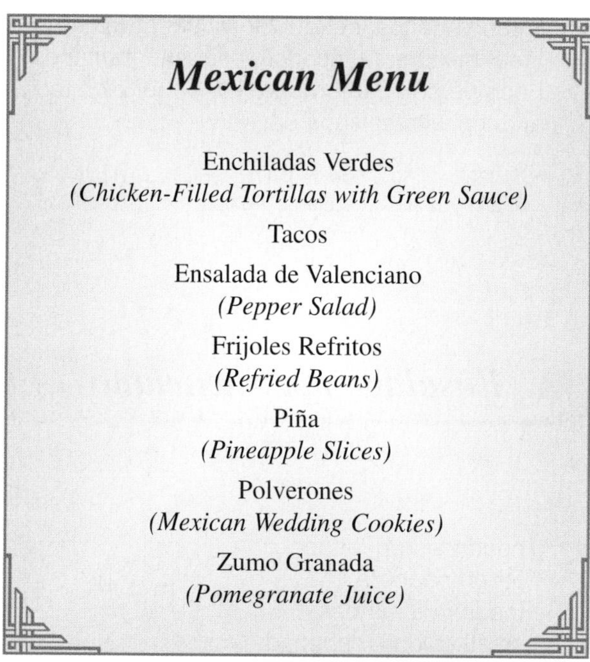

Mexican Menu

Enchiladas Verdes
(Chicken-Filled Tortillas with Green Sauce)
Tacos
Ensalada de Valenciano
(Pepper Salad)
Frijoles Refritos
(Refried Beans)
Piña
(Pineapple Slices)
Polverones
(Mexican Wedding Cookies)
Zumo Granada
(Pomegranate Juice)

Tortillas

(Flat Cornbread)
Makes 12

$2\frac{1}{4}$ cups instant masa harina (corn flour)
1 teaspoon salt
$1\frac{1}{3}$ cups cold water

1. In medium mixing bowl, combine corn flour and salt.
2. Gradually add all but 3 tablespoons of the water.
3. Knead mixture with hands, adding more water (1 tablespoon at a time) until dough no longer sticks to the fingers.
4. Divide the dough in half. With a rolling pin, roll dough between sheets of waxed paper to a thickness of $\frac{1}{16}$ inch.
5. Using a 6-inch plate as a pattern, cut around the plate with a sharp knife or pastry wheel.
6. Place rounds of dough between pieces of waxed paper.
7. Preheat oven to 250°F.
8. Heat a heavy 7- to 8-inch skillet over moderate heat.
9. Cook tortillas one at a time.
10. When lightly browned (about 2 minutes on each side), transfer to foil and keep warm in the oven. Fill as desired.

*Note: Tortillas may be made ahead and refrigerated lightly covered. To rewarm tortillas, brush both sides with water and heat a few minutes in a skillet, one at a time.

Per tortilla: 94 cal. (4% from fat), 2 g protein, 20 g carbohydrate, 0 g fat, 0 mg cholesterol, 2 g fiber, 178 mg sodium.

Enchiladas Verdes

(Chicken-Filled Tortillas with Green Sauce)
Makes 6

1 whole boneless, skinless chicken breast
$\frac{1}{2}$ cup chicken stock
3 ounces Neufchâtel cheese
1 cup evaporated fat free milk
$\frac{1}{3}$ cup finely chopped onions
3 fresh green peppers
$\frac{1}{3}$ cup canned Mexican green tomatoes, drained
1 hot chili (canned) drained, rinsed, and chopped finely
$2\frac{1}{2}$ teaspoons chopped, fresh cilantro
1 egg
dash pepper
$1\frac{1}{2}$ tablespoons shortening
6 tortillas
3 tablespoons grated Parmesan cheese

1. Place chicken breast in small skillet.
2. Pour stock over chicken breast and cover; simmer until chicken is tender, about 20 minutes.
3. Remove chicken to plate and reserve stock.
4. When chicken is cool enough to handle, shred meat and set it aside.
5. In small mixing bowl, beat Neufchâtel cheese until smooth.
6. Add $\frac{1}{2}$ cup evaporated milk, a little at a time.
7. Add onions and chicken, stirring with wooden spoon or rubber spatula. Set aside.
8. Skin peppers. (To skin peppers, place them on a baking sheet in a 350°F oven for 20 to 30 minutes. Turn the peppers every 5 to 8 minutes. When the skins appear to have pulled away from the peppers, remove them from the oven. Place them immediately into a plastic bag for 5 minutes. Slip off skins with a sharp knife.)
9. Remove stem and seeds; coarsely chop peppers and place in blender container.

10. Add tomatoes, hot chili, cilantro and 1/4 cup reserved stock. Blend on high speed until sauce is smooth.
11. Add rest of evaporated milk, egg, and pepper. Blend 10 more seconds; pour into bowl.
12. Preheat oven to 350°F.
13. Grease a small baking dish or 8-inch square cake pan.
14. Melt shortening in small skillet.
15. Fry tortillas one at a time; filling each before frying the next.
16. To fill, place 1/4 cup filling in center of tortilla. Fold one side to center; roll tortilla up completely to form a cylinder.
17. Place filled tortillas side by side in baking dish.
18. When all the tortillas have been filled, pour remaining sauce over them and sprinkle with cheese.
19. Bake about 15 minutes or until cheese has melted. Serve immediately.

Per enchilada: 253 cal. (36% from fat), 19 g protein, 24 g carbohydrate, 10 g fat, 81 mg cholesterol, 2 g fiber, 280 mg sodium.

Tacos

Makes 6

3/4 pound lean ground beef
1 envelope commercial taco or chili seasoning mix
3/4 cup tomato juice
6 tortillas
softened margarine
shredded lettuce
shredded Monterey Jack cheese
coarsely chopped tomatoes
salsa

1. In large skillet, brown ground beef, pouring off fat as it accumulates.
2. When meat is browned, add seasoning mix and tomato juice. Stir well.
3. Simmer, covered, about 10 minutes; stir occasionally.
4. Arrange tortillas on greased baking sheet; brush with margarine.
5. Bake at 400°F 10 to 15 minutes. (Tortillas should begin to set, but they should still be flexible.)
6. Remove from pan and fold in half to form shells.
7. To serve tacos, set out individual bowls of meat mixture, lettuce, cheese, and tomatoes. Each person can prepare his or her own taco and top with salsa, if desired.

Per taco: 282 cal. (50% from fat), 17 g protein, 19 g carbohydrate, 16 g fat, 52 mg cholesterol, 1 g fiber, 440 mg sodium.

Ensalada de Valenciano

(Pepper Salad)
Serves 6

1 head iceberg lettuce
5 green peppers
4 medium tomatoes
2 small onions, chopped
3/4 cup low-calorie French dressing
1 tablespoon chopped parsley

1. Core, rinse, and thoroughly drain lettuce; chill in plastic bag or refrigerator crisper.
2. Roast peppers in a 350°F oven, turning them every 5 minutes. When the skins appear to have pulled away from the peppers, remove them from the oven and place them in a plastic bag for 5 minutes. Peel peppers with a sharp knife; remove seeds and cut in thin strips.
3. Peel and seed tomatoes; dice. Chill peppers and tomatoes.
4. Line 6 salad plates with outer lettuce leaves; shred remaining lettuce and toss with peppers, tomatoes, onion, and dressing.
5. Arrange salad on lettuce-lined plates; sprinkle with parsley.

Per serving: 113 cal. (34% from fat), 3 g protein, 17 g carbohydrate, 5 g fat, 0 mg cholesterol, 5 g fiber, 630 mg sodium.

Frijoles Refritos

(Refried Beans)
Serves 5 to 6

2 cups dried pinto, black, red, or kidney beans (soaked in cold water overnight and drained)
2 tablespoons vegetable shortening
1 onion, finely chopped
3 medium tomatoes, seeded and finely chopped

2 small, fried, hot chilies, crumbled
$^{2}/_{3}$ cup Monterey Jack or Cheddar cheese, crumbled
salt
pepper

1. Place beans in large saucepan and add enough cold water to completely cover beans.
2. Over moderate heat, bring water to a boil. Reduce heat to low, cover pan, and simmer beans until tender, about 1$^{1}/_{2}$ hours. Drain.
3. Puree beans in a blender (or push them through a fine sieve).
4. In a large, heavy skillet, melt shortening.
5. Add onions and cook until lightly browned.
6. Add tomatoes and chilies; cook, stirring frequently, for 5 minutes.
7. Add pureed beans, cheese, and salt and pepper to taste.
8. Cook, stirring occasionally, until cheese melts and beans are hot, about 10 minutes. Serve immediately.

Per serving: 220 cal. (28% from fat), 11 g protein, 29 g carbohydrate, 7 g fat, 10 mg cholesterol, 7 g fiber, 65 mg sodium.

Polverones

(Mexican Wedding Cookies)
Makes 4 dozen cookies

$^{1}/_{2}$ cup margarine
$^{1}/_{2}$ cup shortening
1 teaspoon vanilla
$^{1}/_{2}$ cup confectioner's sugar
2 cups all-purpose flour
$^{3}/_{4}$ cup finely chopped nuts
confectioner's sugar

1. Preheat oven to 425°F.
2. In medium mixing bowl, cream margarine, shortening, and vanilla until fluffy.
3. Mix the $^{1}/_{2}$ cup confectioner's sugar, flour, and nuts together; add to creamed mixture, stirring to form a soft dough.
4. Shape dough into small balls and place on ungreased baking sheet.
5. Bake cookies about 10 minutes or until lightly brown.
6. Roll warm cookies in confectioner's sugar.

Per cookie: 71 cal. (65% from fat), 1 g protein, 5 g carbohydrate, 5 g fat, 0 mg cholesterol, 0 g fiber, 22 mg sodium.

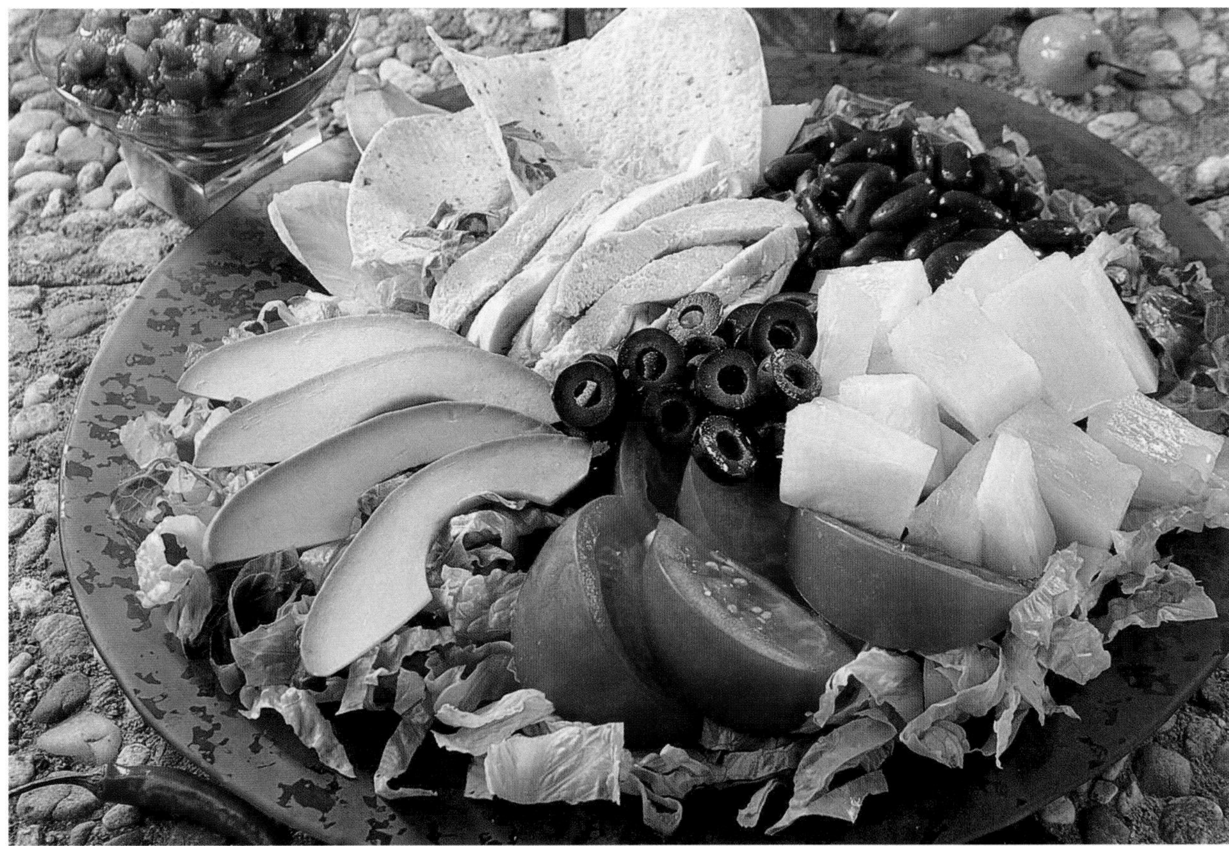

Dole Food Company

Avocados are bland-flavored tropical fruits that often appear in Mexican salads as well as the popular guacamole dip.

South America

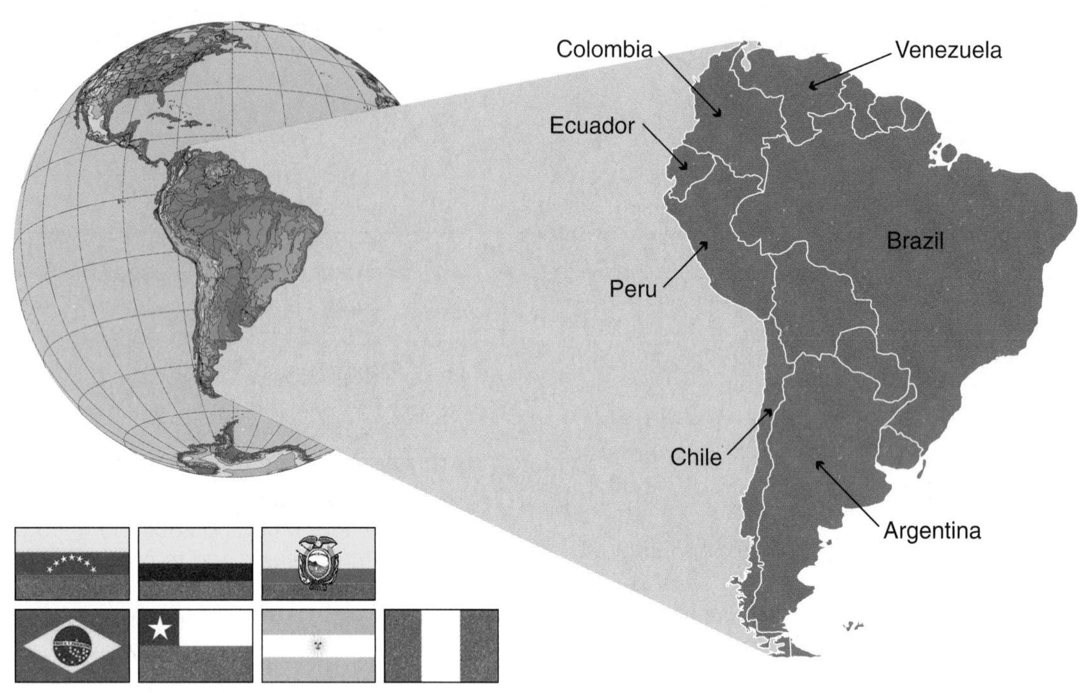

The Atlantic and Pacific Oceans and the Caribbean Sea form the boundaries of South America. South America is nearly twice the size of the United States. It is a land of contrasts—dense rain forests and snowcapped mountains; deserts and lush farmland; large, modern cities and untamed jungles.

Geography and Climate of South America

The geography in South America is varied. Mountains, grasslands, jungles, forests, plateaus, and deserts divide the continent. The Andes Mountains form the longest and second highest mountain chain in the world. These mountains and dense jungles have made travel impossible in many parts of the continent. As a result, each country has developed independently and has preserved a unique culture.

You can find nearly every kind of climate in South America. In parts of Chile, meteorologists have never recorded any rainfall. The area is an arid wasteland. However, rain falls daily in the tropical rain forests of Brazil. Snow and high winds bring bitter cold to the peaks of the Andes, yet the jungles below are hot and humid.

South American Culture

A number of peoples influenced the development of South American culture. These influences can still be seen in the lifestyle of South America today.

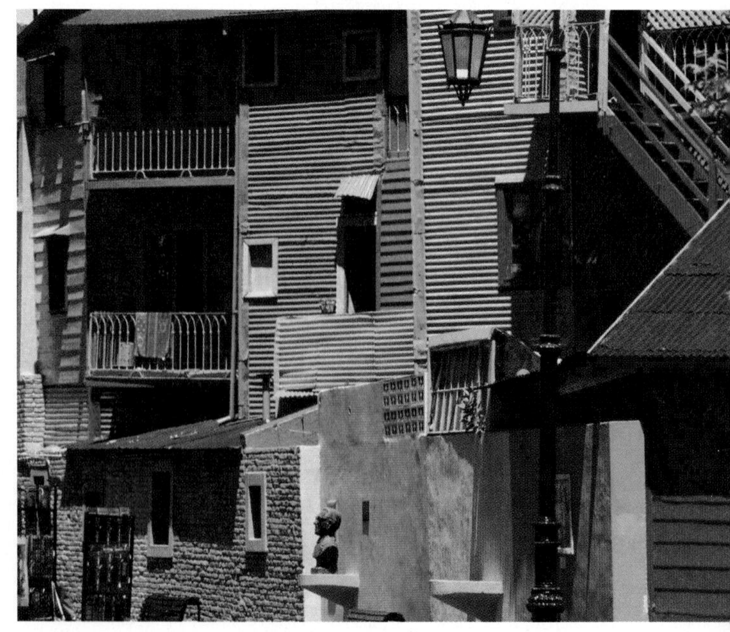

Colorful housing gives neighborhoods in Buenos Aires, Argentina, a unique character.

Influences on South American Culture

When the first explorers came to South America in the sixteenth century, they found the land inhabited by a number of native tribes. One group of Native South Americans, the ***Inca,*** built a large empire in the Andes Mountains. The Inca were advanced in many ways. They built roads and bridges to facilitate travel throughout the empire. They used an irrigation system to increase the productivity of their farmlands.

When Spanish explorers discovered the Incan empire, they were amazed by the level of civilization. Like the explorers in Mexico, however, the explorers of South America were more fascinated by gold and silver. The Incan empire was unable to survive the Spanish conquest. However, Incan influence is still felt in South America today.

Explorers from Portugal landed in the area that is now Brazil. The Portuguese stayed in the area and built large plantations where they grew sugarcane. Today, Portuguese is the official language of Brazil.

The Portuguese brought Africans to Brazil to work in the sugar fields. The Africans influenced the development of South American cuisine. They raised crops of foods from their homeland, including bananas, yams, and coconuts, 28-7. African women used some of their native foods and cooking techniques in the kitchens of the Portuguese.

Modern Culture in South America

Today, South America is in a process of evolution. Most South American countries are

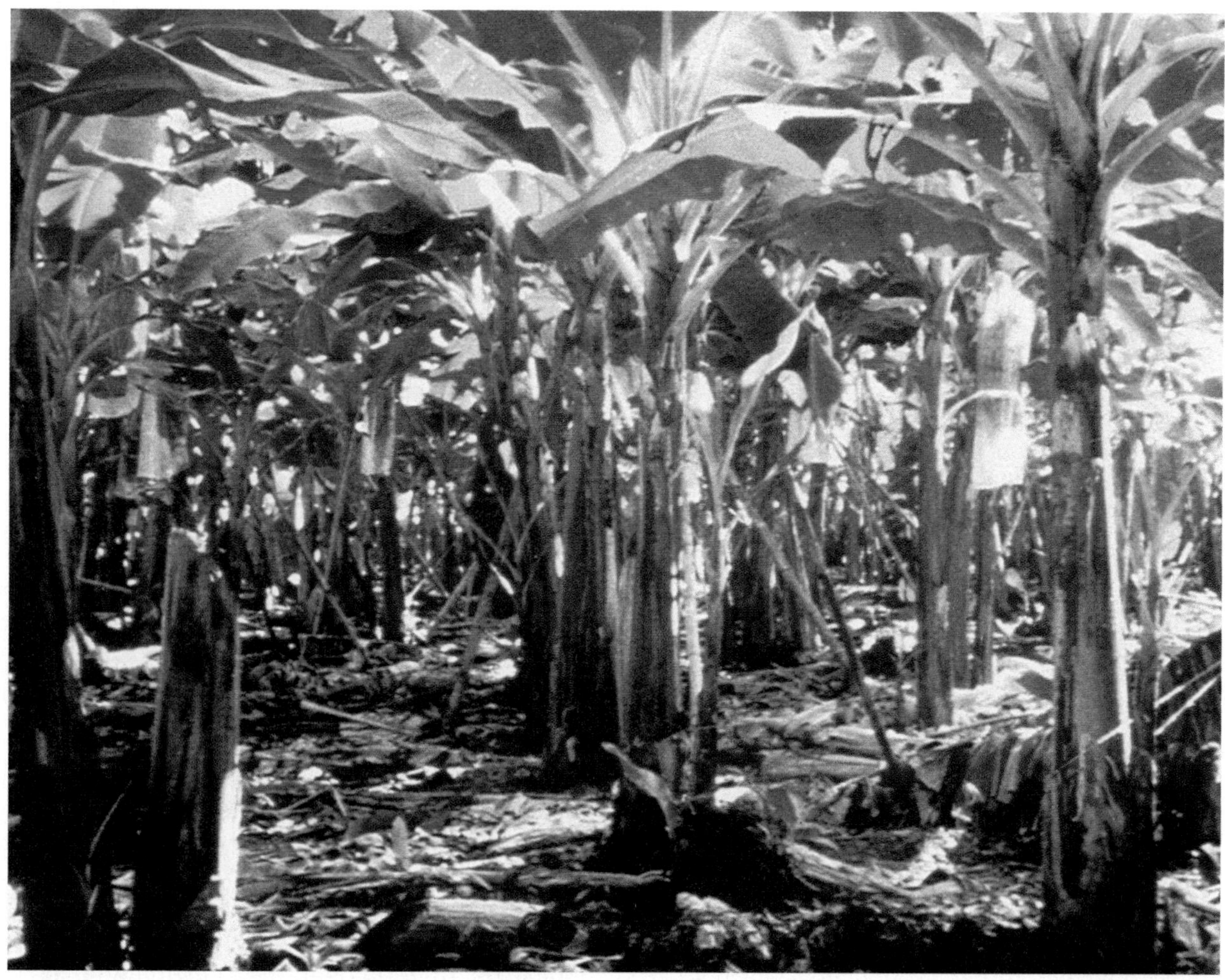

International Banana Association

28-7 *Bananas grow in several South American countries and play an important role in South American cuisine.*

experiencing rapid population growth.

Great economic and technological progress can be seen in skyscrapers, modern highways, and industrial plants. Brasilia, Rio de Janeiro, Caracas, and Buenos Aires are modern cities. Their architecture and transportation systems resemble those of cities in Europe and the United States. However, intermingled with modern buildings are churches that date back to the Spanish conquistadores and the Inca.

South America has both great wealth and great poverty. Some landowners control vast amounts of the most productive farmland. However, most farmers barely survive on small plots with poor soil. The members of the upper classes enjoy the best foods, entertainment, and housing. At the same time, the lower classes are hindered by illiteracy, lack of transportation, antiquated farming methods, and poor wages.

Be a Clever Consumer

Many hotels, restaurants, and shops in other countries may be willing to accept U.S. currency. However, it is more convenient and economical to use local currency when you travel.

The value of U.S. dollars in other countries changes frequently. You may want to exchange some money (perhaps $50) at a bank before leaving home. This will allow you to cover small expenses when you first arrive in another country. However, you should wait until you reach your destination before exchanging most of your money. This will allow you to get a better exchange rate (more foreign currency in exchange for U.S. currency). You will also get a better exchange rate at a bank than you will at a store or hotel.

South American Holidays

Many festivals in South America are blends of Christian celebrations and other beliefs. In Brazil, many holidays combine traditions of African religions with days honoring saints in the Catholic church. In Peru, ancient Incan beliefs are mixed with church holy days.

Many South American festivals last for several days. They are public celebrations with processions through village streets. Music, dancing, parades, and colorful costumes are part of many of these celebrations. Vendors often sell food to the crowds of people who gather to celebrate.

The most elaborate of the South American festivals is Carnival. This is the Brazilian festival that parallels the Mardi Gras festival celebrated in the southern United States. Carnival is held the six days before Ash Wednesday, which is the beginning of Lent in the Christian church. All year, people plan the floats, costumes, and exotic masks that will be part of this celebration.

South American Cuisine

South American cuisine combines influences of native tribes with those of the Spanish, Portuguese, and Africans. Many staple foods, such as corn, potatoes, and manioc, are found throughout the continent, 28-8. (***Manioc,*** known as ***cassava*** in some regions, is a starchy root plant eaten as a side dish and used in flour form in cooking and baking.) However, most food customs have developed on a regional basis because of geographic isolation. Each region reflects cultural influences as well as geographic and climatic ones. The following discussion will give you an overview of some of the unique dishes typical of South America.

Venezuela

The Spanish who explored Venezuela found rich, fertile soil and a temperate climate in the valleys formed by the Andes. The cuisine of this country reflects these two factors. It also reflects the tropical climate found in the jungle lowlands just south of the valleys and the food customs of the Spanish explorers.

Much of Venezuela is inhabited by small farming families. ***Arepa,*** a corn pancake similar to a tortilla, is a traditional Venezuelan bread. It forms the basis of the small farmer's diet. Cooks make arepa by mixing corn flour with water and salt. They shape the stiff dough into balls or patties and toast it on a lightly greased griddle. Although people often eat arepa plain, they also use it to make more elaborate dishes. *Bollos pelones,* for example, are balls of arepa dough stuffed with a meat mixture. These dumplings are then deep-fried or simmered in soup or sauce.

Those people living in the tropical lowlands make good use of the banana, plantain, and

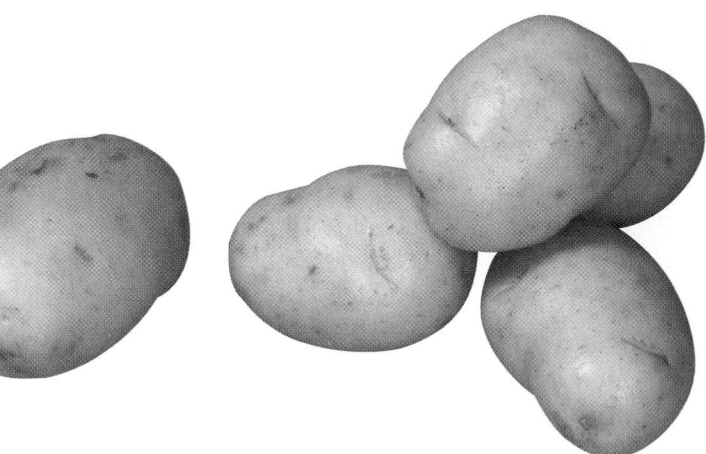

28-8 Potatoes are a staple in the diets of many South American people.

coconut. Bananas and plantains are boiled, fried, baked, and added to stews and soups. Plantains, thinly sliced and fried until crisp, are a popular Venezuelan snack. Banana leaves are used to wrap *hallacas*, Venezuela's national dish, which is cornmeal dough filled with other foods. Candies, puddings, and cakes are made from coconuts. Coconut and coconut milk are also added to stewed meats. A sponge-type cake moistened with muscatel (a type of wine) and covered with coconut cream is a famous Venezuelan dessert.

Colombia

Potatoes, which are grown high in the mountains, are especially important in the diets of northern Colombians. Farther south, cassavas are used instead of potatoes.

Poor Colombians eat little meat. However, stews and thick soups are popular in Colombia. Cooks make one soup, *ajiaco*, with potatoes, chicken, corn, and cassava.

Colombia is an important coffee-producing country. The coffee trees thrive on the cool slopes of the Andes Mountains. The coffee served in Colombia is much stronger than that served in the United States. However, Colombians do not drink as much coffee as people in the United States. See 28-9.

Ecuador

Because Ecuador is a large producer of bananas, local dishes often feature bananas. Ecuadorian people make bananas into flour, which they use to make breads and pastries. They cut firm green bananas and plantains into chips and deep-fry them. The simplest and most common banana dessert is made by slowly frying ripe bananas in butter. As the slices begin to brown, sugar is added little by little until the bananas are brown on both sides. Before serving, the sauteed banana slices are splashed with brandy and dusted with powdered sugar.

Peru

The descendants of the Inca still live in Peru. They have retained many of the customs of their ancestors. Their cuisine reflects both Incan and Spanish traditions.

Since the days of the Inca, the *papa* (potato) has been the staple food of the Peruvian people. The Inca developed over 100 potato varieties. To preserve their potatoes, they freeze-dried them. The cold night air of the Andes quickly froze the potatoes. When the sun came out, the potatoes thawed. At night, they froze once again. The moisture that formed evaporated. Soon the potatoes became hard as

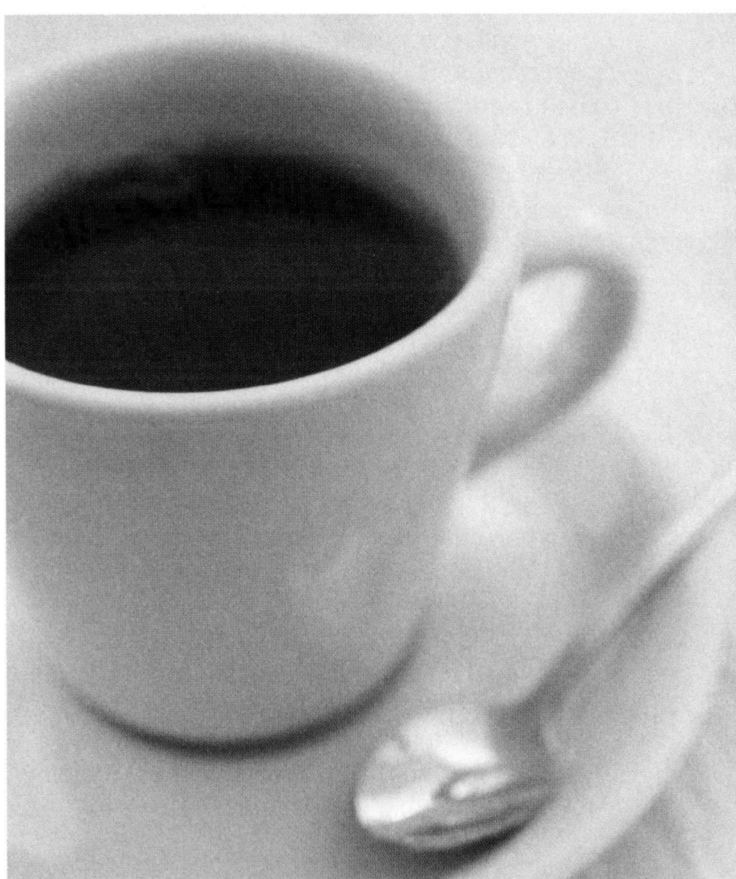

28-9 Much of the coffee consumed in the United States is grown in Colombia.

stone but very lightweight. The Inca could then store the potatoes indefinitely.

The poorest people of Peru eat boiled potatoes alone or with a few local herbs or chilies, which the Peruvians (and Chileans) call ***ají.*** Those who are not quite so poor prepare potatoes in many unusual and delicious ways. One popular potato dish is made by pouring a thick sauce made of cheese, milk, ají, and various local spices over boiled potatoes. Another flavorful potato dish of Incan origin is *causa a la limena.* A mixture of stiff mashed potatoes, olive oil, lemon juice, salt, pepper, chopped onions, and ají is pressed into small molds. The unmolded dish is garnished with hard-cooked eggs, cheese, sweet potatoes, prawns (a shrimplike crustacean), and olives.

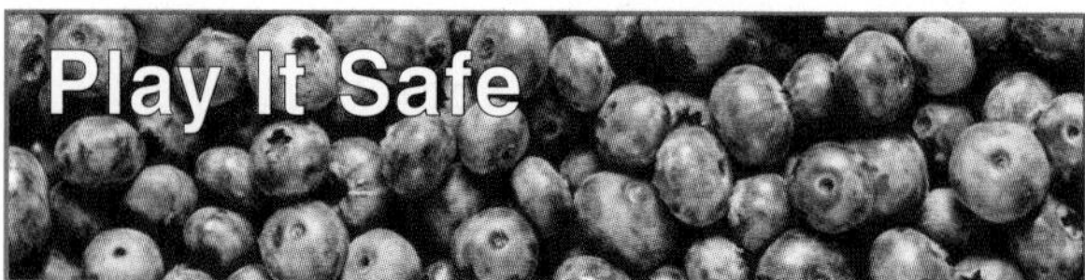

You should avoid drinking tap water or beverages that contain ice when traveling in other countries. Microorganisms in the water can cause diarrhea for people who are not used to drinking it. Bottled water is a safe alternative for drinking. You would also be wise to use bottled water when brushing your teeth.

Peruvians often make *cuy* (guinea pig) into a stew. They also brush cuy with olive oil and garlic and roast it. Vendors on Peruvian streets sell another popular meat dish called *anticuchos.* They marinate small strips of beef heart overnight and thread them on skewers. They baste the meat with a sauce and grill it over hot coals.

Peruvians who live along the coast eat a variety of seafood. Shrimp is especially popular in both appetizers and main dishes. *Chupe,* a thick soup made from milk, vegetables, and shellfish, is served as a main dish.

Peruvians invented ***ceviche,*** a marinated raw fish dish, 28-10. However, people throughout South America enjoy it. Cooks usually make ceviche from *corvinas* (a type of whitefish found off the Peruvian coast), but they can use other types of whitefish. They cut the fish into small cubes. Then they cover it with a marinade made of lime juice, lemon juice, salt, pepper, garlic, onion, and ají. After the fish has marinated for several hours, its texture becomes similar to that of cooked fish. The ceviche is then ready to eat. Peruvians often serve ceviche with corn and sweet potatoes. People in other South American countries often serve it as an appetizer.

Peruvian tamales contain a variety of foods including meat, chicken, sausage, eggs, peanuts, raisins, and olives. Unlike Mexican tamales, they often are somewhat sweet.

Chile

Chile is a long, thin country. The upper third of Chile is arid desert, and the lower third is mountainous. The central region has fertile valleys, irrigated fields, and forests.

Because the land is not suitable for raising cattle or sheep, Chileans eat little meat. Instead, seafood, beans, and small amounts of meat are combined with vegetables in many delicious stews. *Porotos granados,* for example, contains cranberry beans, corn, squash, garlic, and onion.

Another popular dish in Chile is *pastel de choclo.* It is a meat pie made with a sugar-coated

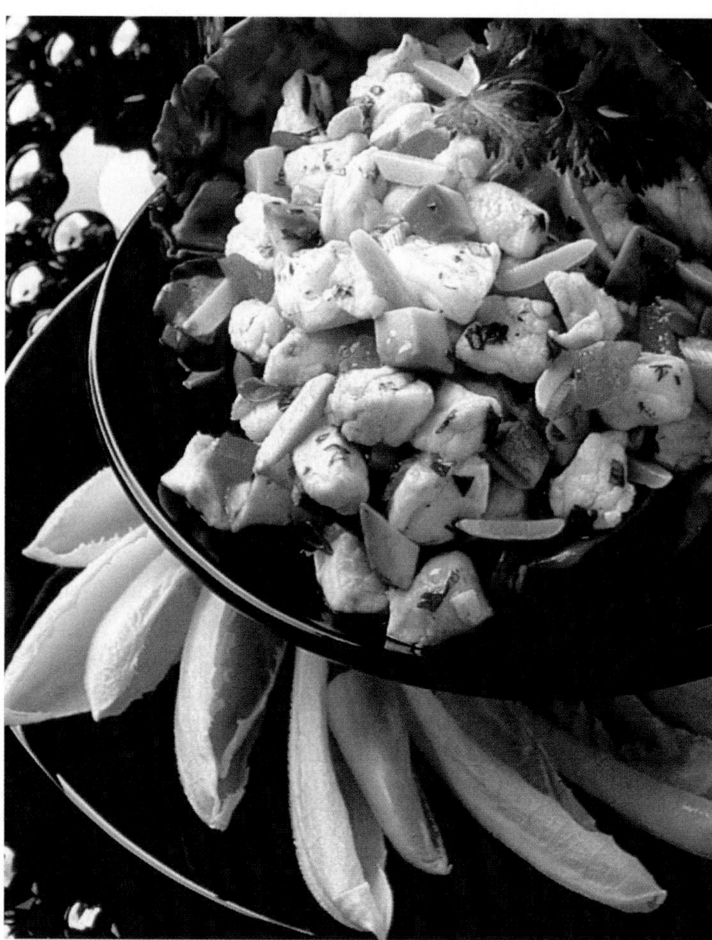

Almond Board of California

28-10 *Although it is Peruvian in origin, ceviche is enjoyed by people throughout South America.*

Q: How can I avoid getting gas when I eat Latin bean dishes?

A: When preparing beans, boil them for 2 to 3 minutes. Let them soak in the boiling liquid for at least an hour. Then drain and rinse the beans before cooking them in fresh water. This preparation method helps remove many of the substances in beans that cause gas.

topping of ground fresh corn. Beef, or a combination of beef and chicken, usually is used in the filling. Raisins and olives may be added. Some cooks also add pepper or ají. However, most Chilean dishes are not peppery.

Of all the South Americans, Chileans probably eat the most seafood. Seafood is both plentiful and inexpensive, and shellfish are particularly popular. Crabs, lobsters, clams, scallops, and sea urchins are used in many dishes. *Chupe de marisco* (scallop stew) is baked in a deep dish. A creamy cheese sauce flavored with paprika, nutmeg, pepper, and onion complements the flavors of scallops and rice.

Argentina

The Pampas are the richest lands in South America. They cover the southeastern part of the continent and reach into the countries of Argentina and Uruguay. Here, large herds of cattle and sheep graze until they are ready for market.

Because it is so readily available, the people of Argentina eat large amounts of meat. Much of the meat is roasted in the style of the gauchos. The ***gauchos*** were nomadic herders of the Pampas during the eighteenth and nineteenth centuries. They put meat from freshly slaughtered cattle on large stakes placed at an angle around a fire. (This prevented the juices from dripping into the coals.) A peppery herb and parsley sauce called *chimichurri* accompanied the freshly roasted meat.

Argentine cooks also prepare meat in other ways. They make one popular dish, metambre, by layering spinach, hard-cooked eggs, carrots, and onions on top of a marinated flank steak. Then they roll the metambre, tie it, and either poach it or roast it until tender.

Argentine appetizers are called ***empanadas.*** They are small turnovers filled with chopped meat, olives, raisins, and onions.

Although most of the foods of Argentina have a strong flavor, mild-flavored squashes and pumpkins have been popular for centuries, 28-11. Cooks use squash to make fritters, soups, and puddings. They sometimes thicken and decorate stews with squash. *Carbonada criolla,* a colorful stew, contains pieces of beef, squash, tomatoes, corn on the cob, and fresh peaches. It sometimes is served in a squash or pumpkin shell.

Humitas are similar to Mexican tamales. Unripe kernels of corn are mixed with onions, tomatoes, salt, pepper, sugar, and cinnamon. Sometimes cheese is also added. Humitas may be cooked with milk until tender and served plain. They may also be rolled into corn husks, tied, and boiled or steamed.

Brazil

Brazilian culture is a mixture of Native South American, Portuguese, and African cultures. The native inhabitants of Brazil were more primitive than the Inca of the Andes. They did not practice agriculture on a wide scale. However, they did produce manioc, which is still a staple food in Brazil.

The Africans brought to Brazil by the early Portuguese made a great impact on Brazilian

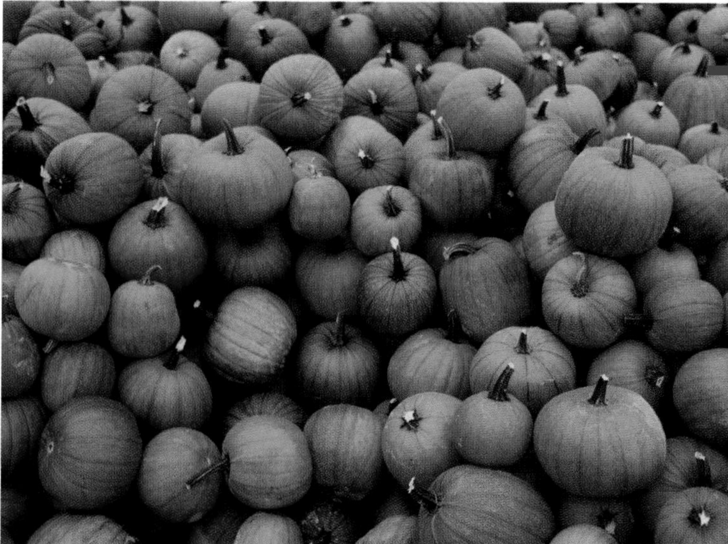

28-11 *Pumpkin adds a mild flavor to some Argentine dishes.*

cuisine. The ***dendé oil*** (palm oil that gives Brazilian dishes a bright yellow-orange color), red pepper, bananas, and coconuts used in many Brazilian dishes were first used by the African cooks.

The African women were skilled cooks and made use of the readily available shrimp and fish. *Vatapa,* for example, is a delicious stew made of pieces of shrimp and fish cooked with coconut milk, palm oil, and pieces of bread. Vatapa is usually served over rice.

The Brazilians serve rice, a second staple food, in a variety of ways. One popular dish is a casserole made of layers of rice, shrimp, ham, chicken, cheese, and tomato. A popular Afro-Brazilian coconut pudding also contains rice.

Beans, a third staple food, are as important to Brazilian cooking as they are to Mexican cooking. Brazilians prefer shiny black beans they can cook to a paste. They use these beans to make ***feijoada completa,*** Brazil's national dish. Feijoada completa is made with meat and beans. It can be simple or elaborate depending on the ingredients used. Traditional feijoada completa includes dried beef and smoked tongue. Other meats, such as fresh beef, pork, bacon, sausage, and pigs' feet, can also be added. The meats are cooked until tender and then arranged on a large platter. The black beans, cooked to a pulp, are served in a separate pot. Bowls of hot sauces, cooked rice, manioc meal, shredded kale or collard greens, and orange slices accompany the beans and meat. See 28-12.

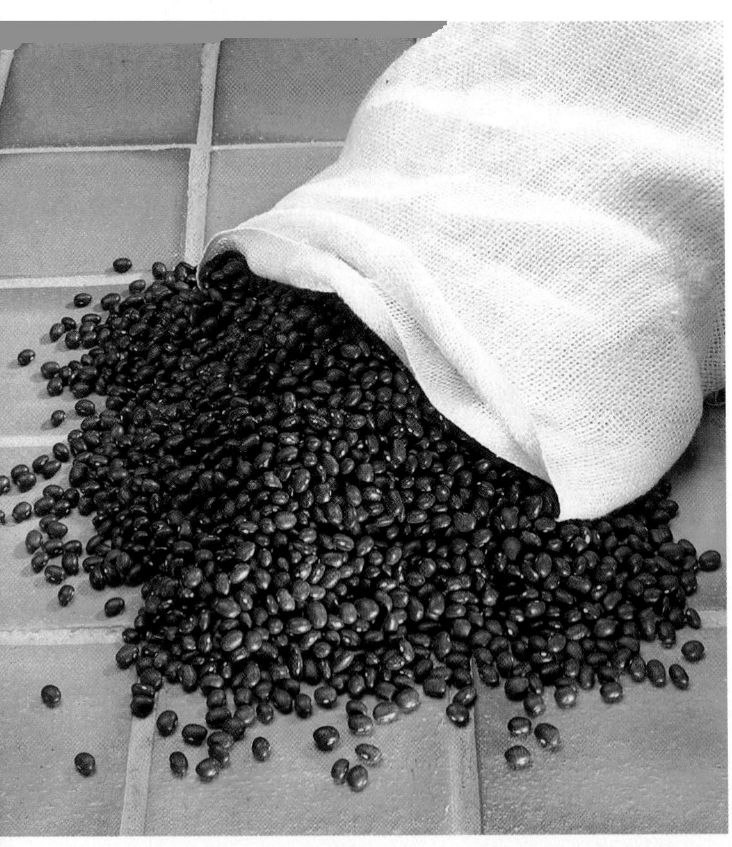

courtesy of W. Atlee Burpee & Co.

28-12 *Black beans are characteristic of Brazilian recipes.*

A Brazilian version of the tamale, called *abara,* is African in origin. Abara is a mixture of cowpeas, shrimp, pepper, and dendé oil rolled into banana leaves and cooked over an open fire.

Cuscuz, a steamed grain dish, is either Arabian or North African in origin. The Brazilians adopted it and developed two different forms of it.

One kind of cuscuz is sweet and is served as a dessert. Cooks mix tapioca, freshly grated coconut, coconut milk, sugar, and water together with boiling water. They pour the mixture into a mold and refrigerate it. Later, they slice and serve the chilled cuscuz. The other type of cuscuz, often called *cuscuz paulista,* is served as a main dish. Cuscuz paulista is made with specially prepared cornmeal mixed with shredded vegetables and meat and a small amount of fat. The mixture is steamed and garnished decoratively.

South American Menu
Empanadas
(Turnovers)
Carbonada Criolla
(Beef Stew)
Couve à Mineira
(Shredded Kale)
Tortillas de Maiz
(Corn Pancakes)
Plàtanos Tumulto
(Broiled Bananas)
Brasileiras
(Brazilian Coconut Cookies)
Café
(Coffee)

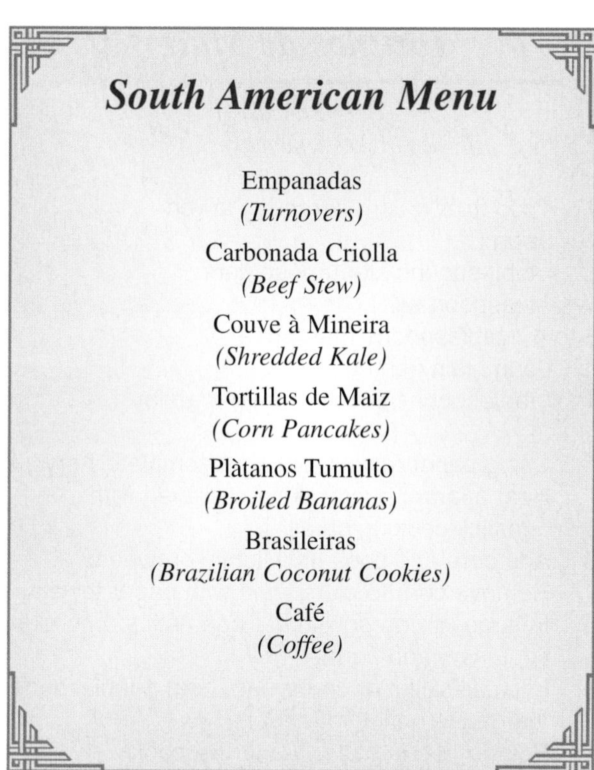

Empanadas

(Turnovers)
Makes about 24

Filling:
1 pound lean ground beef
1 onion, finely chopped
1/2 clove garlic, chopped
2 medium tomatoes
8 large green olives, chopped
1/2 cup raisins
salt
pepper

1. In large, heavy skillet, brown ground beef.
2. Add onions and garlic.
3. When browned, add tomatoes, olives, raisins, and salt and pepper to taste.
4. Simmer mixture uncovered until cooked, about 20 minutes.
5. Remove from heat and refrigerate until you are ready to fill empanadas.

Pastry:
2 cups all-purpose flour
1/2 teaspoon salt
1 teaspoon baking powder
1/2 cup shortening
1/3 cup ice water

1. Sift flour, salt, and baking powder into a large mixing bowl.
2. With pastry blender or two knives, cut shortening into dry ingredients until particles are the size of coarse cornmeal.
3. Add ice water, stirring gently with a fork until dough forms a ball.
4. On lightly floured board or pastry cloth, roll out dough.
5. Using a 2-inch biscuit cutter, cut dough into circles.
6. Place about 1 tablespoon filling in the center of each circle. Fold dough over filling and seal edges well with a little cold water.
7. Bake in a 450°F oven until lightly browned, about 10 to 15 minutes. (For a more authentic dish, empanadas can be fried, a few at a time, in 375°F oil until golden brown.)

Per serving: 126 cal. (50% from fat), 5 g protein, 11 g carbohydrate, 7 g fat, 11 mg cholesterol, 1 g fiber, 95 mg sodium.

Carbonada Criolla

(Beef Stew)
Serves 10

2 tablespoons vegetable oil
2 1/2 pounds beef chuck, cut into 1-inch cubes
3/4 cup coarsely chopped onions
1/2 cup coarsely chopped green pepper
1/2 teaspoon finely chopped garlic
4 1/2 cups beef stock
3 medium tomatoes, seeded and chopped
1/2 teaspoon oregano
1 bay leaf
1 1/4 teaspoons salt
1/2 teaspoon pepper
4 1/2 cups sweet potatoes, cut into 1/2-inch cubes (about 1 1/2 pounds)
4 1/2 cups white potatoes, cut into 1/2-inch cubes (about 1 1/2 pounds)
3/4 pound zucchini, cubed
4 small ears sweet corn, shucked and cut into rounds, 1 inch wide
6 canned peach halves, rinsed in cold water

1. Heat oil in a large Dutch oven.
2. Add meat and brown.
3. Transfer browned meat to a platter and cook onions, green peppers, and garlic until lightly browned.
4. Add beef stock and bring to a boil.
5. Return meat to stock and add tomatoes, oregano, bay leaf, salt, and pepper.
6. Cover Dutch oven and reduce heat to low. Simmer stew for 15 minutes.
7. Remove cover and add sweet potatoes and white potatoes. Simmer for 15 minutes more.
8. Remove cover and add zucchini. Cover and cook 10 minutes more.
9. Remove cover and add corn and peach halves, cover and cook 5 minutes more.

Per serving: 312 cal. (32% from fat), 20 g protein, 34 g carbohydrate, 11 g fat, 53 mg cholesterol, 4 g fiber, 403 mg sodium.

Couve à Mineira

(Shredded Kale)
Serves 6

1 1/2 pounds kale*
2 tablespoons bacon drippings
1/2 teaspoon salt
dash pepper

1. Under running water, carefully wash kale. With a sharp knife, remove any bruised spots and cut tender leaves from tough stems. Discard stems. Shred kale into strips about 1/2 inch wide.
2. In large saucepan, bring 2 quarts water to a boil.
3. Add kale and cook uncovered 3 minutes.
4. Drain kale in a colander, removing as much water as possible.
5. In a large, heavy skillet, melt bacon drippings.
6. When hot, add kale. Cook, stirring frequently, until kale is tender, about 30 minutes. (Kale should still be slightly crisp.)
7. Add salt and pepper and serve immediately.

*Collard greens may be substituted for kale.

Per serving: 58 cal. (62% from fat), 1 g protein, 4 g carbohydrate, 4 g fat, 8 mg cholesterol, 3 g fiber, 193 mg sodium.

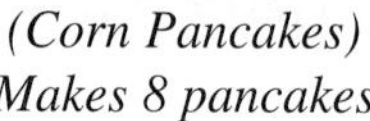

Tortillas de Maiz

(Corn Pancakes)
Makes 8 pancakes

1 cup frozen corn kernels, thawed
1 egg
2 tablespoons all-purpose flour
1/4 teaspoon salt
3 to 4 tablespoons margarine
1/2 cup plain nonfat yogurt
1 1/2 tablespoons chopped fresh parsley

1. Using paper towels, pat corn completely dry.
2. Heat a large, heavy skillet, sprayed with nonstick cooking spray.
3. Add corn and cook until lightly browned.
4. Remove corn to plate lined with paper towels.
5. In large mixing bowl, beat egg until foamy; add flour, salt, and corn.
6. In small skillet or crepe pan, heat 1 tablespoon margarine until it foams.
7. Pour in 1/8 cup batter. As tortilla cooks, gently lift edges to allow uncooked batter to flow underneath.
8. When tortilla is brown on the bottom, flip with spatula and cook other side 1 minute.
9. Slide tortilla onto a heated platter and keep warm in a 225°F oven.
10. Continue making tortillas, adding a teaspoon of margarine before frying each.
11. Serve tortillas topped with 1 tablespoon of yogurt and chopped parsley.

Per tortilla: 79 cal. (55% from fat), 2 g protein, 7 g carbohydrate, 5 g fat, 35 mg cholesterol, 1 g fiber, 137 mg sodium.

Plàtanos Tumulto

(Broiled Bananas)
Serves 6

6 firm, medium bananas
lemon juice
3 tablespoons light brown sugar, packed
3/4 teaspoon cinnamon
3 tablespoons margarine

1. Preheat broiler.
2. Peel bananas and slice in half lengthwise.

3. Place banana halves cut side up on broiler pan; sprinkle with lemon juice.
4. Combine brown sugar and cinnamon in small bowl; cut in margarine until mixture resembles large peas. Sprinkle over banana halves.
5. Place bananas 2 inches from heat and broil until sugar has melted. (Watch carefully.) Serve immediately.

Per serving: 198 cal. (29% from fat), 1 g protein, 34 g carbohydrate, 7 g fat, 0 mg cholesterol, 2 g fiber, 71 mg sodium.

Brasileiras

(Brazilian Coconut Cookies)
Makes about 3 dozen

- 1 cup granulated sugar
- 1/2 cup water
- 4 egg yolks, slightly beaten
- 1/4 cup all-purpose flour
- 2 1/4 cups freshly grated or packaged coconut
- 1/2 teaspoon vanilla

1. In heavy saucepan, combine sugar and water. Cook over moderate heat, stirring until sugar dissolves.
2. Cook syrup undisturbed until candy thermometer reads 230°F. (A small amount of syrup dropped into ice water should immediately form a hard thread.)
3. In small mixer bowl, combine egg yolks and flour until well blended.
4. Add 2 tablespoons of the hot syrup, stirring constantly.
5. Slowly add this mixture to the syrup remaining in the pan, stirring constantly.
6. Add coconut and simmer over low heat, stirring constantly, until mixture becomes thick. (Do not let it boil.)
7. Remove from heat and quickly stir in vanilla. Let mixture cool to room temperature.
8. Preheat oven to 375°F.
9. Shape cookie dough into small balls.
10. Arrange balls 1 inch apart on lightly greased baking sheets.
11. Bake 15 minutes or until cookies are a delicate golden brown.
12. Remove to wire racks to cool.

Per serving: 50 cal. (41% from fat), 1 g protein, 7 g carbohydrate, 2 g fat, 30 mg cholesterol, 1 g fiber, 2 mg sodium.

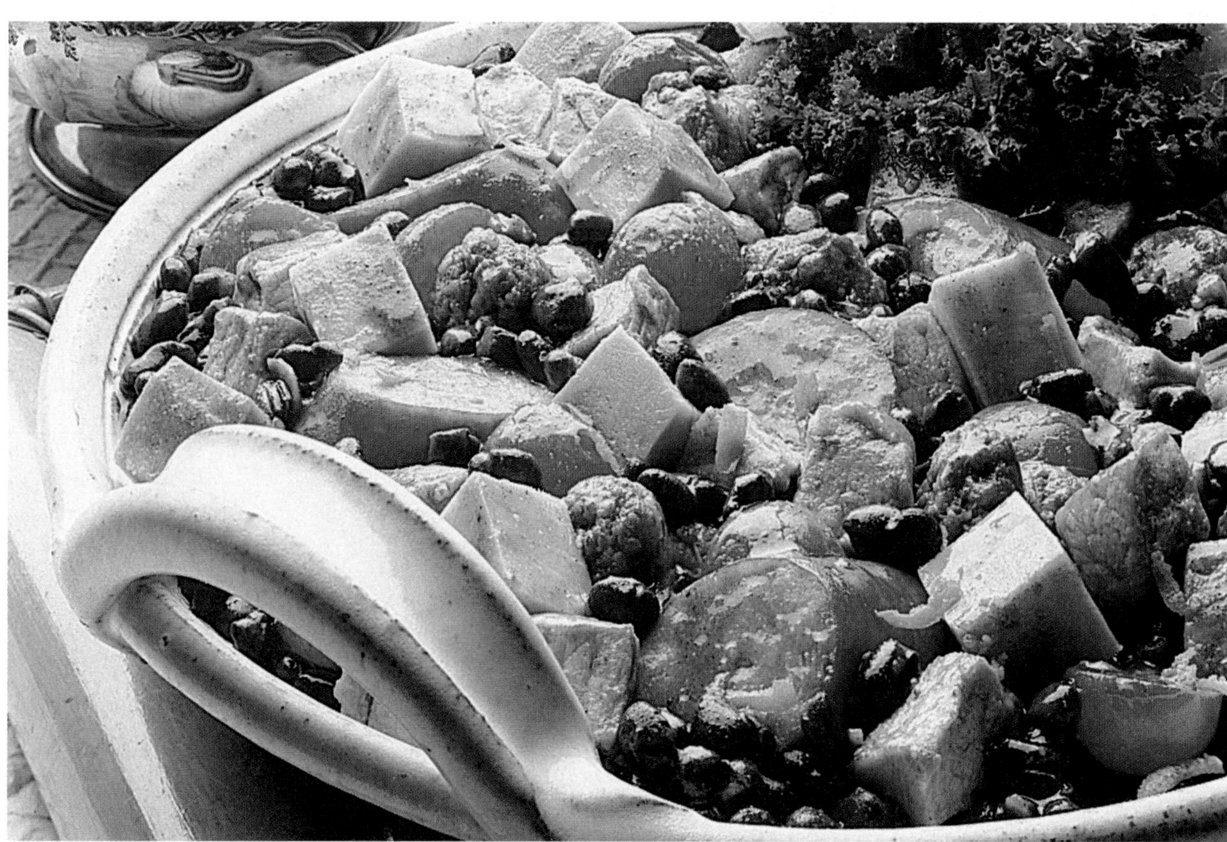

courtesy of National Pork Board

Feijoada completa, a hearty mixture of meat and black beans, is Brazil's national dish.

Chapter 28 Review
Latin America

Summary

The Aztecs and the Spanish conquistadores played a role in Mexico's history. They also contributed to Mexico's cuisine. Many Mexicans are farmers. The corn and beans they grow are important to the economy. These foods are important ingredients in Mexican cuisine, too. Mexican cooks also make much use of peppers, fruits, and vegetables in their cooking. They prepare a variety of flavorful sauces and stews and unique desserts and beverages. Many of these dishes have evolved on a regional basis due to Mexico's varied climate and geography.

Spanish, Portuguese, and African influences are blended with foods of native tribes to form South American cuisine. Throughout the continent, corn, potatoes, and manioc are used as staple foods. However, geographic isolation has caused the way these foods are used to vary from region to region.

Review What You Have Read

Write your answers on a separate sheet of paper.

1. How have climate and geography affected Mexican food customs?
2. The Aztecs and the Spaniards made many contributions to Mexican cuisine. Name four contributions of each.
3. What is a tortilla and how is it made? Describe three Mexican foods made from the tortilla.
4. What are the colors of peppers used in Mexican cooking and how are they used?
5. True or false. Guacamole is a popular spread made from mashed bananas.
6. Describe one type of mole.
7. In Mexico, the main meal of the day is called _____. What foods are usually served at this meal?
8. A corn pancake similar to a tortilla that is a traditional Venezuelan bread is _____.
9. What has been the staple food of the Peruvian people since the days of the Inca? How did the Inca preserve this food?
10. With which South American country are the following words associated: Pampas, gaucho, chimichurri, and carbonada criolla?
    A. Argentina
    B. Brazil
    C. Chile
    D. Venezuela
11. Brazilian culture is a mixture of three cultures. Name them.
12. True or false. Feijoada completa is a Peruvian national dish made with meat and beans.

Build Your Basic Skills

1. **History/writing.** Research the history of the Aztecs and write a two-page report summarizing your findings.
2. **Geography/verbal.** Borrow several travel videos from your local library to learn more about South America. Then participate in a class discussion about how the countries of South America are similar to and different from the United States.

Build Your Thinking Skills

1. **Plan.** Plan and prepare a Mexican meal. Set the mood with appropriate decorations.
2. **Apply.** Apply what you have learned about each of the South American countries you have studied by preparing a buffet of representative foods.

Apply Technology

1. Use the Internet to find out which airlines fly to Mexico and South America. Identify the nearest point of departure as well as three Mexican and three South American destinations. Share your findings in class.
2. Work in a small group to choose a specific aspect of a Latin American country on which you want to focus a presentation. Your group should scan or download images and then use presentation software to create a slide show to present to the class.

Using Workplace Skills

Armando is a Spanish interpreter for a travel agency that serves mainly Latin American clients traveling in the United States. His job is to translate his clients' questions and comments to tour guides and hotel and restaurant staff who do not speak Spanish.

To be an effective worker, Armando needs to display sociability toward his clients. He needs to demonstrate understanding, friendliness, and empathy to people who are in unfamiliar surroundings and are unable to communicate. Put yourself in Armando's place and answer the following questions about your need for and use of this quality:

A. How might your clients be affected if you lack sociability?
B. How might tour guides and hotel and restaurant staff interacting with your clients be affected if you lack sociability?
C. How might your travel agency be affected if you lack sociability?
D. What is another skill you would need in this job? Briefly explain why this skill would be important.

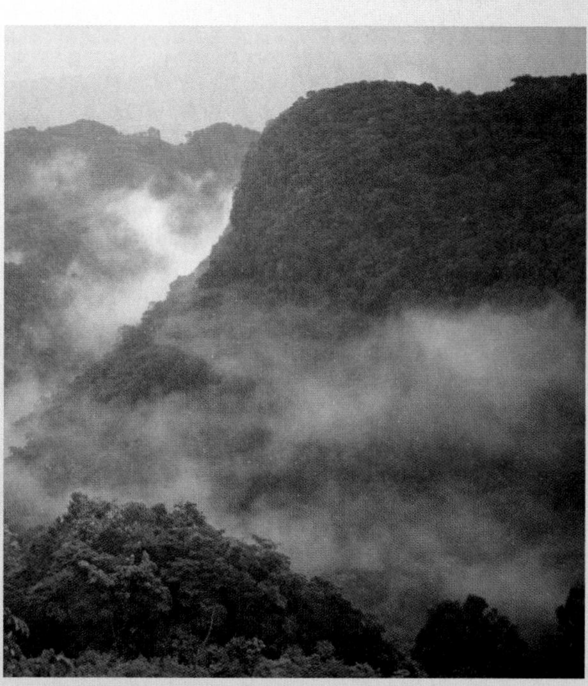

Chapter 29
Europe

Tea Taster
Tastes samples of tea to determine palatability of product or to prepare blending formulas.

Sommelier
Selects, requisitions, stores, sells, and serves wines in a restaurant.

Tour Guide
Arranges transportation and other accommodations for groups of tourists, following planned itinerary, and escorts groups during entire trip, within single area or at specified stopping points of tour.

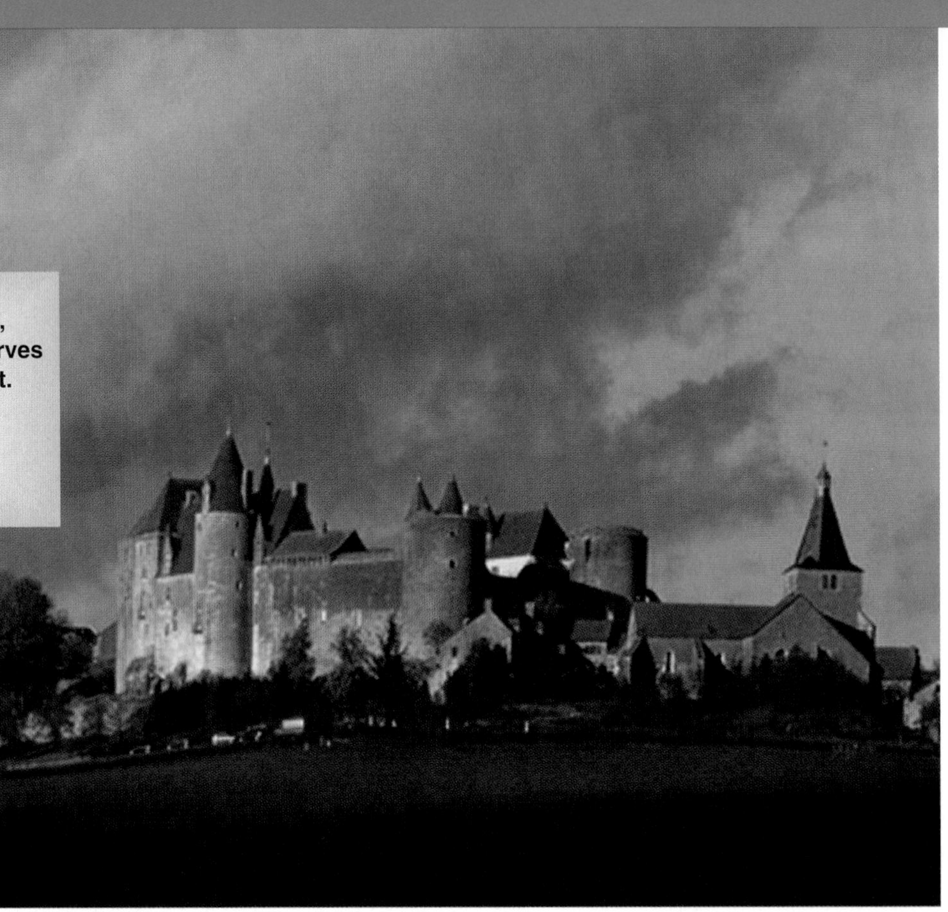

Terms to Know

cockles
fish and chips
pudding basin
tea
haggis
colcannon
haute cuisine
provincial cuisine
nouvelle cuisine
fines herbes
hors d'oeuvres
croissant
crêpe
truffles
escargot
quiche
braten
kartoffelpuffer
sauerkraut
spätzle
strudel
crayfish
smørrebrød
lutefisk
smörgåsbord
husmankost
lingonberry
sauna

Objectives

After studying this chapter, you will be able to

- identify food customs of the British Isles, France, Germany, and the Scandinavian countries.
- explain how and why these customs have evolved.
- prepare foods native to each of these countries.

Europe is the second smallest continent in terms of land area. Despite its small size, it is one of the most heavily populated continents. Nearly one-fifth of the world's people live in Europe.

Europe has been a cultural, political, and economic leader for centuries. Its history is rich and varied.

Because so many countries are part of Europe, you will read about them in two groups. The next chapter will discuss Spain, Italy, and Greece. This chapter will focus on the British Isles, France, Germany, and Scandinavia.

Each European country has a unique cuisine, but some common diet patterns emerge. The diets of Northern European countries include a variety of fruits, vegetables, and breads. However, meals in these countries tend to center around meat, fish, poultry, or game. Dairy products also play an important role in many Northern European cuisines. Rich desserts are popular in these cuisines, too. Together, these characteristics describe a diet that tends to be fairly high in fat.

To include Northern European foods in a healthful diet, choose generous portions of vegetable and grain dishes. Limit portion sizes of meat and dairy foods. Select fruits for dessert often. Enjoy rich desserts only occasionally.

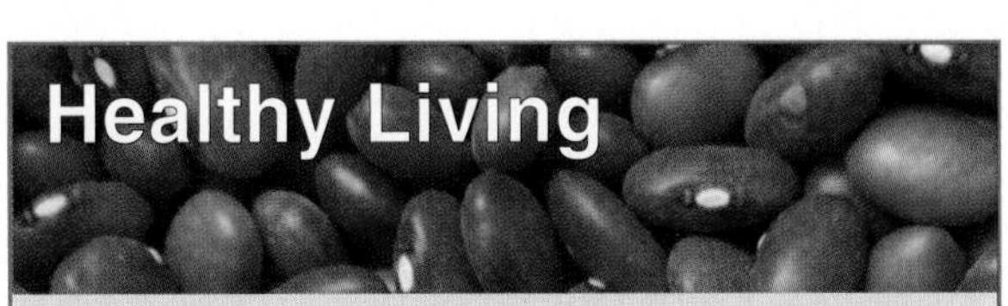

When flying to Europe, or anywhere else, be sure to drink plenty of beverages on the plane. The air on airplanes is dry. An adequate fluid intake will help you prevent dehydration.

Stone walls divide many hillsides in the picturesque Irish countryside into sheep pastures.

British Isles

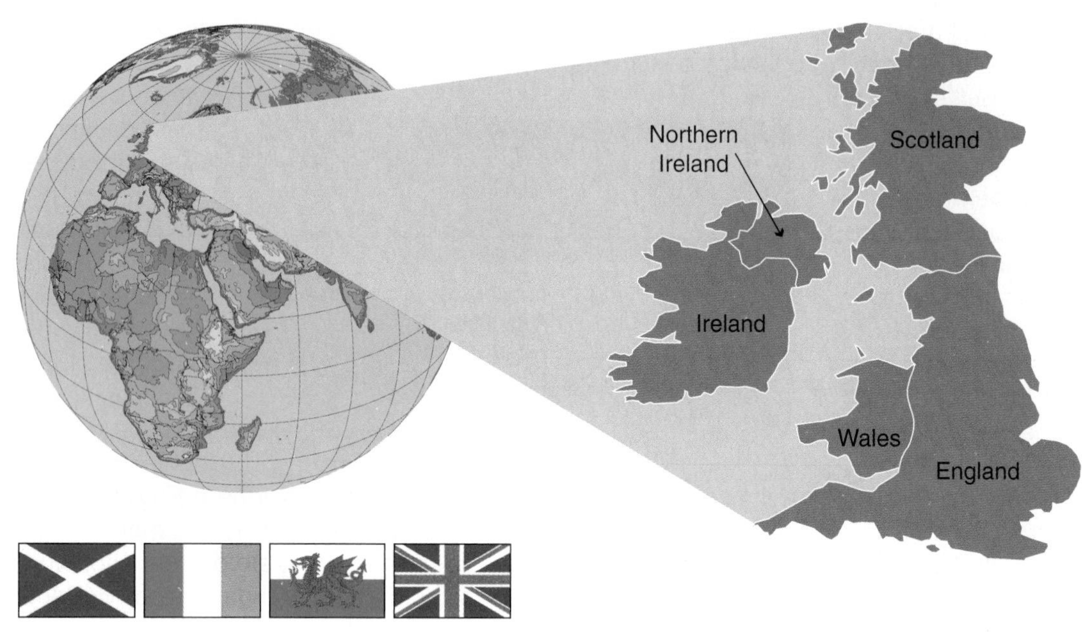

The British Isles are a group of two large islands and several small islands. They are located northwest of mainland Europe. The largest island, Great Britain, includes England, Scotland, and Wales. The second largest island, Ireland, is politically divided between two countries. Northern Ireland is joined with England, Scotland, and Wales to form the United Kingdom of Great Britain and Northern Ireland. The United Kingdom has four political divisions united under a single government. The southern part of the island of Ireland is the country of Ireland, which is an independent nation with its own government.

The people of the British Isles share a common ancestry and culture. Due to geographic isolation, however, each region of the British Isles has separate customs and traditions.

Geography and Climate of the British Isles

The Atlantic Ocean, North Sea, Irish Sea, and English Channel are the bodies of water that surround the British Isles. Much of England is composed of fertile farmlands. The Pennine Chain is a mountain range that runs northward through the center of England to the Scottish border. Southern Scotland is made up of rolling hills. The central lowland region is the location of most of Scotland's population, industry, and farmland. Northern Scotland is a rugged, mountainous area known as the Highlands. Wales can be divided into two parts. North Wales is

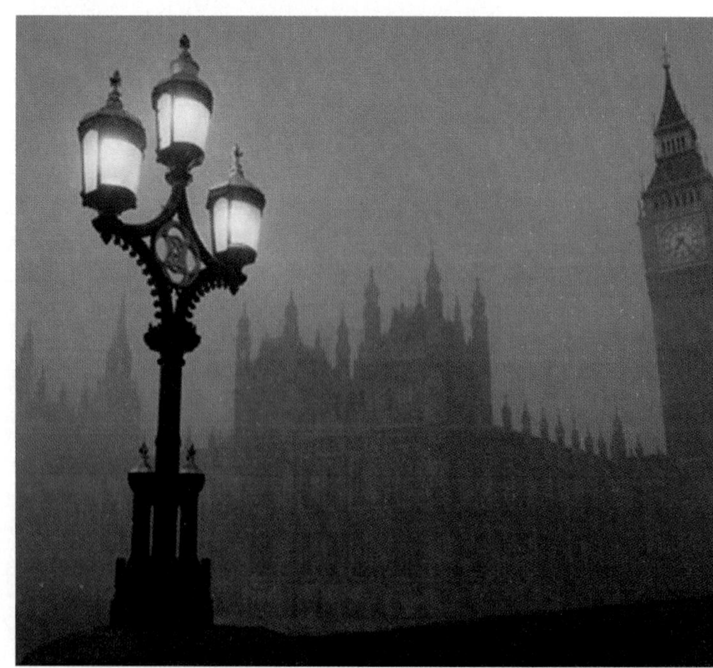

Fog is a common sight on the streets of London.

mountainous country. South Wales is marked by valleys and coastal plains. Much of Ireland is covered with rolling hills and windswept plains. The landscape of Northern Ireland rises into low mountains along the northeast coast.

The weather changes in Britain from hour to hour and from village to village. Fog along the coasts is common, and the air is often raw and bone-chilling.

Culture of the British Isles

The British Isles have a long and colorful history. For centuries, this was the center of one of the world's greatest empires. It was a well-spring of contributions in the areas of art, architecture, and literature. The United Kingdom is still one of the most influential nations on earth.

British History

A number of groups of people shaped the culture of the British Isles. These included the Celts, Romans, Germanic tribes, and Normans. The Celts lived on the British Isles from about 500 B.C. until the Romans invaded some 600 years later.

The Jutes, Angles, and Saxons were Germanic tribes that invaded England from mainland Europe in the A.D. 400s. Eventually, the Angles and Saxons set up kingdoms throughout England. (The name *England* comes from "land of the Angles.") In 1066, William the Conqueror led a Norman army into England. (The Normans were a group of Scandinavian Vikings who had settled in northern France.) Through a military victory William became the new king of England, and Norman influence spread throughout the British Isles.

The English language developed from the Germanic and Norman languages. It is the official language used throughout the United Kingdom. Welsh is a second official language in Wales. Many people in Scotland and Northern Ireland speak a form of an ancient Celtic language called *Gaelic*. Gaelic and English are both official languages in Ireland.

Good Manners Are Good Business

When meeting people from Great Britain, avoid starting a conversation by asking "What do you do?" This would be typical small talk in the United States. However, the British consider this question to be rather personal. You would also be wise to avoid such controversial topics as politics and religion. The British love animals, so try chatting about animals instead.

British Government

Wales was united with England in 1536 under King Henry VIII. In 1707, Scotland was united with England and Wales to form the Kingdom of Great Britain. Ireland became joined with Great Britain in 1801 to form the United Kingdom of Great Britain and Ireland.

Most of the people on the island of Ireland had been Roman Catholic for centuries. During the early 1600s, land on the northern part of the island was given to Protestants. Ongoing conflict existed between the Protestants in the north and the Catholics in the south. In 1921, the British Parliament agreed to the formation of the Irish Free State in southern Ireland. In 1937, this state adopted a new constitution and changed its name to Ireland, or Eire in Gaelic. In 1949, Ireland severed all connections with the United Kingdom and became an independent nation. Northern Ireland remains part of the United Kingdom. However, strife between Protestants and Catholics living in Northern Ireland continues.

London is the capital of the United Kingdom. It is the home of the Houses of Parliament, where British laws are made. The House of Lords and the House of Commons are the two bodies that make up Parliament. The monarchy has no real power. Instead, the head of government is the Prime Minister. The Prime Minister is usually the political party leader with the most members in the House of Commons.

British Agriculture

Much of the land on the British Isles is suitable for growing crops and raising livestock. Wheat, oats, and barley are the key grains grown in the British Isles. Potatoes are also an important crop throughout this area. Ireland has always been known for its excellent cattle, and Irish pedigree bulls are traded all over the world.

Chickens, hogs, and dairy cattle are important sources of food. Sheep are raised for their wool as well as their meat.

Because water surrounds the British Isles, fishing is an important industry. Cod, haddock, and mackerel are among the most important catches. Along the Welsh coast, a type of mussel called ***cockles*** has flourished for hundreds of years. People still go to the shore and dig cockles out of the sand to sell in nearby markets.

Recreation in the British Isles

The people of the British Isles enjoy outdoor activities and sporting events throughout the year. Golf, hiking, mountain climbing, horseback riding, cycling, fishing, and tennis are well-liked activities when the weather is warm. In colder weather, skiing and curling are favorite pastimes. Popular sporting events in the British Isles include soccer, rugby, cricket, and hurling.

In Scotland, the Highland games are an annual recreational event. They are held in different areas throughout the spring, summer, and fall. The games include a variety of events, similar to a track meet.

Throughout the British Isles, a favorite social activity is relaxing with friends in a local public house, or pub. People gather to enjoy a glass of beer, play darts, and talk. See 29-1.

British Holidays

Festivals and holiday traditions are reflections of culture among the people of the British Isles. In Scotland, New Year's Eve is called Hogmanay. It is celebrated with bonfires and feasts. A Scottish tradition centers around the first person to enter a family's home after midnight. This person is called the *first-footer.* The Scots look for the first-footer to carry bread, coal, and money. They believe this means the family will not be hungry, cold, or poor in the coming year. The Scots drink a New Year's toast of sweet or spiced ale from a *wassail bowl.* This name comes from "Waes hael," which is Gaelic for "Be well."

An annual Welsh festival is St. David's Day, which honors the patron saint of Wales. This celebration takes place on March 1. Welsh people pin daffodils (a spring flower) or leeks (a winter vegetable) to their clothes. This symbolizes the passing of winter into spring. St. David's Day feasts feature traditional Welsh foods, such as leek soup, lamb, and Welsh wines and cheeses.

St. Patrick's Day is a national celebration held in honor of Ireland's patron saint. People often dress in green and display shamrocks to observe St. Patrick's Day. Green represents the color of Ireland's countryside. Shamrocks are Ireland's national emblem. This day is celebrated by Irish people throughout the world with food, folk music, and parades. In Ireland, however, St. Patrick's Day is an important religious holiday spent quietly with family and friends.

November 5 is a distinctly English holiday—Guy Fawkes Night. This celebration is named for a man who tried to blow up the Houses of Parliament in 1605. The British gather for fireworks and bonfires. The bonfires are topped with figures made of paper or straw stuffed into old clothes to represent Guy Fawkes.

Cuisine of the British Isles

The cuisine of the British Isles is hearty and filling. Cooks use many locally grown foods. They prepare them in a variety of ways to

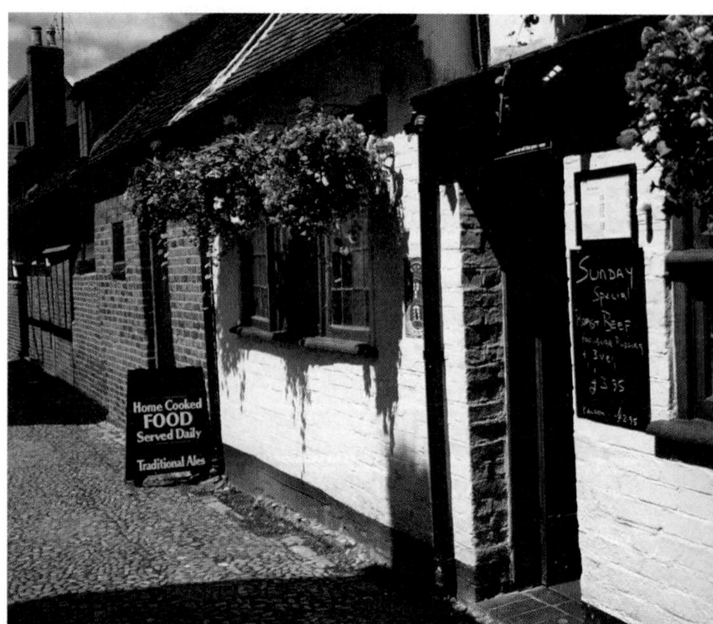

29-1 *Local pubs play an important role in British social life as popular meeting places.*

create dishes that are substantial yet simple and economical.

Development of Cuisine

The early Anglo-Saxons hunted, fished, and gathered nuts and berries for food. They eventually made small gardens and grew grain along the edges of the forests.

Using techniques they had brought from their homelands, the Anglo-Saxons brewed ale from barley. They ground grain for use in baking bread. They made the milk of sheep and cattle into butter and cheese. The Anglo-Saxons also grew apple trees for cider and kept bees for honey. They either roasted the meat from freshly caught game or cooked it in large iron pots. By the eleventh century, the Anglo-Saxons had added puddings and pies to their cuisine.

Several other contributions to British cuisine were made during the reign of William the Conqueror. The Normans prepared delicious breads and pastries. They made some unusual dishes, such as *tripe* (stomach tissue of cattle and oxen). They also used spices and herbs in large quantities.

Norman meals had several courses. Normans served their meat course on *trenchers* (wooden or metal platters or large slices of bread). This was an example of the more refined manners the Normans used.

British Cuisine

The bread, meat, cheese, pies, and puddings of the Anglo-Saxons are still staples of the British diet today. For centuries, England has specialized in a variety of dishes based on these staple foods. Steamed puddings and pickled meats are among the many foods for which British cooks are famous. Savory and sweet pies, crumpets, and a slightly sweet yeast bread called Sally Lunn are also popular British foods, 29-2.

British Main Dishes

The British enjoy beef, pork, lamb, mutton, and wild game. The British perfected the art of roasting centuries ago, and roasting is still popular.

Rivaling the British love of meat is the love of fish. The British eat fresh mackerel, whiting, cod, haddock, Dover sole, halibut, salmon, and many other varieties. They often prepare these fish by baking or poaching. Kippers (split and salted herring) are popular smoked fish.

Shops selling fish and chips are scattered throughout England. ***Fish and chips*** are battered, deep-fried fish fillets served with the British version of French fries. The type of fish vendors use often depends on the particular day's catch. Cod, haddock, and sole are the most popular.

Creative British cooks turn leftovers into a number of popular dishes. *Bubble and squeak* is the name for a cold cooked beef and potato dish. The beef and potatoes are mixed with either cold cabbage or Brussels sprouts and cooked until crisp. *Shepherd's pie* is a mixture of finely chopped meat and leftover vegetables topped with mashed potatoes and baked, 29-3. *Toad in the hole* is made by pouring a thick batter over pieces of leftover meat and baking the mixture.

British Fruits and Vegetables

Apples have grown in England for centuries, and British cooks use apples in many simple but creative ways. Baked apples, apple charlotte,

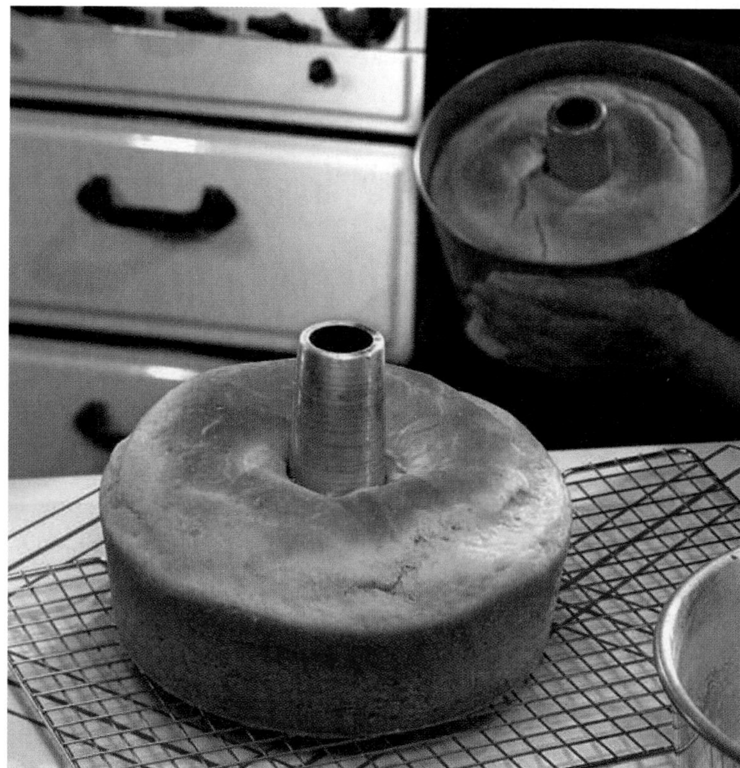

photo courtesy of Fleischmann's Yeast

29-2 Sally Lunn is a rich yeast bread that is made from a batter and has a slightly sweet taste.

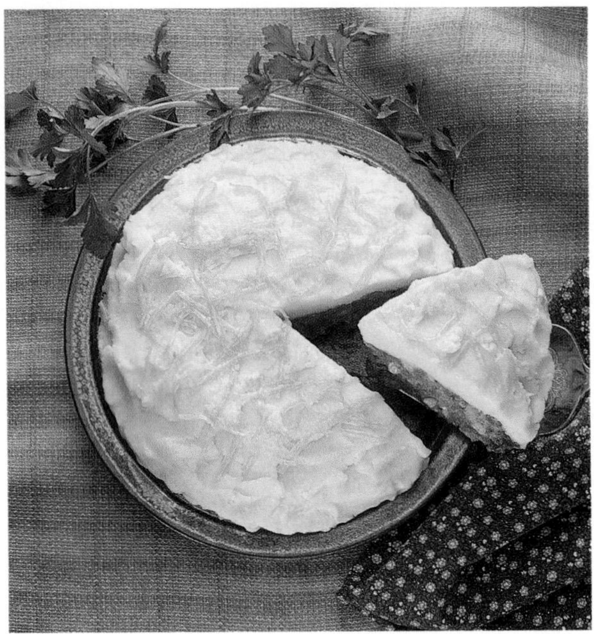

Idaho Potato Commission

29-3 Hearty shepherd's pie is a filling British main dish that can be made from leftovers.

apple crumble, apple pudding, and apple sponge are popular desserts. British people enjoy other fruits, too. They serve fresh strawberries with rich, thick cream. They use a variety of berries as well as apples, plums, and other fruits to make jams, jellies, and preserves.

Carrots, spinach, parsnips, peas, beans, cabbage, cauliflower, onions, and potatoes grow well in British gardens. Sauces appear occasionally, but the British usually serve vegetables right from the garden cooked with just butter and simple seasonings.

British Pies and Puddings

A discussion of British foods would not be complete without mentioning pies and puddings. Both can be either desserts or main dishes.

Steak and kidney pie is one of the best known British pies. Cooks combine slices of kidney with beef chuck and a savory gravy and cover it with a pastry crust. A plum pie dusted with sugar is a popular dessert pie.

The British serve hundreds of sweet puddings. Each pudding begins with the same basic ingredients—milk, sugar, eggs, flour, and butter. Extra ingredients, such as dried fruit, spices, and lemon juice, make each pudding unique.

Most puddings are steamed in a ***pudding basin.*** The traditional basin is a deep, thick-rimmed bowl. A cook pours the pudding mixture into the basin and covers it with a clean cloth. Then the basin goes into a large kettle that is partially filled with water to steam the pudding. See 29-4. Cooks make boiled puddings by wrapping the dough in a piece of floured cloth. Then they tie the cloth at the top and immerse the pudding in a kettle of boiling water.

A *summer pudding* is neither boiled nor steamed. A basin is lined with slices of bread. The lined mold is then filled to the top with sweetened, fresh berries, covered with more bread, weighted, and chilled. During chilling, the bread soaks up the fruit juices. The unmolded pudding often is served with heavy cream.

The *trifle* is another popular British dessert. You might call it a pudding-cake. A mold or serving dish is lined with slices of pound cake spread with a fruit jam. The cake is soaked with sherry. The mold is then filled with layers of custard, fresh fruit, whipped cream, and slivered almonds.

British Meals

Traditional British breakfasts are hearty, including eggs, bacon, fried bread served with marmalade, and tea. People in many parts of

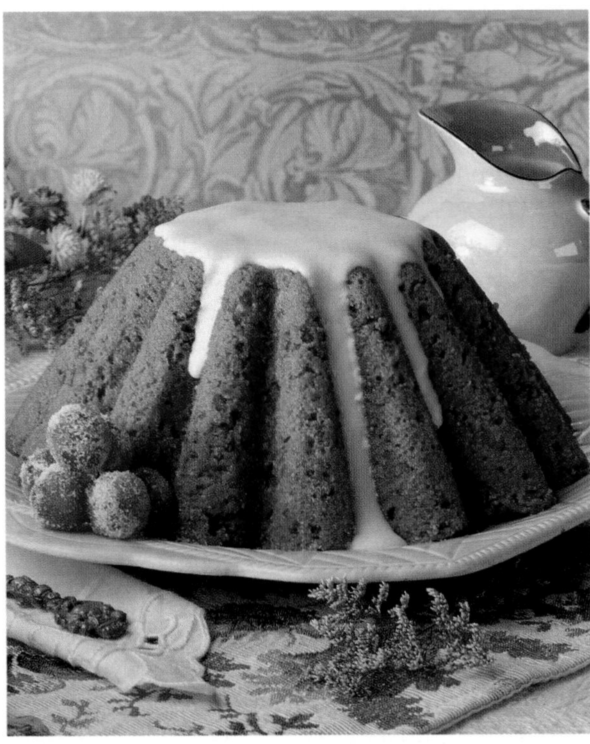

Gold Medal Flour

29-4 Steamed pudding is often served at the end of Christmas dinner in England.

England also eat fruits, main dish pies, ham, smoked fish, and porridge as breakfast foods.

During the week, lunch often is little more than a hearty meat or cheese sandwich and tea. On Sunday, however, lunch is the main meal of the day.

People in all the countries of the British Isles serve tea throughout the day as a beverage. The term ***tea*** also refers to a light meal. In rural areas, for example, the evening meal is called tea. In the cities, where people usually serve dinner in the evening, tea is a snack in the afternoon.

The British serve many foods for tea. A simple tea may consist of tea and a few cookies or a piece of cake. More elaborate teas may include a variety of sandwiches, sausages, cheeses, breads, cakes, and cookies. In England, people often serve crumpets with butter and homemade jam. *Crumpets* are a bread product similar to the English muffin served in the United States. See 29-5.

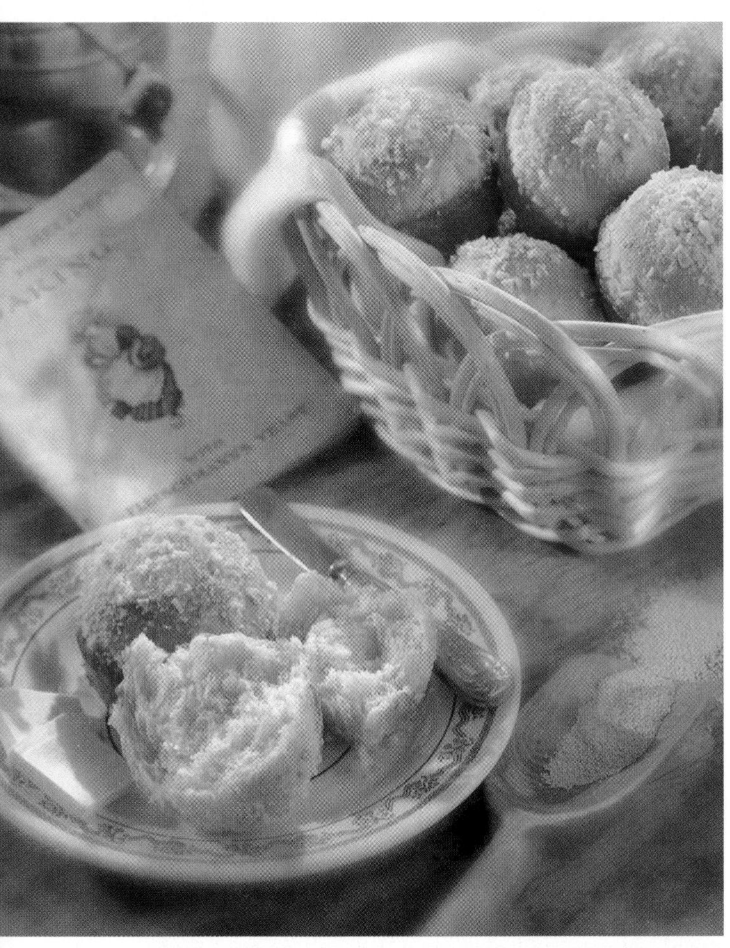

photo courtesy of Fleischmann's Yeast

***29-5** English bath buns, spread with butter and jam, might be served for tea.*

Scottish Cuisine

Oats and barley grow well in Scotland. Both grains have long been staple foods. Cooks often use them to make breads and porridges. Cooks also use oats to prepare the traditional Scottish holiday dish called haggis. ***Haggis*** is a sheep's stomach stuffed with a pudding made from oatmeal and the sheep's organs. Barley is basic to the production of ales and liquors, many of which are exported. Fine Scotch whiskey, for example, is known throughout the world.

Scottish cooks are known for the good, simple, wholesome foods they prepare. Many Scottish dishes contain locally produced beef, lamb, or mutton. Others contain fish caught in coastal waters. Fresh fruits and vegetables, cereal products made of oats and barley, and dairy products may be added. For example, a hearty broth made from meat bones and vegetables often forms the basis for soup. Scotch broth and cock-a-leekie are two traditional Scottish soups. *Scotch broth* is made with lamb and barley; *cock-a-leekie* is made from chicken broth and leeks.

Fishing is an important industry in Scotland. As a result, the Scots eat fish often. Kippers and *finnan haddie* (split and smoked haddock) are especially popular in Scotland.

The Scots eat even heartier breakfasts than the British. They eat large amounts of porridge with *baps* (soft breakfast rolls), kippers, and many steaming cups of tea. Dundee is the birthplace of marmalade, which is eaten throughout the British Isles. Aberdeen is the birthplace of the breakfast sausage.

Scottish cooks consider baking to be one of their greatest skills. Their baking skills are most apparent at high tea, which they serve at around six o'clock. Scottish specialties served at high tea include scones, shortbread, Dundee cake, and black bun. *Scones* are rich, triangle-shaped biscuits. They are usually split in half and spread with butter and marmalade, 29-6. *Shortbread* is a rich, buttery cookie made from flour, sugar, and butter. *Dundee cake* is a rich fruitcake sprinkled with almonds. *Black bun* is a fruitcake covered with pastry. Gingerbread cakes, oatcakes, and brown and white rolls are other favorites.

Welsh Cuisine

Welsh food is similar to the foods of England and Scotland in its simplicity. The

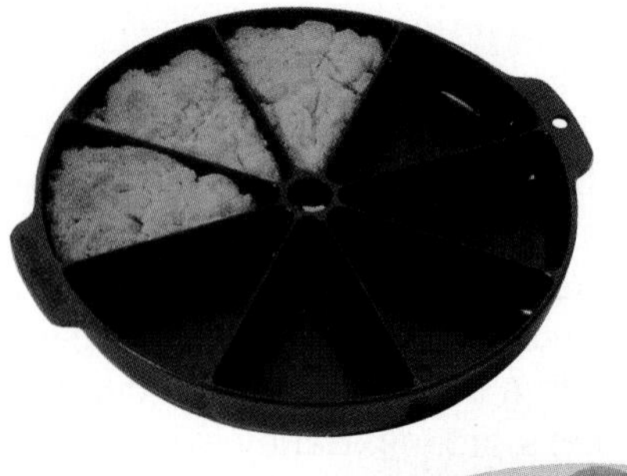

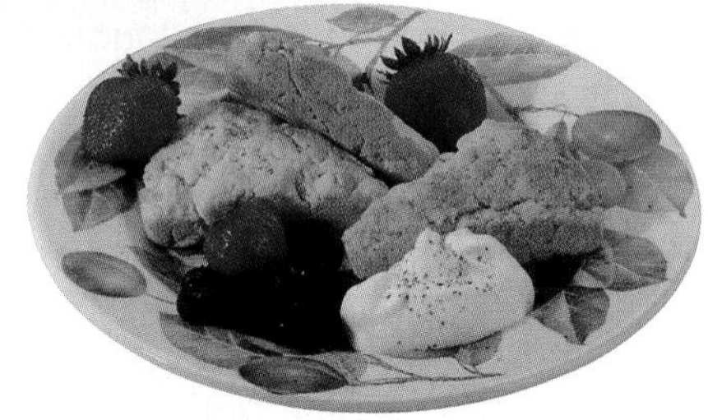

Nordic Ware

29-6 Scones are a specialty of many Scottish bakers.

Welsh use homegrown foods to prepare dishes that are substantial yet plain and economical.

The rugged hills found in much of Wales are suitable for sheep production. The finest spring lambs in the British Isles graze on the grasses in the Brecon Beacons of Wales. Understandably, lamb and mutton are prominent in the Welsh diet. *Cawl* is a hearty soup made from mutton and leeks and other vegetables.

Besides lamb, the Welsh eat beef, pork, veal, and seafood. The Welsh often serve ham boiled. They eat cockles with a dash of vinegar.

The Welsh grow potatoes, carrots, and other vegetables in local gardens and add them to soups and stews. *Tatws slaw* (potatoes mashed with buttermilk) frequently accompanies ham.

The Welsh serve tea in late afternoon or early evening. Various baked goods accompany cups of steaming tea. *Crempog* (buttermilk cakes) and *bara ceirch* (oatcakes spread with butter and eaten with buttermilk) are especially popular. Sponge cake and *bara brith* (a bread filled with currants) are enjoyed as well.

Familiar to many people in the United States is Welsh rabbit (or rarebit). *Welsh rabbit* is toast covered with a rich cheese sauce. One story says this dish got its name because Welsh peasants were too poor to buy meat, even rabbit meat. The closest dish they could afford was this cheese dish, which they nicknamed "Welsh rabbit."

Irish Cuisine

Though the island of Ireland is divided politically, the people share a culinary heritage. Local dishes are still prepared with recipes that have been handed down from generation to generation.

Irish Vegetables

Potatoes have been the mainstay of the Irish diet for centuries. Their importance can best be seen in the results of the 1847 potato crop failure. Thousands of Irish people died, and over a million fled to the United States to escape the "black famine."

In many Irish homes, potatoes are still part of the daily diet. The Irish cook potatoes in a small amount of salted water and serve them with butter. They also use potatoes in soups, stews, breads, rolls, and cakes. Crisp, fried cakes made from grated raw potatoes, flour, salt, and milk are called *boxty*. Potatoes mashed with finely chopped scallions and milk and served with melted butter are called *champ*. Mashed potatoes mixed with chopped scallions, shredded cooked cabbage, and melted butter are called ***colcannon.***

Q: Can potatoes take the place of bread or rice at a meal?

A: Although potatoes are high in starch, they are in the vegetable group. If you replace bread or rice with potatoes, you still need at least six daily servings of grain foods. You also need to choose at least two additional servings of nonstarchy vegetables, such as broccoli, carrots, and tomatoes.

A variety of other vegetables are also grown in small gardens across Ireland. Cabbage, onions, carrots, cauliflower, parsnips, turnips, and peas are plentiful. The Irish may serve these vegetables creamed, baked, or cooked in water. Mushrooms gathered from the fields are sauteed in butter or added to soups and stews.

Garlic and parsley add both color and flavor to meats, poultry, soups, and stews.

Irish Main Dishes

The excellent beef cattle produced in Ireland account for the popularity of *corned beef and cabbage*. This Irish dish is economical because it is made with the beef brisket. The Irish also use beef for roasting, braising, and adding to stews. The Irish steak and kidney stew is similar to the steak and kidney pie served in England.

Sheep thrive in the mountainous areas of Ireland where the land is too poor for farming. The Irish serve the first lamb of the year on Easter Sunday to mark the beginning of spring. They usually roast the leg of lamb. However, they use less tender parts of the animal to make Irish stew. *Irish stew* is pieces of lamb and potatoes in hearty gravy, 29-7.

The Irish eat pork both fresh and cured, but Ireland is best known for its boiled hams. Traditionally, the Irish covered a whole boiled ham with sugar and bread crumbs and studded it with cloves.

The Irish who live close to the sea carry home buckets of seafood from fishing boats on the wharf. Most kinds of seafood are inexpensive because they are readily available. Favorites include crabs, mussels, prawns, and scallops.

Irish Baked Goods

Many people consider Irish breads to be some of the best in the world. Some Irish farm families still bake *soda bread* and *brown bread* every day.

Baking is most important at tea. The Irish sometimes serve eggs, cold meats, and salads at tea. However, they always serve a variety of breads and cakes. They spread soda bread, brown bread, oatcakes, and scones thickly with butter. *Barmbrack,* a light fruitcake served with butter, is one of the most popular Irish cakes. On All Hallows' Eve (October 31), the family baker adds a wedding ring wrapped in paper to the batter before baking. Legend says the person who receives the slice of barmbrack with the ring will marry before the year ends. Two other favorite desserts served for tea are sponge cake and Irish whiskey cake.

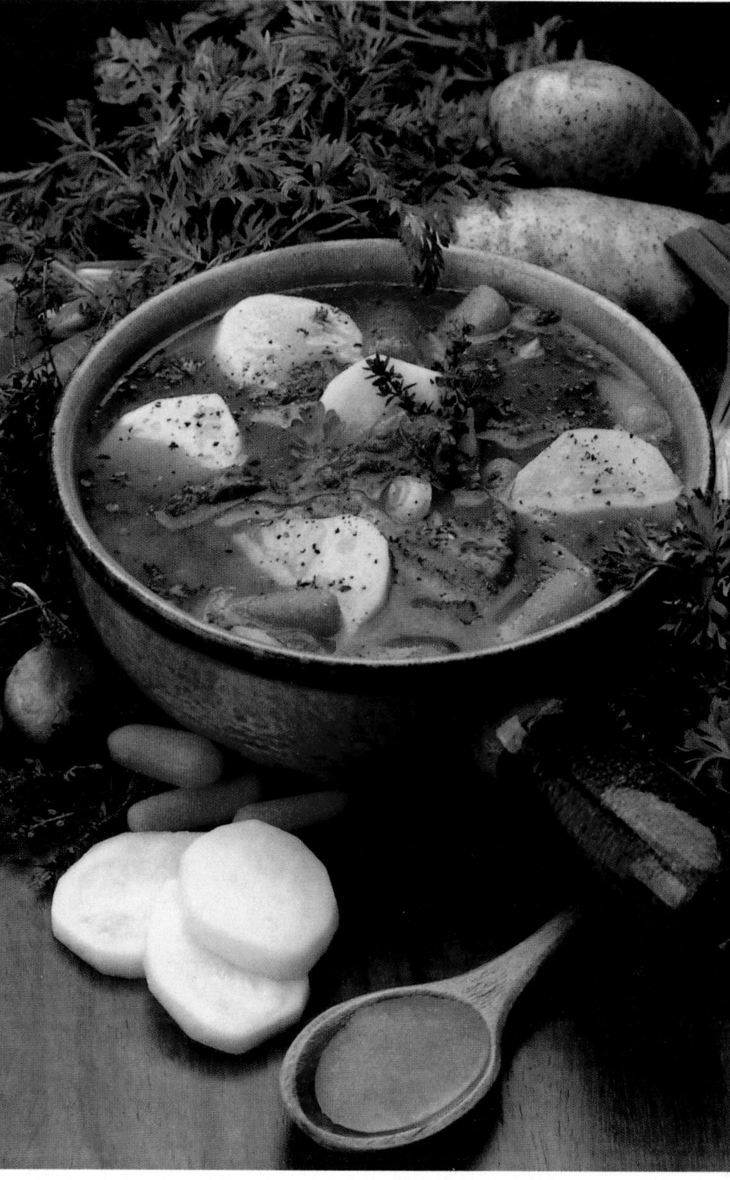

Idaho Potato Commission

29-7 *Irish stew is a savory blend of meat, potatoes, onions, carrots, and seasonings simmered together until tender and flavorful.*

Irish Meals

In Ireland, as in other parts of the British Isles, the day begins with a hearty breakfast. Breakfast commonly includes porridge, eggs, bread, butter, and tea. The Irish serve dinner in the middle of the day. It is the main meal for many people, especially those who live in rural areas. The Irish serve tea at about six o'clock in the evening.

British Menu

Welsh Rabbit
Corned Beef and Cabbage
Parsley-Buttered Potatoes and Carrots
Scones and Marmalade
English Trifle
Tea

Welsh Rabbit

Serves 6

- 2 tablespoons all-purpose flour
- 3/4 cup fat free milk
- 1/8 teaspoon pepper
- 1/4 teaspoon dry mustard
- 1/2 teaspoon Worcestershire sauce
- 1 cup shredded Cheddar cheese
- 6 slices toast, cut diagonally into quarters

1. Combine flour and milk in a small, tightly covered container. Shake until thoroughly blended.
2. Pour flour mixture into a small saucepan. Blend in pepper, mustard, and Worcestershire sauce, stirring until mixture is smooth.
3. Cook over medium heat, stirring constantly, until sauce comes to a boil. Cook and stir for one additional minute until sauce is thick and smooth.
4. Remove sauce from heat and add cheese, stirring constantly until the cheese is melted.
5. Serve over toast pieces. Garnish with hard-cooked egg wedges, parsley, or paprika.

Per serving: 164 cal. (38% from fat), 9 g protein, 16 g carbohydrate, 7 g fat, 20 mg cholesterol, 0 g fiber, 274 mg sodium.

Corned Beef and Cabbage

Serves 8

- 2 pounds corned beef
- 1 sprig thyme
- 1 onion studded with 6 cloves
- 1/4 teaspoon pepper
- 1 bay leaf
- 1 carrot, cut into 8 sticks
- cold water
- 1 small head cabbage, cut into wedges

1. Place beef, thyme, studded onion, pepper, bay leaf, and carrot in a large pot. Cover with cold water. Do not cover the pot.
2. Slowly bring to a boil. Simmer for 3 hours, skimming when necessary.
3. Remove thyme sprig and bay leaf and add cabbage. Simmer for another 10 to 15 minutes or until the cabbage is crisp-tender.
4. Remove corned beef to heated serving platter. Surround with cabbage wedges, carrot sticks, and onion.

Per serving: 261 cal. (59% from fat), 18 g protein, 8 g carbohydrate, 17 g fat, 61 mg cholesterol, 3 g fiber, 162 mg sodium.

Parsley Buttered Potatoes

Serves 6 to 8

- 2 1/2 pounds small new potatoes*
- 2 tablespoons margarine
- fresh parsley, coarsely chopped

1. Carefully scrub potatoes. Remove one strip of peel around the center of each potato.
2. Place potatoes in a large pan filled with cold water. Bring to a boil. Gently simmer 35 to 40 minutes or until potatoes are tender.
3. Drain potatoes well. Add margarine and parsley; stir gently until potatoes are coated. Serve immediately.

*Red potatoes may be substituted for the new potatoes.

Per serving: 124 cal. (25% from fat), 3 g protein, 23 g carbohydrate, 4 g fat, 0 mg cholesterol, 1 g fiber, 49 mg sodium.

Carrots

Serves 6 to 8

- 2 pounds carrots
- 1 1/2 tablespoons margarine
- salt and pepper

1. Wash and peel carrots. Leave carrots whole if small, otherwise slice or dice.

2. Bring a small amount of salted water to a boil in a saucepan; add carrots.
3. Bring water again to a boil. Then reduce heat and let carrots gently simmer until crisp-tender, about 10 to 15 minutes.
4. Drain carrots well and toss with margarine. Season with salt and pepper to taste. Serve immediately.

Per serving: 75 cal. (33% from fat), 2 g protein, 12 g carbohydrate, 3 g fat, 0 mg cholesterol, 4 g fiber, 75 mg sodium.

Scones

Makes 8 scones

2½ cups all-purpose flour
2½ teaspoons baking powder
½ teaspoon salt
1 tablespoon sugar
3 tablespoons margarine
1 egg
1 cup fat free milk

1. Preheat oven to 400°F.
2. Grease a baking sheet and set aside.
3. In a large bowl, combine flour, baking powder, salt, and sugar.
4. Cut in margarine until mixture resembles coarse cornmeal.
5. Beat the egg until frothy, reserving 1 tablespoon.
6. Add the milk to the beaten egg and pour into the flour mixture.
7. Stir dough lightly with a fork until it forms a soft ball.
8. On a floured board, roll the dough into a square ½ inch thick. With a sharp knife, cut the square into quarters. Then cut each quarter diagonally into a triangle.
9. Place the triangles about 1 inch apart on the baking sheet; brush the tops with reserved beaten egg.
10. Bake scones for 15 minutes or until light brown. Serve at once.

Per scone: 207 cal. (23% from fat), 6 g protein, 33 g carbohydrate, 6 g fat, 35 mg cholesterol, 1 g fiber, 306 mg sodium.

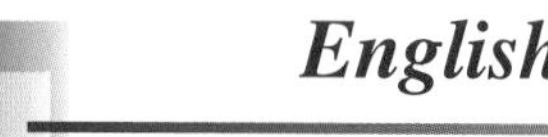

English Trifle

Serves 12

1 pound cake (homemade or packaged)
4 tablespoons raspberry jam
1 cup blanched almonds, halved
2 cups fresh raspberries or 2 packages frozen raspberries, 10 ounces each
2 cups soft custard (See Chapter 16)
2 cups heavy cream
2 tablespoons confectioner's sugar

1. Cut the pound cake into slices, ½ inch thick.
2. Coat about half of the slices with jam and place them, jam side up, along the bottom and sides of a glass bowl.
3. Cut the remaining slices into cubes and scatter the cubes over the jam covered slices.
4. Sprinkle ½ cup of the almonds over the cake.
5. Reserve 12 of the best raspberries. (Drain juice from frozen berries.) Sprinkle the remaining berries over the cake.
6. Using a rubber spatula, gently spread the custard over the fruit.
7. In a small, chilled bowl, whip cream until slightly thick.
8. Add sugar gradually, beating until cream forms soft peaks.
9. Spread half the whipped cream over the custard.
10. Using a pastry bag, pipe the remaining cream decoratively around the edge of the trifle. Garnish with reserved berries and almonds.

Per serving: 436 cal. (59% from fat), 8 g protein, 38 g carbohydrate, 30 g fat, 147 mg cholesterol, 3 g fiber, 179 mg sodium.

France

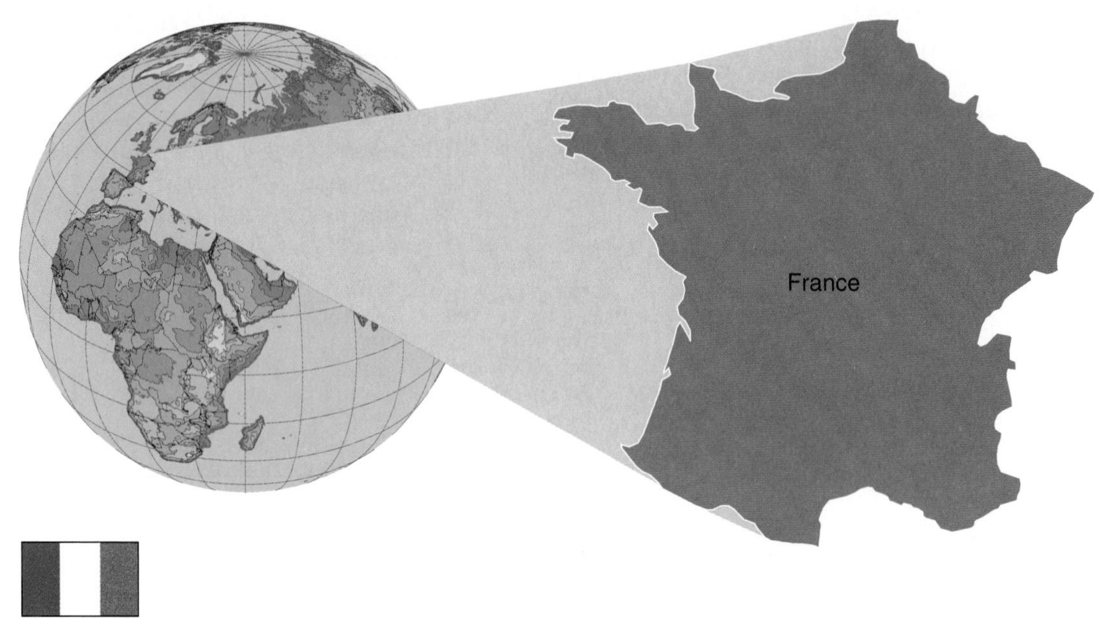

France is the largest country in Western Europe. France also is the oldest unified nation in Europe. It has been an important world power for centuries. The French have had an impact on the development of the entire Western civilization. They have made many contributions in art, science, government, and philosophy.

Geography and Climate of France

The Atlantic Ocean, the Mediterranean Sea, and the English Channel border France. Belgium, Luxembourg, Germany, Switzerland, Italy, and Spain also border France. All these nations have influenced the development of French culture.

The eastern and southwestern areas of France are mountainous. The northern and western parts of the country are rolling plains. Both highlands and lowlands are found in the central provinces.

The climate of France is moderate. In the higher elevations, snow falls during the winter. However, most of the country has cool, rainy weather instead of snow. Throughout much of France, spring is humid, summer is moderate, and autumn is long and sunny. These climatic conditions are especially favorable for the production of the grapes used to make famous French wines.

French Culture

The French are a mixture of many different peoples who originally came to France from

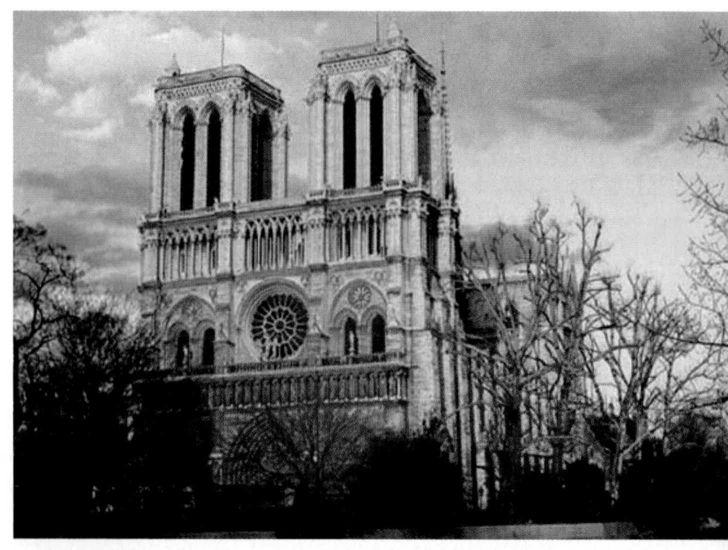

Notre Dame is one of the most famed cathedrals in Europe.

areas throughout Europe. Each group settled in a different part of the country.

In the Middle Ages, France was divided into areas called *domains*. A member of the nobility ruled each domain and peasants worked the land. During the Renaissance, France became a unified country. However, many of the people of France did not think of themselves as French citizens. Instead, they considered themselves citizens of the regions in which they lived, such as Brittany and Burgundy. Today, regional ties continue to be strong in many parts of France, especially in rural areas.

Today, France is a republic headed by a president. Paris, France's largest city and marketing and distribution center, is the seat of government. The official language is French. The greatest percentage of the population is Roman Catholic.

Fishing and agricultural industries are important to France. Fishers catch large amounts of cod, crab, herring, lobster, mackerel, oysters, sardines, shrimp, and tuna along the French coastlines. Grapes grow throughout much of the southern part of the country. They are used in wine production. Cattle provide meat and dairy products. Wheat, corn, oats, and barley are important grain crops. Sugar beets, fruits, vegetables, flax, flowers, and other livestock are also important agricultural commodities.

French Holidays

Joan of Arc Day is a national holiday in France, which is observed on the second Sunday in May. This day is named for a 17-year-old girl who became a French national heroine and a Catholic saint. French people celebrate the holiday held in her honor by decorating the streets with statues and pictures of Joan.

France's national independence day, Bastille Day, is July 14. On this date in 1789, a crowd of French citizens captured a Paris prison called the Bastille. This volatile event signaled the start of the French Revolution. The French celebrate this holiday with parades, parties, dancing, and fireworks.

Many other celebrations throughout the year in France are church holidays. On January 6, the eve of Epiphany, children lay fruit and cake on the church altar for the Christ child. *Mardi Gras* heralds the beginning of Lent with parades of flower-covered floats. *Pâques,* the French name for Easter, comes from the name of the Jewish Passover. On this day, children receive colored candy eggs and chocolate chickens. Corpus Christi is a festival in early June honoring the bread and wine used for Holy Communion. These sacred elements are taken from church altars in gold and silver bowls and carried through the streets. Small altars covered with boughs and flowers are set up at village crossroads. *Noël,* or Christmas, is a time for family reunions, carol singing, and gifts for the children. See 29-8.

French Cuisine

In France, good food and wine are an important part of daily life. In many parts of France, cooks buy food fresh each day, and they take great care in selecting it. The French usually shop in small specialty shops rather than in large supermarkets.

French cooking can be divided into three main classes: haute cuisine, provincial cuisine and nouvelle cuisine. ***Haute cuisine*** is characterized by elaborate preparations, fancy garnishes, and rich sauces. Chefs make lavish use of eggs, cream, and butter in this style of French cooking. Haute cuisine is seen most often in leading restaurants and hotels.

Provincial cuisine is the style of cooking practiced by most French families. Provincial

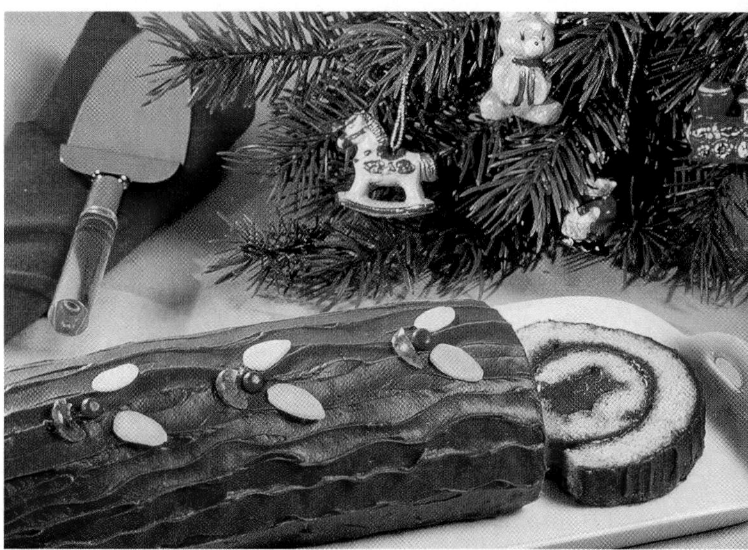

American Egg Board

29-8 *Sponge cake rolled with chocolate filling is decorated to become a traditional French Christmas dessert called a yule log.*

cooks make fewer fancy sauces and lavish creations. Instead, the flavors of locally grown foods are enhanced by simple cooking methods. Many provincial dishes were once regional specialties.

Nouvelle cuisine emphasizes lightness and natural taste in foods. Flavor, color, texture, and presentation are as important in nouvelle cuisine as they are in haute cuisine. However, nouvelle cooks believe the richness and heaviness of haute cuisine spoil the natural flavors of food. The idea behind nouvelle cuisine is to preserve the nutrients and natural taste of foods. Nouvelle cuisine appeals to people who love French food but are concerned about fat and calories.

Nouvelle cooks serve less butter, cream, and other high-calorie foods. They use fewer starches and sauces. When they do serve a sauce, they do not thicken it with flour. Instead, nouvelle cooks use vegetable purees to thicken sauces. Nouvelle cuisine includes more fresh fruits and vegetables. (The vegetables are served nearly raw.) Meat, fish, and poultry are often broiled or poached.

Foundations of French Cooking

Two basic points form the secret of good French cooking. First, the ingredients used must be of top quality. Bread, for example, is baked twice a day in French bakeries to ensure its freshness. Second, successful cooks are very patient. Patience can make the difference between a dish that is good and one that is excellent. Cooks may simmer some sauces for hours to develop the flavors of all their ingredients.

French Sauces

The French use a variety of sauces. A sauce can be used as the basis for a dish or as a finishing touch.

A *roux* is a mixture of butter (or other fat) and flour. It forms the base of all white sauces. When you add milk to a roux, the mixture becomes a *béchamel* sauce. If you add chicken, veal, or fish stock to a roux, the mixture becomes a *velouté* sauce. You can make many variations of these sauces by adding extra ingredients like mustard or cheese.

The classic French brown sauce is called a *demi-glace* sauce. Cooks make it from a slightly thickened stock-based sauce they have simmered for a long time. They add additional stock and flavorings to this basic sauce. They may or may not use a thickening agent, such as a roux.

Hollandaise sauce contains egg yolks, lemon juice, and butter. The cook must warm and gently thicken the beaten egg yolks to prevent curdling. Then the butter must be added slowly to keep the sauce from separating. Hollandaise sauce often accompanies green vegetables such as asparagus, 29-9.

Vinaigrettes are made by combining wine vinegar, oil, and seasonings. Many variations are possible. Vinaigrettes are commonly used as dressings on green salads and as marinades for vegetables.

Butter sauces include *cold flavored butters, white butter sauce,* and *brown butter sauce.* Cooks use them when baking and broiling seafood, when preparing vegetables and poultry, and when making other sauces.

French Seasonings

Herbs are just as important to French cooking as sauces. ***Fines herbes*** is a mixture of fresh chives, parsley, tarragon, and chervil. Many French chefs use this combination of herbs to flavor soups and stews. Marjoram, rosemary, basil, saffron, oregano, fennel, bay leaves, thyme, and savory are also common in French cooking.

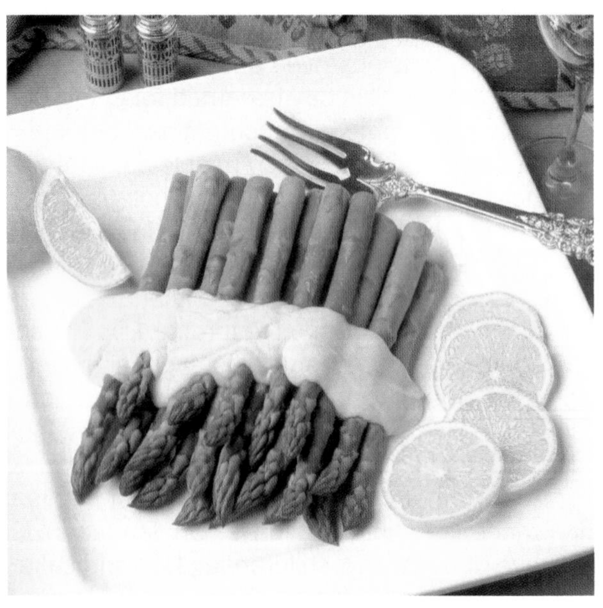

California Asparagus Commission

29-9 *Smooth hollandaise sauce with a tangy hint of lemon is a classic French topping for asparagus.*

Cooks add herbs directly to some dishes. For other dishes, such as stews, they tie herbs in a cheesecloth bag and add it to the liquid. (They remove the bag before serving.)

French Appetizers and Soups

A French meal would not be complete without hors d'oeuvres. ***Hors d'oeuvres*** are small dishes designed to stimulate the appetite. They may be hot or cold, but chefs always plan for them to complement the other menu items.

Soup often follows hors d'oeuvres. French soups fall into four basic categories: consommés, puree soups, cream soups, and velouté soups. *Consommés* have a meat stock base. They are rich and clear and may be served hot or cold. *Puree soups* are made from meat, poultry, fish, or vegetables that have been cooked in liquid and pureed. *Cream soups* generally use a béchamel sauce as a base. Pureed meat, fish, poultry, or vegetables are added to the béchamel sauce along with cream. *Velouté soups* are similar to cream soups. Meat, fish, poultry, or vegetables are added to a velouté sauce. Egg yolks, butter, and cream thicken the soup.

French Main Dishes

Seafood and poultry form the basis of many French main dishes. As a rule, the French eat red meat less often than people in the United States.

Many types of freshwater and saltwater fish are popular in France. Frog legs, crabs, scallops, and mussels are especially popular. Poaching is the preparation technique used most often for fish fillets and whole fish.

The French eat all types of poultry. They often truss and roast chicken, duck, and goose whole with or without a stuffing. They also fricassee chicken and add it to stews. They finely chop and season the meat of game birds, such as pigeons, to make a spread called *pâté*.

The French usually broil beef steaks and serve them with a sauce. They often braise other beef and veal cuts and use some of them in stews. Lamb is particularly popular in the spring. The French consider organ meats of all kinds to be delicacies. See 29-10.

French Vegetables and Salads

Vegetables are an important part of a French meal. The French often serve two or more fresh vegetables with a main dish. They cook vegetables just to the crisp-tender stage and then serve them immediately to preserve their textures.

The French often serve vegetables with just butter and seasonings. Vegetables can also be creamed, braised, glazed, or served with a cheese or hollandaise sauce. Some vegetables, such as spinach, adapt particularly well to soufflés.

The French usually serve a green salad after the main course but before dessert. They often dress it with a vinaigrette sauce. Other salads, such as potato salads and meat salads, are popular additions to lighter and more casual meals. One of the best-known salads of this type is *salade nicoise*. This popular salad is a colorful combination of potatoes, green beans, and tomatoes, served with a vinaigrette sauce.

France is famous for its cheeses, and cheese is an important part of meals. The French serve cheese and fresh fruit after the green salad and before the sweet dessert in a

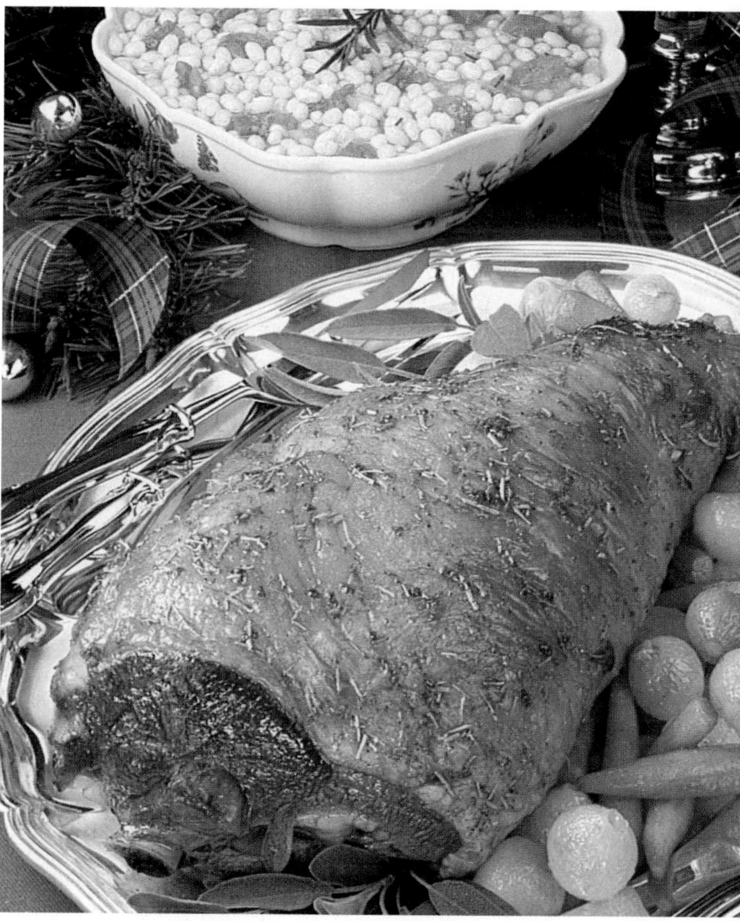

American Lamb Council

29-10 *The French roast lamb with herbs to give it a delicately-seasoned flavor.*

large meal. Many simpler meals include only cheese, sausage, bread, fresh fruit, and wine.

French Baked Goods

The French serve bread at every meal. *Baguette* is the most popular. It contains only yeast, flour, salt, and water. People buy the long, crusty loaves daily from local bakers. Other breads are popular, too. *Brioche* is a rich yeast roll that contains egg. ***Croissants*** are flaky, buttery yeast rolls shaped into crescents, 29-11.

The dessert course may be simple or elaborate. Some of the most elegant desserts in the world originated in France. *Napoleons* are layers of puff pastry separated by creamy fillings. *Éclairs* are slender pastry shells filled with custard or a cream filling and iced. *Baba au rhum* is a yeast cake soaked in a rum syrup. Chocolate, vanilla, liqueur, or fruit-based soufflés are popular. Fruit tarts and crêpes filled with fruit, custard, or other sweet filling are also favorite desserts.

Regional Nature of French Cuisine

French cuisine is regional in nature. A visitor can travel throughout the country and never eat the same dish prepared in the same way twice.

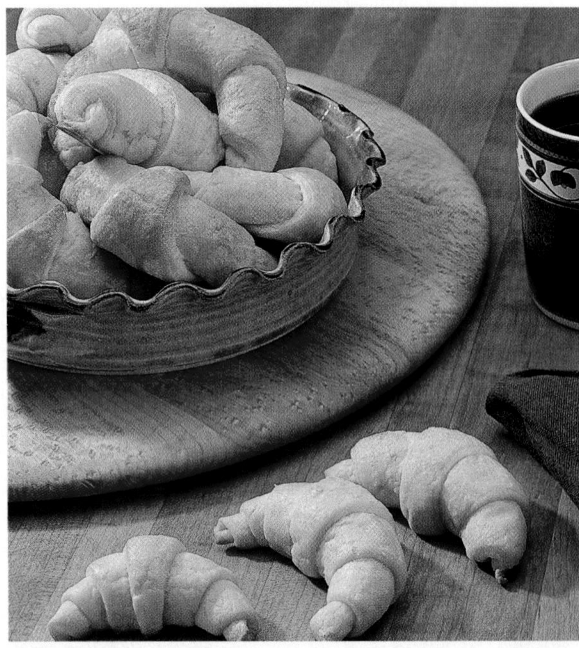

Lesaffre Yeast Corporation, the RED STAR® Yeast Collection

***29-11** Flaky croissants make a delicious, light breakfast but may be served at other meals as well.*

A traveler can even identify certain regions by their local dishes.

Normandy is located in the northwestern corner of France. Cattle graze in the fertile green pastures, and apple orchards dot the countryside. Normandy is known for tender veal, rich cream and butter, and apples. *Calvados*, a liquor made from apple cider, is produced locally for export around the world.

Brittany, Normandy's neighbor to the southwest, is relatively poor. Much of the land is rocky and wooded. Because agriculture is difficult, much of the local food comes from the sea. In early spring, vegetables are harvested from small gardens throughout Brittany. The asparagus, artichokes, and cauliflower are reported to be the best in France. Brittany is also known for its ***crêpes*** (thin, delicate pancakes usually rolled around a filling).

To the southwest, in the *Aquitaine* region, the finest pâté is produced. It is made from expensive goose liver and truffles. ***Truffles*** are a rare type of fungi that grow underground near oak trees. This region is also known for its poultry, veal, and pork.

Cassoulet is a traditional stew of the *Languedoc-Roussillon* region located in southern France. It is made with white beans, goose or chicken, pork, bacon, and herbs.

Provence is a rich agricultural region in southeastern France. Fresh vegetables are used in many colorful dishes. One of the most popular vegetable dishes is *ratatouille.* It is a vegetable casserole containing tomatoes, eggplant, green pepper, zucchini, onions, and seasonings. See 29-12. The olive trees that grow on the sunny slopes along the Mediterranean Sea provide the oil needed to make aioli. (*Aioli* is a regional sauce made from olive oil and garlic.) *Bouillabaisse* (a seafood stew), leg of lamb, grilled fish, and chicken are equally popular. Many of the dishes of Provence are flavored with locally grown herbs.

Burgundy, located in central France, is famous for its vineyards and the wines they produce. Many Burgundy dishes are flavored with the local wines. *Boeuf à la Bourguignonne* (beef Burgundy) is one of the most famous of these dishes. ***Escargots*** (snails eaten as food) are another Burgundy specialty. They often are served in their shells with garlic butter.

For centuries, the people of the *Rhône-Alpes* region have based their diets on local foods. Potatoes grow in the hilly land. The cows that graze on mountain grasses provide milk and

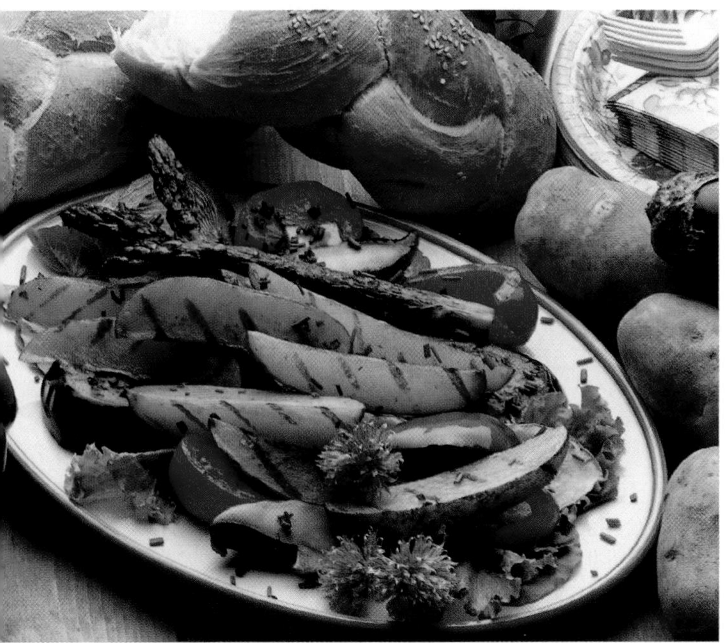

Idaho Potato Commission

29-12 Although ratatouille is typically a casserole, the ingredients may also be combined as a warm salad.

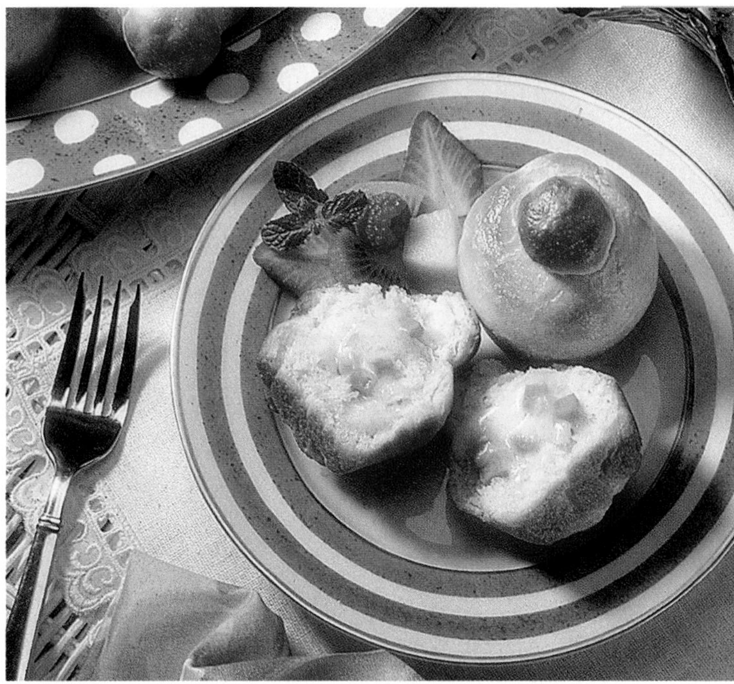

photo courtesy of Fleischmann's Yeast

29-13 Classic French brioches have a rich flavor and characteristic shape.

cheese. Many Alpine dishes combine these three staple foods.

The Germans have influenced the foods of the *Alsace* and *Lorraine* regions. Sausages and smoked hams are popular throughout these regions, as are fruit pies and tarts. Fine white wines are produced in Alsace. ***Quiche,*** a custard tart served in many variations as an appetizer and a main dish, originated in Lorraine. The most famous type of quiche is called *Quiche Lorraine.* It contains grated Swiss cheese, crumbled bacon, and diced onions along with eggs and cream.

Q: What can I use in place of the wine listed in some French recipes?

A: For sweet recipes, replace red and white wine with red and white grape juice, respectively. When making savory dishes, try chicken broth in place of white wine and beef broth in place of red.

French Meals

Most French people eat three meals a day. *Le petit dejeuner* (breakfast) usually is light. The French often have *café au lait* (hot milk and coffee) and brioche or crusty bread with butter and jam. See 29-13

Traditionally, *le dejeuner* (the midday meal) was the main meal of the day. People ate it leisurely. In many parts of France this is still the case. People in the major cities, however, often eat the heavier meal in the evening. A traditional midday meal might include hot or cold hors d'oeuvres, soup, and a main dish. A vegetable, a green salad, bread and butter, dessert, and wine would also be served. If the main dish contains vegetables, a separate vegetable usually would be eliminated.

In France, bread usually remains on the table through the end of the meal. The salad usually is served after the main course, and coffee usually accompanies dessert.

The traditional evening meal is light. Soup, an omelet, bread and butter, fruit, and a beverage are typical supper dishes. City dwellers, however, may eat a more substantial evening meal. Business hours are later in France than they are in the United States. Therefore, the evening meal usually is not served before eight o'clock.

French Menu

Soupe à l'Oignon
(Onion Soup)
Poulet au Citron
(Chicken with Lemon)
Ratatouille
(Vegetable Casserole)
Salade Verte
(Green Salad)
Pain
(French Bread)
Mousse au Chocolat
(Chocolate Mousse)
Café
(Coffee)

Soupe à l'Oignon

(Onion Soup)
Serves 6

5 medium onions
2 tablespoons margarine
dash pepper
6 cups low-sodium beef broth
6 thick slices French bread
3 tablespoons grated Parmesan cheese
3/4 cup shredded Swiss cheese

1. Clean onions, cut into thin slices.
2. In a large, heavy skillet, melt margarine.
3. Add onions and pepper and saute until onions are golden brown and transparent (about 10 minutes).
4. Slowly stir in beef broth. Bring soup to a boil, reduce heat and simmer for 30 minutes.
5. Toast bread slices in the oven.
6. Place one piece of toasted bread in each of six ovenproof soup bowls or use one large tureen; sprinkle with Parmesan cheese.
7. Preheat broiler.
8. Pour soup over bread. Sprinkle Swiss cheese on top.
9. Place soup bowls under broiler and broil until cheese is light brown. Serve soup immediately.

Per serving: 192 cal. (42% from fat), 9 g protein, 18 g carbohydrate, 9 g fat, 11 mg cholesterol, 2 g fiber, 407 mg sodium.

Poulet au Citron

(Chicken with Lemon)
Serves 8

1 tablespoon margarine
1 tablespoon vegetable oil
2 broilers, 2 pounds each, cut-up, skin removed
3/4 teaspoon salt
pepper to taste
2 tablespoons finely chopped parsley
1 tablespoon minced chives
1 teaspoon marjoram
2 teaspoons paprika
grated rind and juice of two lemons
1 cup low-sodium chicken broth
2 tablespoons cornstarch
3 tablespoons cold water

1. Preheat oven to 350°F.
2. Heat margarine and oil together in a large nonstick skillet.
3. Brown chicken pieces.
4. Place chicken in a large casserole or baking pan. Season with salt and pepper, parsley, chives, marjoram, and paprika. Sprinkle with lemon juice and rind.
5. Cover pan tightly, and bake chicken until tender, about 45 minutes. Use a meat thermometer to check the internal temperature of chicken pieces. Breast pieces should reach an internal temperature of 170°F. Wings and thighs should reach an internal temperature of 180°F.
6. Remove chicken to a heated platter.
7. Pour juices into a small saucepan. Add chicken broth and bring to a boil.
8. Quickly whisk in cornstarch dissolved in cold water.
9. Simmer sauce until thickened, about 2 minutes. Serve with chicken.

Per serving: 162 cal. (44% from fat), 19 g protein, 3 g carbohydrate, 8 g fat, 57 mg cholesterol, 0 g fiber, 310 mg sodium.

Ratatouille

(Vegetable Casserole)
Serves 6 to 8

1 medium eggplant
1 teaspoon salt
2 tablespoons vegetable oil
1½ large onions, cut into rings
2 cloves garlic, crushed
2 green peppers, cut into strips
3 medium zucchini, cut into bite-sized pieces
2 medium tomatoes, cut into wedges
1 bay leaf
½ teaspoon thyme
¼ teaspoon salt
pepper to taste

1. Cut eggplant first into thick slices and then into bite-sized pieces. Sprinkle with salt and let eggplant stand 30 minutes. Rinse and pat dry with paper towels.
2. In a large skillet, heat oil. Saute onions and garlic until golden.
3. Add green pepper strips and cook for 2 minutes.
4. Add eggplant and cook for 3 minutes, stirring constantly.
5. Add zucchini and continue stirring and cooking another 3 minutes.
6. Add tomatoes and seasonings. Simmer uncovered for 40 minutes or until vegetables are tender.
7. Remove bay leaf. Ratatouille can be served immediately or refrigerated and reheated later.

Per serving: 98 cal. (46% from fat), 2 g protein, 12 g carbohydrate, 5 g fat, 0 mg cholesterol, 3 g fiber, 273 mg sodium.

Salade Verte

(Green Salad)
Serves 6

6 cups assorted salad greens
1 tablespoon lemon juice
1 tablespoon white wine vinegar
salt
pepper
⅓ cup olive oil

1. Wash salad greens and tear into bite-sized pieces.
2. In small bowl, whisk together lemon juice, wine vinegar, and salt and pepper to taste.
3. Add oil, a few drops at a time while beating with whisk. Continue to beat dressing until all of the oil has been added.
4. Toss greens together in a salad bowl with dressing. (If dressing has separated, shake well before using.)

Per serving: 119 cal. (91% from fat), 1 g protein, 2 g carbohydrate, 12 g fat, 0 mg cholesterol, 1 g fiber, 105 mg sodium.

Pain

(French Bread)
Makes 2 loaves

2¼ cups water
6½ cups all-purpose flour
2 packages active dry yeast
2 teaspoons salt
cornmeal
vegetable oil
cold water

1. In small saucepan, heat water to 120°F.
2. In large mixer bowl, combine 3 cups flour, yeast, and salt.
3. Add warm water and mix by hand or on medium speed of electric mixer for 3 minutes. Gradually add enough remaining flour to form a stiff dough.
4. Turn dough out onto lightly floured board or pastry cloth; knead until smooth and satiny, about 8 to 10 minutes.
5. Place dough in a greased bowl, turning once to grease top. Cover and let rise in a warm place 30 minutes.
6. Punch down and divide into 2 equal parts.
7. Roll each half of dough into a 15 × 8-inch rectangle on a lightly floured board.
8. Beginning with long side, roll dough up tightly, sealing edges and ends well.
9. Place loaves seam side down, diagonally, on a lightly greased baking sheet that has been sprinkled with cornmeal. Brush loaves with oil, cover. Refrigerate 2 to 24 hours.
10. When ready to bake, preheat oven to 400°F.
11. Remove bread from refrigerator, uncover and let stand 10 minutes.
12. Brush bread with water. Slash tops of loaves diagonally at 2-inch intervals just before baking.
13. Bake at 400°F, 35 to 40 minutes.

Per slice: 98 cal. (6% from fat), 3 g protein, 20 g carbohydrate, 1 g fat, 0 mg cholesterol, 1 g fiber, 134 mg sodium.

Mousse au Chocolat

(Chocolate Mousse)
Serves 6

- 1/4 pound semisweet chocolate, broken into chunks
- 4 eggs, separated
- 4 tablespoons margarine, softened
- 4 teaspoons water
- 1/2 cup sugar
- 6 strips orange peel

1. Melt chocolate in the top of a double boiler over barely simmering water.
2. In small bowl of electric mixer, beat egg yolks until thick and lemon-colored (about 10 minutes).
3. Add margarine a tablespoon at a time to chocolate, beating until mixture is smooth.
4. Add the beaten egg yolks and cook, beating constantly, until the mixture has thickened and is smooth, about 5 minutes. (Do not let mixture come to a boil.)
5. Remove pan from the heat. Set top portion of double boiler aside, and cool chocolate mixture to room temperature, about 30 minutes.
6. In a heavy saucepan or double boiler, stir together egg whites, water, and sugar.
7. Cook egg whites over low heat, beating with a portable mixer until the whites stand in soft peaks.
8. Gently fold chocolate mixture into egg whites, folding until no streaks of white are visible.
9. Pour mousse into a pretty bowl or individual serving dishes and refrigerate until set, at least four hours.
10. Garnish mousse with strips of orange peel.

Per serving: 272 cal. (56% from fat), 5 g protein, 29 g carbohydrate, 17 g fat, 145 mg cholesterol, 0 g fiber, 133 mg sodium.

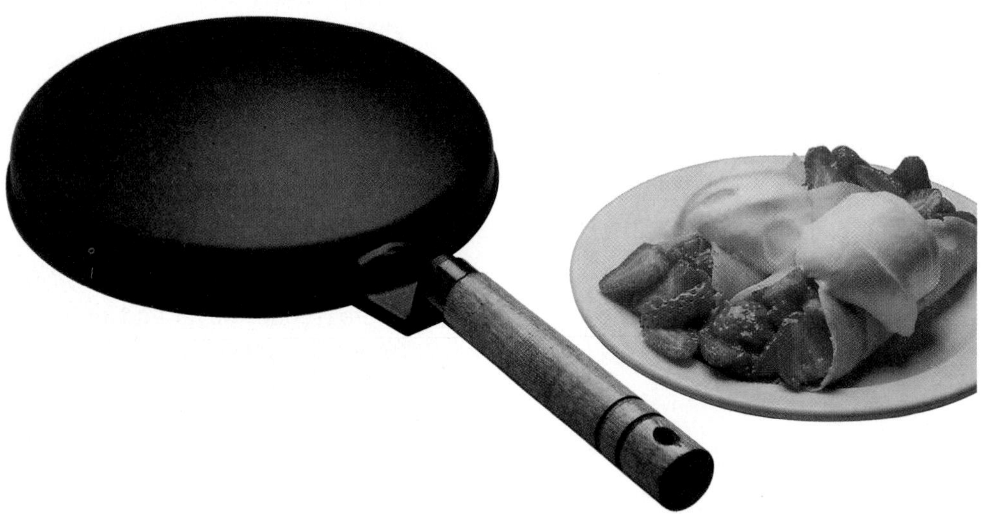

Nordic Ware

Fresh fruit filling turns delicate crêpes into a luscious dessert.

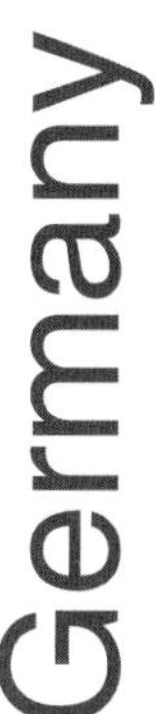

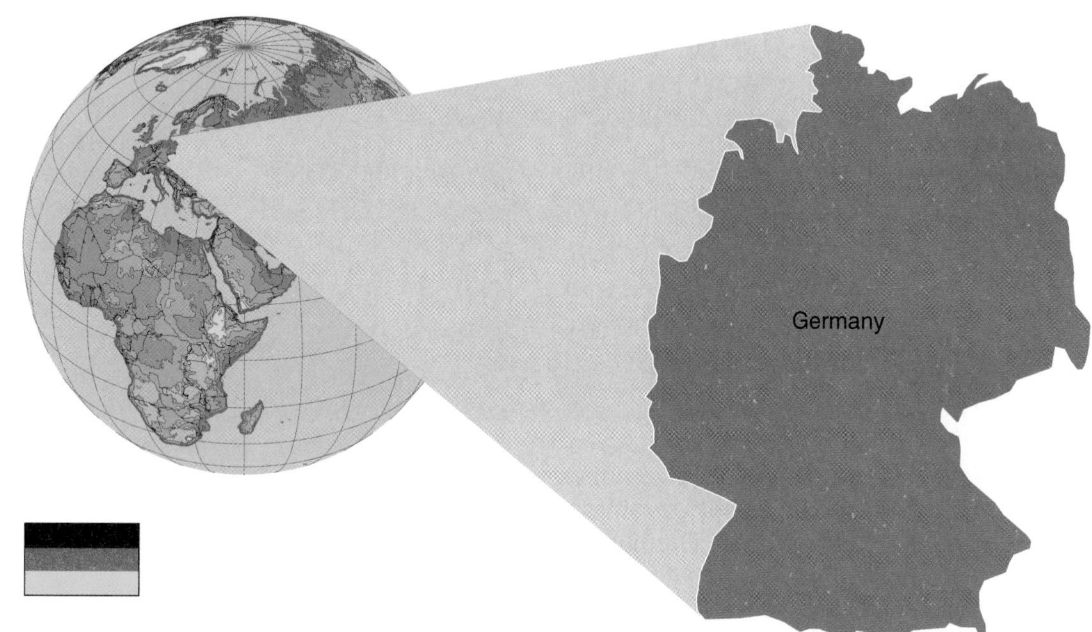

Germany is in the heart of Western Europe. Germany's boundaries have changed several times over the years. Many of these changes were the result of wars.

German culture and cuisine developed with more unity than German politics. Common heritage and ingredients have led to the origin of dishes that are liked throughout Germany. However, Germany also has many regional dishes.

Geography and Climate of Germany

To the north of Germany are the Baltic and North Seas. The Rhine and the Elbe are the most important rivers in Germany.

Lowlands (flat, sandy plains) make up much of the northern part of the country. Highlands are in the central and southern regions. Two other important geographical regions, the Bavarian Alps and the Black Forest, are in southern Germany.

Germany's climate is generally moderate. However, the Baltic region has extremes of temperature. Also, the higher elevations in the southern mountains receive large amounts of snow.

German Culture

After the collapse of the Roman Empire, a series of empires rose and fell. Each one brought new peoples to Germany. Many of these peoples came from what is now Poland, Denmark, Switzerland, Austria, and France.

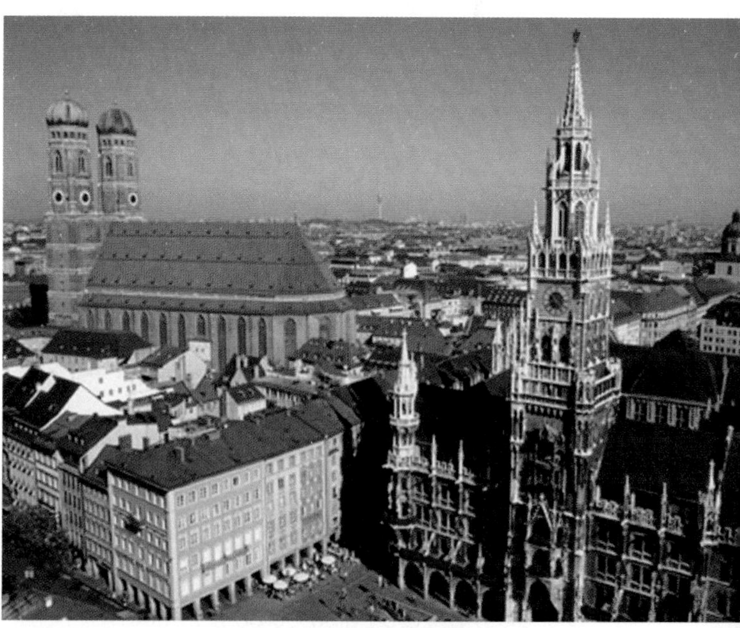

The Marienplatz is a square in the center of Munich, Germany, which is dominated by the Gothic architecture of the New Town Hall.

Until the last half of the nineteenth century, Germany was a loose mixture of states, kingdoms, duchies, and principalities. Following the unification of these territories, Germany became involved in the two World Wars. Both wars left much of the country devastated. World War II resulted in the split of the country. West Germany had a democratic government. East Germany had a communistic government.

For years, the people of both German nations longed to live under a common flag. In 1989, they tore down the Berlin Wall—a symbol of the political division between the countries. In the following year, the two nations were reunited under a single democratic government.

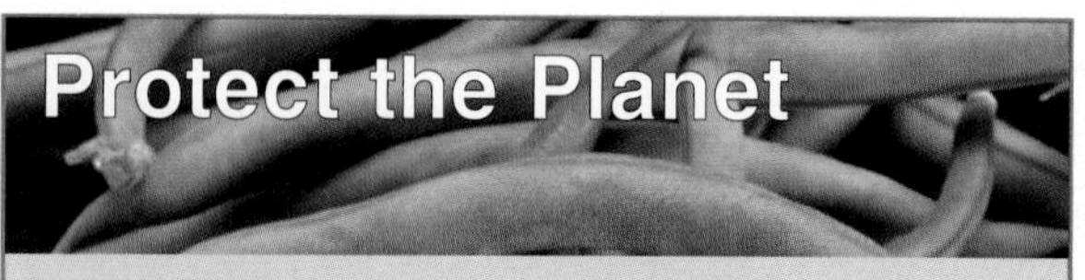

Protect the Planet

Before leaving for a trip, turn off your hot water heater. Empty your refrigerator and set the control on the least cool setting. Turn air conditioning off in the summer and adjust your thermostat to about 55°F (13°C) in the winter. These steps will save energy and energy costs while you are away.

German Agriculture

The northern lowlands and southern highlands of Germany are primarily agricultural. Potatoes and sugar beets are the main crops of the northern lowlands. In addition, farmers grow some rye, oats, wheat, and barley and raise some cattle. The southern highlands are known for their cattle, wheat, and dairy products. Grapes and other fruits grow in the west and southwest regions. Hops grow in Bavaria, the center of the German brewing industry.

German Holidays

The Germans celebrate many church holidays with traditional foods. One of these holidays is St. Martin's Day, which is a harvest festival held on November 11. Roast goose and breads baked in symbolic shapes are among the foods typically served on St. Martin's Day. At dusk, children sing and parade with paper lanterns.

During Advent, the four-week period leading to Christmas, German bakers prepare holiday cakes, cookies, and breads. On December 6, children receive candy and fruit from St. Nicholas. Children also go door to door receiving candy and money from friends and neighbors. Advent ends on Christmas Eve, which is a bigger celebration than Christmas Day. German parents decorate Christmas trees as a surprise for their children. Family members exchange gifts and enjoy a festive meal. The traditional Christmas meal was carp because the church forbade the eating of meat. Today, however, roast turkey, goose, or duck is more common. The Germans observe 12 Days of Christmas, which last until January 6. On this date, German boys dress up in celebration of the kings who visited the infant Jesus.

German Cuisine

German cuisine is characterized by roasted meats, filling side dishes, and delicious baked goods. World-famous beers and fine white wines are also typical German fare.

German Main Dishes

Meat has been the foundation of German cuisine for centuries. The ***braten*** (roast) is Germany's national dish. A variety of traditional German dishes contain pork, beef, veal, and game.

Pork, both fresh and cured, is the most popular of all meats. Hams are roasted, marinated in wine, or cut in slices and then fried and served with a sauce. One of the most popular pork dishes is called *kasseler rippenspeer.* It is a whole smoked pork loin that is roasted. It is served with sauerkraut, apples or chestnuts, peas, white beans, mushrooms, and browned potatoes. See 29-14.

Boiled beef served with a horseradish sauce is one of the most popular beef dishes. *Sauerbraten,* a sweet-sour marinated beef roast, is popular, too. The ingredients used in the marinade vary from one region to another. One method uses red wine, wine vinegar, onion, peppercorns, juniper berries, and bay leaves. Sauerbraten gravy may be thickened and flavored with crushed gingersnaps and raisins.

Hasenpfeffer is rabbit that is first marinated in wine, vinegar, onions, and spices. Then the

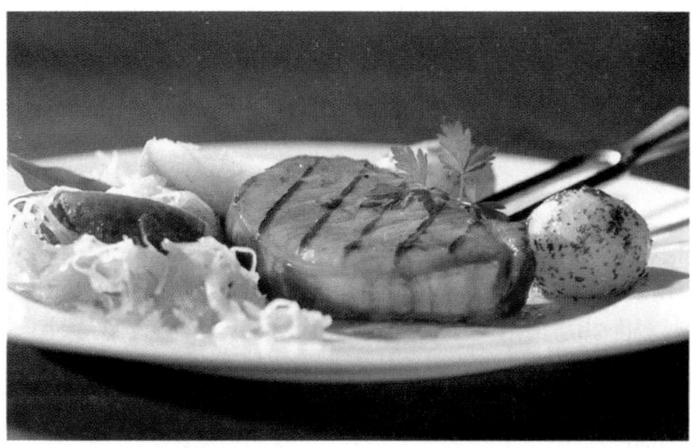

CMA, the German Agricultural Marketing Board, North America

29-14 *Kasseler rippenspeer is a traditional German pork dish.*

meat is stewed in the marinade. Sour cream is often added to the stew for thickening and flavor.

Many German meat dishes have regional origins. One such dish is schnitzel. *Schnitzel* is a breaded, sauteed veal cutlet. Schnitzel originated in Holstein where it is served with a fried egg. Richly flavored, smoked uncooked *Westphalian ham* originated in Westphalia, but it is served throughout Germany.

The German people use leftovers to make hearty soups and one-dish meals. Filling lentil soups and *eintopf,* a popular stew, are both made with leftover meats.

Sausages

A discussion of German meat dishes would not be complete without mentioning sausage. The Germans produce hundreds of types of sausages. Some are ready-to-eat. Others must be grilled, boiled, or fried. Some sausages are smoked, and a few are pickled.

Some sausages bear the names of the cities where they were first produced. *Braunschweiger,* for example, is a type of liver sausage. It was first produced in Braunschweig. The *frankfurt* (hot dog) originated in the German city of Frankfurt. Other well-known German sausages include *blutwurst,* which is blood sausage. *Bratwurst* is sausage made of fresh-ground, seasoned pork that is usually cooked by grilling. *Knockwurst* is smoked, precooked sausage made of beef and pork. *Schinkenwurst* is a ready-to-eat pork sausage that contains pieces of ham.

German Seafood

Open air fish markets scattered throughout northern Germany sell a variety of seafood obtained from the North and Baltic Seas. Smoked eel, enjoyed by many northern Germans, is inexpensive. Herring is prepared in a variety of ways. Salty, sharp, pickled Bismarck herring bears the name of a chancellor who helped unify the German territories.

German Side Dishes

Germans usually serve fruit accompaniments with pork and game dishes. Apples, prunes, raisins, and apricots accompany pork. Tart fruits like currants and *preiselbeeren* (small, cranberry-like fruits) accompany game.

At least one meal a day in Germany includes potatoes. Potatoes cooked in salted water, drained, and steamed until dry are known as *salzkartoffeln.* Salzkartoffeln are served most often as a side dish with melted butter, parsley, and bits of bacon. *Kartoffelsalat* is hot or cold potato salad made with a vinegar dressing and bits of cooked bacon. ***Kartoffelpuffer*** are the famous potato pancakes enjoyed throughout Germany. They are served with mixed stewed fruit or applesauce. *Kartoffelklösse* are potato dumplings. See 29-15.

Sauerkraut, another German specialty, is fermented or pickled cabbage. German cooks usually flavor sauerkraut with caraway, apple, onion, or juniper berries and serve it hot. The

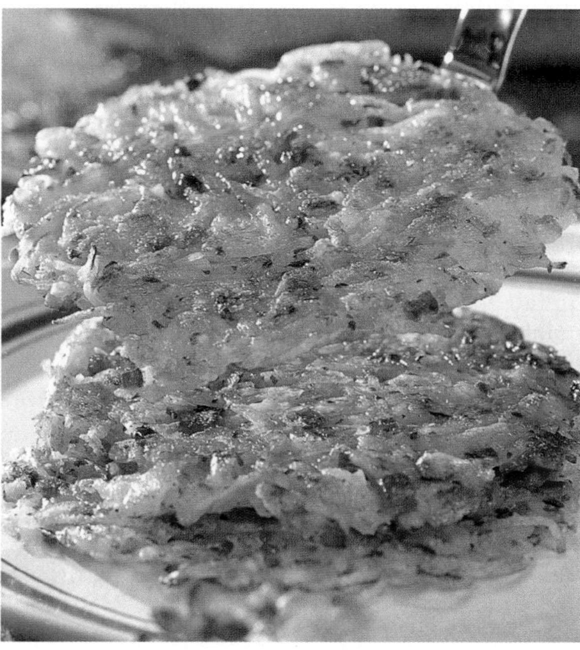

CMA, the German Agricultural Marketing Board, North America

29-15 *Grated potatoes held together with eggs and flour and fried in bacon drippings become German potato pancakes known as kartoffelpuffer.*

Germans often eat sauerkraut with pig's knuckles, spareribs, pork chops, and pork roasts.

The Germans may serve vegetables as side dishes or add them to stews. Cabbage and root vegetables are especially popular during winter months. Asparagus and mushrooms are spring delicacies. Cooks use fresh greens to make delicious salads, which they often serve with a vinegar dressing flavored with bacon.

Spätzle (small dumplings made from wheat flour) are another popular side dish. Cheese spätzle and liver spätzle are just two of the many kinds of spätzle eaten in Germany.

German Baked Goods

The German people serve bread at nearly every meal. Many breads and rolls are produced all over the country, while others are strictly regional. Some breads are baked in round or oblong rolls. Others are made into fanciful shapes and called *gebildbrote* (picture breads).

Rye, pumpernickel, and other dark breads are favorites. Bakers make *pumpernickel* bread from unsifted rye flour. They let it rise and bake for long periods. This allows the natural sugars in the rye to sweeten the bread evenly.

Sweet baked goods are also popular in Germany. Sweet rolls, breads, and coffee cakes are served at coffee time. Snail-shaped *schnecken*, streusel-topped coffee cakes, and *apfelkuchen* (apple cake) are served throughout Germany, 29-16. *Stollen* is a rich yeast bread filled with almonds, raisins, and candied fruit. It usually is served at Christmastime.

German bakers have traditionally made cakes with honey or honey and spices. *Lebkuchen,* one of Germany's best known honey-spice cakes, has a long history. For centuries, the Germans have used decorated lebkuchen to celebrate weddings, birthdays, and anniversaries. Sometimes young men and women have given lebkuchen to their sweethearts as gifts.

Glamorous *torten* (tortes) are made of layers of cake separated by sweet fillings. The most famous German torten is the *Schwarzwälder Kirschtorte* (Black Forest cherry cake). Bakers make this rich dessert with three layers of chocolate sponge cake. They moisten the cake with *Kirschwasser,* which is brandy made from a special variety of cherry. They spread kirsch-flavored whipped cream and cherries between the cake layers. They then decorate the torten with tart cherries, chocolate curls, and more whipped cream.

Another popular German dessert with a regional origin is strudel. ***Strudel*** is paper-thin layers of pastry filled with plums, apples, cherries, or poppy seeds. It usually is sprinkled with confectioners' sugar and served warm. (People in some parts of Germany also make strudel with a protein-based filling and serve it as a main dish.)

German Beverages

Beer drinking is one of Germany's oldest customs. Germans drink beer by itself and with meals. Beer halls are familiar sights in all German cities and towns.

Many wine experts agree the finest table wines are produced in France and Germany. They also agree the best German wines are white wines. Most of the grapes used to make Germany's white wines grow in the valleys bordering the Rhine and Moselle Rivers.

The Germans serve table wines with meals and snacks. Both wine and beer festivals are common in many parts of the country.

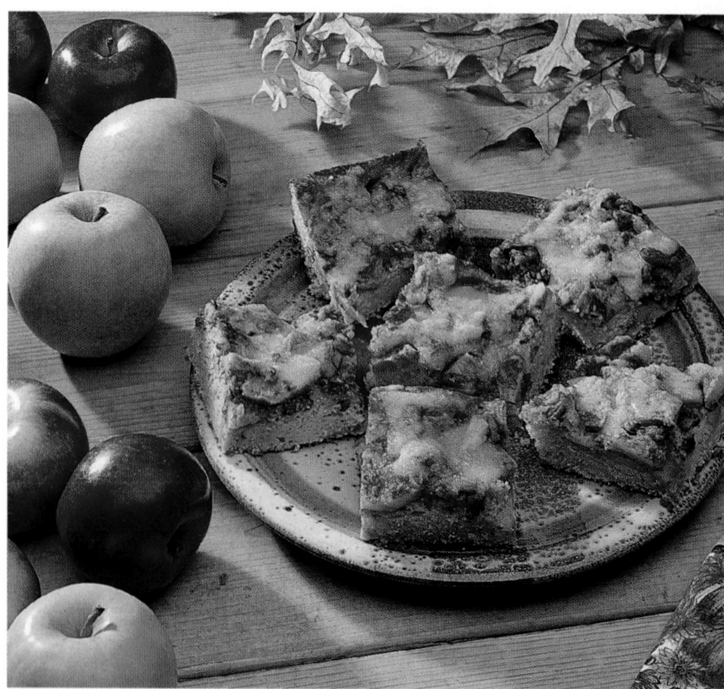

Lesaffre Yeast Corporation, the RED STAR® Yeast Collection

29-16 *Apfelkuchen is a delicious, apple-filled yeast cake topped with a sweet butter sauce.*

German Meals

Traditionally, Germans who could afford to do so ate five meals a day. Many Germans still follow this custom.

Frühstück (breakfast) is hearty. The Germans serve eggs with dark bread and freshly baked crisp rolls. They eat butter and jams with the breads, and serve their coffee with milk. People in northern Germany often serve ham, sausage, and cheese with the eggs.

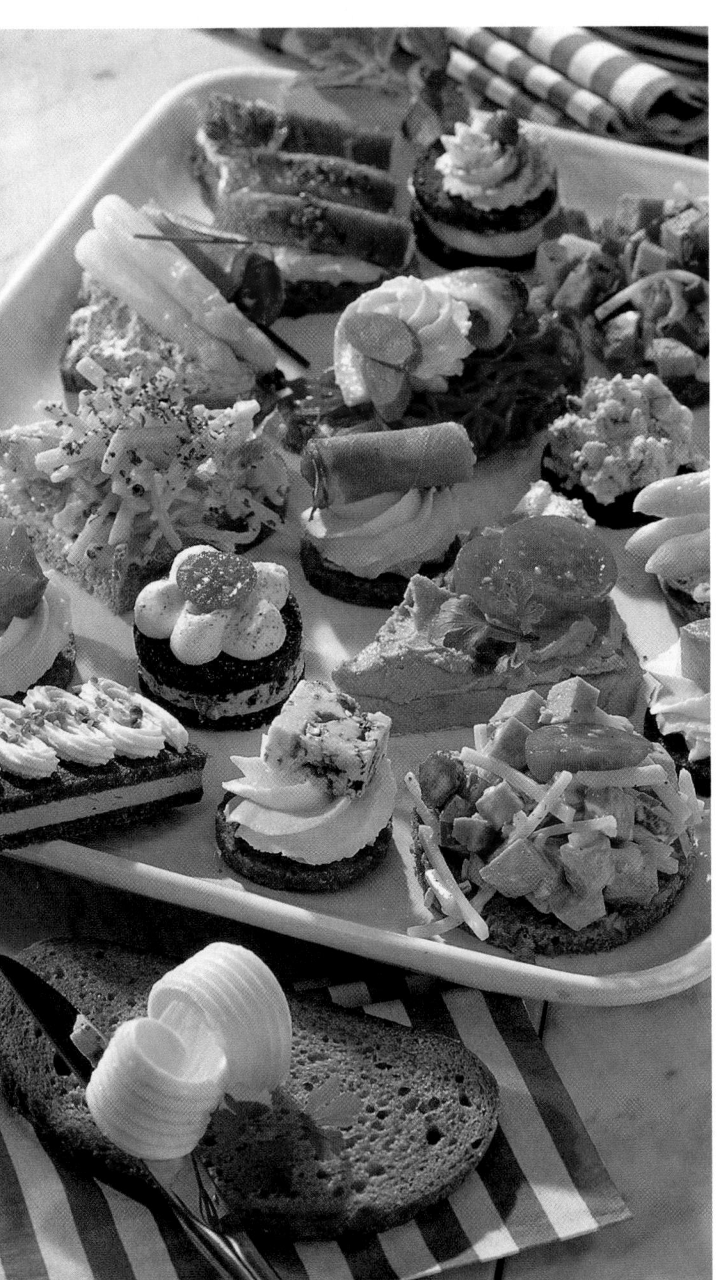

CMA, the German Agricultural Marketing Board, North America

29-17 *A German host might serve these fancy sandwiches in late afternoon for kaffee.*

The Germans eat *zweites frühstück* (second breakfast) during midmorning. Office workers often eat thick sandwiches made of sausage and cheese. Other Germans leave their morning's work for a snack of beer and sausage at a beer hall. Still others prefer fresh pastries at the *bäckerei* (bakery) or cheese sandwiches at the *mölkerei* (dairy).

Mittagessen is the main meal of the day for those Germans who are able to go home at noon. A typical mittagessen might include soup, eintopf, dumplings, and a simple dessert like rote grutze. *Rote grutze* is a pudding made of raspberry, cherry, or red currant juice thickened with cornstarch.

The Germans eat *kaffee* (a sociable snack) in late afternoon. They serve coffee and a variety of small sandwiches, cakes, and rich pastries. Kaffee is important to the Germans, for it is a time to talk with friends. See 29-17.

The Germans usually serve *abendroft* (light supper) in the early evening. Traditionally, abendroft is nothing more than buttered breads served with a variety of cold meats, sausages, and cheeses. For those who cannot eat a hearty meal at noon, however, abendroft is the main meal of the day. An appetizer, soup, main dish, vegetable, bread, and dessert are typical.

German Menu

Sauerbraten
(Marinated Beef in Sweet-Sour Sauce)
Kartoffelpuffer mit Apfelmus
(Potato Pancakes with Applesauce)
Rotkohl
(Red Cabbage)
Grün Salat mit Heiss Speck Socce
(Green Salad with Hot Bacon Dressing)
Pumpernickel
(Rye Bread from Westphalia)
Pflaumenkuchen
(Plum Cake)
Kaffee
(Coffee)

Sauerbraten

(Marinated Beef in Sweet-Sour Sauce)
Serves 8

1 cup water
1 cup vinegar
1/4 cup brown sugar, firmly packed
1 teaspoon salt
1 teaspoon peppercorns
1/2 teaspoon pepper
3 bay leaves
1 medium onion, sliced
2 pounds boneless beef rump roast
1 tablespoon shortening
1/4 cup brown sugar, firmly packed
1/4 cup seedless raisins
6 gingersnaps, broken
1 cup plain nonfat yogurt

1. In a 2- or 3-quart saucepan, combine water, vinegar, 1/4 cup brown sugar, salt, peppercorns, pepper, bay leaves, and onion and bring to a boil.
2. Remove marinade from heat and let cool to room temperature.
3. Place roast in a deep crock or a deep stainless steel (or enameled) pot large enough to hold the meat and marinade.
4. Pour the cooled marinade over the meat. Cover the pan tightly and refrigerate for 24 to 48 hours, turning meat occasionally.
5. Remove meat and pat dry with paper towels.
6. Melt shortening in a large Dutch oven.
7. Add meat and brown on all sides.
8. Add marinade. Cover and simmer meat until tender, about 2 hours.
9. Take meat from Dutch oven and slice; keep warm.
10. Meanwhile strain liquid. Add ¼ cup brown sugar to Dutch oven. Add strained marinade gradually and stir until sugar dissolves.
11. Add raisins and gingersnaps. Cook sauce until smooth and thick, about 5 minutes, stirring constantly.
12. Blend in yogurt. Do not let sauce boil. Serve sauce over sliced meat.

Per serving: 260 cal. (28% from fat), 21 g protein, 27 g carbohydrate, 8 g fat, 58 mg cholesterol, 1 g fiber, 384 mg sodium.

Kartoffelpuffer mit Apfelmus

(Potato Pancakes with Applesauce)
Makes 18 pancakes

2 tablespoons all-purpose flour
1 teaspoon salt
1/2 teaspoon sugar
1/4 teaspoon baking powder
1/8 teaspoon pepper
3 cups grated potatoes (6 medium potatoes)
2 eggs, well beaten
1 tablespoon grated onion
1 tablespoon minced parsley
no-stick cooking spray
applesauce

1. Sift flour, salt, sugar, baking powder, and pepper together in large mixing bowl; set aside.
2. Drain grated potatoes thoroughly. Press potatoes against the sides and bottom of a sieve with spoon to remove excess moisture.
3. Combine eggs, onion, and parsley; add to sifted ingredients.
4. Stir in grated potatoes. Mix thoroughly.
5. Spray heavy nonstick skillet with no-stick cooking spray.
6. For each pancake, drop about 2 tablespoonfuls batter into skillet and spread with the back of the spoon to make a 3-inch round.
7. Fry pancakes until crisp and golden brown. Turn carefully and brown other side.
8. Drain on paper toweling. Serve with applesauce.

Per pancake: 65 cal. (20% from fat), 2 g protein, 12 g carbohydrate, 1 g fat, 30 mg cholesterol, 1 g fiber, 127 mg sodium.

Rotkohl

(Red Cabbage)
Serves 6 to 8

1 head red cabbage (about 2 pounds)
3 1/4 cups water
1/4 cup light brown sugar
3 tablespoons vinegar
3 tablespoons bacon drippings
3/4 teaspoon salt
1 1/2 teaspoons all-purpose flour
1/8 teaspoon allspice
4 whole cloves
dash pepper

1. Coarsely shred cabbage.
2. Put water into 2- to 3-quart saucepan and bring to a boil.
3. Add cabbage, cover, and bring water again to a boil.
4. Reduce heat and gently simmer cabbage until tender, about 10 minutes.
5. Drain cabbage well.
6. Combine brown sugar, vinegar, bacon drippings, salt, flour, allspice, cloves, and pepper.
7. Pour sauce over cabbage; toss well and serve.

Per serving: 110 cal. (52% from fat), 1 g protein, 13 g carbohydrate, 7 g fat, 6 mg cholesterol, 2 g fiber, 252 mg sodium.

Pumpernickel

(Rye Bread from Westphalia)
Makes 2 loaves

6 cups all-purpose flour
2 cups rye flour
2 teaspoons salt
2/3 cup whole bran cereal
1/2 cup yellow cornmeal
1 package plus 1 teaspoon active dry yeast
2 1/4 cups plus 1 tablespoon water
3 tablespoons dark molasses
1 square (1 ounce) unsweetened chocolate
2 1/2 teaspoons softened margarine
1 1/3 cups mashed potatoes (at room temperature)
1 1/2 teaspoons caraway seeds

1. Combine all-purpose and rye flours.
2. In a large mixing bowl, combine 1 1/2 cups of flour mixture, salt, bran cereal, cornmeal, and dry yeast; mix well.
3. In a large saucepan, combine water, molasses, chocolate, and margarine. Heat over low heat until liquid is very warm (120°F to 130°F). (The margarine and chocolate do not have to be completely melted.)
4. Gradually add liquid ingredients to dry ingredients and beat 2 minutes with an electric mixer, at medium speed, scraping bowl occasionally.
5. Add potatoes and 1 cup flour mixture. Beat at high speed 2 minutes, scraping bowl occasionally.
6. Stir in caraway seeds and enough additional flour mixture to make a soft dough.
7. Turn dough out onto lightly floured board or pastry cloth. Knead until smooth and elastic, about 15 minutes.
8. Place dough in greased bowl, turning once to grease top. Cover with a clean towel and let rise in a warm place until doubled in bulk, about 1 hour.
9. Punch dough down and let rise again for 30 minutes.
10. Punch down, and turn out onto lightly floured board or cloth. Divide dough in half and shape each half into a round ball.
11. Place shaped dough in two 8- to 9-inch greased round cake pans. Cover with a clean towel and let rise in a warm place until doubled in bulk, about 45 minutes.
12. Bake breads at 350°F about 50 minutes or until loaves sound hollow when tapped with the knuckles.
13. Remove bread from pans and cool on racks.

Per slice: 140 cal. (8% from fat), 4 g protein, 29 g carbohydrate, 1 g fat, 0 mg cholesterol, 3 g fiber, 186 mg sodium.

Grüner Salat mit Heisser Specksosse

(Green Salad with Hot Bacon Dressing)
Serves 8

2 cups fresh spinach
2 cups iceberg lettuce
2 cups red leaf lettuce
2 cups escarole
1 medium sweet onion cut into rings
1/2 pound bacon finely diced (about 1 1/2 cups)
1/2 cup finely chopped onions
1/4 cup cider vinegar
1/4 cup water
1/2 teaspoon salt
1/4 teaspoon pepper

1. Place greens in a large salad bowl and add onion slices.

2. In a heavy skillet, cook bacon over moderate heat until crisp. Remove bacon from skillet and place on paper towels.
3. Add chopped onions to bacon fat remaining in skillet. Cook onions until soft and transparent, stirring constantly, about 5 minutes.
4. Add vinegar, water, salt, and pepper; cook, stirring constantly for a minute or so.
5. Add bacon and pour over salad greens. Serve immediately. Dressing also may be served alongside the greens, if desired.

Per serving: 85 cal. (43% from fat), 5 g protein, 7 g carbohydrate, 4 g fat, 7 mg cholesterol, 4 g fiber, 289 mg sodium.

Pflaumenkuchen

(Plum Cake)
Serves 8

Topping:
1½ tablespoons all-purpose flour
¾ cup sugar
½ teaspoon cinnamon
2 tablespoons margarine
Cake:
1¼ cups all-purpose flour
1 teaspoon sugar
1 teaspoon baking powder
½ teaspoon salt
¼ cup margarine
1 tablespoon fat free milk
1 egg
3 cups purple plum halves

1. Prepare topping by combining flour, sugar, and cinnamon in small mixing bowl.
2. With pastry blender or two knives, cut in margarine until mixture resembles coarse crumbs. Set aside.
3. Preheat oven to 350°F.
4. Sift flour, sugar, baking powder, and salt onto a large piece of waxed paper; set aside.
5. In large mixer bowl, cream margarine until fluffy.
6. Add dry ingredients and mix well.
7. Gently beat milk and egg together until combined; add to flour mixture.
8. Press dough into a greased 8-inch square pan.
9. Overlap plum halves in neat rows on top of dough; sprinkle with topping.
10. Bake for about 45 to 50 minutes or until cake tests done.
11. Serve warm or at room temperature with ice cream or whipped cream.

Per serving: 287 cal. (28% from fat), 3 g protein, 49 g carbohydrate, 9 g fat, 34 mg cholesterol, 3 g fiber, 280 mg sodium.

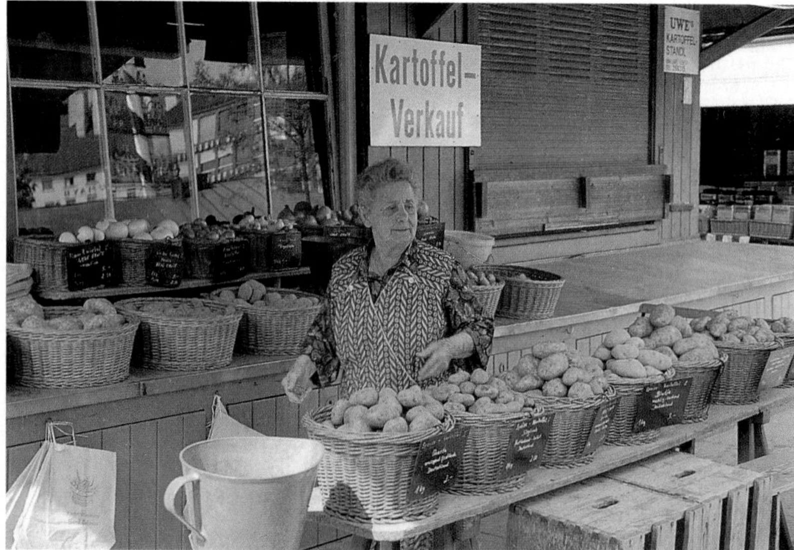

CMA, the German Agricultural Marketing Board, North America

Potatoes have long been a staple in the German diet.

Scandinavia

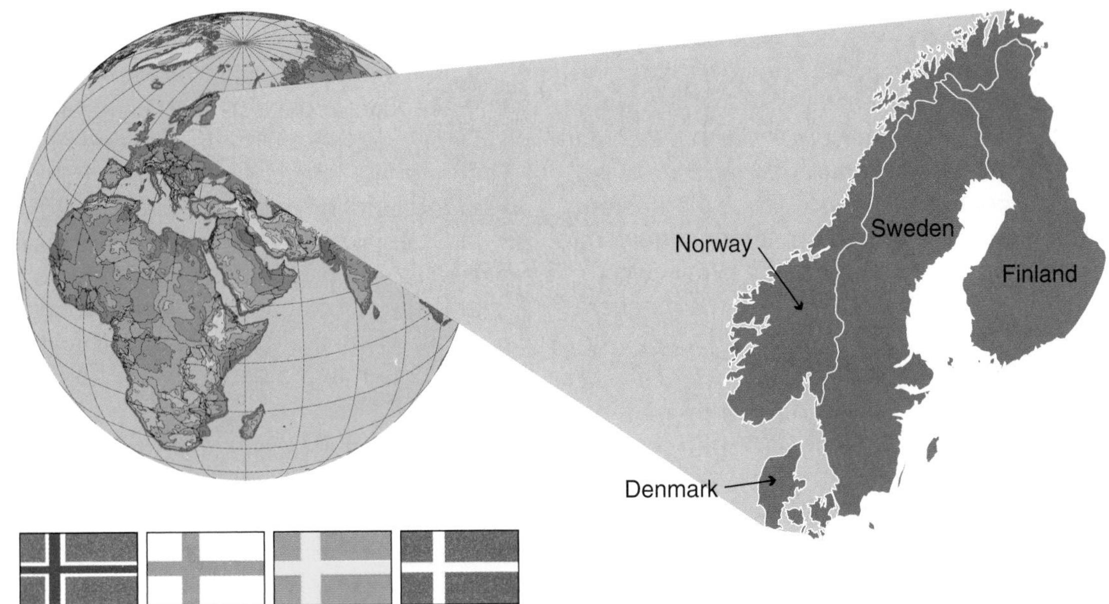

Scandinavia is a land of rugged wilderness and breathtaking beauty. Lakes made centuries ago by glaciers are crystal clear. Dense forests, snowcapped mountains, and lush valleys dot the landscape once ruled by Vikings.

Geography and Climate of Scandinavia

Scandinavia includes the countries of Denmark, Norway, Sweden, and Finland. Norway, Sweden, and Finland are part of a large peninsula that extends above the Arctic Circle. In the northern sections of these three countries, winters are long and severe. Summers are short and cool, thus making the growing season short. Above the Arctic Circle, however, the sun does not set for about two months during the summer. For this reason, the Scandinavian regions above the Arctic Circle are often called the "Land of the Midnight Sun."

Norway is a long, narrow country. Its rocky, mountainous coast makes up much of its land area. Norway is known for its *fjords,* which are slender, deep bays that cut deeply into the land. Norway's greatest wealth is in timber and seafood.

Mountains separate Sweden from Norway, and forests cover much of the northern part of Sweden. The most fertile areas are located in the southern tip of the peninsula.

Glaciers have left much of Finland stony, rough, and dotted with over 60,000 lakes. The

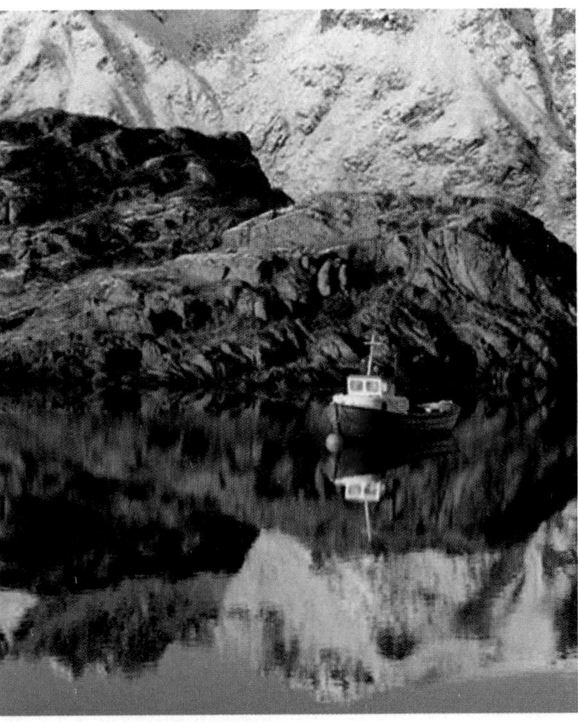

Seas border each of the Scandinavian countries, causing fishing to be an important industry to the people of these nations.

glaciers also formed large marshy areas. These areas give the country its Finnish name, Swomi, which means swamp. Forests cover much of the rest of the land.

Of the four Scandinavian nations, Denmark has the most moderate climate and the least rugged geography. Forests fringe the eastern shore, and irregular hills cut through the central part of the country. The climate is mild with plenty of rainfall. The average winter temperature is 32°F (0°C), which is considerably warmer than the rest of Scandinavia.

Scandinavian Culture

The *Vikings* are the ancestors of the Scandinavian peoples. (The Finns' origins are found in the Central Asian steppes, but Viking influence is present.) The Vikings were both industrious and warlike. They sailed to all parts of the known world during the eighth, ninth, and tenth centuries.

As the Viking Age was ending, the people of Norway, Sweden, Denmark, and Finland began a series of governments. Some of these were joint governments; others were single. These governments lasted into the nineteenth century.

Today, governments in Sweden, Norway, and Denmark differ in form but are similar in effect. Denmark and Norway have constitutional monarchies, and Sweden has a limited monarchy. Finland has a representative government headed by a President. All four nations are peace-loving, and all are known for their advanced forms of social welfare.

Scandinavians, for the most part, have the height, light hair, and blue eyes of their Viking forebears. They are industrious, hard-working people with deep family ties. Scandinavians enjoy singing, dancing, and a variety of sports. They like to ski and ice skate in the winter. They enjoy swimming, sailing, and hiking in the summer.

Scandinavian Agriculture

Many Scandinavians make their living in the large fishing industries found in all four countries. They catch herring, cod, haddock, salmon, and a variety of other fish and shellfish. They sell some locally, but they export much of their catch.

All the Scandinavian countries obtain as many agricultural products as possible from the land. Denmark's climate and geography help make it the most agriculturally prosperous. In Denmark, the climate is mild and about 75 percent of the land can be farmed. (Only 8 percent of the land in Finland and 10 percent of the land in Sweden can be farmed.) Denmark's main wealth is in pigs, cows, and chickens. These animals provide bacon, dairy products, and eggs, which the Danes export. Danish farmers grow grain and other crops for home use and to feed livestock.

Grain and livestock (including dairy cattle) are the main agricultural products of the other Scandinavian countries. Norway also produces large quantities of potatoes.

Scandinavian Holidays

Throughout the year, festivals and holidays are times for merrymaking in Scandinavia, 29-18. One annual event in Denmark is not Danish at all. It is the July 4 celebration of Independence Day in the United States. Like U.S. citizens, Danes enjoy this day by singing, dancing, eating, listening to speeches, and watching fireworks. This event promotes international unity. It also honors values Denmark shares with the United States.

In Norway, as in other Scandinavian countries, Midsummer's Eve is a time to celebrate.

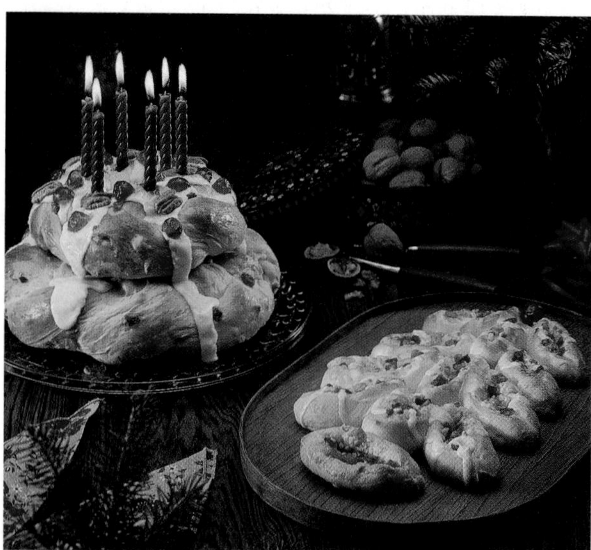

Lesaffre Yeast Corporation, the RED STAR® Yeast Collection

29-18 *Food, like this Swedish Saint Lucia crown, is an important part of many Scandinavian holidays.*

This festival, which is held on June 23, really falls at the beginning of summer in Scandinavia. In the part of Norway that lies above the Arctic Circle, the sun never sets at this time of year. Norwegians welcome the sunshine and warm weather by dancing around a maypole. New potatoes with dill are a traditional food at Midsummer celebrations. Fresh strawberries are a classic Midsummer dessert.

A traditional Swedish festival is Lucia Day, which is December 13. Before dawn, young girls dress in long white robes with red sashes. Wearing crowns of candles on their heads, they awaken their families with a traditional song. They serve hot coffee, saffron buns called *lussekatter,* and gingerbread biscuits called *pepparkakor.*

In Finland, July 21 marks the beginning of an annual tradition—the crayfish party. ***Crayfish*** are crustaceans related to the lobster. The Finns drop the crayfish one-by-one into a pot of boiling water flavored with fresh dill. As they cook, the crayfish turn bright red. The Finns serve them with toast, butter, schnapps, and beer. The atmosphere at these parties is casual and fun as guests feast on this summer treat.

Scandinavian Cuisine

Three major factors have affected Scandinavian cuisine. The first of these is geography. The geography of Scandinavia has made it hard to produce food. (Denmark is an exception.) Scandinavians have had to work to gain enough food from the water, forests, and tillable land.

Human isolation is the second factor affecting Scandinavian cuisine. Mountains and seas have separated the Scandinavian countries from most of Europe. As a result, other European countries have had little impact on Scandinavian cuisine. Geography has also kept the Scandinavian people apart from one another. Therefore, many local and regional dishes can be found.

The third factor affecting Scandinavian cuisine is climate. The Scandinavian climate includes long winters. The growing seasons are short. Therefore, much effort has to be put into preserving food. Pickled, dried, and salted foods are common.

The basic diets of the Danes, Norwegians, Swedes, and Finns are all rather plain and hearty, 29-19. However, preparation and serving methods differ.

Danish Foods

Of all Scandinavian foods, Danish foods are the richest. The Danes use butter, cream, cheese, eggs, pork, and chicken in large quantities. Fish is not nearly as popular in Denmark as it is in the other Scandinavian countries.

The Danes are famous for their smørrebrød, which is literally translated as *buttered bread.* ***Smørrebrød*** are open-faced sandwiches usually made with thin, sour rye bread spread thickly with butter. (Soft white bread is used for smørrebrød with shellfish toppings.) Toppings can be nearly any type of meat, fish, cheese, or vegetable. Danish blue cheese with raw egg yolk is a typical topping. Sliced roast pork garnished with dried fruit and smoked salmon and scrambled eggs garnished with chives are also popular toppings.

The Danes frequently accompany their smørrebrød with glasses of chilled aquavit. *Aquavit* is a clean, potent spirit distilled from grain and potatoes and flavored with caraway seeds. It is served throughout Denmark, Sweden, and Norway.

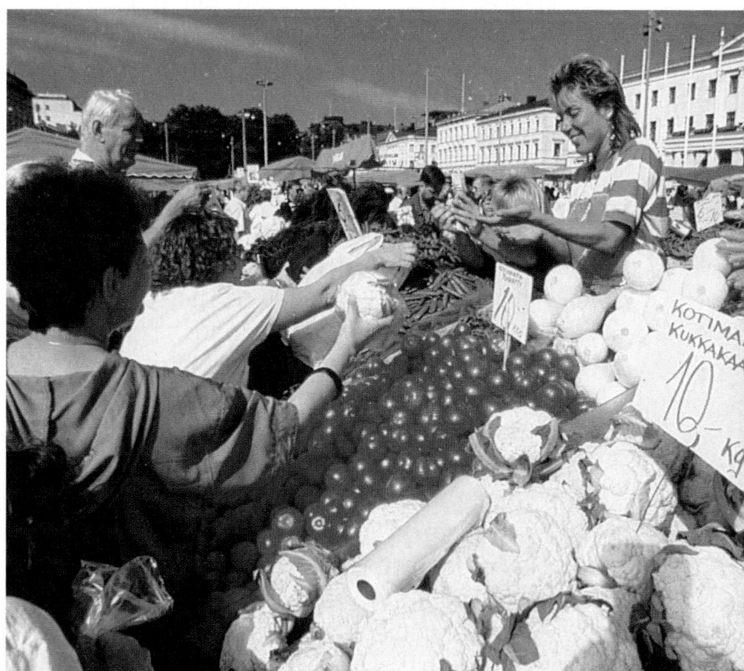

Finnish Tourist Board

29-19 *Locally grown vegetables add color and nutrients to hearty Scandinavian cuisine.*

Danish cheeses are exported and used in Danish homes to make smørrebrød. Tybo, Danbo, Danish brie, havarti, Danish blue, and Danish Camembert are particularly well known.

Danes eat a great deal of pork. They often stuff pork roasts with dried fruits. They mix ground pork with ground veal to make *frikadeller* (meat patties). The Danes use pork liver to make liver paste, which is an important part of the Danish cold table. This cold table, which is a buffet similar to the Swedish smörgåsbord, is called *koldebord.*

Most Danes love desserts. Fruit pudding, apple cake, rum pudding, and pancakes wrapped around ice cream are favorites.

The Danes often begin their day with a substantial breakfast. This meal consists of several dairy products, such as yogurt, sour milk served with cereal, and ymer. Ymer is a high-protein milk product. This may be followed with cheese, bread, a boiled egg, juice, milk, strong coffee, and weinerbrød. *Weinerbrød* are layers of buttery pastry filled with fruit or custard and sprinkled with sugar or nuts. The famous smørrebrød are eaten for lunch. Dinner may include a roast, vegetables, bread, and a rich fruit and cream dessert.

Norwegian Food

Norwegians begin the day with a big breakfast. They may eat herring, eggs, bacon, potatoes, cereals, breads, pastries, fruit, juice, buttermilk, and coffee.

The Norwegians work from early in the morning to midafternoon. Norwegians enjoy foods that are quick to prepare, yet filling and nourishing. Such foods include hearty soups like Bergen fish soup and rich desserts like sour cream waffles. *Lefse,* a thin potato pancake, is also a traditional Norwegian food.

Because of their nearness to the sea, Norwegians have relied on seafood as a staple in their diets, 29-20. Herring (smoked, pickled, and fresh), halibut, cod, and salmon are all popular. The Norwegians often poach fish or add it to nourishing stews and soups. ***Lutefisk*** (dried cod that have been soaked in a lye solution before cooking) is a traditional Norwegian fish dish.

The Norwegians raise goats and sheep on their mountainous land. They use goats' milk to make cheese. They use lamb and mutton in a variety of dishes. The Norwegians make a stew called *får i kål* from mutton and cabbage. One of the most popular smoked meat dishes is *fenalår,* which the Norwegians make from smoked mutton.

Danish cooks use sweet and whipped cream, but Norwegian cooks traditionally use sour cream. Soups, sauces, salads, and meat dishes are all likely to contain sour cream. Sour cream spread on bread or crackers is a popular snack.

Norwegians take great pride in their baked goods. They serve many traditional cookies and cakes at Christmastime. *Krumkaker* are thin, delicate cookies baked on a special iron and rolled around a wooden spoon while still warm. The cooled cookies are eaten plain or filled with whipped cream and fruit. *Rosettes* are light and airy cookies cooked on the ends of special irons in hot fat. *Fattigman,* diamond-shaped cookies, are also fried in fat. *Kringla* are rich with sour cream or buttermilk and tied in figure eights or knots.

Swedish Food

The famous smörgåsbord originated in Sweden where it is served in private homes as well as in restaurants. A ***smörgåsbord*** is a buffet that includes a wide variety of hot and cold dishes. The word *smörgåsbord* means bread and butter table. However, smörgåsbords

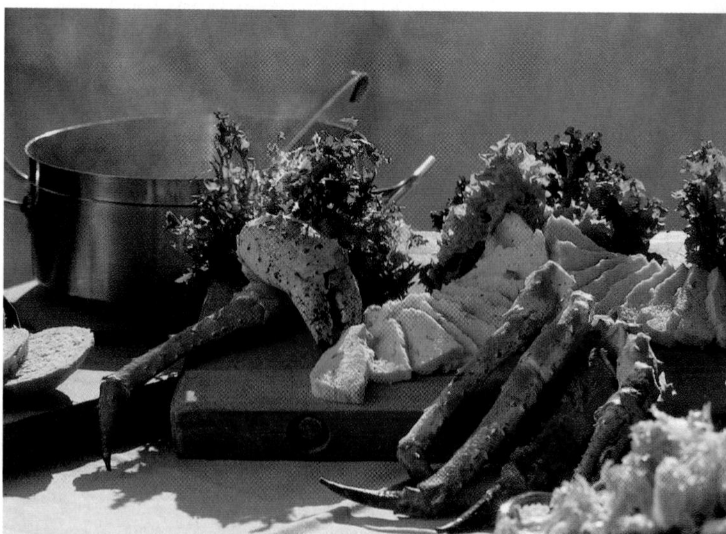

Terje Rakke/NTR/East Norway

29-20 *Seafood plays an important role in the diet and the economy of Norway.*

can be elegant and may include 30 or more dishes, depending on the occasion. Typical smörgåsbord dishes include herring dishes; cold fish, meats, and salads; hot meats, eggs, or fish; breads; cheeses; and desserts. Diners return to the smörgåsbord several times to partake of the different courses.

Generally, people save the smörgåsbord for large gatherings and special occasions. The traditional, everyday style of cooking, called ***husmankost,*** is very simple. Visitors in Swedish homes are likely to see rich yellow pea soup and salt pork served for supper. Traditionally, these foods are followed by Swedish pancakes and ***lingonberries*** (tart, red berries) for dessert.

Baked brown beans, herring and sour cream, fried pork sausages, pickled beets, and fruit soups are other traditional Swedish foods.

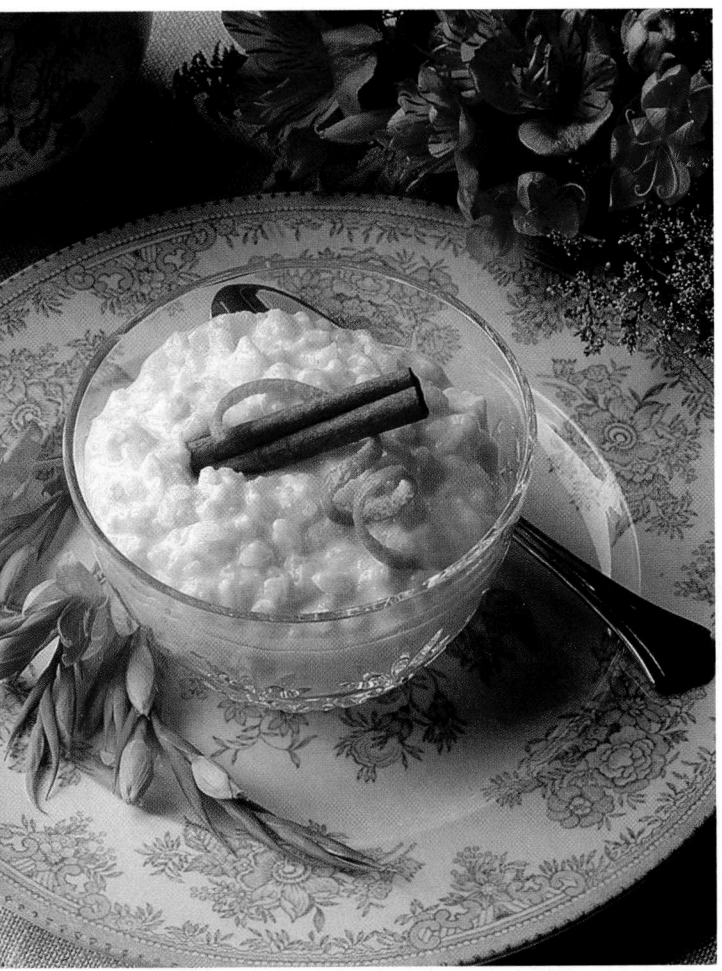

USA Rice Federation

29-21 *Milk makes this Swedish rice pudding nutritious as well as rich and creamy.*

Nyponsoppa is a fruit soup made with rose hips (the orange seed capsules of the rose). It is served with whipped cream and almonds and is a Swedish specialty.

Reindeer is not exclusively Swedish, for reindeer herds roam the northern sections of Norway and Finland as well as Sweden. Reindeer flesh has a mild, wild flavor. Shaving reindeer meat into hot fat and frizzling it is one popular preparation method.

Some Swedes consider dessert to be the best part of a meal, 29-21. Ostkaka and spettekaka are two of their favorites. They make *ostkaka,* a rich puddinglike cake, from milk, heavy cream, eggs, sugar, rennet, and flour. Strawberries, lingonberries, or raspberries are common accompaniments. *Spettekaka* is a delicate cake made of eggs, sugar, and flour. Swedish bakers slowly pour the batter onto a cone-shaped spit placed in front of a fire. As they rotate the cone, the batter dries in layers and forms a pattern.

Finnish Food

In Finland, forests are everywhere. The Finns gather raspberries, strawberries, lingonberries, arctic cloudberries, Finnish cranberries, and mesimarja from the forests. (Finnish cranberries are smaller than those grown in the United States. *Mesimarja* are small, delicate fruits similar to raspberries.) The Finns use berries to make liqueurs, puddings, tarts, and snows (light puddings containing beaten egg whites). One popular fruit pudding is called *vatkattu marjapuuro.* Finnish cooks make it by whipping fruit juice, sugar, and a cereal product similar to farina until light and fluffy.

Finnish foods are hearty, often in a primitive way. *Vorshmack,* which is ground mutton, salt herring, and beef combined with onions and garlic, is a traditional Finnish dish. Pork gravy, black sour rye bread, and rutabagas and other root vegetables help warm the Finns during the bitter winters. The Finns add mushrooms to soups, sauces, salads, gravies, and stews. They make porridges and gruels from whole grains, just as their ancestors did centuries ago. *Mämmi* is a pudding made of molasses, bitter orange peel, rye flour, and rye malt. The Finns serve it at Easter with sweet cream.

At one time, the Finns lived under Russian rule. As a result, some Russian foods have become part of Finnish cuisine. Two of the most popular Finnish dishes with Russian origins are pasha and piirakka. *Pasha* is a type of cheesecake and *piirakka* are pastries or pies. The Finns fill piirakka with meat, fish, vegetables, and fruits. They serve the piirakka as appetizers, side dishes, or desserts.

A Finnish tradition is the sauna. The ***sauna*** is a steam bath in which water is poured on hot stones to create steam. Finns follow the heat of the sauna with a quick dip in a chilly lake or swimming pool. They serve snacks during the sauna. They often serve salty fish to help replace the salt lost through sweat during the sauna. After the sauna, the Finns eat a light meal. Grilled sausages, piirakka, poached salmon, salads, and Finnish rye bread are popular after-sauna supper dishes. The Finns may serve chilled vodka or beer with the meal.

Q: Isn't sitting in a sauna supposed to help you lose weight?

A: Sitting in a sauna is not a recommended weight-loss technique. Any weight loss is temporary due to water lost through sweat. Excessive sweating causes dehydration, so be sure to drink plenty of fluids before and after spending time in a sauna.

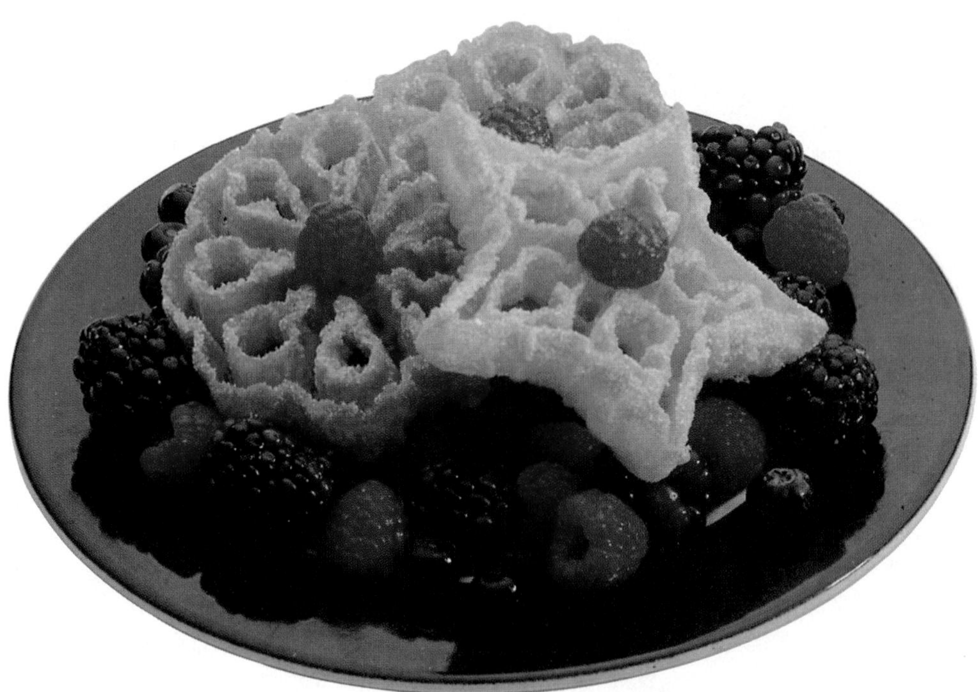

Nordic Ware

Light, airy rosettes are popular Norwegian Christmas cookies.

Scandinavian Menu

Sill med Kremsaus
(Herring in Cream Sauce)

Kesäkeitto
(Summer Soup)

Frikadeller
(Danish Meat Patties)

Brunede Kartofler
(Caramelized Potatoes)

Syltede Rødbeder
(Pickled Beets)

Limpa
(Swedish Rye Bread)

Kringla
(Double-Ring Twist Biscuits)

Fattigman
(Poor Man's Cookies)

Kaffe
(Coffee)

Sill med Kremsaus

(Herring in Cream Sauce)
Serves 6

$1\frac{1}{2}$ cups coarsely chopped herring (salt, pickled, or Bismark herring)
2 tablespoons finely chopped onion
2 tablespoons fresh dill, divided
dash pepper
3 tablespoons white wine vinegar, divided
2 chilled hard-cooked egg yolks
1 teaspoon prepared mustard
1 tablespoon vegetable oil
$3\frac{1}{2}$ tablespoons evaporated fat free milk

1. In a small mixing bowl, combine herring, onion, 1 tablespoon dill, pepper, and $1\frac{1}{2}$ tablespoons white wine vinegar; set aside.
2. In another bowl, mash egg yolks with a wooden spoon.
3. Add mustard, remaining $1\frac{1}{2}$ tablespoons vinegar, and oil, beating until smooth.
4. Gradually add evaporated fat free milk, beating constantly, until sauce is the thickness of heavy cream.
5. Pour sauce over herring mixture and refrigerate, covered, at least two hours.
6. Garnish with remaining fresh dill just before serving.

Per serving: 168 cal. (73% from fat), 16 g protein, 2 g carbohydrate, 11 g fat, 114 mg cholesterol, 0 g fiber, 108 mg sodium.

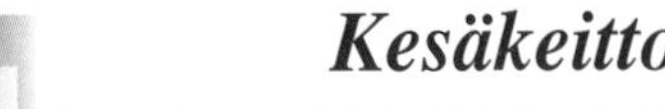

Kesäkeitto

(Summer Soup)
Serves 6 to 8

1 cup fresh green peas*
1 small head cauliflower, separated into small florets
5 small carrots, diced
2 small potatoes, diced
$\frac{1}{2}$ pound fresh string beans, cut into narrow strips*
4 cups cold water
$\frac{1}{4}$ pound fresh spinach, finely chopped
2 tablespoons all-purpose flour
1 cup fat free milk
$\frac{1}{4}$ cup evaporated fat free milk
1 egg yolk
salt and white pepper to taste
chopped parsley

1. With the exception of the spinach, place vegetables in a large saucepan, cover with cold water, and simmer until just tender, about 5 minutes.
2. Add spinach and cook another 5 minutes.
3. Remove from heat and strain liquid into a bowl; set aside.
4. Place vegetables in a second bowl.
5. Combine flour and milk in a covered jar or blender container. Shake or blend until smooth.
6. Pour flour mixture into the saucepan used for the vegetables. Cook over medium heat, stirring constantly until sauce comes to a boil. Cook and stir for one additional minute until sauce is thick and smooth.
7. Add hot vegetable stock slowly, stirring constantly.
8. In a small bowl combine the evaporated fat free milk and egg yolk.
9. Add a few tablespoons of hot soup to the egg mixture, beating constantly. Then add the warmed egg mixture to the hot soup.

10. Add vegetables and bring soup to a simmer. Simmer uncovered over low heat for 3 to 5 minutes.
11. Taste and add salt and pepper as needed.
12. Pour into a tureen and garnish with chopped parsley.

*If fresh peas, string beans, or spinach are not available, substitute frozen June peas, French-style green beans, and chopped spinach. Adjust cooking time accordingly.

Per serving: 148 cal. (6% from fat), 7 g protein, 28 g carbohydrate, 1 g fat, 46 mg cholesterol, 7 g fiber, 362 mg sodium.

Frikadeller

(Danish Meat Patties)
Makes about 15 meat patties

- 1/2 pound ground pork shoulder or fresh ham
- 1/2 pound ground shoulder of veal
- 1/2 cup flour
- 2 eggs
- 1 large onion, chopped
- salt and pepper to taste
- 2/3 cup fat free milk
- margarine for frying

1. In a large bowl, mix the meats with the flour, eggs, onion, salt, and pepper.
2. Add milk gradually and mix thoroughly. Let the mixture stand 15 minutes to allow the flour to absorb the milk.
3. Shape the mixture into small meat patties.
4. Melt margarine in an electric skillet or frying pan over medium heat.
5. Fry patties about 5 minutes on each side. Use a meat thermometer to be sure the internal temperature has reached 160°F.
6. Drain on paper towels.

Per meat patty: 98 cal. (50% from fat), 7 g protein, 5 g carbohydrate, 5 g fat, 58 mg cholesterol, 0 g fiber, 40 mg sodium.

Brunede Kartofler

(Caramelized Potatoes)
Serves 6

- 2 pounds small red potatoes
- 1/4 cup sugar
- 2 tablespoons melted margarine

1. Scrub potatoes carefully. Do not remove skins.
2. Fill a heavy 2- to 3-quart saucepan with water and bring it to a boil.
3. Add potatoes and simmer 15 to 20 minutes or until potatoes are tender.
4. Cool potatoes slightly; slip off skins.
5. In a large, heavy skillet, melt sugar. Use a low heat and stir sugar constantly until it turns into light brown syrup. (Heat must be low or sugar will scorch.)
6. Add melted margarine.
7. Add potatoes, a few at a time, shaking pan to coat all sides with syrup. Serve immediately.

Per serving: 216 cal. (17% from fat), 3 g protein, 43 g carbohydrate, 4 g fat, 0 mg cholesterol, 3 g fiber, 54 mg sodium.

Syltede Rødbeder

(Pickled Beets)
(Makes 2 1/2 cups)

- 1/4 cup cider vinegar
- 1/4 cup white vinegar
- 1/2 cup sugar
- 1/2 teaspoon salt
- dash pepper
- 2 1/2 cups thinly sliced canned beets

1. In a 1 1/2- to 2-quart stainless steel saucepan, combine all ingredients but beets. Boil briskly for 2 minutes.
2. While marinade boils, place beets in a deep stainless steel or glass bowl.
3. Pour hot marinade over beets; let cool for 20 minutes, uncovered.
4. Cover bowl and refrigerate at least 12 hours, stirring occasionally.

Per ½-cup serving: 105 cal. (0% from fat), 1 g protein, 28 g carbohydrate, 0 g fat, 0 mg cholesterol, 2 g fiber, 466 mg sodium.

Limpa

(Swedish Rye Bread)
Makes 2 loaves

- 1 package active dry yeast
- 1 3/4 cups warm water (105°F to 115°F)
- 1/2 cup light brown sugar, packed
- 1/2 cup light molasses
- 1 1/2 teaspoons salt
- 2 tablespoons shortening
- 1 tablespoon grated orange peel

1/2 cup dark seedless raisins
2 1/2 cups rye flour
3 1/2 to 4 cups all-purpose flour

1. In a large bowl, dissolve yeast in warm water.
2. Add brown sugar, molasses, salt, shortening, orange peel, raisins, and rye flour; beat well.
3. Add enough all-purpose flour to make a soft dough.
4. Turn dough out onto a lightly floured board or pastry cloth. Cover; let rest 10 minutes.
5. Knead dough until smooth and elastic, about 10 minutes.
6. Place dough in a lightly greased bowl, turning once to grease surface. Cover with a towel. Let dough rise in a warm place until doubled in bulk (about 1 1/2 to 2 hours).
7. Punch dough down. Turn dough out on lightly floured board or cloth and divide into 2 portions.
8. Shape each portion into a ball; cover, let rest 10 minutes.
9. Pat balls of dough into 2 round loaves and place on a greased baking sheet. Cover loaves and let rise in a warm place until double (about 1 1/2 to 2 hours).
10. Bake loaves at 375°F for 25 to 30 minutes.
11. Remove bread from pans to cooling racks. For a soft crust, butter tops of loaves while hot.

Per slice: 119 cal. (8% from fat), 3 g protein, 25 g carbohydrate, 1 g fat, 0 mg cholesterol, 2 g fiber, 107 mg sodium.

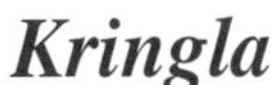

Kringla

(Double-Ring Twist Biscuits)
Makes about 24 cookies

1 cup sugar
1 cup plain nonfat yogurt
1 cup sour milk
1 egg
1 teaspoon baking soda
pinch salt
1/2 teaspoon cinnamon
1 1/2 to 2 cups all-purpose flour

1. Preheat oven to 375°F.
2. Combine sugar, yogurt, sour milk, egg, baking soda, salt, and cinnamon in a large bowl.
3. Add enough flour to make a fairly stiff dough.
4. Roll dough between palms to form pencil-sized rolls; shape rolls into figure eights.
5. Place cookies on lightly greased baking sheet and bake until lightly browned, about 10 to 12 minutes.

Per cookie: 92 cal. (4% from fat), 2 g protein, 20 g carbohydrate, 0 g fat, 12 mg cholesterol, 0 g fiber, 51 mg sodium.

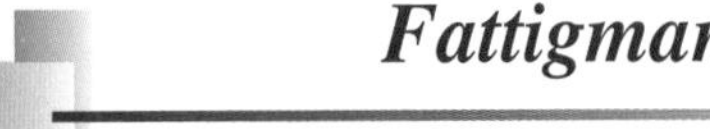

Fattigman

(Poor Man's Cookies)
Makes about 3 dozen cookies

4 eggs
1/2 cup sugar
dash salt
4 tablespoons evaporated fat free milk
1 1/2 cups all-purpose flour
shortening or oil for frying
sugar

1. Beat eggs, sugar, and salt until thick and light.
2. Add evaporated milk and enough flour to make a soft dough.
3. Cut dough into diamond shapes and fry in hot shortening (375°F).
4. While warm, sprinkle cookies with sugar.

Per cookie: 53 cal. (13% from fat), 2 g protein, 10 g carbohydrate, 1 g fat, 31 mg cholesterol, 0 g fiber, 10 mg sodium.

Chapter 29 Review

Europe

Summary

The British Isles include the countries of England, Scotland, Wales, Northern Ireland, and Ireland. These countries have a common climate and culture. However, each has unique aspects to its cuisine. Roasted meats, baked apples, main dish pies, and steamed puddings are among the popular foods in England. Simple, wholesome foods of the Scots often include such basic ingredients as oats, barley, lamb, and fish. The hearty fare of Wales is similar to that of its neighbors. Potatoes are the staple of the Irish diet. Tea is a popular beverage throughout the British Isles. It is also the name of a light meal served in the late afternoon or early evening.

France has long been known for its fine cuisine. French cooks use three main cooking styles: haute cuisine, provincial cuisine, and nouvelle cuisine. A variety of sauces and delicate seasonings characterize French cooking. Local dishes are popular throughout the various regions of France.

German cuisine is filling and flavorful. Roasted meats and a variety of sausages are common main dishes in Germany. Potatoes, sauerkraut, and dumplings are popular as hearty side dishes. Delicious breads as well as sweet rolls and cakes are the pride of German bakers. Of course, people throughout the world know Germany for its beers and wines.

Denmark, Norway, Sweden, and Finland are all part of Scandinavia. Much of Scandinavia is characterized by rugged terrain. This has made farming difficult in many areas and has isolated one region from another. Scandinavia is also typified by a cold climate. These factors have all affected the development of Scandinavian cuisine. Danish foods tend to be rich, often containing butter, cream, cheese, eggs, and pork. The Norwegians eat much fish and use sour cream in many of their recipes. Special occasions in Sweden often feature a smörgåsbord, but the everyday style of cooking is much simpler. Some Finnish dishes have Russian origins, and many include berries, mushrooms, and potatoes gathered from local forests.

Review What You Have Read

Write your answers on a separate sheet of paper.

1. What annual festival is celebrated in Wales on March 1, and what foods are traditionally served on this day?
2. What are four staples of the British diet that were introduced by the Anglo-Saxons?
3. What foods might be served for a traditional breakfast in England?
4. True or false. Haggis is an Irish porridge made with potatoes and cabbage.
5. Define *haute cuisine, provincial cuisine,* and *nouvelle cuisine.*
6. Name and describe three types of French sauces.
7. True or false. The French serve the salad as a first course.
8. Name three foods that are eaten in the Provence region of France.
9. Describe three popular German potato dishes.
10. True or false. German bakers have traditionally made their cakes with molasses.
11. How do German meal patterns differ from those in the United States?
12. What are two specific toppings commonly eaten on Danish smørrebrød?
13. Describe three kinds of Norwegian cookies.
14. What dishes are typically included at a smörgåsbord?
15. What do Finns often snack on during a sauna and why?

Build Your Basic Skills

1. **Verbal.** Investigate the celebration of a German holiday. Share your findings about traditional customs, decorations, and foods in a brief oral report.
2. **Math.** Europeans use the metric system of measurement. List the metric equivalents for each ingredient in the British, French, German, or Scandinavian recipes found in this chapter. You may wish to refer to Chapter 13, "Getting Started in the Kitchen," for more information on metric measurements.

Build Your Thinking Skills

1. **Organize.** Work with a small group to organize the thorough research of one of the regions of France. Each member of the group should be responsible for a different part of the research. Research topics should include the geography, agriculture, culture, and cuisine of the region. Coordinate your research findings as your group presents a team report to the class.
2. **Create.** Create a Scandinavian dessert buffet. Be sure to include Danish pastries, Norwegian cookies, Swedish rice pudding, and Finnish vatkattu marjapuuro.

Apply Technology

1. Use a computer and the table function in word processing software to create a two-column survey form. The first column should be headed *Rank,* and the second column should be headed *Attractions.* Leave the first column blank and list 10 popular European attractions in the second column.
2. Give printouts of the European attractions survey form created in the preceding activity to five friends. Ask your friends to write the rank of each attraction in the first column, with 1 being the favorite attraction. Then use a computer to tally the results of the survey and sort the attractions according to ascending numbers. Discuss the results in class.

Using Workplace Skills

Ian owns a small travel agency called European Excursions. In addition to managing the business, Ian serves as the main tour guide. He arranges transportation and meal and lodging accommodations for groups of tourists traveling throughout Europe. He also accompanies the tour groups on their trips. He makes sure the groups follow their schedules and reach planned stopping points along the way.

To be an effective worker, Ian needs to display honesty and integrity. He knows he could make a bigger profit by booking groups into lower-class hotels or second-rate restaurants. However, Ian wants his business to have a reputation for giving tour groups the best value for their travel dollar. Imagine you are a client in one of Ian's tour groups. Answer the following questions about Ian's need for and use of the qualities of honesty and integrity:

A. Suppose you didn't know anything about Ian's character and business philosophy. How would you assume you would be treated by the owner of a travel agency who was arranging your vacation?
B. How would Ian's obvious honesty and integrity make you feel once you were on your trip?
C. What impact would Ian's behavior have if you were planning a second European trip or talking to a friend who was planning a European trip?
D. What is another skill Ian would need in this job? Briefly explain why this skill would be important.

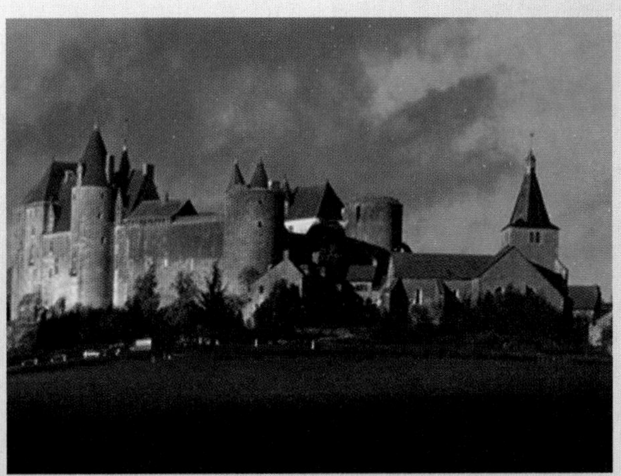

Chapter 30
Mediterranean Countries

International Airplane-Flight Attendant
Performs a variety of personal services to provide for safety and comfort of international airline passengers during flight.

Press Tender
Tends battery of presses that automatically mix ingredients, and knead and extrude dough for use in making macaroni products.

Italian Chef
Supervises, coordinates, and participates in activities of cooks and other kitchen personnel engaged in preparing and cooking Italian foods in hotel, restaurant, or other establishment.

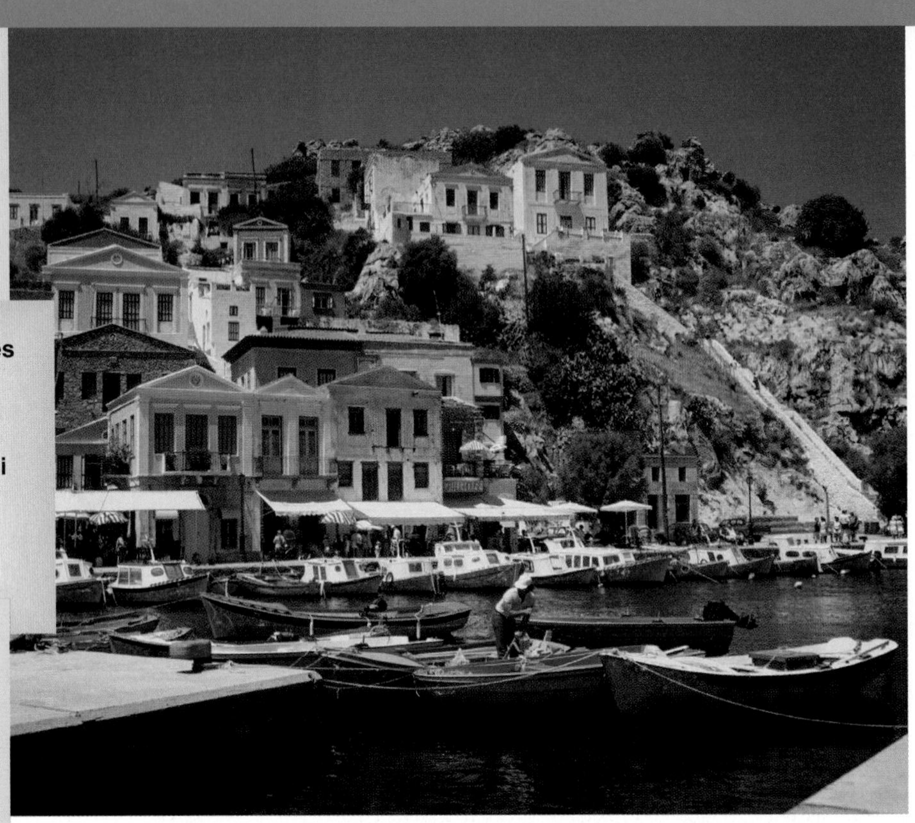

Terms to Know

eggplant
del pueblo
tapas
gazpacho
chorizo
paella
sangria
al dente
risotto
minestrone
antipasto
taverna
avgolemono
phyllo
mezedhes

Objectives

After studying this chapter, you will be able to

- describe the food customs of Spain, Italy, and Greece.
- discuss how geography, climate, and culture have influenced these customs.
- prepare foods that are native to each of these countries.

The Mediterranean Sea is a warm, salty body of water that lies south of Europe. The Mediterranean region supports crops like citrus fruit, olives, grapes, wheat, barley, peaches, and apricots. The sea itself harbors a variety of fish as well as sponges and coral. For ages, people in the Mediterranean region have harvested these products and the sea salt to earn a living.

The climate in this region is balmy with plenty of sunshine throughout the year. The winters are mild with average rainfall. The summers are hot and dry. This weather makes the Mediterranean a popular vacation area.

Three European countries that lie along the Mediterranean Sea are Spain, Italy, and Greece. Because of their similar climates and resources, the cuisines of these countries resemble one another. Vegetables like tomatoes, eggplant, and green peppers are used in many dishes in each of these countries. (***Eggplant*** is a fleshy, oval-shaped vegetable with a deep purple skin.) Seafood is also common in each of these cuisines.

As you read about Spain, Italy, and Greece, you will recognize how their food customs are similar. You will also note unique aspects of each cuisine.

In recent years, nutrition experts have focused much attention on the health benefits of the traditional Mediterranean diet. Rates of cancer and heart disease are low in this part of the world. Diet seems to play a key role in these positive health statistics.

A number of features add to the healthfulness of the Mediterranean diet. The most notable characteristic is the broad use of plant foods. Fruits such as grapes, oranges, figs, and melons grow well in the warm Mediterranean climate. They, rather than rich desserts, are often served at the end of Mediterranean meals. Tomatoes, eggplant, peppers, legumes, onions, and garlic form the basis of many dishes. Pasta, rice, and/or bread are staples at most meals. Olive oil, which has no cholesterol and is high in monounsaturated fats, is the main cooking fat in the Mediterranean. People in this region tend to eat much seafood but only limited portions of meat. These characteristics define a diet that is fairly low in fat. The variety of plant foods in the Mediterranean diet provides vitamins, minerals, fiber, and other helpful plant substances.

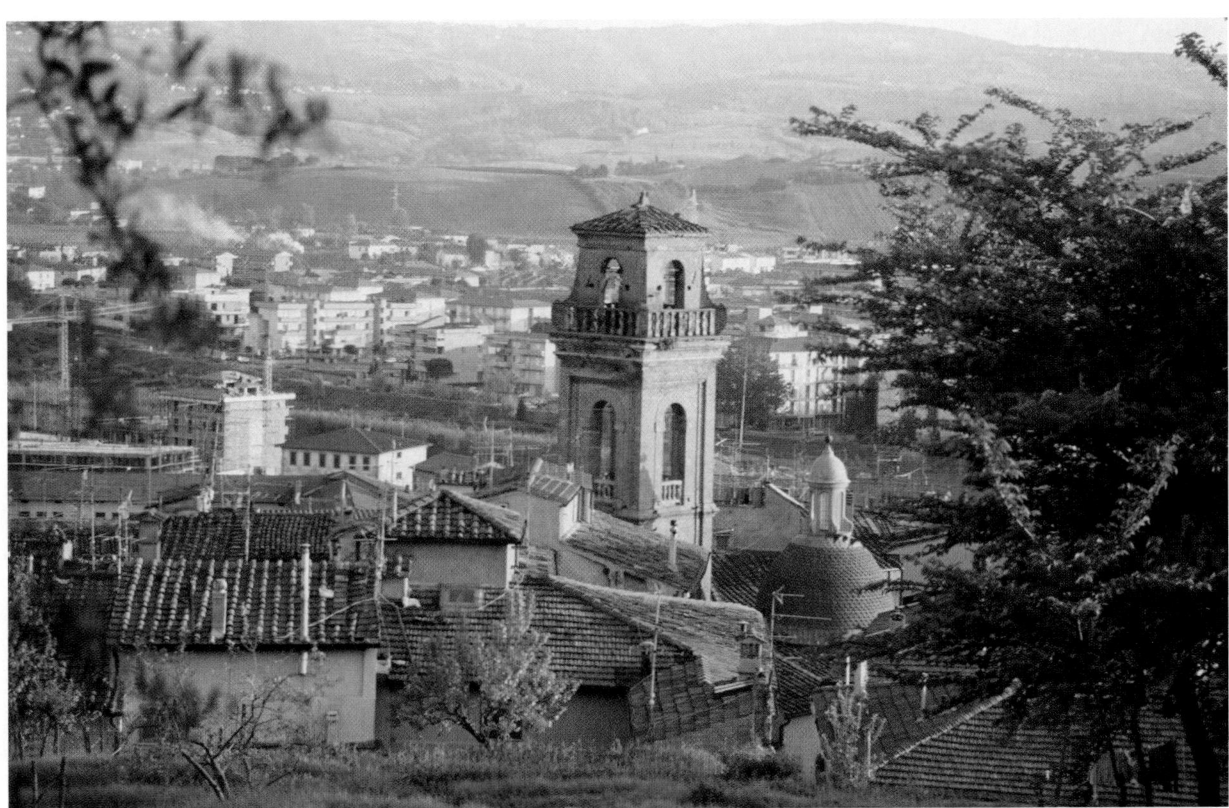
The Tuscany region of Italy is known for its rural beauty and distinct Mediterranean cuisine.

Spain

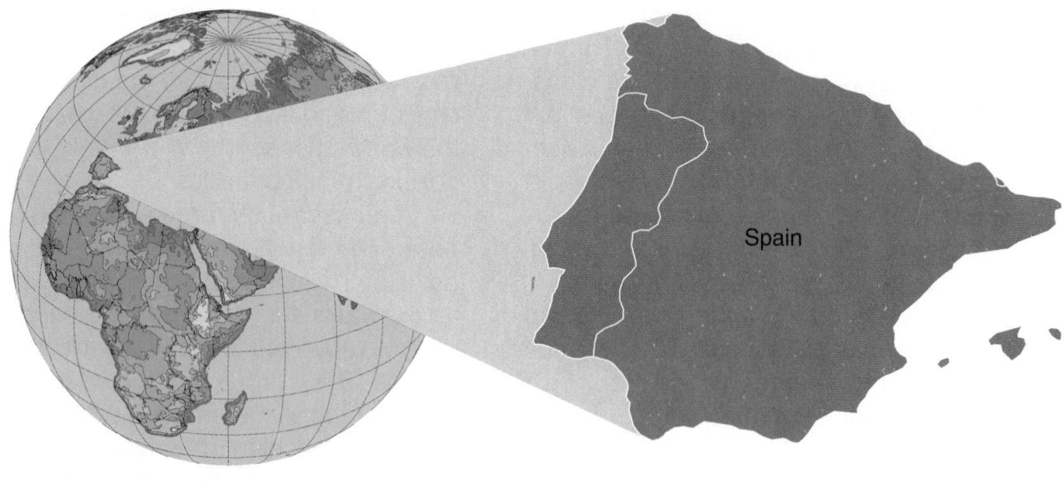

The Iberian Peninsula lies between the Mediterranean Sea and the Atlantic Ocean. This land mass forms the southwestern corner of Europe. Spain and Portugal share the peninsula. Spain occupies the largest part.

Geography and Climate of Spain

The two main geographic features of Iberia are water and mountains. Water nearly surrounds the peninsula, and several mountain ranges crisscross the land.

Most Spaniards live along the coast of the Bay of Biscay and the Mediterranean Sea. There the land is fertile and agriculture is prosperous.

In the North, the Pyrenees separate Spain from France and the rest of Europe. Four other mountain ranges divide the rest of the land into isolated units. Within the circle formed by the mountain ranges is the Meseta. The *Meseta* is a large plateau. It occupies more than half of the total area of Spain.

Spain has a surprising range of climates for a country that is relatively small. Much of Spain has a Mediterranean climate with hot, dry summers, mild winters, and light rainfall. Northern Spain has cool summers with mild, damp winters. The Meseta of central Spain has the most severe climate with extremes of both heat and cold. The southernmost tip of Spain is semidesert with virtually no winter.

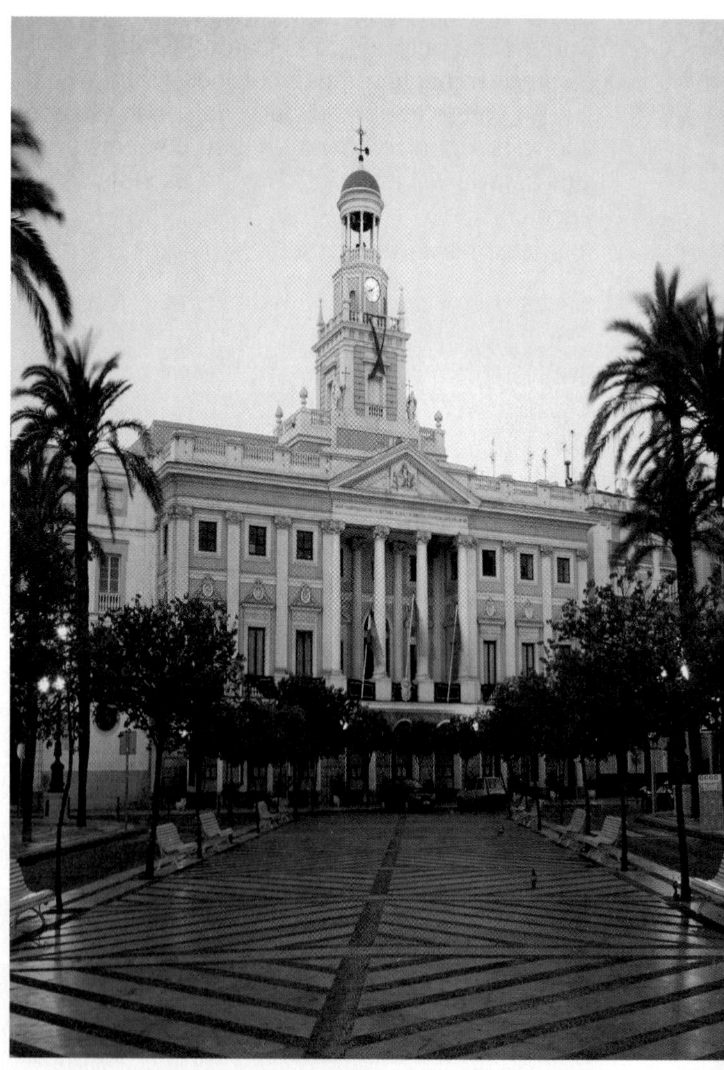

The town hall in Cadiz, Spain is a stately example of classic Spanish architecture.

Spanish Culture

Spain has a rich cultural heritage. This heritage has influenced life in the country today.

Influences on Spanish Culture

The Romans ruled Spain for a period of six centuries beginning in the 200s B.C. During this time, cities were built, the Spanish language developed, and Christianity became the official religion.

Roman rule was followed by a Germanic government under the Visigoths. Then in A.D. 711, the Moors, a Muslim people from northern Africa, crossed into Spain and started taking control. Some graceful palaces and beautiful mosques built by the Moors can still be seen in Spain today.

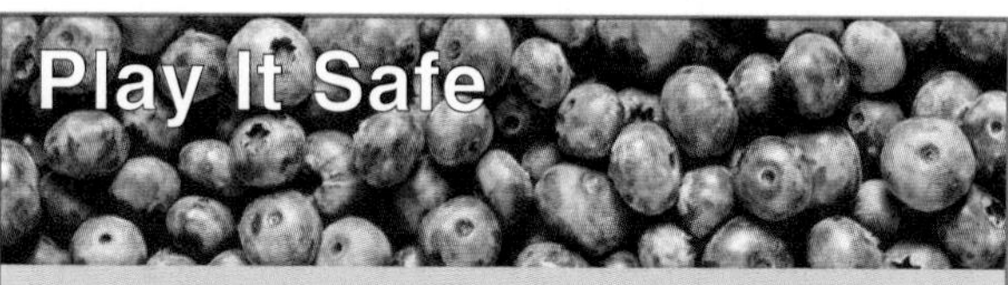

To reduce losses in the event of theft, avoid carrying large amounts of currency when you travel. Traveler's checks and credit cards are a safer bet.

By the fifteenth century, Christian kingdoms that had formed in northern sections of Spain threatened Moorish rule. In 1479, the Christian kingdoms became united under King Ferdinand and Queen Isabella. During the reign of Ferdinand and Isabella, explorers journeyed to the New World and claimed land for Spain.

The Spanish Empire began to decline in 1588 with the defeat of the Spanish Armada, a fleet of armed ships. Following this defeat, France began attacking Spain. To ease relations, the king of Spain formed an alliance with France that lasted until 1789.

The 1800s in Spain were marked by frequent periods of unrest. In 1931, the Spanish Republic was proclaimed. In 1936, however, the Spanish Civil War broke out. Three years later when this brutal war ended, the Spanish Republic became a dictatorship under Francisco Franco. Following Franco's death in 1975, a democratic government was established in Spain.

Spanish Agriculture

Many Spaniards make their living fishing or farming. There are some large landowners in Spain. However, most people live on their own small farms. Wheat, olives, barley, oats, rye, potatoes, rice, beans, grapes, and honey are Spain's primary crops. Valencian oranges grown in Spain are among the best oranges in the world. Farmers raise sheep on the Meseta and in mountainous areas. They raise some cattle in grassy areas.

The land along the southeastern Mediterranean coast is the "gardenland" of Spain. Once arid, the Moors built extensive irrigation systems there. Today, almonds, oranges, lemons, figs, dates, melons, pomegranates, and sugarcane thrive. Spain's two most popular wines are also produced there. See 30-1.

Spanish Celebrations

Annual Spanish celebrations include some unique traditions. One interesting custom is part of the New Year's Eve celebration. People pop a grape into their mouths each time the clock strikes at midnight. Twelve grapes represent twelve months of good luck.

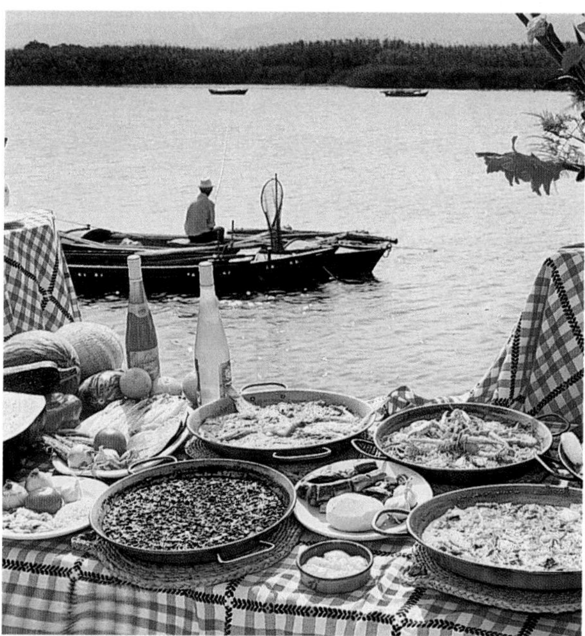

Tourist Office of Spain

30-1 *Spanish cooks combine fish from the Mediterranean Sea with locally grown fruits, vegetables, and grains to create Spain's unique cuisine.*

Q: Is olive oil more healthful than butter or margarine?

A: Using olive oil while staying within recommended daily limits for fats is a healthful choice. Olive oil is lower in saturated and *trans* fatty acids than butter and stick margarine. It is also higher in monounsaturated fatty acids, which have been linked to a lower risk of heart disease.

Bullfights are part of the festivities during the annual feast day observed for the patron saint of each town. Besides bullfighting, feast days are celebrated with parades, bonfires, and beauty contests.

A well-known Spanish festival is the *Fiesta of San Fermin,* which is held in Pamplona each July. As part of this celebration, a herd of bulls is set loose to run through the streets of the town. Young men run ahead of the bulls to a bull ring where they take part in amateur bullfights.

Spanish Cuisine

Spanish cuisine can best be described as ***del pueblo,*** or *food of the people*. It is simple for the most part. Its goodness relies on fresh ingredients and basic preparation methods.

History of Spanish Cuisine

Spanish cuisine began centuries ago with the Romans. The Romans contributed olive oil and garlic. Spanish cooks still use these two ingredients in many dishes.

The occupation by the Moors led to several culinary advances. The Moors brought citrus fruits, peaches, and figs. They introduced the cultivation of rice. They also grew a number of spices, including saffron, pepper, nutmeg, and anise. The Romans knew of the almond. However, it was the Moors who planted large almond groves and often used almonds in cooking.

The next phase of Spanish cooking resulted from the settlement of the New World. Spain's colonies provided tomatoes, chocolate, potatoes, and sweet and hot peppers.

Invasion by various enemy groups and Spain's rugged terrain further affected the development of food customs. These two factors helped divide the country into distinct culinary regions.

Characteristics of Spanish Cuisine

Today, each of Spain's regions still clings to its style of cooking. However, cooks throughout the country use similar ingredients and cooking methods.

Spaniards made many contributions to Mexican cuisine. However, Spanish cooking differs from the spicy cooking of Mexico. Throughout Spain, tomatoes, onions, and garlic form the base of many sauces. Garlic, pepper, and paprika flavor many main dishes, soups, and salads. Olive oil replaces butter in most recipes. Parsley serves as more than a garnish. In *salsa verde*, for example, large amounts of parsley add flavor as well as color. Spaniards eat raw almonds as appetizers. They use toasted almonds in sauces, cookies, cakes, pastries, and appetizers. See 30-2.

A traditional Spanish cooking method is to slowly simmer foods in earthenware pots. Cooks gently move the pots back and forth across the flame as they slowly stir the food inside. They often use the natural juices when cooking meat, fish, or poultry as the base for a sauce. They add other ingredients only to heighten the natural flavors of these juices.

Spanish cooks like to mix two or more food flavors in a single dish. They prepare mixtures of meat and fish; fish and vegetables; and meat, fish, and rice. One of the best examples of this method of mixing flavors is the *cocido.* Vegetables, beef, lamb, ham, poultry, and a spicy sausage cook together in a large pot. Spaniards first eat the thick soup in large bowls. Then they follow with the tender meats, poultry, and vegetables as a separate course.

Spanish Appetizers

Spanish meals often begin with ***tapas*** (appetizers). Friends at a sidewalk cafe may

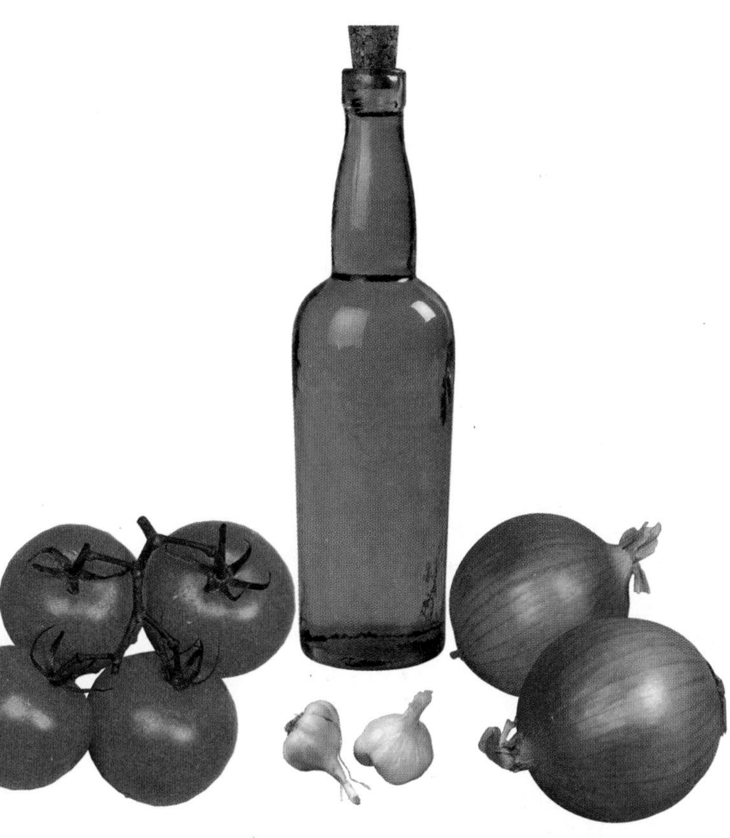

30-2 Tomatoes, olive oil, onions, and garlic are key ingredients in many Spanish recipes.

also enjoy sharing tapas. Tapas may be as simple as a few olives or toasted almonds. However, some are more fancy and require hours to prepare. Scallops, prawns, pickled herring, ham, marinated mushrooms, and anchovies are popular tapas that are simple to prepare. Fancier tapas include *buñuelitos,* which are small fritters. They are prepared by deep-frying small pieces of vegetables, meat, poultry, or fish that have been coated with a batter. *Empanadillas* are small pastries filled with chopped meat, fish, or poultry. They can be eaten hot or cold. *Banderillas* are colorful tapas served on long toothpicks. *Pinchos* are grilled foods.

Spanish Salads and Soups

A salad often follows the tapas. Sometimes it is little more than lettuce and tomato with a simple oil and vinegar dressing. Other times, it may be an attractive arrangement of raw vegetables on a plate.

Soups are popular throughout Spain. One of the heartiest soups is a fish soup called *sopa al cuarto de hora,* or 15-minute soup. It is made with mussels, prawns, whitefish, rice, peas, hard-cooked eggs, saffron, salt, pepper, and meat broth. All the ingredients cook together for 15 minutes—just long enough to blend the flavors.

People throughout Spain enjoy garlic soup. Cooks prepare one of the simplest versions by slowly sauteing two cloves of garlic in olive oil. Once the garlic browns, a few slices of bread, salt, pepper, and water are added. Then the soup cooks for just a few minutes. Other versions include a small amount of minced ham and tomatoes.

Another popular Spanish soup is ***gazpacho.*** This soup is often made with coarsely pureed tomatoes, onions, garlic, cucumbers, and green peppers; olive oil; and vinegar. It can be thick or thin, served icy cold or at room temperature. See 30-3.

Spanish Main Dishes

Most culinary experts agree that few cooks can prepare seafood as well as the Spaniards. Mussels, shrimp, and crab are popular shellfish in Spain. Tuna, hake, sole, squid, and cod are also caught off Spain's coasts. Cooks bake, fry, and poach fish and shellfish. In some parts of Spain, they serve seafood with *all-i-oli* (garlic mayonnaise).

Although methods for cooking meat are not as refined as those for seafood, Spain produces some excellent meat dishes. Veal, lamb, and pork are the most popular meats. The lean, dark Spanish pig is used in many ways. Raw ham, which is air cured high in the mountains, is a specialty. Filet of cured pork is sliced thinly and served as an appetizer. However, the best known pork product is ***chorizo,*** a dark sausage with a spicy, smoky flavor.

People throughout Spain eat poultry. Although Spaniards eat pigeon, pheasant, and partridge, chicken is by far the most popular type of poultry. Cooks stew and roast chicken. They also use it in the famous Spanish dish called paella. ***Paella*** is a Spanish rice dish that has many variations. All versions of paella, however, are colorful and delicious. The version most often seen in the United States contains chicken, shrimp, mussels, whitefish, peas, and rice. It is flavored with saffron, salt, pepper, and pimiento.

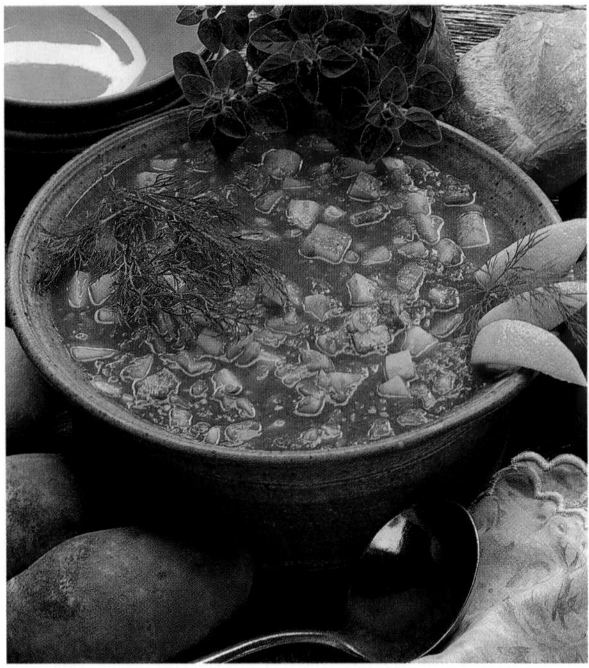

Idaho Potato Commission

***30-3** Classic Spanish ingredients, including olive oil, garlic, onions, and tomatoes, are used to make this delicious gazpacho.*

Spanish Accompaniments

The Spanish serve bread with soups, salads, and main dishes. A variety of breads are popular. *Pan de Santa Teresa* (fried cinnamon bread) is a sweet bread similar to French toast. *Picatostes* (fried sugar breads) are more like a pastry. They are served as an afternoon snack with coffee.

Tortillas (Spanish omelets) may be served as a separate course or as an accompaniment. Spanish cooks use a variety of fillings for tortillas. Potato, onion, white bean, and eggplant are the most popular. Sometimes cooks pile several tortillas with different fillings on top of one another. They serve them the way people serve pancakes in the United States.

Spaniards generally serve vegetables as a separate course. However, potatoes or grilled tomatoes may accompany a main dish. Vegetables served alone are often cooked in a tomato sauce or coated with a batter and deep-fried. Two or more vegetables are often combined and cooked in liquid. Many Spanish vegetable dishes contain artichokes, cauliflower, and eggplant. Spaniards also enjoy dried beans, lentils, and chickpeas, which they call *pulses.* Dried beans often appear in one-dish meals with meat, poultry, and fish.

Spanish Desserts

Simple desserts like fresh fruit, dried figs, cheese, or almonds often follow a meal. Spaniards usually save fancy cakes, cookies, pastries, and other rich desserts for guests. They may also serve these desserts as afternoon snacks. Rice pudding, sponge cake, and *flan* (caramel custard) are especially popular.

Spanish cakes and pastries contain very little baking powder or butter. However, they do contain many eggs and powdered almonds. They are flavored with cinnamon, anise, and orange and lemon peel. Spaniards fry rather than bake many cakes and pastries. This is because most Spanish homes did not have ovens until recent years.

Spanish Meals

Spanish meals are similar to Mexican meals with the same names. The people of Spain begin each day with *desayuno* (breakfast). They may just have coffee or a chocolate drink. Sometimes they have bread and jam or a sweet roll. *Churro,* a thin pastry fried in deep fat, is especially popular at breakfast. See 30-4.

People who have slept late or workers who find themselves hungry around 11 o'clock eat a second morning meal, *almuerzo.* It is more substantial than desayuno. This meal varies depending on locale and personal taste. It may include an omelet, grilled sausage, fried squid, open-faced sandwiches, fish, or lamb chops.

The *comida* is the main meal of the day. Spaniards eat this meal in the middle of the afternoon, around two or three o'clock. Most businesses close to escape the hottest part of the day, and workers come home to eat. A main course of fish, poultry, or meat usually follows salad or soup. Fruit or another light dessert ends the meal.

Spaniards serve *merienda* around six o'clock. It usually is a light snack of cakes and cookies or bread and jam. If a family has visitors, however, the meal may be more substantial.

Dusk is a pleasant time of day in Spain. The sidewalk cafés fill with people, and the odors of the tapas drift out to the streets. Around nine o'clock, the streets empty, and everyone goes

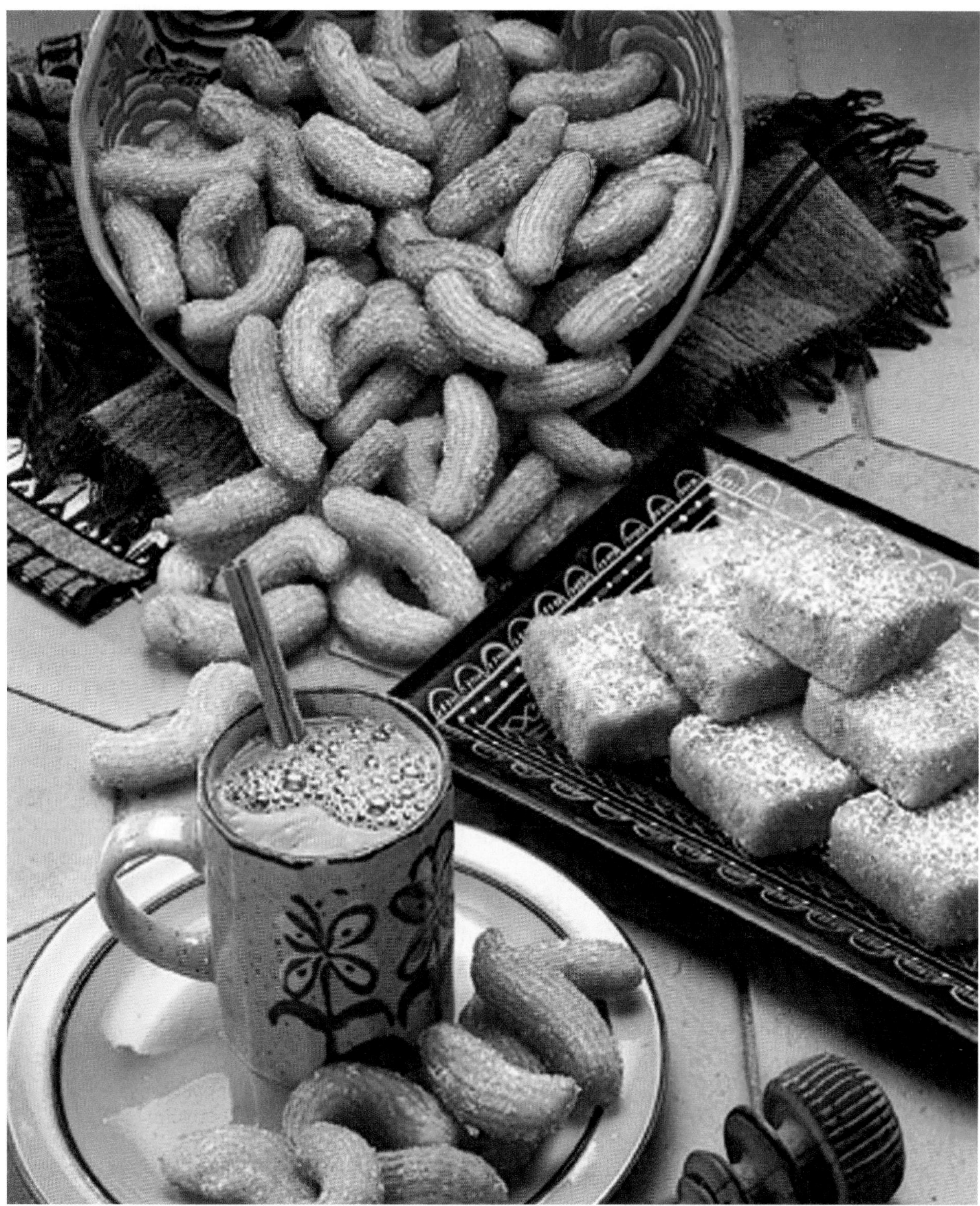

Mazola Corn Oil

30-4 Deep-fried churros are a popular Spanish breakfast food.

home for *cena* (supper). Cena is a light meal similar to almuerzo.

Wine is Spain's national drink, and both the rich and poor serve it with every meal. Two popular Spanish wines are Malaga and sherry. *Malaga* has a brown color and a sweet taste. *Sherry* has a characteristic nutlike flavor. Restaurants and taverns throughout Spain serve ***sangria,*** a wine-based punch. There are many versions of the punch, but they all include red wine, fruit juice, and sparkling water.

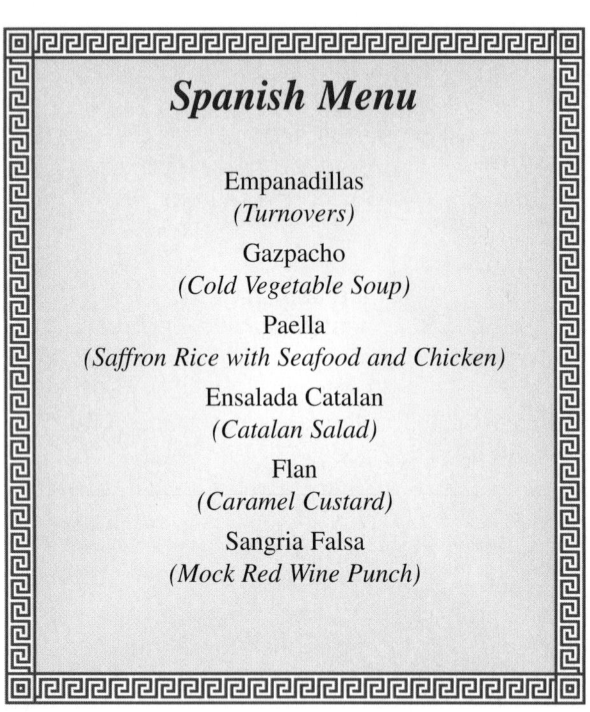

Spanish Menu

Empanadillas
(Turnovers)
Gazpacho
(Cold Vegetable Soup)
Paella
(Saffron Rice with Seafood and Chicken)
Ensalada Catalan
(Catalan Salad)
Flan
(Caramel Custard)
Sangria Falsa
(Mock Red Wine Punch)

Empanadillas

(Turnovers)
Makes 40

Pastry:
3 cups all-purpose flour
1 teaspoon salt
1/2 cup olive oil
1/2 cup cold water
Filling:
2 tablespoons olive oil
2 small onions, chopped
2 small tomatoes, peeled and chopped
1 clove garlic, minced
2 hard-cooked eggs
3/4 cup diced, cooked chicken
1 egg, beaten (optional)

1. Mix flour and salt together in a large mixing bowl.
2. Add 1/2 cup oil and water.
3. With fingers, mix dough until it forms a ball. Let dough rest while preparing the filling.
4. Heat 2 tablespoons oil in large skillet until very hot (but not smoking).
5. Add onions and saute until golden.
6. Add tomatoes and garlic and continue cooking vegetables until the liquid has evaporated.
7. In small bowl, mash hard-cooked eggs.
8. Add mashed eggs and chicken to skillet. Cook mixture 2 to 3 minutes, stirring occasionally; remove from heat. Taste filling and add salt and pepper, if needed.
9. Preheat oven to 425°F.
10. On a lightly floured board, roll pastry to a thickness of 1/8 inch. Cut circles from pastry with a 3-inch biscuit cutter.
11. Place a rounded tablespoon of filling on one half of each circle. Fold the other half of the dough over the filling and press edges together with a fork to seal.
12. Place turnovers on lightly greased baking sheet and brush surface with beaten egg, if desired.
13. Bake turnovers until brown and crisp, about 25 minutes.

Per turnover: 77 cal. (47% from fat), 2 g protein, 8 g carbohydrate, 4 g fat, 16 mg cholesterol, 0 g fiber, 60 mg sodium.

Gazpacho

(Cold Vegetable Soup)
Serves 8

1 quart low-sodium chicken broth
4 medium tomatoes, chopped
2 cucumbers, peeled and chopped
1 large onion, sliced
1/2 green pepper, chopped
2 cups bread cubes
2 tablespoons wine vinegar
1 clove garlic, minced
1 teaspoon sugar
dash cayenne
Garnish:
1 1/4 cups bread cubes (1/4 inch)
1/3 cup chopped onion
1/2 cup chopped green peppers
1/2 cup peeled and chopped tomato

1. In a large bowl, combine chicken broth, tomatoes, cucumbers, onion, green pepper, bread cubes, vinegar, garlic, sugar, and cayenne.
2. Puree mixture in a blender, 2 cups at a time.
3. Chill thoroughly.
4. Just before serving, stir soup lightly. Pour into a tureen or individual soup bowls. Pass garnishes separately.

Per serving: 85 cal. (11% from fat), 4 g protein, 16 g carbohydrate, 1 g fat, 0 mg cholesterol, 3 g fiber, 169 mg sodium.

Paella

(Saffron Rice with Seafood and Chicken)
Serves 10

12 medium-sized canned shrimp
7 small hard-shelled clams
1/2 pound garlic-seasoned smoked pork sausage
1 2-pound chicken, cut into serving-sized pieces, skin removed
3/4 teaspoon garlic salt
dash pepper
1/2 cup olive oil
1/4 pound lean boneless pork, cut into 1/2-inch cubes
1/2 cup chopped onions
1 large green pepper, cleaned and cut
1 large tomato, peeled and finely chopped
2 cloves garlic, crushed
3 cups uncooked long grain rice
1/4 teaspoon ground saffron
6 cups water
3/4 cup frozen peas, thoroughly defrosted

1. Drain and rinse shrimp; place in small bowl and set aside.
2. Scrub clams with stiff brush under cold running water. Place clams on plate and set aside.
3. Prick sausage in several places with a fork. Place in a large, heavy skillet and cover with cold water.
4. Bring water to a boil, then reduce heat to low. Simmer sausage uncovered for 5 minutes.
5. Drain sausage well and slice into rounds about 1/4 inch thick; set aside.
6. Rinse chicken and pat dry with paper towels. Season with garlic salt and pepper.
7. Heat 1/4 cup olive oil in large skillet until very hot but not smoking.
8. Add chicken pieces, a few at a time, and fry until golden brown.
9. Remove browned pieces to a plate lined with paper towels and continue cooking the rest of the chicken.
10. Add sausage slices to skillet and quickly brown; transfer to a plate lined with paper towels and drain.
11. Remove oil from skillet and wipe skillet with paper towels.
12. Add 1/4 cup fresh olive oil and heat until hot but not smoking.
13. Add pork cubes and brown quickly.
14. Add onions, green peppers, tomatoes, and garlic. Cook vegetables and meat, stirring constantly, until most of the liquid has evaporated. (This is called a sofrito.) Set aside.
15. Preheat oven to 400°F.
16. In an ovenproof skillet or casserole, which is at least 14 inches wide and 2 inches deep, add the sofrito, rice, and saffron.
17. Bring the 6 cups of water to a boil and pour into skillet.
18. Bring mixture to a boil, stirring constantly.
19. Remove from heat immediately and taste for seasonings.
20. Arrange shrimp, clams, sausage, and chicken over the top of the rice. Sprinkle peas over meats and seafood.
21. Place pan or skillet on bottom rack in oven and bake for 25 to 30 minutes or until the liquid has been absorbed. (Do not stir the paella.)
22. When paella is cooked, remove it from oven and place a clean kitchen towel over the top. Let the paella rest about 5 minutes. Serve immediately.

Note: All of the ingredients can be prepared a short time ahead. The oven should be preheated one-half hour before paella is to be served.

Per serving: 418 cal. (22% from fat), 30 g protein, 49 g carbohydrate, 10 g fat, 94 mg cholesterol, 3 g fiber, 539 mg sodium.

Ensalada Catalana

(Catalan Salad)
Serves 6

1/2 head romaine lettuce
3 medium tomatoes
1 large sweet onion
1 green pepper
1 red pepper
1/4 cup green olives
1/4 cup pitted black olives
olive oil
wine vinegar

1. Clean romaine under cool running water. Separate and dry leaves. Break into bite-sized pieces.
2. Wash tomatoes, slice into wedges.
3. Peel onion; cut into rings.
4. Wash and clean green and red peppers; cut into thin rings.
5. Set six chilled salad plates on a tray. Make a bed of romaine on each plate.

6. Attractively arrange the rest of the ingredients on the top of the lettuce.
7. Serve salads with olive oil and wine vinegar.

Per serving: 107 cal. (71% from fat), 2 g protein, 7 g carbohydrate, 9 g fat, 0 mg cholesterol, 3 g fiber, 145 mg sodium.

Sangria Falsa

(Mock Red Wine Punch)
Serves 8

1 lemon, cut into slices
1 orange, cut into slices
1 lime, cut into slices
2 bottles red grape juice, well chilled
1 bottle club soda, well chilled
ice cubes

1. In large pitcher, combine fruits and grape juice. Refrigerate until ready to serve.
2. Just before serving, add club soda. Serve sangria immediately over ice.

Per serving: 136 cal. (1% from fat), 0 g protein, 35 g carbohydrate, 0 g fat, 0 mg cholesterol, 1 g fiber, 31 mg sodium.

Flan

(Caramel Custard)
Serves 8

1/2 cup sugar
2 tablespoons water
2 cups fat free milk
2 cups evaporated fat free milk
6 eggs
pinch salt
3/4 cup sugar
1 1/2 teaspoons vanilla

1. To caramelize mold: In small, heavy saucepan combine ½ cup sugar and water. Cook over moderate heat, stirring constantly, until the sugar melts and turns a golden brown.
2. Quickly pour syrup into a 6-cup mold (or 8 custard cups), which has been warmed by placing it in hot water. Turn mold or custard cups in all directions so syrup coats both bottom and sides. Set aside.
3. In a large saucepan, combine milk and evaporated milk and heat to just below boiling.
4. Remove from heat and cool slightly.
5. Preheat oven to 350°F.
6. In a mixer bowl, beat eggs and salt slightly.
7. Add 3/4 cup sugar gradually as you continue beating.
8. Add combined milks slowly, beating constantly, then add vanilla.
9. Pour custard into the mold. Place mold in a larger pan; fill the pan with very hot water to about 1/2 inch from the top of the mold.
10. Bake about 1 hour (25 to 30 minutes for custard cups), until a knife inserted near the center comes out clean.
11. Cool custard 10 minutes, then refrigerate until well chilled.
12. To unmold, run a knife between the custard and mold. Place a serving dish on top of mold and invert. Custard should slide out.

Per serving: 254 cal. (14% from fat), 12 g protein, 42 g carbohydrate, 4 g fat, 164 mg cholesterol, 0 g fiber, 193 mg sodium.

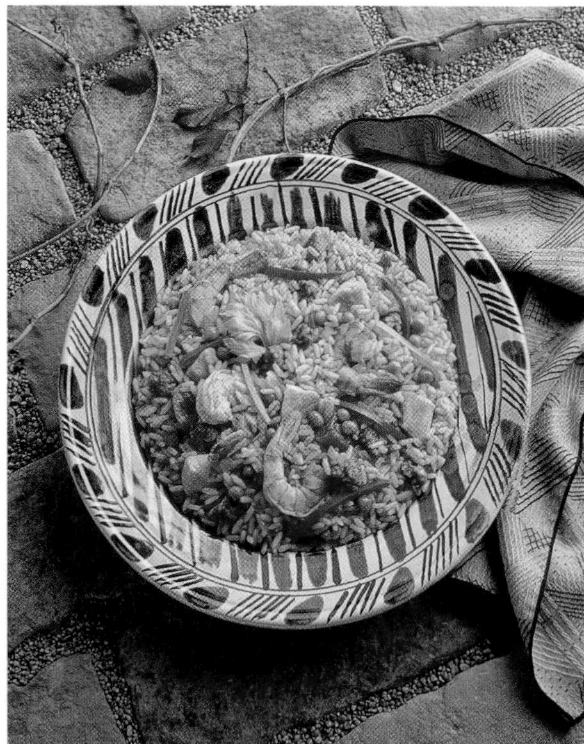

USA Rice Federation

Paella is a colorful Spanish rice dish made with chicken and a variety of shellfish.

Italy

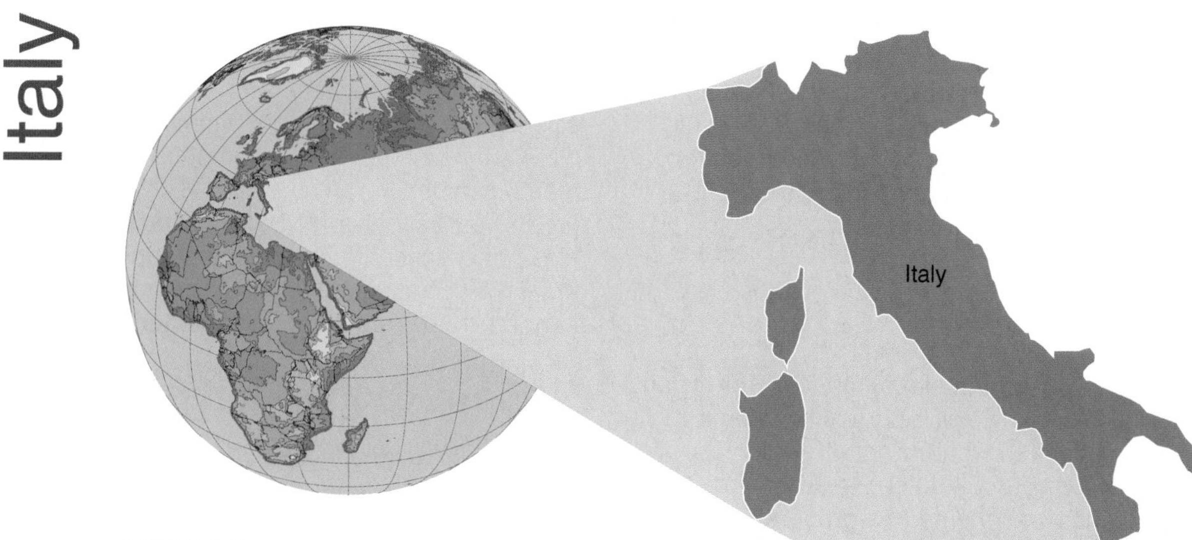

Italy's warm, sunny climate and awesome scenery make it a popular vacation spot. Italy's remarkable art, architecture, and history appeal to culture lovers. Of course, everyone enjoys Italy's delicious food.

Geography and Climate of Italy

Italy is a rather small country. Many islands and a boot-shaped peninsula that juts into the Mediterranean Sea make up Italy. Italy's expansive coastline makes seafood important in Italian cuisine.

Much of Italy is mountainous. The rugged Italian Alps form a semicircular barrier in the North, shutting out neighboring countries. The Apennines run in a bow shape, dividing the peninsula in half. Between the Alps and the Apennines lies the Po Valley, which is a rich agricultural area. Narrow coastal plains that border both sides of the peninsula are also suitable for agriculture. Farming takes place in small valleys formed by the mountains, too.

Italy has three distinct geographic regions. Northern Italy has great beauty and rich land. The fertile Po River basin makes the Po Valley the most productive farming area in the country. Central Italy is mountainous and hilly. Grain, grapes, and olives grow on the terraced hillsides. Southern Italy is poor in terms of natural resources. However, olives, tomatoes, and mozzarella cheese are important agricultural products of this region.

Italy's climate is as variable as its geography. Much of Italy has a Mediterranean

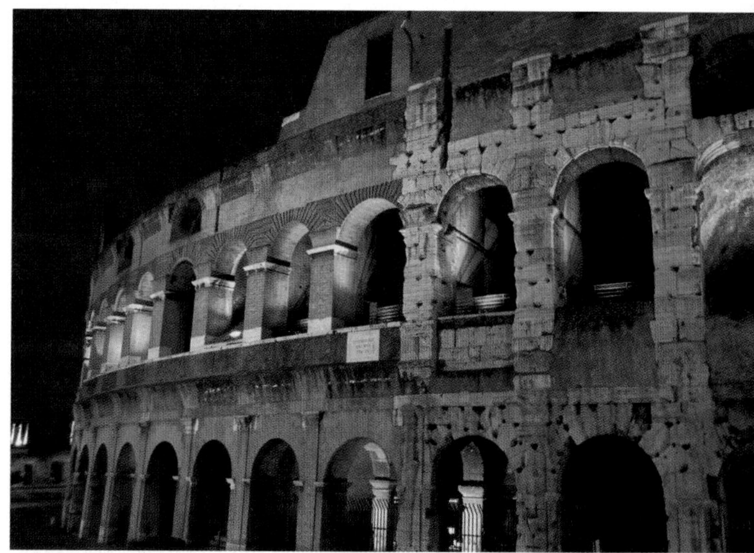

The Colosseum in Rome is one of the world's most famous landmarks.

climate. Summers are sunny and dry with most of the rainfall occurring in the winter. In the North, however, temperatures are cooler, and rain can come during any season. As a result, Italy has a range of vegetation. Pine trees grow in the North. Citrus fruits grow in the South.

Italian Culture

Italy has been the site of many major historical and cultural events. At one time, Rome ruled the Western world. Centuries later, Italy led the rest of Europe in the Renaissance. The Renaissance was a time of a great rebirth in art and learning.

Influences on Italian Culture

A number of factors have influenced Italian culture. The early inhabitants, the rise and fall of the Roman Empire, and the Catholic Church all have had an impact.

The Roman Empire

Around 1000 B.C. the Etruscans developed a refined society in Northern and Central Italy. About the same time, the Greeks colonized Southern Italy and the island of Sicily.

At the height of Etruscan and Greek power, the Latins were farmers on the hills bordering the Tiber River. Gradually, the Latins gained power. They made Rome their capital. Rome prospered and in time became the head of the mighty Roman Empire. During the Roman Empire's Golden Age, Rome ruled Europe, northern Africa, and western Asia. Roman culture spread throughout the Empire.

The fall of the Western Roman Empire (the part located in Europe) began in A.D. 330. This was when Emperor Constantine moved his capital from Rome to Constantinople. Before long, waves of barbarians came from the North. They first invaded Northern Italy and later destroyed the city of Rome.

The Renaissance

As civil rule declined in the Roman Empire, the Roman Catholic Church slowly gained power. The Church met the people's need for leadership. The structure of the Church became more governmental. Then in the fifth century, the Bishop of Rome became the Pope.

With the support of the papacy and wealthy Italian families, the *Renaissance* began in Italy in the fourteenth century. Arts, literature, and science flourished. The movement spread all through Europe. It lasted into the seventeenth century.

As the Renaissance began to fade, struggles between local rulers and the papacy tore at the Italian city-states. Italy finally became independent in the late nineteenth century.

Modern Culture in Italy

Italy has been involved in wars of modern times. However, its republican form of government is at peace today. Italy is aligned with nations of the Western world. Agricultural and industrial growth are under way.

Italian Agriculture

Agriculture is vital to Italy's economy. About half of the nation's land is used for farming. In many areas, farmers cannot use machines to do farm work. Therefore, they must do it by hand.

The richest and most productive farmland is located in Northern Italy in the Po River Valley. Leading crops are wheat, corn, rice, sugar beets, and flax. The many dairy herds make this region the largest cheese-producing region in the country. Olive trees thrive in Southern Italy. Farmers grow vegetables and fruits for local use and for export to other European countries.

Vineyards are scattered throughout the country. They supply grapes for Italy's large wine industry, 30-5. Italian wine makers produce a variety of red, white, and sparkling wines for domestic use and export.

Italian Holidays

Almost all Italians are Roman Catholics. Many Italian holidays celebrate events in the church. *Pasqua*, or Easter, is one important holiday. A number of foods are used to celebrate this holy day that ushers in spring. Cakes and breads made with fruits and nuts are baked in shapes such as doves. People serve lamb as a symbol of spring. Eggs symbolize life, and wheat symbolizes the resurrection of Christ.

Italians hold harvest festivals in the late summer and early fall. These events celebrate the gathering of important foods. At an olive festival, farmers and workers who have brought in the olive crop sit at a long outdoor table.

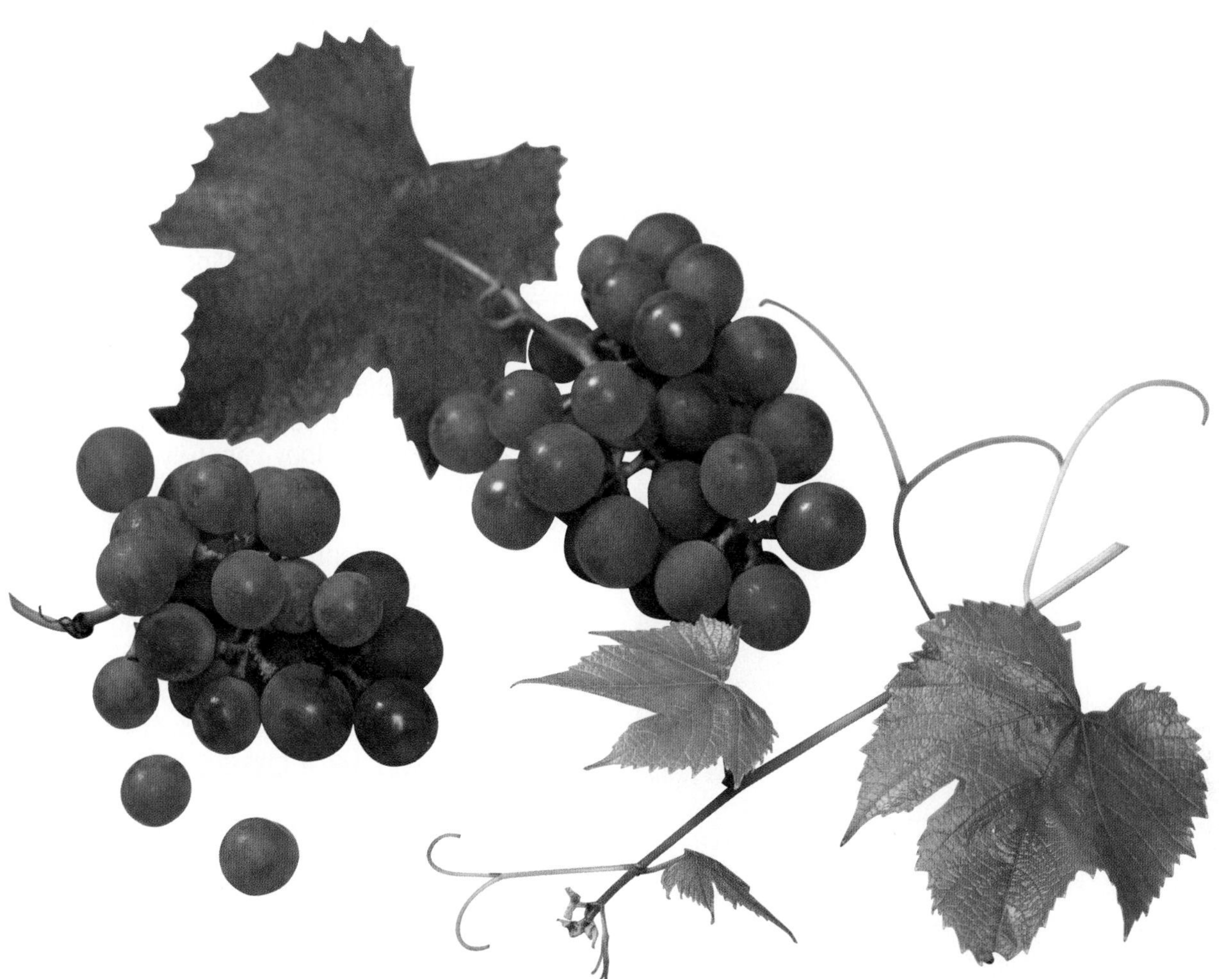

30-5 As the key ingredient in Italian wines, grapes are an important agricultural product in Italy.

They feast on a meal of pasta, olives, and wine. At fishing festivals held in coastal towns, people enjoy eating seafood barbecued along the shore.

On November 2, Italians celebrate *Festa Dei Morti,* or All Souls' Day. On this day, they pay respect to dead relatives by visiting cemeteries to place flowers and candles on the graves. People may also leave buns, fruit-shaped candies, and lentils in their kitchens at night. They believe the souls of their relatives will enter the home through an open window and enjoy the food.

Christmas is a special time of celebration in Italy. Some people travel to Rome to hear the Pope deliver a Christmas sermon. Many families decorate trees and display nativity scenes depicting the birth of Christ. Children receive gifts from *Babbo Natale,* or Father Christmas. Italians refrain from eating meat on Christmas Eve, but they enjoy a meal of roast meat on Christmas Day. See 30-6.

Italian Cuisine

During the Renaissance, Italian cooking became the "mother cuisine." It is the source of many Western cuisines.

History of Italian Cuisine

The beginning of Italian cuisine belongs to the Greeks. Ancient Rome was known for its elaborate feasts. Romans paid high prices for Greek chefs because good food was a status symbol.

Cooking declined somewhat after the fall of the Roman Empire. Cooking and food experienced a rebirth during the Renaissance. Many

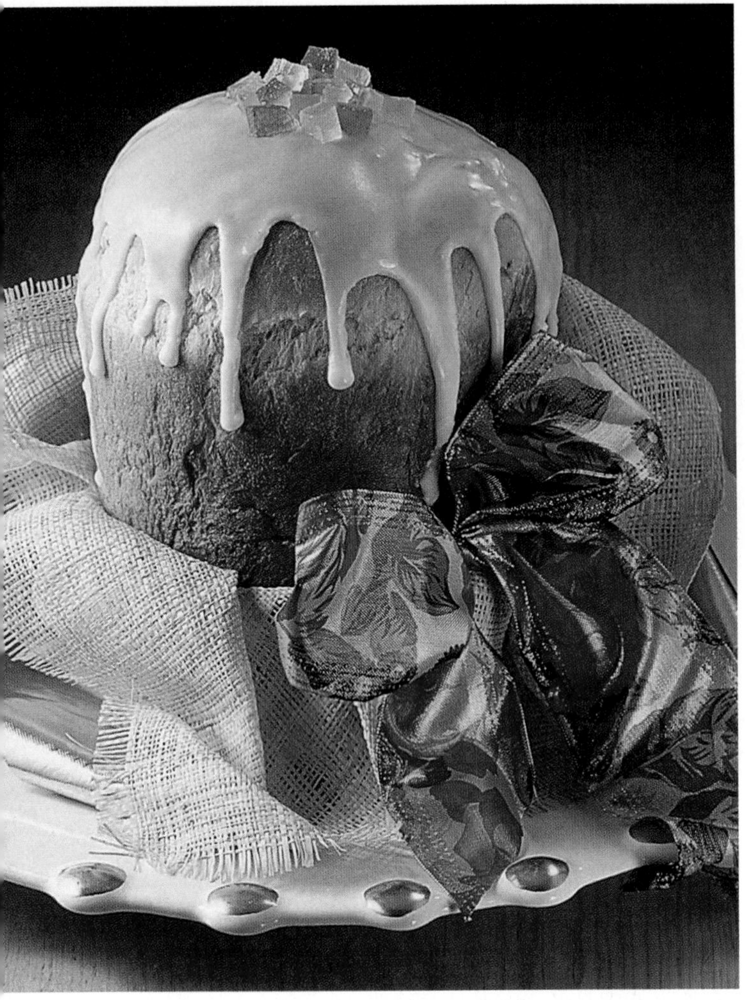

photo courtesy of Fleischmann's Yeast

***30-6** Panettone is a glazed, fruited bread that is often served at Italian Christmas celebrations.*

people say the French have the greatest Western cuisine. However, even the French grudgingly give Italy credit for laying the foundation for haute cuisine. Catherine de Medici, an Italian, brought her cooks to France when she married the future French king, Henri II. These cooks taught new cooking skills to the French. They also introduced new foods like peas, haricot beans, artichokes, and ice cream.

Characteristics of Italian Cuisine

Italian food, as a whole, is lively, interesting, colorful, and varied, yet it is basically simple. The Italians believe in keeping the natural flavors of food, and they insist on fresh, high-quality ingredients. Many Italian cooks shop daily so foods will be as fresh as possible. They do not indulge in convenience foods. If a particular food is too costly or out of season, an Italian cook substitutes whatever is available.

Italian cooks use many kinds of herbs, spices, and other seasonings. They stock their kitchens with parsley, marjoram, sweet basil, thyme, sage, rosemary, tarragon, bay leaves, oregano, and mint. Other commonly used flavorings include cloves, saffron, coriander, celery, onions, shallots, garlic, vinegar, olives, and lemon juice.

Fresh fruits and vegetables are as important to the Italian kitchen as herbs and spices. Those who live in the country grow many of the fruits and vegetables they use. City dwellers make trips to the local market each day. There, they select the ripest and freshest tomatoes, artichokes, peas, beans, and other produce.

Italian cooks prepare many dishes on top of the range, either by simmering or frying. Because fuel is relatively expensive, they use the oven as little as possible.

Italian Staple Foods

People throughout Italy eat pasta. Pasta refers to any paste made from wheat flour that is dried in various shapes, 30-7. Pasta may be made from just flour and water. However, pasta may have added ingredients like eggs. It may be made at home, or it may be made commercially.

Italians serve pasta in many ways, but they always serve it cooked ***al dente*** (slightly resistant to the bite). They may serve it with butter, a sprinkling of cheese, or a variety of sauces. They may add it to soups or stews or stuff it with meat, poultry, vegetables, or cheese.

After pasta, Italy's most important staple food is seafood. Every locale with a coastline has developed unique methods of preparing and serving fish. Sole, sea bass, anchovies, sardines, mackerel, tuna, eel, squid, and octopus are some of the varieties of fish caught. Equally popular are the shellfish, including oysters, clams, mussels, spiny lobsters, shrimp, and crayfish.

Rice is both an important agricultural product and a staple food. Italians cook the rice so the grains remain separate with a slight firmness.

Pork, lamb, veal, and beef are produced and eaten in Italy. Sausage, wild game, and poultry are equally popular. Meat is relatively expensive, so many Italian dishes rely on meat extenders. The sauces for many pasta dishes contain little meat. If large cuts of meat are served, they usually are roasted.

Italian Dairy Products

Among the best-known Italian cheeses sold in the United States are Parmesan, mozzarella, Romano, ricotta, provolone, and Gorgonzola. Some varieties of cheese, such as Parmesan, are named after their place of origin.

The Italians introduced ice cream to the rest of Europe. There are two basic varieties. *Granita* is a light sherbet made with powdery ice and coffee or fruit-flavored syrup. *Gelati* is made with milk. It resembles the vanilla and chocolate ice creams familiar to people in the United States.

Italian Beverages

Caffe espresso is a rich, dark, flavorful coffee served throughout Italy. It is made in a special type of coffeemaker called a *caffettiera*. Darkly roasted, finely ground coffee beans must be used. (This type of coffee is often called *French roast* in stores in the United States.)

Even more important to the Italians than caffe espresso is *vino* (wine). Even children drink it. Mild burgundy or Chianti usually replaces water at Italian meals.

Regional Italian Specialties

Thanks to modern transportation, people throughout Italy can now buy foods that were once strictly regional. Pizza, for example, originated in Naples, 30-8. Today it is eaten all over Italy and much of the rest of the world as well. Despite this, Italian cooking is regional cooking. Most culinary experts agree the best regional foods are still found within their home regions.

Geography and climate create a culinary division between the North and South. Northern

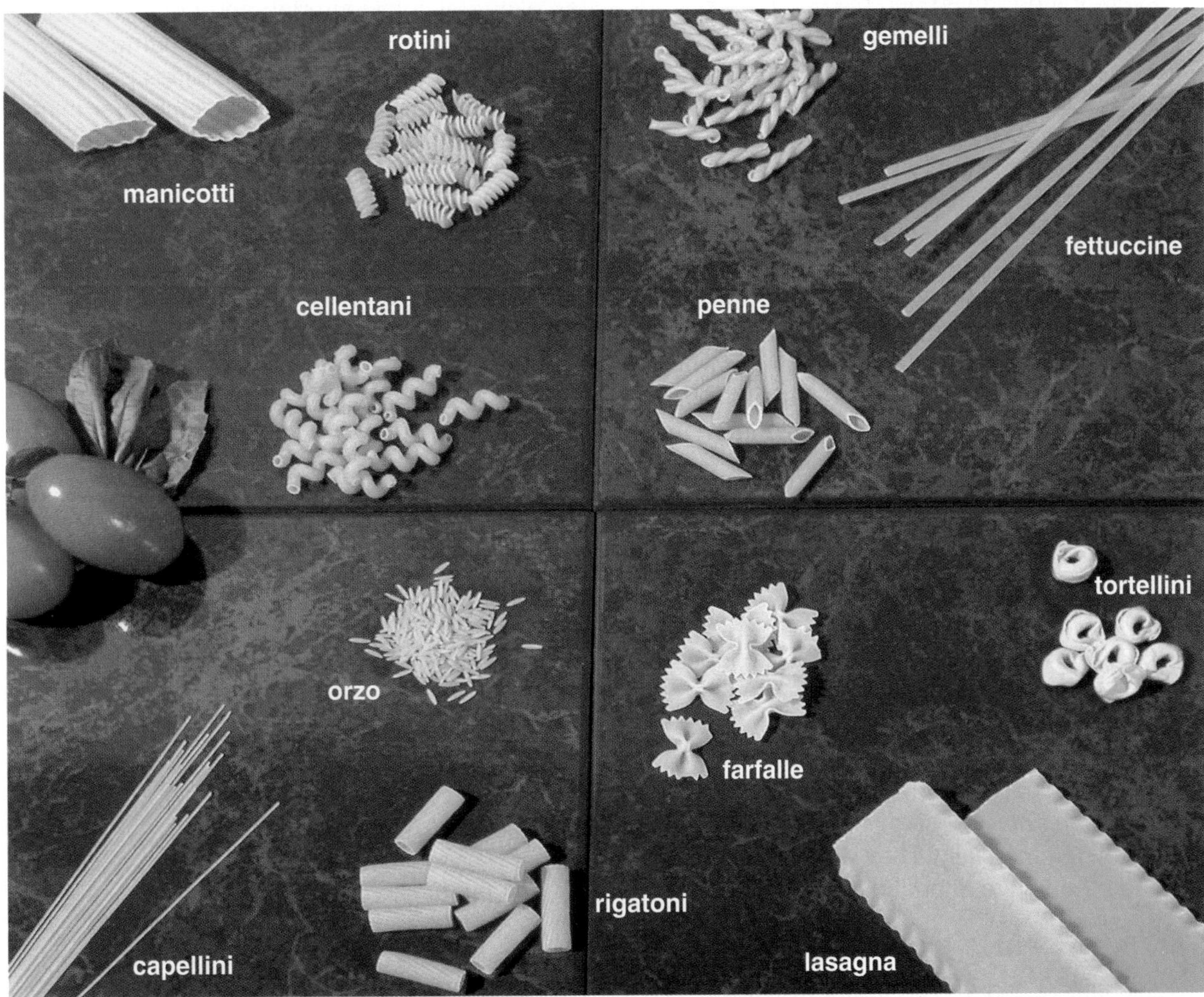

Jack Klasey

30-7 Varied pasta shapes form the base for countless Italian entrees.

Q: Should I choose egg-free pasta instead of egg noodles?

A: The addition of egg does make egg noodles a bit higher in fat and cholesterol than other pasta products. However, the amounts can fit easily into a healthful diet. Therefore, unless you are on a low-cholesterol diet, feel free to choose either type of pasta.

Italy has more resources than Southern Italy. Meat is easier to obtain and less expensive. Dairy products are more common. Foods are not as heavily spiced as they are in the South. Cooks use delicate sauces instead of heavier tomato sauces.

Most of the farming and grazing land in Southern Italy is of poor quality. This region is rather sparsely populated and many of the people are poor. Meat is expensive and eaten in small amounts. Dairy products, except for cheese, are rare. Most foods are hearty, filling, and economical. Southern Italian cooking is the cooking with which most people in the United States are familiar. This is because most Italian restaurants in the United States are Neapolitan, and Naples is the heart of Southern Italian cooking.

Cooking fats and pasta varieties also differ between the North and the South. Northern Italy is too cold to raise olive trees but has excellent grazing land for dairy cattle. Southern Italy is warm enough for olive trees but has poor grazing land. Therefore, butter is the favored cooking fat in the North. In the South, cooks prefer olive oil.

Northern Italy is the home of the fat, ribbon-shaped groups of pastas called *pasta bolognese.* These pastas usually are made at home and contain egg. Southern Italy is the home of the tubular-shaped groups of pastas called *pasta naploetania.* These pastas are usually produced commercially. They do not contain egg, and they have a longer shelf life.

Specialties of Northern Italy

The specialties of Northern Italy include the simple *minestras* (soups) of the Friuli-Venezia region. The elegant stuffed pastas and rich meat sauces of the city of Bologna are also part of this fare.

The North is known for its sausages and other pork products. Bologna's *mortadella* is one of the best-known Italian sausages in the United States. It is made with beef and pork and seasoned with pepper and garlic. Delicately-flavored *Parma ham* is a popular appetizer.

In the North, people often serve risottos, gnocchi, and polenta instead of pasta. ***Risottos*** are rice dishes made with butter, chopped onion, stock or wine, and Parmesan cheese. They may have meats and vegetables added, 30-9. Because many of the northern regions lie along the sea, risottos in this area often contain seafood. *Gnocchi* are dumplings. They may be made of potatoes or wheat flour. *Polenta* is a porridge made of cornmeal. It sometimes is combined with butter and cheese and served as a filling side dish.

In several of the northeastern regions, Austrian influences are evident. Foods such as *apfelstrudel* (apple strudel) and *crauti* (sauerkraut) have retained their original names.

Other Northern Italian specialties popular in the United States are chicken cacciatore, minestrone soup, and osso buco. *Pollo alla cacciatore* (chicken hunter-style) is prepared by simmering pieces of chicken with tomatoes and mushrooms. ***Minestrone*** is a satisfying soup made with onions, carrots, zucchini, celery, cabbage, rice (or pasta), and seasonings. It is served with Parmesan cheese. *Osso buco* is the portion of a calf's leg between the knee and hock. It is served with the marrow that fills the

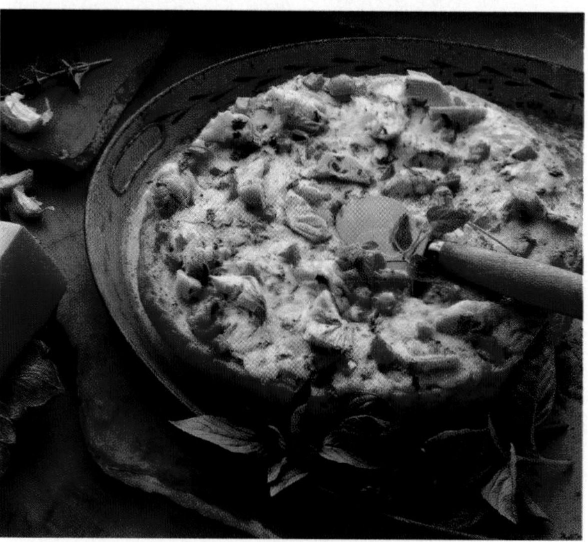

30-8 *Pizza has its roots in Naples, Italy.*

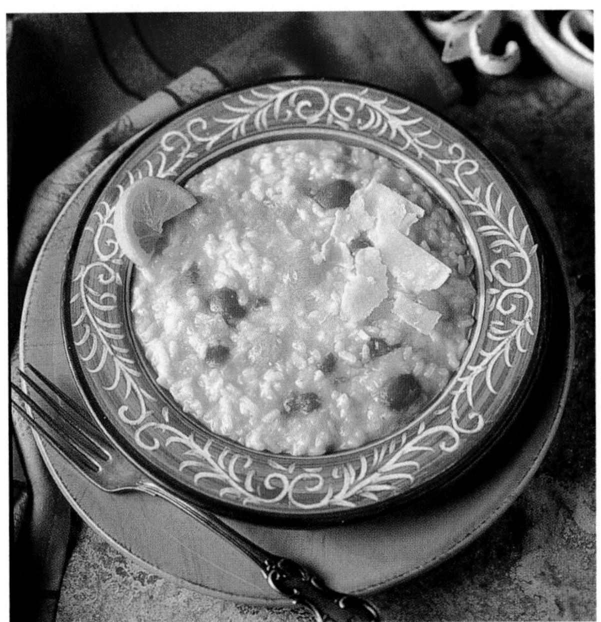

USA Rice Federation

***30-9** Tomatoes, shallots, and lemon zest flavor this tasty risotto.*

center of the bone. The flavorful marrow is eaten with rice.

Famous Northern Italian sweets include zabaglione and panettone. *Zabaglione* is fluffy egg custard flavored with Marsala wine. *Panettone* is a sweet cake filled with fruit and nuts. It is often served for breakfast.

Specialties of Central Italy

Several of Central Italy's specialties have Roman origins. Roman cooks serve spaghetti in at least 25 ways. Of these, people in the United States may be most familiar with the spaghetti dish called *spaghetti alla carbonara.* The sauce for this dish contains eggs, pork, pepper, and cheese.

Of all meats, Romans enjoy lamb the most. Cooks rub young lambs with garlic, rosemary, pepper, and salt. Then they cover the lambs with rosemary and roast them until tender.

The Romans must be given credit for inventing cheesecake. The early Romans made their *crostata di ricotta* (cheese pie) without any sweetening. It contained flour, cheese, and eggs. Today's cooks sweeten crostata di ricotta with sugar and flavor it with candied fruits, almonds, and vanilla.

In the rich countryside of Tuscany, home-grown vegetables, beans, and charcoal-grilled meats are specialties. Tuscan cooks add beans to minestras. They also cook beans with garlic and tomatoes or flavor them with sage and cheese. They prepare beans *nel fiasco* by cooking them with garlic, water, and olive oil in an empty wine flask. Tuscan cooks grill large beefsteaks on gridirons. The steaks are sprinkled with coarse salt and pepper to make *bistecca alla fiorentina.*

Cenci and panforte are sweets with Central Italian origins. *Cenci* are deep-fried pastry strips shaped like bows. *Panforte* is a honey cake flavored with cinnamon and cloves.

Specialties of Southern Italy

Southern Italian cooks serve pasta with rich tomato sauces, 30-10. They may flavor the sauces with meat, seafood, or vegetables. Spaghetti and lasagne are the southern pastas with which people in the United States are most familiar. However, Southern Italian cooks do not limit themselves to just these varieties. Fusilli (pulled out spirals), orecchietta (little ears), and ricci di donna (ladies' curls) are equally popular. Large tubular pastas like cannelloni and rigatoni are used as well.

With pasta, the Southern Italians love rich tomato sauces. The traditional Neapolitan tomato sauce is simple. Cooks combine fresh tomatoes with fried onions, larded filet of beef, and a sprig of basil. The mixture simmers in an

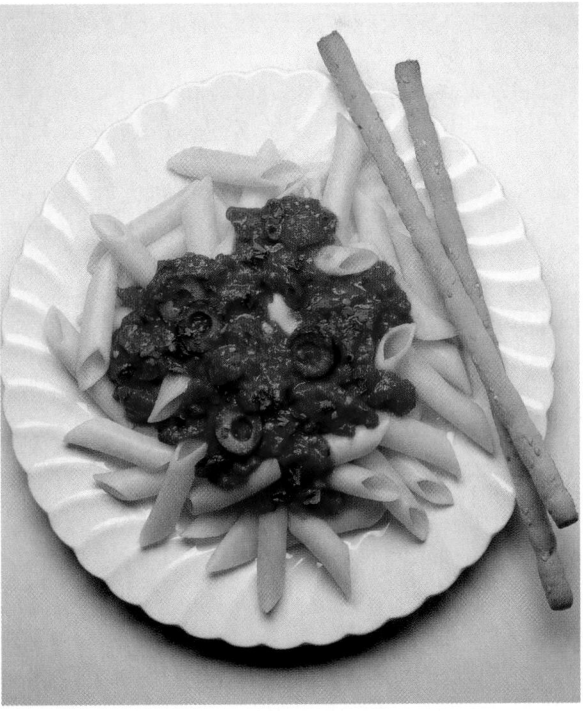

photography compliments of Ronzoni pasta

***30-10** Tubular pastas topped with rich tomato sauces are typical of Southern Italy.*

earthenware pot for several hours to bring out all the flavors.

One popular Neapolitan dish is *stuffed lasagne*. Long, wide noodles are layered with cheeses and meats. Cheeses include ricotta, mozzarella, and grated Parmesan. The filling may contain pieces of sausage, minced pork, strips of ham, and hard-cooked egg slices. A thick tomato sauce is poured over the mixture and the lasagne is baked until bubbly.

Tomatoes and mozzarella cheese are two of Southern Italy's major agricultural products. They are also key ingredients in the popular Neapolitan dish called *pizza*. The Italians make many kinds of pizza. All pizzas contain tomato sauce, cheese, and a crust made from yeast dough. Sausage, anchovies, mushrooms, green peppers, olives, and other ingredients are optional.

Good Manners Are Good Business

It would be ungracious for you to refuse an invitation to dine in the home of an Italian business associate. When you go, you might take flowers as a gift for your host. Avoid taking chrysanthemums, however, as Italians consider them to be funeral flowers. You are probably safest with a mixed bouquet, which should contain an odd number of flowers.

Other Southern Italian specialties feature vegetables. *Soffritti* is lightly fried onions and other vegetables mixed with a small amount of meat. *Eggplant Napoli* is eggplant layered with tomato sauce and cheese. *Zucchini Parmesan* is sliced zucchini and cubed tomatoes tossed with Parmesan cheese.

USA Dry Pea & Lentil Council

30-11 *Parmesan cheese and Italian sausage flavor this hearty Italian soup.*

Italian Meals

Like many Europeans, Italians typically eat a light breakfast and a hearty noon meal. The noon meal is the largest meal of the day and people usually eat it at home.

The well-known ***antipasto*** is an appetizer course that often begins the meal. Foods in an antipasto may include salami, Parma ham, anchovies, and hard-cooked eggs. Celery, radishes, pickled beets, black olives, marinated red peppers, and stuffed tomatoes are popular antipasto foods, too. Regardless of the selection of foods, the tray must have both color and taste appeal.

Minestra (soup) may follow or replace the antipasto at the start of a meal. Each region has its favorite soups. One common soup is *pasta in brodo,* which is a simple broth with pasta. See 30-11.

A main course of a meat, poultry, or fish dish usually follows the soup. Italians often roast their meat, and lamb is particularly popular when roasted. Poultry often is served in a sauce, whereas fish is baked or broiled. (If meat is too costly, a large serving of pasta may replace the main dish. Pasta is usually served with a sauce containing small pieces of meat or fish.) A vegetable or salad usually accompanies the main dish. Salads always contain tomatoes and other vegetables.

Fruit and cheese end a typical meal. Italians reserve fancier desserts for special occasions.

The evening meal usually is light. Soup, omelets, and risottos are popular supper dishes. Bread, wine, and a simple fruit dessert complete the meal.

Italian Menu

Antipasto
(Appetizers)

Minestrone
(Vegetable Soup)

Pollo alla Cacciatore
(Chicken Hunter-Style)

Fettuccine Verde
(Green Noodles)

Panne
(Italian Bread)

Spumoni with Cenci
(Three-Flavored Ice Cream with Deep-Fried Sweet Pastry)

Caffe Espresso
(Rich Coffee)

Antipasto

(Appetizers)

Many different foods can appear in an antipasto. Regardless of the number of types of foods chosen, however, all antipasto ingredients should be attractively arranged on the serving platter. The following foods frequently are part of an antipasto.

Anchovy fillets
Artichoke hearts
Black olives
Celery hearts
Finocchio (Italian celery)
Peperoncini (small green peppers pickled in vinegar)
Prosciutto (smoky-flavored Italian ham)
Provolone cheese
Radishes
Salami
Sauteed cold mushrooms marinated in vinegar and oil
Sliced hard-cooked eggs
Sliced tomatoes
Sweet red peppers

Minestrone

(Vegetable Soup)
Serves 8

2 quarts low-sodium chicken bouillon
1 3/4 cups canned Italian peeled tomatoes
1 medium onion, chopped
2 ribs celery, cut into 1-inch pieces
1/4 cup chopped parsley
1/2 teaspoon oregano
1/8 teaspoon pepper
1 clove garlic, minced
1 3/4 cups canned chickpeas, rinsed and drained
1 cup cubed zucchini
1 cup fresh or thoroughly defrosted frozen peas
1 cup diced carrots
1 cup chopped cabbage
1/2 cup uncooked white rice or orzo pasta
1/2 cup grated Parmesan cheese
chopped fresh parsley

1. In kettle, combine bouillon, tomatoes, onion, celery, 1/4 cup parsley, oregano, pepper, and garlic. Simmer, stirring occasionally, 20 to 30 minutes.
2. Add chickpeas, zucchini, peas, carrots, cabbage, and rice or pasta; simmer an additional 20 to 25 minutes or until vegetables and rice or pasta are tender.
3. Before serving, taste soup and adjust seasonings if needed.
4. Pour soup into large tureen or individual soup bowls. Pass bowls of grated Parmesan cheese and chopped parsley separately.

Per serving: 123 cal. (22% from fat), 9 g protein, 19 g carbohydrate, 3 g fat, 4 mg cholesterol, 3 g fiber, 359 mg sodium.

Pollo alla Cacciatore

(Chicken Hunter-Style)
Serves 6

1 4-pound broiler
1/2 cup all-purpose flour
1/2 teaspoon salt
1/4 teaspoon pepper
2 tablespoons olive oil
2 medium onions, chopped
1 clove garlic, finely minced
1 cup canned whole tomatoes, low sodium
1 cup sliced green pepper
1 1/2 cups sliced mushrooms

1. Rinse chicken; pat dry with paper towels. Cut into serving-sized pieces and remove skin.
2. Combine flour, salt, and pepper.
3. Coat chicken pieces with seasoned flour.
4. In large skillet, heat oil until hot but not smoking.
5. Add chicken pieces, a few at a time, and fry until golden brown.
6. Combine onions, garlic, tomatoes, and green peppers in a mixing bowl; add to chicken.
7. Cover skillet and simmer chicken slowly until tender, about 40 minutes.
8. Add mushrooms and simmer an additional 10 to 15 minutes.
9. Use a meat thermometer to check the internal temperature of chicken pieces. Breast pieces should reach an internal temperature of 170°F. Wings and thighs should reach an internal temperature of 180°F.
10. Taste; add additional seasonings if needed. Serve immediately.

Per serving: 267 cal. (37% from fat), 27 g protein, 14 g carbohydrate, 11 g fat, 76 mg cholesterol, 2 g fiber, 274 mg sodium.

Fettuccine Verde

(Green Noodles)
Serves 8

2 packages frozen chopped spinach, 10 ounces each
2 cups all-purpose flour
½ teaspoon salt
2 eggs
6 to 8 quarts water
2 tablespoons margarine, softened

1. In medium saucepan, cook spinach in a small amount of simmering salted water until tender. Drain well and squeeze dry.
2. Using fine blade of food processor, grind spinach 2 or 3 times.
3. Transfer chopped spinach to mixing bowl. Add flour, salt, and eggs.
4. Using hands, mix to form a soft dough.
5. Turn dough out onto a floured board and knead until smooth and no longer sticky, adding additional flour if needed.
6. Roll dough very thin into a rectangle. Cover with damp towels and let stand 1 hour.
7. Starting at the narrow end closest to you, fold dough over and over until it is about 3 inches wide.
8. Using a sharp knife, cut folded dough into very thin strips, about ¼ inch wide.
9. Unroll strips on flat surface and let dry 2 to 3 hours or overnight.
10. When ready to cook, bring water to boil in large kettle. Add noodles and simmer until tender.
11. When noodles are tender, drain well. Toss with margarine and serve immediately.

Per serving: 174 cal. (26% from fat), 7 g protein, 27 g carbohydrate, 5 g fat, 53 mg cholesterol, 3 g fiber, 242 mg sodium.

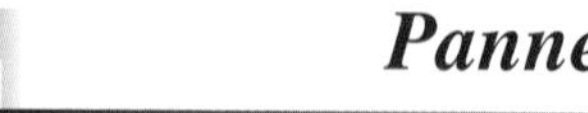

Panne

(Italian Bread)
Makes 2 loaves

4½ to 5½ cups all-purpose flour
1 tablespoon sugar
1½ teaspoons salt
2 envelopes active dry yeast
1 tablespoon softened margarine
1¾ cups very warm water (120°F to 130°F)
cornmeal
olive oil
1 egg white
1 tablespoon cold water

1. In large mixing bowl, combine 1½ cups flour, sugar, salt, and dry yeast.
2. Work in margarine.
3. Gradually add warm water and beat 2 minutes on medium speed of electric mixer, scraping bowl occasionally.
4. Add ¾ cup flour and beat 2 more minutes on high speed.
5. Stir in enough additional flour to make a stiff dough.
6. Turn dough out onto lightly floured board or pastry cloth. Knead until smooth and elastic, about 8 to 10 minutes.
7. Place dough in greased bowl and turn once to grease top. Cover with plastic wrap and a clean towel and let rest 20 minutes.
8. Divide dough in half and shape into two long loaves. (Shape by rolling each piece into an oblong. Beginning at wide end, roll tightly like a jelly roll and seal edges well.)
9. Place loaves on lightly greased baking sheets that have been sprinkled with cornmeal. Brush loaves lightly with olive oil and cover with plastic wrap. Refrigerate dough 2 to 24 hours.
10. When ready to bake, remove dough from refrigerator. Uncover dough carefully and let stand at room temperature 10 minutes.
11. Meanwhile, preheat oven to 425°F.

12. Slash loaves diagonally 4 to 5 times with a sharp knife.
13. Bake for 20 minutes.
14. Remove from oven and brush with beaten egg white mixed with water.
15. Return to oven and bake an additional 5 to 10 minutes or until loaves are golden brown and sound hollow when tapped with the knuckles.
16. Remove to cooling racks.

Per slice: 73 cal. (8% from fat), 2 g protein, 14 g carbohydrate, 1 g fat, 0 mg cholesterol, 1 g fiber, 106 mg sodium.

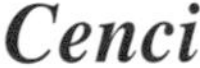

Cenci

(Deep-Fried Sweet Pastry)
Makes about 4 dozen pastries

2 cups all-purpose flour
2 whole eggs
2 egg yolks
1 teaspoon rum extract
1 tablespoon sugar
vegetable shortening for frying
confectioner's sugar

1. Place flour in a large mixing bowl. Make a well in the center and add the eggs, egg yolks, rum extract, and 1 tablespoon sugar.
2. Using a fork or fingers, mix until soft dough forms.
3. Turn dough out onto a lightly floured board or pastry cloth. Knead until dough is smooth, adding more flour if needed.
4. Refrigerate for one hour.
5. Heat 4 inches of shortening to 350°F.
6. Roll the dough until paper thin.
7. Cut into strips six inches long and 1/2 inch wide. Tie the strips into loose knots and fry until golden brown.
8. Drain on absorbent paper and sprinkle with confectioner's sugar. Serve immediately.

Per pastry: 40 cal. (37% from fat), 1 g protein, 5 g carbohydrate, 2 g fat, 23 mg cholesterol, 0 g fiber, 14 mg sodium.

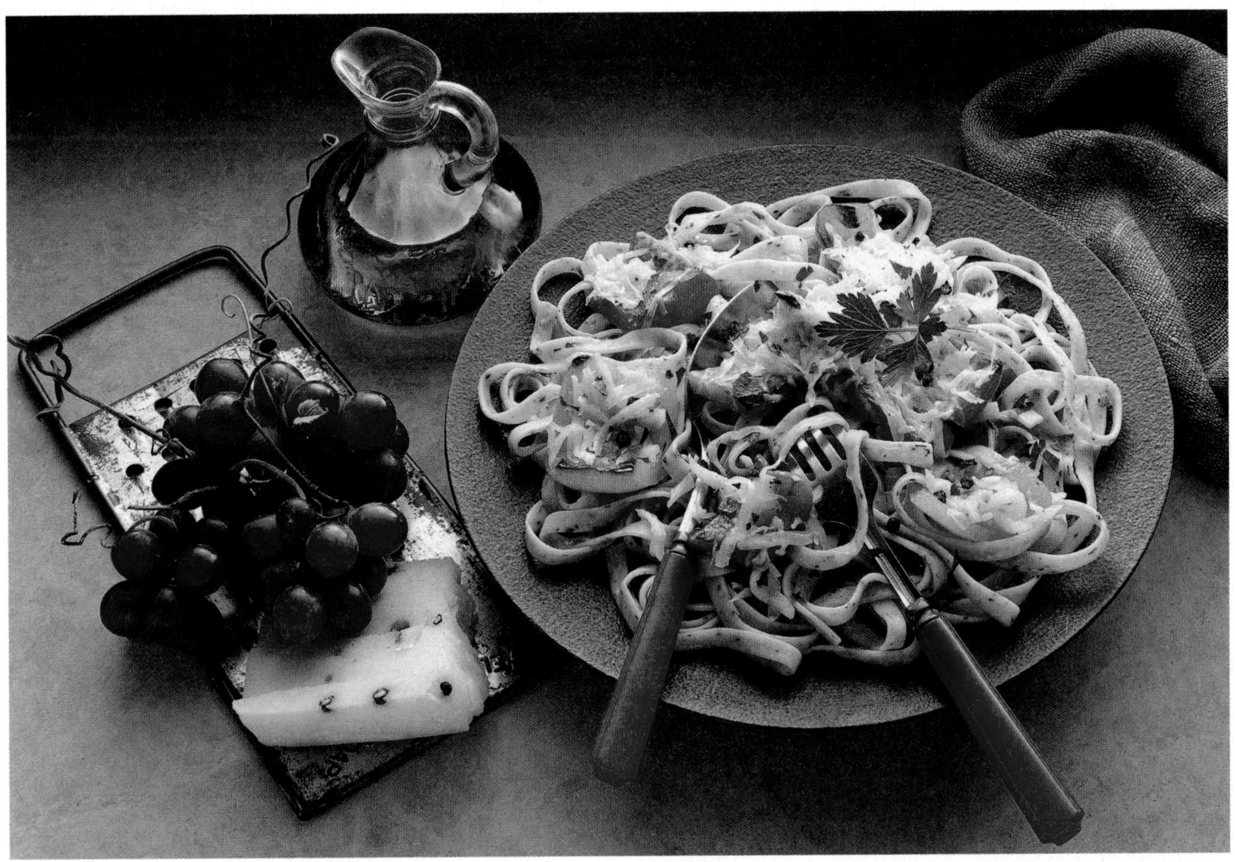

Pasta is a staple food that is served daily in some Italian homes.

Greece

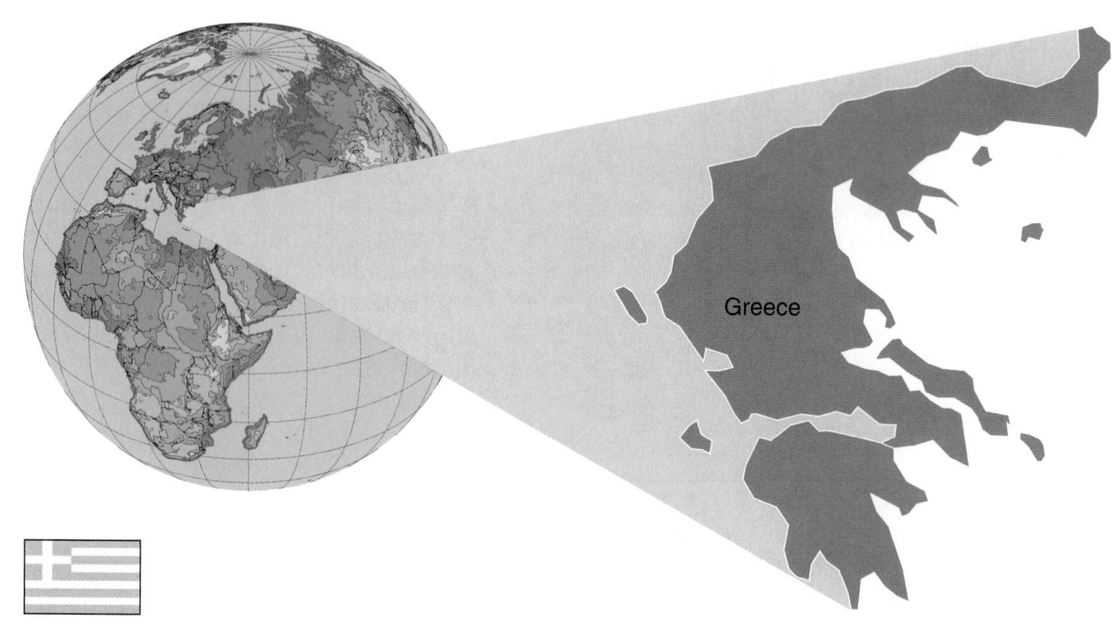

Greece is a land of terraced gardens, busy seaports, and ancient temples. In this sunny land, the art, literature, science, and philosophy that form the basis of Western civilization began. Parts of Greek culture, such as some Greek foods, have their roots in the older civilization of the Middle East. The foods moussaka and baklava are examples.

Geography and Climate of Greece

Greece forms the southern tip of Europe's Balkan Peninsula. The country is made up of one large landmass and many islands.

The geography of Greece is varied. Mountain ridges form the jagged coastline. To the east lie Mount Olympus and another strip of mountains separated by fertile valleys. The mountainous land with its stony, dry soil makes farming difficult. However, olive trees and grapevines, with their deep roots, can be cultivated in this terrain. Sheep thrive on the short grasses of the more mountainous areas.

The short, swift rivers of Greece are not useful for transportation. However, the Greeks do travel by way of the seas that surround much of their homeland.

Greece has mild winters and warm, sunny summers. Rainfall rarely exceeds 20 inches (50 cm) per year, and most of the rain falls in the winter. Because Greece has little or no frost, subtropical fruits and flowers can be grown.

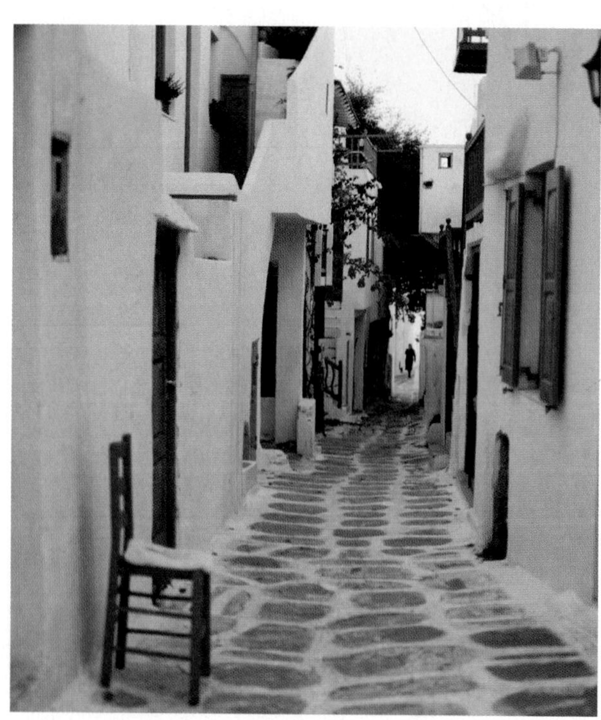

Quiet, cobble-stoned alleys are a common sight in small Greek towns.

Greek Culture

Greek history spans centuries. It usually is divided into two stages: the history of *Ancient Greece* and the history of *Modern Greece*. (Ancient Greece is sometimes called *Classical Greece*.)

> **Be a Clever Consumer**
>
> When traveling to an unfamiliar area, you may want to look into package tours. However, be sure to read all information carefully before signing any contracts or paying any money. Be sure you know exactly what your package includes. Find out about cancellation policies, too. Canceling a prepaid trip often means losing a large portion of the money you paid.

Ancient Greek Culture

Achievements in art, literature, science, and philosophy mark the history of Ancient Greece. The philosophers Socrates, Aristotle, and Plato and the jurist Solon were products of Ancient Greece. The dramatists Sophocles, Aristophanes, and Euripides and the scientist Hippocrates were from this culture, too. This is also the era that produced examples of classical architecture, such as the Parthenon in Athens.

Ancient Greece was divided into *city-states*. These were self-governing political units consisting of a city and surrounding territory. Although Ancient Greece never became unified, two of the city-states, Athens and Sparta, became seats of power. Athens was democratic, and the Athenians originated the basic concepts of Western law. Sparta, on the other hand, was not democratic. Spartans lived a strict, military life with stern laws. The Spartan ideal was individual sacrifice for community welfare.

The city-states fell to the Roman Empire. After the seat of Roman government moved to Constantinople, Greece lost much of its importance. Invaders later overran Greece, and by the fifteenth century, the Turks had control of all of Greece.

Turkey ruled Greece until the nineteenth century. Turkey granted liberty to a large part of the Greek peninsula in 1829. Then the Greeks began their fight to regain those parts of their country that remained under foreign rule.

Modern Greek Culture

Just under half of the Greek population lives in urban areas. The people of Greece share a common language, Greek, and a common religion. The majority of Greeks belong to the Greek Orthodox Church.

Greece is a relatively poor country. Many Greeks are farmers, despite the lack of fertile farmland. They produce wheat and corn on small acreages. They raise vegetables in terraced gardens. Grapes, olives, and citrus fruits grow in more fertile areas. Goats and sheep, which graze in the mountains, provide milk, cheese, and meat. Farming is difficult, and many families are able to provide only enough food for themselves. With new agricultural methods, however, food production in Greece's fertile areas has increased tremendously in recent years.

The Greek people are skilled mariners, and Greek ships carry cargo to ports all over the world. Fishing is an important industry on the islands and in coastal areas. Much of the seafood that is caught is eaten in Greece. However, some is exported along with olive oil and raisins.

In small communities, the ***tavernas*** are cafés that serve as public meeting places. Guests who gather in the tavernas often order glasses of retsina or ouzo. (*Retsina* is a resin-flavored wine. *Ouzo* is a strong spirit with the flavor of anise.) Often, someone will play a mandolin-like instrument called a *bouzoukia* while the other guests talk, play games, or dance. See 30-12.

Greek Holidays

Religious holidays hold great importance in Greece. People devote much time and energy to their celebration. Many of these celebrations involve special food traditions.

The year of Greek celebrations begins with Saint Basil's Day, which is also New Year's Day. On this day (rather than on Christmas) Greek people exchange gifts. Children receive a Saint Basil's cake, which is covered with almonds and walnuts and has a coin baked inside. Eating something sweet on New Year's Day is believed to bring a sweet year.

Easter is the most important religious holiday in Greece. A seven-week fast characterizes the Lenten season that precedes Easter. The fast is broken on Holy Saturday (the day before Easter) with a dish called *mayeritsa*. This is the internal organs of a lamb cooked in a seasoned

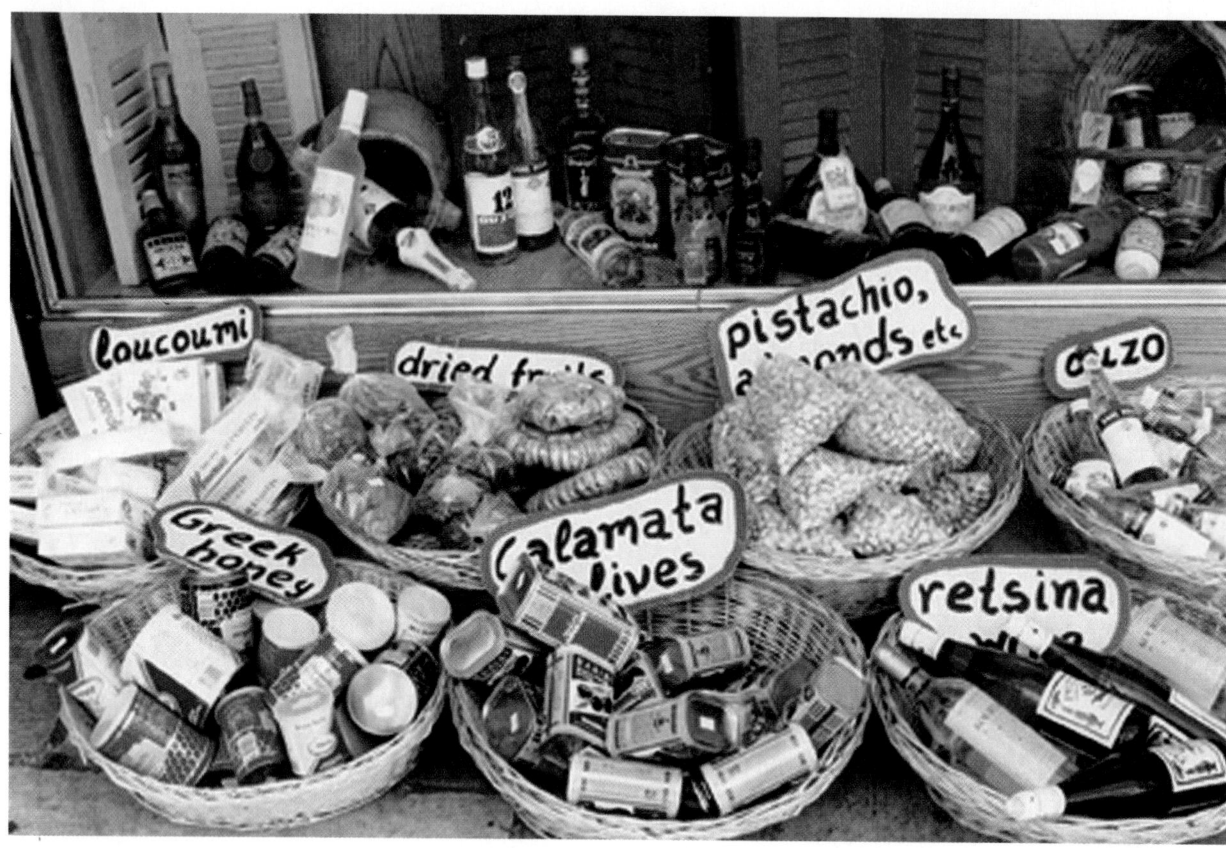

John F. Flanagan

30-12 Retsina and ouzo are sold in Greek shops as well as tavernas.

broth. After midnight on Holy Saturday, people watch displays of fireworks. Then early the next morning, the rest of the lamb is roasted whole and served for Easter dinner.

Each village and town in Greece has a patron saint. The feast day for the local patron saint is a holiday. On the feast day and the evening before, people go to a church service. Then the feast day is celebrated with food, wine, singing, and dancing. Some people wear traditional Greek clothes for the celebration.

Many Greek towns also hold annual harvest festivals. For example, the town of Megara has a fish festival in the spring.

Greek Cuisine

For thousands of years, the Greeks have been developing their cuisine. Early records show that the Greeks cooked foods while the rest of the world ate raw foods. Early Greek foods included roast lamb with capers, wild rice with saffron, and honey cakes. As Greek civilization spread throughout the Mediterranean, so did Greek cuisine. The Greeks taught the Romans how to cook, and a Greek named Hesiod wrote one of the first cookbooks.

Greek cooking has a rich and varied past. A pre-Greek people living in the Stone Age brought foods like lamb and beans to Greece. Other foods, like olives, grapes, and seafood, are native to the area. Invading groups of peoples added their food customs to these native foods. The many Greek pasta dishes, for example, are Italian in origin. Layers of pasta, ground lamb, and cheese covered with a rich custard and baked is called *pastitsio.* Kebabs, yogurt, Greek coffee, and rich sweet pastries are Turkish in origin. (*Kebabs* are pieces of meat, poultry, fish, vegetables, or fruits threaded onto skewers and broiled.)

Greek Staple Foods

A number of foods are basic to Greek cooking. Greek cooks make liberal use of lemon juice, tomatoes, and green peppers. ***Avgolemono,*** one of the most popular Greek sauces, is a mixture of egg yolks and lemon juice. The Greeks use it to flavor soups and stews. They serve it with vegetables and fish, too. Greek cooks stuff tomatoes and green peppers with meat and other vegetables. They also thread them on skewers and broil them and add them to soups and stews. Tomato sauces are used with both meat and fish dishes.

Greek cooks use many herbs and spices to bring out the natural flavors of lamb, fish, and vegetables. The most widely used herbs and spices include cinnamon, basil, dill, bay leaves, garlic, and oregano.

The Greeks serve eggplant as a side dish or add it to main dishes, 30-13. Cooks prepare *moussaka* by layering slices of eggplant, ground lamb, and cheese. (They often cook the lamb with tomato paste, wine, cinnamon, and onion.) They pour a rich cream sauce over the meat, vegetable, and cheese mixture before baking.

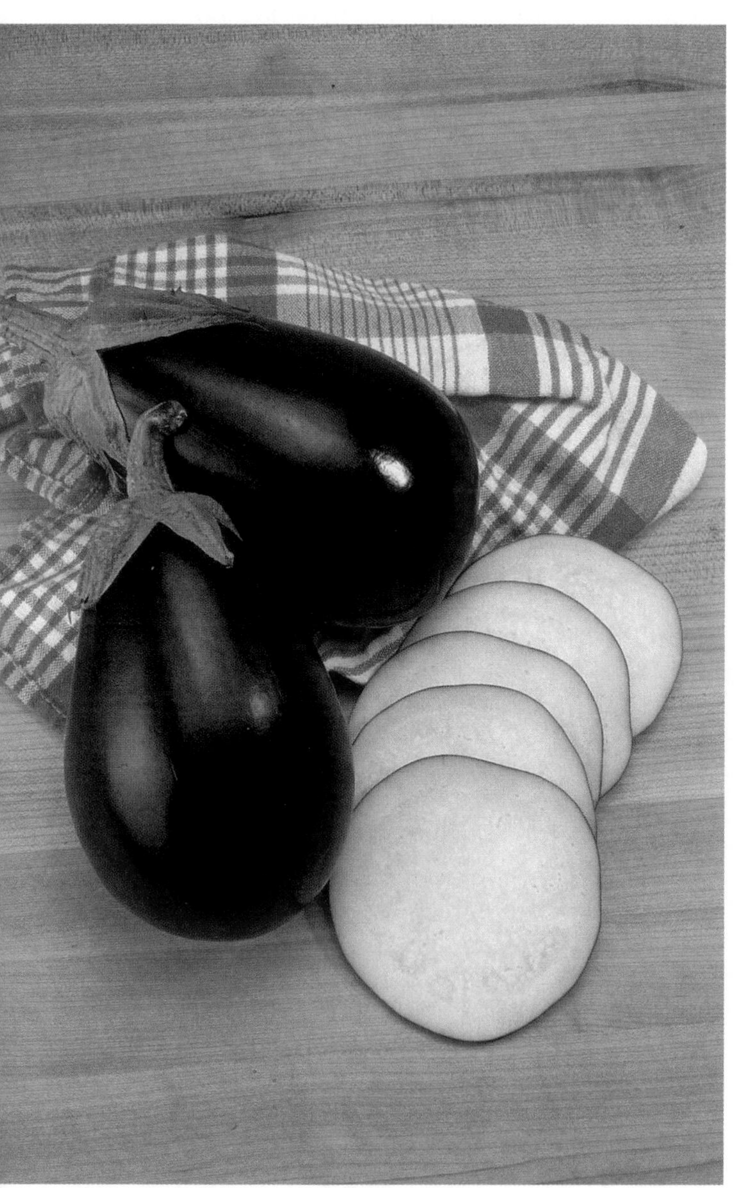

courtesy of W. Atlee Burpee & Co.

***30-13** Eggplant is a staple food in Greece that is an ingredient in many recipes.*

Lamb

Sheep have been raised in Greece since prehistoric times. Greek cooks roast lamb whole or thread it onto skewers and broil it. They also grind and layer it with other ingredients in casseroles. They use lamb as a filling for vegetables and add it to soups and stews, too.

Seafood

Because of Greece's location, seafood is an important part of the Greek diet. Fishers catch red mullet, crawfish, cuttlefish, sea bass, red snapper, swordfish, squid, and shrimp in the Mediterranean Sea.

Greek cooks prepare freshly caught seafood simply, usually by baking or broiling. They often bake fresh vegetables, such as tomatoes and zucchini, with the fish. Squid is particularly popular. Fresh squid stuffed with rice, onions, nuts, and seasonings is poached and served as a favorite main dish. Raw squid served with raw green beans or artichokes is eaten as an appetizer. Another popular appetizer or snack is *taramasalata,* a pâté made from fish roe (eggs).

Olives

Olives grow in abundance in Greece. Their many sizes, shapes, and colors often amaze people from the United States. The flavor of olive oil dominates Greek cuisine. People throughout Greece eat olives as appetizers and snacks or add them to other dishes. The popular *salata horiatiki* (rural salad) contains olives, a variety of greens, tomatoes, and feta cheese. (*Feta cheese* is a slightly salty, crumbly, white cheese made from goat's milk.)

Honey

Greek honey is world famous. In Ancient Greece, people used honey to make *melamacarons* (honey cakes), which they offered as gifts to the gods. Today, Greek bakers prepare the same honey cakes to celebrate the New Year. Honey is the basic sweetener used in the preparation of many Greek desserts, pastries, and cakes, 30-14.

Although the Greeks enjoy sweets, they usually serve sweets only on special occasions. The Greeks make many of their desserts with ***phyllo,*** a paper-thin pastry made with flour and

Q: Isn't honey a better choice for a sweetener than sugar?

A: Nutritionally speaking, honey and sugar are almost identical. There are no health benefits of choosing one over the other.

water. Some Greek cooks still make phyllo; others prefer to buy sheets of phyllo ready-made. *Baklava* is thin layers of phyllo filled with nuts and soaked with a honey syrup. *Galat oboureko* is phyllo layered with rich custard, honey, and nuts. *Kopenhai* is a nut cake with phyllo.

Other popular sweets contain flour, eggs, and oil rather than phyllo. They are deep-fried and are similar to fritters. *Diples,* for example, are small thin sheets of dough that are rolled with two forks as they are fried. They may be coated with a honey and nut syrup flavored with cinnamon.

Greek Meals

The Greeks appreciate simple pleasures. Their meals reflect this simplicity.

Breakfast is often no more than a slice of dry bread and a cup of warm milk. Sometimes, eggs or cheese accompanies the bread.

Both lunch and dinner are hot meals. The Greeks eat lunch at noon and dinner late in the evening.

Early evening is generally the most pleasant and enjoyable time of day. Many Greek families go for an evening walk. Some choose to sit at small outdoor cafes and enjoy a variety of appetizers called ***mezedhes.*** Olives, feta cheese, pistachio nuts, garlic-flavored sausage, shrimp, and hard-cooked eggs are popular mezedhes. Ouzo and conversation accompany this early snack.

Later, families gather at home for the evening meal. This meal might include either baked or broiled fish, a vegetable, and bread. Fresh fruit would complete the meal.

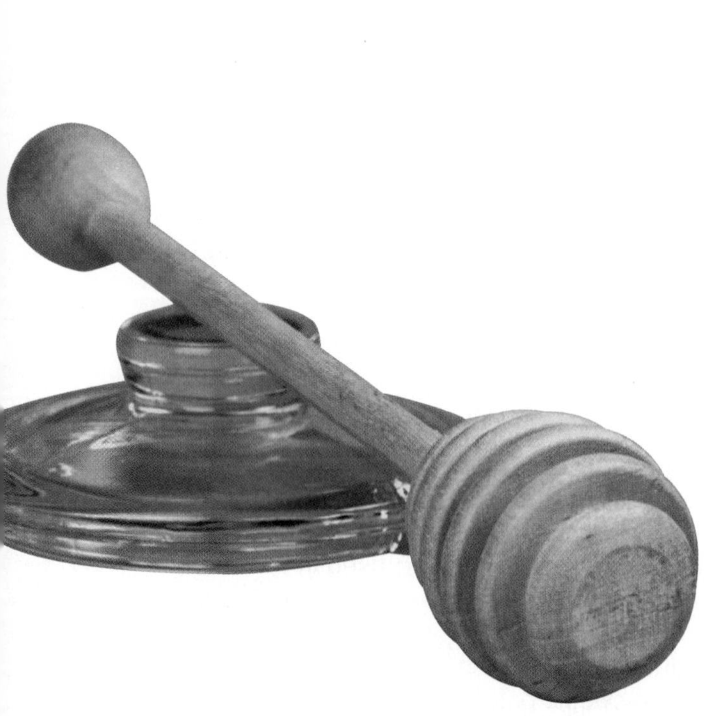

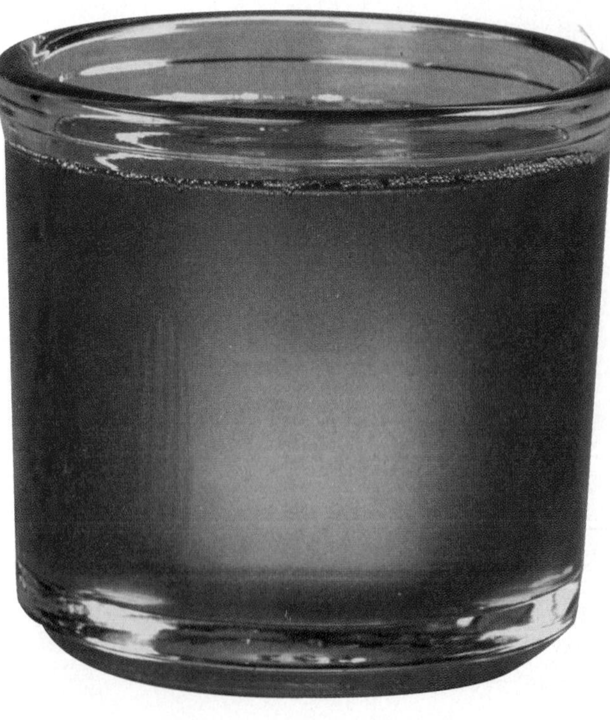

30-14 *For centuries, the Greeks have used honey to sweeten baked goods.*

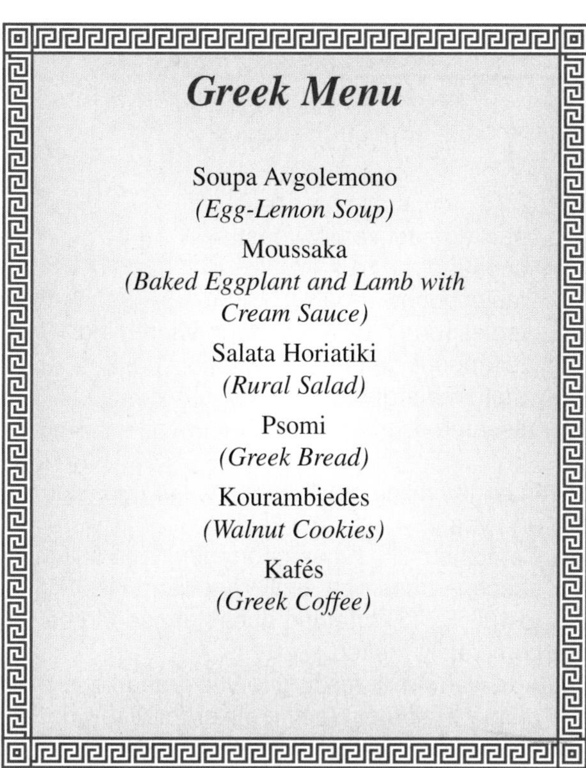

Greek Menu

Soupa Avgolemono
(Egg-Lemon Soup)
Moussaka
(Baked Eggplant and Lamb with Cream Sauce)
Salata Horiatiki
(Rural Salad)
Psomi
(Greek Bread)
Kourambiedes
(Walnut Cookies)
Kafés
(Greek Coffee)

Soupa Avgolemono

(Egg-Lemon Soup)
Serves 6 to 8

- 8 cups low-sodium chicken bouillon
- 1/2 cup uncooked white rice
- 3 eggs
- 2 to 3 tablespoons lemon juice
- salt
- pepper
- finely chopped parsley

1. In a large saucepan, bring chicken bouillon to a boil.
2. Add rice and simmer until tender.
3. Pour contents of saucepan through a strainer, catching excess bouillon in a large liquid measure. Set rice and bouillon aside.
4. Put eggs and lemon juice into blender container. Cover and process at high speed until frothy.
5. Remove cover and slowly pour the hot bouillon into the egg mixture while processing at low speed.
6. Pour soup into saucepan; add rice. Cook over low heat until thoroughly heated. Do not let soup boil.
7. Season soup with salt and pepper. Serve immediately garnished with parsley.

Per serving: 114 cal. (28% from fat), 5 g protein, 16 g carbohydrate, 4 g fat, 137 mg cholesterol, 0 g fiber, 43 mg sodium.

Salata Horiatiki

(Rural Salad)
Serves 6

- 6 cups assorted salad greens
- 3 medium tomatoes, washed and cut into wedges
- 1/2 cup chopped green onion
- 1 medium cucumber, washed and sliced thinly
- 1/3 cup olive oil
- 2 tablespoons lemon juice
- 2 teaspoons sugar
- 1/2 teaspoon salt
- few dashes pepper
- 1 1/2 ounces feta cheese
- 6 canned anchovy filets, drained
- 6 whole pitted ripe olives
- crumbled dry oregano

1. Wash greens and pat dry.
2. In a large salad bowl, combine greens with tomatoes, onions, and cucumber.
3. In a small bowl, mix olive oil, lemon juice, sugar, salt, and pepper to taste. Toss with greens mixture.
4. Crumble cheese coarsely and sprinkle over salad in a ring.
5. Wrap each anchovy around an olive and place inside ring of cheese.
6. Sprinkle oregano over all.

Per serving: 178 cal. (76% from fat), 4 g protein, 9 g carbohydrate, 15 g fat, 10 mg cholesterol, 3 g fiber, 474 mg sodium.

Moussaka

(Baked Eggplant and Lamb with Cream Sauce)
Serves 12

- 3 medium eggplants
- salt
- 2 pounds ground lamb
- 3 onions, chopped
- 2 tablespoons tomato paste
- 1/2 cup tomato sauce
- 1/4 cup parsley, chopped
- salt and pepper to taste

$^1/_2$ cup water
dash cinnamon
$^1/_2$ cup grated Parmesan cheese
$^1/_2$ cup bread crumbs
3 tablespoons all-purpose flour
3 cups fat free milk
dash nutmeg
4 egg yolks, lightly beaten
2 tablespoons olive oil
$^1/_4$ cup grated Parmesan cheese

1. Remove $^1/_2$-inch wide strips of peel lengthwise from eggplants, leaving $^1/_2$ inch peel between the strips.
2. Cut eggplant into thick slices. Sprinkle slices with salt and let stand between two heavy plates while browning meat and making sauce.
3. In large skillet, saute ground lamb and onions until meat is browned.
4. Add tomato paste, tomato sauce, parsley, salt, pepper, and water. Simmer until liquid is absorbed; cool.
5. Add cinnamon, $^1/_2$ cup cheese, and half of the bread crumbs to meat mixture. Set aside.
6. Combine flour and milk in a covered jar or blender container. Shake or blend until smooth.
7. Pour milk mixture into a heavy saucepan. Cook over medium heat, stirring constantly until sauce comes to a boil. Cook and stir for one additional minute until sauce is thick and smooth; add nutmeg.
8. Stir a little of the hot sauce into beaten egg yolks, then stir egg mixture into sauce and cook over very low heat for 2 minutes, stirring constantly. Set aside.
9. Preheat oven to 350°F.
10. In large skillet, heat oil.
11. Brown eggplant slices on both sides.
12. Grease a 13-by-9-inch baking dish and sprinkle bottom with remaining bread crumbs. Cover with layer of eggplant slices, then a layer of meat. Repeat layering until all eggplant and meat have been used, finishing with a layer of eggplant.
13. Cover eggplant and meat with sauce, sprinkle with $^1/_4$ cup grated cheese and bake 1 hour or until hot and bubbly.

Per serving: 300 cal. (48% from fat), 21 g protein, 18 g carbohydrate, 16 g fat, 126 mg cholesterol, 4 g fiber, 273 mg sodium.

Psomi

(Greek Bread)
Makes 2 loaves

$3^3/_4$ to $4^1/_4$ cups all-purpose flour
1 package active dry yeast
$1^1/_3$ cups fat free milk
2 tablespoons sugar
1 tablespoon plus 1 teaspoon shortening
$1^1/_2$ teaspoons salt
melted margarine
sesame seeds

1. In large mixing bowl, combine $1^1/_2$ cups flour and yeast.
2. Combine milk, sugar, shortening, and salt in saucepan and heat until very warm (120°F to 130°F). (Shortening does not need to be completely melted.)
3. Add warm milk mixture to yeast and flour. Beat on low speed of electric mixer (or with wooden spoon) $^1/_2$ minute (75 strokes) scraping the sides of the bowl often.
4. Beat an additional 3 minutes at high speed (900 strokes). Add enough additional flour to make a soft dough.
5. Turn dough out onto lightly floured board or pastry cloth and knead until smooth and elastic (about 8 to 10 minutes).
6. Place dough in lightly greased bowl, turning once to grease top. Cover with a clean towel and let rise in a warm place until doubled in bulk (about $1^1/_2$ hours).
7. Punch dough down and divide in half. Shape each half into a round loaf.
8. Place loaves on a lightly greased baking sheet. Brush tops with melted margarine and sprinkle with sesame seeds. Cover with a clean towel and let rise in a warm place until almost doubled in bulk (about 1 hour).
9. Bake loaves at 375°F until they are golden brown and sound hollow when gently tapped with the knuckles.
10. Remove breads to cooling racks and cool thoroughly before storing.

Per slice: 65 cal. (10% from fat), 2 g protein, 13 g carbohydrate, 1 g fat, 0 mg cholesterol, 0 g fiber, 106 mg sodium.

Kourambiedes

(Walnut Cookies)
Makes 3 dozen cookies

- 3/4 pound margarine
- 3 tablespoons confectioner's sugar
- 1/2 teaspoon vanilla
- 1 1/2 teaspoons baking powder
- 3 1/2 cups all-purpose flour, minus 1 tablespoon
- 1/2 cup finely chopped walnuts
- 1/2 cup confectioner's sugar

1. Melt margarine in small saucepan and cool to lukewarm.
2. Preheat oven to 350°F.
3. In large mixing bowl, combine melted margarine, 3 tablespoons sugar, vanilla, and baking powder; stir with a wooden spoon until mixed.
4. Add flour, 1/4 cup at a time, beating well after each addition.
5. Add walnuts, stirring until mixed.
6. On a lightly floured board, roll about 2 tablespoons of dough into an S-shaped rope, 6 inches long and 1/4 inch thick. Repeat with remaining dough.
7. Place cookies 1 inch apart on baking sheet. Bake until light brown, about 15 minutes.
8. Sprinkle with remaining confectioner's sugar.

Per cookie: 130 cal. (60% from fat), 2 g protein, 12 g carbohydrate, 9 g fat, 0 mg cholesterol, 0 g fiber, 102 mg sodium.

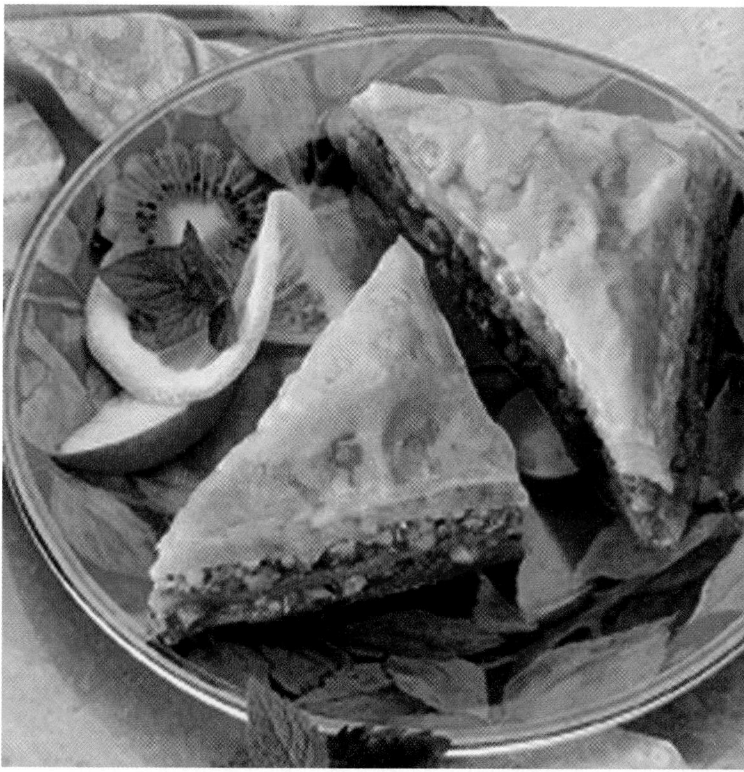

Grecian Delight Foods, Inc.

Crunchy nuts packed between layers of phyllo and drenched with honey syrup form the rich Greek dessert called baklava.

Chapter 30 Review
Mediterranean Countries

Summary

The mild climate of the Mediterranean region is favorable for the growth of a bounty of fruits and vegetables. These foods, along with fish from the sea, appear in a variety of dishes throughout Spain, Italy, and Greece. Despite common ingredients, however, each of these countries has a distinct cuisine.

Spanish cuisine is simple and colorful, focusing on the natural flavors of fresh ingredients. Spaniards enjoy an assortment of tapas at the beginnings of meals or while socializing with friends. Attractive salads and flavorful soups are popular throughout Spain. Main dishes such as cocido and paella include a variety of ingredients cooked together to produce a blend of flavors. Breads, tortillas, vegetables, and desserts round out Spanish meals.

Italy was the center of the Roman Empire, the birthplace of the Renaissance, and the home of the Roman Catholic Church. The foods of Italy are as notable as its cultural heritage. Italian cuisine focuses on fresh fruits and vegetables, a variety of seasonings, and rangetop cooking methods. Pasta, rice, and seafood are staples of the Italian diet.

The cuisine in each of Italy's three main geographic regions has distinct features. In Northern Italy, foods are cooked in butter, and homemade, ribbon-shaped pastas are popular. This region is also known for its soups, sausages, and risottos. The Central region is known for roasted lamb and cheesecake from Rome and grilled meats and bean dishes from Tuscany. In the South, cooks use olive oil and tubular pastas. This region is the home of rich tomato sauces, stuffed lasagne, and pizza.

Greek cuisine has been evolving for centuries. Staple foods of the Greek diet include lamb, seafood, olives, and honey. Lemon juice, tomatoes, green peppers, garlic, and eggplant also appear in many Greek dishes. Greek cooks flavor their foods with a number of herbs and spices.

Review What You Have Read

Write your answers on a separate sheet of paper.

1. Name three culinary advances the Moors made to Spanish cuisine.
2. Spanish meals often begin with appetizers called _____.
3. What is the difference between tortillas in Spain and tortillas in Mexico?
4. Why is Italian cuisine known as the "mother cuisine"?
5. Describe three ways Italians may serve pasta.
6. True or false. Northern Italian cooks favor olive oil for cooking, but Southern Italian cooks prefer butter.
7. List the courses that would make up a typical noon meal in Italy. Give an example of a food that might be served for each course.
8. Name three dishes invading groups of people contributed to Greek cuisine and two foods that are native to Greece.
9. Which of the following foods would most likely be served as a main dish in Greece?
   A. Avgolemono.
   B. Diples.
   C. Moussaka.
   D. Taramasalata.
10. What is the basic sweetener used in the preparation of many Greek desserts, pastries, and cakes?

Build Your Basic Skills

1. **Reading/writing.** Research the similarities and differences between Spanish and Mexican cuisine. Summarize your findings in a two-page written report.
2. **History.** Prepare a time line illustrating major events in Italian history from the Roman Empire to today. Explain to the class the significance of one of the events shown on your time line.

Build Your Thinking Skills

1. **Analyze.** Working in lab groups, research and prepare a regional version of paella. Each group should choose a different version. Serve all the paellas buffet-style. Analyze the major differences that are apparent among the dishes.
2. **Combine.** Divide the class into four groups. Then combine information and efforts to turn your classroom into a Greek taverna. One group should find appropriate music and learn a traditional Greek dance to teach the rest of the class. One group should be responsible for decorations. One group should learn a few Greek games to teach the rest of the class. The fourth group should choose a menu of Greek appetizers and find recipes to distribute. Each group should prepare one of the appetizer recipes.

Apply Technology

1. Go to a weather information Web site to find out the weather forecast for a specific Mediterranean location. Share your findings in class.
2. Use a computer and language translation software to translate the phrase "Celebrate the taste of the Mediterranean" into Greek, Italian, and Spanish. Then print banners of the English phrase and the three translations. Use the banners as classroom decorations on days when your class is sampling Mediterranean foods.

Using Workplace Skills

Antonio is an Italian chef at a trendy new restaurant called Pasta Roma. He supervises a number of cooks and assistants as they prepare a variety of popular Italian dishes. He also orders ingredients and sees they are stored properly. He sets up workstations for the cooks and makes sure each station includes the necessary equipment.

To be an effective worker, Antonio needs skill in organizing and distributing the resources of materials and facilities. In a small group, answer the following questions about Antonio's need for and use of this skill:

A. What are some specific material and facility resources Antonio would need to organize? How would he need to distribute these resources?
B. How might the cooks and assistants Antonio supervises be affected if Antonio lacked skill in organizing and distributing resources?
C. How might the patrons of Pasta Roma be affected if Antonio lacked skill in organizing and distributing resources?
D. What is another skill Antonio would need in this job? Briefly explain why this skill would be important.

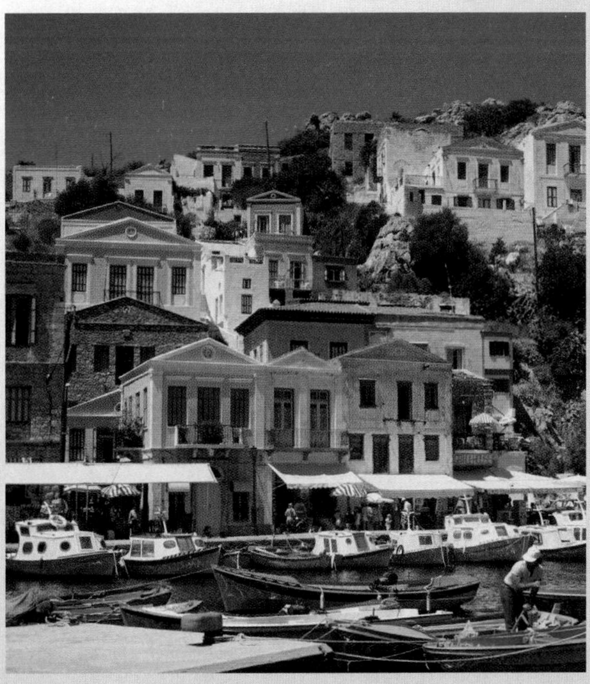

Chapter 31
Middle East and Africa

Foreign Correspondent
Collects and analyzes information about newsworthy events to write news stories for publication or broadcast.

Travel Clerk
Plans itinerary and schedules travel accommodations for military and civilian personnel and dependents according to travel orders, using knowledge of routes, types of carriers, and travel regulations.

Moshgiach
Supervises workers engaged in storing, preparing, and cooking meats, poultry, and other foods in restaurants, catering halls, hospitals, or other establishments to ensure observance of Hebrew dietary laws and customs.

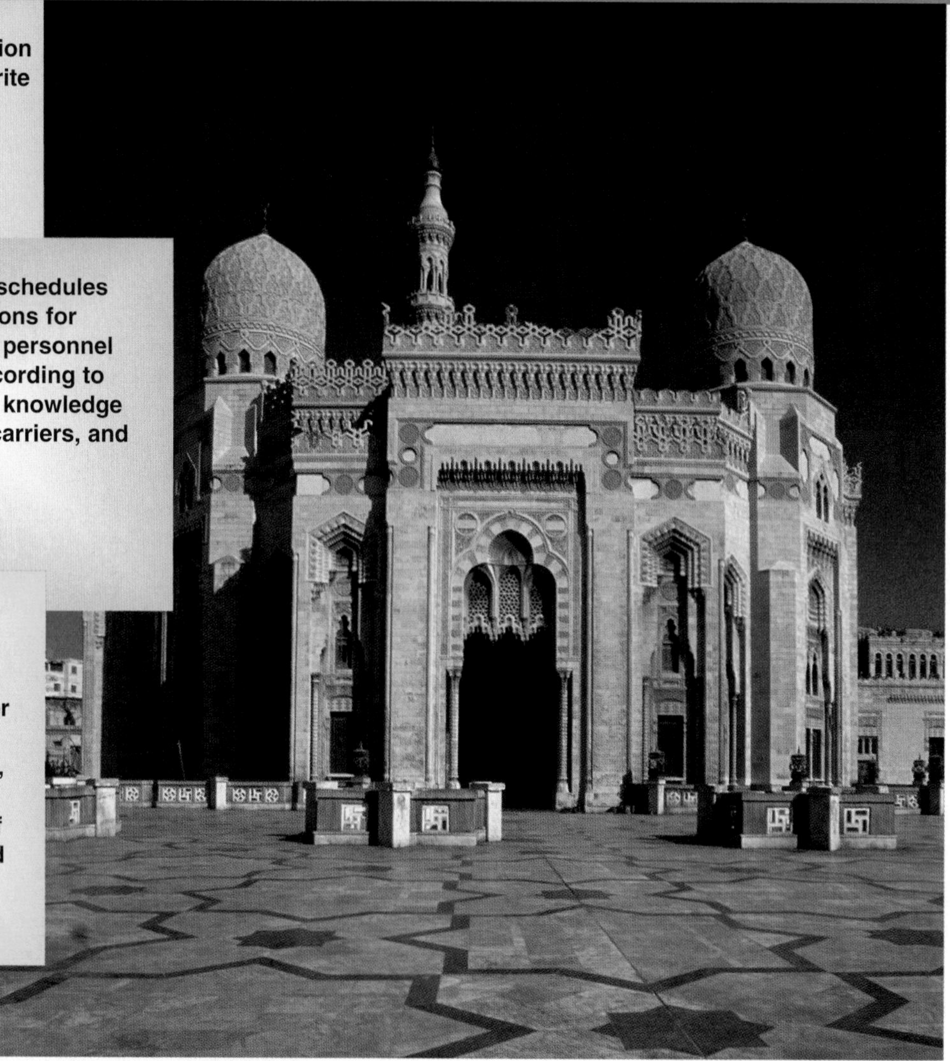

Terms to Know

Halal
Haram
bulgur
mazza
chelo kebab
kibbutzim
matzo
kashrut
kosher
shohet
milchig foods
fleishig foods
pareve foods
felafel
cacao
pita bread
injera
teff
wat

Objectives

After studying this chapter, you will be able to

- describe the food customs of the Middle East and Africa.
- discuss how geography, climate, and culture have influenced these customs.
- prepare foods that are native to each of these countries or regions.

The Middle East and Africa cover a large area. These regions are home to people of several races and many nationalities. They speak a number of major languages and hundreds of dialects.

Geographical features in the Middle East and Africa vary widely. In Egypt, the hot, dry, sandy desert stretches for miles. In Eastern Africa, rugged, snow-capped mountains rise above the arid plains. Along the equator, tropical rain forests boast lush vegetation.

The climate limits the types of foods that are available in each of the countries in this area. Strict religious doctrines also restrict the foods that many Middle Eastern and African people can eat. These factors have caused a number of distinct cuisines to emerge in these regions.

Cooking styles vary. However, there are some similarities in foods from this part of the world. For instance, many foods eaten in Israel originated in other Middle Eastern countries and parts of Africa.

The cuisines of these regions are nutritious. Cooks in the Middle East and Africa use only limited amounts of meat. A starchy food, such as cassava, rice, plantains, or some type of bread, accompanies every meal. Meals also include a wide variety of vegetables and fruits. These mealtime staples are rich in complex carbohydrates, vitamins, minerals, and fiber. Because frying is a favored cooking method, some dishes can be high in fat. However, many foods are prepared by lowfat cooking methods, such as broiling and stewing. By practicing balance when planning menus, all Middle Eastern and African foods can fit into a healthful diet.

As you read about these regions, you will become more familiar with their cultures, climates, and customs. You will begin to identify differences and similarities in their cuisines.

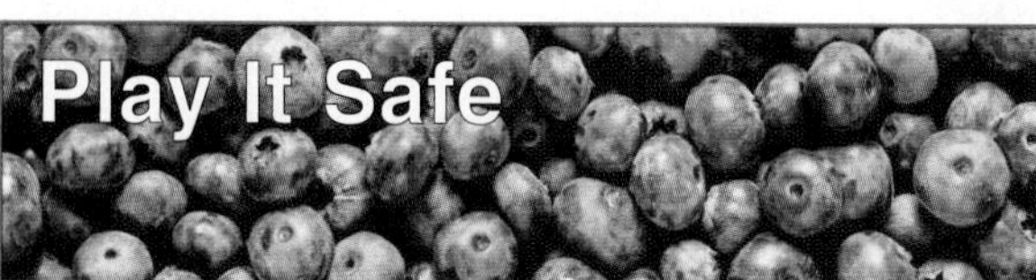

Play It Safe

Before leaving for a trip, contact the post office to have your mail held. Also stop delivery of any newspapers you receive. Set timers to turn lights on and off and play the TV or radio. Arrange to have someone care for your lawn, too. Making these arrangements will create the appearance that someone is in your home. This will make your home seem less inviting to would-be intruders.

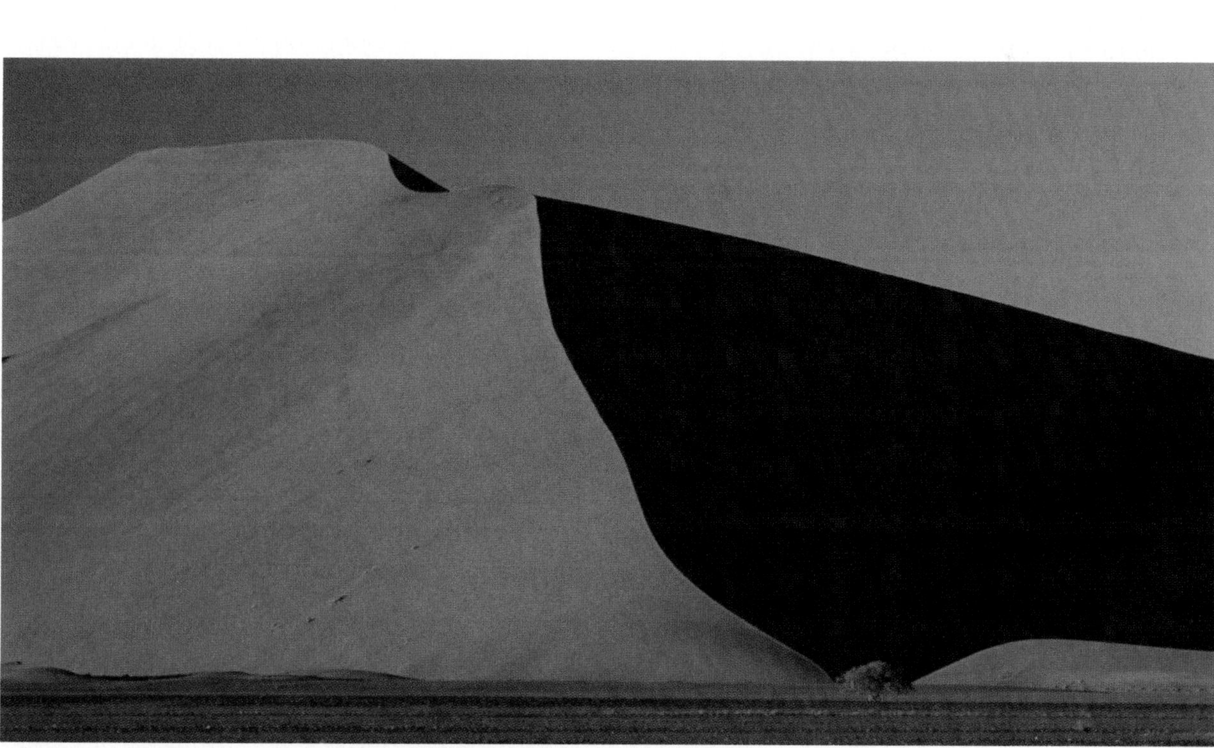

Desert regions are common throughout much of the Middle East and Africa.

Middle East

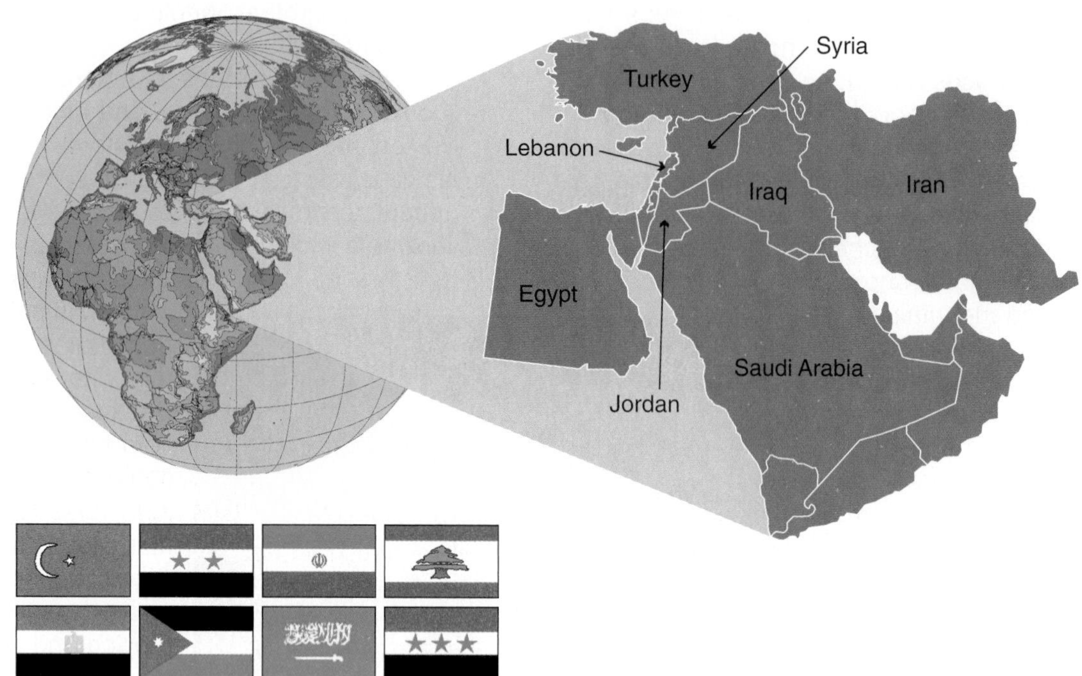

The Middle East forms a large horseshoe from the eastern edge of the Mediterranean Sea to North Africa. This land is the cradle of civilization. Christianity, Judaism, and Islam began in this region. This is where the Byzantine, Persian, Arab, and Ottoman Empires flourished.

The exact boundaries of the Middle East are sometimes disputed. However, the countries of Iran, Iraq, Syria, Lebanon, Jordan, Egypt, and Saudi Arabia form its center. (Israel is also part of the Middle East, but because its cuisine has unique qualities, Israel will be discussed separately.) Turkey, which lies just to the north and east, shares some characteristics with its Middle Eastern neighbors.

Geography and Climate of the Middle East

Mountains, high plateaus, and deserts are important geographical features of the Middle East. Much of the land is arid and barren. However, fertile oases are scattered throughout the region.

Seven major bodies of water border the nations that form the core of the Middle East. Three of the world's most famous rivers, the Nile, Tigris, and Euphrates, are in this region. The lands along the banks are among the world's richest. Coastal lands and inland mountain valleys are also excellent farming areas.

Rainfall varies in the Middle East. Areas in southern Egypt may not have rain for 10 to 20 years. However, some coastal regions may have 20 to 30 inches (50 to 70 cm) of rain during one season. As a whole, much of the Middle East is hot and dry. Therefore, irrigation is essential. When rain does fall, it is often so heavy that flooding occurs.

The climate along the Mediterranean coasts is subtropical with warm, dry summers and mild, rainy winters. Mountain valleys have hot, dry summers and cool winters. Desert areas have daytime temperatures above 100°F (38°C) and little if any rain.

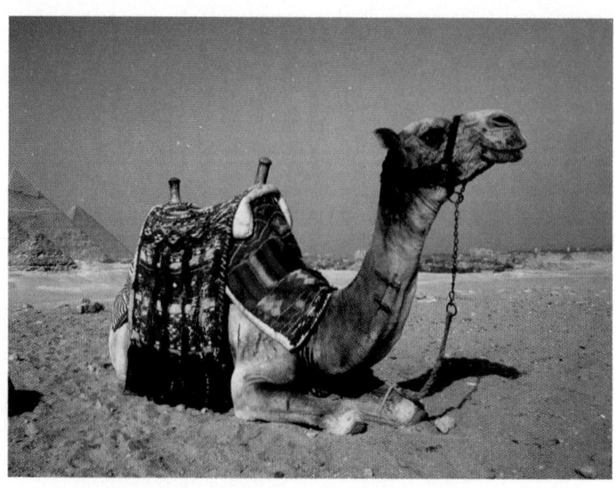

Camels serve as a food source and a means of transportation for some people in the Middle East.

Middle Eastern Culture

Egypt has one of the world's oldest civilizations. Thousands of years before the birth of Christ, the Egyptians had reached a high level of civilization. They had an orderly government and a written language. They traded with other parts of the world and built great structures of stone.

Ancient Empires of the Middle East

Much of the history of the Middle East centers around large empires that rose to power, weakened, and fell. The first of the four greatest Middle Eastern empires was the Persian Empire. Today, the country of Iran is all that remains of this once mighty empire. The Byzantine Empire formed when the Roman Empire split into East and West. Its headquarters were in Constantinople, which later became the capital of the Ottoman Empire. The followers of the prophet Muhammad formed the Arab Empire. People in Middle Eastern countries where Islam is the primary faith still speak the Arabic language. Eventually, the Ottoman Turks combined parts of the Persian, Byzantine, and Arab Empires to form the Ottoman Empire. As a result, Turkish foods and customs are evident in many parts of the Middle East.

Middle Eastern Agriculture

Today, many Middle Easterners make their living as farmers or herders. Sheep, goats, and camels graze on the short, stubby grasses of the arid regions. They supply meat, milk (used to make yogurt and cheese), and hides. Camels also serve as pack animals.

A variety of crops grow in areas where there are irrigation systems or where there is enough rain. Wheat and barley are the major grain crops. Corn grows in some areas. Citrus fruits, Persian melons, olives, bananas, figs, grapes, and other fruits grow in the subtropical climate of the coastal regions. Other important food crops include sugar beets and rice. Families grow vegetables for home use on small plots of land.

Religion in the Middle East

More than 90 percent of the people living in the Middle East practice the same religion. This religion is Islam, and those people who follow it are called *Muslims*. Islam is based on the teachings of the prophet Muhammad. Islam greatly affects the lifestyle and food choices of the Muslims.

The *Koran* is a book of sacred writings in the Islamic religion. It specifies foods Muslims should and should not eat. It forbids the eating of animals that have died from disease, strangulation, or beating. Only animals that have been slaughtered by a proper ritual are considered edible. The Koran also forbids Muslims to eat pork and drink wine and other alcoholic beverages. Foods considered lawful according to the Islamic religion are called ***Halal.*** Foods that are forbidden are called ***Haram.*** See 31-1.

Middle Eastern Holidays

With the large Muslim population, it is not surprising that many Middle Eastern celebrations are Muslim holidays. Each country may have different names for and ways of celebrating these holidays.

The first month of the Muslim year is called *Muharram*. This is also the name given to the 10-day Muslim New Year Festival. The last day of this festival is another Muslim holiday called *Ashura*. This day commemorates the death of the martyr Husain, who was the grandson of the prophet Muhammad. It also celebrates the safe landing of Noah's ark. On Ashura, Muslim people eat a pudding of the same name. This pudding is made with dates, raisins, figs, and nuts as was a legendary pudding made by Noah's wife.

Another Muslim observance is the *Fast of Ramadan*. Ramadan is the ninth month of the Muslim calendar, and the fast lasts the entire month. Muslims are to abstain from food and

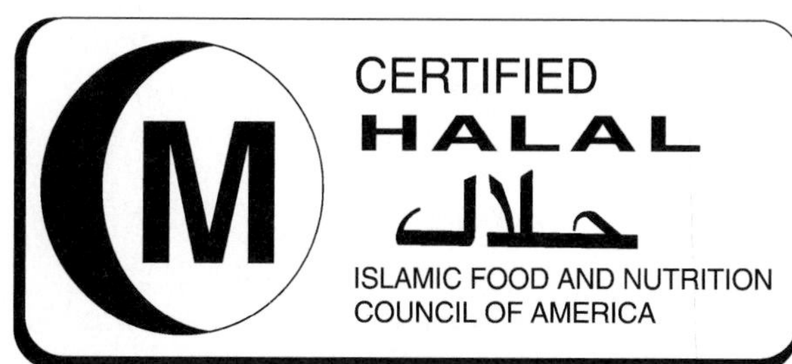

31-1 *This symbol on a food product label assures Muslims the food is Halal, or in keeping with Islamic dietary laws.*

drink throughout the day. Each night they may break the fast. In some regions the fast is broken with a light meal, in other areas, people feast during the night. *Id-al-Fitr* is a three-day celebration that marks the end of the Fast of Ramadan.

Another Muslim holiday is *Maulid an-Nabi.* This is a nine-day celebration of Muhammad's birthday. Fairs, parades, and community feasting may be part of the observance.

Middle Eastern Cuisine

Middle Eastern cuisine, which is sometimes called Eastern Mediterranean cuisine, has been developing for centuries. As traders crossed the deserts and one group of people conquered another, recipes were exchanged and modified. As a result, it is often difficult to determine the exact origin of a particular dish.

Foods Found Throughout the Middle East

Basic to all Middle Eastern cooking are five ingredients: garlic, lemon, green pepper, eggplant, and tomato. These ingredients appear again and again in dishes served throughout the area. Also basic is the taboo against eating pork. Both Judaism and Islam forbid their followers to eat the meat of swine. See 31-2.

Both olives and olive oil are common in Middle Eastern cuisine. Olives come in a variety of shapes, sizes, and colors. People eat them as appetizers and snacks. They use olive oil in place of butter or lard for cooking. Fresh olive oil gives a special flavor to Middle Eastern foods.

Spice caravans were once a common sight in the Middle East. Therefore, it seems only natural to expect cooks to use spices liberally. Middle Eastern foods are not spicy hot. Instead, spices and herbs add delicate flavor to foods.

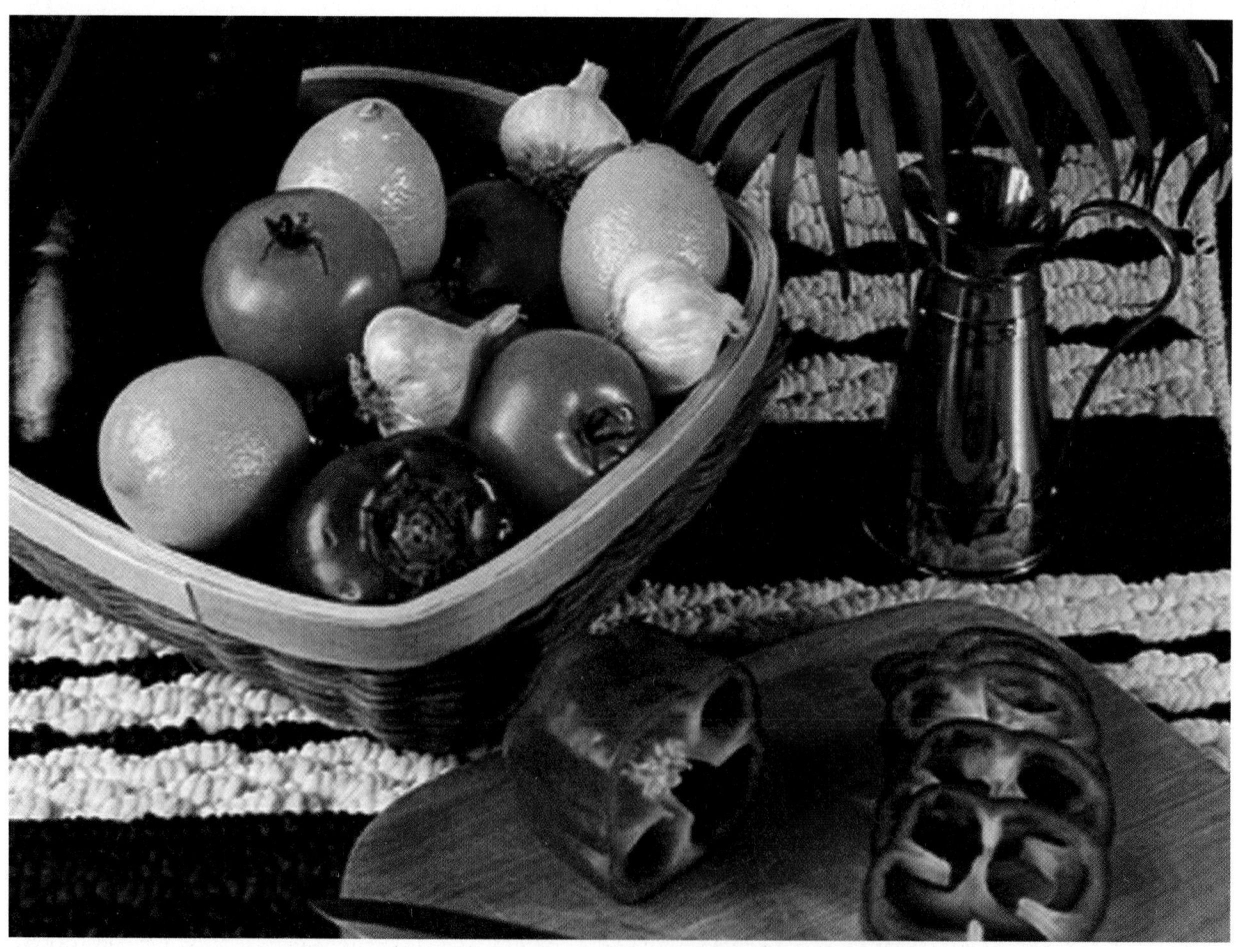

Jack Klasey

31-2 *These five basic ingredients add flavor and color to a number of Middle Eastern dishes.*

Q: Do herbs and spices have any nutritional value?

A: Herbs and spices do not provide proteins, carbohydrates, or minerals. However, some seasonings have been found to contain phytochemicals that health experts believe may help prevent some kinds of cancer.

In the Middle East, lamb is the staple meat. It is often roasted whole. Chunks of lamb sometimes are threaded on skewers and served as *shish kebabs* or added to hearty stews. Ground lamb is used to make dolmas. *Dolmas* are a mixture of ground meat and seasonings wrapped in grape leaves or stuffed into vegetables.

Middle Eastern yogurt is curdled milk with a tangy flavor. It is not at all like the yogurt eaten in the United States. People throughout the Middle East eat it as a side dish, snack, and dessert. They also use it to make cakes and hot and cold soups. In some areas, people serve diluted yogurt as a beverage.

Middle Eastern Grains and Legumes

Wheat, beans, rice, lentils, and chickpeas are the staple grains and legumes of the Middle East. Middle Easterners use wheat flour to make bread. Middle Eastern people serve bread at every meal and often buy it from the village baker twice a day.

Middle Eastern people also serve wheat as bulgur. ***Bulgur*** is a grain product made from whole wheat that has been cooked, dried, partly debranned, and cracked. Middle Easterners add bulgur to soups, stews, stuffings, and salads. They also serve it as a side dish with ground lamb, 31-3. *Felafel* is a deep-fried mixture of bulgur, ground chickpeas, and spices. Street vendors sell felafel and people eat it much as people in the United States eat hot dogs.

Rice is as popular as bulgur, and in Iran, it is even more popular. People in the Middle East often serve rice plain. However, they may cook it with tomato juice or saffron and make it into a seasoned rice dish called *pilav*.

Middle Eastern Dessert and Coffee

Middle Eastern people, as a group, enjoy sweets and rich desserts. However, they usually eat these foods as snacks or serve them on special holidays. They eat fruit at the end of most meals. Quince, pomegranates, figs, and melons are particularly popular.

People throughout most of the Middle East drink coffee. (Iran is an exception. There, tea is the main beverage.) All Middle Eastern coffee is strong, but it can be prepared in several ways. People who make khave (Turkish-style coffee) use a long-handled pot with a wide bottom and thin neck. They combine and heat water, coffee, and sugar just until the mixture begins to foam. They quickly remove the pot from the heat. Then they return the pot to the heat once or twice to again build up the foam. Finally, they pour the foaming liquid into small cups and top it with the remaining coffee, grounds and all. More sugar can be added if desired. *Arab-style coffee* rarely contains sugar. People who make this type of coffee bring it to a boil only once. They pour it into a second pot to get rid of the grounds and sediment. They may add cloves and cardamom seeds before serving.

Turkish Foods

Many people do not regard Turkey as part of the Middle East. However, it lies next to three Middle Eastern countries. Therefore, the influence of Turkish cuisine is found throughout this

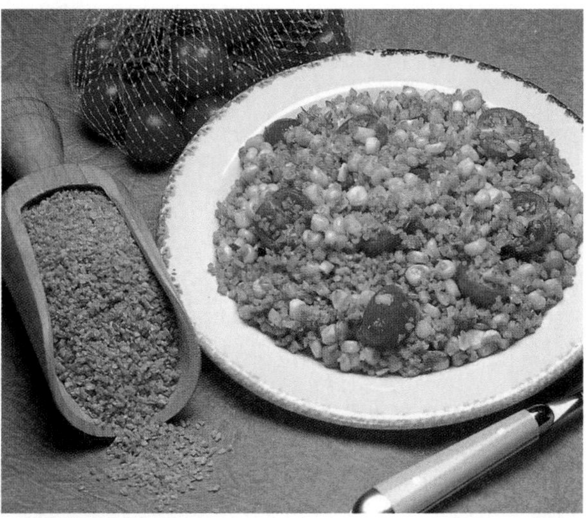

Wheat Foods Council

31-3 *Bulgur is a filling Middle Eastern side dish made from wheat.*

region. Any discussion of Middle Eastern cuisine would be lacking if it did not include information about Turkish foods.

The waters that border Turkey on three sides provide a variety of fish and shellfish. Seafood vendors in Istanbul sell lobster, salty red caviar, jumbo shrimp, mussels, haddock, bass, and mackerel.

Lamb is the most readily available and most popular meat. Lamb cubes marinated in a mixture of olive oil, lemon juice, and onions are threaded onto skewers and charcoal broiled. Rice, sliced tomatoes, and bread often accompany this dish, which is called *shish kebab.* Another type of kebab, the *döner kebab,* is a large cone made of thin pieces of lamb. As the cone rotates over a bed of charcoal, the outside slices of meat become crisp and flavorful. Turkish cooks slice these crisp pieces from the cone with large knives. They serve the meat with a salad, onion rings, cucumbers, and tomato slices. By the time they serve one helping, the next layer of meat has become crisp. See 31-4.

Stuffed vegetables, cacik, and pilav are other common Turkish foods. Cacik is slices of cucumber in a yogurt sauce flavored with mint; *pilav* is seasoned rice. Turkish cooks may serve pilav plain or mix it with currants, nuts, and tomato sauce.

Snacking is popular in Turkey. Nuts, pumpkin seeds, and toasted chickpeas are favorite snack foods. Vendors in the streets of Istanbul sell crisp bracelets of bread from long poles. Other vendors look like walking refreshment stands. Each carries a container of sweet, fruit-flavored syrup, a jug of water, and a rack of glasses. The vendor mixes a little of the syrup with some of the water and sells the beverage by the glass.

Sweets are popular in Turkey. *Halva* is a candylike sweet made from farina or semolina and sugar. *Baklava* is a sweet pastry made from phyllo, nuts, and honey. *Kurabiye* is a rich butter cookie. *Rahat lokum* (Turkish delight) is a candylike sweet made from grape jelly coated with powdered sugar. Other sweets have even more exotic names. The "vizier's finger" is a sweet roll fried in olive oil until crisp. A "lady's navel" is a deep-fried fritter with a depression in the center. "Sweetheart's lips" are rounds of

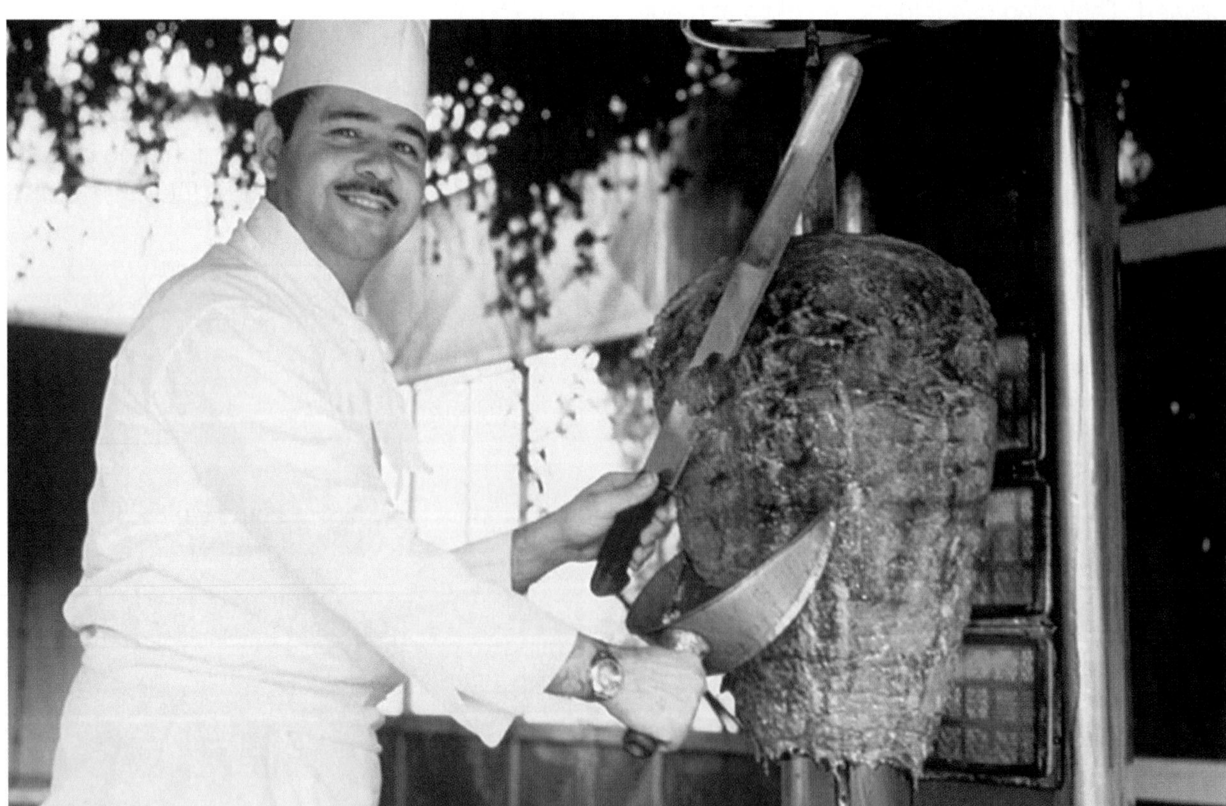

Turkish Tourism Office, Washington, DC

31-4 *As this döner kebab rotates near a heat source, the outer layer of the lamb meat becomes crisp and tasty. The cook then slices off pieces of the meat to serve as a popular Turkish food.*

dough filled with nuts and folded in a way that resembles human lips.

Foods of the Arab States

The countries of Lebanon, Iraq, Jordan, Syria, Saudi Arabia, and Egypt are often called the *Arab States.* The Arab States include the area once called the *Fertile Crescent.* This is where people first learned to grow crops.

People can buy a variety of spices at bazaars throughout the Arab world. Vendors scoop cinnamon, cumin, ginger, coriander, allspice, and hot peppers onto pieces of paper, which they roll into cones. Arab cooks add spices to many dishes. They use rose water and orange-flower water to flavor their sweets.

No Arab meal is complete without ***mazza*** (appetizers). *Arak,* an anise-flavored liqueur, is usually served with the mazza. One kind of mazza, called *tabbouleh,* is actually a salad. It is made of chopped tomatoes, radishes, green and white onions, parsley, mint, and bulgur. People break off pieces of *shrak* (a flat bread) and use them to scoop up the tabbouleh.

Islam law forbids the eating of pork, but the Arabs enjoy both camel and lamb. Camel, boiled in sour milk until it is tender, is popular among the nomadic Bedouin people. Most other Arabs prefer lamb.

Kibbi (called *kibbi* in Syria, *kobba* in Jordan, and *kubba* in Iraq) is a popular Arab lamb dish. Arab cooks pound raw lamb and bulgur into a paste and shape it into flat patties or hollow balls. They fry the patties. They stuff the hollow balls with ground lamb, pine nuts, rice, or vegetables and either bake or broil them.

Arab cooks love both color and pattern, and they use both lavishly. For example, they often garnish hummus with red pepper, green parsley, and brown cumin. *Hummus* is a mixture of chickpeas and sesame paste, 31-5. They serve torshi the way people serve pickle relish in the United States. *Torshi* is a mixture of pickled turnips, onions, peppers, eggplant, cucumbers, and occasionally beets. They use saffron to give a bright gold color to a variety of dishes.

Along the eastern Mediterranean coastline, fishers catch a variety of fish daily. Cooks quickly clean mullet, sea bass, turbot, swordfish, cod, sardines, and other fish. Then they bake or poach the fish or cook them over charcoal. Restaurants that line the riverbanks of the Tigris serve smoked shabait (a kind of trout).

Bedouins are a nomadic group of Arabs. In the tent of a Bedouin *sheikh,* or chief, it is customary to dine on the rug-covered floor. The sheikh's family members serve trays covered with Arab bread, rice, pine nuts, almonds, and lamb. According to Arab custom, diners must eat the food with the right hand only. At the end of the meal, coffee and tea are served in small cups.

Iranian Foods

The Persians (predecessors of the present day Iranians) laid the foundation for Middle Eastern cooking. Scholars believe that wine, cheese, sherbet, and ice cream were first made in Persia. The Persians were also the first to extract the essence of roses and combine exotic herbs and spices with foods.

For centuries, rice has been the staple food of the Iranians. They serve many kinds of rice dishes. All these dishes belong to one of two groups: chelo or polo. *Chelo* is plain boiled, buttered rice served with *khoresh* (a topping made of varied sauces, vegetables, fruits, and meats). *Polo* is similar to pilaf in that all the accompaniments cook with the rice.

Iran's national dish is called ***chelo kebab.*** The kebab consists of thin slices of marinated, charcoal-broiled lamb. Diners combine three accompaniments with the chelo: a pat of

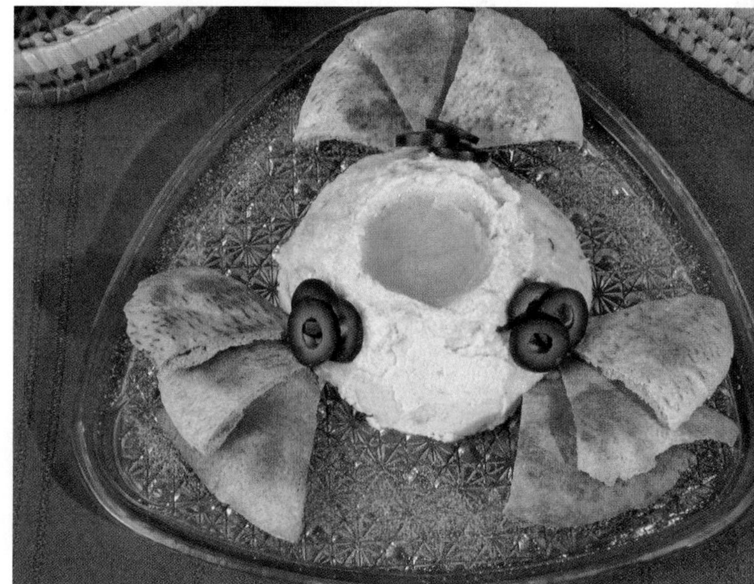

Jack Klasey

31-5 *Ground chickpeas and sesame paste are used to make hummus, which is a spread that is often served with pita bread.*

butter, a raw egg, and a bowl of sumac.

Iran's proximity to the Caspian Sea with its many sturgeon makes caviar a bargain. (*Caviar* is the processed eggs of a large fish, often the sturgeon.) Over 95 percent of the world's caviar comes from the Caspian Sea. See 31-6.

Iranians use yogurt to make a variety of hot and cold soups. One popular version contains grated cucumber and is served with a topping of raisins and fresh mint leaves. When combined with plain or carbonated water, yogurt becomes a refreshing drink.

Iranians are not quite as fond of rich pastries as other Middle Easterners. They eat fresh fruits instead. Iran produces some of the finest Persian melons, watermelons, peaches, pomegranates, apricots, quinces, dates, pears, and grapes. Iranians often eat these fruits plain. However, sometimes they slice and sweeten the fruits and serve them with crushed ice or make them into sherbets.

Good Manners Are Good Business

Follow the lead of your host when dining with a Middle Eastern business associate. Be ready to eat with your fingers if he or she does so. Also, remember to eat only with your right hand.

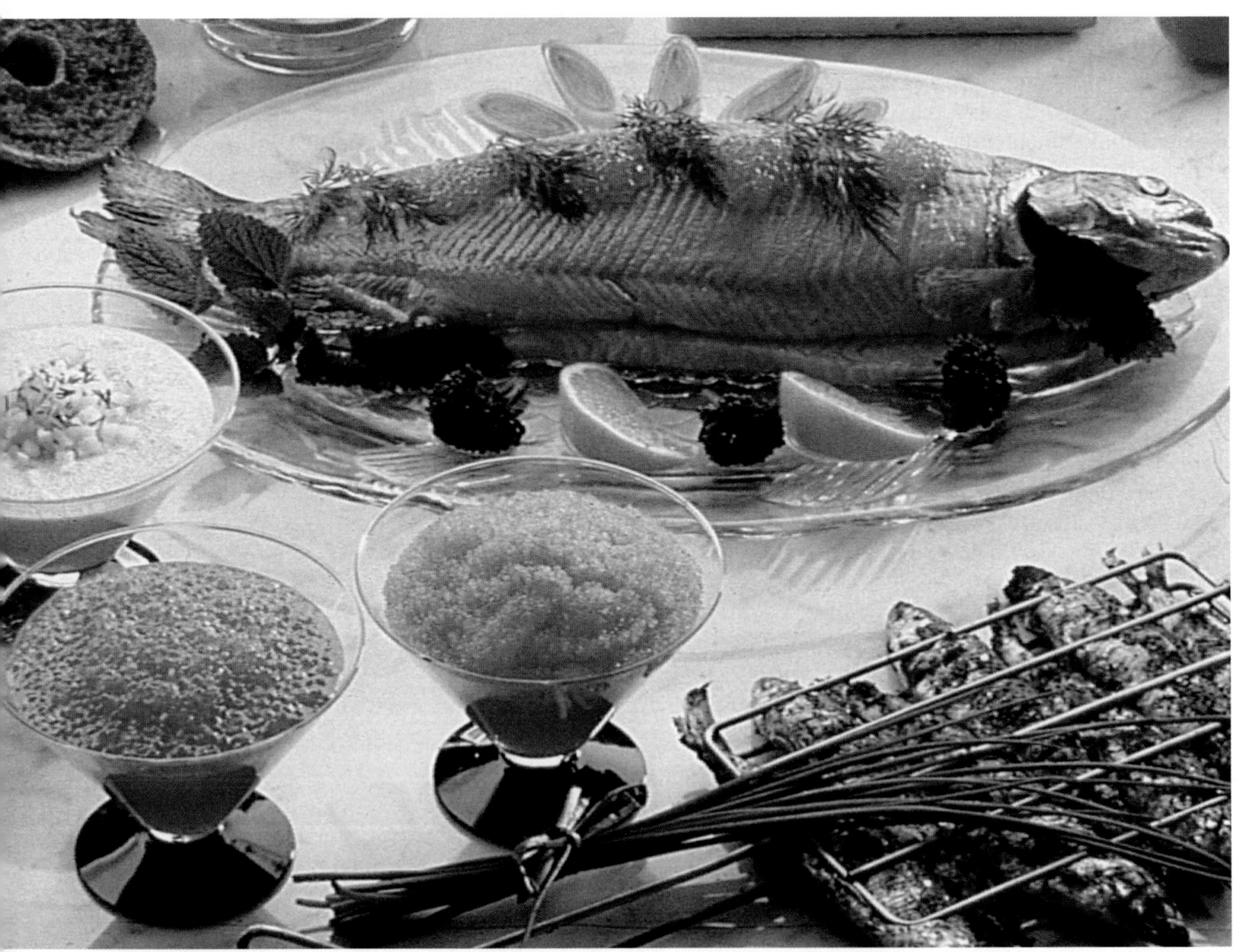

Finnish Tourist Board

31-6 *Much of the caviar consumed throughout the world comes from the Caspian Sea, which borders Iran.*

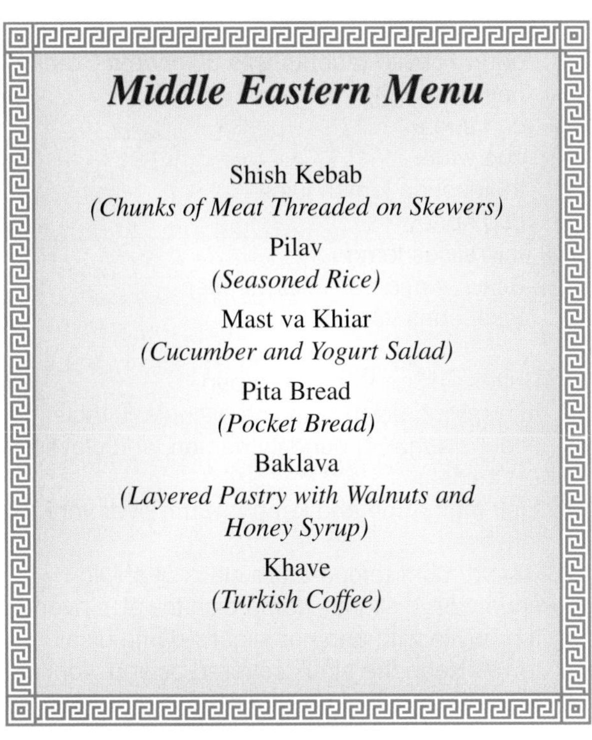

Shish Kebabs

(Chunks of Meat Threaded on Skewers)
Serves 8

1 large onion
4 tablespoons olive oil
1/2 cup lemon juice
1 teaspoon salt
1/2 teaspoon pepper
1/2 teaspoon garlic powder
2 pounds lean, boneless lamb cut into 2-inch cubes
4 large tomatoes, quartered
4 large green peppers, cut into chunks
1/4 cup evaporated fat free milk

1. Remove papery covering from onion and slice into rings.
2. Put onion rings into deep pan. Add oil, lemon juice, salt, pepper, and garlic powder.
3. Add lamb cubes to marinade and stir well. Cover and place in refrigerator for at least 4 hours, turning lamb occasionally.
4. Preheat broiler.
5. Thread lamb cubes on eight long skewers.
6. Thread tomato quarters and green pepper chunks on two more skewers.
7. Place skewers of meat side by side along the length of a deep roasting pan. Brush meat with evaporated milk.
8. Broil 4 inches from the heat, turning occasionally, until meat reaches the desired degree of doneness, about 10 minutes for pink lamb and 15 minutes for well-done lamb.
9. Add vegetables to roasting pan about a third of the way through the cooking period. Watch carefully and remove when tender. Serve lamb with broiled vegetables and pilav.

Per serving: 157 cal. (42% from fat), 16 g protein, 7 g carbohydrate, 7 g fat, 50 mg cholesterol, 2 g fiber, 133 mg sodium.

Pilav

(Seasoned Rice)
Serves 6 to 8

2 tablespoons margarine
1 1/2 cups uncooked white rice
3 cups low-sodium chicken stock
salt
pepper
1 tablespoon melted margarine

1. In heavy saucepan, melt 2 tablespoons margarine.
2. Add rice and stir for several minutes to evenly coat rice with fat. (Do not let rice brown.)
3. Add chicken stock and salt and pepper to taste.
4. Bring mixture to a boil, stirring constantly.
5. Cover pan, reduce heat, and simmer rice slowly for 20 minutes or until all the liquid has been absorbed.
6. Add melted margarine, stir with a fork.
7. Let rice stand, covered with a clean towel, for 20 minutes before serving.

Per serving: 224 cal. (24% from fat), 3 g protein, 38 g carbohydrate, 6 g fat, 0 mg cholesterol, 1 g fiber, 160 mg sodium.

Mast va Khiar

(Cucumber and Yogurt Salad)
Serves 8

2 medium cucumbers
4 tablespoons finely chopped green pepper
3 tablespoons finely chopped green onion
2 tablespoons dried tarragon or dill
1 teaspoon lime juice
1/2 teaspoon salt
2 cups plain nonfat yogurt

1. Wash cucumbers and peel.
2. Slice each cucumber in half lengthwise. Scoop out seeds and chop cucumber coarsely.

3. Put cucumber in a deep bowl and add green pepper, green onion, tarragon or dill, lime juice, and salt. Mix well.
4. Add yogurt and stir to coat vegetables.
5. Chill at least one hour before serving.

Per serving: 40 cal. (4% from fat), 4 g protein, 6 g carbohydrate, 0 g fat, 1 mg cholesterol, 0 g fiber, 178 mg sodium.

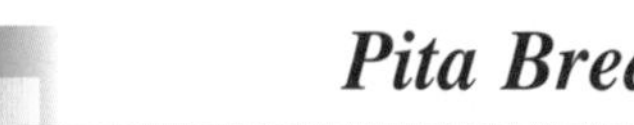

Pita Bread

(Pocket Bread)
Makes 18

5 to 6 cups all-purpose flour
1 package active dry yeast
2 cups water
2 tablespoons sugar
1½ teaspoons salt

1. In large mixing bowl, stir together 2 cups flour and yeast.
2. Heat water, sugar, and salt over low heat until warm (105°F to 115°F), stirring to blend.
3. Add liquid ingredients to flour mixture and beat until smooth, about 2 minutes on medium speed of electric mixer.
4. Add 1 cup flour and beat 1 minute more.
5. Stir in enough additional flour to make a moderately stiff dough.
6. Turn dough out onto lightly floured board or pastry cloth and knead until smooth and satiny, about 18 to 20 minutes.
7. Divide dough into 18 portions. Roll each into a 3-inch circle.
8. Place circles on lightly greased baking sheet. Cover with a clean towel and let rise in warm place until doubled, about 45 minutes.
9. Bake on middle shelf of preheated 450°F oven, 10 to 12 minutes or until lightly browned. Cool.

Per pita: 133 cal. (2% from fat), 4 g protein, 28 g carbohydrate, 0 g fat, 0 mg cholesterol, 1 g fiber, 179 mg sodium.

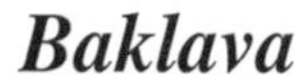

Baklava

(Layered Pastry with Walnuts and Honey Syrup)
Makes about 3 dozen pieces

4 cups walnuts, finely chopped
5 tablespoons sugar
1 teaspoon ground cinnamon
dash ground cloves
¾ cup margarine
1 pound phyllo (about 20 to 30 sheets Greek pastry dough)
1 cup sugar
1 cup water
1 tablespoon lemon juice
½ cup honey
4 thin slices lemon
3-inch cinnamon stick, broken
2 teaspoons vanilla

1. Butter a 13 × 9 × 2-inch pan.
2. In a mixing bowl, combine walnuts, 5 tablespoons sugar, ground cinnamon, and cloves; set aside.
3. Melt margarine and keep it warm over very low heat.
4. Unfold room temperature stack of phyllo sheets on a slightly damp dish towel. Cover the phyllo with another slightly damp dish towel. Keep the stack covered as you work.
5. Place 2 sheets of phyllo pastry in the prepared pan, folding edges to fit pan. Brush evenly with melted margarine. Place another sheet of phyllo in the pan and brush it with margarine. Continue layering phyllo sheets and brushing them with margarine until 5 sheets have been used.
6. Sprinkle 1 cup nut mixture over the buttered top sheet. Place 5 more sheets of phyllo over the nut layer, brushing each sheet with margarine. Repeat this step three more times, using all the nut mixture and ending with 5 sheets of phyllo brushed with margarine on top.
7. Preheat oven to 350°F.
8. With a very sharp knife, cut the baklava diagonally into diamond-shaped pieces.
9. Sprinkle any remaining margarine over the top.
10. Bake baklava for 30 minutes.
11. Reduce heat to 300°F and continue to bake for 45 minutes more.
12. While baklava is baking, prepare syrup. In medium saucepan, combine 1 cup sugar, water, lemon juice, honey, lemon slices, and cinnamon stick. Bring to a boil, stirring until sugar is dissolved.
13. Simmer syrup uncovered for 10 minutes.
14. Remove lemon slices and cinnamon stick. Add vanilla. Set syrup aside to cool.
15. As soon as baklava comes out of the oven, pour the syrup over the hot pastry. Allow the pastry to set for several hours before serving.

Per serving: 196 cal. (55% from fat), 3 g protein, 20 g carbohydrate, 12 g fat, 0 mg cholesterol, 1 g fiber, 107 mg sodium.

Israel

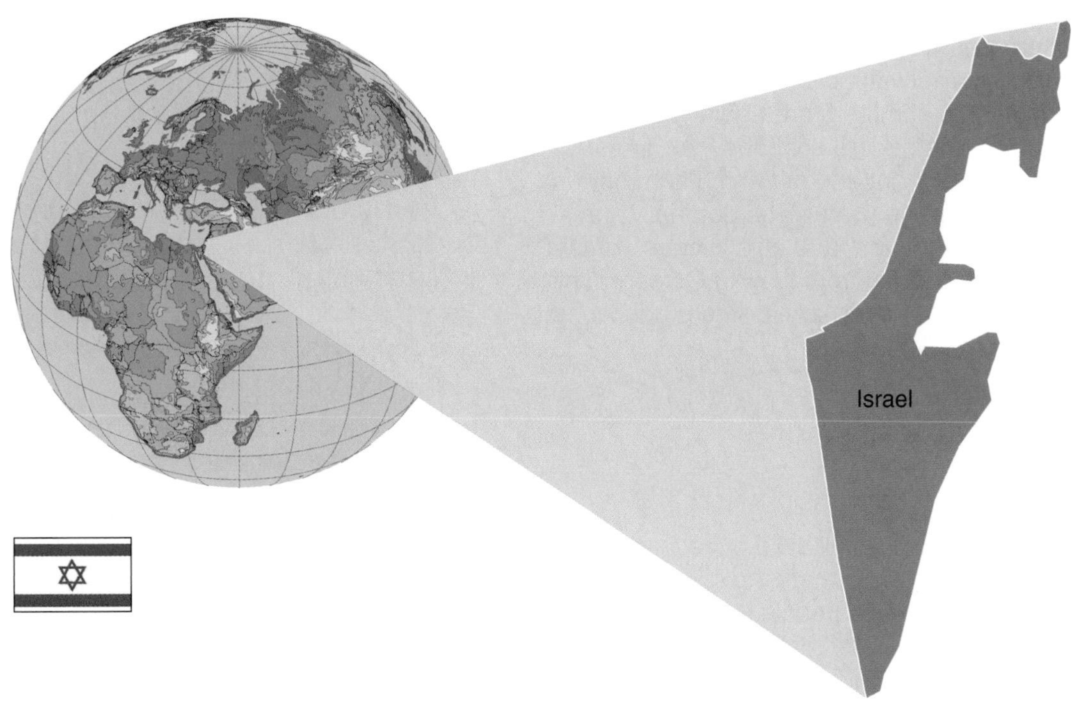

To Jewish people throughout the world, the date May 14, 1948, has a special meaning. On this date, the state of Israel was established. Israel was founded on the land that had been called Palestine for centuries. This land was the birthplace of the Jews. For the first time in more than 2,000 years, Jews were able to govern themselves.

Since 1948, Israel has grown at a tremendous rate. Irrigation systems and modern farming techniques have increased agricultural production. Heavy industry flourishes in Haifa, Israel's largest seaport. As the home of many talented writers, artists, and musicians, Israel also has flourished as a cultural center.

Geography and Climate of Israel

The Mediterranean Sea forms Israel's western border. The northern part of the country borders Syria and Lebanon. There the land rises from a fertile coastal plain to the hills of Galilee. Galilee's scattered green valleys are suitable for agriculture. To the east is the Jordan River, which separates Israel from Jordan. To the south lies the triangular Negev Desert bordered by Egypt and the Red Sea.

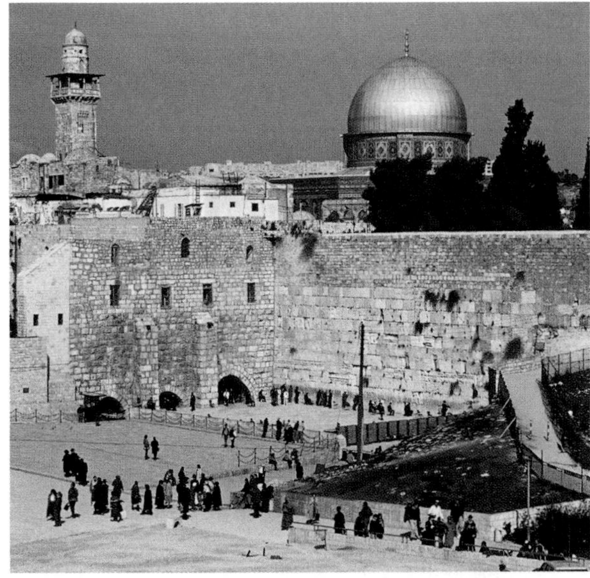

Jerusalem is considered a holy city by Jewish, Christian, and Muslim people throughout the world.

Israel has four climatic regions. Along the Mediterranean Sea, summers are warm, and winters are mild with occasional rain. In the central highlands, summers are again warm and dry, but the winters are cold and wet. The Negev Desert is hot and dry in the summer and cool and dry in the winter. The Jordan Valley has hot, dry summers and mild winters. Almost no rain falls in Israel from May to October. This makes irrigation necessary for the production of most crops.

Q: How does kosher salt differ from table salt?

A: Kosher salt is coarser and flakier than table salt. Many chefs prefer these properties when making a salt crust on meat or adding a pinch of salt for flavor. However, these properties keep kosher salt from being a good choice for baking.

Israeli Culture

Periods of peace followed by revolts, invasions, and foreign rule mark the history of Palestine. The Jewish population gradually dwindled. Some Jews were killed or sold into slavery. Some fled to nearby Middle Eastern countries and to other countries around the world. The Jews were physically separated from their homeland and from one another. Even so, they were able to keep their identity and religion. Jews around the world waited for the time when they could return to the place of their birth.

The movement of Jews back into Palestine began in the second half of the nineteenth century. However, the present state of Israel was not declared until 1948. Since that time, territorial disputes with neighboring Arabs have marked Israeli history. Even so, growth and progress continue at a rapid rate.

Almost all the fruits and vegetables eaten in Israel are grown there. Guavas, citrus fruits, mangoes, dates, bananas, avocados, and melons are some of the most popular fruits. Cattle, sheep, poultry, and fish are also available from local sources. Cattle breeds that are suitable for the semiarid land are raised. Fresh fish and ducks are scientifically raised on farm ponds.

Many of the farms in Israel operate as collective communities called ***kibbutzim.*** Members of a kibbutz own their property collectively and live together in a cluster of dwellings. They receive no wages for their work, but all their needs are met. Food, clothing, medical care, and entertainment are supplied. Children who live in a kibbutz are educated communally according to age. A kibbutz may have from 30 to 2,000 members and may or may not have a few small industries.

Jerusalem, Israel's capital, has been an important city to people of many nationalities and religions for centuries. Jerusalem is called the "Holy City" by Christians, Jews, and Muslims.

Israeli Holidays

Holidays are an important part of the culture in Israel. Over 80 percent of Israel's citizens are Jewish, so most of the holidays revolve around the Jewish faith. These celebrations always begin and end at sunset. Many of them involve special food traditions. For instance, *Rosh Hashanah* begins a period called the Ten Days of Repentance. This holiday celebrates the Jewish New Year. On this day, Jews in Israel eat sweet foods, such as sliced apples, honey cookies, and sweet potato pudding. They hope eating these foods will bring a new year that is sweet and happy. The last of the Ten Days of Repentance is called *Yom Kippur*. This is the holiest day of the year. Jewish people spend the day at the synagogue fasting, praying, and reading.

Chanukah is an eight-day festival in December. It commemorates the regaining of Jewish control of the Temple in Jerusalem. Chanukah is sometimes called the Festival of Lights. During this holiday, families light candles in a nine-branched candlestick called a *menorah*. Traditional Chanukah foods include *latkes* (potato pancakes) and *sufganiyah* (doughnuts).

Pesakh, or Passover, is celebrated for eight days in the spring. It commemorates the Jews' freedom from slavery in Egypt thousands of years ago. On the first evening of Passover, families share the *seder*. This is a traditional meal of specific foods, each with a symbolic meaning. Bitter herbs, such as horseradish, are eaten as a symbol of the bitterness of slavery. Parsley represents the coming of spring. ***Matzo*** is an unleavened bread. It reminds the Jews their ancestors had no time to let bread rise when they were fleeing Egypt. A roasted egg and a shank of lamb symbolize beasts given to God as sacrifices. A dish of salt water stands for the tears of the Hebrew slaves. *Charoset*, a mixture of nuts, apples, and wine, represents the cement the slaves used to build cities for the Egyptians. See 31-7.

Israeli Cuisine

When the Jews fled from Palestine, they settled in many parts of the world. Thus Jewish cuisine is multinational. This is most noticeable in Israel. For there, people of 80 nationalities have added their foods to the area's native Middle Eastern cuisine. Borscht, sauerbraten, and shish kebab might be listed in an Israeli cookbook along with kreplach, challah, and blintzes.

Besides this mixture of native and ethnic Jewish foods, Israeli cooks have developed totally new dishes. These dishes are based on foods readily available in Israel. Many of them contain fish, poultry, and fresh fruit.

Jewish Dietary Laws

People in most Israeli homes and restaurants observe the Jewish ***kashrut*** (dietary laws). Foods prepared according to the dietary laws are considered ***kosher.***

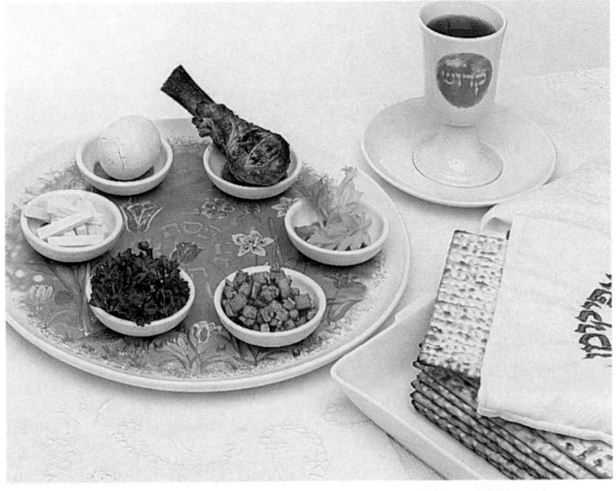

The B. Manischewitz Company, Jersey City, NJ

31-7 Jewish people eat a ceremonial seder meal on the first evening of Passover. Each of the traditional foods on the seder plate has a special symbolism.

The first of these laws concerns foods that are suitable for eating. Only animals that have cloven (split) hoofs and chew their cud are considered fit to eat. Therefore, Jews cannot eat pigs because pigs do not chew their cud. Fish must have both scales and fins. Therefore, people cannot eat shellfish. They can eat domestic fowl, but not wild fowl. Cooks must carefully check vegetables and cereals to be sure they are free of insects. They must break eggs into a separate dish and inspect them for blood spots before using them. Manufactured products must not contain any nonkosher ingredients.

Other dietary laws describe the proper methods of slaughter. According to these laws, a ***shohet*** (licensed slaughterer) must slaughter all animals and fowl.

There are distinctions between ***milchig*** (dairy) and ***fleishig*** (meat) ***foods.*** People cannot cook or eat milchig and fleishig foods together. For this reason, kosher kitchens contain two complete sets of eating, serving, and food preparation utensils. Cooks use one set for milchig foods. They use the other set for fleishig foods. People may eat fleishig foods after milchig foods—but only if they thoroughly cleanse their mouth first. They cannot eat milchig foods for three hours after fleishig foods.

Foods that are neither milchig nor fleishig are called ***pareve foods.*** Pareve foods include eggs, fruits, vegetables, cereals, fish, and baked goods made with vegetable shortening, 31-8. Except for fish, pareve foods can be prepared and eaten with both milk and meat dishes.

Traditional Jewish Dishes

For centuries, soups have played an important part in Jewish cooking. They are hot, filling, and relatively inexpensive. Soups may be clear or thick. Chicken soup is perhaps the best-known clear soup. Lentil soup is perhaps the best-known thick soup. Other popular soups include borscht, barley and bean, and fruit soup.

Jewish cooks serve many Jewish soups with *knaidlach* or *mandlen.* Both are similar to dumplings and are frequently made with *matzo meal* (meal made from matzos).

Gefilte fish is another popular Jewish dish. A variety of freshwater fish may be used to make gefilte fish. However, pike, carp, and whitefish are most common. The cook forms a minced

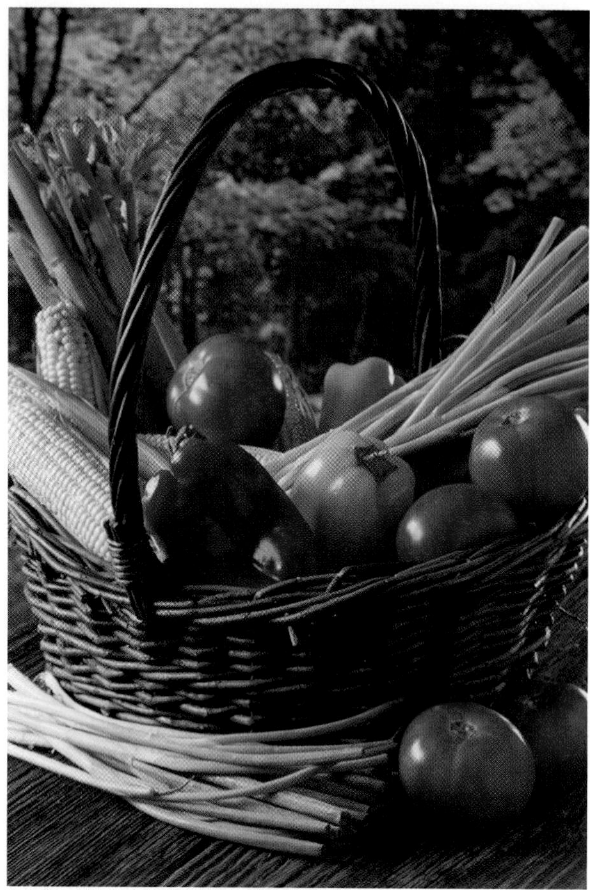

31-8 Vegetables are considered pareve foods according to Jewish dietary laws, so they can accompany either dairy products or meat.

fish mixture into balls the size of small dumplings. Then he or she either bakes the gefilte fish or simmers it in fish stock with a few vegetables.

Chicken is both versatile and economical. Cooks boil and roast chicken and use it to make soup. Other popular Jewish chicken dishes include gizzards simmered in seasoned gravy. Chopped chicken liver and neck skin stuffed with seasoned bread crumbs are well-liked chicken dishes, too.

Homemade noodles and dumplings are frequent additions to soups, main dishes, and puddings. They are also used to make the popular kreplach. *Kreplach* are squares of noodle dough stuffed with a filling made of meat, cheese, potato, chicken, or chicken liver. Kreplach may also be stuffed with kasha, which is cooked, coarsely ground, hulled buckwheat.

Kugels, which resemble puddings, may contain vegetables, fruits, noodles, rice, or fish. A kugel may be a separate course or a side dish. Sweet kugels are often served for dessert.

Tzimmes are combinations of meats, vegetables, and fruits. Although the cook's imagination determines the choice of ingredients, long, slow cooking improves the flavor of all tzimmes.

Blintzes, knishes, latkes, and challah have been Jewish specialties for centuries. *Blintzes* are thin pancakes similar to French crêpes. Blintzes are browned on one side only. Then they are filled with a cheese or fruit filling and folded like a napkin with the browned side up. Knishes are dumplings. They may be filled with potato, cheese, meat, or chicken. *Latkes* (pancakes) can be made from matzo meal, buckwheat, or wheat flour. However, potato latkes, which are similar to German potato pancakes, are particularly popular. *Challah* is a braided, rich egg bread. Jewish people often serve it at holiday meals. See 31-9.

Middle Eastern Foods

Many of the foods found in Israel originated in other Middle Eastern countries. One of these foods, felafel, has become one of Israel's national dishes. ***Felafel*** is a mixture of ground chickpeas, bulgur, and spices that is formed into balls and deep-fried. The warm balls of felafel are tucked inside a half slice of Arab bread and served with a salad.

A variety of salads and colorful, spicy hot hashes have North African origins. *Couscous,* for example, is a thick, steamed semolina porridge flavored with chicken and spices.

Leben is an Israeli delicacy. It is a type of cheese made from sour milk. Jewish people often serve it with crackers as an appetizer.

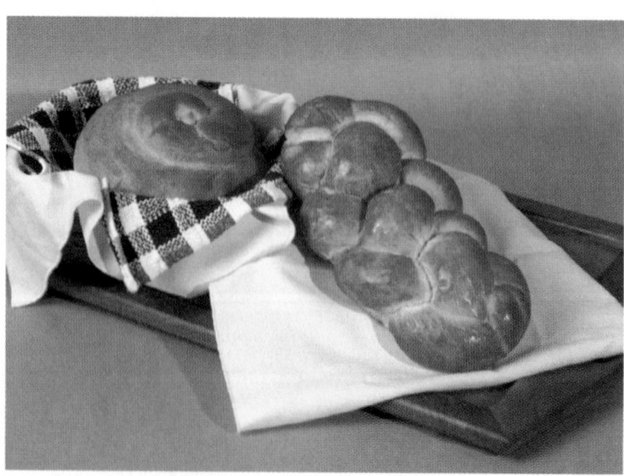

Jack Klasey

31-9 *Challah is a traditional Jewish holiday bread.*

Israeli Additions

The citrus fruits, figs, dates, almonds, grapes, and melons that grow abundantly in Israel have inspired many new dishes. Turkey pieces coated with flour, browned, and stewed in orange juice with peas and mushrooms is uniquely Israeli. Avocado halves stuffed with a mixture of walnuts, pistachios, sour cherries, and marinated herring is a new native dish, too.

Some desserts are also uniquely Israeli. For instance, sabra liqueur has the flavor of the Jaffa orange. Jewish cooks use it to make a rich dessert. They dip chocolate cookies into hot, strong coffee. Then they arrange the cookies in layers with whipped cream flavored with the liqueur. After chilling, the dessert is cut into pieces and served like a cake.

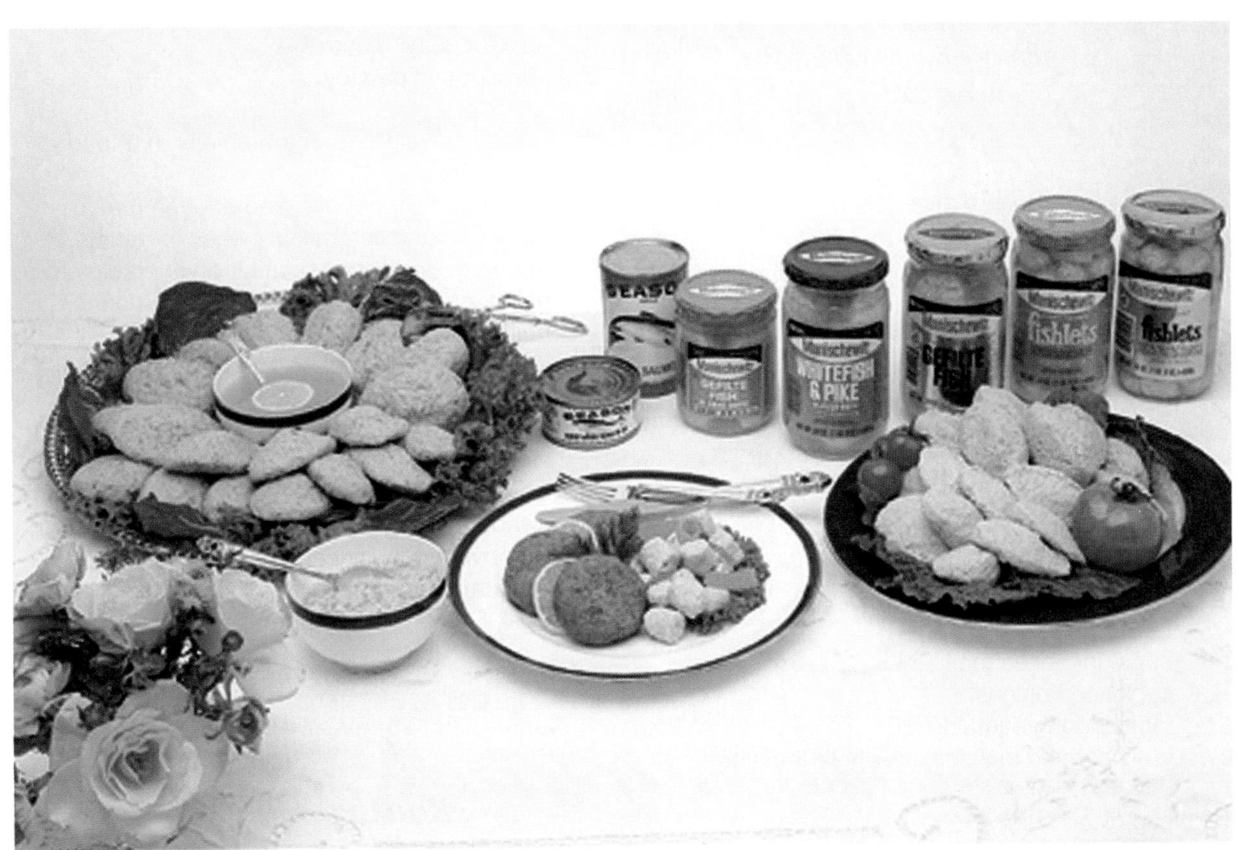

The B. Manischewitz Company, Jersey City, NJ

Baked gefilte fish is a popular Jewish dish.

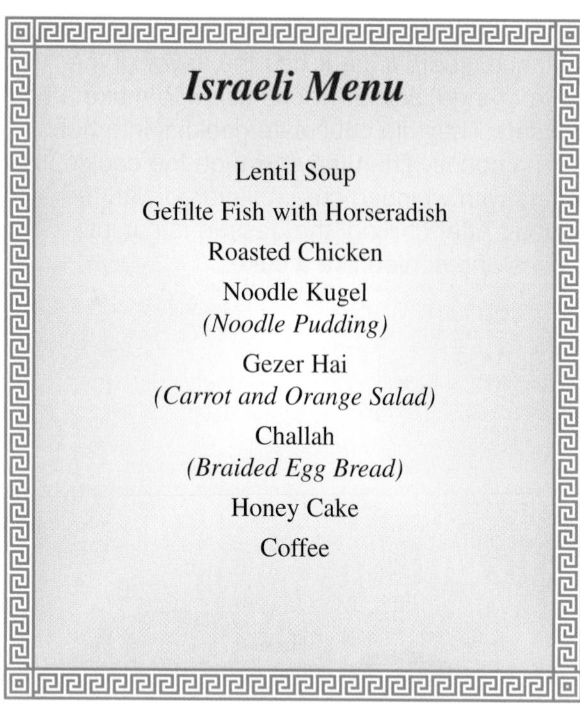

Israeli Menu

Lentil Soup
Gefilte Fish with Horseradish
Roasted Chicken
Noodle Kugel
(Noodle Pudding)
Gezer Hai
(Carrot and Orange Salad)
Challah
(Braided Egg Bread)
Honey Cake
Coffee

Lentil Soup

Serves 6 to 8

1¹/₄ cups uncooked lentils
1 cup sliced onions
1 tablespoon vegetable oil
2¹/₂ cups canned low-sodium whole tomatoes, mashed slightly
1 cup diced celery
³/₄ cup diced carrots
³/₄ cup diced parsnips
³/₄ cup chopped green pepper
6 cups cold water
³/₄ teaspoon salt
¹/₂ teaspoon pepper

1. Wash and sort lentils. Set aside.
2. In Dutch oven or large saucepan, saute onions in oil until browned.
3. Add lentils, tomatoes, celery, carrots, parsnips, green pepper, water, and seasonings. Bring to a boil.
4. Reduce heat and cover pan. Simmer soup about 40 minutes, or until lentils are very tender.

Per serving: 205 cal. (13% from fat), 11 g protein, 35 g carbohydrate, 3 g fat, 0 mg cholesterol, 16 g fiber, 339 mg sodium.

Gefilte Fish

Makes 6 to 8 appetizer servings

1 pound skinless whitefish fillets
1 medium onion
1 egg
¹/₂ teaspoon salt
¹/₄ teaspoon pepper
2 to 3 tablespoons matzo meal
4 cups vegetable stock
1 medium onion, chopped
1 carrot, diced
1 stalk celery, diced
2 teaspoons parsley

1. Grind fish with one of the onions in a food processor.
2. Add egg, salt, pepper, and enough matzo meal to make fish mixture easy to handle.
3. In a large saucepan, combine vegetable stock, onion, carrot, celery, and parsley. Bring to a boil, then reduce heat to a simmer.
4. With wet hands, shape fish mixture into balls, using about ¹/₄ cup mixture for each.
5. Gently lower the fish balls into the simmering stock.
6. Cover and simmer for 1 hour and 10 minutes without stirring.
7. Remove fish balls carefully to a bowl. Strain stock and pour it over the fish balls.
8. Chill. Serve with horseradish.

Per serving: 177 cal. (36% from fat), 20 g protein, 8 g carbohydrate, 7 g fat, 93 mg cholesterol, 1 g fiber, 267 mg sodium.

Roasted Chicken

Serves 8

2 roasting chickens, 2 pounds each
margarine, softened
salt and pepper

1. Preheat oven to 350°F.
2. Remove heart, liver, and giblets from chickens.
3. Rinse chickens under cool running water. Pat dry with paper towels.
4. Place chickens breast side up on rack in roasting pan.
5. Rub skin with margarine. Sprinkle with salt and pepper.
6. Roast, uncovered, about 1¹/₂ hours or until meat thermometer inserted into the thickest part of the thigh reads 180°F.

7. Carve chickens and remove skin before serving.

Per serving: 165 cal. (44% from fat) 21 g protein, 0 g carbohydrate, 8 g fat, 65 mg cholesterol, 0 g fiber, 96 mg sodium.

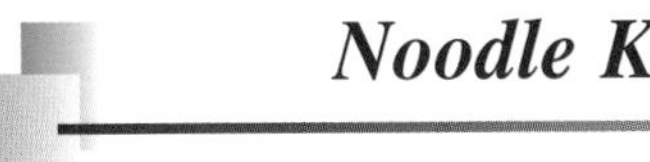

Noodle Kugel

(Noodle Pudding)
Serves 8

3	eggs
4	tablespoons light brown sugar
1/4	teaspoon nutmeg
1/2	teaspoon cinnamon
4	cups cooked wide egg noodles
2/3	cup seedless raisins
1/2	cup sliced blanched almonds
1	tablespoon lemon juice
2	tablespoons melted margarine
3	tablespoons bread crumbs

1. Preheat oven to 350°F.
2. In large bowl, beat eggs until foamy.
3. Add brown sugar, nutmeg, and cinnamon and continue beating until well mixed.
4. Fold in noodles, raisins, almonds, lemon juice, and melted margarine.
5. Pour into a 1½-quart greased casserole or ring mold.
6. Sprinkle with bread crumbs.
7. Bake for 50 minutes or until browned.

Per serving: 277 cal. (34% from fat), 8 g protein, 39 g carbohydrate, 11 g fat, 128 mg cholesterol, 3 g fiber, 83 mg sodium.

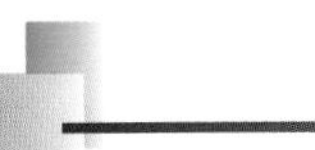

Gezer Hai

(Carrot and Orange Salad)
Serves 8

1	cup fresh orange juice
1/4	teaspoon ground ginger
1/4	teaspoon salt
2	tablespoons lemon juice
1	tablespoon honey
4	cups coarsely grated carrots
2	navel oranges
	salad greens

1. In small bowl, mix together orange juice, ginger, salt, lemon juice, and honey.
2. Pour over carrots, cover, and refrigerate for at least an hour.
3. When ready to serve, peel and section oranges.
4. Line 8 small salad plates with salad greens.
5. Top greens with grated carrots.
6. Garnish with orange sections. Serve at once.

Per serving: 72 cal. (0% from fat), 2 g protein, 17 g carbohydrate, 0 g fat, 0 mg cholesterol, 4 g fiber, 98 mg sodium.

Challah

(Braided Egg Bread)
Makes 2 loaves

4 1/2 to 5 1/2	cups all-purpose flour
2	tablespoons sugar
1 1/2	teaspoons salt
1	package active dry yeast
1/3	cup softened margarine
	pinch powdered saffron (optional)
1	cup very warm water (120°F to 130°F)
3	eggs (at room temperature)
1	teaspoon cold water
1	teaspoon poppy seeds

1. In large mixing bowl, combine 1 1/4 cups flour, sugar, salt, and dry yeast.
2. Work in softened margarine with pastry blender or two knives.
3. Dissolve saffron in the very warm water. Gradually add water to dry ingredients, beating on medium speed of electric mixer for 2 minutes, scraping bowl occasionally.
4. Divide one of the eggs and set aside the yolk. Add the egg white and the other two eggs to the dough mixture along with 1/2 cup flour. Beat at high speed for 2 minutes.
5. Stir in enough additional flour to form a stiff dough.
6. Turn dough out onto a lightly floured board or pastry cloth. Knead until smooth and elastic, about 8 to 10 minutes.
7. Place dough in greased bowl, turning once to grease top.
8. Cover with a clean towel and let rise in a warm place until doubled in bulk, about 1 hour.
9. Punch dough down and divide it in half. Divide each half into three strips. Place strips side by side on a lightly greased baking sheet and braid, pinching ends to seal.
10. Braid the second loaf.
11. Beat together reserved egg yolk with 1 teaspoon cold water.
12. Brush loaves with egg wash and sprinkle with poppy seeds.

13. Let rise in a warm place until doubled in bulk, about 1 hour.
14. Bake at 400°F for 20 to 25 minutes or until loaves sound hollow when tapped with knuckles.
15. Remove loaves from baking sheets and place on cooling racks.

Per slice: 92 cal. (25% from fat), 2 g protein, 14 g carbohydrate, 3 g fat, 26 mg cholesterol, 1 g fiber, 129 mg sodium.

Honey Cake

Serves 12

2 tablespoons vegetable oil
1 cup sugar
3 eggs
2/3 cup cold strong coffee
1 cup honey
3 cups cake flour
2 teaspoons baking powder
1 teaspoon baking soda
1 teaspoon cinnamon
1/2 teaspoon ginger
1/2 teaspoon nutmeg
1/2 cup blanched almonds, chopped (reserve a few for the top)
1/2 cup seedless raisins

1. Preheat oven to 350°F.
2. In large mixer bowl, combine oil, sugar, and eggs. Beat until light and fluffy.
3. In small bowl, combine coffee and honey.
4. Sift together flour, baking powder, baking soda, cinnamon, ginger, and nutmeg.
5. Add dry ingredients alternately with liquid ingredients to egg mixture.
6. Fold in almonds and raisins.
7. Pour batter into a greased and floured 9-inch tube pan.
8. Sprinkle batter with the reserved almonds.
9. Bake for 45 minutes to 1 hour, or until toothpick inserted in center comes out clean.

Per piece: 332 cal. (18% from fat), 5 g protein, 66 g carbohydrate, 7 g fat, 69 mg cholesterol, 2 g fiber, 143 mg sodium.

Africa

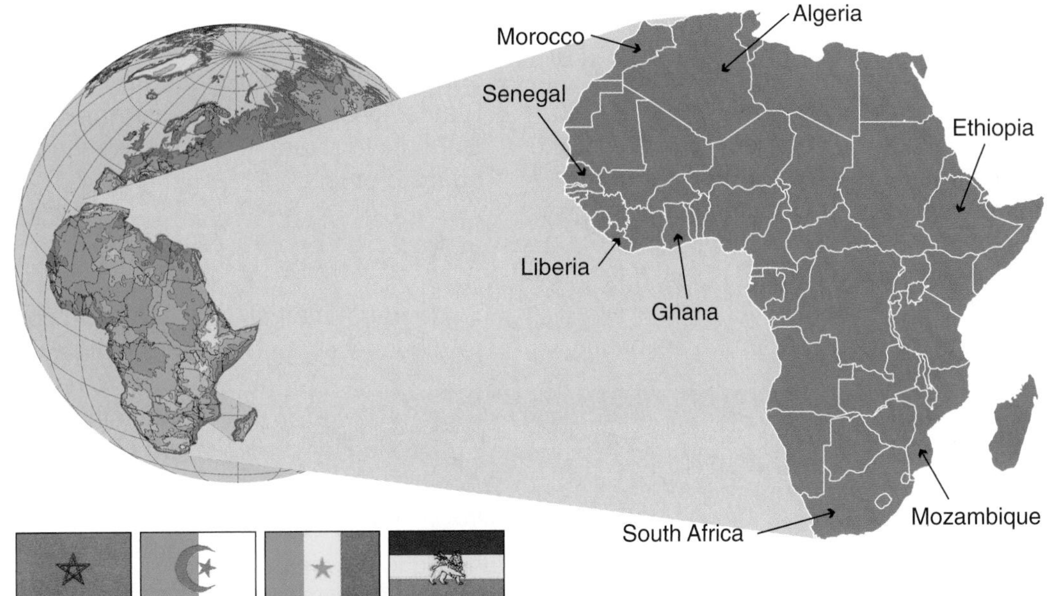

Africa is the second largest continent; only Asia is larger. Africa shares the title of warmest continent with South America. The geographic extremes of Africa range from sandy deserts to tropical forests.

The countries of Africa are as varied as its geography. Much of Africa is in a state of political, economic, and cultural development. Therefore, Africa does not have a typical cuisine. Each African nation has unique foods.

Climate and Geography of Africa

Since the equator runs through the middle of Africa, both the extreme northern and southern countries have subtropical climates. Summers are dry, with the highest monthly average temperature above 72°F (22°C). Monthly winter temperatures average above

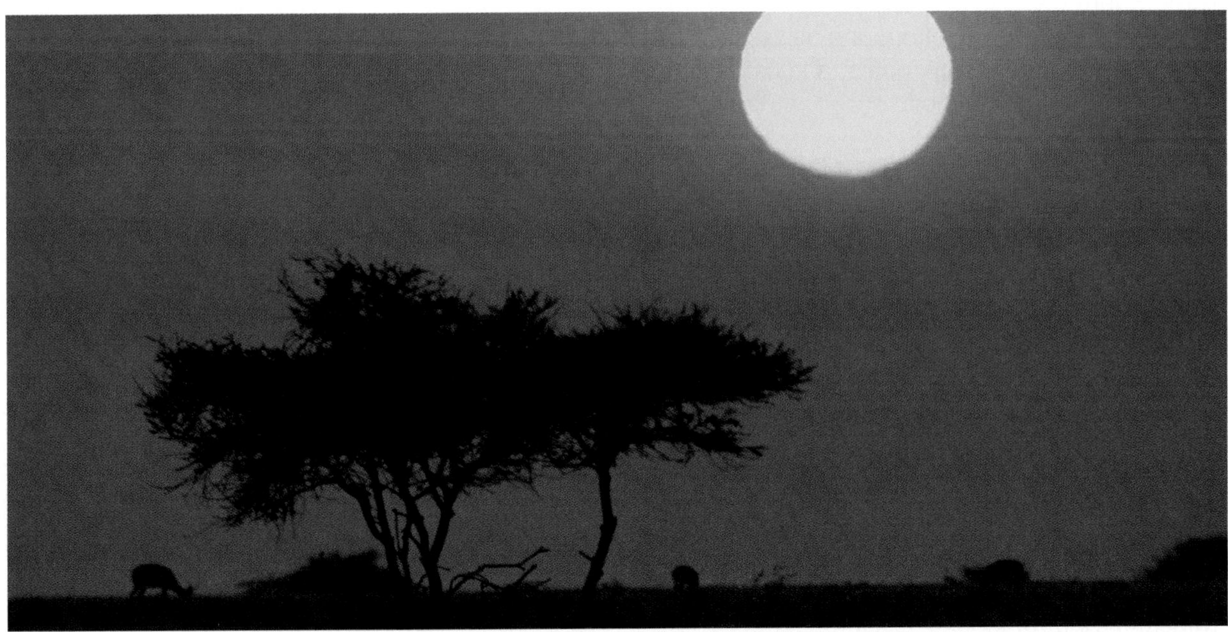

Wide open African plains have an untouched, natural beauty.

50°F (10°C). In these areas, grains such as millet, teff, and sorghum grow well.

Along the equator in central and western Africa, temperatures range between 64°F (18°C) and 80°F (27°C) year round. This area has rainfall throughout the year. In these tropical, humid sections, root crops and vegetables are grown. Other products include palm oil, groundnuts (peanuts), bananas, dates, figs, plantains, citrus fruits, sugarcane, coffee, and cacao. (***Cacao*** is a plant that produces beans that are ground into cocoa or made into chocolate.)

The majority of the people in Africa live on the savannas, or grasslands. These are the broad areas above and below the equatorial belt. They receive less precipitation and have greater temperature ranges. Raising crops is difficult and unprofitable on the savannas because the soil is poor. The soil has little *humus,* a substance formed by decayed matter. Humus holds water near the ground surface, within reach of plant roots.

North and south of the savannas are the deserts. Average summer temperatures may reach 98°F (37°C) and winter temperatures never drop below 59°F (15°C). Rain, when it falls, is brief. In the deserts, there are places called oases where water is available. Groups of people known as nomads move from one oasis to another. They herd sheep, goats, and camels as was done in primitive times.

Healthy Living

When on a long airplane flight, try to prop up your feet. This will allow increased circulation in your legs and reduce your risk of getting swollen feet and ankles.

African Culture

Native Africans make up over 70 percent of Africa's population. Over five million people of European descent also live in Africa.

More than 800 languages are spoken in Africa. Most Africans speak a local language in their home village. They also speak an interchange language to communicate with people outside their village.

Over half the people in Africa have not had an opportunity to attend school. Therefore, few Africans can read or write. This has made it hard for African governments to communicate modern ideas to their people. To help solve this problem, African governments send some students to schools in Europe and the United States. In payment, the governments expect students to return to their native lands and help educate others.

African Holidays

Many of the holidays in African countries are religious festivals. Therefore, holidays vary from region to region, depending on the main form of religion. Muslims in Africa observe such events as the Fast of Ramadan. Christmas and Easter are celebrated by African Christians. Besides these holy days, New Year festivals are popular in Africa. Many areas hold harvest festivals in the autumn. Independence day celebrations are also common in Africa. The people celebrate the days their nations gained freedom from the European countries that colonized them. These festivals often involve parades, speeches, parties, and fireworks. Music, dancing, and the wearing of masks are part of many African festivals, too.

African Cuisine

Each African country has unique dishes. However, similarities exist among the foods of a region. For instance, *akla* is a popular snack food in Ghana, a country in western Africa. It is made of cowpeas, which are cooked, mashed, formed into balls, and fried. This dish, known by many other names, is also found in other west African countries.

Most African people do not have refrigerators. Cooks who live in cities are likely to take daily trips to the market to buy fresh ingredients. Those who live in rural areas often grow the fruits and vegetables they need.

A wide variety of fruits and vegetables grow in Africa. A *papaya* is a small melonlike fruit. A guava is a small fruit with many seeds. A *plantain* is like a banana, but it is much larger and has a bland flavor. *Cassava* is a root vegetable much like a sweet potato. *Okra,* which also grows in the United States, is a native African vegetable. See 31-10.

Some of the breads and pastries prepared in Africa are kesra, brik, and pita. *Kesra* is a round oven bread made in mountain villages. A *brik* is a pastry that is filled and then deep-fried. ***Pita bread*** is found throughout Africa as well as the Middle East. It is a flat, round, hollow bread. When cut in half, each half opens like a pocket and can be filled with meat or vegetables.

The French influenced the foods of the North African countries of Morocco, Senegal, and Algeria. In the ninteenth century, the French invaded these countries and brought their European customs to the region. A common meat in Algeria is lamb. It is usually grilled or stewed. *Mechoui* is lamb that has smoldered and cooked over a fire for many hours. The smoked head of a sheep is a delicacy.

Ghana is located on the midwestern coast of the African continent. This has made seafood an important ingredient in many of the spicy soups and stews served in this country. These main dishes are usually served with a starchy side dish, such as boiled yams, cassava, or plantains. These starchy vegetables may also be boiled and pounded into a dish called *fufu,* which is similar to dumplings.

Another country along the western coast is Liberia. Freed slaves from the United States founded Liberia in the late 1800s after the Civil War. The food of Liberia is similar to soul food in the United States. It is a combination of American and African cooking.

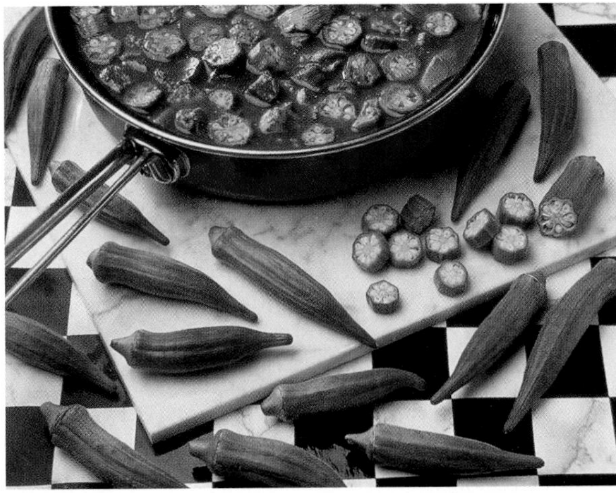

courtesy of W. Atlee Burpee & Co.

31-10 *Okra is a green, pod-shaped vegetable that was brought to the United States from Africa.*

One of the oldest countries in Africa is Ethiopia, which is located in the East. Christianity is the predominant religion in Ethiopia. Therefore, Ethiopian cuisine is not bound by the many religious dietary restrictions found in neighboring Muslim countries. Ethiopia's main dish is ***injera,*** which is a large sourdoughlike pancake made from teff. ***Teff*** is a milletlike grain grown only in Africa and the Middle East. Injera is served with ***wat,*** a spicy sauce or stew. Diners tear the injera into pieces, roll it around in the wat, and eat it with their fingers.

South Africa is an African country with many contrasts. Dutch, French, German, and British colonists brought foods to South Africa from their home nations. These European foods have been blended with native foods over the years.

Portuguese influence can be seen in the foods of Mozambique, a country in southeastern Africa. Chicken is cooked the Portuguese way with tomatoes and wine. Hot curries are another food typical of Mozambique.

Q: Where can I buy teff?

A: Teff is sold by some specialty grain suppliers and health food stores. If you can't find teff, you can substitute equal parts of wheat and rye flours. However, this mixture will not have the characteristic nutty flavor of teff.

African Meals

In urban areas of Africa, some people follow a daily meal pattern that includes breakfast, lunch, and dinner. However, people in rural areas are more likely to follow the traditional pattern of eating just two meals a day. Both meals, the first at midday and the second in the evening, are quite similar. They typically consist of a main dish soup or stew and a starchy accompaniment, such as rice or bread, 31-11.

Snacking is popular in Africa. In city streets, vendors sell such foods as fried plantains and broiled meat to satisfy hunger between meals.

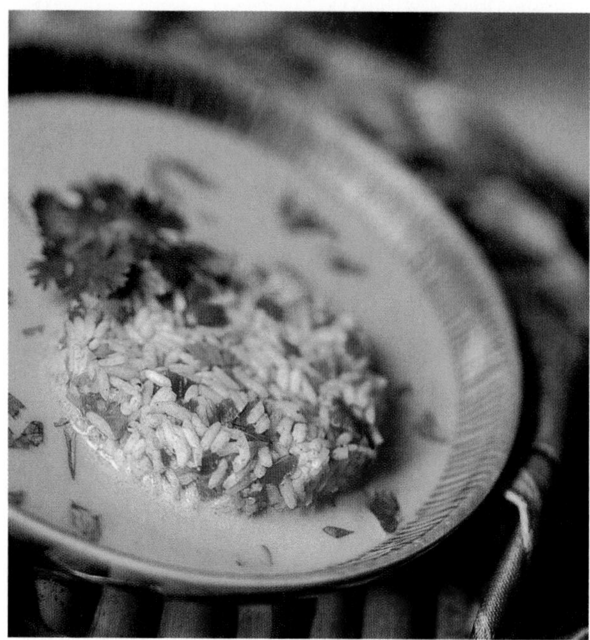

USA Rice Federation

31-11 *This African peanut soup is served with spicy rice that is molded into a rounded shape.*

Africans often serve meals on low tables with pillows, folded carpets, or the floor used as seats. Food is often served in the brass or earthenware vessels in which it was cooked. The food is usually arranged on one large tray and placed in the center of the table. Then each household member takes his or her individual share. Although diners do not use knives and forks, they may use spoons. However, they use the fingers of their right hands to eat most foods. They use flat breads to sop up the stews and sauces.

In most of Africa, a hand-washing ritual takes place before meals. A servant or member of the household brings in a long-necked pitcher of water and a bowl or basin. This person pours water over the hands of each household member and catches it in the basin. He or she then offers a small towel to dry the hands. Since diners eat most of the food with their fingers, this ritual is usually repeated after the meal.

African Menu

Meat on a Stick
(East Africa)
Spinach Stew
(West Africa)
Rice
Salatat Fijl wa Latsheen
(Radish and Orange Salad - North Africa)
Melktert
(Milk Pie - South Africa)
Coffee

Meat on a Stick

Serves 8

$^{3}/_{4}$ teaspoon cayenne pepper
1 teaspoon garlic salt
1 pound round steak
1 medium onion

1. Place 8 12-inch bamboo skewers in a 13 × 9-inch oblong pan. Cover with water and allow to soak for 30 minutes.
2. Cut round steak into 1-inch cubes.
3. Cut onion into 1-inch chunks.
4. Combine cayenne pepper and garlic salt in a resealable plastic bag.
5. Toss steak cubes, a few at a time, into the bag with the seasonings. Seal and shake to coat. Remove coated cubes from the bag and set aside while repeating coating process with remaining cubes.
6. Alternately thread steak cubes and onion chunks onto skewers.
7. Place skewers under broiler. Broil 4 to 5 minutes. Turn; broil another 4 to 5 minutes until meat is cooked and onions are browned.

Per serving: 72 cal. (38% from fat), 11 g protein, 1 g carbohydrate, 3 g fat, 28 mg cholesterol, 0 g fiber, 168 mg sodium.

Spinach Stew

Serves 6

1 medium onion, chopped
2 tablespoons peanut oil
1 medium tomato, cubed
6 tablespoons tomato paste, unsalted
1 10-ounce package frozen chopped spinach, thawed
1 12-ounce can corned beef hash
1 teaspoon cayenne pepper
$4^{1}/_{2}$ cups hot, cooked rice

1. In a large, nonstick skillet, saute onion in peanut oil over medium heat until tender.
2. Add tomatoes and tomato paste. Cook, stirring gently, until tomatoes are tender, about 5 minutes.
3. Add spinach, corned beef hash, and cayenne pepper. Reduce heat to low, cover, and cook for 30 minutes.
4. Serve over rice.

Per serving: 416 cal. (30% from fat), 21 g protein, 51 g carbohydrate, 14 g fat, 48 mg cholesterol, 2 g fiber, 615 mg sodium.

Salatat Fijl wa Latsheen

(Radish and Orange Salad)
Serves 6

6 seedless oranges
$^{1}/_{3}$ cup lemon juice
3 tablespoons sugar
$^{1}/_{4}$ teaspoon salt
1 bunch radishes
$^{1}/_{4}$ teaspoon cinnamon

1. Peel and section oranges into a large bowl.
2. In a separate bowl, combine lemon juice, sugar, and salt. Stir until sugar and salt are dissolved.
3. Wash and coarsely grate radishes.
4. Toss radishes and lemon juice mixture with the orange sections.
5. Sprinkle with cinnamon and serve immediately.

Per serving: 89 cal. (0% from fat), 1 g protein, 23 g carbohydrate, 0 g fat, 0 mg cholesterol, 3 g fiber, 101 mg sodium.

Melktert

(Milk Pie)

Serves 6

1 3/4 cups fat free milk
1 tablespoon butter
1 cinnamon stick
1 small orange, peeled and cut into pieces
1/4 cup sugar
1/3 cup flour
1/4 cup fat free milk
2 eggs, beaten
pastry for one single-crust, 9-inch pie
1 1/2 teaspoons sugar
1/4 teaspoon cinnamon

1. In a 2-quart heavy saucepan, combine 1 3/4 cups milk, butter, cinnamon stick, and orange pieces. Bring to a boil.
2. Remove from heat. Remove cinnamon stick and orange pieces with a slotted spoon.
3. Combine 1/4 cup sugar with the flour. Add 1/4 cup milk and stir until smooth.
4. Stir flour mixture into the milk in the sauce pan. Place over low heat and cook, stirring constantly, until thickened.
5. Remove from the heat. Stir a small amount of the hot liquid into the beaten eggs. Then add the eggs to the hot mixture, mixing well.
6. Pour the pudding into a pastry lined pie plate.
7. Bake at 450°F for 20 minutes.
8. Reduce heat to 350°F and bake for another 10 minutes.
9. Combine 1 1/2 teaspoons sugar with the cinnamon and sprinkle over the top of the pie. Serve warm.

Per serving: 303 cal. (39% from fat), 8 g protein, 40 g carbohydrate, 13 g fat, 78 mg cholesterol, 1 g fiber, 283 mg sodium.

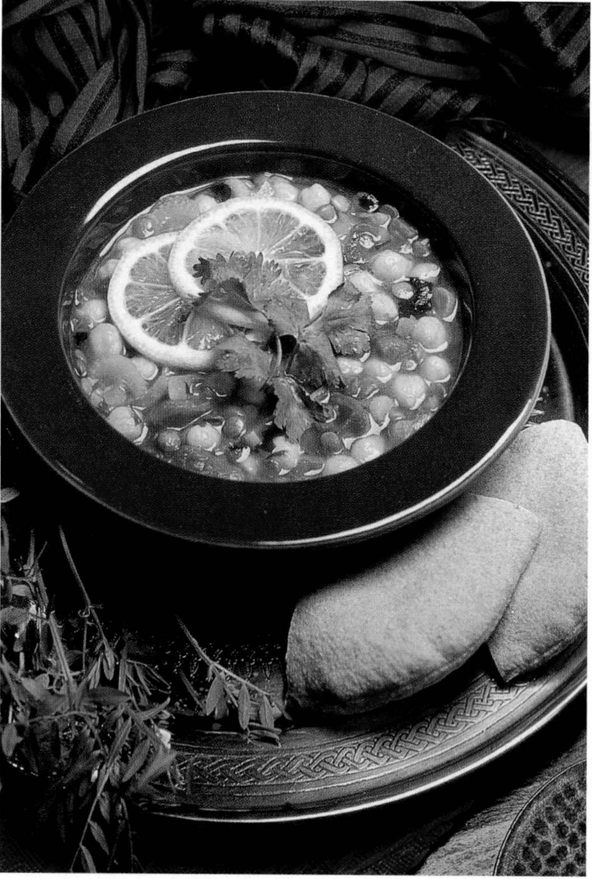

USA Dry Pea & Lentil Council

This colorful Moroccan soup is flavored with a variety of herbs and spices.

Chapter 31 Review
Middle East and Africa

Summary

The climate throughout much of the Middle East and Africa is hot and dry. Irrigation is essential for growing crops in many Middle Eastern and African countries. Religion is an important part of the culture in this part of the world. Religious laws as well as the climate have an impact on the foods of this region.

A number of ingredients and foods are common throughout the Middle East. However, unique dishes are found in each Middle Eastern country. Lamb is the staple meat of this region and bulgur and rice are often served as side dishes. Fish is popular in coastal countries. Middle Eastern cooks use a variety of spices to season foods. Fruits and rich pastries are common desserts. Coffee is a favorite beverage, although Iranians prefer tea.

Israel has a rather eclectic cuisine. Jewish people from many parts of the world have made contributions to the foods of Israel. The neighboring Middle Eastern and African countries have had an influence, too. Of course, Jewish dietary laws also affect many foods.

The Islamic religion influences food habits throughout much of Africa. European countries that colonized various parts of Africa also left their mark on the cuisine. Although each African country has unique dishes, some foods are common all over the continent. Such foods include a variety of fruits and vegetables and several breads and pastries.

Review What You Have Read

Write your answers on a separate sheet of paper.

1. How do Muslims observe the Fast of Ramadan?
2. List the five ingredients basic to all Middle Eastern cooking.
3. True or false. Both Islam and Judaism forbid their followers to eat poultry.
4. Describe three Turkish sweets.
5. Which of the following is an Arabian mazza?
   A. Hummus.
   B. Kibbi.
   C. Tabbouleh.
   D. Torshi.
6. Name and describe the two types of rice dishes served in Iran.
7. Explain the symbolism of five foods eaten as part of the seder shared by Jewish families during Passover.
8. Match the following terms and definitions associated with Jewish dietary laws:
   ___ Someone who, in accordance with Jewish dietary laws, is licensed to slaughter all animals and fowl used as food.
   ___ Foods that are prepared according to Jewish dietary laws.
   ___ Dairy foods.
   ___ Meat foods.
   ___ Fruits, vegetables, cereal, fish, and baked goods made with vegetable shortening.
   A. fleishig
   B. Halal
   C. kosher
   D. milchig
   E. pareve
   F. shohet
9. Name four foods used to stuff kreplach.
10. Most of the world's chocolate is made from a plant grown in Africa called _____.
11. What is injera? How is it served and eaten?
12. On what do Africans sit during a meal?

Build Your Basic Skills

1. **Reading/verbal.** Many spices grow in the Middle East. Make a list of five spices that come from this area. Find both Middle Eastern and American recipes that include each of these spices. Compare the two types of recipes. Discuss in class what foods are typically flavored with these spices in each cuisine.
2. **Reading/writing.** Use library resources to read about the establishment of the state of Israel. Summarize your findings in a brief written report.

Build Your Thinking Skills

1. **Analyze.** Investigate the average annual rainfall in various regions of the Middle East. Analyze how rainfall affects agricultural production in these regions.
2. **Trace.** Work in a small group to trace the specific food customs of one African country. Use visual aids to give a presentation about the ingredients, cooking methods, eating habits, and meal patterns in your chosen country. Each member of the group should be responsible for a different part of the presentation. Following the group presentations, each group should prepare a dish typical of their country to serve as part of an African banquet

Apply Technology

1. Go to a news Web site to find a recent story from the Middle East. Make a printout of the story to share with the class.
2. Use a computer and the table function in word processing software to make a table comparing Islam, Judaism, and Christianity.

Using Workplace Skills

Abira is a foreign correspondent in the Middle East for NWN, a cable news network. She must gather information about newsworthy events and analyze it for accuracy. Sometimes this involves a lot of effort and perseverance as she tracks down sources of information and confirms facts. Then she uses credible information to write news stories for broadcast on her network.

To be an effective worker, Abira needs to display responsibility. In a small group, answer the following questions about Abira's need for and use of this quality:

A. In what kinds of situations would the quality of responsibility be especially important to Abira?
B. How might Abira's information sources respond if she failed to display responsibility?
C. How might the viewers of Abira's broadcasts be affected if she failed to display responsibility?
D. What is another skill Abira would need in this job? Briefly explain why this skill would be important.

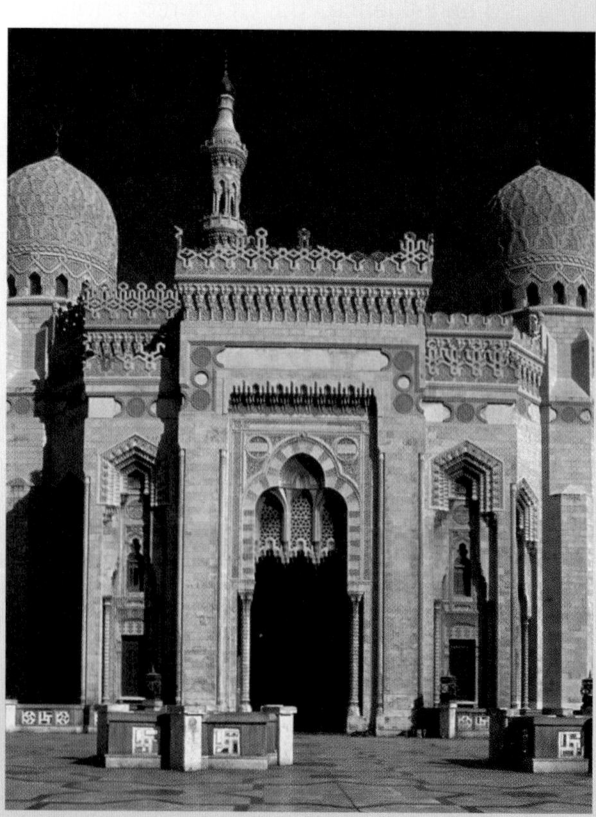

Chapter 32
Asia

Travel Agent
Plans itineraries and arranges accommodations and other travel services for customers of travel agency.

Japanese Translator
Translates documents and other materials from Japanese into one or more other languages.

Chinese-Style Food Cook
Plans menus and cooks Chinese-style dishes, dinners, desserts, and other foods, according to recipes.

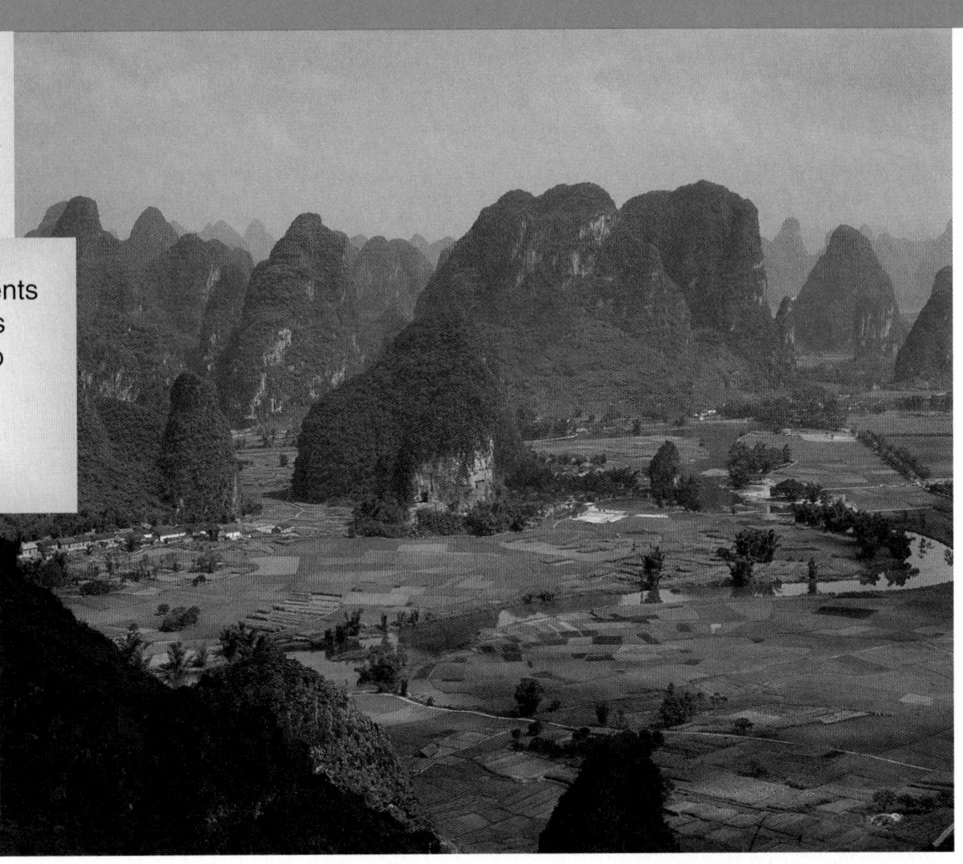

Terms to Know

kasha
zakuska
caviar
schi
borscht
beef stroganov
paskha
kulich
caste system
curry
ghee
masala
chapatis
tandoori
korma
vindaloo
chasnidarth
dynasty
wok
congee
chopsticks
gohan
soybean
tofu
sukiyaki
tsukemono
kaiseka
nihon-cha

Objectives

After studying this chapter, you will be able to

- ❑ describe how geography, climate, and culture have influenced the food customs of Russia, India, China, and Japan.
- ❑ name foods that are native to each of these countries.
- ❑ use recipes to prepare foods that are native to each of these countries.

Asia is the largest continent in the world. It covers nearly a third of the earth's total land surface. Asia is also the home of over three-fifths of the world's people. Deserts, jungles, swamps, and mountains cover much of Asia. Therefore, most of its people are crowded into small areas that can better support crops.

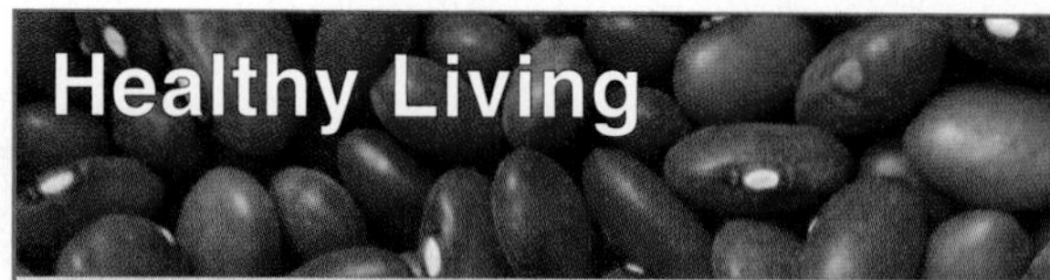

Healthy Living

When you are traveling, be sure to start every day with a good breakfast. Do not skip lunch, either. Sightseeing requires energy. You might want to keep some bread and fruit in your travel tote. This will allow you to grab a quick bite while you are on the go.

When people in the rest of the world were making crude tools, people in Asia were becoming highly advanced. Asian art, architecture, and technology laid the groundwork for the later development of Western civilization.

Russia, India, China, and Japan dominate the Asian continent in area and population. (The largest portion of Russia lies in Asia. The smaller portion lies in Europe.) Interest in these nations, however, goes far beyond size and population statistics. Each of these nations has a unique culture. The culture of Russia is a mixture of Eastern and Western influences. The cultures of India, Japan, and China are far different from those of any Western nation. Despite growing Western influence, many of the customs and traditions of these countries have been preserved.

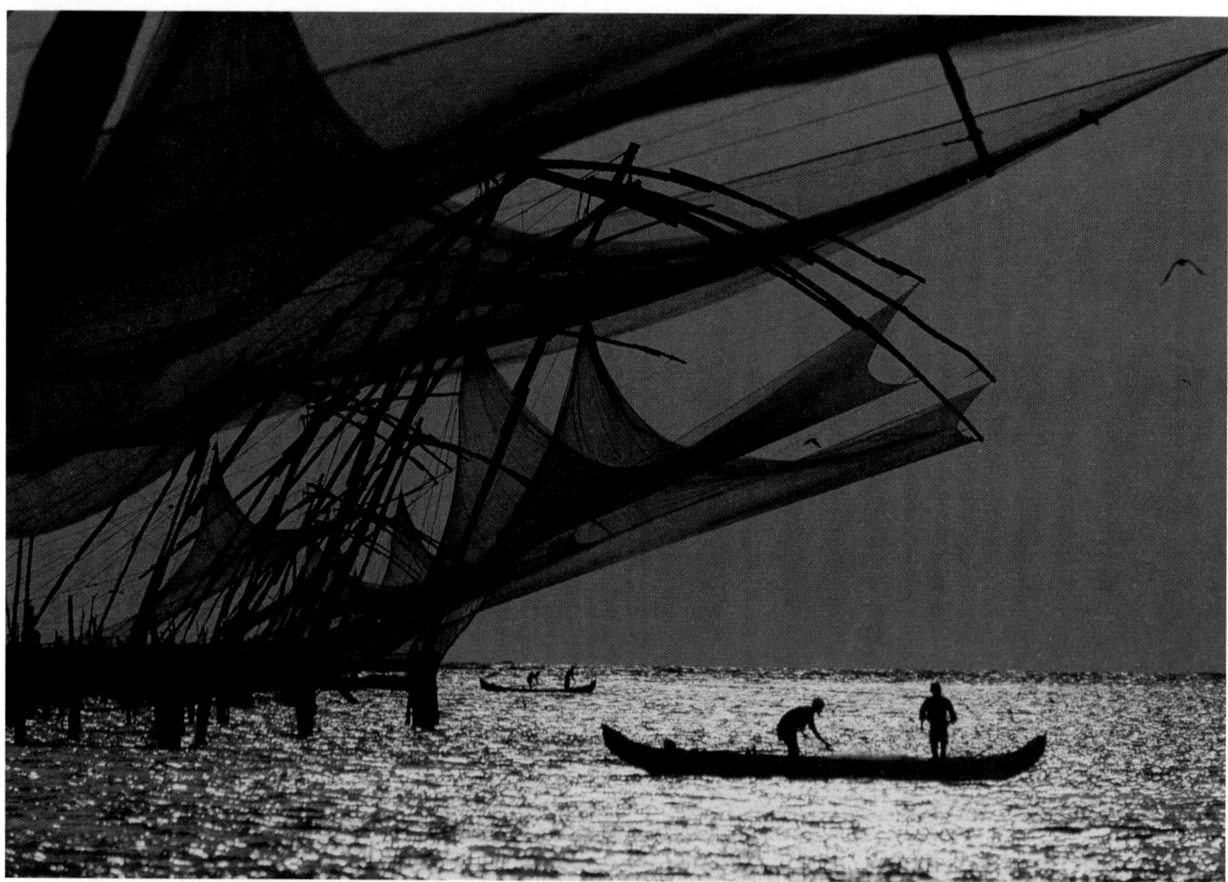

Asia is home to some of the world's largest and most modern cities. However, life in some rural areas is much the same as it was years ago.

Russia

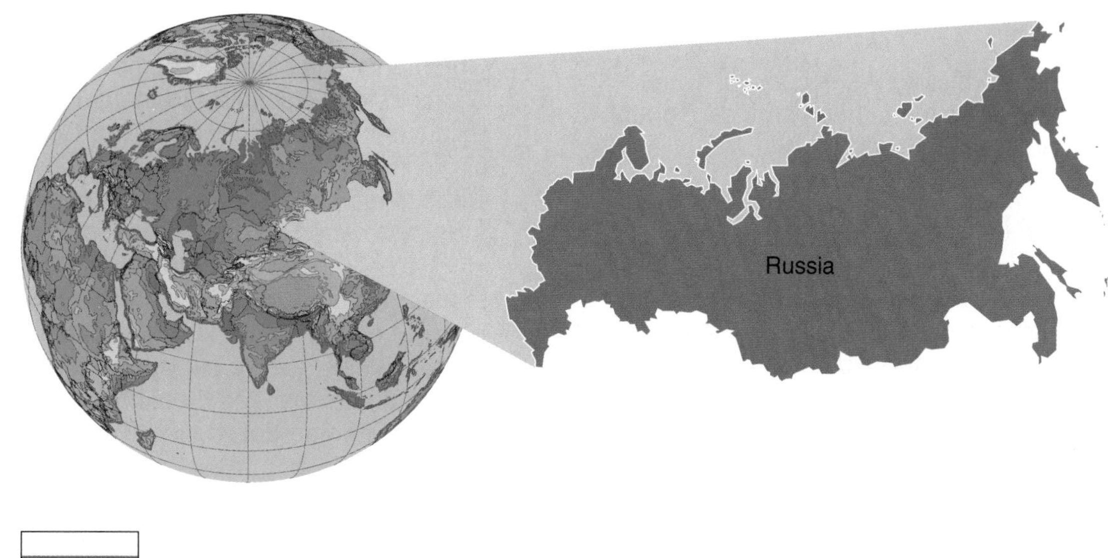

Inside Russia's borders are vast natural resources. Forests provide timber. Thousands of rivers provide power, food, water, and transportation. A large population representing a range of cultures has added to the diversity of Russian cuisine.

Geography and Climate of Russia

Russia is the largest country in the world. It is almost twice the size of the United States. Most of Russia is a vast lowland, but mountains are important, too. The Ural Mountains divide Europe from Asia. The other important mountain ranges form a large arc along the southern and southwestern borders. The rivers of Russia are important transportation arteries. Because many of the rivers run north and south, canals have been built to improve east-west transportation.

The climate in a large portion of Russia is marked by short, cool summers; long, severe winters; and light precipitation. Much of the European part of Russia (including Moscow) has short, mild summers. The winters are long and cold, and precipitation is moderate. In the northern Arctic regions, summers are short and chilly, and winters are long and bitterly cold. Temperatures of -94°F (-70°C) have been recorded in northeastern Siberia. The Pacific Ocean brings monsoons to the far southeastern portion of the country.

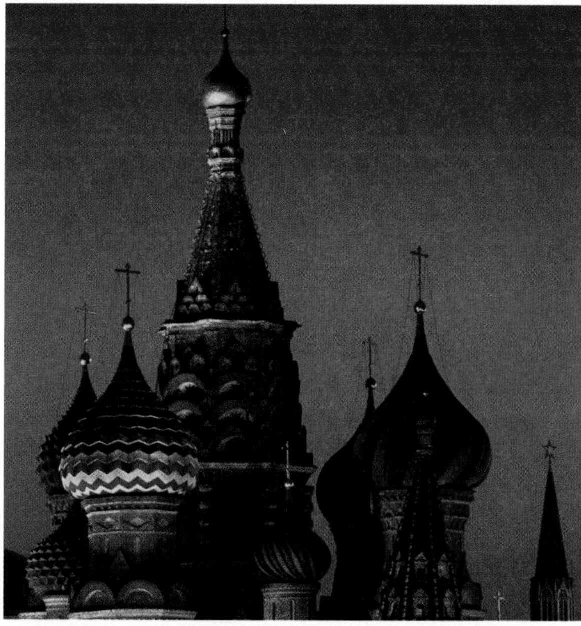

The colorful onion domes of St. Basil's Cathedral in Moscow are a classic example of Russian Orthodox architecture.

Russian Culture

Russian history dates back for centuries. However, Russia has been an independent country for only a few years.

Influences on Russian Culture

Little is known about Russia's early history. However, during the eighth and ninth centuries, the Russ civilization began to develop. In the tenth century, a ruler named Vladimir worked to unite the land of Russ.

During the thirteenth century, Mongolian Tatars invaded from the south. Their customs had an influence on Russian culture. During their rule, Moscow became an important political center.

In 1547, Ivan the Terrible became the first czar of Russia. (The word *czar* means ruler.) He fought against the Tatars and ended their rule. Ivan's military successes led to territorial growth. In 1613, the Romanov family began a rule of the Russian Empire that lasted until 1917.

In 1917, Vladimir Lenin led a revolutionary group, called the *Bolsheviks,* that took control of the government. Following a civil war, the Union of Soviet Socialist Republics (U.S.S.R., or Soviet Union) was formed.

Modern Culture in Russia

With the establishment of the U.S.S.R., a communist dictatorship replaced rule by the czars. The Communist Party controlled the government until 1991. In that year, the Communist Party was dissolved. The Soviet Union was broken up into 15 independent countries, one of which is Russia.

Russian Agriculture

Wheat is Russia's major grain crop, followed by rye, barley, oats, and corn. Other important crops include sugar beets, sunflower seeds, and flax. Fruit and vegetable crops are not as varied as they are in the United States. However, hardy fruits and vegetables, such as cabbage, potatoes, and apples, grow where climate and soil are suitable.

Russian Holidays

The Communist government had a great impact on the celebration of holidays in Russia. Many traditional holidays are linked to the Russian Orthodox church. During the years of Communist rule, the government closed churches and discouraged the celebration of religious holidays. With the fall of Communism, churches reopened. Religious holidays, such as Christmas and Easter, regained importance in the lives of the Russian people.

Two of Russia's winter festivals involve some special food traditions. Most Russian people consider New Year to be the best holiday. Children receive candy and gifts from Grandfather Frost and the Snow Maiden, who arrive in a horse-drawn sled. Families get together to enjoy a meal that includes borscht, beef stroganov, pickled tomatoes, and salads. Festival of Winter is a period of several weeks during which parks are decorated with lights and Christmas trees. People stroll through the parks and enjoy blinis and tea purchased from vendors. *Blinis* are pancakes made from buckwheat flour. Russians fry them in butter and serve them with butter and sour cream, caviar, smoked fish, or jam. Their round shape symbolizes the sun and the coming of spring.

Russian Cuisine

Russian cuisine is, for the most part, hearty and filling. The Russian diet is also nutritious, with bread and other grain products forming the foundation, 32-1. Vegetables frequently appear in healthful soups and side dishes. Russians make more liberal use of meat and dairy products than many of their Asian neighbors. Although these foods add a balance of nutrients, they also increase the amount of fat in the diet. Serving moderate portions will help keep fat under control. Smoked and pickled foods, which are linked with certain types of cancer, should be enjoyed in limited amounts, too.

Contributions to Russian Cuisine

Russian cuisine has Slavic origins. The first Slavs depended on the forests, mountains, and waters for most of their food. Cream sauces and the queen cake are examples of Scandinavian foods contributed by these early people. (*Queen cake* is apples and cherries baked between layers of sweet pastry and topped with meringue.)

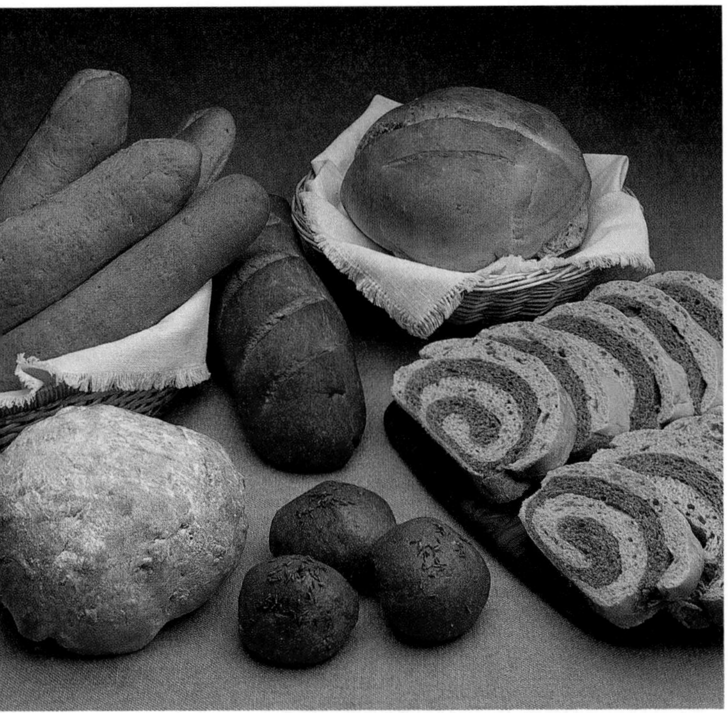

Lesaffre Yeast Corporation, the RED STAR® Yeast Collection

32-1 Russian farmers grow a lot of rye, and hearty rye breads are a staple of the Russian diet.

The next major contribution to Russian cuisine came from the Mongols. The Mongols taught the Slavs how to broil meat and how to make sauerkraut, yogurt, kumys, and curd cheese. (*Kumys* is a mild alcoholic beverage.) The Mongols also introduced tea drinking and the *samovar* (a special piece of equipment used to make Russian tea).

The czars staged elaborate banquets and introduced European foods to Russia. For instance, Peter the Great brought French soups and Dutch cheeses to the Russian court. He also introduced the custom of serving fruit preserves with meat.

Staple Foods of Russian Peasants

Few Russians ate like the czars. Most people were peasants who ate foods they could grow themselves or obtain from the forests or rivers. Bread, kasha, and soup formed the basis of their diets.

Peasant bread was dark, nourishing, and filling. Peasants usually made it from rye flour because they could grow rye in the short, cool growing season.

Kasha was another staple food. The peasants usually made ***kasha*** from buckwheat, but they also used other grains. They first fried the raw grain. Then they simmered it until tender. The peasants could eat the kasha alone. However, those who could afford to do so added vegetables, meat, eggs, or fish.

The third staple food of the peasants was soup. Cabbage, beet, and fish soups were the most common.

Some peasant families had enough money to have a small vegetable garden and some livestock. The garden supplied potatoes, cabbage, cucumbers, beets, carrots, and turnips. A cow provided milk and milk products. Chickens gave eggs, and hogs and cattle provided meat.

Modern Russian Cuisine

The Russian cuisine of today combines native Russian foods with foods of neighboring European and Asian countries.

Russian Appetizers and Soups

Zakuska (appetizers), such as smoked salmon, pickled herring, fish in aspic, and sliced cold meats, begin many Russian meals. Pâtés, salads, cheese, pickles, and breads are also among the many foods that appear on a zakuska table. However, the star of the table is always caviar.

Caviar is the processed, salted roe (eggs) of large fish. The roe of the sturgeon are used most often. Russians serve their fine black caviar on small pieces of white bread.

Soup usually follows the zakuska. ***Schi*** (cabbage soup) is one of the most popular Russian soups. Cooks obtain different flavors by varying the vegetables and broth. ***Borscht*** (beet soup) can be thin and clear or thick with chunks of beets and other vegetables, 32-2. Russians often top borscht with a dollop of sour cream. Other popular soups include *ouba,* which is a clear fish broth. *Rasolnik* is a mixture of vegetables garnished with chopped veal or lamb kidneys. *Solianka* contains meat or fish and salted cucumber.

Russian Main Dishes

Many Russian meat dishes have regional origins. *Shashlik* (cubes of marinated lamb grilled on skewers), for example, developed in Georgia (a country that borders Turkey).

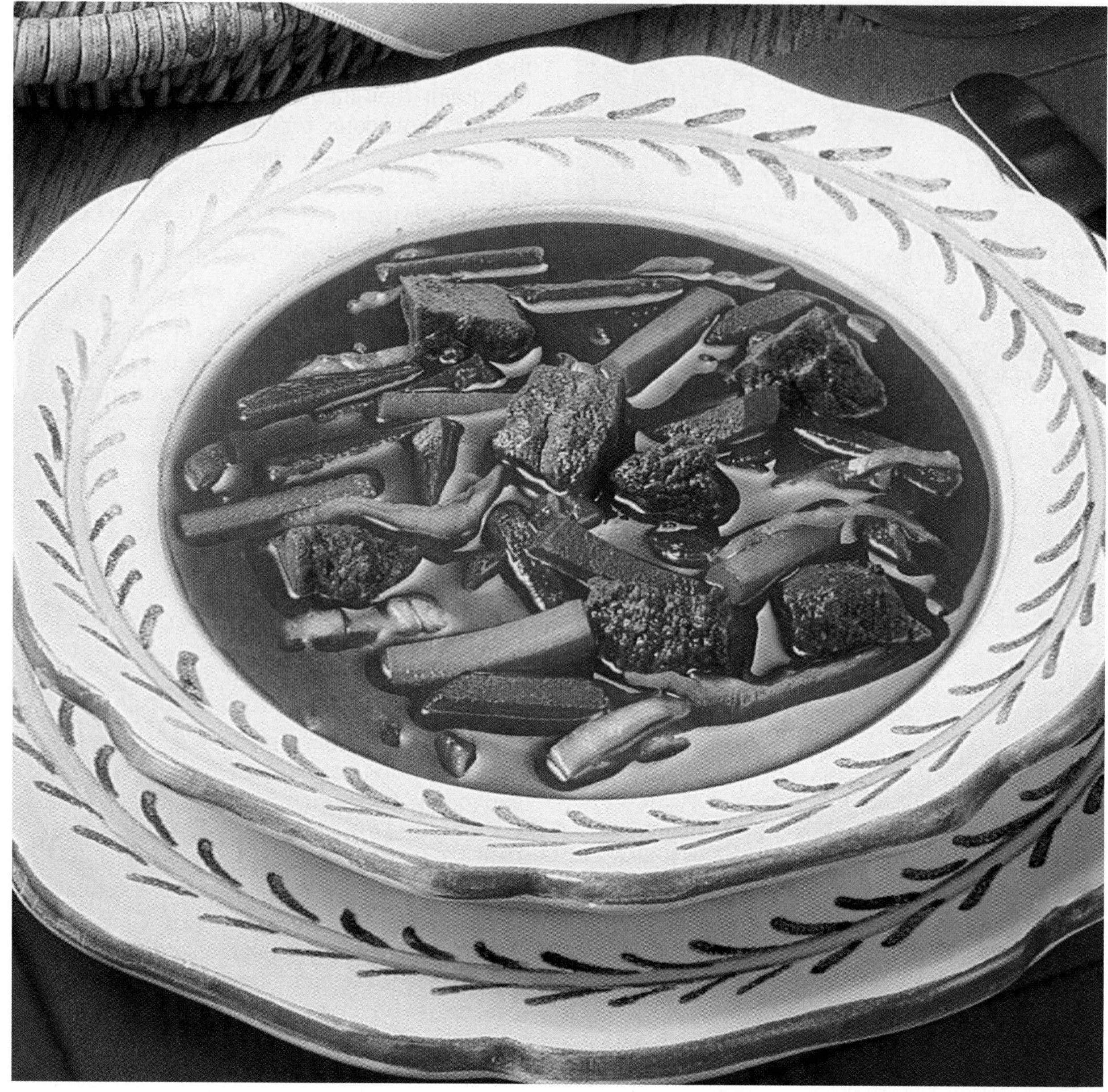

courtesy of National Cattlemen's Beef Association and Cattlemen's Beef Board

32-2 *Beets give borscht its vivid red color.*

One of the best-known Russian meat dishes was created for a Russian count of the late nineteenth century. ***Beef stroganov*** is made with tender strips of beef, mushrooms, and a seasoned sour cream sauce.

Other Russian main dishes are made with chicken. *Chakhokhbili* is stewed chicken with tomato sauce, onions, vinegar, wine, peppers, and olives. *Kurnik* is a chicken and rice pie and kotmis satsivi is roasted chicken with walnut sauce. *Kotlety po-kyivskomu* (chicken Kiev) is pounded chicken breasts wrapped around pieces of sweet butter. The rolls of chicken are then breaded and deep-fried until golden brown. When a fork pierces the golden coating, the butter spurts out and serves as a sauce.

More than 100 types of fish live in the waters that border Russia. Sturgeon, pike, carp, bream, salmon, and trout were favorites of the Russian czars. A branch of Russian cuisine developed around these and other varieties of fish. In one region, sturgeon and swordfish are prepared on skewers. White-fleshed fish are served in aspic, and crisp fish cakes are eaten with a mustard sauce.

Russian Side Dishes

Russian vegetable dishes have always changed with the seasons. During the cold winters, rutabagas and other root vegetables, potatoes, pickles, dried mushrooms, and sauerkraut are eaten. During the summers, asparagus, peas, and fresh cabbage are more common.

Cereals are available year-round. Because they are both filling and inexpensive, they serve as staples in the Russian diet. Russian cooks use cereals to make dark breads, white breads, and sweet breads. They use cereals to make kasha, which is still popular in Russia. Russians may serve kasha plain or add it to soups. They may combine it with other foods and serve it as a side dish or a puddinglike dessert. Russian cooks use flour doughs to make noodles, dumplings, and pirozhki. *Pirozhki* are pastries filled with protein-based or sweet fillings.

Milk and milk products are an important part of Russian cooking. Russian cooks use *smetana* (sour cream) on top of borscht and in cakes, pastries, salads, sauces, and main dishes. They also use *prostokvasa* (sour milk), *kefir* (a type of yogurt), and *koumys* (sour mare's milk).

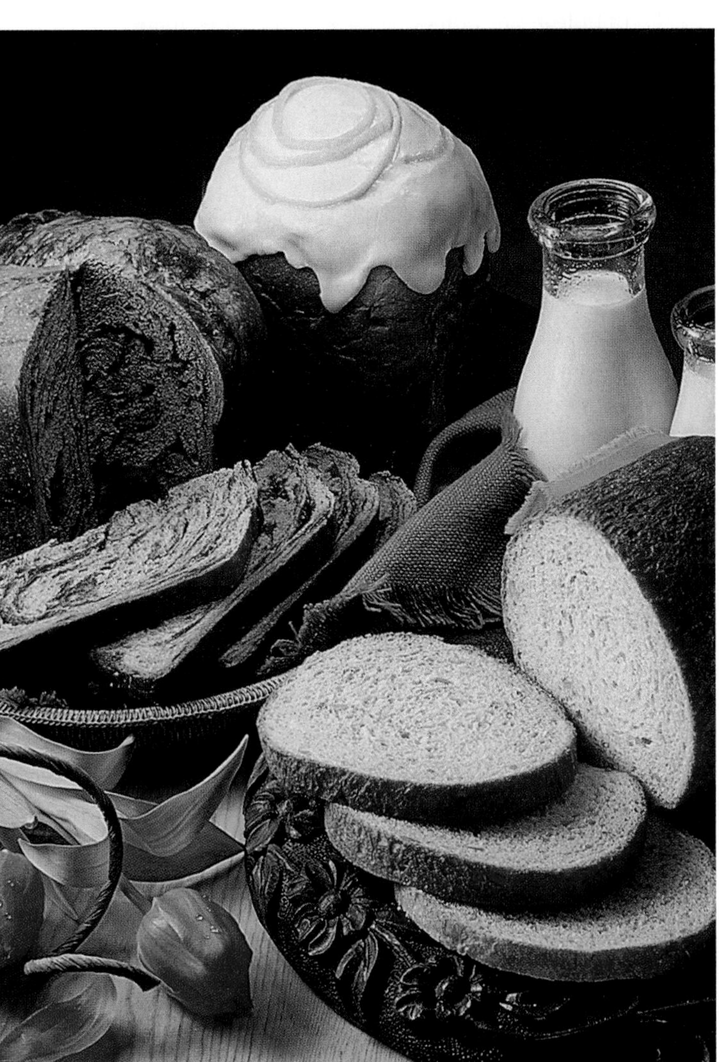

photo courtesy of Fleischmann's Yeast

32-3 *Kulich is a Russian Easter bread that gets flavor and texture from the additions of candied fruits and nuts.*

Russian Desserts

Russian desserts have varied origins. Some Russian desserts, like *charlotte* russe (ladyfinger mold with cream filling) and fruit tarts, were favorites of the czars. Other desserts, like *kisel* (pureed fruit), were eaten by the peasants. Many desserts are strictly regional in origin. These include *samsa* (sweet walnut fritters) and *medivnyk* (honey cake).

Two of the most popular Russian desserts are part of the Easter celebrations of the Russian Orthodox Church. ***Paskha*** is a rich cheesecake. It is molded into a pyramid and decorated with the letters *XB*. These are the initials of the Greek phrase *Christos voskres,* meaning Christ has risen. ***Kulich*** is a tall, cylindrical yeast bread filled with fruits and nuts. Russians always serve kulich by first removing the top half of the cake and placing it on a serving plate. Then they slice the rest of the cake and arrange the slices around the mushroom-shaped top. See 32-3.

Russian Meals

The average Russian family eats three meals a day. Breakfast generally is simple. Kasha with milk, bread, butter, jam, hot tea, and an occasional egg are typical.

Lunches may be eaten in factory cafeterias or the fields. They may consist of a hearty soup, thick slices of bread with a little cheese or sausage, and tea. In wealthier families, a fish or meat course and vegetables may follow the soup.

Dinner is the main meal of the day. Russians serve a small assortment of zakuska with glasses of vodka or *kvas* (similar to European beers). They often follow zakuska with soup. Then they serve the main course of meat, poultry, or fish. Potatoes, vegetables, and bread usually accompany the main course. A simple dessert, such as kisel and hot tea, follows.

Russian Menu

Pirozhki
(Small Pastries Filled with Meat)
Borscht
(Beet Soup)
Kotlety Po-Kyivskomu
(Chicken Kiev)
Kartoplia Solimkoi
(Deep-Fried Straw Potatoes)
Màslo Garókh
(Buttered Peas)
Chernyi Khlib
(Black Bread)
Paskha
(Easter Cheese Pyramid)
Tchai
(Tea)

Pirozhki

(Small Pastries Filled with Meat)
Makes 20

Pastry:
2 cups all-purpose flour
¼ teaspoon salt
¼ cup margarine, cut into small pieces
¼ cup vegetable shortening
4 to 6 tablespoons ice water

1. Sift flour and salt into mixing bowl.
2. Using pastry blender, two knives, or fingers, cut in margarine and shortening until mixture resembles coarse cornmeal.
3. Add ice water, stirring gently with fork, until dough forms a ball.
4. Wrap dough in waxed paper and refrigerate at least one hour.
5. On lightly floured board or pastry cloth, roll dough into a strip about 11 × 3 inches. Fold the dough into thirds, turn pastry around, and again roll into a lengthwise strip about 11 × 3 inches. Fold into thirds, turn and roll again. Repeat this process two more times, ending with folded dough.
6. Wrap dough in waxed paper and refrigerate for at least 1 hour while filling is prepared.

Filling:
2 tablespoons margarine
1¼ cups finely chopped onion
¾ pound lean ground beef
1 hard-cooked egg, chopped
3 tablespoons chopped fresh dill
½ teaspoon salt
dash pepper

1. In medium skillet, melt margarine.
2. Add onions and saute until golden brown.
3. Add meat. Cook over moderate heat, stirring occasionally, until no pink remains.
4. Remove meat from heat and allow to cool for 15 minutes. On cutting board, chop meat mixture as finely as possible or run through grinder with fine blade.
5. In large bowl, mix meat with egg, dill, salt, and pepper.
6. Preheat oven to 400°F.
7. On floured board or pastry cloth, roll dough to a thickness of ⅛ inch. With a floured 3-inch biscuit cutter, cut out as many rounds as you can. Reroll scraps.
8. Place 2 tablespoons of filling in the center of each round. Fold one side to center. Fold two ends of dough about ½ inch toward center. Fold remaining edge to center and seal.
9. Place pirozhki side by side, seam sides down, on lightly greased baking sheet.
10. Bake 30 minutes or until golden brown.

Per pastry: 137 cal. (56% from fat), 5 g protein, 10 g carbohydrate, 9 g fat, 24 mg cholesterol, 1 g fiber, 133 mg sodium.

Borscht

(Beet Soup)
Serves 6

2 pounds beef brisket
8 medium beets, coarsely grated
4 medium onions, sliced
2 medium tomatoes, coarsely chopped
2 tablespoons sugar
2 tablespoons lemon juice
1½ teaspoons salt
⅛ teaspoon pepper
½ pound white cabbage, shredded
sour cream

1. Fill a large Dutch oven with water. Add brisket, beets, onions, and tomatoes; simmer until meat is tender, about 1½ hours.
2. Remove meat. Add sugar, lemon juice, salt, and pepper to stock. Stir until sugar has dissolved.
3. Add cabbage and simmer an additional 25 minutes.
4. Skim fat.
5. Shred meat and add to soup.
6. Pour soup into large tureen and serve immediately with dollops of sour cream. (Soup may also be served cold, if desired.)

Per serving: 310 cal. (26% from fat), 36 g protein, 22 g carbohydrate, 9 g fat, 104 mg cholesterol, 4 g fiber, 723 mg sodium.

Kotlety Po-Kyivskomu

(Chicken Kiev)
Serves 6

6 boneless, skinless chicken breast halves
6 tablespoons chilled margarine
salt
pepper
1½ teaspoons chopped parsley
¼ cup fat free milk
2 eggs, beaten
½ cup all-purpose flour
1½ cups dry bread crumbs
vegetable oil for deep-frying

1. Place chicken breasts, one at a time, between two sheets of waxed paper. Flatten with a meat mallet until ¼ inch thick.
2. Cut margarine into 6 equal pieces. Shape each into a cylinder. Wrap in waxed paper and chill.
3. Place one piece of chilled margarine on each breast. Sprinkle with salt, pepper, and parsley.
4. Roll chicken breast around margarine and seasonings; carefully seal edges with toothpicks.
5. Beat milk and eggs until smooth.
6. Dredge rolled chicken breast in flour, dip in milk mixture; then roll in bread crumbs. Repeat coating process until all rolls have been coated. Chill until ready to cook.
7. Heat oil to 375°F. Fry chicken rolls until golden brown. Remove toothpicks and serve immediately.

Per serving: 433 cal. (43% from fat), 34 g protein, 27 g carbohydrate, 20 g fat, 161 mg cholesterol, 2 g fiber, 421 mg sodium.

Kartoplia Solimkoi

(Deep-Fried Straw Potatoes)
Serves 6

6 medium-sized baking potatoes
vegetable oil for deep-frying
½ teaspoon salt

1. Peel potatoes and cut into strips about 2½ inches long and ⅛ inch thick.
2. Place strips in a bowl. Fill the bowl with ice water and set aside until potatoes are ready to be fried. Then, drain potatoes in a colander and place on paper towels. Using more paper towels, pat potatoes until they are thoroughly dry.
3. In large saucepan, heat oil to 375°F.
4. Place potatoes in frying basket and fry for about 15 seconds, occasionally shaking basket to keep potatoes from sticking. Potatoes should be a pale golden brown.
5. Drain well on paper towels. (Potatoes can rest up to an hour.)
6. Just before serving, reheat oil to 385°F.
7. Put potatoes in basket and fry 15 more seconds or until crisp and brown.
8. Drain, transfer to a platter, and sprinkle with salt. Serve immediately.

Per serving: 135 cal. (29% from fat), 2 g protein, 23 g carbohydrate, 4 g fat, 0 mg cholesterol, 1 g fiber, 172 mg sodium.

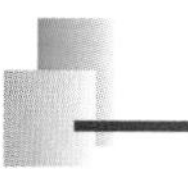

Màslo Garókh

(Buttered Peas)
Serves 6

water
½ teaspoon salt
1½ pounds shelled, fresh peas*
1 tablespoon margarine

1. In medium saucepan, bring a small amount of salted water to a boil.
2. Add peas and gently simmer until tender.
3. Drain; add margarine and serve immediately.

*Two 10-ounce packages of frozen peas may be substituted for the fresh peas.

Per serving: 83 cal. (22% from fat), 4 g protein, 12 g carbohydrate, 2 g fat, 0 mg cholesterol, 5 g fiber, 290 mg sodium.

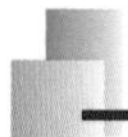

Chernyi Khlib

(Black Bread)
Makes 2 loaves

- 4 cups rye flour
- 3 cups all-purpose flour
- 1 teaspoon sugar
- 2 teaspoons salt
- 2 cups whole bran cereal
- 1½ tablespoons caraway seeds, crushed
- 2 teaspoons instant coffee
- 1 teaspoon onion powder
- ½ teaspoon fennel seed, crushed
- 2 packages active dry yeast
- 2½ cups water
- ¼ cup vinegar
- ¼ cup molasses
- 1 square unsweetened chocolate, 1 ounce
- ¼ cup margarine
- 1 egg white
- 1 teaspoon cold water

1. On a sheet of waxed paper, combine rye flour and all-purpose flour.
2. In a large mixer bowl, combine 2⅓ cups mixed flour, sugar, salt, bran cereal, caraway seeds, instant coffee, onion powder, fennel seed, and dry yeast.
3. In medium saucepan, combine 2½ cups water, vinegar, molasses, chocolate, and margarine. Heat over low heat until very warm (120°F to 130°F). (Margarine and chocolate do not need to melt).
4. Gradually add warm liquids to dry ingredients in mixer bowl and beat on medium speed of electric mixer 2 minutes, scraping bowl occasionally.
5. Add ½ cup of mixed flour and beat on high speed 2 minutes.
6. Add enough remaining mixed flour to form a soft dough.
7. Turn dough out onto a lightly floured board or pastry cloth. Cover with a clean towel and let rest 15 minutes.
8. Knead dough until smooth and elastic, about 10 to 15 minutes. (Dough will still be a little sticky.)
9. Place dough in greased bowl, turning to grease top. Cover with a clean towel and let rise in a warm place until doubled in bulk, about 1 hour.
10. Punch dough down; turn out onto lightly floured board. Divide in half and shape each half into a ball about 5 inches in diameter.
11. Place each ball in a greased 8-inch round cake pan. Cover with a clean towel and let rise in a warm place until doubled in bulk, about 1 hour.
12. Bake at 350°F for 45 to 50 minutes or until loaves sound hollow when gently tapped with knuckles.
13. Remove to cooling rack and brush tops with egg white that has been mixed with 1 teaspoon water.

Per slice: 130 cal. (16% from fat), 4 g protein, 26 g carbohydrate, 3 g fat, 0 mg cholesterol, 5 g fiber, 206 mg sodium.

Paskha

(Easter Cheese Pyramid)
Serves 18

- 2 cups sweet butter, softened
- 2 cups granulated sugar
- 3 pounds pot cheese
- ¾ cup orange juice concentrate
- ⅓ cup toasted slivered almonds, chopped
- 1 cup mixed candied fruit, chopped

1. In a large mixing bowl, cream butter and sugar until light and fluffy.
2. Gradually beat in pot cheese and continue beating until mixture is very smooth and creamy.
3. Add orange juice concentrate, almonds, and candied fruit.
4. Line a new 6-inch clay flower pot (one with a hole in the bottom) with several layers of cheesecloth.*
5. Turn cheese mixture into pot and pack tightly.
6. Cover with cheesecloth and place pot in a shallow pan. Put weights on top. Refrigerate for 24 hours, pouring off the liquid that accumulates every few hours.
7. To serve, unmold paskha onto a serving platter and remove cheesecloth. Garnish with candied fruits.

*Flower pot should have a 9-cup capacity.

Per serving: 395 cal. (57% from fat), 10 g protein, 34 g carbohydrate, 25 g fat, 67 mg cholesterol, 1 g fiber, 310 mg sodium.

India

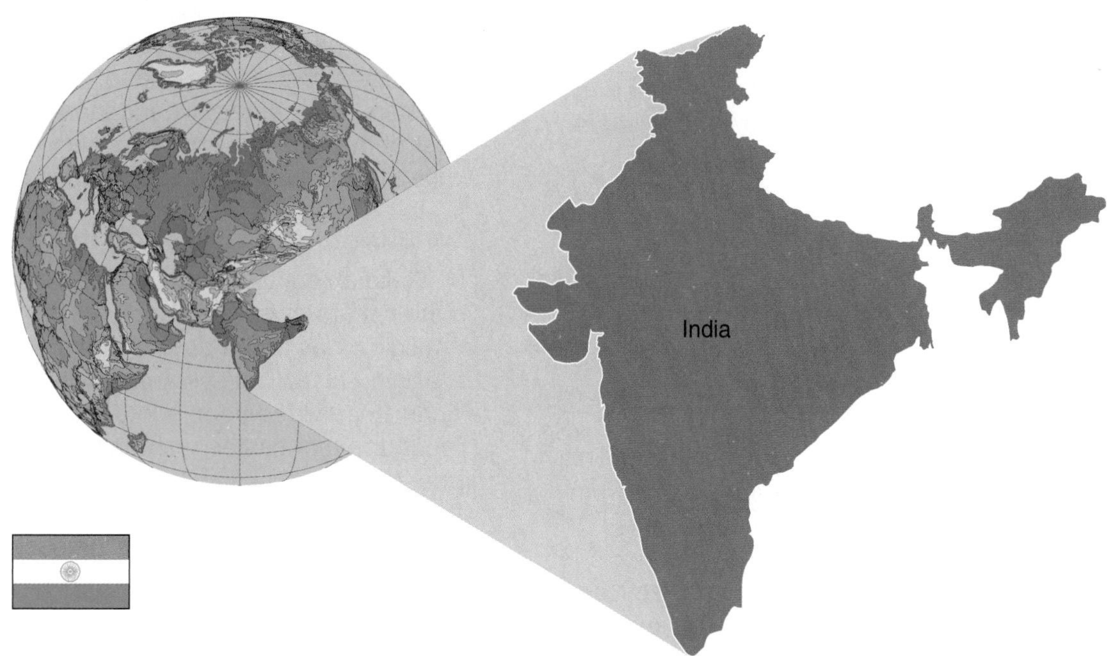

The local people call it Bharat. The English call it India. Both names belong to the seventh largest country in the world. It is a beautiful country with mountains, jungles, rich valleys, and miles of coastline.

Geography and Climate of India

India is located on a peninsula of southern Asia. The Himalayan Mountains form one of three distinct geographical areas in India. The mountains form a natural barrier from the rest of Asia. The hilly regions beneath the mountains are forests or grazing lands.

The plains formed by the Indus, Ganges, and Brahmaputra rivers are the second geographical area. The rich, deep soil of the Ganges River basin allows farmers to plant two crops each year.

The third geographical area lies to the south of the fertile river plains. It is a large plateau called the *Deccan,* which covers most of the peninsula. Agriculture is possible in level areas of the Deccan where rainfall or irrigation systems provide enough moisture.

India has a tropical climate. Cool weather lasts only from about December to March. The monsoon season lasts from June until the end of September. (*Monsoons* are storms with high winds and heavy rains.) The monsoon rains provide needed moisture for the dry earth. In just a short time, however, they can force rivers to flood their banks.

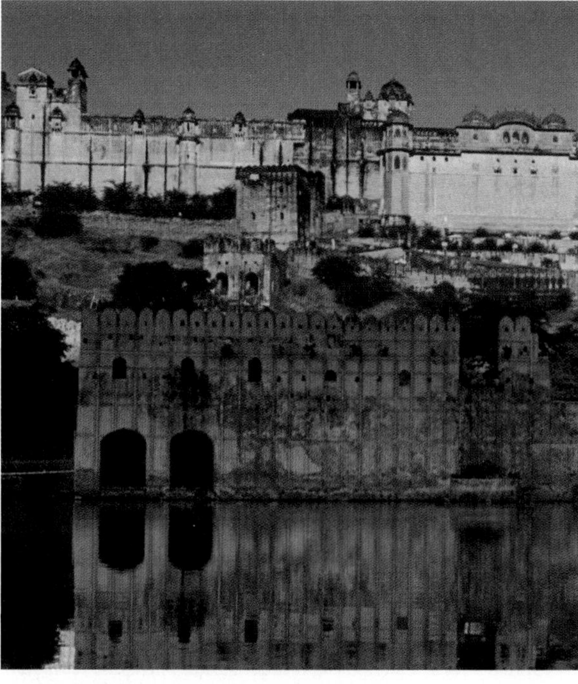

The reflection of the beautiful Amber Fort near Jaipur, India, appears in the still waters of Maotha Lake below.

Indian Culture

The people of India belong to a variety of races and religions. Most Indians are Hindus. Muslims are the next largest group. Small groups of Christians, Sikhs, Jains, Buddhists, and Parsees also live in India.

Indians speak over 700 languages and dialects. This variety is the result of foreign invasions that lasted many centuries.

Influences on Indian Culture

A series of invasions helped shape Indian culture centuries ago. The Aryans came from the north and conquered the Indians. The Persians, Huns, Arabs, Turks, and Mongols followed. During the Persian rule, India actively traded with ports in the Persian Gulf and the Mediterranean and Red Seas. During Mongol rule, Islam became an important religion. Great cities like Delhi were founded, and beautiful monuments like the Taj Mahal were built, 32-4.

During the sixteenth century, European nations began struggling to gain political power in India. In 1848, Great Britain took control and made India the center of its Indian Empire.

Following World War I, many Indian people began to demand home rule. Mahatma Gandhi became the leader of those Indians who wanted an independent nation. Gandhi developed a program of passive resistance and noncooperation with the government. In this way, he was able to transform the outbursts of social discontent into a passive revolutionary movement.

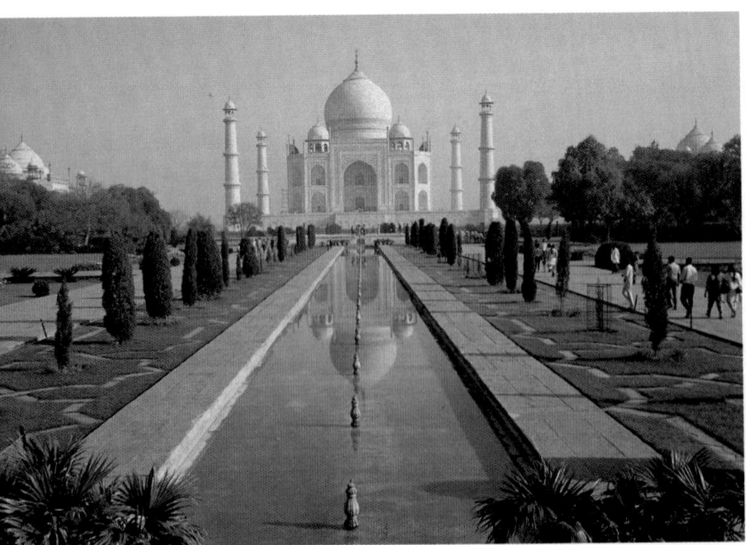

***32-4** Many people traveling to India make a point of visiting the beautiful Taj Mahal.*

In 1947, British rule ended, and India and Pakistan emerged as two independent nations. Most of the Muslims chose to live in Pakistan, while the Hindus chose to remain in India.

Religion and Holidays in India

Religion continues to play an important role in the culture of India's people. A key influence of religion was in the development of the ***caste system.*** This social system, which evolved from Hinduism, divided people into groups, or castes. The four major castes were the *Brahmins* (priests), *Kshatriyas* (warriors), *Vaisyas* (farmers), and *Sudras* (laborers). Below the Sudras were the outcasts, or "untouchables." The untouchables were forced to live away from the rest of the people. They were even forbidden to use public roads or bridges.

Today, many of the old caste restrictions have been relaxed. It is now illegal to view anyone as untouchable. Caste divisions are observed mainly for choosing marriage partners.

Another way religion influences Indian culture is in the celebration of holidays. Three popular festivals honor Hindu gods. The *Pongal Harvest Festival* is a time of thanksgiving for the winter harvest of rice, an important crop in India. It honors Surya, the sun god, for helping to ripen the rice. Hindu families offer a special rice pudding to Surya before eating it themselves. *Janmashtami* celebrates the birthday of one of the most popular Hindu gods, Krishna. The traditions of this holiday include going to the temple and bathing a statue of Krishna. The statue is bathed with clarified butter mixed with milk, sugar, and honey. The people in the temple then eat the sweet mixture with which they washed the statue. The *Ganesha Festival* is named for an elephant-headed god. Hindu people ask Ganesha to bring them success when they start new projects. During the festival, people place statues of Ganesha in their homes and present offerings of candy and fruit to it.

Indian Agriculture

Over 70 percent of India's people are farmers. Rice is India's major crop. Wheat, barley, millet, corn, and sorghum are grown in areas lacking the moisture needed for rice. Other important crops are chickpeas, beans, peas, and other legumes; sugarcane; and tea.

Smaller quantities of coffee, coconuts, and spices are also grown. See 32-5.

Indians raise more cattle than any other type of livestock. Cows provide some milk, but Indians primarily use cattle as work animals. They also raise smaller numbers of goats, hogs, sheep, and water buffalo and export the hides and skins.

Indian Cuisine

Indian cuisine gets a high rating on the nutrition scale. Many Indian dishes are vegetarian. Even those dishes that include meat generally do so in small amounts. This plant-based diet, which centers on grains, vegetables, and legumes, is high in fiber. It includes a variety of seasonings, which researchers believe may offer health benefits. The Indian diet is also rich in vitamins, minerals, and many other nutrients. However, the fat content of some dishes can be high due to the liberal use of fat in cooking.

Geography and climate have influenced India's cuisine. Geographically, the major division occurs between the North and the South. Invading groups of people, especially the Mongols, influenced Northern India. The Mongols brought the meat-based cuisine of their central Asian home. This cuisine developed in the royal kitchens and became characterized by foods that are rich and heavily seasoned.

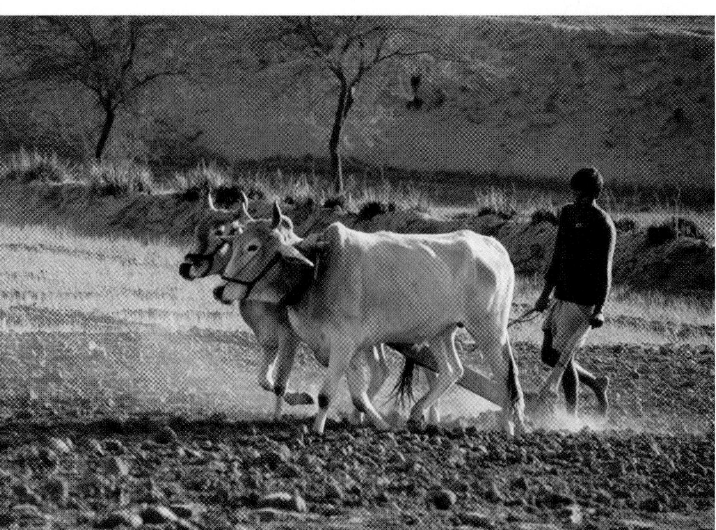

32-5 Many of India's farmers rely on the assistance of animals and manual tools to till the land.

Foreigners had less influence on Southern India. Its foods are hotter and not as subtle or refined as those of the North.

Climate has played a large part in the development of the two styles of Indian cooking. The heavy rainfall of the South allows large crops of rice, fruits, and vegetables to grow. In the drier North where wheat grows, bread sometimes replaces rice.

Influence of Religion on Indian Cuisine

Religion has been a third major influence on the development of Indian cuisine. Most Indian people are either Hindu or Muslim. Therefore, the dietary restrictions of these two religions have been most influential.

Many Hindu taboos concern food. Hindus cannot eat beef because they consider the cow to be sacred. Most Hindus are vegetarians. However, some Hindus, usually members of lower castes, eat mutton, poultry, goat, and fish. A member of the diner's caste must prepare these foods with cooking utensils belonging to that caste. In addition, food cannot be organically altered. (Artificial color and chemical processes used as preservatives are allowed.)

Although Muslims cannot eat pork, they do eat beef, mutton, lamb, fish, and poultry. These animal foods are more common in Northern India where most Indian Muslims live.

Indian Vegetable Dishes

Vegetable dishes are common in Indian cooking. This is especially true in the South where many people are vegetarians. There, *pulses* (legumes) are an important source of protein.

One way Indian cooks prepare pulses is to combine them with other vegetables in filling stews. Another way they serve pulses is by mashing or pureeing them with spices to make *dal.* Dal may be thinned and eaten as soup. It may also be poured over rice or served as a dipping sauce for bread.

Indian cooks prepare many vegetable dishes by frying the vegetables with spices. They shape mashed vegetables into balls, deep-fry them, and serve them with a sauce. They skin eggplant; flavor it with oil, pepper, and lemon; and grill it. *Raita,* a salad made of yogurt, vegetables, and seasonings, is a cool accompaniment to spicy dishes. *Rayata*, a potato salad flavored with yogurt, cucumber, tomatoes, cumin, and paprika, is served as a main dish.

Indian Main Dishes

Rice is a staple food throughout much of India. Rice often is served as a side dish. However, it sometimes is used in a variety of main dishes and desserts. Rice also is served as part of a group of dishes called curries. See 32-6.

Literally, ***curry*** is a variation of a word meaning sauce. It describes a type of stew. Curry can be prepared in many ways depending on the region. One common curry is prepared by pounding a variety of spices. The powdered spices are added to pickled fruit and the mixture is cooked with sugar and vinegar. The curry may be combined with vegetables, meat, poultry, or fish and accompanied by a variety of condiments.

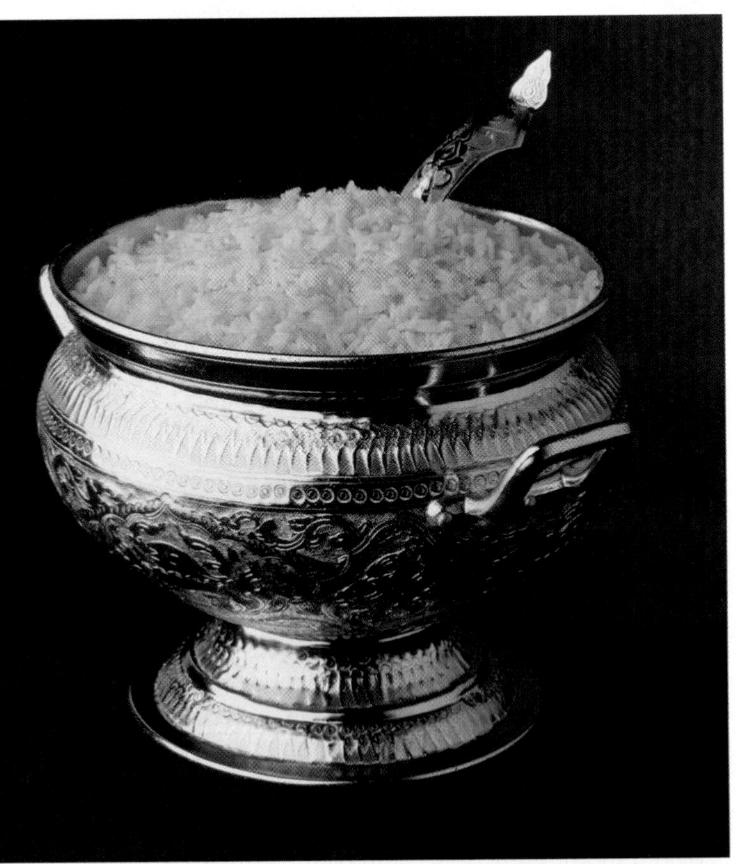

32-6 *Rice may become part of almost any course in an Indian meal.*

India's many miles of coastline provide a variety of fish. Fish are dried, marinated, and smoked. One specialty is a marinated fish prepared by layering fillets of fish with spices, salt, and tamarind pulp. *Bombil,* a small, nearly transparent fish, is caught in large quantities. When dried, it can be stored for long periods. *Pomfret* often is stuffed with a mixture of spices. It is then wrapped in a banana leaf and steamed, baked, or fried.

Q: Is brown rice really better for you than white rice?

A: Enriched white rice is actually higher in iron and some of the B vitamins than brown rice. However, brown rice provides about four times as much fiber as white rice. Also, nutrition experts recommend you choose brown rice and other whole grains regularly to get the benefits of nonnutrient substances they contain.

Shellfish are also widely available in India. Shrimp and prawns are baked, grilled, or used in curries. Cooks often coat these crustaceans with a spicy batter and deep-fry them. Crabs and lobsters are shredded; mixed with coconut milk, eggs, and spices; and fried in butter.

Most Indian meat dishes are made with goat or mutton. Few Indians eat pork, and beef is both scarce and expensive. Indians prepare meat in many ways. Meat braised in yogurt, cream, or a mixture of the two is called *korma. Bhona* is meat that is first sauteed and then baked. Kebabs are made from mutton that has been spiced, minced, and grilled. *Koftas* are spicy meatballs.

Chicken dishes are also popular in parts of India. People in the North marinate chicken in a mixture of yogurt and spices and roast it on a spit. People in the South add chicken to a spicy, coconut-flavored curry. See 32-7.

Indians cook many dishes in oil or fat. ***Ghee*** (Indian clarified butter) is the preferred cooking fat. Ghee is prepared by simmering butter and

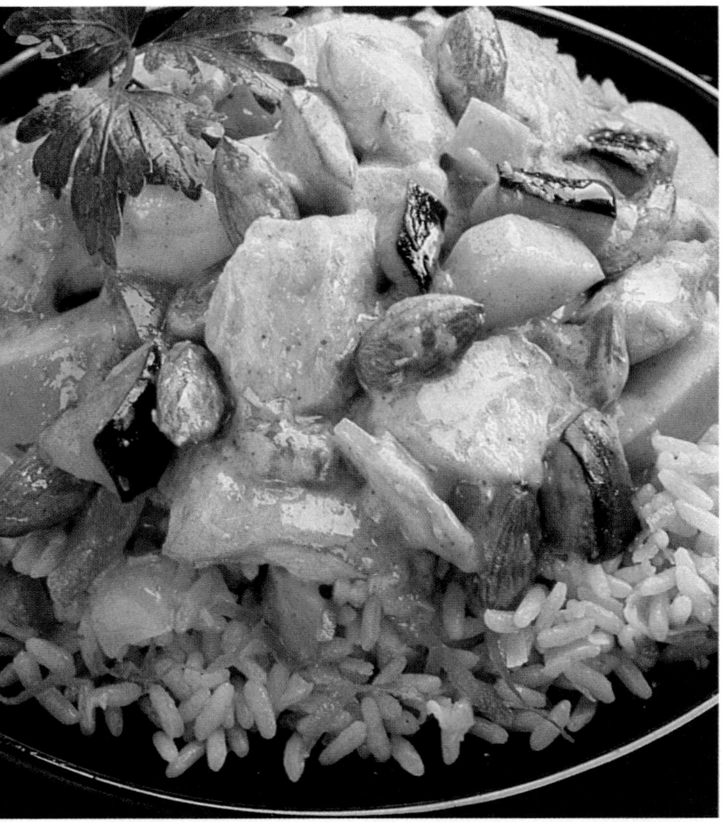

Almond Board of California

32-7 This rich, flavorful chicken curry is served over rice.

then straining it to remove solids that could cause rancidity during storage.

Indian Seasonings

The essence of Indian cooking lies in mastering the art of using spices. ***Masala*** is a mixture of spices used to make curry. The combination of spices can vary. However, each ingredient of the masala must retain its identity without overpowering the other flavors.

The spicy dishes of the coastal South use *wet masalas.* These are prepared by mixing the spices with vinegar, coconut milk, or water. They must be used immediately. Northern Indians use *dry masalas.* Dry masalas contain no liquid and cooks can prepare them ahead and store them for a short time.

Saffron, fenugreek, cumin seed, coriander seed, turmeric, and fennel seed are basic to Indian cooking. Other seasonings essential to Indian cooking are garlic, onions, and hot chili peppers. Spices add color as well as flavor to Indian dishes. Saffron and turmeric give rice and potato dishes a bright yellow color. Red and green chilies add vivid color to curries.

Fresh herbs add flavor to Indian foods. They are also used to make *chutneys* (condiments containing fruits, onions, spices, and herbs) and sauces. Coriander leaves, mint, and sweet basil are the most popular fresh herbs.

Indian Breads

Indians eat several kinds of *roti,* or bread. Most Indian breads are made from wheat, and they are unleavened and round. The most common is ***chapatis,*** a flat bread. Indian bakers make *naan* with yeast or baking powder and bake it in an Indian oven called a *tandoor.* When bakers make *paratha,* they roll and fold it several times so layers form when the bread bakes. Indians often stuff paratha with a meat or vegetable mixture.

Indian Sweets

Indians make many of their sweets from milk. Cooks simmer the milk into a thickened mass called *mawa.* They cook the mawa with sugar and add flavorings, such as almonds and coconut.

Another group of confections is made from semolina, chickpea flour, wheat flour, or corn flour. *Halva,* one type of flour-based sweet, is made from semolina.

Indian Cooking Techniques

A number of cooking techniques characterize Indian cuisine. ***Tandoori,*** the simplest cooking technique, is used most often in Northern India. It requires a clay oven called a *tandoor.* Tandoori chicken, lamb on skewers, and naan are three traditional foods prepared by this method.

Korma is the second major cooking technique. Foods prepared in this fashion are braised, usually in yogurt. Lamb traditionally is prepared in this way.

Vindaloo is the third major technique. Foods prepared in this way have a hot, slightly sour flavor created by combining vinegar with spices.

Chasnidarth is the fourth major technique. This simply is an Indian version of the Chinese sweet and sour.

Indian Meals

During Indian meals, all dishes are served at one time. The serving dishes usually are placed on a thalis. A *thalis* is a large, round tray, which is often made of brass, stainless steel, or silver. (In some parts of India, a banana leaf replaces the thalis.) See 32-8.

Rice generally is placed in the center of the thalis. Chutneys, pickles, yogurt, and other condiments surround it. The main dishes are placed around the edges of the tray. Diners help themselves to the food by using their fingers.

In middle-class Indian homes, the main meal of the day usually includes a meat or fish dish. (Vegetarian families would omit this dish.) Several vegetable dishes or rice or lentils and bread are also included. Occasionally, *samosas* (small pastries stuffed with vegetables, fish, or meat) may be served as an appetizer. If sweets are served, Indians eat them with the meal rather than afterward.

Family etiquette requires that diners wash their hands and rinse their mouths following a meal. They frequently follow this ritual with paan. *Paan* is a betel leaf spread with lime paste and wrapped around chopped betel nuts. As people chew it, it acts as a mouth freshener and digestive aid.

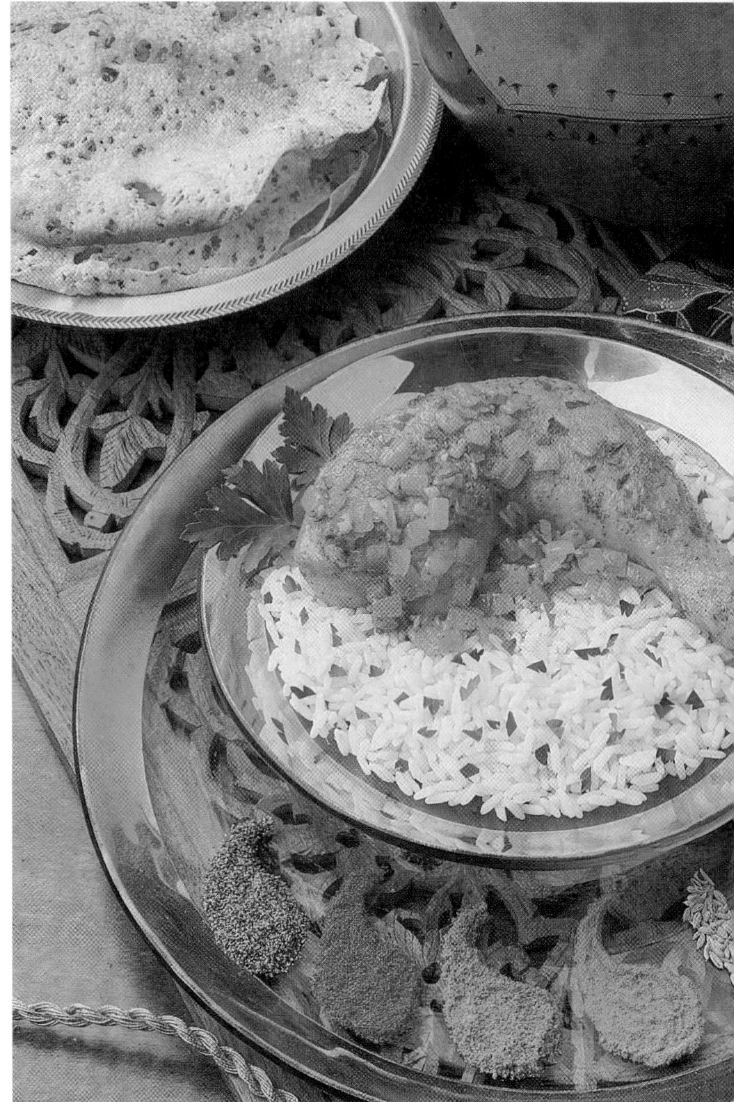

USA Rice Federation

32-8 *Indian serving dishes are generally placed on a round tray called a thalis.*

Indian Menu

Samosas
(Savory Stuffed Pastries)
Chatni
(Mixed Fruit Chutney)
Raita
(Yogurt with Vegetables)
Dal
(Lentil Puree)
Chapatis
(Unleavened Bread)
Pongal Rice
(Rice Pudding)
Tea

Ghee

(Clarified Butter)
Makes about ¾ cup

½ pound sweet butter

1. In a heavy saucepan, melt butter over very low heat.
2. When butter has melted, increase heat just enough to bring it to a boil.
3. Stir once and reduce the heat to very low. Simmer the butter, uncovered, for 50 minutes.
4. Line a strainer with 3 or 4 thicknesses of cheesecloth.
5. Carefully strain the clear liquid ghee through the cheesecloth. Make sure none of the solids in the bottom of the pan go through the cheesecloth.
6. Pour the ghee into a jar, cover, and store in a cool place.

Per tablespoon: 100 cal. (100% from fat), 0 g protein, 0 g carbohydrate, 11 g fat, 31 mg cholesterol, 0 g fiber, 2 mg sodium.

Garam Masala

(Indian Spice Mixture)

24 large cardamom seeds
2 ounces coriander seeds
2 ounces black peppercorns
1½ ounces caraway seeds
½ ounce whole cloves
½ ounce ground cinnamon

1. Remove skin from the cardamom seeds.
2. Grind cardamom seeds, coriander seeds, peppercorns, caraway seeds, and cloves until fine.
3. Add cinnamon and mix thoroughly.
4. Seal in airtight container.

Samosas

(Savory Stuffed Pastries)
Makes about 30

Pastry:
1½ cups all-purpose flour
1 tablespoon vegetable oil
¾ teaspoon salt
½ cup warm water

1. In medium mixer bowl, blend flour, oil, salt, and water until soft dough forms.
2. Turn dough out onto lightly floured board. Knead until dough is smooth and elastic, about 10 minutes.
3. Cover and set aside while preparing filling.

Filling:
1 tablespoon ghee
1 clove garlic, chopped
1 teaspoon chopped ginger root
1 medium onion, chopped
1½ cups mashed potatoes
½ cup cooked peas
1 teaspoon garam masala
1 tablespoon fresh coriander or mint
vegetable oil for frying

1. In a large skillet, heat ghee over medium heat. Add garlic, ginger root, and onion. Saute until vegetables are tender.
2. Remove from heat. Stir in mashed potatoes and peas. Season with garam masala and coriander or mint.

3. Using fingers, shape tablespoons of pastry dough into small balls. Roll each ball into a flat circle about 6 inches in diameter.
4. Cut each circle in half. Place 1 teaspoon of filling on one side of each half circle.
5. Moisten the edge of the pastry with water. Fold dough over to form a triangle and press edges together to seal.
6. In a deep saucepan, heat vegetable oil to 375°F.
7. Fry samosas a few at a time until golden brown.
8. Drain on absorbent paper. Serve immediately.

Per samosa: 50 cal. (36% from fat), 1 g protein, 7 g carbohydrate, 2 g fat, 1 mg cholesterol, 1 g fiber, 90 mg sodium.

Chatni

(Mixed Fruit Chutney)
Serves 8

1/2 pound cooking plums
1/2 pound cooking apples
1/2 pound pears or apricots
1 clove garlic
1/4 ounce fresh ginger root
2 teaspoons garam masala
1 teaspoon caraway seeds
1 teaspoon salt
2 tablespoons raisins
1 1/2 teaspoons chili powder
1/2 cup brown sugar
1 cup vinegar

1. Peel fruit, core or pit, and cut into small pieces.
2. Mince garlic and ginger root.
3. Put fruit, garlic, and ginger in large saucepan.
4. Add garam masala, caraway seeds, salt, raisins, and chili powder. Bring mixture to a boil and simmer over moderate heat for 35 minutes, stirring frequently.
5. Remove from heat, stir in sugar and vinegar, and cool. Serve cold as an accompaniment.

Per serving: 106 cal. (4% from fat), 1 g protein, 29 g carbohydrate, 1 g fat, 0 mg cholesterol, 2 g fiber, 278 mg sodium.

Raita

(Yogurt with Vegetables)
Serves 6 to 8

3 medium cucumbers
3 tablespoons chopped onions
1 teaspoon salt
3 medium firm ripe tomatoes
3 tablespoons chopped coriander
3 cups plain nonfat yogurt
1 tablespoon cumin

1. With a small sharp knife, peel cucumbers. Slice them lengthwise into halves. Scoop out the seeds. Make lengthwise slices about 1/8 inch thick. Then cut slices crosswise into 1/2-inch pieces.
2. In medium mixer bowl, combine cucumbers, onions, and salt and mix thoroughly. Let rest at room temperature for five minutes.
3. Squeeze cucumbers and onions gently to remove the excess liquid and transfer to a clean bowl.
4. Add the tomato and coriander and toss together thoroughly.
5. Combine the yogurt and cumin. Pour over the vegetables.
6. Refrigerate until ready to serve.

Per serving: 93 cal. (10% from fat), 7 g protein, 14 g carbohydrate, 1 g fat, 2 mg cholesterol, 1 g fiber, 386 mg sodium.

Dal

(Lentil Puree)
Serves 6

1 1/2 cups dried lentils
3 cups water
2 tablespoons ghee or butter
3 cloves garlic, crushed
1/2 teaspoon ground ginger
1 teaspoon coriander seeds
3/4 teaspoon salt
1/2 teaspoon cayenne pepper

1. Wash and sort lentils.
2. Place lentils and water in a large saucepan. Bring to a boil over medium-high heat.

3. Reduce heat, cover, and simmer until lentils are very tender, about 20 minutes.
4. In large skillet, heat ghee or melt butter.
5. Add the garlic, ginger, and coriander seeds. Stir over medium heat for about 3 minutes.
6. Add lentils and any remaining cooking water to skillet. Mash lentils until smooth as you stir them into the seasonings. Add water as needed to reach desired consistency for dipping.
7. Add salt and cayenne pepper.
8. Serve hot with chapatis for dipping.

Per serving: 152 cal. (24% from fat), 9 g protein, 21 g carbohydrate, 4 g fat, 10 mg cholesterol, 8 g fiber, 294 mg sodium.

Chapatis

(Unleavened Bread)
Makes 8

2 cups whole wheat flour
1/2 teaspoon salt
4 tablespoons margarine
3/4 cup water
1 tablespoon ghee

1. Mix flour and salt together in mixing bowl.
2. With pastry blender, two knives, or fingers, cut margarine into dry ingredients until particles are the size of small peas.
3. Add 1/4 cup water all at once. Mix with fingers, gradually adding enough additional water to form a soft dough.
4. Turn dough out onto a lightly floured board or pastry cloth. Knead dough until smooth and elastic, about 10 minutes.
5. Place dough in bowl, cover and let stand at room temperature 30 minutes.
6. Turn dough out onto floured surface. Divide into 8 pieces. Roll each piece into a thin circle about 5 inches in diameter.
7. Meanwhile, heat a heavy skillet over moderate heat.
8. Put chapatis, one at a time, in skillet. When small blisters appear on surface, turn and cook other side until golden.
9. Remove from skillet. Brush with ghee and keep warm in 200°F oven until all chapatis are cooked. Serve warm.

Per piece: 163 cal. (40% from fat), 4 g protein, 21 g carbohydrate, 8 g fat, 4 mg cholesterol, 6 g fiber, 201 mg sodium.

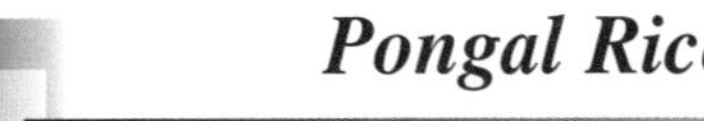

Pongal Rice

(Rice Pudding)
Serves 6 to 8

1/2 cup uncooked rice
1 cup water
6 cups fat free milk
3/4 cup sugar
1/4 teaspoon cardamom
1/4 teaspoon cinnamon
1/4 cup raisins
1/4 cup slivered, blanched almonds

1. Place rice and water in a medium saucepan. Bring to a boil over high heat.
2. Reduce heat, cover, and simmer for 5 minutes. Drain.
3. In a large, heavy saucepan, heat milk over medium heat until steaming, but not boiling.
4. Add rice. Reduce heat to low and simmer, stirring frequently, for 45 minutes.
5. Stir in sugar and continue simmering for 15 more minutes, until pudding is thick.
6. Remove pudding from heat. Stir in cardamom, cinnamon, raisins, and almonds.
7. Pour pudding into serving dishes. Chill well before serving.

Per serving: 291 cal. (12% from fat), 12 g protein, 52 g carbohydrate, 4 g fat, 5 mg cholesterol, 1 g fiber, 147 mg sodium.

China

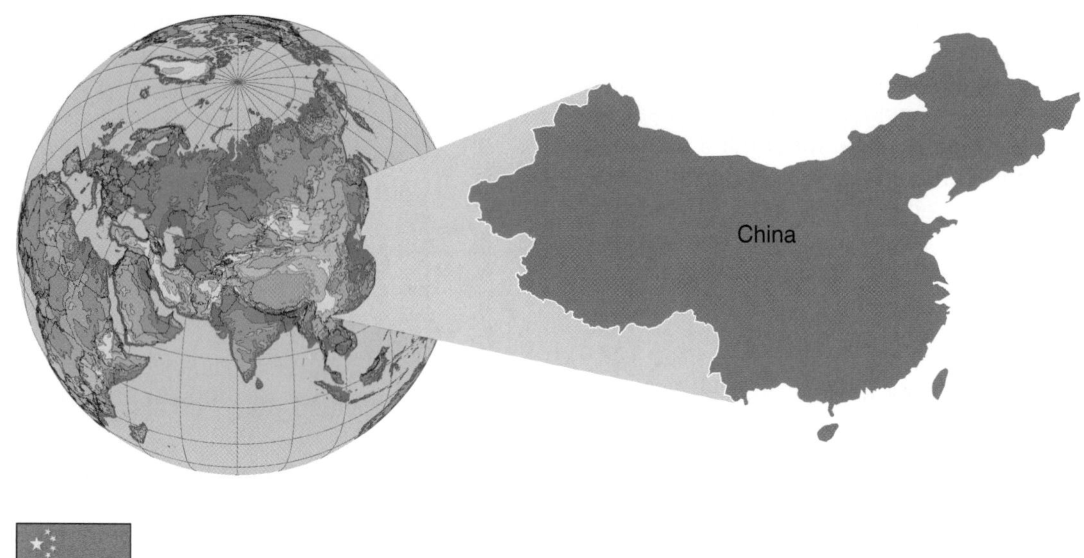

The People's Republic of China (commonly called China) is the home of one of the oldest civilizations. In modern history, China has gone through many changes. Some of these changes have affected the nation's diet. However, the roots of Chinese cuisine date back centuries.

Geography and Climate of China

China is the third largest country in the world. It occupies nearly one-fourth of Asia. Geographical features have kept China isolated for much of its history.

The Pacific Ocean and the South China Sea form China's coastlines. Western China is mountainous. The Himalayan and Tien Shan Mountains are most familiar to the Western world. Much of western and southwestern China is barren. The mountains are too high and rugged, and the valleys are too cold and dry for food production.

Eastern China is more suitable for human life. The mountains and hills are lower, and the rolling plains are fairly level. The wide valleys formed by China's great rivers have rich soil. Historically, most of China's people have crowded within this geographic area.

Because China's borders extend so far north and south, there are extremes in climate. In China's northernmost regions, the ground stays frozen two-thirds of the year. Subarctic conditions keep temperatures below zero for months at a time. Rainfall is scarce. In the southernmost provinces, however, the climate is subtropical with ample rainfall.

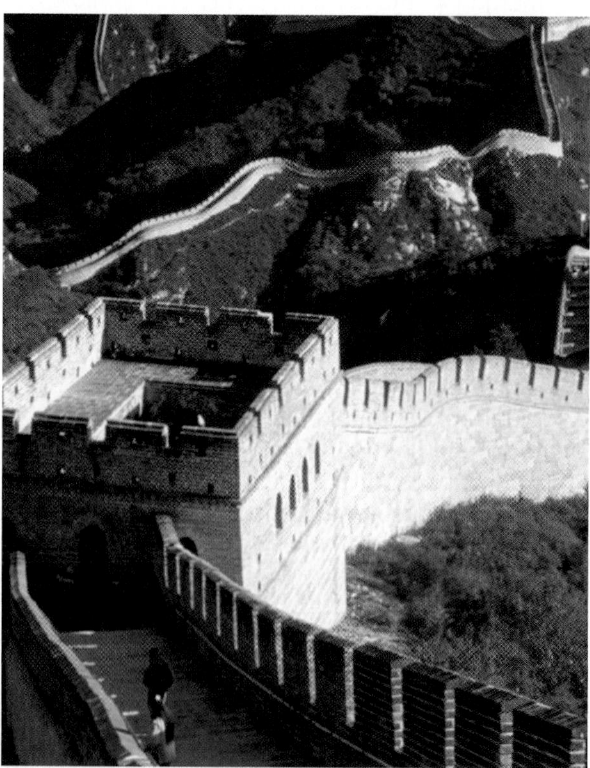

The Great Wall of China, which stretches about 4,000 miles, is an ancient feat of engineering.

The monsoons that come off the Pacific Ocean bring dust storms to the North. They also bring undependable rainfall to much of the eastern third of the country. Both drought and flooding are common.

Chinese Culture

China has a population larger than any other nation. Many notable achievements have taken place in China throughout the ages. The Chinese are credited with numerous inventions, including paper, gunpowder, and the magnetic compass. They built the Great Wall, which stretches about 4,000 miles through northern China. The Chinese also created beautiful works of art and made important contributions in literature.

Influences on Chinese Culture

A series of dynasties ruled China for over 3,000 years. (A ***dynasty*** is a chain of rulers with the same ancestry.) For centuries, a repeated pattern occurred in which a dynasty would come to power, rule, gradually weaken, and be overthrown. Periods of division sometimes followed the fall of a dynasty. Then in time, another dynasty would rise to power and reunify China.

Chinese history is marked by two key invasions of foreign people. Kublai Khan led Mongol invaders into China. He established the Yuan dynasty, which ruled in the thirteenth and fourteenth centuries. In the seventeenth century, invaders from Manchuria established the Qing dynasty. This was China's last dynasty. It ruled until 1912, when the Republic of China was established.

Modern Culture in China

The Chinese Republic lasted until 1949. Then, the Chinese Communists gained control. They named the country the People's Republic of China. The leaders of the former Chinese Republic were forced to flee to the nearby island of Taiwan.

In pre-Communist days, most Chinese were Buddhists, Taoists, or Confucianists. Smaller groups of Chinese Christians and Muslims lived in scattered groups. Today, most people do not openly practice religion in China.

Chinese Agriculture

Today most of China's people are farmers, just as they were thousands of years ago. Some small family farms still exist. There, the farming methods are primitive. Farmers do nearly all the work by hand or with the help of a single water buffalo or donkey. The government controls other farms and operates them as communes.

China's chief agricultural product is rice. Other important products include wheat, corn, millet, sorghum, oats, rye, barley, soybeans, tea, and sugarcane. Chinese celery, turnips, radishes, and eggplant are the most important vegetable crops. The Chinese also grow pears, grapes, oranges, apricots, kumquats, lychee nuts, and figs where weather permits.

The Chinese raise few beef or dairy cattle. Instead, they raise pigs, chickens, ducks, geese, and other small animals that can eat scraps, 32-9. A few sheep and goats graze in mountainous and grassy areas. China's waters provide an abundance of fish.

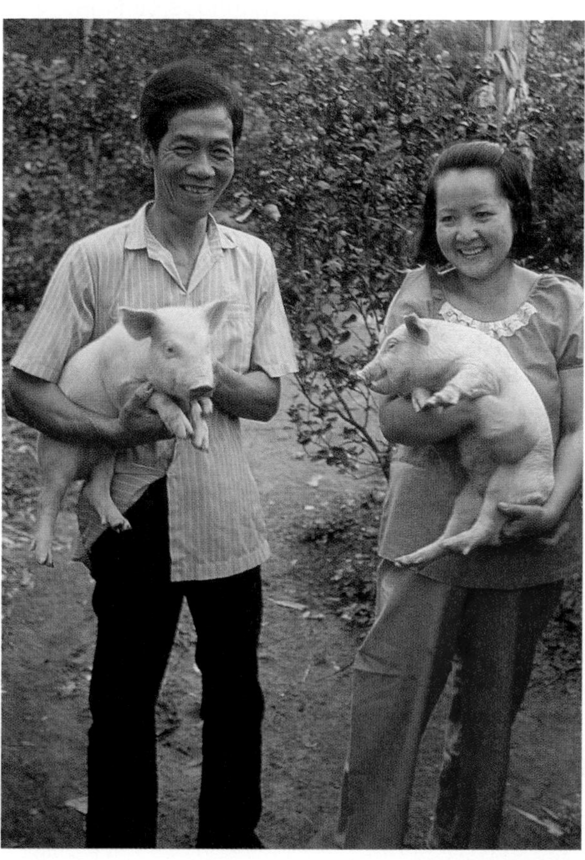

Heifer Project International

32-9 *Pigs provide a good source of nutrition and income without requiring grazing room or costly feed.*

Chinese Holidays

The most widely celebrated festival in China is the *Spring Festival,* which recognizes the new year. The Chinese zodiac follows a 12-year cycle, with each year being named for a different animal. Each new year is welcomed with a special dinner of festive foods, including candied fruits and dumplings.

The *Dragon Boat Festival* falls in midsummer. People used to throw rice cakes into the river to appease a mythical dragon. Now they recognize this occasion by holding boat races and eating rice cakes that have been wrapped in bamboo leaves.

The *Moon Festival* comes in midautumn. The Chinese celebrate this festival by eating moon cakes, which are pastries filled with bean paste or lotus seeds. Adults sit outside and enjoy the full moon while children parade through the streets with lanterns.

Chinese Cuisine

The Chinese enjoy a nutritious cuisine. Their meals include large amounts of rice and vegetables but only small amounts of meat. They stir-fry, steam, or simmer many of their dishes. This combination of healthful ingredients and light cooking methods makes Chinese cuisine fairly low in fat. However, it is high in vitamins, minerals, and fiber. One nutritional drawback of the Chinese diet is the high sodium level that results from liberal use of soy sauce.

Besides nourishing the body, Chinese cuisine delights the senses. An old Chinese proverb describes a well-prepared dish as one that smells appetizing as it is brought to the table. The dish must stimulate the appetite by its harmonious color combinations. The food must taste delicious and sound pleasing as it is being chewed. Today, the best Chinese dishes still live up to these high standards.

Chinese Ingredients

In the past, many Chinese ingredients were difficult to obtain in the United States. Today, most large cities have specialty shops that stock Chinese foods.

The ingredients described in 32-10 often appear in Chinese recipes. Besides these ingredients, Chinese cooks use many seasonings. Important seasonings include ginger root, scallions, garlic, sugar, bean paste, and fermented black bean. Monosodium glutamate (MSG), hot pepper, sesame seed oil, star anise, Chinese peppercorns, and five spice powder are also common.

Preparing Ingredients

The Chinese spend more time preparing food to be cooked than they spend cooking. Because most Chinese dishes cook so quickly, cooks must assemble all the ingredients in advance.

Much of the preparation time involves slicing, chopping, shredding, dicing, and mincing vegetables and meats. You can prepare many ingredients hours or even days in advance and refrigerate them until use.

Chinese Cooking Utensils

Of all Chinese cooking utensils, the wok is the most versatile. A ***wok*** looks like a metal bowl with sloping sides. Some woks have covers. A metal ring makes it possible to use a wok on a gas or electric range.

Woks are ideal for stir-frying because they conduct heat evenly and rapidly. There are few foods that cannot be cooked in a wok. Other cooking methods, such as deep-frying, can also be done in a wok. If you do not have a wok, you can use a heavy, smooth skillet for this type of cooking.

A second piece of Chinese cooking equipment is the *steamer.* A steamer looks like a round, shallow basket with openings. Steamers often are sold in sets of five so several foods can steam at the same time. Most Chinese steamers are made from bamboo. In the United States, aluminum steamers are more common.

A third cooking tool is the *cleaver.* Because the Chinese eat with chopsticks, cooks must cut all the ingredients into pieces that diners can handle easily. Small pieces of food also cook more evenly and rapidly. Chinese cooks use cleavers to perform all cutting tasks as well as crushing and pounding tasks. They use the wide, flat sides of cleaver blades to scoop and transfer food.

A number of other tools will come in handy when preparing Chinese foods. A *curved*

Basic Ingredients Used in Chinese Cooking
bamboo shoots. Cream-colored vegetable that adds a crisp, chewy texture to foods.
bean curd. Gelatinous, cream-colored cake made from soybeans that is a major source of protein in the Chinese diet.
bean sprouts. Sprout of the mung bean.
bean threads (cellophane noodles). Thin, smooth, and translucent noodles.
black mushrooms. Very dark mushrooms that are sold dried.
Chinese cabbage (bok choy). Type of cabbage with a white celerylike stalk topped with green leaves that is used for cooking and stewing.
Chinese pea pods. Tender, crisp, green, pod-shaped vegetable.
golden needles. Parts of the tiger lily plants that look like brown shriveled stems.
hoisin sauce. Dark, thick sauce that is made from beans, salt, spices, and sugar that is used in cooking and at the table.
oyster sauce. Dark brown sauce that is made from oysters and seasonings and is used with dark-colored dishes and as a dipping sauce.
soy sauce. Brown sauce made from soybeans, wheat, flour, salt, and water.
water chestnuts. Round, cream-colored vegetables that can be purchased canned or fresh.
winter melon. Large melon with pale green skin and white flesh that is cooked with vegetables and meat or added to soup.
wood ears. Type of brown fungus that grows on trees.

***32-10** Some of these Chinese ingredients are available in most supermarkets. Others can be found at Asian specialty stores.*

spatula that fits the shape of the pan is ideal for stirring and turning foods in the wok. *Long chopsticks* are useful for loosening and mixing food. A *wire-mesh strainer* helps lift deep-fried foods out of hot oil. A *ladle* can be used to serve foods and spoon liquids over ingredients in the wok. A *bamboo brush* is helpful for cleaning the wok. See 31-11.

Chinese Cooking Methods

The Chinese use four main cooking methods: stir-frying, steaming, deep-frying, and simmering. Less often, they also use roasting as a cooking method.

Stir-Frying

Stir-frying is the most common Chinese cooking method. Meat, poultry, fish, and vegetables can be stir-fried. You must cut all ingredients into uniform pieces so they will cook evenly.

To stir-fry foods, heat a small amount of oil in the wok. When the oil becomes hot, add the ingredients that need the longest cooking time. Then add the ingredients that cook more quickly. Stir continuously throughout the cooking period. When the vegetables are crisp-tender, the dish is ready to serve. (Sometimes you might add a little stock or water and seasonings to form a sauce.)

Stir-fried foods cook rapidly, so you must watch them carefully. Stir-fried foods retain their color, texture, flavor, and nutrients. You must serve them immediately, however, or they will lose their texture and flavor. Never overfill a wok. If you are serving more than a few people, you will need to prepare several batches of the same dish.

Steaming

Steaming is the second most common cooking method in China. Because most

Chinese do not have ovens, steaming replaces baking. You can steam meats, poultry, dumplings, bread, and rice. The kettle used for steaming must be large enough to allow the steam to circulate freely around the food. (The water never should touch the food.) Like stir-frying, steaming is economical. Because you can steam several dishes at the same time, you save energy.

Deep-Frying

Deep-frying seals in juices and gives foods a crisp coating. Meat, poultry, egg rolls, and wontons are often deep-fried.

Foods to be deep-fried are first cut into cubes. You can coat the cubes with cornstarch or dip them in a flour and egg batter. (Sometimes you might marinate the cubes before coating them.) Plunge the coated food into hot fat a few pieces at a time. Drain all deep-fried foods on absorbent paper.

Simmering

You may prepare Chinese soups and large pieces of meat by *simmering,* 32-12. In this method of cooking, you cook the ingredients in simmering liquid over low heat. If you use a clear liquid, such as chicken broth, this method is called *clear-simmering*.

Roasting

The Chinese occasionally use several other cooking methods. Of these methods, *roasting* is most popular. The Chinese sometimes roast pork and poultry. They first rub the meat or bird with oil and/or marinate it. A quick searing over an open flame makes the skin crisp. Then they place the meat or bird on a rack or hang it on a hook to roast slowly. Of all roasted dishes, *Peking duck* is the best known. The Chinese roll slices of the crisp duck skin and tender flesh inside thin pancakes with scallions and hoisin sauce.

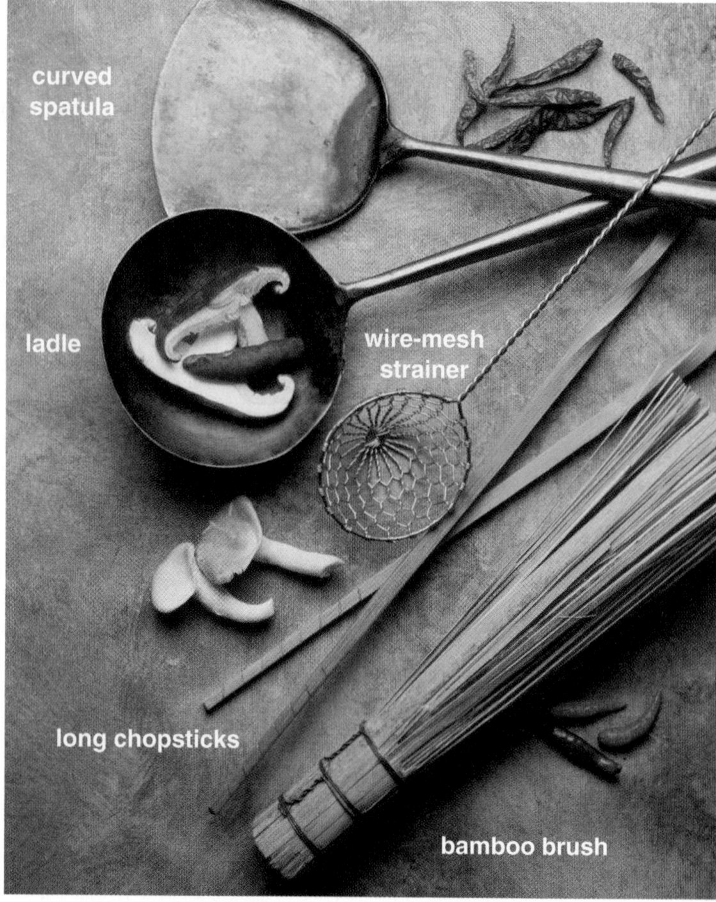

32-11 *These Chinese utensils are especially helpful when preparing foods in a wok.*

Traditional Chinese Foods

From basic ingredients and cooking methods, the Chinese prepare a variety of traditional foods.

Chinese Grain Products

For centuries, rice has been the backbone of the southern Chinese diet. This is mainly because rice is both inexpensive and filling.

The Chinese use glutinous, short-grain rice to make rice flour and translucent rice noodles. They use rice flour to make pastries and dumplings. They serve long-grain rice as a side dish and use it to make the main dish called *fried rice*. For this dish, Chinese cooks mix rice with meat, poultry, or fish; eggs; vegetables; and seasonings.

The Chinese prepare most rice by steaming. When ready to serve, the rice should be fluffy with firm, distinct grains.

In some parts of China, noodles or flat pancakes made from wheat flour are used in place of rice. One type of noodle is called *lo mein*. It is made from flour and eggs and resembles spaghetti.

The Chinese also use wheat flour to make the skins or wrappers for *wontons* (dumplings) and *egg rolls*. The dough for both contains wheat flour and eggs. The Chinese usually fill egg rolls and wontons with a mixture of minced vegetables and meat, poultry, or shellfish. They prepare wontons by steaming, deep-frying, or

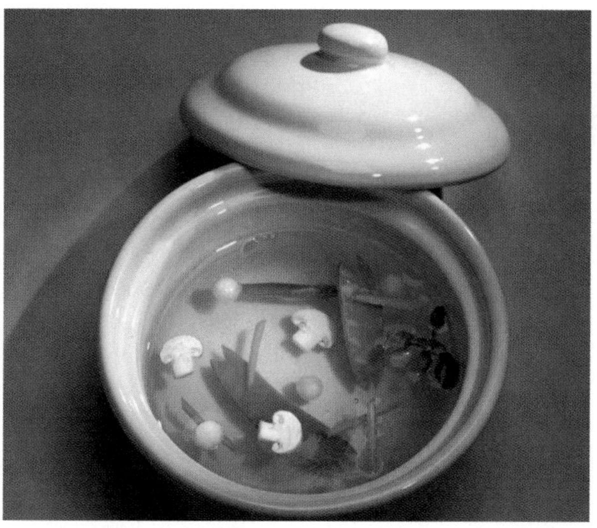

32-12 Simmering helps develop the subtle flavors of Chinese soups.

boiling them in soups. Egg rolls usually are deep-fried.

Chinese Vegetables

Vegetables are used to a greater extent than meat in the Chinese diet. The Chinese grow many varieties of vegetables. These include Chinese cabbage, broccoli, spinach, pea pods, radishes, mushrooms, and cauliflower, 32-13. The Chinese eat vegetables alone, in salads, and in soups. They also use vegetables to stretch small amounts of meat, fish, and poultry. Vegetables help make Chinese cooking economical and nutritious.

Q: Is it true that drinking tea has health benefits?

A: Tea contains phytochemicals called bioflavonoids. These substances act as antioxidants, which protect certain compounds in the body from the damaging effects of oxygen. Antioxidants have been shown to reduce the risks of cancer and heart disease.

Chinese Main Dishes

Although the Chinese eat chicken and duck, they eat little beef. This is partly because beef is scarce and not very good. Also, some religions forbid the eating of beef. Religions may forbid the eating of pork as well. Sweet and sour pork is a popular dish among those allowed to eat pork. *Sweet and sour pork* is a mixture of deep-fried pork cubes, pineapple, and vegetables in a sweet-sour sauce.

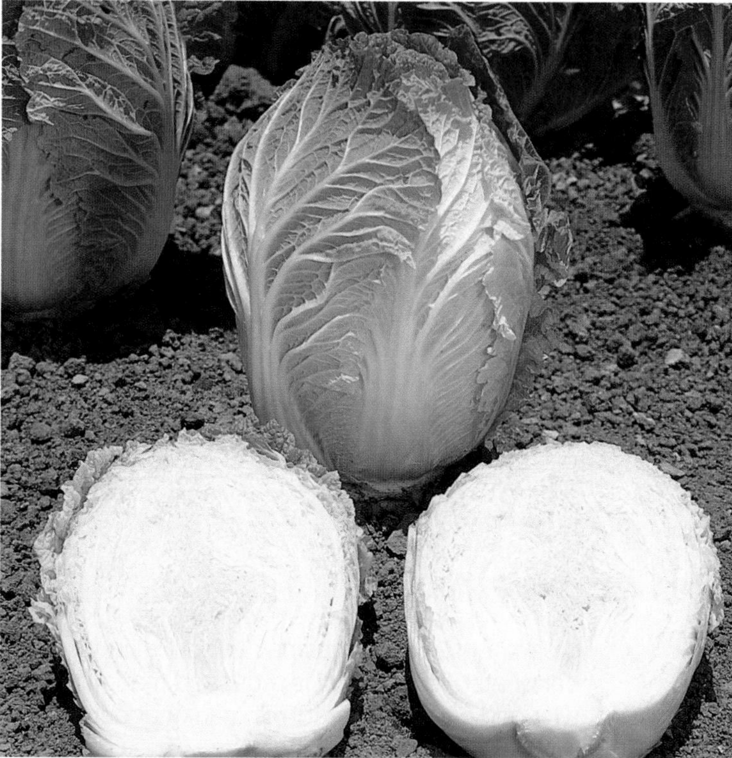

courtesy of W. Atlee Burpee & Co.

32-13 Chinese cabbage has larger leaves, a lighter color, and a milder flavor than green cabbage.

Fish are more important to the Chinese diet than meat. Many kinds of fresh- and saltwater fish and shellfish are available. The Chinese preserve some fish by drying. This allows them to transport the fish inland or store it for times of need.

The Chinese also like eggs, which they consider a sign of good luck. The Chinese eat both chicken eggs and duck eggs, but they prefer chicken eggs. They use eggs in soups, such as egg drop soup. (*Egg drop soup* is seasoned chicken broth containing beaten eggs.) They also use eggs in main dishes, such as fried rice and egg foo yung. (*Egg foo yung* is the Chinese version of an omelet.) The Chinese scramble, steam, and smoke eggs, too.

Chinese Soups

Soups are popular throughout China. Some soups, such as *Chinese noodle soup,* are very light. Others, such as velvet-corn soup, are heavier. The Chinese use exotic ingredients to make *shark fin soup* and *bird nest soup*.

Most Chinese soups are accompaniments rather than filling main dishes. Soup is the only dish the Chinese eat without chopsticks. They use spoons instead.

Good Manners Are Good Business

In the United States, people are often coached to accept a portion of all the foods offered to them. Following this practice at a Chinese business dinner, however, could cause you to offend your host. As a sign of his or her generosity, your host is likely to repeatedly refill your empty dish. He or she will probably offer plain rice as the next-to-last course. Eating the rice would indicate that you are still hungry. This would make your host feel as though he or she had failed to meet your needs. You would be wise to refuse the rice course.

Chinese Desserts

Chinese cooks use few dairy products. Chinese recipes rarely call for milk, cheese, butter, or cream. However, some Chinese people now eat ice cream, and they sometimes serve Peking dust at banquets. *Peking dust* is a dessert made of whipped cream covered with chestnut puree and garnished with nuts.

Sweet desserts are much less common in China than in other Asian countries. The Chinese reserve sweet desserts for banquets. Then they serve the desserts in the middle of the meal rather than at the end. Fresh or preserved fruits, almond cookies, almond float, and eight treasure rice pudding are popular desserts. (*Almond float* is cubes of almond-flavored gelatin garnished with fruit. *Eight treasure rice pudding* is a molded rice pudding made with candied or dried fruits.)

Chinese Tea

Tea is China's national drink. The Chinese serve black teas, oolong teas, and green teas. (In China, black tea is called *red tea* because black is an unlucky color.) Some teas are scented with fragrant blossoms. The Chinese never add cream, lemon, or sugar to their tea. They usually serve tea at the end of meals. They also offer tea to arriving and departing guests as a sign of hospitality. See 32-14.

Chinese Meals

The Chinese eat three meals a day. Breakfast may be just a bowl of ***congee*** (a thick porridge made from rice or barley), rice, or boiled noodles. More well-to-do families often serve the congee with several salty side dishes. They may also serve hot sesame muffins, Chinese doughnuts, or pastries bought from a nearby street vendor.

Lunch and dinner are similar. At both meals, all the dishes are served at once. The soup is placed in the center of the table. Four other dishes of pork, chicken, or fish, with or without vegetables, and one vegetable dish surround the soup. Rice always accompanies the main dishes.

Although the Chinese eat few sweets, they do enjoy snacks. *Dim sum* (steamed dumplings) are delicate pastries filled with meat, fish, vegetables, or occasionally a sweet fruit. Most are steamed, but a few are deep-fried.

At a Chinese table, each person's cover is set with a rice bowl, soup spoon, and shallow soup bowl. A shallow sauce dish, a larger dish for main dishes, and a tea cup are also placed at each cover. The Chinese use ***chopsticks*** as their eating utensils for all dishes except soup and finger foods.

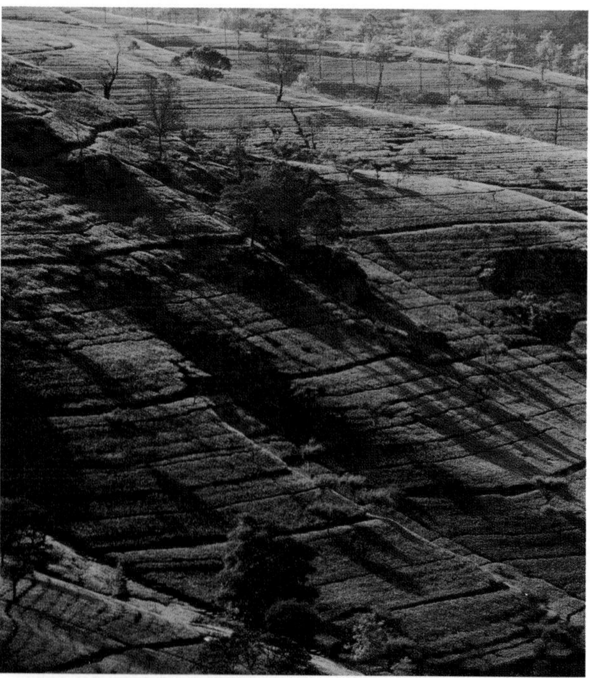

32-14 Tea is often grown on terraced hillsides to increase the amount of farmable land.

Chinese Menu

Ch'un-Chuan
(Egg Rolls)
Tan-Hau-T'ang
(Egg Drop Soup)
T'ien-Suan-Ku-Lao-Jou
(Sweet and Sour Pork)
Chao-Hsueh-Tou
(Stir-Fried Snow Peas with Chinese Mushrooms and Bamboo Shoots)
Pai-Fan
(Steamed Rice)
Preserved Kumquats
Hsing-Jen-Ping
(Almond Cookies)
Ch'a
(Tea)

Ch'un-Chuan

(Egg Rolls)
Makes 16 to 18 egg rolls

- 1/2 pound ground pork
- 1 1/2 teaspoons cornstarch
- dash pepper
- 1 tablespoon light brown sugar
- 1 tablespoon low-sodium soy sauce
- 3 tablespoons vegetable oil
- 2 cups shredded cabbage
- 1 cup finely chopped celery
- 3 cups raw bean sprouts, washed and drained
- 1/4 cup sliced mushrooms
- 1 tablespoon cornstarch
- 2 tablespoons cold water
- 1 1-pound package commercial egg roll wrappers
- 3 cups oil for frying

1. In medium mixing bowl, combine pork, cornstarch, pepper, brown sugar, and soy sauce. Let stand while heating oil.
2. Heat 1 tablespoon oil in wok or large skillet over high heat for 30 seconds.
3. Swirl oil over bottom and sides of wok and heat another 30 seconds. (If oil begins to smoke, reduce heat to moderate.)
4. Add pork and fry 2 minutes stirring constantly. (Meat should lose its reddish color.) Put meat in bowl and set aside.
5. Add the remaining 2 tablespoons of oil to the wok.
6. Add cabbage, celery, and bean sprouts, stir-fry 3 minutes.
7. Add mushrooms, stir-fry another 2 minutes.
8. Return pork to wok. Continue cooking and stirring over moderate heat until liquid comes to a boil.
9. Remove meat and vegetables. Remove all but 3 tablespoons of the cooking liquid from the wok.
10. Mix cornstarch with cold water. Add to cooking liquid and stir until slightly thickened.
11. Return meat and vegetables to wok to glaze with sauce and then transfer entire contents of wok to shallow pan. Cover and refrigerate until cool enough to handle, about 20 minutes.
12. Place one egg roll wrapper diagonally on the surface in front of you.
13. Use fingers to shape about 1/4 cup of cooled filling into a cylinder about 4 inches long. Place the cylinder parallel to the edge of your work surface in the center of the wrapper.
14. Fold the corner of the wrapper closest to you over the filling. Fold the two side corners toward the center like an envelope. Brush a little water on the top corner. Then roll the egg roll toward the top corner and seal well.
15. Place filled egg rolls on a baking sheet and cover with a slightly damp towel.
16. Place 3 cups of oil in a wok or deep saucepan. Heat oil to 375°F.
17. Fry egg rolls, 5 at a time, until crisp and golden brown, about 3 or 4 minutes.
18. Place cooked egg rolls on a plate lined with paper towels to drain while you finish frying. Serve immediately or keep warm for a short time in a 225°F oven.

Per egg roll: 124 cal. (31% from fat), 6 g protein, 16 g carbohydrate, 4 g fat, 27 mg cholesterol, 1 g fiber, 132 mg sodium.

Tan-Hau-T'ang

(Egg Drop Soup)
Serves 5 to 6

- 5 cups lowfat chicken broth
- 3/4 cup minced, cooked chicken
- 1 tablespoon cornstarch

3 tablespoons cold water
2 eggs, lightly beaten
2 scallions, finely chopped

1. In a large saucepan, bring chicken broth to a boil.
2. Reduce heat to moderate and add chicken. Simmer 5 minutes.
3. Mix cornstarch with cold water. Add to soup, stirring until soup thickens and becomes clear.
4. Slowly pour in eggs and stir once, gently. Turn off the heat.
5. Transfer soup to a heated tureen and garnish with chopped scallions.

Per serving: 60 cal. (45% from fat), 6 g protein, 3 g carbohydrate, 3 g fat, 87 mg cholesterol, 0 g fiber, 188 mg sodium.

T'ien-Suan-Ku-Lao-Jou

(Sweet and Sour Pork)
Serves 5 to 6

2 eggs, lightly beaten
1 teaspoon low-sodium soy sauce
1/2 cup cornstarch
1/2 cup flour
1/2 cup lowfat chicken broth
1 pound lean pork, trimmed and cut into 1-inch cubes
3 cups vegetable oil for frying

Sauce:
2 tablespoons vegetable oil
3 green onions, finely chopped
3 medium green peppers, cleaned, seeded, and cut into strips
2 cups canned pineapple chunks, drained (reserve juice)
3 tablespoons brown sugar
1/2 teaspoon ground ginger
3/4 cup reserved pineapple juice
4 1/2 tablespoons cider vinegar
1 1/2 tablespoons red wine vinegar
3 tablespoons reduced-sodium soy sauce
1 1/2 tablespoons cornstarch dissolved in
2 tablespoons cold water

1. In large bowl, prepare coating batter by combining eggs, 1 teaspoon soy sauce, 1/2 cup cornstarch, flour, and chicken broth. Set aside.
2. Prepare and assemble all other ingredients.
3. Just before cooking, add pork cubes to coating batter. With fork or chopsticks, stir to coat cubes evenly.
4. Preheat oven to 250°F.
5. Put 3 cups oil into wok or very large skillet. Over high heat, heat oil to 375°F.
6. Add pork cubes, a few at a time, fry until crisp and golden.
7. Remove pork to paper towel-lined baking pan to drain. Then, put pork in baking dish and keep warm in oven.
8. Pour remaining oil from wok or skillet. Add 2 tablespoons fresh oil and heat over high heat for 30 seconds.
9. Add green onions and green peppers to wok or skillet. Stir-fry about 2 to 3 minutes.
10. Add pineapple and stir-fry an additional minute.
11. Add brown sugar, ginger, pineapple juice, cider vinegar, red wine vinegar, and soy sauce. Cook until bubbly.
12. Add dissolved cornstarch to sauce. Cook, stirring constantly, until sauce thickens and becomes clear.
13. Pour sauce over fried pork cubes and serve immediately.

Per serving: 494 cal. (42% from fat), 18 g protein, 60 g carbohydrate, 23 g fat, 121 mg cholesterol, 2 g fiber, 477 mg sodium.

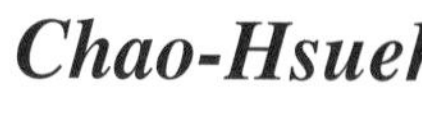

Chao-Hsueh-Tou

(Stir-Fried Snow Peas with Chinese Mushrooms and Bamboo Shoots)
Serves 6

2/3 cup dried Chinese mushrooms
1 1/2 pounds fresh snow peas (or thoroughly defrosted frozen snow peas)
2 tablespoons vegetable oil
1 cup canned bamboo shoots, rinsed and sliced thinly
2 teaspoons sugar
1 1/2 tablespoons low-sodium soy sauce

1. In a small bowl, combine mushrooms with 1/2 cup boiling water. Let soak 15 minutes.
2. Drain, squeezing excess water from mushrooms with fingers. (Reserve soaking liquid.)
3. Cut off stems and cut mushrooms into quarters.
4. Remove tips from fresh snow peas and string from pods.
5. In wok or heavy skillet, heat the oil over high heat.
6. Add mushrooms and bamboo shoots and stir-fry for 2 minutes.

7. Add snow peas, sugar, 2 tablespoons of the reserved soaking liquid, and soy sauce. Cook over high heat, stirring constantly, until water evaporates, about 2 to 3 minutes.
8. Transfer contents of wok to a serving dish and serve immediately.

Per serving: 92 cal. (49% from fat), 3 g protein, 8 g carbohydrate, 5 g fat, 0 mg cholesterol, 2 g fiber, 262 mg sodium.

Pai-Fan

(Steamed Rice)
Serves 6

1 cup uncooked long grain rice
2 cups cold water

1. Put rice and cold water in heavy saucepan and bring to a boil. Stir once or twice.
2. Cover pan, reduce heat to low and simmer 15 minutes.
3. Remove from heat and let rest 5 minutes. (Do not uncover pan.)
4. Remove cover and fluff rice with chopsticks or a fork. Serve immediately.

Per serving: 112 cal. (1% from fat), 2 g protein, 25 g carbohydrate, 0 g fat, 0 mg cholesterol, 1 g fiber, 2 mg sodium.

Hsing-Jen-Ping

(Almond Cookies)
Makes 5 dozen cookies

4 cups all-purpose flour
1 1/2 cups sugar
1/2 teaspoon baking powder
1 teaspoon salt
1 cup shortening
1 egg, beaten
1 tablespoon water
1 teaspoon almond extract
5 dozen blanched whole almonds
1 egg yolk
2 tablespoons fat free milk

1. Preheat oven to 375°F.
2. In large mixing bowl, combine flour, sugar, baking powder, and salt.
3. With pastry blender or two knives, cut in shortening until particles are the size of small peas.
4. In small bowl, combine egg, water, and almond extract.
5. Add egg mixture to flour mixture all at once. Mix well.
6. Knead dough in the bowl for 1 minute.
7. Roll dough into small balls. Place 2 inches apart on ungreased baking sheets.
8. Flatten dough balls to about 3/8-inch thickness. Top each cookie with a blanched almond and brush with egg glaze made by combining the egg yolk with milk.
9. Bake cookies until lightly browned, about 12 minutes.

Per cookie: 93 cal. (46% from fat), 1 g protein, 11 g carbohydrate, 5 g fat, 9 mg cholesterol, 1 g fiber, 40 mg sodium.

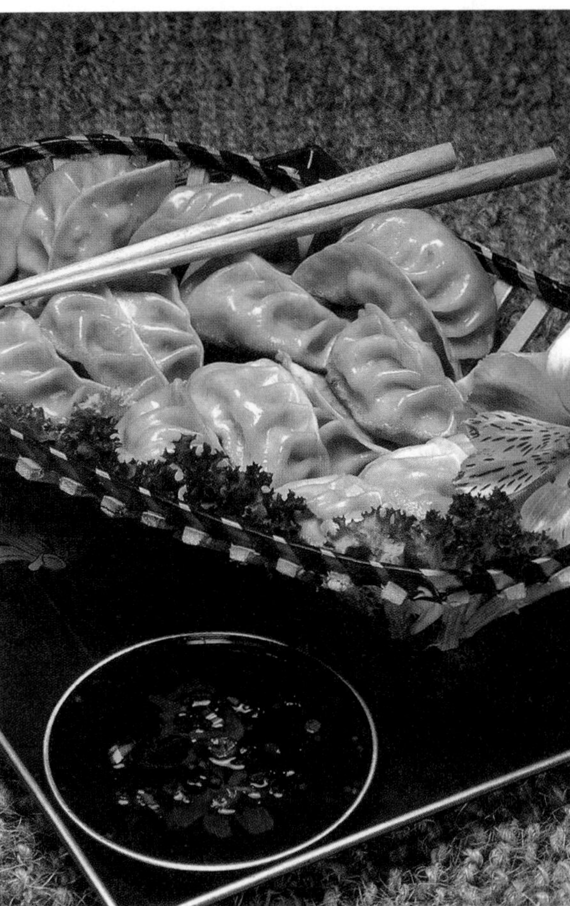

Wheat Foods Council

Chinese pot stickers are small, stuffed dumplings that are fried, boiled, or steamed and served with a dipping sauce.

Japan

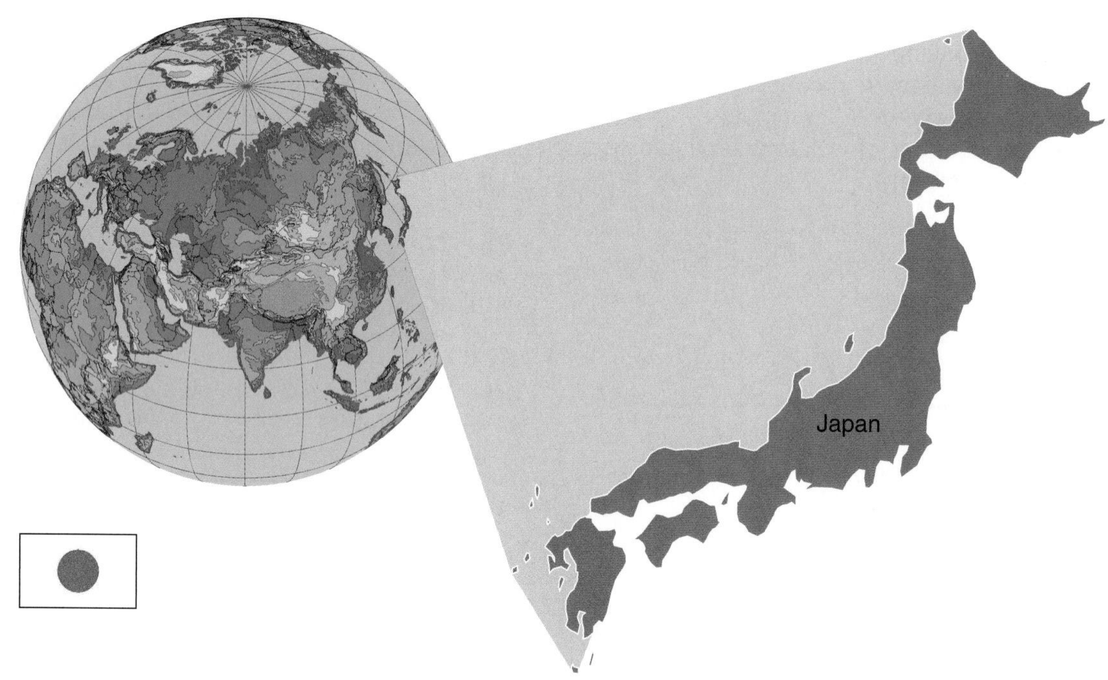

Japan has successfully adapted to Western ways without losing its sense of identity. Industrial growth after World War II brought many changes to cities like Tokyo. However, Japan's traditional values are still alive today. These values include respect for family, love of nature, and belief in hard work. The Japanese word *sappari* means "clean, light, and sparkling with honesty." Sappari still describes the Japanese people, their country, and their cuisine.

Geography and Climate of Japan

Japan is a nation of islands. Three-fourths of Japan's total land area is mountainous or hilly. The mountains have made farming difficult and have caused crowded living conditions in the few lowlands.

Swift-flowing rivers and crystal clear lakes dot Japan's landscape. Many of the rivers end in picturesque waterfalls. Others bring the water used to irrigate rice fields. A few provide hydroelectric power.

Because the islands cover such a large latitude, Japan has a variety of climates. The southern part of the country is subtropical. Summers are hot and humid, and winters are mild. The bulk of the population lives in this area. Their housing, clothing, and farming methods are suited to a warm climate.

Hokkaido, Japan's northernmost island, has cold winters. Temperatures fall below freezing

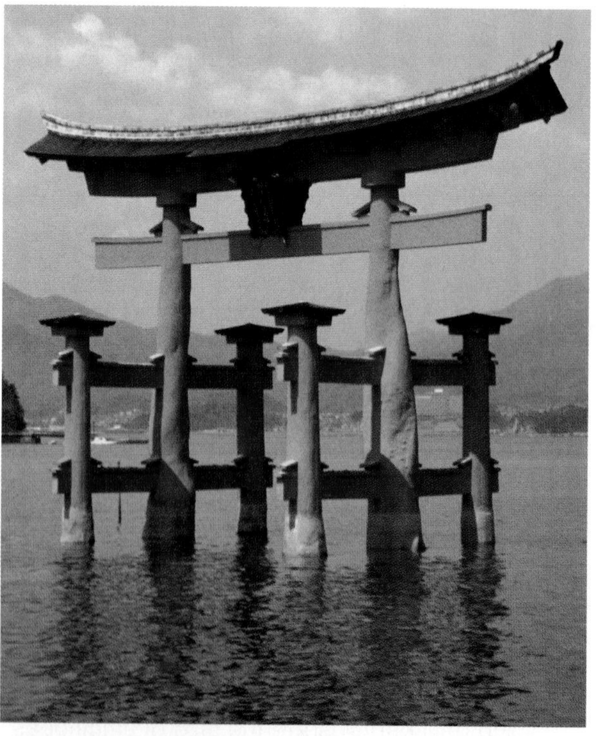

The Gateway at Miyajima Island is said to welcome spirits as they come to visit a historic Buddhist shrine on the Japanese island.

for at least four months during the winter, and snowfall is heavy.

Japan receives more than adequate moisture. Seasonal winds, called *monsoons*, bring rain in summer and snow in winter. During September, severe storms, called *typhoons*, bring heavy rains and damaging winds.

Japanese Culture

The exact origin of the Japanese people is uncertain. However, archaeologists believe the first inhabitants came from the arid steppes of northern Asia.

Influences on Japanese Culture

The imperial family that set up the first state in Japan is thought to have consolidated scattered clans. This happened around A.D. 4. The imperial family, headed by an emperor, actively ruled Japan until 1192. Then, a military government took over, and the emperor became a figurehead. Military rule under the shoguns lasted for nearly 700 years.

The first *Occidentals* (Westerners) arrived in Japan in the sixteenth century. The Portuguese were the first to arrive. Jesuit missionaries and, later, groups of Spanish, Dutch, and English traders followed the Portuguese. The Japanese ruling class encouraged both trade and Christianity.

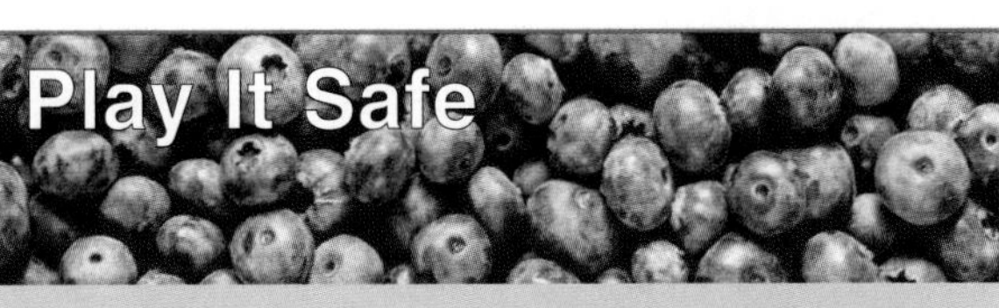

Becoming lost in an unfamiliar place is not only frightening, it can also be dangerous. This problem can be further complicated if you are unable to communicate with the local people. You should carry the name and address of the place you are staying with you. (When visiting a country that uses a different alphabet, ask someone who knows the language to write it for you.) You can show the address to taxi drivers or others who might be helping you with directions.

In the early seventeenth century, the shoguns began to see Occidental influence as a threat to their power. As a result, they closed Japan's doors to the rest of the world. Japanese ports remained closed to most foreign ships for two centuries.

In 1867 the shogun gave up his power. With the emperor again in control, class distinction ended and feudalism was abolished. Two years later, a constitutional monarchy was established.

Modern Culture in Japan

Japan experienced a tremendous period of expansion toward the end of the nineteenth century. By the end of World War I, Japan was recognized as one of the world's great powers. Japanese military strength continued to grow, and the government became a military dictatorship.

Following their defeat in World War II, Japan began to rebuild. In the decades that followed, Japan experienced rapid industrial growth. Today, Japan plays a major role in world affairs.

Japanese Agriculture

Rice is Japan's most important crop. Over half the tillable land is used for rice production. In the far south, Japanese farmers can grow two crops each year. Other important crops include sweet potatoes, wheat, and sugar beets.

The Japanese raise tea bushes on terraced hillsides. They grow mandarin oranges and strawberries in the South. They grow peaches, pears, persimmons, cherries, apples, and other hearty fruits in the North. The Japanese also grow beans, large radishes, cucumbers, lettuce, onions, cabbage, turnips, carrots, and spinach. They grow many varieties of peas, squash, and pumpkins, too.

Land has always been scarce, and the teachings of Buddhism forbid the eating of meat. Therefore, the Japanese have traditionally raised little livestock. In recent years, however, livestock production has increased. This is partly due to the abandonment of Buddhist dietary laws. Also, a taste for eggs, milk, meat, and poultry has been developing among the Japanese people.

Seafood provides most of the protein in the Japanese diet. Japan's fishing industry is one of the world's largest. Sardines, salmon, herring, cuttlefish, yellowtail, and other kinds of fish, as well as seaweed, live in coastal waters. The Japanese freeze or can some of the seafood catch for export.

Japanese Festivals

Festivals are an important part of Japanese culture, 32-15, and foods are an important part of many festivals. The biggest celebration in Japan is the New Year festival. The Japanese eat long noodles on New Year's Eve as a symbol for living a long life. They also make offerings of rice cakes to the New Year god.

Soybeans play a symbolic role in a second Japanese New Year celebration called *Setsubun*. This holiday takes place in early February—the time of the new year according to Japan's archaic lunar calendar. Japanese people still celebrate this event by eating one soybean for each year they have lived. They also throw handfuls of roasted soybeans in and around their homes to chase away demons. Celebrities stand near shrines and throw soybeans into crowds of people. People who catch the beans are believed to be blessed with good fortune throughout the following year.

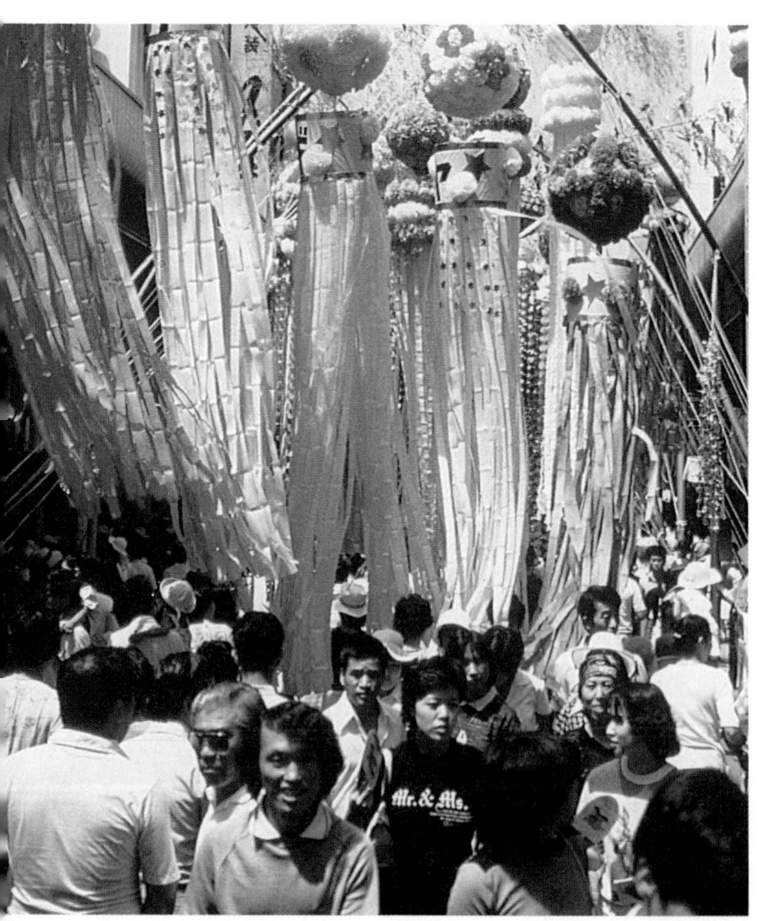

Japan National Tourist Organization

***32-15** The streets of Japanese cities become especially crowded during festival celebrations.*

A third annual tradition in Japan is the welcoming of spring with Cherry Blossom celebrations. The cherry blossom is Japan's national flower. Families enjoy picnicking under the blooming trees. People also recognize this time of year by eating cherry blossom cakes. These cakes are made of cooked, sweetened azuki beans wrapped in a pounded rice mixture to look like cherry blossoms.

Japanese Cuisine

Japan's staple foods can be easily obtained from the sea and the country's limited land resources. Rice, which forms the basis of the Japanese diet, is rich in complex carbohydrates. Soybeans and fish are the main sources of protein. These foods keep the cuisine lower in fat, saturated fat, and cholesterol than a cuisine based on meat. Vegetables, fruits, and seaweed supply vitamins, minerals, and fiber. Light cooking methods help retain the nutritional value of Japanese staple foods. However, the Japanese diet is rather high in sodium due to the popularity of soy sauce as a flavoring agent.

An important element of Japanese cuisine is subtlety of taste. Cooks achieve this subtlety through the careful selection of ingredients and cooking methods.

Another important element is aesthetic appearance. Japanese cooks place great emphasis on the color, shape, and arrangement of food on a serving dish. Many times an arrangement may suggest a particular season or mood. For instance, a cook might arrange ingredients to represent the mountains, rivers, trees, and flowers of a Japanese spring. Such a dish might be served at the spring fish festival.

Basic Japanese Ingredients

Ingredients commonly used in Japanese cooking include sesame oil, mild rice vinegar, daikon, mirin, and sake, 32-16. *Kanpyo,* gobo, and shirataki are common ingredients, too. Kanpyo is strips of dried gourd. *Gobo* is burdock root, and *shirataki* is a mixture made from a yamlike tuber. The Japanese also use salt, pepper, sugar, chives, onions, mustard, scallions, and other familiar seasonings. However, four ingredients are basic to Japanese cookery: rice, soybeans, fish, and seaweed.

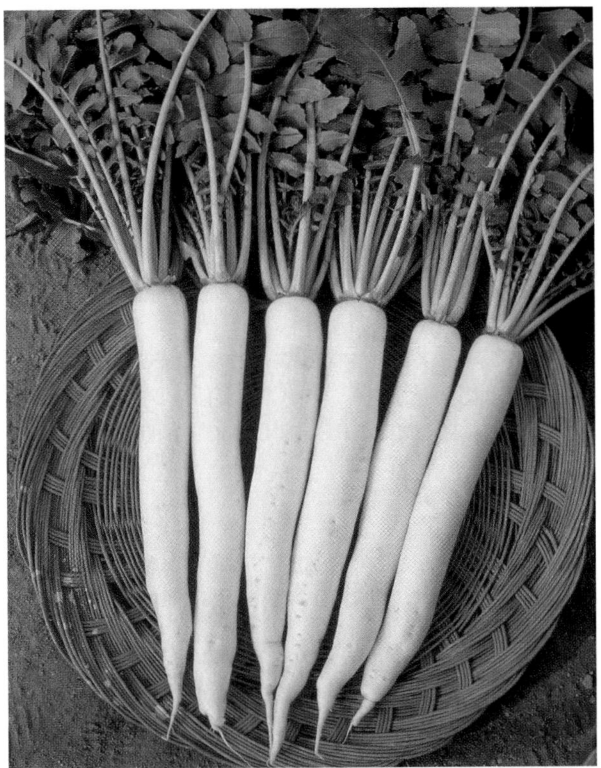

courtesy of W. Atlee Burpee & Co.

32-16 Daikon is a giant white radish that is a traditional ingredient in Japanese cuisine.

Rice

Rice is so important to the Japanese diet that the Japanese word for meal is ***gohan,*** which means rice. Japanese rice is a short-grain variety. Cooks usually steam it and serve it plain. Sometimes they cook rice with other ingredients or serve it with a sauce. Two other products, *sake* (Japanese rice wine) and *mirin* (sweet wine), are obtained from rice.

Soybeans

The Chinese introduced the soybean to the Japanese. The ***soybean*** is a legume with seeds that are rich in protein and oil. The Japanese use soybeans in many forms.

Miso is a fermented soybean paste. The Japanese use miso in a soup they serve for breakfast. It may also be an ingredient in a marinade used to prepare fish and vegetables.

Tofu is a custardlike cake made from soybeans. It has a very mild flavor. The Japanese may roll tofu in cornstarch and deep-fry it. They may scramble it with eggs. They may also saute, boil, or broil it. Sometimes, they add tofu to soups. *Sumashi* (clear broth with tofu and shrimp) is an example.

Shoyu, Japanese soy sauce, contains wheat or barley, salt, water, and malt along with soybeans. Shoyu is an all-purpose seasoning in the Japanese kitchen. (Chinese soy sauce is heavier and does not make a suitable substitute.)

Fish

Tuna, bass, flounder, cod, mackerel, ayu (sweet fish), carp, and squid are popular in Japan. The Japanese also eat many varieties of shellfish and more unusual subtropical species. *Katsuo* (dried bonito) is an essential ingredient of *dashi,* a Japanese fish stock. *Fugu* (blowfish) is a Japanese delicacy. Fugu contains a lethal toxin that can kill a diner unless the fish has been properly cleaned. Licensed fugu chefs perform this task.

Japanese cooks demand that all fish and shellfish must be fresh. Therefore, they do not kill shellfish until minutes before cooking. They keep freshwater varieties that will be eaten raw alive until serving time.

Two of the most popular fish dishes are sashimi and sushi. *Sashimi* are raw fillets of fish eaten alone or with a sauce. *Sushi* are balls of cooked rice flavored with vinegar. They are served with strips of raw or cooked fish, eggs, vegetables, or seaweed. Sashimi and sushi restaurants and snack bars are found throughout Japan. See 32-17.

Seaweed

The Japanese use seaweed from the surrounding oceans in both fresh and dried forms. They roll *nori,* a dried variety of seaweed, around fish or rice. They also use it as a garnish. The Japanese use *konbu* (dried kelp) in dashi. They use other varieties of seaweed as flavorings, garnishes, and vegetables in soups.

Japanese Vegetables and Fruits

Japanese farmers grow many vegetables. Traditional Japanese vegetables include *daikon,* which is a giant white radish. *Negi* is a thin Japanese leek. *Wasabi* is Japanese horseradish, and *bakusai* is Chinese cabbage. Lotus roots and shoots, edible chrysanthemum leaves, burdock, spinach, ginger root, and bamboo shoots are also popular. Many types of peas, beans, ferns, and mushrooms are common, too.

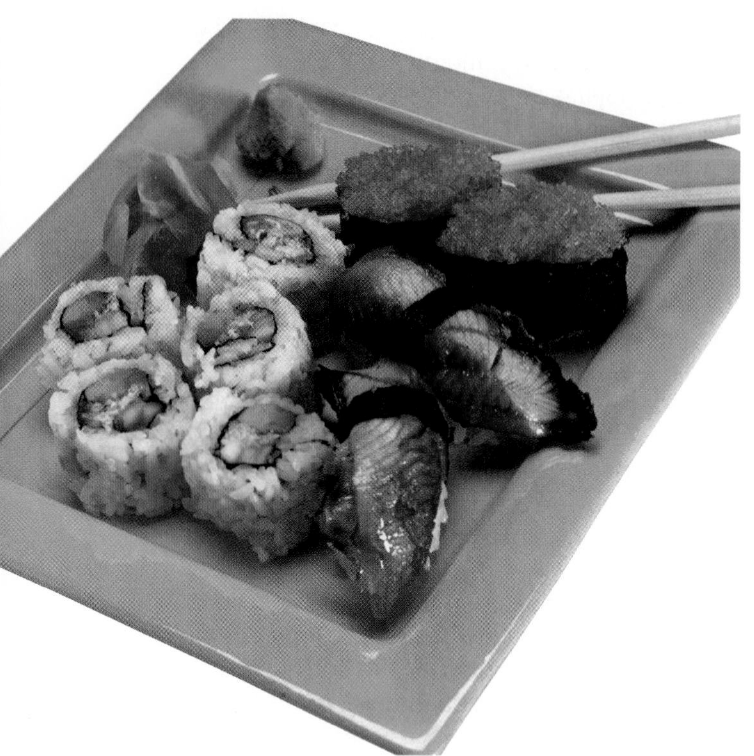

32-17 *Sushi and sashimi are served at restaurants throughout Japan.*

Japanese cooks often mix vegetables together in salads. Japan has two kinds of salads: *aemono* (mixed foods) and *sunomono* (vinegared foods). Aemono salads contain several raw or cooked vegetables in a thick dressing. Sunomono salads contain crisp, raw vegetables and cold, cooked fish or shellfish. They are served with a thin dressing made of rice vinegar, sugar, and soy sauce. *Namusu* (vegetables in a vinegar dressing) is an example.

Japanese fruits are plentiful. Persimmons and many types of oranges grow in Japan. One of the best-known oranges is the *mikan,* or mandarin orange. Apples, pears, cherries, strawberries, plums, and melons also grow well.

Japanese Main Dishes

Meat traditionally was not part of the Japanese diet. Today, however, meat appears on many Japanese tables. Because it is costly, the Japanese usually serve meat in small amounts with other foods.

Although the Japanese eat both pork and beef, their beef is famous. The tenderness of the meat results in part from the treatment the cattle receive. Japanese farmers feed the animals bran, beans, rice, and beer. They massage each steer daily with *shochu* (Japanese gin).

Poultry production in Japan has grown in recent years. Chickens are less costly to raise, so they appear more often in Japanese recipes than meat. Eggs are becoming more popular, too. *Tamago dashimaki* is the Japanese version of an omelet.

Q: Is there a link between soy foods and increased or decreased cancer risk?

A: Many studies on soy-cancer links have been conducted, but more research is needed. Some findings have been conflicting. For now, nutrition experts recommend soy foods, like all foods, be eaten in moderation as part of a varied diet.

Japanese Cooking Methods

In Japan, cooks always cut food into small pieces before cooking. This makes the food easy to pick up with chopsticks. (The Japanese use knives only for food preparation. They do not place knives on the table.)

Japanese cooks boil a variety of foods, including meat, poultry, seafood, and vegetables. The cooking liquid may be a strongly flavored stock or a mild broth. Foods cooked in boiling liquid are called *nimono.* Examples of nimono are *kimini* (sake-seasoned shrimp with egg yolk glaze) and *kiriboshi daikon* (chicken simmered with white radish threads).

Steaming is the simplest of all cooking methods. *Mushimono* (steamed foods) retain their fresh flavors, colors, and nutrients. Japanese cooks use two steaming methods. *Mushi* foods are foods cooked on a plate suspended over boiling water. *Chawan mushi* foods are foods steamed in an egg custard. Mushi foods are mild in flavor, so the Japanese usually serve them with a dipping sauce. Chawan mushi foods are richer in flavor and usually are served without a sauce.

The Japanese use frying to prepare *tempura*. Japanese cooks prepare tempura by coating vegetables, meat, poultry, and seafood in a light batter. Then they quickly fry the coated pieces in oil. See 32-18. Other Japanese *agemono* (fried foods) are deep-fried in oil. All Japanese agemono are light and delicate. They are never greasy or heavy.

The Japanese usually use broiling for meat, poultry, and fish. One popular *yakimono* (broiled food) is beefsteak. It is dipped in a mixture of soy sauce and mirin and grilled over charcoal. Beef teriyaki and yakitori are two types of yakimono popular in the United States. *Beef teriyaki* is slices of beef glazed with a special sauce. *Yakitori* is chicken, scallions, and chicken livers broiled on a skewer.

Japanese cooks prepare many dishes at the table. They use one or a combination of the above cooking methods. Sukiyaki combines two cooking methods—*nabemono* (dishes cooked at the table) and *nimono* (foods cooked in boiling liquid). ***Sukiyaki*** is a popular Japanese dish made of thinly sliced meat, bean curd, and vegetables cooked in a sauce. Cooks prepare all the raw ingredients in the kitchen. Then they cook the beef and vegetables with their accompanying sauce in a skillet at the table. Another method of preparing food at the table uses the hibachi. A *hibachi* is a small grill that can be freestanding or built into the center of the table.

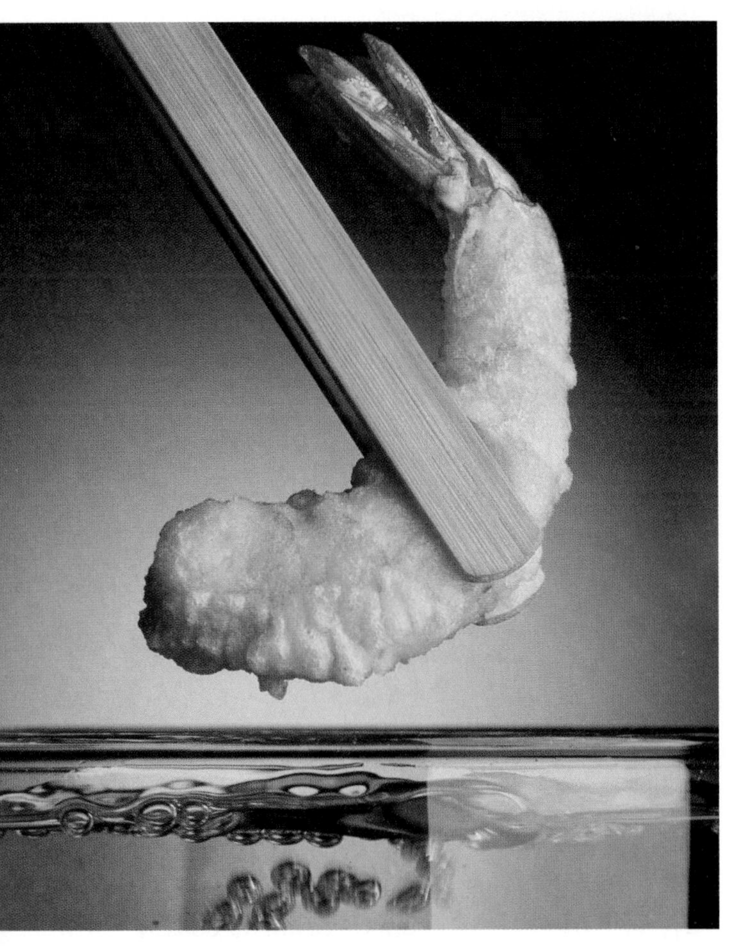

32-18 Like other foods prepared in the tempura style, this shrimp is lightly battered before being fried in oil.

Japanese Eating Customs

The Japanese do not use napkins. Instead, small, soft towels called *oshibori* are brought to the table at the beginnings and ends of meals. The oshibori are warm, damp, and fragrant. The Japanese use them to wipe their faces and hands.

Bowls used for hot foods are served covered. Diners usually remove the cover of the individual rice bowl first. This indicates that rice is Japan's most honored food. The Japanese do not eat rice all at once. Instead, they eat it with the other foods in much the same way people in the United States eat bread. The Japanese must use both hands to place a rice bowl on a tray for refilling. To use one hand is a breach of courtesy.

The Japanese drink soup from a cup rather than spooning it from a bowl. They remove the cup from the table and hold it in the left hand. Then they hold their chopsticks in the right hand to secure the food. The oldest guest always picks up his or her chopsticks first as a token of respect. After use, diners return their chopsticks to the chopstick rest.

To show appreciation for the cook's skill, it is quite proper to smack the lips or make sucking sounds. Guests often exchange sake cups with their host as a sign of respect.

Japanese Meals

Japanese meals are made up of many light dishes. The quantities served are much smaller than those served in the West. See 32-19.

In the morning, some Japanese people eat eggs and other breakfast foods popular in the United States. In many parts of Japan, however, people eat more traditional breakfast foods. Such foods include umeboshi and miroshiru. *Umeboshi* is a tiny, red, pickled plum. *Miroshiru*

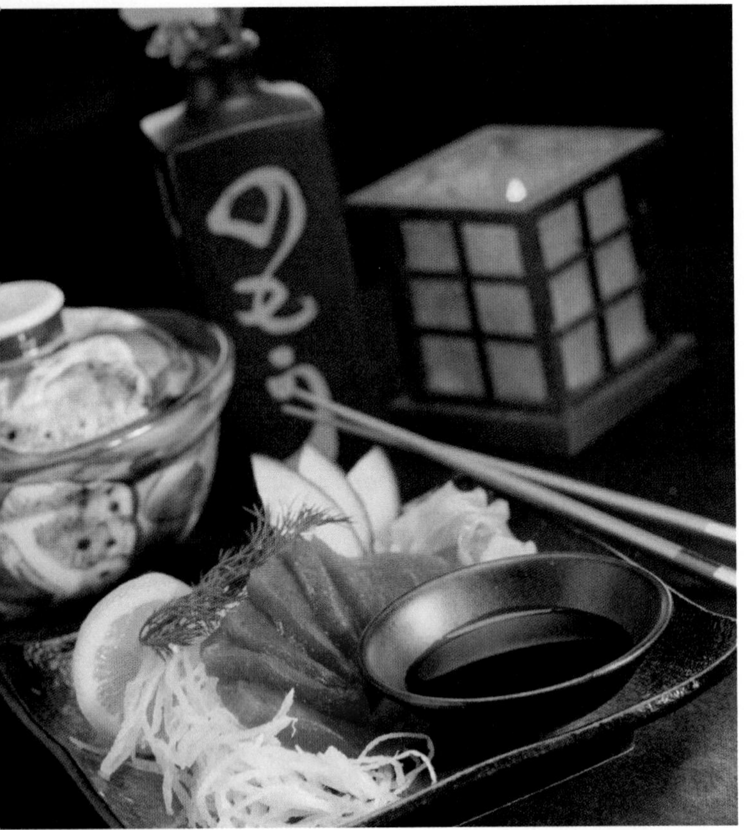

32-19 *Japanese meals emphasize the quality of food rather than the quantity.*

is a hearty soup made of dashi, miso, and rice. Japanese breakfast foods also include rice, which is often sprinkled with *nori* (a type of dried seaweed).

Japanese families may serve a carefully prepared lunch if family members come home at noon or they are expecting guests. Otherwise, Japanese cooks usually prepare simple lunches. The morning rice is reheated and served with leftover vegetables and meat or a simple sauce.

The evening meal is much more elaborate. Because businesses stay open later in Japan than in the United States, the meal usually is served later. The young children eat their meal first. The Japanese prepare children's versions of many popular foods. An example is *kushizashi* (meats, fowl, and vegetables grilled on a skewer). Cooks make kushizashi with hot peppers for adults. However, they use milder scallions when preparing the dish for children.

The Japanese usually serve all the dishes in the main meal together. They usually serve broiled or fried meat, poultry, or fish as a main course. Although the main course can vary, rice, soup, and tsukemono must be served. ***Tsukemono*** (soaked foods) are lightly pickled pieces of daikon, cucumber, melon, eggplant, and other vegetables. The Japanese eat them with rice near the end of the meal.

The Japanese rarely eat sweet desserts. They reserve sweets for special occasions. Instead, most meals end with fresh fruit.

Another meal enjoyed by the Japanese is ***kaiseka.*** This is a delicate meal that may be served after the tea ceremony. Tea is Japan's national drink. The Japanese serve green teas, which they call ***nihon-cha.*** The Japanese perform the tea ceremony just as their ancestors did hundreds of years ago. Each step of the ceremony is done according to established rules. Each movement the host makes is designed to bring pleasure to the guest. Harmony must exist among all the elements of the ceremony and among all the people present. Simple tea ceremonies may last just 40 minutes. Those that include kaiseka may last as long as four hours. See 32-20.

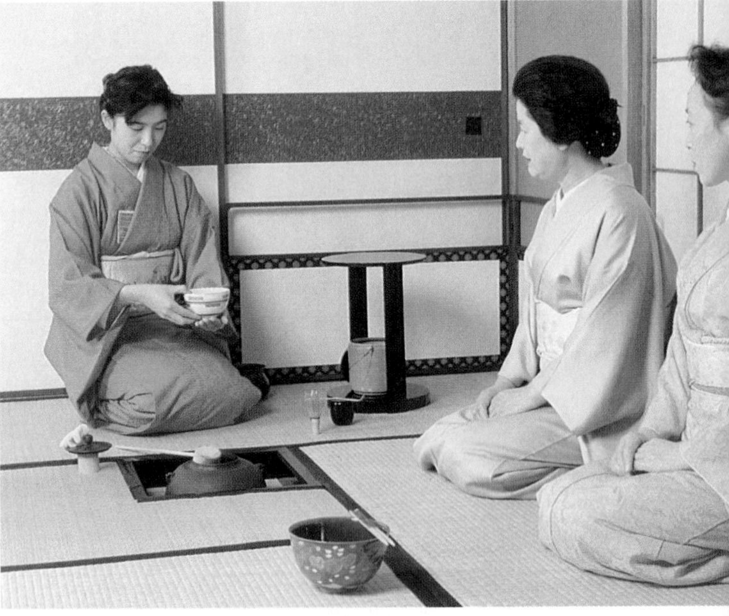

Japan National Tourist Organization

32-20 *The tea ceremony is a ritual that has been performed in Japan for hundreds of years.*

Japanese Menu

Sumashi Wan
(Clear Broth with Tofu and Shrimp)
Sukiyaki
(Beef and Vegetables Cooked in Seasoned Liquid)
Namasu
(Vegetables in a Vinegar Dressing)
Gohan
(Steamed Rice)
Snow Peas
Mikan
(Mandarin Oranges)
Nihon-Cha
(Green Tea)

Sumashi Wan

(Clear Broth with Tofu and Shrimp)
Serves 6

2 cups water
1 cake tofu, 6 ounces, cut into 6 equal squares
1 cup water
salt
7 spinach leaves (or 1/2 package frozen leaf spinach thoroughly defrosted and separated into leaves)
4 cups clam broth
2 cups lowfat chicken broth
6 small canned shrimp

1. In small saucepan, bring 2 cups of water to a boil.
2. Add tofu and let water return to a simmer.
3. Remove from heat immediately and cover. Set aside until ready to serve soup.
4. In a second saucepan, bring 1 cup lightly salted water to a boil.
5. Add spinach and cook just until tender.
6. Drain immediately and rinse under cold running water. Remove excess moisture with paper towels and set aside.
7. Wash saucepan. Combine clam broth and chicken broth and bring to a boil.
8. Meanwhile, set six soup bowls on a tray. Place a spinach leaf, a shrimp, and a cube of tofu in the bottom of each.
9. Pour broth into bowls, filling each about 3/4 full and being careful not to disturb garnish. (Pour broth down the sides of the bowls.) Serve immediately.

Per serving: 50 cal. (41% from fat), 5 g protein, 2 g carbohydrate, 2 g fat, 7 mg cholesterol, 0 g fiber, 169 mg sodium.

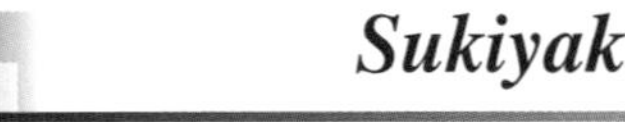

Sukiyaki

(Beef and Vegetables Cooked in Seasoned Liquid)
Serves 4 to 6

1 pound beef tenderloin or sirloin steak
1 cup water
8 ounces shirataki (long noodlelike threads) or cooked vermicelli
2 medium onions, sliced crosswise
5 leeks, split lengthwise and cut in 1 1/2-inch lengths
3/4 pound fresh mushrooms, washed and sliced
5 stalks celery, cut diagonally into 1/4-inch slices
1 pound fresh spinach, cleaned (or 1 package frozen leaf spinach, thoroughly defrosted)
1/2 pound tofu, cut into cubes
1/2 cup low-sodium soy sauce
2 tablespoons sugar
1 1/2 cups low-sodium beef broth
1/4 cup margarine

1. Slice beef cross-grained into paper-thin slices, 1 × 2 inches. (Slightly frozen meat is easier to slice.) Trim fat. Arrange slices attractively on a plate, cover with plastic wrap, and refrigerate.
2. Bring one cup of water to a boil.
3. Add shirataki and return water to a boil.
4. Drain and slice shirataki into thirds.
5. Arrange shirataki, vegetables, and tofu attractively on a serving platter, cover with plastic wrap, and refrigerate.
6. Combine soy sauce, sugar, and beef broth in a small bowl. Cover and refrigerate.
7. To cook sukiyaki, heat two tablespoons margarine in a wok over moderately high heat or an electric skillet preheated to 425°F.
8. Add half of the beef slices and cook until meat loses its pink color. Push meat to the side.
9. Add half of the onions and leeks and cook until transparent and lightly browned. (Turn meat as needed.) Push vegetables to the side.

10. Add half of the mushrooms and half of the celery in two groups. Stir-fry 2 to 3 minutes.
11. Add half the sauce and simmer about 5 minutes. Turn all foods occasionally.
12. Add half of the spinach and cook 1 minute.
13. Add half of the noodles or vermicelli and tofu. (These will absorb the broth.) Serve immediately or keep warm in a 225°F oven while you cook the remaining half of the ingredients.

Per serving: 474 cal. (23% from fat), 28 g protein, 66 g carbohydrate, 12 g fat, 26 mg cholesterol, 7 g fiber, 992 mg sodium.

Namasu

(Vegetables in a Vinegar Dressing)
Serves 6

1/2 pound daikon or white turnip, peeled and shredded
1 medium carrot, scraped and shredded
1 teaspoon salt
1 cup cold water
1/4 cup preflaked, dried bonito
1 tablespoon white vinegar
2 teaspoons sugar
monosodium glutamate (MSG), optional

1. In small bowl, combine daikon, carrot, salt, and water. Stir to mix and let stand 30 minutes.
2. Put dried bonito in a small pan and heat over low heat for 3 to 4 minutes to dry further.
3. Transfer bonito to a blender container and grind to a fine powder.
4. Drain carrot and daikon. Squeeze dry and put in mixing bowl.
5. Add vinegar, sugar, and two pinches of monosodium glutamate. Mix well and add powdered bonito. Serve at room temperature.

Per serving: 38 cal. (5% from fat), 5 g protein, 4 g carbohydrate, 0 g fat, 8 mg cholesterol, 1 g fiber, 451 mg sodium.

Gohan

(Steamed Rice)
Makes 3 cups

1 cup uncooked short-grain rice
2 cups cold water

1. Place rice and water in a large, heavy saucepan.
2. Bring water to a boil, reduce heat to low and cook rice covered for about 15 minutes, or until rice has absorbed all the liquid.
3. Remove from heat. Let the rice rest, undisturbed, 5 minutes.
4. Remove cover, fluff with fork, and serve.

Per serving: 112 cal. (1% from fat), 2 g protein, 25 g carbohydrate, 0 g fat, 0 mg cholesterol, 1 g fiber, 2 mg sodium.

Snow Peas

Serves 6

1 1/2 pounds snow peas (or two 10 ounce packages frozen snow peas)
water
salt

1. Snap ends from fresh snow peas and remove center rib. Rinse in cool water.
2. In a medium saucepan, bring small amount of salted water to a boil.
3. Add snow peas and return water to a boil. Simmer peas until crisp-tender.
4. Drain and serve immediately.

Per serving: 46 cal. (4% from fat), 3 g protein, 8 g carbohydrate, 0 g fat, 0 mg cholesterol, 1 g fiber, 86 mg sodium.

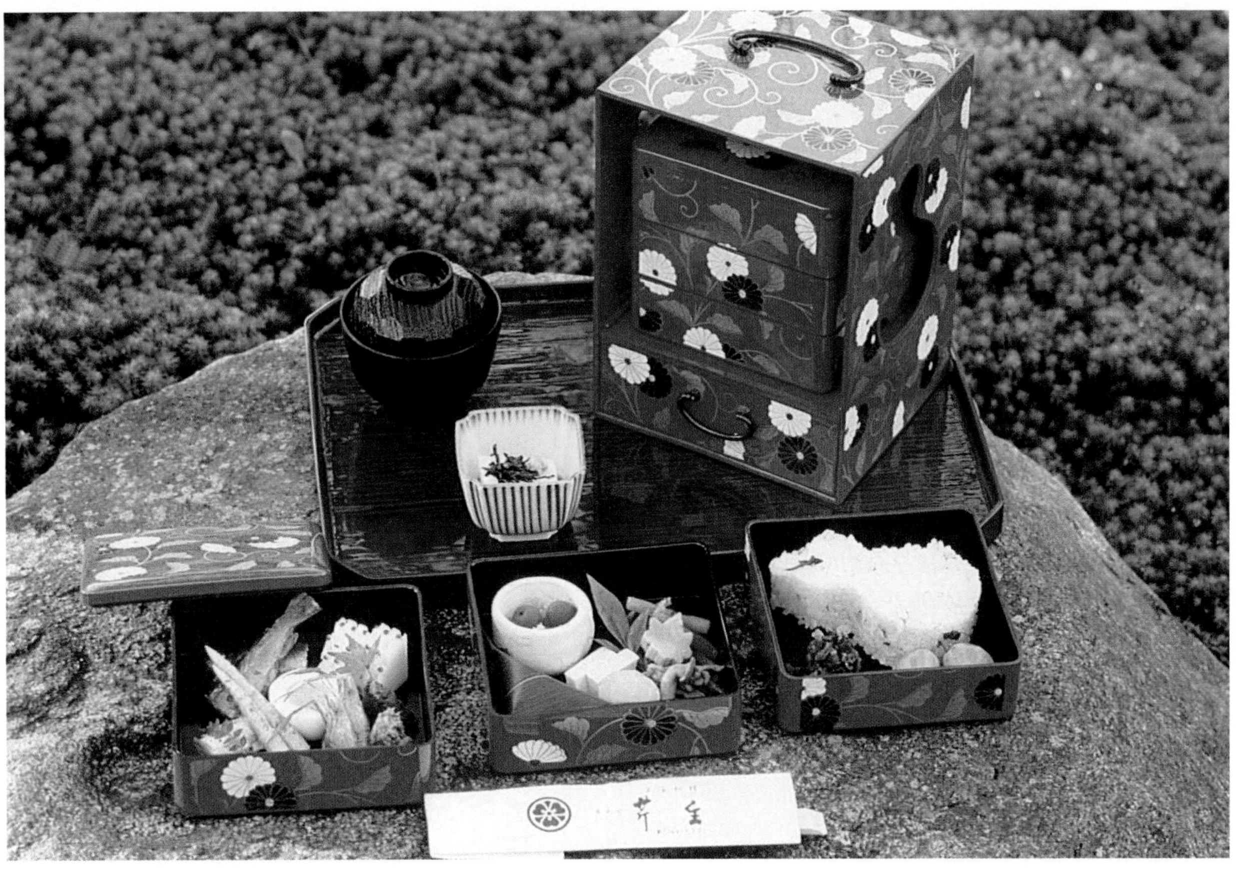

Japan National Tourist Organization

The color, shape, and arrangement of these foods reflect the importance Japanese cooks place on aesthetic appearance.

Chapter 32 Review
Asia

Summary

Russia, India, China, and Japan have cuisines that differ greatly from the cuisine of the United States. The cuisines of these countries also differ greatly from one another.

Russian cuisine was influenced by the Slavs and Mongols. The czars also made a number of contributions. In the days of the Russian Empire, however, most Russians were peasants. The staple foods of their diet were bread, kasha, and soup. Today, Russian meals often begin with appetizers, called zakuska. A hearty soup, such as schi or borscht, and a meat, fish, or poultry main dish would follow. Rye bread, potatoes, and a seasonal vegetable would accompany the main dish. A simple dessert of pureed fruit might round out the meal.

Religious dietary restrictions play a major role in the cuisine of India. Different climates and influences have created some specific distinctions between the cuisines of Northern and Southern India. Four basic cooking techniques are used to prepare Indian cuisine: tandoori, korma, vindaloo, and chasnidarth. Curry is a dish found throughout India. However, cooks in different regions prepare and season it in different ways.

Chinese foods contain some unique ingredients. A few special utensils, including a wok, are helpful for preparing Chinese foods. Most Chinese foods are prepared by stir-frying, steaming, deep-frying, or simmering. Rice is a staple of the Chinese diet. Vegetables also play an important role. Vegetables and meat or poultry are cut into small pieces to make them easier to eat with chopsticks.

Four ingredients are basic to Japanese cuisine: rice, soybeans, fish, and seaweed. Many Japanese foods feature vegetables with smaller amounts of meat, poultry, or fish. The Japanese often boil, steam, fry, or broil their foods. The aesthetic appearance of foods is an important aspect of Japanese cuisine. The Japanese also follow some specific eating customs. Many of these are observed in the traditional tea ceremony.

Review What You Have Read

Write your answers on a separate sheet of paper.

1. What are four contributions the Mongols made to Russian cuisine?
2. Name and describe two Russian soups.
3. Name and describe two Russian desserts.
4. In general, how does the cuisine of Northern India differ from the cuisine of Southern India?
5. Many Indian dishes are cooked in a clarified butter called _____.
6. Which of the following Indian cooking techniques involves braising foods in yogurt?
   A. Chasnidarth.
   B. Korma.
   C. Tandoori.
   D. Vindaloo.
7. What is China's chief agricultural product?
8. Choose four important ingredients in Chinese cooking and briefly define each.
9. What is the most versatile of all Chinese cooking utensils?
10. Why have the Japanese traditionally raised little livestock?
11. Name and describe three food products made from soybeans in Japan.
12. Describe two Japanese eating customs.

Build Your Basic Skills

1. **Reading/verbal.** Use library resources to research one of the Russian czars. Prepare an oral report for the class.
2. **Writing.** Investigate the major differences between Hinduism and Buddhism. Summarize your findings in a written report.

Build Your Thinking Skills

1. **Compare.** Prepare ghee. Fry potatoes in lard, vegetable shortening, margarine, and ghee. Compare differences in browning and flavor.
2. **Evaluate.** Design an evaluation form for a tea tasting. Then complete the form as you taste and compare several varieties of tea popular in China.
3. **Demonstrate.** Work with a small group to research the traditional Japanese tea ceremony. Each member of the group should be responsible for demonstrating one aspect of the ceremony in a presentation to the class.

Apply Technology

1. Use Internet resources to find out more about the culture in one of the Asian countries covered in the chapter. Prepare visual aids to use as you share your findings in an oral report. Also share the Web site addresses you found most interesting.
2. Use a computer to set up a table comparing traditional foods and cooking methods of China and Japan.

Using Workplace Skills

Chen is a Chinese-style food cook at Szechwan East, a small Chinese carryout owned by his uncle. Chen's uncle takes telephone orders and collects payment from customers when they come in to pick up the orders. Chen works in the small kitchen with his aunt and two cousins to prepare foods items. Chen and his family members must avoid getting in one another's way as they work together to quickly fill orders.

To be an effective worker, Chen needs skill in working as a member of a team. Put yourself in Chen's place and answer the following questions about his need for and use of this skill:

A. What are some tasks of a Chinese-style food cook that might especially require teamwork skills when working in a small kitchen?
B. How might your aunt and cousins be affected if you lack skill in working as a member of a team?
C. How might customers of Szechwan East be affected if you lack skill in working as a member of a team?
D. What is another skill you would need in this job? Briefly explain why this skill would be important.

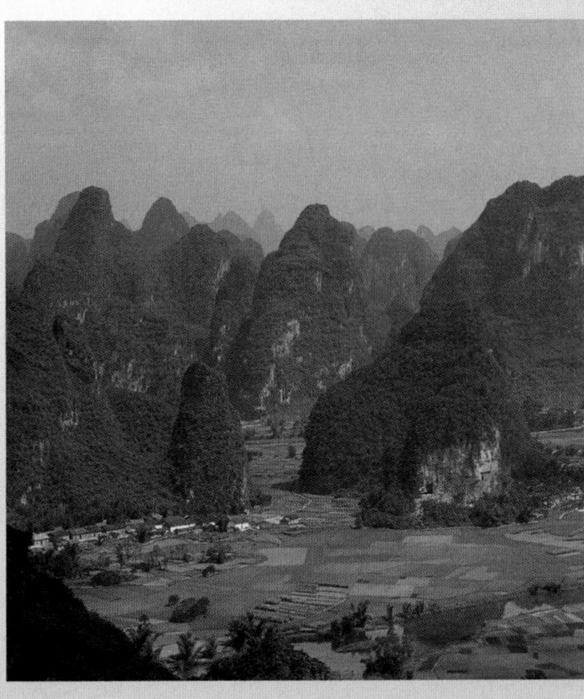

Appendix A Canada's Food Guide

Health Canada Santé Canada

CANADA'S Food Guide TO HEALTHY EATING

FOR PEOPLE FOUR YEARS AND OVER

Enjoy a variety of foods from each group every day.

Choose lower-fat foods more often.

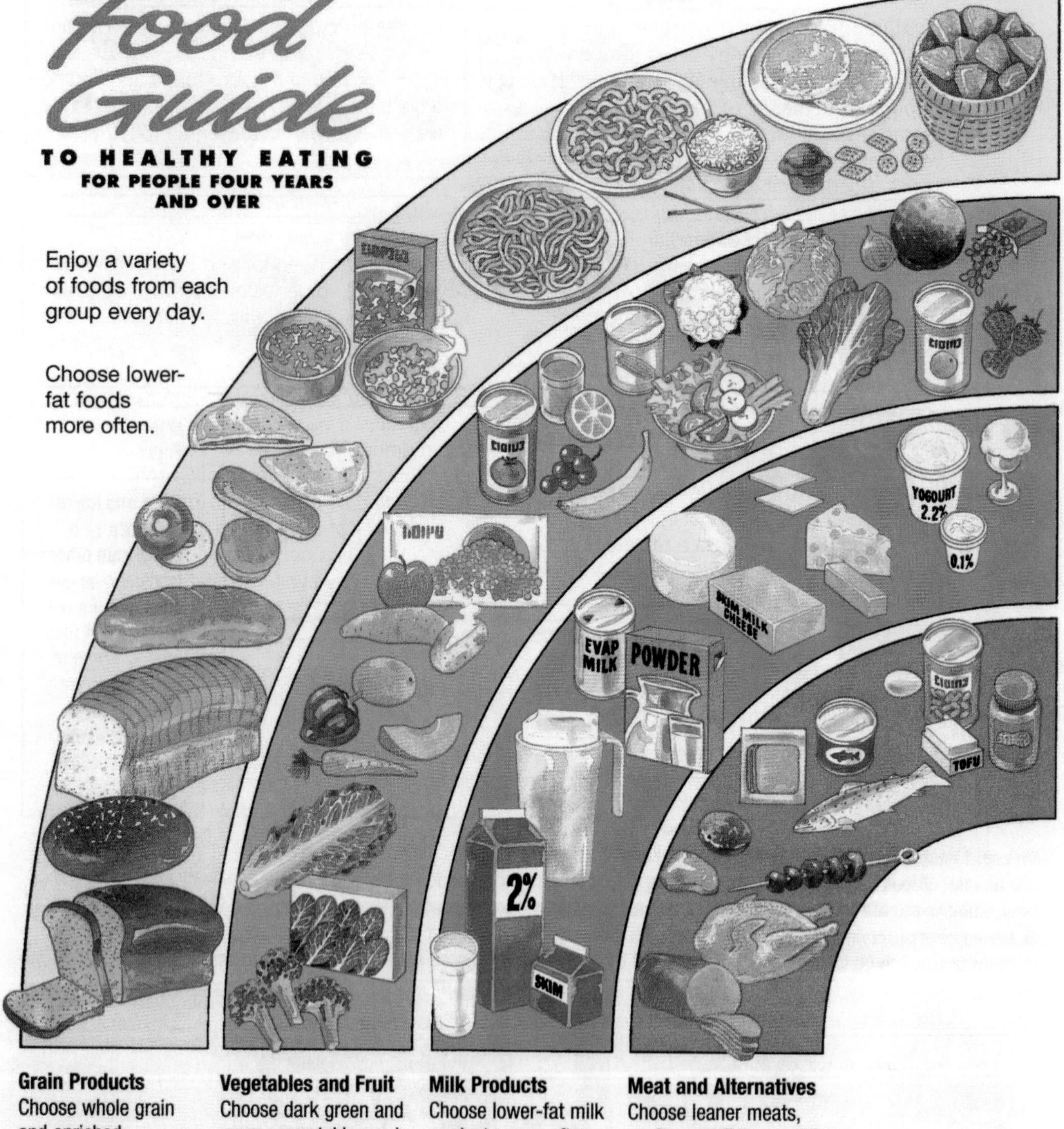

Grain Products
Choose whole grain and enriched products more often.

Vegetables and Fruit
Choose dark green and orange vegetables and orange fruit more often.

Milk Products
Choose lower-fat milk products more often.

Meat and Alternatives
Choose leaner meats, poultry and fish, as well as dried peas, beans and lentils more often.

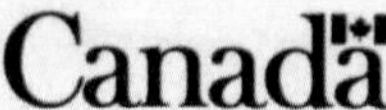

Grain Products

5–12

SERVINGS PER DAY

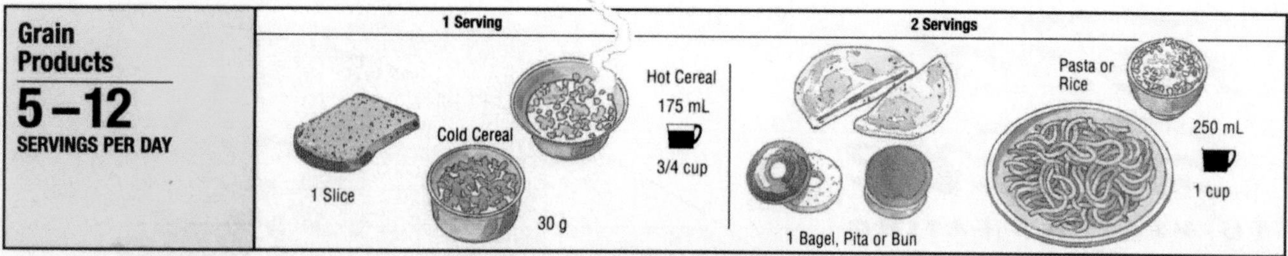

Vegetables and Fruit

5–10

SERVINGS PER DAY

1 Serving
1 Medium Size Vegetable or Fruit
Fresh, Frozen or Canned Vegetables or Fruit
125 mL
1/2 cup
Salad
250 mL
1 cup
Juice
125 mL
1/2 cup

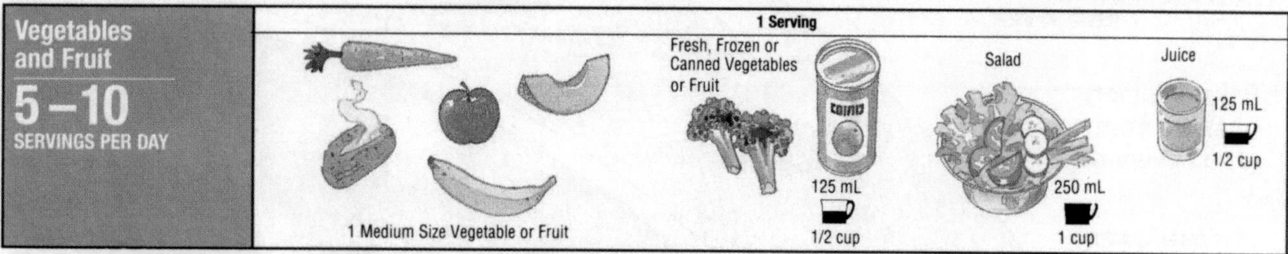

Milk Products

SERVINGS PER DAY

Children 4–9 years: 2–3
Youth 10–16 years: 3–4
Adults: 2–4
Pregnant and Breast-feeding Women 3–4

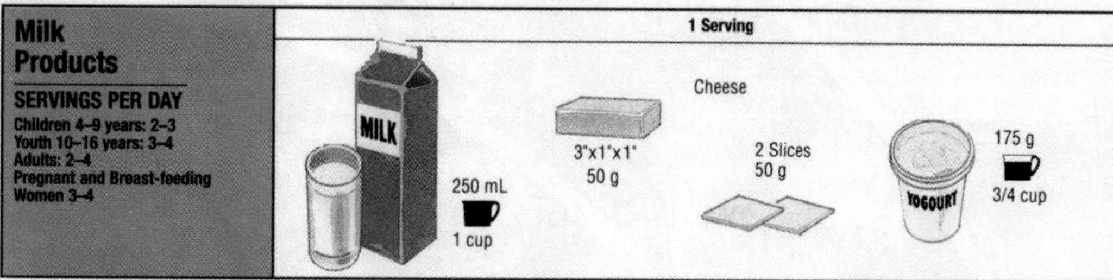

Meat and Alternatives

2–3

SERVINGS PER DAY

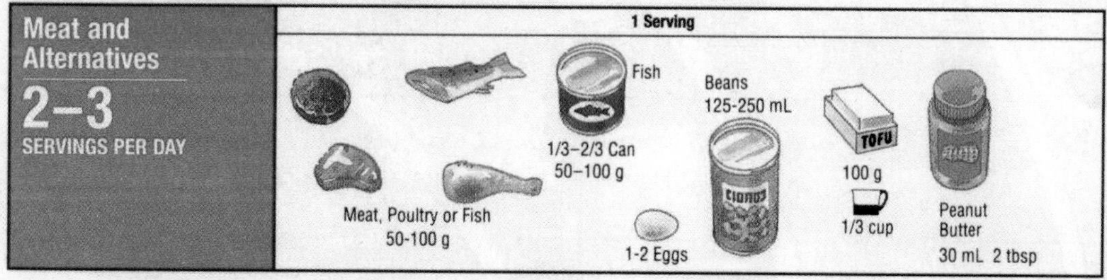

Other Foods

Taste and enjoyment can also come from other foods and beverages that are not part of the 4 food groups. Some of these foods are higher in fat or Calories, so use these foods in moderation.

Different People Need Different Amounts of Food

The amount of food you need every day from the 4 food groups and other foods depends on your age, body size, activity level, whether you are male or female and if you are pregnant or breast-feeding. That's why the Food Guide gives a lower and higher number of servings for each food group. For example, young children can choose the lower number of servings, while male teenagers can go to the higher number. Most other people can choose servings somewhere in between.

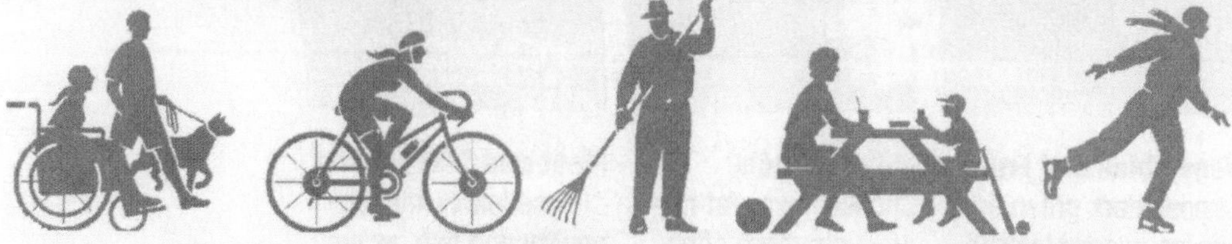

Consult *Canada's Physical Activity Guide to Healthy Active Living* to help you build physical activity into your daily life.

Enjoy eating well, being active and feeling good about yourself. That's
VITALIT

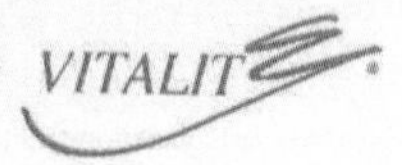

Cat. No. H39-252/1992E ISBN 0-662-19648-1

Appendix B Recommended Nutrient Intakes

Reference Heights and Weights for Children and Adults in the United States		
Life-Stage Group	**Median Reference Height (inches)**	**Median Reference Weight (pounds)**
Infants		
2-6 mo	24	13
7-12 mo	28	20
Children		
1-3 yr	34	27
4-8 yr	45	44
Male		
9-13 yr	57	79
14-18 yr	68	134
19-30 yr	70	154
Female		
9-13 yr	57	81
14-18 yr	64	119
19-30 yr	64	126

Food and Nutrition Board, Institute of Medicine, The National Academies

Dietary Reference Intakes: Energy		
Life-Stage Group	**Energy[a] (kcal)**	
	Males	**Females**
Infants		
0-6 mo	570	520
7-12 mo	743	676
Children		
1-2 yr	1,046	992
3-8 yr	1,742	1,642
Adolescents and Adults		
9-13 yr	2,279	2,071
14-18 yr	3,152	2,368
>18 yr	3,067[b]	2,403[b]
Pregnancy		
14-18 yr		
1st trimester		2,368
2nd trimester		2,708
3rd trimester		2,820
19-50 yr		
1st trimester		2,403[b]
2nd trimester		2,743[b]
3rd trimester		2,855[b]
Lactation		
14-18 yr		
1st 6 mo		2,698
2nd 6 mo		2,768
19-50 yr		
1st 6 mo		2,733[b]
2nd 6 mo		2,803[b]

Food and Nutrition Board, Institute of Medicine, The National Academies

a The intake that meets the average energy expenditure of healthy, moderately active individuals at the reference height, weight, and age. (See height and weight table.)

b Subtract 10 kcal/day for males and 7 kcal/day for females for each year of age above 19 years.

Dietary Reference Intakes: Macronutrients				
Life-Stage	**Carbohydrates (g)**	**Total Fiber (g)**	**Total Fat (g)**	**Protein[a] (g)**
Infants				
0-6 mo	60	ND[b]	31	9.1
7-12 mo	95	ND	30	13.5
Children				
1-3 yr	130	19	ND	13
4-8 yr	130	25	ND	19
Males				
9-13 yr	130	31	ND	34
14-18 yr	130	38	ND	52
19-30 yr	130	38	ND	56
31-50 yr	130	38	ND	56
51-70 yr	130	30	ND	56
>70 yr	130	30	ND	56
Females				
9-13 yr	130	26	ND	34
14-18 yr	130	26	ND	46
19-30 yr	130	25	ND	46
31-50 yr	130	25	ND	46
51-70 yr	130	21	ND	46
>70 yr	130	21	ND	46
Pregnancy				
14-18 yr	175	28	ND	+25[c]
19-50 yr	175	28	ND	+25[c]
Lactation				
14-18 yr	210	29	ND	+25[d]
19-50 yr	210	29	ND	+25[d]

Food and Nutrition Board, Institute of Medicine, The National Academies

NOTE: This table presents Recommended Dietary Allowances (RDAs) in unshaded boxes and Adequate Intakes (AIs) in shaded boxes. RDAs and AIs may both be used as goals for individual intake. RDAs are set to meet the needs of almost all (97 to 98 percent) individuals in a group. For healthy human milk-fed infants, the AI is the mean intake. The AI for other life-stage and gender groups is believed to cover needs of all healthy individuals in the group, but lack of data or uncertainty in the data prevent being able to specify with confidence the percentage of individuals covered by this intake.

a AI or RDA for reference individuals. (See height and weight table.) The RDA for men and women is 0.8 g/kg (0.36 g/lb) body weight/day of protein.

b ND = not determined.

c The RDA for pregnancy is 25 g/day protein in addition to the RDA of the nonpregnant woman. This added amount is recommended only for the second half of pregnancy. For the first half of pregnancy, the protein requirements are the same as those of the nonpregnant woman.

d In addition to the RDA of the nonlactating adolescent or woman.

Dietary Reference Intakes: Vitamins

Life-Stage Group	Biotin (μg/d)	Folate (μg/d)[a]	Niacin (mg/d)[d]	Pantothenic Acid (mg/d)	Riboflavin (mg/d)	Thiamin (mg/d)	Vitamin A (μg/d)	Vitamin B_6 (mg/d)	Vitamin B_{12} (μg/d)	Vitamin C (mg/d)	Vitamin D (μg/d)[f,g]	Vitamin E (mg/d)[h]	Vitamin K (μg/d)
Infants													
0-6 mo	5	65	2	1.7	0.3	0.2	400	0.1	0.4	40	5	4	2.0
7-12 mo	6	80	4	1.8	0.4	0.3	500	0.3	0.5	50	5	6	2.5
Children													
1-3 yr	8	150	6	2	0.5	0.5	300	0.5	0.9	15	5	6	30
4-8 yr	12	200	8	3	0.6	0.6	400	0.6	1.2	25	5	7	55
Males													
9-13 yr	20	300	12	4	0.9	0.9	600	1.0	1.8	45	5	11	60
14-18 yr	25	400	16	5	1.3	1.2	900	1.3	2.4	75	5	15	75
19-30 yr	30	400	16	5	1.3	1.2	900	1.3	2.4	90	5	15	120
31-50 yr	30	400	16	5	1.3	1.2	900	1.3	2.4	90	5	15	120
51-70 yr	30	400	16	5	1.3	1.2	900	1.7	2.4[e]	90	10	15	120
>70 yr	30	400	16	5	1.3	1.2	900	1.7	2.4[e]	90	15	15	120
Females													
9-13 yr	20	300	12	4	0.9	0.9	600	1.0	1.8	45	5	11	60
14-18 yr	25	400[b]	14	5	1.0	1.0	700	1.2	2.4	65	5	15	75
19-30 yr	30	400[b]	14	5	1.1	1.1	700	1.3	2.4	75	5	15	90
31-50 yr	30	400[b]	14	5	1.1	1.1	700	1.3	2.4	75	5	15	90
51-70 yr	30	400	14	5	1.1	1.1	700	1.5	2.4[e]	75	10	15	90
>70 yr	30	400	14	5	1.1	1.1	700	1.5	2.4[e]	75	15	15	90
Pregnancy													
≤18 yr	30	600[c]	18	6	1.4	1.4	750	1.9	2.6	80	5	15	75
19-30 yr	30	600[c]	18	6	1.4	1.4	770	1.9	2.6	85	5	15	90
31-50 yr	30	600[c]	18	6	1.4	1.4	770	1.9	2.6	85	5	15	90
Lactation													
≤18 yr	35	500	17	7	1.6	1.5	1,200	2.0	2.8	115	5	19	75
19-30 yr	35	500	17	7	1.6	1.5	1,300	2.0	2.8	120	5	19	90
31-50 yr	35	500	17	7	1.6	1.5	1,300		2.8	120	5	19	90

Food and Nutrition Board, Institute of Medicine, The National Academies

NOTE: This table represents Recommended Dietary Allowances (RDAs) in unshaded boxes and Adequate Intakes (AIs) in shaded boxes. RDAs and AIs may both be used as goals for individual intake. RDAs are set to meet the needs of almost all (97 to 98 percent) individuals in a group. For healthy human milk-fed infants, the AI is the mean intake. The AI for other life-stage and gender groups is believed to cover needs of all healthy individuals in the group, but lack of data or uncertainty in the data prevent being able to specify with confidence the percentage of individuals covered by this intake.

[a] As dietary folate equivalents (DFE). 1 DFE = 1 μg food folate = 0.6 μg of folic acid (from fortified food supplement) consumed with food – 0.5 μg of synthetic (supplemental) folic acid taken on an empty stomach.

[b] In view of evidence linking folate intake with neural tube defects in the fetus, it is recommended that all women capable of becoming pregnant consume 400 μg of synthetic folic acid from fortified foods and/or supplements in addition to intake of food folate from a varied diet.

[c] It is assumed that women will continue consuming 400 mg of folic acid until their pregnancy is confirmed and they enter prenatal care, which ordinarily occurs after the end of the periconceptional period—the critical time for formation of the neural tube.

[d] As niacin equivalents (NE). 1 mg of niacin = 60 mg of tryptophan; 0-6 months = preformed niacin (not NE).

[e] Because 10 to 30 percent of older people may malabsorb food-bound B_{12}, it is advisable for those older than 50 years to meet their RDA mainly by consuming foods fortified with B_{12} or a supplement containing B_{12}.

[f] As cholecalciferol. 1 mg cholecalciferol = 40 IU vitamin D.

[g] In the absence of adequate exposure to sunlight.

[h] As α-tocopherol, which includes RRR-α-tocopherol, the only form of α-tocopherol that occurs naturally in foods, and the 2*R*-stereoisomeric forms of α-tocopherol (*RRR-*, *RSR-*, *RRS-*, and *RSS*-α-tocopherol) that occur in fortified foods and supplements. Does not include the 2*S*-stereoisomeric forms of α-tocopherol (*SRR-*, *SSR-*, *SRS-*, and *SSS*-α-tocopherol), also found in fortified foods and supplements.

Dietary Reference Intakes: Minerals								
Life-Stage Group	**Calcium (mg/d)**	**Fluoride (mg/d)**	**Iodine (µg/d)**	**Iron (mg/d)**	**Magnesium (mg/d)**	**Phosphorus (mg/d)**	**Selenium (mg/d)**	**Zinc (mg/d)**
Infants								
0-6 mo	210	0.01	110	0.27	30	100	15	2
7-12 mo	270	0.5	130	11	75	275	20	3
Children								
1-3 yr	500	0.7	90	7	80	460	20	3
4-8 yr	800	1	90	10	130	500	30	5
Males								
9-13 yr	1,300	2	120	8	240	1250	40	8
14-18 yr	1,300	3	150	11	410	1250	55	11
19-30 yr	1,000	4	150	8	400	700	55	11
31-50 yr	1,000	4	150	8	420	700	55	11
51-70 yr	1,200	4	150	8	420	700	55	11
>70 yr	1,200	4	150	8	420	700	55	11
Females								
9-13 yr	1,300	2	120	8	240	1250	40	8
14-18 yr	1,300	3	150	15	360	1250	55	9
19-30 yr	1,000	3	150	18	310	700	55	8
31-50 yr	1,000	3	150	18	320	700	55	8
51-70 yr	1,200	3	150	8	320	700	55	8
>70 yr	1,200	3	150	8	320	700	55	8
Pregnancy								
≤ 18 yr	1,300	3	220	27	400	1250	60	12
19-30 yr	1,000	3	220	27	350	700	60	11
31-50 yr	1,000	3	220	27	360	700	60	11
Lactation								
≤ 18 yr	1,300	3	290	10	360	1250	70	13
19-30 yr	1,000	3	290	9	310	700	70	12
31-50 yr	1,000	3	290	9	320	700	70	12

Food and Nutrition Board, Institute of Medicine, The National Academies

NOTE: This table represents Recommended Dietary Allowances (RDAs) in unshaded boxes and Adequate Intakes (AIs) in shaded boxes. RDAs and AIs may both be used as goals for individual intake. RDAs are set to meet the needs of almost all (97 to 98 percent) individuals in a group. For healthy human milk-fed infants, the AI is the mean intake. The AI for other life-stage and gender groups is believed to cover needs of all healthy individuals in the group, but lack of data or uncertainty in the data prevent being able to specify with confidence the percentage of individuals covered by this intake.

Upper Tolerable Intake Levels (UL[a])										
Nutrient	**0-6 mo**	**7-12 mo**	**1-3 yr**	**4-8 yr**	**9-13 yr**	**14-18 yr**	**19-30 yr**	**31-50 yr**	**51-70 yr**	**> 70 yr**
Vitamins										
Biotin	ND[b]	ND	ND	ND	ND	ND	ND	ND	ND	ND
Folate	ND	ND	300 μg	400 μg	600 μg	800 μg	1,000 μg	1,000 μg	1,000 μg	1,000 μg
Niacin	ND	ND	10 mg	15 mg	20 mg	30mg	35 mg	35 mg	35 mg	35 mg
Pantothenic Acid	ND	ND	ND	ND	ND	ND	ND	ND	ND	ND
Riboflavin	ND	ND	ND	ND	ND	ND	ND	ND	ND	ND
Thiamin	ND	ND	ND	ND	ND	ND	ND	ND	ND	ND
Vitamin A	600 μg	600 μg	600 μg	900 μg	1,700 μg	2,800 μg	3,000 μg	3,000 μg	3,000 μg	3,000 μg
Vitamin B_6	ND	ND	30 mg	40 mg	60 mg	80 mg	100 mg	100 mg	100 mg	100 mg
Vitamin B_{12}	ND	ND	ND	ND	ND	ND	ND	ND	ND	ND
Vitamin C	ND	ND	400 mg	650 mg	1,200 mg	1,800 mg	2,000 mg	2,000 mg	2,000 mg	2,000 mg
Vitamin D	25 μg	25 μg	50 μg	50 μg	50 μg	50 μg	50 μg	50 μg	50 μg	50 μg
Vitamin E	ND	ND	200 mg	300 mg	600 mg	800 mg	1,000 mg	1,000 mg	1,000 mg	1,000 mg
Vitamin K	ND	ND	ND	ND	ND	ND	ND	ND	ND	ND
Minerals										
Calcium	ND	ND	2,500 mg	2,500 mg	2,500 mg	2,500 mg	2,500 mg	2,500 mg	2,500 mg	2,500 mg
Fluoride	0.7 mg	0.9 mg	1.3 mg	2.2 mg	10 mg	10 mg	10 mg	10 mg	10 mg	10 mg
Iodine	ND	ND	200 μg	300 μg	600 μg	900 μg	1,100 μg	1,100 μg	1,100 μg	1,100 μg
Iron	40 mg	40 mg	40 mg	40 mg	40 mg	45 mg	45 mg	45 mg	45 mg	45 mg
Magnesium	ND	ND	65 mg	110 mg	350 mg	350 mg	350 mg	350 mg	350 mg	350 mg
Phosphorus	ND	ND	3,000 mg	3,000 mg	4,000 mg	4,000 mg[c]	4,000 mg[c]	4,000 mg[c]	4,000 mg	3,000 mg
Selenium	45 μg	60 μg	90 μg	150 μg	280 μg	400 μg	400 μg	400 μg	400 μg	400 μg
Zinc	4 mg	5 mg	7 mg	12 mg	23 mg	34 mg	40 mg	40 mg	40 mg	40 mg

Food and Nutrition Board, Institute of Medicine, The National Academies

a The UL represents the maximum level of daily nutrient intake that is likely to pose no risk of adverse effects. Unless otherwise specified, the UL represents total intake from food, water, and supplements. Due to lack of suitable data, ULs could not be established for biotin, pantothenic acid, riboflavin, thiamin, vitamin B_{12}, or vitamin K. In the absence of ULs, extra caution may be warranted in consuming levels above recommended intakes. UL values are the same for males and females in all life-stage groups. UL values are also unaffected by pregnancy and lactation unless otherwise noted.

b Not determinable due to lack of data of adverse effects in this age group and concern with regard to lack of ability to handle excess amounts. Source of intake should be from food only to prevent high levels of intake.

c 3,500 mg during pregnancy.

SOURCES: The tables in this appendix are adapted from the following DRI reports: *Dietary Reference Intakes for Calcium, Phosphorus, Magnesium, Vitamin D, and Fluoride (1997); Dietary Reference Intakes for Thiamin, Riboflavin, Niacin, Vitamin B_6, Folate, Vitamin B_{12}, Pantothenic Acid, Biotin, and Choline (1998); Dietary Reference Intakes for Vitamin C, Selenium, and Carotenoids (2000); Dietary Reference Intakes for Vitamin A, Vitamin K, Arsenic, Boron, Chromium, Copper, Iodine, Iron, Manganese, Molybdenum, Nickel, Silicon, Vanadium, and Zinc (2001); and Dietary Reference Intakes for Energy, Carbohydrates, Fiber, Fat, Protein, and Amino Acids (Macronutrients) (2002).* These reports may be accessed through the National Academies Press Web site at nap.edu.

Appendix C Nutritive Values of Foods

(Tr indicates nutrient present in trace amount.)

Item No. (A)	Foods, approximate measures, units, and weight (weight of edible portion only) (B)		Water (C)	Food energy (D)	Protein (E)	Fat (F)	Saturated fat (G)	Cholesterol (H)	Carbohydrate (I)	Dietary fiber (J)	Calcium (K)	Iron (L)	Potassium (M)	Sodium (N)	Vitamin A (O)	Thiamin (P)	Riboflavin (Q)	Niacin (R)	Vitamin C (S)
Beverages		Grams	Percent	Calories	Grams	Grams	Grams	Milligrams	Grams	Grams	Milligrams	Milligrams	Milligrams	Milligrams	Micrograms	Milligrams	Milligrams	Milligrams	Milligrams
Carbonated:[2]																			
Club soda	12 fl. oz.	355	100	0	0	0	0.0	0	0	0	18	Tr	0	78	0	0.00	0.00	0.0	0
Cola type:																			
Regular	12 fl. oz.	369	89	160	0	0	0.0	0	41	0	11	0.2	7	18	0	0.00	0.00	0.0	0
Diet, artificially sweetened	12 fl. oz.	355	100	Tr	0	0	0.0	0	Tr	0	14	0.2	7	[3]32	0	0.00	0.00	0.0	0
Ginger ale	12 fl. oz.	366	91	125	0	0	0.0	0	32	0	11	0.1	4	29	0	0.00	0.00	0.0	0
Grape	12 fl. oz.	372	88	180	0	0	0.0	0	46	0	15	0.4	4	48	0	0.00	0.00	0.0	0
Lemon-lime	12 fl. oz	372	89	155	0	0	0.0	0	39	0	7	0.4	4	33	0	0.00	0.00	0.0	0
Orange	12 fl. oz.	372	88	180	0	0	0.0	0	46	0	15	0.3	7	52	0	0.00	0.00	0.0	0
Pepper type	12 fl. oz.	369	89	160	0	0	Tr	0	41	0	11	0.1	4	37	0	0.00	0.00	0.0	0
Root beer	12 fl. oz.	370	89	165	0	0	0.0	0	42	0	15	0.2	4	48	0	0.00	0.00	0.0	0
Cocoa and chocolate-flavored beverages. See Dairy Products																			
Coffee:																			
Brewed	6 fl. oz.	180	100	Tr	Tr	Tr	0.0	0	Tr	0	4	Tr	124	2	0	0.00	0.02	0.4	0
Instant, prepared (2 tsp. powder plus 6 fl. oz. water)	6 fl. oz.	182	99	Tr	Tr	Tr	0.0	0	1	0	2	0.1	71	Tr	0	0.00	0.03	0.6	0
Fruit drinks, noncarbonated:																			
Canned:																			
Fruit punch drink	6 fl. oz.	190	88	85	Tr	0	0.0	0	22	0	15	0.4	48	15	2	0.03	0.04	Tr	[4]61
Grape drink	6 fl. oz.	187	86	100	Tr	0	0.0	0	26	Tr	2	0.3	9	11	Tr	0.01	0.01	Tr	[4]64
Pineapple-grapefruit juice drink	6 fl. oz.	187	87	90	Tr	Tr	Tr	0	23	Tr	13	0.9	97	24	6	0.06	0.04	0.5	[4]110
Frozen:																			
Lemonade concentrate:																			
Undiluted	6-fl.-oz. can	219	49	425	Tr	Tr	Tr	0	112	1	9	0.4	153	4	4	0.04	0.07	0.7	66
Diluted with 4 1/3 parts water by volume	6 fl. oz.	185	89	80	Tr	Tr	Tr	0	21	Tr	2	0.1	30	1	1	0.01	0.02	0.2	13
Limeade concentrate:																			
Undiluted	6-fl.-oz. can	218	50	410	Tr	Tr	Tr	0	108	1	11	0.2	129	Tr	Tr	0.02	0.02	0.2	26
Diluted with 4-1/3 parts water by volume	6 fl. oz	185	89	75	Tr	Tr	0.0	0	20	Tr	2	Tr	24	Tr	Tr	Tr	Tr	Tr	4
Fruit juices. See type under Fruits and Fruit Juices.																			
Milk beverages. See Dairy Products.																			
Tea:																			
Brewed	8 fl. oz.	240	100	Tr	Tr	Tr	0.0	0	Tr	0	0	Tr	36	1	0	0.00	0.03	Tr	0
Instant, powder, prepared:																			
Unsweetened (1 tsp. powder plus 8 fl. oz. water)	8 fl. oz.	241	100	Tr	Tr	Tr	0.0	0	1	0	1	Tr	61	1	0	0.00	0.02	0.1	0
Sweetened (3 tsp. powder plus 8 fl. oz. water)	8 fl. oz.	262	91	85	Tr	Tr	Tr	0	22	0	1	Tr	49	Tr	0	0.00	0.04	0.1	0
Dairy Products																			
Butter. See Fats and Oils																			
Cheese:																			
Cheddar:																			
Cut pieces	1 oz.	28	37	115	7	9	0.6	30	Tr	0	204	0.2	28	176	86	0.01	0.11	Tr	0
	1 in.^{3}	17	37	70	4	6	3.6	18	Tr	0	123	0.1	17	105	52	Tr	0.06	Tr	0
Shredded	1 cup	113	37	455	28	37	23.8	119	1	0	815	0.8	111	701	342	0.03	0.42	0.1	0
Cottage (curd not pressed down):																			
Creamed (cottage cheese, 4% fat):																			
Large curd	1 cup	225	79	235	28	10	6.4	34	6	0	135	0.3	190	911	108	0.05	0.37	0.3	Tr
Small curd	1 cup	210	79	215	26	9	6.0	31	6	0	126	0.3	177	850	101	0.04	0.34	0.3	Tr
Lowfat (2%)	1 cup	226	79	205	31	4	2.8	19	8	0	155	0.4	217	918	45	0.05	0.42	0.3	Tr

(A)	(B)		(C)	(D)	(E)	(F)	(G)	(H)	(I)	(J)	(K)	(L)	(M)	(N)	(O)	(P)	(Q)	(R)	(S)
Uncreamed (cottage cheese dry curd, less than 1/2% fat)	1 cup	145	80	125	25	1	1.4	10	3	0	46	0.3	47	19	12	0.04	0.21	0.2	0
Cream	1 oz.	28	54	100	2	10	6.2	31	1	0	23	0.3	34	84	124	Tr	0.06	Tr	0
Mozzarella, made with:																			
Whole milk	1 oz.	28	54	80	6	6	3.7	22	1	0	147	0.1	19	106	68	Tr	0.07	Tr	0
Part skim milk (low moisture)	1 oz.	28	49	80	8	5	3.1	15	1	0	207	0.1	27	150	54	0.01	0.10	Tr	0
Parmesan, grated:																			
Tablespoon	1 tbsp.	5	18	25	2	2	1.0	4	Tr	0	69	Tr	5	93	9	Tr	0.02	Tr	0
Ounce	1 oz.	28	18	130	12	9	5.4	22	1	0	390	0.3	30	528	49	0.01	0.11	0.1	0
Swiss	1 oz.	28	37	105	8	8	5.0	26	1	0	272	Tr	31	74	72	0.01	0.10	Tr	0
Pasteurized process cheese:																			
American	1 oz.	28	39	105	6	9	5.6	27	Tr	0	174	0.1	46	406	82	0.01	0.10	Tr	0
Swiss	1 oz.	28	42	95	7	7	4.6	24	1	0	219	0.2	61	388	65	Tr	0.08	Tr	0
Pasteurized process cheese:																			
food, American	1 oz.	28	43	95	6	7	4.4	18	2	0	163	0.2	79	337	62	0.01	0.13	Tr	0
spread, American	1 oz.	28	48	80	5	6	3.8	16	2	0	159	0.1	69	381	54	0.01	0.12	Tr	0
Cream, sweet:																			
Half-and-half (cream and milk)	1 cup	242	81	315	7	28	17.3	89	10	0	254	0.2	314	98	259	0.08	0.36	0.2	2
	1 tbsp.	15	81	20	Tr	2	1.1	6	1	0	16	Tr	19	6	16	0.01	0.02	Tr	Tr
Light, coffee, or table	1 cup	240	74	470	6	46	28.8	159	9	0	231	0.1	292	95	437	0.08	0.36	0.1	2
	1 tbsp.	15	74	30	Tr	3	1.8	10	1	0	14	Tr	18	6	27	Tr	0.02	Tr	Tr
Whipping, unwhipped (volume about double when whipped):																			
Light	1 cup	239	64	700	5	74	46.1	265	7	0	166	0.1	231	82	705	0.06	0.30	0.1	1
	1 tbsp.	15	64	45	Tr	5	2.9	17	Tr	0	10	Tr	15	5	44	Tr	0.02	Tr	Tr
Heavy	1 cup	238	58	820	5	88	54.7	326	7	0	154	0.1	179	89	1,002	0.05	0.26	0.1	1
	1 tbsp.	15	58	50	Tr	6	3.4	21	Tr	0	10	Tr	11	6	63	Tr	0.02	Tr	Tr
Whipped topping, (pressurized)	1 cup	60	61	155	2	13	8.3	46	7	0	61	Tr	88	78	124	0.02	0.04	Tr	0
	1 tbsp.	3	61	10	Tr	1	0.6	2	Tr	0	3	Tr	4	4	6	Tr	Tr	Tr	0
Cream, sour	1 cup	230	71	495	7	48	29.9	102	10	0	268	0.1	331	123	448	0.08	0.34	0.2	2
	1 tbsp.	12	71	25	Tr	3	1.8	5	1	0	14	Tr	17	6	23	Tr	0.02	Tr	Tr
Cream products, imitation (made with vegetable fat):																			
Whipped topping:																			
Frozen	1 cup	75	50	240	1	19	16.4	0	17	0	5	0.1	14	19	[5]65	0.00	0.00	0.0	0
	1 tbsp.	4	50	15	Tr	1	1.1	0	1	0	Tr	Tr	1	1	[5]3	0.00	0.00	0.0	0
Pressurized	1 cup	70	60	185	1	16	13.2	0	11	0	4	Tr	13	43	[5]33	0.00	0.00	0.0	0
	1 tbsp.	4	60	10	Tr	1	0.8	0	1	0	Tr	Tr	1	2	[5]2	0.00	0.00	0.0	0
Ice cream. See Milk desserts, frozen.																			
Ice milk. See Milk desserts, frozen.																			
Milk:																			
Fluid:																			
Whole (3.3% fat)	1 cup	244	88	150	8	8	5.1	33	11	0	291	0.1	370	120	76	0.09	0.40	0.2	2
Lowfat (2%):																			
No milk solids added	1 cup	244	89	120	8	5	2.9	18	12	0	297	0.1	377	122	139	0.10	0.40	0.2	2
Milk solids added, label claim less than 10 g of protein per cup	1 cup	245	89	125	9	5	2.9	18	12	0	313	0.1	397	128	140	0.10	0.42	0.2	2
Lowfat (1%):																			
No milk solids added	1 cup	244	90	100	8	3	1.6	10	12	0	300	0.1	381	123	144	0.10	0.41	0.2	2
Milk solids added, label claim less than 10 g of protein per cup	1 cup	245	90	105	9	2	1.5	10	12	0	313	0.1	397	128	145	0.10	0.42	0.2	2
Nonfat (skim):																			
No milk solids added	1 cup	245	91	85	8	Tr	0.3	4	12	0	302	0.1	406	126	149	0.09	0.34	0.2	2
Milk solids added, label claim less than 10 g of protein per cup	1 cup	245	90	90	9	1	0.4	5	12	0	316	0.1	418	130	149	0.10	0.43	0.2	2
Buttermilk	1 cup	245	90	100	8	2	1.3	9	12	0	285	0.1	371	257	20	0.08	0.38	0.1	2
Canned:																			
Condensed, sweetened	1 cup	306	27	980	24	27	16.8	104	166	0	868	0.6	1,136	389	248	0.28	1.27	0.6	8
Evaporated:																			
Whole milk	1 cup	252	74	340	17	19	11.6	74	25	0	657	0.5	764	267	136	0.12	0.80	0.5	5
Nonfat milk	1 cup	255	79	200	19	1	0.3	9	29	0	738	0.7	845	293	298	0.11	0.79	0.4	3
Dried:																			
Nonfat, instantized:																			
Envelope, 3.2 oz., net wt.[6]	1 envelope	91	4	325	32	1	0.4	17	47	0	1,120	0.3	1,552	499	[7]646	0.38	1.59	0.8	5

Nutritive Values of Foods – Continued
(Tr indicates nutrient present in trace amount.)

Item No. (A)	Foods, approximate measures, units, and weight (weight of edible portion only) (B)		Water (C)	Food energy (D)	Protein (E)	Fat (F)	Saturated fat (G)	Cholesterol (H)	Carbohydrate (I)	Dietary fiber (J)	Calcium (K)	Iron (L)	Potassium (M)	Sodium (N)	Vitamin A (O)	Thiamin (P)	Riboflavin (Q)	Niacin (R)	Vitamin C (S)
		Grams	Percent	Calories	Grams	Grams	Grams	Milligrams	Grams	Grams	Milligrams	Milligrams	Milligrams	Milligrams	Micrograms	Milligrams	Milligrams	Milligrams	Milligrams
Milk beverages:																			
Chocolate milk (commercial):																			
Regular	1 cup	250	82	210	8	8	5.2	31	26	3	280	0.6	417	149	73	0.09	0.41	0.3	2
Lowfat (2%)	1 cup	250	84	180	8	5	3.1	17	26	3	284	0.6	422	151	143	0.09	0.41	0.3	2
Lowfat (1%)	1 cup	250	85	160	8	3	1.5	7	26	3	287	0.6	425	152	148	0.10	0.42	0.3	2
Cocoa and chocolate-flavored beverages:																			
Powder containing nonfat dry milk	1 oz.	28	1	100	3	1	0.7	1	22	Tr	90	0.3	223	139	Tr	0.03	0.17	0.2	Tr
Powder without nonfat dry milk	3/4 oz.	21	1	75	1	1	0.4	0	19	1	7	0.7	136	56	Tr	Tr	0.03	0.1	Tr
Eggnog (commercial)	1 cup	254	74	340	10	19	11.3	149	34	0	330	0.5	420	138	203	0.09	0.48	0.3	4
Malted milk:																			
Chocolate:																			
Powder	3/4 oz.	21	2	85	1	1	0.5	1	18	Tr	13	0.4	130	49	5	0.04	0.04	0.4	0
Shakes, thick:																			
Chocolate	10-oz. container	283	72	335	9	8	6.5	30	60	Tr	374	0.9	634	314	59	0.13	0.63	0.4	0
Vanilla	10-oz. container	283	74	315	11	9	5.3	33	50	Tr	413	0.3	517	270	79	0.08	0.55	0.4	0
Milk desserts, frozen:																			
Ice cream, vanilla:																			
Regular (about 11% fat):																			
Hardened	1/2 gal.	1,064	61	2,155	38	115	72.4	476	254	1	1,406	1.0	2,052	929	1,064	0.42	2.63	1.1	6
	1 cup	133	61	270	5	14	9.0	59	32	Tr	176	0.1	257	116	133	0.05	0.33	0.1	1
Soft serve (frozen custard)	1 cup	173	60	375	7	23	12.9	153	38	Tr	236	0.4	338	153	199	0.08	0.45	0.2	1
Ice milk, vanilla:																			
Hardened (about 4% fat)	1/2 gal.	1,048	69	1,470	41	45	27.7	146	232	1	1,409	1.5	2,117	836	419	0.61	2.78	0.9	6
	1 cup	131	69	185	5	6	3.5	18	29	Tr	176	0.2	265	105	52	0.08	0.35	0.1	1
Soft serve (about 3% fat)	1 cup	175	70	225	8	5	2.8	13	38	Tr	274	0.3	412	163	44	0.12	0.54	0.2	1
Sherbet (about 2% fat)	1/2 gal.	1,542	66	2,160	17	31	17.9	113	469	0	827	2.5	1,585	706	308	0.26	0.71	1.0	31
	1 cup	193	66	270	2	4	2.2	14	59	0	103	0.3	198	88	39	0.03	0.09	0.1	4
Yogurt:																			
With added milk solids:																			
Made with lowfat milk:																			
Fruit-flavored[8]	8-oz. container	227	74	230	10	2	1.6	10	43	1	345	0.2	442	133	25	0.08	0.40	0.2	1
Plain	8-oz. container	227	85	145	12	4	2.3	14	16	0	415	0.2	531	159	36	0.10	0.49	0.3	2
Made with nonfat milk	8-oz. container	227	85	125	13	Tr	0.3	4	17	0	452	0.2	579	174	5	0.11	0.53	0.3	2
Eggs																			
Eggs, large (24 oz. per dozen):																			
Raw:																			
Whole, without shell	1 egg	50	75	80	6	6	1.6	274	1	0	28	1.0	65	69	78	0.04	0.15	Tr	0
White	1 white	33	88	15	3	Tr	0.0	0	Tr	0	4	Tr	45	50	0	Tr	0.09	Tr	0
Yolk	1 yolk	17	49	65	3	6	1.6	272	Tr	0	26	0.9	15	8	94	0.04	0.07	Tr	0
Cooked:																			
Fried in butter	1 egg	46	68	95	6	7	1.9	278	1	0	29	1.1	66	162	94	0.04	0.14	Tr	0
Hard-cooked, shell removed	1 egg	50	75	80	6	6	1.6	274	1	0	28	1.0	65	69	78	0.04	0.14	Tr	0
Poached	1 egg	50	74	80	6	6	1.6	273	1	0	28	1.0	65	146	78	0.03	0.13	Tr	0
Scrambled (milk added) in butter. Also omelet	1 egg	64	73	110	7	8	2.2	282	2	0	54	1.0	97	176	102	0.04	0.18	Tr	Tr
Fats and Oils																			
Butter (4 sticks per lb.):																			
Tablespoon (1/8 stick)	1 tbsp.	14	16	100	Tr	11	7.1	31	Tr	0	3	Tr	4	[9]116	[10]106	Tr	Tr	Tr	0
Pat (1 in. square, 1/3 in. high; 90 per lb.	1 pat	5	16	35	Tr	4	2.5	11	Tr	0	1	Tr	1	[9]41	[10]38	Tr	Tr	Tr	0
Fats, cooking (vegetable shortenings)	1 cup	205	0	1,810	0	205	51.5	0	0	0	0	0.0	0	0	0	0.00	0.00	0.0	0
	1 tbsp.	13	0	115	0	13	3.3	0	0	0	0	0.0	0	0	0	0.00	0.00	0.0	0

(A)	(B)		(C)	(D)	(E)	(F)	(G)	(H)	(I)	(J)	(K)	(L)	(M)	(N)	(O)	(P)	(Q)	(R)	(S)
Margarine:																			
Imitation (about 40% fat), soft	8-oz. container	227	58	785	1	88	14.5	0	1	0	40	0.0	[11]57	2,178	[12]2,254	0.01	0.05	Tr	Tr
	1 tbsp.	14	58	50	Tr	5	0.9	0	Tr	0	2	0.0	4	[11]134	[12]139	Tr	Tr	Tr	Tr
Regular (about 80% fat):																			
Hard (4 sticks per lb.):																			
Tablespoon (1/8 stick)	1 tbsp.	14	16	100	Tr	11	1.8	0	Tr	0	4	Tr	6	[11]132	[12]139	Tr	0.01	Tr	Tr
Pat (1 in. square, 1/3 in. high; 90 per lb.)	1 pat	5	16	35	Tr	4	0.8	0	Tr	0	1	Tr	2	[11]47	[12]50	Tr	Tr	Tr	Tr
Soft	8-oz. container	227	16	1,625	2	183	30.7	0	1	0	60	0.0	[11]86	2,449	[12]2,254	0.02	0.07	Tr	Tr
	1 tbsp.	14	16	100	Tr	11	1.9	0	Tr	0	4	0.0	5	[11]151	[12]139	Tr	Tr	Tr	Tr
Spread (about 60% fat):																			
Hard (4 sticks per lb.):																			
Tablespoon (1/8 stick)	1 tbsp.	14	37	75	Tr	9	2.0	0	0	0	3	0.0	4	[11]139	[12]139	Tr	Tr	Tr	Tr
Pat (1 in. square, 1/3 in. high; 90 per lb.)	1 pat	5	37	25	Tr	3	0.7	0	0	0	1	0.0	1	[11]50	[12]50	Tr	Tr	Tr	Tr
Soft	8-oz. container	227	37	1,225	1	138	29.1	0	0	0	47	0.0	[11]68	2,256	[12]2,254	0.02	0.06	Tr	Tr
	1 tbsp.	14	37	75	Tr	9	1.8	0	0	0	3	0.0	4	[11]139	[12]139	Tr	Tr	Tr	Tr
Oils, salad or cooking:																			
Corn	1 cup	218	0	1,925	0	218	29.4	0	0	0	0	0.0	0	0	0	0.00	0.00	0.0	0
	1 tbsp.	14	0	125	0	14	1.8	0	0	0	0	0.0	0	0	0	0.00	0.00	0.0	0
Safflower	1 cup	218	0	1,925	0	218	19.8	0	0	0	0	0.0	0	0	0	0.00	0.00	0.0	0
	1 tbsp.	14	0	125	0	14	1.3	0	0	0	0	0.0	0	0	0	0.00	0.00	0.0	0
Soybean oil, hydrogenated (partially hardened)	1 cup	218	0	1,925	0	218	31.4	0	0	0	0	0.0	0	0	0	0.00	0.00	0.0	0
	1 tbsp.	14	0	125	0	14	2.0	0	0	0	0	0.0	0	0	0	0.00	0.00	0.0	0
Sunflower	1 cup	218	0	1,925	0	218	25.0	0	0	0	0	0.0	0	0	0	0.00	0.00	0.0	0
	1 tbsp.	14	0	125	0	14	1.5	0	0	0	0	0.0	0	0	0	0.00	0.00	0.0	0
Salad dressings:																			
Commercial:																			
Blue cheese	1 tbsp.	15	32	75	1	8	1.5	3	1	Tr	12	Tr	6	164	10	Tr	0.02	Tr	Tr
French:																			
Regular	1 tbsp.	16	35	85	Tr	9	1.5	0	1	Tr	2	Tr	2	188	Tr	Tr	Tr	Tr	Tr
Low calorie	1 tbsp.	16	75	25	Tr	2	0.1	0	2	Tr	6	Tr	3	306	Tr	Tr	Tr	Tr	Tr
Italian:																			
Regular	1 tbsp.	15	34	80	Tr	9	1.0	0	1	Tr	1	Tr	5	162	3	Tr	Tr	Tr	Tr
Low calorie	1 tbsp.	15	86	5	Tr	Tr	0.2	0	2	Tr	1	Tr	4	136	Tr	Tr	Tr	Tr	Tr
Mayonnaise:																			
Regular	1 tbsp.	14	15	100	Tr	11	1.6	8	Tr	0	3	0.1	5	80	12	0.00	0.00	Tr	0
Imitation	1 tbsp.	15	63	35	Tr	3	0.5	4	2	0	Tr	0.0	2	75	0	0.00	0.00	0.0	0
Tartar sauce	1 tbsp.	14	34	75	Tr	8	1.5	4	1	Tr	3	0.1	11	182	9	Tr	Tr	0.0	Tr
Thousand island:																			
Regular	1 tbsp.	16	46	60	Tr	6	1.0	4	2	Tr	2	0.1	18	112	15	Tr	Tr	Tr	0
Low calorie	1 tbsp.	15	69	25	Tr	2	0.2	2	2	Tr	2	0.1	17	150	14	Tr	Tr	Tr	0
Prepared from home recipe:																			
Cooked type	1 tbsp.	16	69	25	1	2	0.5	9	2	Tr	13	0.1	19		20	0.01	0.02	Tr	Tr
Vinegar and oil	1 tbsp.	16	47	70	0	8	1.5	0	Tr	0	0	0.0	1	Tr	0	0.00	0.00	0.0	0
Fish and Shellfish																			
Clams:																			
Raw, meat only	3 oz.	85	82	65	11	1	0.1	43	2	0	59	2.6	154	102	26	0.09	0.15	1.1	9
Crabmeat, canned	1 cup	135	77	135	23	3	0.3	135	1	0	61	1.1	149	1,350	14	0.11	0.11	2.6	0
Fish sticks, frozen, reheated, (stick, 4 by 1 by 1/2 in.)	1 fish stick	28	52	70	6	3	0.9	26	4	Tr	11	0.3	94	53	5	0.03	0.05	0.6	0
Haddock, breaded, fried[14]	3 oz.	85	61	175	17	9	3.2	75	7	1	34	1.0	270	123	20	0.06	0.10	2.9	0
Halibut, broiled, with butter and lemon juice	3 oz.	85	67	140	20	6	0.5	62	Tr	0	14	0.7	441	103	174	0.06	0.07	7.7	1
Salmon:																			
Canned (pink), solids and liquid	3 oz.	85	71	120	17	5	1.7	34	0	0	[15]167	0.7	307	443	18	0.03	0.15	6.8	0
Sardines, Atlantic, canned in oil, drained solids	3 oz.	85	62	175	20	9	1.7	85	0	0	[15]371	2.6	349	425	56	0.03	0.17	4.6	0
Scallops, breaded, frozen, reheated	6 scallops	90	59	195	15	10	2.5	70	10	Tr	39	2.0	369	298	21	0.11	0.11	1.6	0
Shrimp:																			
Canned, drained solids	3 oz.	85	70	100	21	1	0.2	128	1	0	98	1.4	1	1,955	15	0.01	0.03	1.5	0
French fried (7 medium)[16]	3 oz.	85	55	200	16	10	3.8	168	11	Tr	61	2.0	189	384	26	0.06	0.09	2.8	0
Tuna, canned, drained solids:																			
Oil pack, chunk light	3 oz.	85	61	165	24	7	1.3	55	0	0	7	1.6	298	303	20	0.04	0.09	10.1	0
Water pack, solid white	3 oz.	85	63	135	30	1	0.2	48	0	0	17	0.6	255	468	32	0.03	0.10	13.4	0

Nutritive Values of Foods – Continued
(Tr indicates nutrient present in trace amount.)

Item No. (A)	Foods, approximate measures, units, and weight (weight of edible portion only) (B)		Water (C)	Food energy (D)	Protein (E)	Fat (F)	Saturated fat (G)	Cholesterol (H)	Carbohydrate (I)	Dietary fiber (J)	Calcium (K)	Iron (L)	Potassium (M)	Sodium (N)	Vitamin A (O)	Thiamin (P)	Riboflavin (Q)	Niacin (R)	Vitamin C (S)
Fruits and Fruit Juices		Grams	Percent	Calories	Grams	Grams	Grams	Milligrams	Grams	Grams	Milligrams	Milligrams	Milligrams	Milligrams	Micrograms	Milligrams	Milligrams	Milligrams	Milligrams
Apples:																			
Raw:																			
Unpeeled, without cores:																			
2-3/4-in. diam. (about 3 per lb. with cores)	1 apple	138	84	80	Tr	Tr	0.1	0	21	3	10	0.2	159	Tr	7	0.02	0.02	0.1	8
Peeled, sliced	1 cup	110	84	65	Tr	Tr	0.1	0	16	2	4	0.1	124	Tr	5	0.02	0.01	0.1	4
Dried, sulfured	10 rings	64	32	155	1	Tr	Tr	0	42	6	9	0.9	288	[18]56	0	0.00	0.10	0.6	2
Apple juice, bottled or canned[19]	1 cup	248	88	115	Tr	Tr	Tr	0	29	Tr	17	0.9	295	7	Tr	0.05	0.04	0.2	[20]2
Applesauce, canned:																			
Sweetened	1 cup	255	80	195	Tr	Tr	Tr	0	51	3	10	0.9	156	8	3	0.03	0.07	0.5	[20]4
Unsweetened	1 cup	244	88	105	Tr	Tr	Tr	0	28	3	7	0.3	183	5	7	0.03	0.06	0.5	[20]3
Apricots:																			
Raw, without pits (about 12 per lb. with pits)	3 apricots	106	86	50	1	Tr	Tr	0	12	2	15	0.6	314	1	277	0.03	0.04	0.6	11
Canned (fruit and liquid):																			
Heavy syrup pack	1 cup	258	78	215	1	Tr	Tr	0	55	3	23	0.8	361	10	317	0.05	0.06	1.0	8
Juice pack	1 cup	248	87	120	2	Tr	Tr	0	31	3	30	0.7	409	10	419	0.04	0.05	0.9	12
Dried:																			
Uncooked (28 large or 37 medium halves per cup)	1 cup	130	31	310	5	1	Tr	0	80	6	59	6.1	1,791	13	941	0.01	0.20	3.9	3
Apricot nectar, canned	1 cup	251	85	140	1	Tr	Tr	0	36	2	18	1.0	286	8	330	0.02	0.04	0.7	[20]2
Avocados, raw, whole, without skin and seed:																			
California (about 2 per lb. with skin and seed)	1 avocado	173	73	305	4	30	4.5	0	12	6	19	2.0	1,097	21	106	0.19	0.21	3.3	14
Bananas, raw, without peel:																			
Whole (about 2-1/2 per lb. with peel)	1 banana	114	74	105	1	1	0.2	0	27	2	7	0.4	451	1	9	0.05	0.11	0.6	10
Blackberries, raw	1 cup	144	86	75	1	1	0.3	0	18	6	46	0.8	282	Tr	24	0.04	0.06	0.6	30
Blueberries:																			
Raw	1 cup	145	85	80	1	1	Tr	0	20	4	9	0.2	129	9	15	0.07	0.07	0.5	19
Frozen, sweetened	10-oz. container	284	77	230	1	Tr	0.1	0	62	6	17	1.1	170	3	12	0.06	0.15	0.7	3
Cantaloupe. See Melons																			
Cherries:																			
Sour, red, pitted, canned, water pack	1 cup	244	90	90	2	Tr	0.1	0	22	2	27	3.3	239	17	184	0.04	0.10	0.4	5
Sweet, raw, without pits and stems	10 cherries	68	81	50	1	1	0.1	0	11	Tr	10	0.3	152	Tr	15	0.03	0.04	0.3	5
Cranberry juice cocktail, bottled, sweetened	1 cup	253	85	145	Tr	Tr	0.1	0	38	Tr	8	0.4	61	10	1	0.01	0.04	0.1	[21]108
Cranberry sauce, sweetened, canned, strained	1 cup	277	61	420	1	Tr	Tr	0	108	3	11	0.6	72	80	6	0.04	0.06	0.3	6
Dates:																			
Whole, without pits	10 dates	83	23	230	2	Tr	0.2	0	61	6	27	1.0	541	2	4	0.07	0.08	1.8	0
Fruit cocktail, canned, fruit and liquid:																			
Heavy syrup pack	1 cup	255	80	185	1	Tr	Tr	0	48	3	15	0.7	224	15	52	0.05	0.05	1.0	5
Juice pack	1 cup	248	87	115	1	Tr	Tr	0	29	3	20	0.5	236	10	76	0.03	0.04	1.0	7
Grapefruit:																			
Raw, without peel, membrane and seeds (3-3/4 in. diam., 1 lb. 1 oz., whole, with refuse)	1/2 grapefruit	120	91	40	1	Tr	Tr	0	10	1	14	0.1	167	Tr	[22]1	0.04	0.02	0.3	41
Grapefruit juice:																			
Canned:																			
Unsweetened	1 cup	247	90	95	1	Tr	Tr	0	22	Tr	17	0.5	378	2	2	0.10	0.05	0.6	72
Sweetened	1 cup	250	87	115	1	Tr	Tr	0	28	Tr	20	0.9	405	5	2	0.10	0.06	0.8	67
Frozen concentrate, unsweetened																			
Diluted with 3 parts water by volume	1 cup	247	89	100	1	Tr	0.1	0	24	Tr	20	0.3	336	2	2	0.10	0.05	0.5	83
Grapes, European type (adherent skin), raw:																			
Thompson seedless	10 grapes	50	81	35	Tr	Tr	0.1	0	9	Tr	6	0.1	93	1	4	0.05	0.03	0.2	5
Grape juice:																			
Canned or bottled	1 cup	253	84	155	1	Tr	0.1	0	38	2	23	0.6	334	8	2	0.07	0.09	0.7	[20]Tr
Frozen concentrate, sweetened:																			
Diluted with 3 parts water by volume	1 cup	250	87	125	Tr	Tr	0.1	0	32	Tr	10	0.3	53	5	2	0.04	0.07	0.3	[21]60
Lemons, raw, without peel and seeds (about 4 per lb. with peel and seeds)	1 lemon	58	89	15	1	Tr	Tr	0	5	2	15	0.3	80	1	2	0.02	0.01	0.1	31

(A)	(B)		(C)	(D)	(E)	(F)	(G)	(H)	(I)	(J)	(K)	(L)	(M)	(N)	(O)	(P)	(Q)	(R)	(S)
Lemon juice:																			
Canned or bottled, unsweetened	1 cup	244	92	50	1	1	0.1	0	16	1	27	0.3	249	[23]51	4	0.10	0.02	0.5	61
Frozen, single-strength, unsweetened	6 fl. oz. can	244	92	55	1	1	0.1	0	16	1	20	0.3	217	2	3	0.14	0.03	0.3	77
Lime juice:																			
Canned, unsweetened	1 cup	246	93	50	1	1	0.1	0	16	1	30	0.6	185	[23]39	4	0.08	0.01	0.4	16
Melons, raw, without rind and cavity contents:																			
Cantaloupe, orange-fleshed (5 in. diam., 2-1/3 lb., whole, with rind and cavity contents)	1/2 melon	267	90	95	2	1	0.1	0	22	2	29	0.6	825	24	861	0.10	0.06	1.5	113
Honeydew (6-1/2 in. diam., 5-1/4 lb., whole, with rind and cavity contents)	1/10 melon	129	90	45	1	Tr	Tr	0	12	1	8	0.1	350	13	5	0.10	0.02	0.8	32
Nectarines, raw, without pits (about 3 per lb. with pits)1 nectarine	1 nectarine	136	86	65	1	1	0.1	0	16	2	7	0.2	288	Tr	100	0.02	0.06	1.3	7
Oranges, raw:																			
Whole, without peel and seeds (2-5/8 in. diam., about 2-1/2 per lb., with peel and seeds)	1 orange	131	87	60	1	Tr	Tr	0	15	3	52	0.1	237	Tr	27	0.11	0.05	0.4	70
Orange juice:																			
Raw, all varieties	1 cup	248	88	110	2	Tr	0.1	0	26	Tr	27	0.5	496	2	50	0.22	0.07	1.0	124
Canned, unsweetened	1 cup	249	89	105	1	Tr	Tr	0	25	Tr	20	1.1	436	5	44	0.15	0.07	0.8	86
Frozen concentrate:																			
Diluted with 3 parts water by volume	1 cup	249	88	110	2	Tr	Tr	0	27	Tr	22	0.2	473	2	19	0.20	0.04	0.5	97
Orange and grapefruit juice, canned	1 cup	247	89	105	1	Tr	Tr	0	25	Tr	20	1.1	390	7	29	0.14	0.07	0.8	72
Peaches:																			
Raw:																			
Whole, 2-1/2 in. diam., peeled, pitted (about 4 per lb. with peels and pits)	1 peach	87	88	35	1	Tr	Tr	0	10	2	4	0.1	171	Tr	47	0.01	0.04	0.9	6
Canned, fruit and liquid:																			
Heavy syrup pack	1 cup	256	79	190	1	Tr	Tr	0	51	3	8	0.7	236	15	85	0.03	0.06	1.6	7
Juice pack	1 cup	248	87	110	2	Tr	Tr	0	29	4	15	0.7	317	10	94	0.02	0.04	1.4	9
Dried:																			
Uncooked	1 cup	160	32	380	6	1	0.1	0	98	12	45	6.5	1,594	11	346	Tr	0.34	7.0	8
Frozen, sliced, sweetened 10 oz. container	10-oz container	284	75	265	2	Tr	Tr	0	68	4	9	1.1	369	17	81	0.04	0.10	1.9	[21]268
	1 cup	250	75	235	2	Tr	Tr	0	60	4	8	0.9	325	15	71	0.03	0.09	1.6	[21]236
Pears:																			
Raw, with skin, cored:																			
Bartlett, 2-1/2 in. diam. (about 2-1/2 per lb. with cores and stems)	1 pear	166	84	100	1	1	Tr	0	25	4	18	0.4	208	Tr	3	0.03	0.07	0.2	7
Bosc, 2-1/2 in. diam. (about 3 per lb. with cores and stems)	1 pear	141	84	85	1	1	Tr	0	21	3	16	0.4	176	Tr	3	0.03	0.06	0.1	6
Canned, fruit and liquid:																			
Heavy syrup pack	1 cup	255	80	190	1	Tr	Tr	0	49	5	13	0.6	166	13	1	0.03	0.06	0.6	3
Juice pack	1 cup	248	86	125	1	Tr	Tr	0	32	5	22	0.7	238	10	1	0.03	0.03	0.5	4
Pineapple:																			
Raw, diced	1 cup	155	87	75	1	1	Tr	0	19	2	11	0.6	175	2	4	0.14	0.06	0.7	24
Canned, fruit and liquid:																			
Heavy syrup pack:																			
Crushed, chunks, tidbits	1 cup	255	79	200	1	Tr	Tr	0	52	1	36	1.0	265	3	4	0.23	0.06	0.7	19
Juice pack:																			
Chunks or tidbits	1 cup	250	84	150	1	Tr	Tr	0	39	2	35	0.7	305	3	10	0.24	0.05	0.7	24
Pineapple juice, unsweetened, canned	1 cup	250	86	140	1	Tr	Tr	0	34	Tr	43	0.7	335	3	1	0.14	0.06	0.6	27
Plums, without pits:																			
Raw:																			
2-1/8 in. diam. (about 6-1/2 per lb. with pits)	1 plum	66	85	35	1	Tr	Tr	0	9	1	3	0.1	114	Tr	21	0.03	0.06	0.3	6
Canned, purple, fruit and liquid:																			
Heavy syrup pack	1 cup	258	76	230	1	Tr	Tr	0	60	3	23	2.2	235	49	67	0.04	0.10	0.8	1
Juice pack	1 cup	252	84	145	1	Tr	Tr	0	38	3	25	0.9	388	3	254	0.06	0.15	1.2	7
Prunes, dried:																			
Uncooked	4 extra large or 5 large prunes	49	32	115	1	Tr	Tr	0	31	4	25	1.2	365	2	97	0.04	0.08	1.0	2
Cooked, unsweetened, fruit and liquid	1 cup	212	70	225	2	Tr	Tr	0	60	14	49	2.4	708	4	65	0.05	0.21	1.5	6
Prune juice, canned or bottled	1 cup	256	81	180	2	Tr	Tr	0	45	3	31	3.0	707	10	1	0.04	0.18	2.0	10
Raisins, seedless:																			
Cup, not pressed down	1 cup	145	15	435	5	1	0.2	0	115	5	71	3.0	1,089	17	1	0.23	0.13	1.2	5

Nutritive Values of Foods – Continued

(Tr indicates nutrient present in trace amount.)

Item No. (A)	Foods, approximate measures, units, and weight (weight of edible portion only) (B)		Water (C)	Food energy (D)	Protein (E)	Fat (F)	Saturated fat (G)	Cholesterol (H)	Carbohydrate (I)	Dietary fiber (J)	Calcium (K)	Iron (L)	Potassium (M)	Sodium (N)	Vitamin A (O)	Thiamin (P)	Riboflavin (Q)	Niacin (R)	Vitamin C (S)
			Nutrients in Indicated Quantity																
		Grams	Percent	Calories	Grams	Grams	Grams	Milligrams	Grams	Grams	Milligrams	Milligrams	Milligrams	Milligrams	Micrograms	Milligrams	Milligrams	Milligrams	Milligrams
Raspberries:																			
Raw	1 cup	123	87	60	1	1	Tr	0	14	5	27	0.7	187	Tr	16	0.04	0.11	1.1	31
Frozen, sweetened	10-oz. container	284	73	295	2	Tr	Tr	0	74	5	43	1.8	324	3	17	0.05	0.13	0.7	47
Rhubarb, cooked, added sugar	1 cup	240	68	280	1	Tr	Tr	0	75	5	348	0.5	230	2	17	0.04	0.06	0.5	8
Strawberries:																			
Raw, capped, whole	1 cup	149	92	45	1	1	Tr	0	10	2	21	0.6	247	1	4	0.03	0.10	0.3	84
Tangerines:																			
Raw, without peel and seeds (2-3/8 in. diam., about 4 per lb., with peel and seeds)	1 tangerine	84	88	35	1	Tr	Tr	0	9	1	12	0.1	132	1	77	0.09	0.02	0.1	26
Watermelon, raw, without rind and seeds:																			
Piece (4 by 8 in wedge with rind and seeds; 1/16 of 32-2/3 lb. melon, 10 by 16 in.)	1 piece	482	92	155	3	2	0.6	0	35	1	39	0.8	559	10	176	0.39	0.10	1.0	46
Grain Products																			
Bagels, plain or water, enriched, 3-1/2 in. diam.[24]	1 bagel	68	29	200	7	2	0.1	0	38	2	29	1.8	50	245	0	0.26	0.20	2.4	0
Biscuits, baking powder, 2 in. diam. (enriched flour, vegetable shortening):																			
From home recipe	1 biscuit	28	28	100	2	5	1.2	Tr	13	Tr	47	0.7	32	195	3	0.08	0.08	0.8	Tr
From mix	1 biscuit	28	29	95	2	3	0.8	Tr	14	1	58	0.7	56	262	4	0.12	0.11	0.8	Tr
From refrigerated dough	1 biscuit	20	30	65	1	2	2.0	1	10	Tr	4	0.5	18	249	0	0.08	0.05	0.7	0
Breads:																			
Cracked-wheat bread (3/4 enriched wheat flour, 1/4 cracked wheat flour):[25]																			
Slice (18 per loaf)	1 slice	25	35	65	2	1	0.2	0	12	2	16	0.7	34	106	Tr	0.10	0.09	0.8	Tr
French or Vienna bread, enriched:[25]																			
Slice:																			
French, 5 by 2-1/2 by 1 in.	1 slice	35	34	100	3	1	0.2	0	18	1	39	1.1	32	203	Tr	0.16	0.12	1.4	Tr
Vienna, 4-3/4 by 4 by 1/2 in.	1 slice	25	34	70	2	1	0.2	0	13	1	28	0.8	23	145	Tr	0.12	0.09	1.0	Tr
Italian bread, enriched:																			
Slice, 4-1/2 by 3-1/4 by 3/4 in.	1 slice	30	32	85	3	Tr	0.3	0	17	1	5	0.8	22	176	0	0.12	0.07	1.0	0
Pita bread, enriched, white, 6-1/2 in. diam.	1 pita	60	31	165	6	1	0.1	0	33	1	49	1.4	71	339	0	0.27	0.12	2.2	0
Pumpernickel (2/3 rye flour, 1/3 enriched wheat flour):[25]																			
Slice, 5 by 4 by 3/8 in.	1 slice	32	37	80	3	1	0.1	0	16	1	23	0.9	141	177	0	0.11	0.17	1.1	0
Raisin bread, enriched:[25]																			
Slice (18 per loaf)	1 slice	25	33	65	2	1	0.3	0	13	1	25	0.8	59	92	Tr	0.08	0.15	1.0	Tr
Rye bread, light (2/3 enriched wheat flour, 1/3 rye flour):[25]																			
Slice, 4-3/4 by 3-3/4 by 7/16 in.	1 slice	25	37	65	2	1	0.2	0	12	2	20	0.7	51	175	0	0.10	0.08	0.8	0
Wheat bread, enriched:[25]																			
Slice (18 per loaf)	1 slice	25	37	65	2	1	0.2	0	12	1	32	0.9	35	138	Tr	0.12	0.08	1.2	Tr
White bread, enriched:[25]																			
Slice (18 per loaf)	1 slice	25	37	65	2	1	0.2	0	12	1	32	0.7	28	129	Tr	0.12	0.08	0.9	Tr
Slice (22 per loaf)	1 slice	20	37	55	2	1	0.2	0	10	1	25	0.6	22	101	Tr	0.09	0.06	0.7	Tr
Cubes	1 cup	30	37	80	2	1	0.2	0	15	1	38	0.9	34	154	Tr	0.14	0.09	1.1	Tr
Crumbs, soft	1 cup	45	37	120	4	2	0.3	0	22	1	57	1.3	50	231	Tr	0.21	0.14	1.7	Tr
Whole-wheat bread:[25]																			
Slice (16 per loaf)	1 slice	28	38	70	3	1	0.3	0	13	2	20	1.0	50	180	Tr	0.10	0.06	1.1	Tr
Bread stuffing (from enriched bread), prepared from mix:																			
Dry type	1 cup	140	33	500	9	31	2.4	0	50	4	92	2.2	126	1,254	273	0.17	0.20	2.5	0

(A)	(B)		(C)	(D)	(E)	(F)	(G)	(H)	(I)	(J)	(K)	(L)	(M)	(N)	(O)	(P)	(Q)	(R)	(S)
Moist type	1 cup	203	61	420	9	26	3.0	67	40	4	81	2.0	118	1,023	256	0.10	0.18	1.6	0
Breakfast cereals:																			
Hot type, cooked:																			
Corn (hominy) grits:																			
Regular and quick, enriched	1 cup	242	85	145	3	Tr	0.1	0	31	5	0	[27]1.5	53	[28]0	[29]0	[27]0.24	[27]0.15	[27]2.0	0
Instant, plain	1 pkt.	137	85	80	2	Tr	Tr	0	18	Tr	7	[27]1.0	29	[34]3	0	[27]0.18	[27]0.08	[27]1.3	0
Cream of Wheat®:																			
Regular, quick, instant	1 cup	244	86	140	4	Tr	0.1	0	29	1	[30]54	[30]10.9	46	[31, 32]5	0	[30]0.24	[30]0.07	[30]1.5	0
Mix'n Eat, plain	1 pkt.	142	82	100	3	Tr	Tr	0	21	Tr	[30]20	[30]8.1	38	[24]1	[30]376	[30]0.43	[30]0.28	[30]5.0	0
Malt-O-Meal®	1 cup	240	88	120	4	Tr	Tr	0	26	1	5	[30]9.6	31	[33]2	0	[30]0.48	[30]0.24	[30]5.8	0
Oatmeal or rolled oats:																			
Regular, quick, instant, nonfortified	1 cup	234	85	145	6	2	0.4	0	25	4	19	1.6	131	[34]2	4	0.26	0.05	0.3	0
Instant, fortified:																			
Plain	1 pkt.	177	86	105	4	2	0.3	0	18	3	[27]163	[27]6.3	99	[27]285	[27]453	[27]0.53	[27]0.28	[27]5.5	0
Ready-to-eat:																			
All-Bran® (about 1/3 cup)	1 oz.	28	3	70	4	1	0.1	0	21	10	23	[30]4.5	350	320	[30]375	[30]0.37	[30]0.43	[30]5.0	[30]15
Cap'n Crunch® (about 3/4 cup)	1 oz.	28	3	120	1	3	2.2	0	23	1	5	[27]7.5	37	213	4	[27]0.50	[27]0.55	[27]6.6	0
Cheerios® (about 1-1/4 cup)	1 oz.	28	5	110	4	2	0.3	0	20	2	48	[30]4.5	101	307	[30]375	[30]0.37	[30]0.43	[30]5.0	[30]15
Corn Flakes (about 1-1/4 cup):																			
Toasties®	1 oz.	28	3	110	2	Tr	Tr	0	24	1	1	[27]0.7	33	297	[30]375	[30]0.37	[30]0.43	[30]5.0	0
40% Bran Flakes:																			
Kellogg's® (about 3/4 cup)	1 oz.	28	3	90	4	1	0.1	0	22	6	14	[30]8.1	180	264	[30]375	[30]0.37	[30]0.43	[30]5.0	0
Froot Loops® (about 1 cup)	1 oz.	28	3	110	2	1	0.2	0	25	1	3	[30]4.5	26	145	[30]375	[30]0.37	[30]0.43	[30]5.0	[30]15
Golden Grahams® (about 3/4 cup)	1 oz.	28	2	110	2	1	2.9	Tr	24	1	17	[30]4.5	63	346	[30]375	[30]0.37	[30]0.43	[30]5.0	[30]15
Grape-Nuts® (about 1/4 cup)	1 oz.	28	3	100	3	Tr	Tr	0	23	3	11	1.2	95	197	[30]375	[30]0.37	[30]0.43	[30]5.0	0
Honey Nut Cheerios® (about 3/4 cup)	1 oz.	28	3	105	3	1	0.1	0	23	1	20	[30]4.5	99	257	[30]375	[30]0.37	[30]0.43	[30]5.0	[30]15
Nature Valley® Granola (about 1/3 cup)	1 oz.	28	4	125	3	5	5.0	0	19	2	18	0.9	98	58	2	0.10	0.05	0.2	0
Product 19® (about 3/4 cup)	1 oz.	28	3	110	3	Tr	Tr	0	24	1	3	[30]18.0	44	325	[30]1,501	[30]1.50	[30]1.70	[30]20.0	[30]60
Raisin Bran:																			
Kellogg's® (about 3/4 cup)	1 oz.	28	8	90	3	1	0.2	0	21	5	10	[30]3.5	147	207	[30]288	[30]0.28	[30]0.34	[30]3.9	0
Rice Krispies® (about 1 cup)	1 oz.	28	2	110	2	Tr	Tr	0	25	Tr	4	[30]1.8	29	340	[30]375	[30]0.37	[30]0.43	[30]5.0	[30]15
Shredded Wheat (about 2/3 cup)	1 oz.	28	5	100	3	1	0.2	0	23	4	11	1.2	102	3	0	0.07	0.08	1.5	0
Special K® (about 1-1/3 cup)	1 oz.	28	2	110	6	Tr	Tr	Tr	21	Tr	8	[30]4.5	49	265	[30]375	[30]0.37	[30]0.43	[30]5.0	[30]15
Frosted Flakes,																			
Kellogg's® (about 3/4 cup)	1 oz.	28	3	110	1	Tr	Tr	0	26	1	1	[30]1.8	18	230	[30]375	[30]0.37	[30]0.43	[30]5.0	[30]15
Golden Crisps® (about 3/4 cup)	1 oz.	28	3	105	2	1	Tr	0	25	1	3	[30]1.8	42	75	[30]375	[30]0.37	[30]0.43	[30]5.0	[30]15
Total® (about 1 cup)	1 oz.	28	4	100	3	1	0.1	0	22	4	48	[30]18.0	106	352	[30]1,501	[30]1.50	[30]1.70	[30]20.0	[30]60
Wheaties® (about 1 cup)	1 oz.	28	5	100	3	Tr	0.1	0	23	3	43	[30]4.5	106	354	[30]375	[30]0.37	[30]0.43	[30]5.0	[30]15
Buckwheat flour, light, sifted	1 cup	98	12	340	6	1	0.2	0	78	6	11	1.0	314	2	0	0.08	0.04	0.4	0
Cakes prepared from cake mixes with enriched flour:[35]																			
Angel food:																			
Piece, 1/12 of cake	1 piece	53	38	125	3	Tr	0.1	0	29	1	44	0.2	71	269	0	0.03	0.11	0.1	0
Coffeecake, crumb:																			
Piece, 1/6 of cake	1 piece	72	30	230	5	7	1.3	47	38	1	44	1.2	78	310	32	0.14	0.15	1.3	Tr
Devil's food with chocolate frosting:																			
Piece, 1/16 of cake	1 piece	69	24	235	3	8	3.2	37	40	2	41	1.4	90	181	31	0.07	0.10	0.6	Tr
Cupcake, 2-1/2 in. diam.	1 cupcake	35	24	120	2	4	1.9	19	20	1	21	0.7	46	92	16	0.04	0.05	0.3	Tr
Gingerbread:																			
Piece, 1/9 of cake	1 piece	63	37	175	2	4	1.6	1	32	2	57	1.2	173	192	0	0.09	0.11	0.8	Tr
Yellow with chocolate frosting:																			
Whole, 2-layer cake, Piece, 1/16 of cake	1 piece	69	26	235	3	8	3.3	36	40	20	63	1.0	75	157	29	0.08	0.10	0.7	Tr
Cakes prepared from home recipes using enriched flour:																			
Carrot, with cream cheese frosting:[36]																			
Piece, 1/16 of cake	1 piece	96	23	385	4	21	5.5	74	48	1	44	1.3	108	279	15	0.11	0.12	0.9	1
Fruitcake, dark:[36]																			
Piece, 1/32 of cake, 2/3 in. arc	1 piece	43	18	165	2	7	0.5	20	25	2	41	1.2	194	67	13	0.08	0.08	0.5	16
Plain sheet cake:[37]																			
Without frosting:																			
Piece, 1/9 of cake	1 piece	86	25	315	4	12	3.3	61	48	Tr	55	1.3	68	258	41	0.14	0.15	1.1	Tr
With uncooked white frosting:																			
Piece, 1/9 of cake	1 piece	121	21	445	4	14	2.9	70	77	1	61	1.2	74	275	71	0.13	0.16	1.1	Tr

Nutritive Values of Foods – Continued

(Tr indicates nutrient present in trace amount.)

Item No. (A)	Foods, approximate measures, units, and weight (weight of edible portion only) (B)		Water (C)	Food energy (D)	Protein (E)	Fat (F)	Saturated fat (G)	Cholesterol (H)	Carbohydrate (I)	Dietary fiber (J)	Calcium (K)	Iron (L)	Potassium (M)	Sodium (N)	Vitamin A (O)	Thiamin (P)	Riboflavin (Q)	Niacin (R)	Vitamin C (S)
				Nutrients in Indicated Quantity															
		Grams	Percent	Calories	Grams	Grams	Grams	Milligrams	Grams	Grams	Milligrams	Milligrams	Milligrams	Milligrams	Micrograms	Milligrams	Milligrams	Milligrams	Milligrams
Pound:[38]																			
Slice, 1/17 of loaf	1 slice	30	22	120	2	5	0.3	32	15	Tr	20	0.5	28	96	60	0.05	0.06	0.5	Tr
Cakes, commercial, made with enriched flour:																			
Pound:																			
Slice, 1/17 of loaf	1 slice	29	24	110	2	5	3.2	64	15	Tr	8	0.5	26	108	41	0.06	0.06	0.5	0
Snack cakes:																			
Devil's food with creme filling (2 small cakes per pkg.)	1 small cake	28	20	105	1	4	0.9	15	17	Tr	21	1.0	34	105	4	0.06	0.09	0.7	0
Sponge with creme filling (2 small cakes per pkg.)	1 small cake	42	19	155	1	5	0.5	7	27	Tr	14	0.6	37	155	9	0.07	0.06	0.6	0
White with white frosting:																			
Piece, 1/16 of cake	1 piece	71	24	260	3	9	2.8	3	42	1	33	1.0	52	176	12	0.20	0.13	1.7	0
Yellow with chocolate frosting:																			
Piece, 1/16 of cake	1 piece	69	23	245	2	11	3.3	38	39	1	23	1.2	123	192	30	0.05	0.14	0.6	0
Cheesecake:																			
Piece, 1/12 of cake	1 piece	92	46	280	5	18	10.6	170	26	2	52	0.4	90	204	69	0.03	0.12	0.4	5
Cookies made with enriched flour:																			
Brownies with nuts:																			
Commercial, with frosting, 1-1/2 by 1-3/4 by 7/8 in.	1 brownie	25	13	100	1	4	1.1	14	16	1	13	0.6	50	59	18	0.08	0.07	0.3	Tr
Chocolate chip:																			
Commercial, 2-1/4 in. diam., 3/8 in. thick	4 cookies	42	4	180	2	9	3.1	5	28	1	13	0.8	68	140	15	0.10	0.23	1.0	Tr
From refrigerated dough, 2-1/4 in. diam., 3/8 in. thick	4 cookies	48	5	225	2	11	3.2	22	32	1	13	1.0	62	173	8	0.06	0.10	0.9	0
Oatmeal with raisins, 2-5/8 in. diam., 1/4 in. thick	4 cookies	52	4	245	3	10	1.7	2	36	2	18	1.1	90	148	12	0.09	0.08	1.0	0
Peanut butter cookie, from home recipe, 2-5/8 in. diam.[25]	4 cookies	48	3	245	4	14	2.1	0	28	1	21	1.1	110	142	5	0.07	0.07	1.9	0
Sandwich type (chocolate or vanilla), 1-3/4 in. diam., 3/8 in. thick	4 cookies	40	2	195	2	8	1.7	0	29	1	12	1.4	66	189	0	0.09	0.07	0.8	0
Sugar cookie, from refrigerated dough, 2-1/2 in. diam., 1/4 in. thick	4 cookies	48	4	235	2	12	2.8	29	31	Tr	50	0.9	33	261	11	0.09	0.06	1.1	0
Vanilla wafers, 1-3/4 in. diam., 1/4 in. thick	10 cookies	40	4	185	2	7	1.4	25	29	8	16	0.8	50	150	14	0.07	0.10	1.0	0
Corn chips	1 oz. package	28	1	155	2	9	1.3	0	16	1	35	0.5	52	233	11	0.04	0.05	0.4	1
Cornmeal:																			
Degermed, enriched:																			
Dry form	1 cup	138	12	500	11	2	0.3	0	108	10	8	5.9	166	1	61	0.61	0.36	4.8	0
Cooked	1 cup	240	88	120	3	Tr	0.1	0	26	4	2	1.4	38	0	14	0.14	0.10	1.2	0
Crackers:[39]																			
Cheese:																			
Plain, 1 in. square	10 crackers	10	4	50	1	3	0.9	6	6	Tr	11	0.3	17	112	5	0.05	0.04	0.4	0
Sandwich type (peanut butter)	1 sandwich	8	3	40	1	2	0.4	1	5	Tr	7	0.3	17	90	Tr	0.04	0.03	0.6	0
Graham, plain, 2-1/2 in. square	2 crackers	14	5	60	1	1	0.4	0	11	Tr	6	0.4	36	86	0	0.02	0.03	0.6	0
Saltines[40]	4 crackers	12	4	50	1	1	0.3	4	9	Tr	3	0.5	17	165	0	0.06	0.05	0.6	0
Snack-type, standard	1 round cracker	3	3	15	Tr	1	0.1	0	2	Tr	3	0.1	4	30	Tr	0.01	0.01	0.1	0
Wheat, thin	4 crackers	8	3	35	1	1	0.7	0	5	1	3	0.3	17	69	Tr	0.04	0.03	0.4	0
Croissants, made with enriched flour, 4-1/2 by 4 by 1-3/4 in.	1 croissant	57	22	235	5	12	6.7	13	27	1	20	2.1	68	452	13	0.17	0.13	1.3	0
Danish pastry, made with enriched flour:																			
Plain without fruit or nuts:																			
Round piece, about 4-1/4 in. diam., 1 in. high	1 pastry	57	27	220	4	12	2.3	49	26	Tr	60	1.1	53	218	17	0.16	0.17	1.4	Tr
Fruit, round piece	1 pastry	65	30	235	4	13	2.3	56	28	0	17	1.3	57	233	11	0.16	0.14	1.4	Tr
Doughnuts, made with enriched flour:																			
Cake type, plain, 3-1/4 in. diam., 1 in. high	1 doughnut	50	21	210	3	12	1.9	20	24	1	22	1.0	58	192	5	0.12	0.12	1.1	Tr
Yeast-leavened, glazed, 3-3/4 in. diam., 1-1/4 in. high	1 doughnut	60	27	235	4	13	3.5	21	26	1	17	1.4	64	222	Tr	0.28	0.12	1.8	0

(A)	(B)		(C)	(D)	(E)	(F)	(G)	(H)	(I)	(J)	(K)	(L)	(M)	(N)	(O)	(P)	(Q)	(R)	(S)
English muffins, plain, enriched	1 muffin	57	42	140	5	1	0.1	0	27	2	96	1.7	331	378	0	0.26	0.19	2.2	0
French toast, from home recipe	1 slice	65	53	155	6	7	2.0	112	17	Tr	72	1.3	86	257	32	0.12	0.16	1.0	Tr
Macaroni, enriched, cooked (cut lengths, elbows, shells):																			
Firm stage (hot)	1 cup	130	64	190	7	1	0.1	0	39	2	14	2.1	103	1	0	0.23	0.13	1.8	0
Muffins made with enriched flour, 2-1/2 in. diam., 1-1/2 in. high:																			
From home recipe:																			
Blueberry[25]	1 muffin	45	37	135	3	5	1.1	19	20	7	54	0.9	47	198	9	0.10	0.11	0.9	1
Bran[36]	1 muffin	45	35	125	3	6	1.2	24	19	3	60	1.4	99	189	30	0.11	0.13	1.3	3
From commercial mix (egg and water added):																			
Blueberry	1 muffin	45	33	140	3	5	0.7	45	22	1	15	0.9	54	225	11	0.10	0.17	1.1	Tr
Bran	1 muffin	45	28	140	3	4	1.1	28	24	4	27	1.7	50	385	14	0.08	0.12	1.9	0
Corn	1 muffin	45	30	145	3	6	1.3	42	22	2	30	1.3	31	291	16	0.09	0.09	0.8	Tr
Noodles (egg noodles), enriched, cooked	1 cup	160	70	200	7	2	0.5	50	37	2	16	2.6	70	3	34	0.22	0.13	1.9	0
Noodles, chow mein, canned	1 cup	45	11	220	6	11	2.0	5	26	2	14	0.4	33	450	0	0.05	0.03	0.6	0
Pancakes, 4 in. diam.:																			
Buckwheat, from mix (with buckwheat and enriched flours), egg and milk added	1 pancake	27	58	55	2	2	0.5	20	6	1	59	0.4	66	125	17	0.04	0.05	0.2	Tr
Plain:																			
From mix (with enriched flour), egg, milk, and oil added	1 pancake	27	54	60	2	2	0.1	16	8	Tr	36	0.7	43	160	7	0.09	0.12	0.8	Tr
Piecrust, made with enriched flour and vegetable shortening, baked:																			
From home recipe, 9 in. diam.	1 pie shell	180	15	900	11	60	15.5	0	79	3	25	4.5	90	1,100	0	0.54	0.40	5.0	0
From mix, 9 in. diam.	Piecrust for 2-crust pie	320	19	1,485	20	93	27.6	0	141	6	131	9.3	179	2,602	0	1.06	0.80	9.9	0
Pies, piecrust made with enriched flour, vegetable shortening, 9 in. diam.:																			
Apple:																			
Piece, 1/6 of pie	1 piece	158	48	405	3	18	3.3	0	60	3	13	1.6	126	476	5	0.17	0.13	1.6	2
Blueberry:																			
Piece, 1/6 of pie	1 piece	158	51	380	4	17	4.6	0	55	2	17	2.1	158	423	14	0.17	0.14	1.7	6
Cherry:																			
Piece, 1/6 of pie	1 piece	158	47	410	4	18	4.7	0	61	2	22	1.6	166	480	70	0.19	0.14	1.6	0
Creme:																			
Piece, 1/6 of pie	1 piece	152	43	455	3	23	7.4	8	59	0	46	1.1	133	369	65	0.06	0.15	1.1	0
Custard:																			
Piece, 1/6 of pie	1 piece	152	58	330	9	17	4.2	169	36	2	146	1.5	208	436	96	0.14	0.32	0.9	0
Lemon meringue:																			
Piece, 1/6 of pie	1 piece	140	47	355	5	14	2.2	143	53	2	20	1.4	70	395	66	0.10	0.14	0.8	4
Peach:																			
Piece, 1/6 of pie	1 piece	158	48	405	4	17	4.4	0	60	2	16	1.9	235	423	115	0.17	0.16	2.4	5
Pecan:																			
Piece, 1/6 of pie	1 piece	138	20	575	7	32	5.2	95	71	5	65	4.6	170	305	54	0.30	0.17	1.1	0
Pumpkin:																			
Piece, 1/6 of pie	1 piece	152	59	320	6	17	4.2	109	37	6	78	1.4	243	325	416	0.14	0.21	1.2	0
Pies, fried:																			
Apple	1 pie	85	43	255	2	14	6.5	14	31	2	12	0.9	42	326	3	0.09	0.06	1.0	1
Cherry	1 pie	85	42	250	2	14	2.0	13	32	2	11	0.7	61	371	19	0.06	0.06	0.6	1
Popcorn, popped:																			
Air-popped, unsalted	1 cup	8	4	30	1	Tr	Tr	0	6	1	1	0.2	20	Tr	1	0.03	0.01	0.2	0
Popped in vegetable oil, salted	1 cup	11	3	55	1	3	0.5	0	6	1	3	0.3	19	86	2	0.01	0.02	0.1	0
Sugar syrup coated	1 cup	35	4	135	2	1	1.3	0	30	2	2	0.5	90	Tr	3	0.13	0.02	0.4	0
Pretzels, made with enriched flour:																			
Twisted, dutch, 2-3/4 by 2-5/8 in.	1 pretzel	16	3	65	2	1	0.1	0	13	Tr	4	0.3	16	258	0	0.05	0.04	0.7	0
Twisted, thin, 3-1/4 by 2-1/4 by 1/4 in.	10 pretzels	60	3	240	6	2	0.4	0	48	2	16	1.2	61	966	0	0.19	0.15	2.6	0
Rice:																			
Brown, cooked, served hot	1 cup	195	70	230	5	1	0.4	0	50	4	23	1.0	137	0	0	0.18	0.04	2.7	0
White, enriched:																			
Commercial varieties, all types:																			
Cooked, served hot	1 cup	205	73	225	4	Tr	0.2	0	50	1	21	1.8	57	0	0	0.23	0.02	2.1	0
Instant, ready-to-serve, hot	1 cup	165	73	180	4	0	0.1	0	40	1	5	1.3	0	0	0	0.21	0.02	1.7	0

Nutritive Values of Foods – Continued

(Tr indicates nutrient present in trace amount.)

Item No. (A) / Foods, approximate measures, units, and weight (weight of edible portion only) (B)			Water (C)	Food energy (D)	Protein (E)	Fat (F)	Saturated fat (G)	Cholesterol (H)	Carbohydrate (I)	Dietary fiber (J)	Calcium (K)	Iron (L)	Potassium (M)	Sodium (N)	Vitamin A (O)	Thiamin (P)	Riboflavin (Q)	Niacin (R)	Vitamin C (S)
		Grams	Percent	Calories	Grams	Grams	Grams	Milligrams	Grams	Grams	Milligrams	Milligrams	Milligrams	Milligrams	Micrograms	Milligrams	Milligrams	Milligrams	Milligrams
Rolls, enriched:																			
Commercial:																			
Dinner, 2-1/2 in. diam., 2 in. high	1 roll	28	32	85	2	2	0.7	Tr	14	1	33	0.8	36	155	Tr	0.14	0.09	1.1	Tr
Frankfurter and hamburger (8 per 11-1/2 oz. pkg.)	1 roll	40	34	115	3	2	0.5	Tr	20	1	54	1.2	56	241	Tr	0.20	0.13	1.6	Tr
Hard, 3-3/4 in. diam., 2 in. high	1 roll	50	25	155	5	2	0.3	Tr	30	1	24	1.4	49	313	0	0.20	0.12	1.7	0
Hoagie or submarine, 11-1/2 by 3 by 2-1/2 in.	1 roll	135	31	400	11	8	0.9	Tr	72	4	100	3.8	128	683	0	0.54	0.33	4.5	0
Spaghetti, enriched, cooked:																			
Firm stage, "al dente," served hot	1 cup	130	64	190	7	1	0.1	0	39	2	14	2.0	103	1	0	0.23	0.13	1.8	0
Toaster pastries	1 pastry	54	13	210	2	6	0.8	0	38	1	104	2.2	91	248	52	0.17	0.18	2.3	4
Tortillas, corn	1 tortilla	30	45	65	2	1	0.1	0	13	2	42	0.6	43	1	8	0.05	0.03	0.4	0
Waffles, made with enriched flour, 7 in. diam.:																			
From mix, egg and milk added	1 waffle	75	42	205	7	8	1.7	59	27	1	179	1.2	146	515	49	0.14	0.23	0.9	Tr
Wheat flours:																			
All-purpose or family flour, enriched:																			
Sifted, spooned	1 cup	115	12	420	12	1	0.2	0	88	3	18	5.1	109	2	0	0.73	0.46	6.1	0
Cake or pastry flour, enriched, sifted, spooned	1 cup	96	12	350	7	1	0.1	0	76	2	16	4.2	91	2	0	0.58	0.38	5.1	0
Self-rising, enriched, unsifted, spooned	1 cup	125	12	440	12	1	0.2	0	93	3	331	5.5	113	1,349	0	0.80	0.50	6.6	0
Whole-wheat, from hard wheats, stirred	1 cup	120	12	400	16	2	0.4	0	85	15	49	5.2	444	4	0	0.66	0.14	5.2	0
Legumes, Nuts, and Seeds																			
Almonds, shelled:																			
Slivered, packed	1 cup	135	4	795	27	70	6.7	0	28	13	359	4.9	988	15	0	0.28	1.05	4.5	1
Beans, dry:																			
Cooked, drained:																			
Lima	1 cup	190	64	260	16	1	0.2	0	49	14	55	5.9	1,163	4	0	0.25	0.11	1.3	0
Canned, solids and liquid:																			
White with:																			
Pork and tomato sauce	1 cup	255	71	310	16	7	1	10	48	12	138	4.6	536	1,181	33	0.20	0.08	1.5	5
Red kidney	1 cup	255	76	230	15	1	Tr	0	42	5	74	4.6	673	968	1	0.13	0.10	1.5	0
Black-eyed peas, dry, cooked (with residual cooking liquid)	1 cup	250	80	190	13	1	0.2	0	35	12	43	3.3	573	20	3	0.40	0.10	1.0	0
Brazil nuts, shelled	1 oz.	28	3	185	4	19	4.6	0	4	2	50	1.0	170	1	Tr	0.28	0.03	0.5	Tr
Carob flour	1 cup	140	3	255	6	Tr	0.1	0	126	41	390	5.7	1,275	24	Tr	0.07	0.07	2.2	Tr
Cashew nuts, salted:																			
Dry roasted	1 cup	137	2	785	21	63	12.5	0	45	4	62	8.2	774	[41]877	0	0.27	0.27	1.9	0
Roasted in oil	1 cup	130	4	750	21	63	12.4	0	37	4	53	5.3	689	[42]814	0	0.55	0.23	2.3	0
Chestnuts, European (Italian), roasted, shelled	1 cup	143	40	350	5	3	0.6	0	76	9	41	1.3	847	3	3	0.35	0.25	1.9	37
Chick-peas, cooked, drained	1 cup	163	60	270	15	4	0.4	0	45	8	80	4.9	475	11	Tr	0.18	0.09	0.9	0
Coconut:																			
Dried, sweetened, shredded	1 cup	93	13	470	3	33	44.6	0	44	13	14	1.8	313	244	0	0.03	0.02	0.4	1
Filberts (hazelnuts), chopped	1 cup	115	5	725	15	72	5.3	0	18	9	216	3.8	512	3	8	0.58	0.13	1.3	1
	1 oz.	28	5	180	4	18	1.3	0	4	2	53	0.9	126	1	2	0.14	0.03	0.3	Tr
Lentils, dry, cooked	1 cup	200	72	215	16	1	0.1	0	38	5	50	4.2	498	26	4	0.14	0.12	1.2	0
Macadamia nuts, roasted in oil, salted	1 cup	134	2	960	10	103	15.3	0	17	12	60	2.4	441	[43]348	1	0.29	0.15	2.7	0
Mixed nuts, with peanuts, salted:																			
Dry roasted	1 oz.	28	2	170	5	15	3.1	0	7	3	20	1.0	169	[44]190	Tr	0.06	0.06	1.3	0
Roasted in oil	1 oz.	28	2	175	5	16	4.0	0	6	3	31	0.9	165	[44]185	1	0.14	0.06	1.4	Tr
Peanuts, roasted in oil, salted	1 cup	145	2	840	39	71	9.8	0	27	10	125	2.8	1,019	[45]626	0	0.42	0.15	21.5	0
Peanut butter	1 tbsp.	16	1	95	5	8	1.5	0	3	1	5	0.3	110	75	0	0.02	0.02	2.2	0
Peas, split, dry, cooked	1 cup	200	70	230	16	1	0.2	0	42	6	22	3.4	592	26	8	0.30	0.18	1.8	0
Pecans, halves	1 cup	108	5	720	8	73	5.8	0	20	5	39	2.3	423	1	14	0.92	0.14	1.0	2
	1 oz.	28	5	190	2	19	1.5	0	5	1	10	0.6	111	Tr	4	0.24	0.04	0.3	1
Pistachio nuts, dried, shelled	1 oz.	28	4	165	6	14	1.7	0	7	3	38	1.9	310	2	7	0.23	0.05	0.3	Tr

(A)	(B)		(C)	(D)	(E)	(F)	(G)	(H)	(I)	(J)	(K)	(L)	(M)	(N)	(O)	(P)	(Q)	(R)	(S)
Refried beans, canned	1 cup	290	72	295	18	3	1.0	0	51	14	141	5.1	1,141	1,228	0	0.14	0.16	1.4	17
Sesame seeds, dry, hulled	1 tbsp.	8	5	45	2	4	2.9	0	1	3	11	0.6	33	3	1	0.06	0.01	0.4	0
Soy products:																			
Tofu, piece 2-1/2 by 2-3/4 by 1 in.	1 piece	120	85	85	9	5	0.9	0	3	1	108	2.3	50	8	0	0.07	0.04	0.1	0
Sunflower seeds, dry, hulled	1 oz.	28	5	160	6	14	1.9	0	5	2	33	1.9	195	1	1	0.65	0.07	1.3	Tr
Walnuts:																			
Black, chopped	1 cup	125	4	760	30	71	4.5	0	15	6	73	3.8	655	1	37	0.27	0.14	0.9	Tr
English or Persian, pieces or chips	1 cup	120	4	770	17	74	6.7	0	22	5	113	2.9	602	12	15	0.46	0.18	1.3	4
Meat and Meat Products																			
Beef, cooked:[46]																			
Cuts braised, simmered, or pot roasted:																			
Relatively fat such as chuck blade:																			
Lean and fat, piece, 2-1/2 by 2-1/2 by 3/4 in.	3 oz.	85	43	325	22	26	11.6	87	0	0	11	2.5	163	53	Tr	0.06	0.19	2.0	0
Relatively lean, such as bottom round:																			
Lean and fat, piece, 4-1/8 by 2-1/4 by 1/2 in.	3 oz.	85	54	220	25	13	3.6	81	0	0	5	2.8	248	43	Tr	0.06	0.21	3.3	0
Ground beef, broiled, patty, 3 by 5/8 in.:																			
Lean	3 oz.	85	56	230	21	16	7.0	74	0	0	9	1.8	256	65	Tr	0.04	0.18	4.4	0
Regular	3 oz.	85	54	245	20	18	7.9	76	0	0	9	2.1	248	70	Tr	0.03	0.16	4.9	0
Liver, fried, slice, 6-1/2 by 2-3/8 by 3/8 in.[47]	3 oz.	85	56	185	23	7	3.0	410	7	0	9	5.3	309	90	[48]9,120	0.18	3.52	12.3	23
Roast, oven cooked, no liquid added:																			
Relatively fat, such as rib:																			
Lean and fat, 2 pieces, 4-1/8 by 2-1/4 by 1/4 in.	3 oz.	85	46	315	19	26	14.3	72	0	0	8	2.0	246	54	Tr	0.06	0.16	3.1	0
Relatively lean, such as eye of round:																			
Lean and fat, 2 pieces, 2-1/2 by 2-1/2 by 3/8 in.	3 oz.	85	57	205	23	12	6.2	62	0	0	5	1.6	308	50	Tr	0.07	0.14	3.0	0
Steak:																			
Sirloin, broiled:																			
Lean and fat, piece, 2-1/2 by 2-1/2 by 3/4 in.	3 oz.	85	53	240	23	15	8.7	77	0	0	9	2.6	306	53	Tr	0.10	0.23	3.3	0
Beef, canned, corned	3 oz.	85	59	185	22	10	7.0	80	0	0	17	3.7	51	802	Tr	0.02	0.20	2.9	0
Beef, dried, chipped	2.5 oz.	72	48	145	24	4	0.5	46	0	0	14	2.3	142	3,053	Tr	0.05	0.23	2.7	0
Lamb, cooked:																			
Chops, (3 per lb. with bone):																			
Lean and fat	2.2 oz.	63	44	220	20	15	3.5	77	0	0	16	1.5	195	46	Tr	0.04	0.16	4.4	0
Leg, roasted:																			
Lean and fat, 2 pieces, 4-1/8 by 2-1/4 by 1/4 in.	3 oz.	85	59	205	22	13	7.8	78	0	0	8	1.7	273	57	Tr	0.09	0.24	5.5	0
Rib, roasted:																			
Lean and fat, 3 pieces, 2-1/2 by 2-1/2 by 1/4 in.	3 oz.	85	47	315	18	26	14.5	77	0	0	19	1.4	224	60	Tr	0.08	0.18	5.5	0
Pork, cured, cooked:																			
Bacon:																			
Regular	3 medium slices	19	13	110	6	9	3.3	16	Tr	0	2	0.3	92	303	0	0.13	0.05	1.4	6
Canadian-style	2 slices	46	62	85	11	4	1.3	27	1	0	5	0.4	179	711	0	0.38	0.09	3.2	10
Ham, light cure, roasted:																			
Lean and fat, 2 pieces, 4-1/8 by 2-1/4 by 1/4 in.	3 oz.	85	58	205	18	14	6.8	53	0	0	6	0.7	243	1,009	0	0.51	0.19	3.8	0
Ham, canned, roasted, 2 pieces, 4-1/8 by 2-1/4 by 1/4 in.	3 oz.	85	67	140	18	7	3.2	35	Tr	0	6	0.9	298	908	0	0.82	0.21	4.3	[49]19
Luncheon meat:																			
Canned, spiced or unspiced, slice, 3 by 2 by 1/2 in.	2 slices	42	52	140	5	13	4.6	26	1	0	3	0.3	90	541	0	0.15	0.08	1.3	Tr
Cooked ham (8 slices per 8 oz. pkg.):																			
Regular	2 slices	57	65	105	10	6	1.9	32	2	0	4	0.6	189	751	0	0.49	0.14	3.0	[49]16
Extra lean	2 slices	57	71	75	11	3	0.9	27	1	0	4	0.4	200	815	0	0.53	0.13	2.8	[49]15
Pork, fresh, cooked:																			
Chop, loin (cut 3 per lb. with bone):																			
Broiled:																			
Lean and fat	3.1 oz.	87	50	275	24	19	4.6	84	0	0	3	0.7	312	61	3	0.87	0.24	4.3	Tr
Ham (leg), roasted:																			
Lean and fat, piece, 2-1/2 by 2-1/2 by 3/4 in.	3 oz	85	53	250	21	18	0.7	79	0	0	5	0.9	280	50	2	0.54	0.27	3.9	Tr
Rib, roasted:																			
Lean and fat, piece, 2-1/2 by 3/4 in.	3 oz.	85	51	270	21	20	6.7	69	0	0	9	0.8	313	37	3	0.50	0.24	4.2	Tr
Shoulder cut, braised:																			
Lean and fat, 3 pieces, 2-1/2 by 2-1/2 by 1/4 in.	3 oz.	85	47	295	23	22	9.6	93	0	0	6	1.4	286	75	3	0.46	0.26	4.4	Tr
Sausages																			
Bologna, slice (8 per 8 oz. pkg.)	2 slices	57	54	180	7	16	3.2	31	2	0	7	0.9	103	581	0	0.10	0.08	1.5	[49]12
Braunschweiger, slice (6 per 6 oz. pkg.)	2 slices	57	48	205	8	18	3.1	89	2	0	5	5.3	113	652	2,405	0.14	0.87	4.8	[49]6

Nutritive Values of Foods – Continued

(Tr indicates nutrient present in trace amount.)

Item No. (A) Foods, approximate measures, units, and weight (weight of edible portion only)	(B)		Water (C)	Food energy (D)	Protein (E)	Fat (F)	Saturated fat (G)	Cholesterol (H)	Carbohydrate (I)	Dietary fiber (J)	Calcium (K)	Iron (L)	Potassium (M)	Sodium (N)	Vitamin A (O)	Thiamin (P)	Riboflavin (Q)	Niacin (R)	Vitamin C (S)
		Grams	Percent	Calories	Grams	Grams	Grams	Milligrams	Grams	Grams	Milligrams	Milligrams	Milligrams	Milligrams	Micrograms	Milligrams	Milligrams	Milligrams	Milligrams
Brown and serve (10-11 per 8 oz. pkg.), browned	1 link	13	45	50	2	5	1.7	9	Tr	0	1	0.1	25	105	0	0.05	0.02	0.4	0
Frankfurter (10 per 1 lb. pkg.), cooked (reheated)	1 frankfurter	45	54	145	5	13	4.9	23	1	0	5	0.5	75	504	0	0.09	0.05	1.2	[49]12
Salami:																			
Dry type, slice (12 per 4 oz. pkg.)	2 slices	20	35	85	5	7	2.5	16	1	0	2	0.3	76	372	0	0.12	0.06	1.0	[49]5
Sandwich spread (pork, beef)	1 tbsp.	15	60	35	1	3	0.9	6	2	Tr	2	0.1	17	152	1	0.03	0.02	0.3	0
Veal, medium fat, cooked, bone removed:																			
Cutlet, 4-1/8 by 2-1/4 by 1/2 in., braised or broiled	3 oz.	85	60	185	23	9	7.6	109	0	0	9	0.8	258	56	Tr	0.06	0.21	4.6	0
Rib, 2 pieces, 4-1/8 by 2-1/4 by 1/4 in., roasted	3 oz.	85	55	230	23	14	6.1	109	0	0	10	0.7	259	57	Tr	0.11	0.26	6.6	0
Mixed Dishes and Fast Foods																			
Mixed dishes:																			
Beef and vegetable stew, from home recipe	1 cup	245	82	220	16	11	4.9	71	15	2	29	2.9	613	292	568	0.15	0.17	4.7	17
Beef potpie, from home recipe, baked, piece, 1/3 of 9 in. diam. pie[51]	1 piece	210	55	515	21	30	8.4	42	39	3	29	3.8	334	596	517	0.29	0.29	4.8	6
Chicken a la king, cooked, from home recipe	1 cup	245	68	470	27	34	12.7	221	12	1	127	2.5	404	760	272	0.10	0.42	5.4	12
Chicken chow mein:																			
Canned	1 cup	250	89	95	7	Tr	0.0	8	18	2	45	1.3	418	725	28	0.05	0.10	1.0	13
Chili con carne with beans, canned	1 cup	255	72	340	19	16	3.4	28	31	4	82	4.3	594	1,354	15	0.08	0.18	3.3	8
Chop suey with beef and pork, from home recipe	1 cup	250	75	300	26	17	5.7	68	13	4	60	4.8	425	1,053	60	0.28	0.38	5.0	33
Macaroni (enriched) and cheese:																			
Canned[52]	1 cup	240	80	230	9	10	4.2	24	26	1	199	1.0	139	730	72	0.12	0.24	1.0	Tr
From home recipe[38]	1 cup	200	58	430	17	22	8.9	44	40	1	362	1.8	240	1,086	232	0.20	0.40	1.8	1
Spaghetti (enriched) in tomato sauce with cheese:																			
Canned	1 cup	250	80	190	6	2	0.0	3	39	2	40	2.8	303	955	120	0.35	0.28	4.5	10
From home recipe	1 cup	250	77	260	9	9	2.0	8	37	2	80	2.3	408	955	140	0.25	0.18	2.3	13
Spaghetti (enriched) with meatballs and tomato sauce:																			
Canned	1 cup	250	78	260	12	10	2.1	23	29	6	53	3.3	245	1,220	100	0.15	0.18	2.3	5
From home recipe	1 cup	248	70	330	19	12	3.3	89	39	8	124	3.7	665	1,009	159	0.25	0.30	4.0	22
Fast food entrees:																			
Cheeseburger:																			
Regular	1 sandwich	112	46	300	15	15	6.7	44	28	0	135	2.3	219	672	65	0.26	0.24	3.7	1
4 oz. patty	1 sandwich	194	46	525	30	31	10.2	104	40	0	236	4.5	407	1,224	128	0.33	0.48	7.4	3
Chicken, fried. See Poultry and Poultry Products.																			
Enchilada	1 enchilada	230	72	235	20	16	15.0	19	24	0	322	11.0	2,180	4,451	352	0.18	0.26	Tr	Tr
English muffin, egg, cheese, and bacon	1 sandwich	138	49	360	18	18	8.6	213	31	1	197	3.1	201	832	160	0.46	0.50	3.7	1
Fish sandwich:																			
Regular, with cheese	1 sandwich	140	43	420	16	23	6.2	56	39	Tr	132	1.8	274	667	25	0.32	0.26	3.3	2
Large, without cheese	1 sandwich	170	48	470	18	27	5.6	91	41	Tr	61	2.2	375	621	15	0.35	0.23	3.5	1
Hamburger:																			
Regular	1 sandwich	98	46	245	12	11	3.2	32	28	0	56	2.2	202	463	14	0.23	0.24	3.8	1
4 oz. patty	1 sandwich	174	50	445	25	21	9.7	71	38	0	75	4.8	404	763	28	0.38	0.38	7.8	1
Pizza, cheese, 1/8 of 15 in. diam. pizza[51]	1 slice	120	46	290	15	9	2.9	56	39	2	220	1.6	230	699	106	0.34	0.29	4.2	2
Taco	1 taco	81	55	195	9	11	4.6	21	15	1	109	1.2	263	456	57	0.09	0.07	1.4	1
Poultry and Poultry Products																			
Chicken:																			
Fried, flesh, with skin:[53]																			
Batter dipped:																			
Breast, 1/2 breast (5.6 oz. with bones)	4.9 oz.	140	52	365	35	18	4.9	119	13	Tr	28	1.8	281	385	28	0.16	0.20	14.7	0

(A)	(B)		(C)	(D)	(E)	(F)	(G)	(H)	(I)	(J)	(K)	(L)	(M)	(N)	(O)	(P)	(Q)	(R)	(S)
Drumstick (3.4 oz. with bones)	2.5 oz.	72	53	195	16	11	3.0	62	6	Tr	12	1.0	134	194	19	0.08	0.15	3.7	0
Roasted, flesh only:																			
Breast, 1/2 breast (4.2 oz. with bones and skin)	3.0 oz.	86	65	140	27	3	0.9	73	0	0	13	0.9	220	64	5	0.06	0.10	11.8	0
Drumstick, (2.9 oz. with bones and skin)	1.6 oz.	44	67	75	12	2	1.4	41	0	0	5	0.6	108	42	8	0.03	0.10	2.7	0
Chicken liver, cooked	1 liver	20	68	30	5	1	1.6	126	Tr	0	3	1.7	28	10	983	0.03	0.35	0.9	3
Duck, roasted, flesh only	1/2 duck	221	64	445	52	25	9.2	197	0	0	27	6.0	557	144	51	0.57	1.04	11.3	0
Turkey, roasted, flesh only:																			
Dark meat, piece, 2-1/2 by 1-5/8 by 1/4 in.	4 pieces	85	63	160	24	6	4.0	72	0	0	27	2.0	246	67	0	0.05	0.21	3.1	0
Light meat, piece, 4 by 2 by 1/4 in.	2 pieces	85	66	135	25	3	2.7	59	0	0	16	1.1	259	54	0	0.05	0.11	5.8	0
Poultry food products:																			
Chicken:																			
Canned, boneless	5 oz.	142	69	235	31	11	3.1	88	0	0	20	2.2	196	714	48	0.02	0.18	9.0	3
Frankfurter (10 per 1-lb. pkg.)	1 frankfurter	45	58	115	6	9	2.5	45	3	0	43	0.9	38	616	17	0.03	0.05	1.4	0
Roll, light (6 slices per 6 oz. pkg.)	2 slices	57	69	90	11	4	1.1	28	1	0	24	0.6	129	331	14	0.04	0.07	3.0	0
Turkey:																			
Gravy and turkey, frozen	5 oz. package	142	85	95	8	4	1.0	26	7	Tr	20	1.3	87	787	18	0.03	0.18	2.6	0
Loaf, breast meat (8 slices per 6 oz. pkg.)	2 slices	42	72	45	10	1	0.5	17	0	0	3	0.2	118	608	0	0.02	0.05	3.5	[54]0
Patties, breaded, battered, fried (2.25 oz.)	1 patty	64	50	180	9	12	2.7	40	10	Tr	9	1.4	176	512	7	0.06	0.12	1.5	0
Roast, boneless, frozen, seasoned, light and dark meat, cooked	3 oz.	85	68	130	18	5	2.2	45	3	0	4	1.4	253	578	0	0.04	0.14	5.3	0
Soups, Sauces, and Gravies																			
Soups:																			
Canned, condensed:																			
Prepared with equal volume of milk:																			
Clam chowder, New England	1 cup	248	85	165	9	7	2.9	22	17	1	186	1.5	300	992	40	0.07	0.24	1.0	3
Cream of chicken	1 cup	248	85	190	7	11	4.6	27	15	Tr	181	0.7	273	1,047	94	0.07	0.26	0.9	1
Cream of mushroom	1 cup	248	85	205	6	14	5.1	20	15	1	179	0.6	270	1,076	37	0.08	0.28	0.9	2
Tomato	1 cup	248	85	160	6	6	2.9	17	22	1	159	1.8	449	932	109	0.13	0.25	1.5	68
Prepared with equal volume of water:																			
Bean with bacon	1 cup	253	84	170	8	6	1.5	3	23	9	81	2.0	402	951	89	0.09	0.03	0.6	2
Beef broth, bouillon, consomm	1 cup	240	98	15	3	1	0.3	Tr	Tr	0	14	0.4	130	782	0	Tr	0.05	1.9	0
Beef noodle	1 cup	244	92	85	5	3	1.1	5	9	1	15	1.1	100	952	63	0.07	0.06	1.1	Tr
Chicken noodle	1 cup	241	92	75	4	2	0.7	7	9	1	17	0.8	55	1,106	71	0.05	0.06	1.4	Tr
Chicken rice	1 cup	241	94	60	4	2	0.5	7	7	1	17	0.7	101	815	66	0.02	0.02	1.1	Tr
Clam chowder, Manhattan	1 cup	244	90	80	4	2	0.4	2	12	1	34	1.9	261	1,808	92	0.06	0.05	1.3	3
Pea, green	1 cup	250	83	165	9	3	1.8	0	27	5	28	2.0	190	988	20	0.11	0.07	1.2	2
Vegetable beef	1 cup	244	92	80	6	2	0.9	5	10	Tr	17	1.1	173	956	189	0.04	0.05	1.0	2
Vegetarian	1 cup	241	92	70	2	2	0.3	0	12	Tr	22	1.1	210	822	301	0.05	0.05	0.9	1
Dehydrated:																			
Prepared with water:																			
Chicken noodle	1 pkt. (6 fl. oz.)	188	94	40	2	1	0.3	2	6	Tr	24	0.4	23	957	5	0.05	0.04	0.7	Tr
Tomato vegetable	1 pkt. (6 fl. oz.)	189	94	40	1	1	0.4	0	8	1	6	0.5	78	856	14	0.04	0.03	0.6	5
Sauces:																			
From dry mix:																			
Cheese, prepared with milk	1 cup	279	77	305	16	17	9.3	53	23	1	569	0.3	552	1,565	117	0.15	0.56	0.3	2
From home recipe:																			
White sauce, medium[55]	1 cup	250	73	395	10	30	6.4	32	24	Tr	292	0.9	381	888	340	0.15	0.43	0.8	2
Ready to serve:																			
Barbecue	1 tbsp.	16	81	10	Tr	Tr	Tr	0	2	Tr	3	0.1	28	130	14	Tr	Tr	0.1	1
Soy	1 tbsp.	18	68	10	2	0	Tr	0	2	0	3	0.5	64	1,029	0	0.01	0.02	0.6	0
Gravies:																			
Canned:																			
Beef	1 cup	233	87	125	9	5	2.7	7	11	1	14	1.6	189	117	0	0.07	0.08	1.5	0
Chicken	1 cup	238	85	190	5	14	3.4	5	13	Tr	48	1.1	259	1,373	264	0.04	0.10	1.1	0
Mushroom	1 cup	238	89	120	3	6	0.8	0	13	Tr	17	1.6	252	1,357	0	0.08	0.15	1.6	0
From dry mix:																			
Brown	1 cup	261	91	80	3	2	0.8	2	14	Tr	66	0.2	61	1,147	0	0.04	0.09	0.9	0
Chicken	1 cup	260	91	85	3	2	0.5	3	14	Tr	39	0.3	62	1,134	0	0.05	0.15	0.8	3
Sugars and Sweets																			
Candy:																			
Caramels, plain or chocolate	1 oz.	28	8	115	1	3	3	1.9	22	Tr	42	0.4	54	64	Tr	0.01	0.05	0.1	Tr

Nutritive Values of Foods – Continued

(Tr indicates nutrient present in trace amount.)

Item No. (A)	Foods, approximate measures, units, and weight (weight of edible portion only) (B)		Water (C)	Food energy (D)	Protein (E)	Fat (F)	Saturated fat (G)	Cholesterol (H)	Carbohydrate (I)	Dietary fiber (J)	Calcium (K)	Iron (L)	Potassium (M)	Sodium (N)	Vitamin A (O)	Thiamin (P)	Riboflavin (Q)	Niacin (R)	Vitamin C (S)
			Nutrients in Indicated Quantity																
		Grams	Percent	Calories	Grams	Grams	Grams	Milligrams	Grams	Grams	Milligrams	Milligrams	Milligrams	Milligrams	Micrograms	Milligrams	Milligrams	Milligrams	Milligrams
Chocolate:																			
Milk, plain	1 oz.	28	1	145	2	9	5.2	6	16	1	50	0.4	96	23	10	0.02	0.10	0.1	Tr
Milk, with almonds	1 oz.	28	2	150	3	10	4.8	5	15	2	65	0.5	125	23	8	0.02	0.12	0.2	Tr
Milk, with peanuts	1 oz.	28	1	155	4	11	3.4	5	13	2	49	0.4	138	19	8	0.07	0.07	1.4	Tr
Milk, with rice cereal	1 oz.	28	2	140	2	7	4.5	6	18	1	48	0.2	100	46	8	0.01	0.08	0.1	Tr
Semisweet, small pieces (60 per oz.)	1 cup or 6 oz.	170	1	860	7	61	29.8	0	97	10	51	5.8	593	24	3	0.10	0.14	0.9	Tr
Sweet (dark)	1 oz.	28	1	150	1	10	5.9	0	16	2	7	0.6	86	5	1	0.01	0.04	0.1	Tr
Fudge, chocolate, plain	1 oz.	28	8	115	1	3	1.5	1	21	Tr	22	0.3	42	54	Tr	0.01	0.03	0.1	Tr
Gum drops	1 oz.	28	12	100	Tr	Tr	0.0	0	25	0	2	0.1	1	10	0	0.00	Tr	Tr	0
Hard	1 oz.	28	1	110	0	0	0.0	0	28	0	Tr	0.1	1	7	0	0.10	0.00	0.0	0
Jelly beans	1 oz.	28	6	105	Tr	Tr	0.0	0	26	0	1	0.3	11	7	0	0.00	Tr	Tr	0
Marshmallows	1 oz.	28	17	90	1	0	0.0	0	23	Tr	1	0.5	2	25	0	0.00	Tr	Tr	0
Custard, baked	1 cup	265	77	305	14	15	6.2	278	29	0	297	1.1	387	209	146	0.11	0.50	0.3	1
Gelatin dessert prepared with gelatin dessert powder and water	1/2 cup	120	84	70	2	0	0.0	0	17	0	2	Tr	Tr	55	0	0.00	0.00	0.0	0
Honey, strained or extracted	1 cup	339	17	1,030	1	0	0.0	0	279	Tr	17	1.7	173	17	0	0.02	0.14	1.0	3
	1 tbsp.	21	17	65	Tr	0	0.0	0	17	Tr	1	0.1	11	1	0	Tr	0.01	0.1	Tr
Jams and preserves	1 tbsp.	20	29	55	Tr	Tr	0.0	0	14	Tr	4	0.2	18	2	Tr	Tr	0.01	Tr	Tr
Jellies	1 tbsp.	18	28	50	Tr	Tr	Tr	0	13	Tr	2	0.1	16	5	Tr	Tr	0.01	Tr	1
Popsicle, 3 fl. oz. size	1 popsicle	95	80	70	0	0	0.0	0	18	0	0	Tr	4	11	0	0.00	0.00	0.0	0
Puddings:																			
Canned:																			
Chocolate	5 oz. can	142	68	205	3	11	1.0	1	30	1	74	1.2	254	285	31	0.04	0.17	0.6	Tr
Vanilla	5 oz. can	142	69	220	2	10	0.8	1	33	Tr	79	0.2	155	305	Tr	0.03	0.12	0.6	Tr
Dry mix, prepared with whole milk:																			
Chocolate:																			
Instant	1/2 cup	130	71	155	4	4	2.4	14	27	2	130	0.3	176	440	33	0.04	0.18	0.1	1
Rice	1/2 cup	132	73	155	4	4	2.3	15	27	1	133	0.5	165	140	33	0.10	0.18	0.6	1
Vanilla:																			
Instant	1/2 cup	130	73	150	4	4	2.3	15	27	Tr	129	0.1	164	375	33	0.04	0.17	0.1	1
Sugars:																			
Brown, pressed down	1 cup	220	2	820	0	0	0.0	0	212	0	3	0.1	7	5	0	0.00	0.00	0.0	0
White:																			
Granulated	1 cup	200	1	770	0	0	0.0	0	199	0	Tr	Tr	Tr	Tr	0	0.00	0.00	0.0	0
	1 tbsp.	12	1	45	0	0	0.0	0	12	0	Tr	Tr	Tr	Tr	0	0.00	0.00	0.0	0
Powdered, sifted, spooned into cup	1 cup	100	1	385	0	0	0.0	0	99	0	6	0.8	85	36	Tr	Tr	0.02	0.1	0
Syrups:																			
Chocolate-flavored syrup or topping:																			
Thin type	2 tbsp.	38	37	85	1	Tr	0.2	0	21	1	38	0.5	82	42	13	0.02	0.08	0.1	0
Fudge type	2 tbsp.	38	25	125	2	5	2.2	0	22	Tr	274	10.1	1,171	38	0	0.04	0.08	0.8	0
Table syrup (corn and maple)	2 tbsp.	42	25	122	0	0	0.0	0	212	0	187	4.8	757	97	0	0.02	0.07	0.2	0
Vegetables and Vegetable Products																			
Alfalfa seeds, sprouted, raw	1 cup	33	91	10	1	Tr	Tr	0	1	1	11	0.3	26	2	5	0.03	0.04	0.2	3
Asparagus, green:																			
Cooked, drained:																			
From raw:																			
Cuts and tips	1 cup	180	92	45	5	1	0.2	0	8	4	43	1.2	558	7	149	0.18	0.22	1.9	49
From frozen:																			
Cuts and tips	1 cup	180	91	50	5	1	0.2	0	9	4	41	1.2	392	7	147	0.12	0.19	1.9	44
Bamboo shoots, canned, drained	1 cup	131	94	25	2	1	0.1	0	4	3	10	0.4	105	9	1	0.03	0.03	0.2	1

(A)	(B)		(C)	(D)	(E)	(F)	(G)	(H)	(I)	(J)	(K)	(L)	(M)	(N)	(O)	(P)	(Q)	(R)	(S)
Beans:																			
Lima, immature seeds, frozen, cooked, drained:																			
Thick-seeded types (Ford-hooks)	1 cup	170	74	170	10	1	0.2	0	32	12	37	2.3	694	90	32	0.13	0.10	1.8	22
Snap:																			
Cooked, drained:																			
From raw (cut and French style)	1 cup	125	89	45	2	Tr	Tr	0	10	4	58	1.6	374	4	[57]83	0.09	0.12	0.8	12
From frozen (cut)	1 cup	135	92	35	2	Tr	Tr	0	8	4	61	1.1	151	18	[58]71	0.06	0.10	0.6	11
Canned, drained solids (cut)	1 cup	135	93	25	2	Tr	Tr	0	6	2	35	1.2	147	[59]339	[60]47	0.02	0.08	0.3	6
Beets:																			
Canned, drained solids, diced or sliced	1 cup	170	91	55	2	Tr	Tr	0	12	4	26	3.1	252	[61]466	2	0.02	0.07	0.3	7
Beet greens, leaves and stems, cooked, drained	1 cup	144	89	40	4	Tr	Tr	0	8	4	164	2.7	1,309	347	734	0.17	0.42	0.7	36
Broccoli:																			
Cooked, drained:																			
From raw:																			
Spears, cut into 1/2 in. pieces	1 cup	155	90	45	5	Tr	Tr	0	9	2	177	1.8	253	17	218	0.13	0.32	1.2	97
From frozen:																			
Chopped	1 cup	185	91	50	6	Tr	Tr	0	10	5	94	1.1	333	44	350	0.10	0.15	0.8	74
Brussels sprouts, cooked, drained:																			
From frozen	1 cup	155	87	65	6	1	0.2	0	13	6	37	1.1	504	36	91	0.16	0.18	0.8	71
Cabbage, common varieties:																			
Raw, coarsely shredded or sliced	1 cup	70	93	15	1	Tr	Tr	0	4	1	33	0.4	172	13	9	0.04	0.02	0.2	33
Cooked, drained	1 cup	150	94	30	1	Tr	0.1	0	7	4	50	0.6	308	29	13	0.09	0.08	0.3	36
Cabbage, red, raw, coarsely shredded or sliced	1 cup	70	92	20	1	Tr	Tr	0	4	2	36	0.3	144	8	3	0.04	0.02	0.2	40
Carrots:																			
Raw, without crowns and tips, scraped:																			
Whole, 7-1/2 by 1-1/8 in., or strips, 2-1/2 to 3 in. long	1 carrot or 18 strips	72	88	30	1	Tr	Tr	0	7	2	19	0.4	233	25	2,025	0.07	0.04	0.7	7
Cooked, sliced, drained:																			
From frozen	1 cup	146	90	55	2	Tr	Tr	0	12	6	41	0.7	231	86	2,585	0.04	0.05	0.6	4
Cauliflower:																			
Raw, (flowerets)	1 cup	100	92	25	2	Tr	Tr	0	5	2	29	0.6	355	15	2	0.08	0.06	0.6	72
Cooked, drained:																			
From frozen (flowerets)	1 cup	180	94	35	3	Tr	Tr	0	7	4	31	0.7	250	32	4	0.07	0.10	0.6	56
Celery, pascal type, raw:																			
Stalk, large outer, 8 by 1-1/2 in. (at root end)	1 stalk	40	95	5	Tr	Tr	Tr	0	1	1	14	0.2	114	35	5	0.01	0.01	0.1	3
Collards, cooked, drained:																			
From frozen (chopped)	1 cup	170	88	60	5	1	0.2	0	12	6	357	1.9	427	85	1,017	0.08	0.20	1.1	45
Corn, sweet:																			
Cooked, drained:																			
From raw, ear 5 by 1-3/4 in.	1 ear	77	70	85	3	1	0.2	0	19	2	2	0.5	192	13	[63]17	0.17	0.06	1.2	5
From frozen:																			
Ear, trimmed to about 3-1/2 in. long	1 ear	63	73	60	2	Tr	0.1	0	14	2	2	0.4	158	3	[63]13	0.11	0.04	1.0	3
Kernels	1 cup	165	76	135	5	Tr	Tr	0	34	4	3	0.5	229	8	[63]41	0.11	0.12	2.1	4
Canned:																			
Cream style	1 cup	256	79	185	4	1	0.2	0	46	4	8	1.0	343	[64]730	[63]25	0.06	0.14	2.5	12
Whole kernel, vacuum pack	1 cup	210	77	165	5	1	0.2	0	41	4	11	0.9	391	[65]571	[63]51	0.09	0.15	2.5	17
Cucumber, with peel, slices, 1/8 in. thick (large, 2-1/8 in. diam.; small, 1-3/4 in. diam.)	6 large or 8 small slices	28	96	5	Tr	Tr	Tr	0	1	Tr	4	0.1	42	1	1	0.01	0.01	0.1	1
Eggplant, cooked, steamed	1 cup	96	92	25	1	Tr	0.1	0	6	4	6	0.3	238	3	6	0.07	0.02	0.6	1
Kale, cooked, drained:																			
From frozen, chopped	1 cup	130	91	40	4	1	Tr	0	7	2	179	1.2	417	20	826	0.06	0.15	0.9	33
Lettuce, raw:																			
Butterhead, as Boston types:																			
Head, 5 in. diam.	1 head	163	96	20	2	Tr	Tr	0	4	4	52	0.5	419	8	158	0.10	0.10	0.5	13
Crisphead, as iceberg:																			
Head, 6 in. diam.	1 head	539	96	70	5	1	Tr	0	11	4	102	2.7	852	49	178	0.25	0.16	1.0	21
Wedge, 1/4 of head	1 wedge	135	96	20	1	Tr	Tr	0	3	1	26	0.7	213	12	45	0.06	0.04	0.3	5
Pieces, chopped or shredded	1 cup	55	96	5	1	Tr	Tr	0	1	1	10	0.3	87	5	18	0.03	0.02	0.1	2
Mushrooms:																			
Raw, sliced or chopped	1 cup	70	92	20	1	Tr	Tr	0	3	Tr	4	0.9	259	3	0	0.07	0.31	2.9	2
Canned, drained solids	1 cup	156	91	35	3	Tr	Tr	0	8	4	17	1.2	201	663	0	0.13	0.03	2.5	0

Nutritive Values of Foods – Continued

(Tr indicates nutrient present in trace amount.)

Item No. (A)	Foods, approximate measures, units, and weight (weight of edible portion only) (B)		Water (C)	Food energy (D)	Protein (E)	Fat (F)	Saturated fat (G)	Cholesterol (H)	Carbohydrate (I)	Dietary fiber (J)	Calcium (K)	Iron (L)	Potassium (M)	Sodium (N)	Vitamin A (O)	Thiamin (P)	Riboflavin (Q)	Niacin (R)	Vitamin C (S)
		Grams	Percent	Calories	Grams	Grams	Grams	Milligrams	Grams	Grams	Milligrams	Milligrams	Milligrams	Milligrams	Micrograms	Milligrams	Milligrams	Milligrams	Milligrams
Onions:																			
Raw:																			
Chopped	1 cup	160	91	55	2	Tr	Tr	0	12	3	40	0.6	248	3	0	0.10	0.02	0.2	13
Cooked (whole or sliced), drained	1 cup	210	92	60	2	Tr	Tr	0	13	2	57	0.4	319	17	0	0.09	0.02	0.2	12
Onion rings, breaded, par-fried, frozen, prepared	2 rings	20	29	80	1	5	1.7	0	8	Tr	6	0.3	26	75	5	0.06	0.03	0.7	Tr
Parsley:																			
Freeze-dried	1 tbsp.	0.4	2	Tr	Tr	Tr	Tr	0	Tr	1	1	0.2	25	2	25	Tr	0.01	Tr	1
Peas, edible pod, cooked, drained	1 cup	160	89	65	5	Tr	0.1	0	11	4	67	3.2	384	6	21	0.20	0.12	0.09	77
Peas, green:																			
Canned, drained solids	1 cup	170	82	115	8	1	0.2	0	21	6	34	1.6	294	[66]372	131	0.21	0.13	1.2	16
Frozen, cooked, drained	1 cup	160	80	125	8	Tr	Tr	0	23	8	38	2.5	269	139	107	0.45	0.16	2.4	16
Peppers:																			
Hot chili, raw	1 pepper	45	88	20	1	Tr	Tr	0	4	1	8	0.5	153	3	[67]484	0.04	0.04	0.4	109
Sweet (about 5 per lb., whole), stem and seeds removed:																			
Raw	1 pepper	74	93	20	1	Tr	Tr	0	4	1	4	0.9	144	2	[68]39	0.06	0.04	0.4	[69]95
Potatoes, cooked:																			
Baked (about 2 per lb., raw):																			
With skin	1 potato	202	71	220	5	Tr	0.1	0	51	5	20	2.7	844	16	0	0.22	0.07	3.3	26
Flesh only	1 potato	156	75	145	3	Tr	Tr	0	34	2	8	0.5	610	8	0	0.16	0.03	2.2	20
Boiled (about 3 per lb., raw):																			
Peeled after boiling	1 potato	136	77	120	3	Tr	Tr	0	27	2	7	0.4	515	5	0	0.14	0.03	2.0	18
French fried, strip, 2 to 3-1/2 in. long, frozen:																			
Oven heated	10 strips	50	53	110	2	4	3.8	0	17	1	5	0.7	229	16	0	0.06	0.02	1.2	5
Fried in vegetable oil	10 strips	50	38	160	2	8	2.5	0	20	2	10	0.4	366	108	0	0.09	0.01	1.6	5
Potato products, prepared:																			
Au gratin:																			
From dry mix	1 cup	245	79	230	6	10	6.4	12	31	4	203	0.8	537	1,076	76	0.05	0.20	2.3	8
Hashed brown, from frozen	1 cup	156	56	340	5	18	7.0	0	44	3	23	2.4	680	53	0	0.17	0.03	3.8	10
Mashed:																			
From home recipe:																			
Milk and margarine added	1 cup	210	76	225	4	9	2.2	4	35	4	55	0.5	607	620	42	0.18	0.08	2.3	13
Potato chips	10 chips	20	3	105	1	7	3.1	0	10	1	5	0.2	260	94	0	0.03	Tr	0.8	8
Pumpkin:																			
Canned	1 cup	245	90	85	3	1	0.4	0	20	6	64	3.4	505	12	5,404	0.06	0.13	0.9	10
Radishes, raw, stem ends, rootlets cut off	4 radishes	18	95	5	Tr	Tr	Tr	0	1	Tr	4	0.1	42	4	Tr	Tr	0.01	0.1	4
Spinach:																			
Raw, chopped	1 cup	55	92	10	2	Tr	Tr	0	2	2	54	1.5	307	43	369	0.04	0.10	0.4	15
Cooked, drained:																			
From frozen (leaf)	1 cup	190	90	55	6	Tr	Tr	0	10	4	277	2.9	566	163	1,479	0.11	0.32	0.8	23
Canned, drained solids	1 cup	214	92	50	6	1	0.2	0	7	6	272	4.9	740	[72]683	1,878	0.03	0.30	0.8	31
Squash, cooked:																			
Summer (all varieties), sliced, drained	1 cup	180	94	35	2	1	0.2	0	8	2	49	0.6	346	2	52	0.08	0.07	0.9	10
Winter (all varieties), baked, cubes	1 cup	205	89	80	2	1	0.3	0	18	6	29	0.7	896	2	729	0.17	0.05	1.4	20
Sweet potatoes:																			
Cooked (raw, 5 by 2 in.; about 2-1/2 per lb.):																			
Baked in skin, peeled	1 potato	114	73	115	2	Tr	Tr	0	28	4	32	0.5	397	11	2,488	0.08	0.14	0.7	28
Candied, 2-1/2 by 2 in. piece	1 piece	105	67	145	1	3	1.4	8	29	2	27	1.2	198	74	440	0.02	0.04	0.4	7
Canned:																			
Vacuum pack, piece 2-3/4 by 1 in.	1 piece	40	76	35	1	Tr	Tr	0	8	1	9	0.4	125	21	319	0.01	0.02	0.3	11
Tomatoes:																			
Raw, 2-3/5 in. diam. (3 per 12 oz. pkg.)	1 tomato	123	94	25	1	Tr	0.1	0	5	1	9	0.6	255	10	139	0.07	0.06	0.7	22
Canned, solids and liquid	1 cup	240	94	50	2	1	0.1	0	10	2	62	1.5	530	[73]391	145	0.11	0.07	1.8	36

(A)	(B)		(C)	(D)	(E)	(F)	(G)	(H)	(I)	(J)	(K)	(L)	(M)	(N)	(O)	(P)	(Q)	(R)	(S)
Tomato juice, canned	1 cup	244	94	40	2	Tr	Tr	0	10	1	22	1.4	537	[74]881	136	0.11	0.08	1.6	45
Tomato products, canned:																			
Paste	1 cup	262	74	220	10	2	0.3	0	49	11	92	7.8	2,442	[75]170	647	0.41	0.50	8.4	111
Puree	1 cup	250	87	105	4	Tr	Tr	0	25	6	38	2.3	1,050	[76]50	340	0.18	0.14	4.3	88
Sauce	1 cup	245	89	75	3	Tr	Tr	0	18	3	34	1.9	909	[77]1,482	240	0.16	0.14	2.8	32
Turnip greens, cooked, drained:																			
From frozen (chopped)	1 cup	164	90	50	5	1	0.2	0	8	7	249	3.2	367	25	1,308	0.09	0.12	0.8	36
Vegetable juice cocktail, canned	1 cup	242	94	45	2	Tr	Tr	0	11	1	27	1.0	467	883	283	0.10	0.07	1.8	67
Vegetables, mixed:																			
Canned, drained solids	1 cup	163	87	75	4	Tr	Tr	0	15	3	44	1.7	474	243	1,899	0.08	0.08	0.9	8
Frozen, cooked, drained	1 cup	182	83	105	5	Tr	Tr	0	24	5	46	1.5	308	64	778	0.13	0.22	1.5	6
Water chestnuts, canned	1 cup	140	86	70	1	Tr	Tr	0	17	1	6	1.2	165	11	1	0.02	0.03	0.5	2

[1]Value not determined.
[2]Mineral content varies depending on water source.
[3]Blend of aspartame and saccharin; if only sodium saccharin is used, sodium is 75 mg; if only aspartame is used, sodium is 23 mg.
[4]With added ascorbic acid.
[5]Vitamin A value is largely from beta-carotene used for coloring.
[6]Yields 1 qt. of fluid milk when reconstituted according to package directions.
[7]With added vitamin A.
[8]Carbohydrate content varies widely because of amount of sugar added and amount and solids content of added flavoring. Consult the label if more precise values for carbohydrate and calories are needed.
[9]For salted butter; unsalted butter contains 12 mg sodium per stick, 2 mg per tbsp., or 1 mg per pat.
[10]Values for vitamin A are year-round average.
[11]For salted margarine.
[12]Based on average vitamin A content of fortified margarine. Federal specifications for fortified margarine require a minimum of 15,000 IU per pound.
[14]Dipped in egg, milk, and breadcrumbs; fried in vegetable shortening.
[15]If bones are discarded, value for calcium will be greatly reduced.
[16]Dipped in egg, breadcrumbs, and flour; fried in vegetable shortening.
[18]Sodium bisulfite used to preserve color; unsulfited product would contain less sodium.
[19]Also applies to pasteurized apple cider.
[20]Without added ascorbic acid. For value with added ascorbic acid, refer to label.
[21]With added ascorbic acid.
[22]For white grapefruit; pink grapefruit have about 310 IU or 31 RE.
[23]Sodium benzoate and sodium bisulfite added as preservatives.
[24]Egg bagels have 44 mg cholesterol and 22 IU or 7 RE vitamin A per bagel.
[25]Made with vegetable shortening.
[27]Nutrient added.
[28]Cooked without salt. If salt is added according to label recommendations, sodium content is 540 mg.
[29]For white corn grits. Cooked yellow grits contain 145 IU or 14 RE.
[30]Value based on label declaration for added nutrients.
[31]For regular and instant cereal. For quick cereal, phosphorus is 102 mg and sodium is 142 mg.
[32]Cooked without salt. If salt is added according to label recommendations, sodium content is 390 mg.
[33]Cooked without salt. If salt is added according to label recommendations, sodium content is 324 mg.
[34]Cooked without salt. If salt is added according to label recommendations, sodium content is 374 mg.
[35]Excepting angel food cake, cakes were made from mixes containing vegetable shortening and frostings were made with margarine.
[36]Made with vegetable oil.
[37]Cake made with vegetable shortening; frosting with margarine.
[38]Made with margarine.
[39]Crackers made with enriched flour except for rye wafers and whole-wheat wafers.
[40]Made with lard.
[41]Cashews without salt contain 21 mg sodium per cup or 4 mg per oz.
[42]Cashews without salt contain 22 mg sodium per cup or 5 mg per oz.
[43]Macadamia nuts without salt contain 9 mg sodium per cup or 2 mg per oz.
[44]Mixed nuts without salt contain 3 mg sodium per oz.
[45]Peanuts without salt contain 22 mg sodium per cup or 4 mg per oz.
[46]Outer layer of fat was removed to within approximately 1/2 inch of the lean. Deposits of fat within the cut were removed.
[47]Fried in vegetable shortening.
[48]Value varies widely.
[49]Contains added sodium ascorbate. If sodium ascorbate is not added, ascorbic acid content is negligible.
[51]Crust made with vegetable shortening and enriched flour.
[52]Made with corn oil.
[53]Fried in vegetable shortening.
[54]If sodium ascorbate is added, product contains 11 mg ascorbic acid.
[55]Made with enriched flour, margarine, and whole milk.
[57]For green varieties; yellow varieties contain 101 IU or 10 RE.
[59]For regular pack; special dietary pack contains 3 mg sodium.
[60]For green varieties; yellow varieties contain 142 IU or 14 RE.
[61]For regular pack; special dietary pack contains 78 mg sodium.
[63]For yellow varieties; white varieties contain only a trace of vitamin A.
[64]For regular pack; special dietary pack contains 8 mg sodium.
[65]For regular pack; special dietary pack contains 6 mg sodium.
[66]For regular pack; special dietary pack contains 3 mg sodium.
[67]For red peppers; green peppers contain 350 IU or 35 RE.
[68]For green peppers; red peppers contain 4,220 IU or 422 RE.
[69]For green peppers; red peppers contain 141 mg ascorbic acid.
[72]With added salt; if none is added, sodium content is 58 mg.
[73]For regular pack; special dietary pack contains 31 mg sodium.
[74]With added salt; if none is added, sodium content is 24 mg.
[75]With no added salt; if salt is added, sodium content is 2,070 mg.
[76]With no added salt; if salt is added, sodium content is 998 mg.
[77]With salt added.

Glossary

Note: See also the Glossary of Food Preparation Terms on pages 235–237 in Chapter 13, "Getting Started in the Kitchen." Numbers in parentheses refer to the chapter in which each term is defined.

A

abdominal thrust. A procedure used to save choking victims. (6)

Aboriginal. One of the first, or native, inhabitants of a land. (27)

absorption. The process of taking nutrients into the body and making them part of the body. (2)

Adequate Intake (AI). A recommended nutrient intake value, based on observations or experiments, that is set for nutrients for which no RDA can be determined. (3)

aerobic activity. A physical activity that speeds heart rate and breathing, promoting cardiovascular health. (5)

agriculture. The use of knowledge and skill to tend soil, grow crops, and raise livestock. (1)

ají. The Peruvian and Chilean term for chilies. (28)

a la carte. Type of menu in which each menu item is individually priced. (25)

al dente. Italian term describing the way pasta is cooked so its texture is slightly resistant to the bite. (30)

alternative. An option a person might choose when making a decision. (1)

American (family style) service. Style of meal service in which diners pass serving dishes from hand to hand around the table and serve themselves. (25)

amino acid. A chemical compound that serves as a building block of proteins. (2)

anemia. A condition resulting from deficiencies of various nutrients, which is characterized by a reduced number of red blood cells in the bloodstream. (2)

anorexia nervosa. An eating disorder characterized by self-starvation. (5)

anthocyanin. A reddish-blue pigment found in vegetables. (15)

antipasto. An Italian appetizer course. (30)

appetite. A psychological desire to eat. (1)

appetizer. Light food or beverage that begins a meal and is designed to stimulate the appetite. (25)

arcing. Sparking that occurs in a microwave oven when metal comes in contact with the oven walls. (13)

arepa. A corn pancake similar to a tortilla that is a traditional Venezuelan bread. (28)

artificial light. Light that comes from electrical fixtures. (8)

artificial sweetener. A product that sweetens food without providing the calories of sugar. (1)

ascorbic acid. A food additive that prevents color and flavor loss and adds nutritive value; another name for vitamin C. (26)

aseptic packaging. A commercial method of packaging food in which a food and its packaging material are sterilized separately and then the food is packed in the container in a sterile chamber. (26)

avgolemono. A popular Greek sauce made from a mixture of egg yolks and lemon juice. (30)

Aztecs. The original inhabitants of Mexico. (28)

B

bacteria. Single-celled or noncellular microorganisms that live almost everywhere. (6)

basal metabolism. The amount of energy the human body needs to stay alive and carry on vital processes. (5)

batter. Flour-liquid mixture with a consistency ranging from thin to thick, depending on the proportion of dry to liquid ingredients. (23)

beading. Golden droplets of moisture that sometimes appear on the surface of a meringue. (18)

beef. Meat obtained from mature cattle over 12 months of age. (19)

beef stroganov. A popular Russian meat dish made with tender strips of beef, mushrooms, and a seasoned sour cream sauce. (32)

beriberi. A disease of the nervous system resulting from a thiamin deficiency, which is characterized by numbness in the ankles and legs followed by severe cramping and paralysis. (2)

berries. Classification of fruits, including strawberries, raspberries, and grapes, that are small and juicy and have thin skins. (16)

beverageware. Drinking glasses of many shapes and sizes used for a variety of purposes. (8)

binge eating disorder. An eating disorder characterized by repeated episodes of uncontrolled eating of large amounts of food. (5)

bisque. A rich, thickened cream soup. (17)

blend. Several varieties of coffee beans mixed to produce a particular flavor and aroma (13); combination of spices and herbs. (22)

blue plate service. Type of meal service in which the plates are filled in the kitchen, carried to the dining area, and served. (25)

body composition. Proportions of bone, muscle, fat, and other tissues that make up body weight. (5)

body mass index (BMI). A calculation involving a person's weight and height measurements used by health professionals to define overweight and obesity. (5)

borscht. Russian beet soup. (32)

botulism. Foodborne illness caused by eating foods containing the spore-forming bacteria *Clostridium botulinum.* (26)

bouillon. Clear broth made from strained, clarified stock. (22)

bouquet garni. Small group of herbs tied together in a cheesecloth bag and added to a food during cooking for flavor. Parsley, thyme, and bay leaf usually are used. (22)

bran. The outer protective covering of a kernel of grain. (14)

brand name. The name a manufacturer puts on products so people will know that company makes the products. (12)

braten. German term for roast, which is Germany's national dish. (29)

budget. A plan for managing income and expenses. (11)

buffet service. Style of meal service in which a large table or buffet holds the utensils, dinnerware, flatware, napkins, and serving dishes from which guests serve themselves. (25)

bulgur. Grain product made from whole wheat that has been cooked, dried, partly debranned, and cracked. (31)

bulimia nervosa. An eating disorder characterized by repeated eating binges followed by inappropriate behaviors to prevent weight gain. (5)

C

cacao. A plant that produces beans that are ground into cocoa or made into chocolate. (31)

caffeine. A compound found in products like coffee, tea, chocolate, and cola beverages that acts as a stimulant. (13)

Cajun cuisine. Hearty fare of rural Southern Louisiana that reflects the foods and cooking methods of the Acadians, French, Native Americans, Africans, and Spanish. (27)

calorie. The unit used to measure the energy value of foods. (5)

candling. Process by which eggs are quality-graded. (18)

canning. A food preservation process that involves sealing food in airtight containers. (26)

carbohydrate. One of the six basic types of nutrients that is the body's chief source of energy. (2)

career ladder. A career made up of a series of related jobs, each of which builds on the skills learned in the previous job. (7)

carotene. Chemical substance found in dark green and yellow fruits and vegetables that can be converted into vitamin A by the body; chemical substance that gives yellow vegetables and fruits their yellow-orange color. (15)

cassava. A starchy root plant eaten as a side dish and used in flour form in cooking and baking in South America. (28)

casserole. A baking dish with high sides (10); combination of foods baked in a single dish. (22)

caste system. A social system in India that evolved from Hinduism and divided people into groups, or castes. (32)

catering. Business in which food and beverages are prepared for small and large parties, banquets, weddings, and other large gatherings. (7)

caviar. The processed, salted roe (eggs) of large fish, most often sturgeon. (32)

cereal. Starchy grain that is suitable to use as food. (14)

ceviche. A marinated raw fish dish served throughout South America. (28)

chapatis. A flat bread that is common in India. (32)

chasnidarth. A major cooking technique in Indian cuisine that resembles Chinese sweet and sour. (32)

chelo kebab. Iran's national dish, which consists of thin slices of marinated, charcoal-broiled lamb served with plain rice accompanied by a pat of butter, a raw egg, and a bowl of ground sumac. (31)

chiffon cake. Cake that is a combination of a shortened and unshortened cake; cake that contains fat and beaten egg whites. (24)

chilies. Term used in Mexico for hot peppers. (28)

chlorophyll. Green pigment found in green plants (including vegetables) that can be adversely affected by heat. (15)
cholesterol. A fatlike substance that occurs naturally in the body and is found in every cell but occurs only in foods of animal origin. (2)
chopsticks. Chinese eating utensils. (32)
chorizo. A dark sausage with a spicy, smoky flavor. (30)
chowder. Cream soup that contains pieces of seafood, vegetables, poultry, or meat and is made from unthickened milk. (17)
citrus fruits. Classification of fruits, including oranges, lemons, and grapefruit, that have a thick outer rind and thin membranes separating the flesh into segments. (16)
coagulate. To thicken or form a congealed mass. (Proteins are coagulated by heat and can cause a mixture to thicken.) (19)
coagulum. Clumps of a protein food. (18)
cockles. A type of mussel common along the coast of Wales. (29)
colander. A perforated bowl used to drain fruits, vegetables, and pasta. (10)
colcannon. An Irish dish made with mashed potatoes mixed with chopped scallions, shredded cooked cabbage, and melted butter. (29)
collagen. Protein constituent of connective tissue in meat. Collagen is tough and elastic but can be softened by cooking. (19)
combination oven. An oven that can do two types of cooking, such as conventional and convection. (9)
comida. The main meal of the day in Mexico and Spain. (28)
comparison shopping. Evaluating different brands, sizes, and forms of a product before making a purchase decision. (12)
compromise service. Style of meal service in which part of the food is served from the kitchen and part is served at the table. (25)
congee. A thick porridge made from rice or barley often served for breakfast in China. (32)
conquistador. Spanish conqueror who invaded Mexico during the early 1500s. (28)
conservation. The planned use of a resource to avoid waste. (11)
consommé. Clear, rich-flavored soup made from strained and clarified stock. (22)
contaminant. A potentially harmful substance that has accidentally gotten into food. (6)
convection cooking. Method of cooking in which foods are baked or roasted in a stream of heated air. (9)
convenience food. Food product that has had some amount of service added to it. (11)
cooking losses. Fat, water, and other volatile substances that are retained in pan drippings or cooking liquid when meats are cooked. (19)
cooking time. The total amount of time food in a microwave oven is exposed to microwave energy. (13)
course. A part of a meal made up of all the foods served at one time. (11)
cover. The amount of space needed by each person at a dining table; area on a table that contains the linen, dinnerware, flatware, and glassware needed by one person. (8)
crayfish. A crustacean related to the lobster. (29)
Creole cuisine. Style of food popular in the Southern United States that combines cooking techniques of the French with ingredients of the Africans, Caribbeans, Spanish, and Native Americans. (27)
crêpe. A thin, delicate pancake that is usually rolled around a filling. (29)
crisp-tender. Term used to describe vegetables that have been cooked to the proper degree of doneness. (15)
croissant. A flaky, buttery French yeast roll shaped into a crescent. (29)
cross-contamination. The transfer of harmful bacteria from one food to another food. (6)
crustacean. Shellfish with a segmented body that is covered by a crustlike shell. (21)
crystalline candy. Type of candy with very small and fine sugar crystals, which give it a smooth and creamy texture. (24)
culture. The customs and beliefs of a racial, religious, or social group. (1)
curd. Solid portion of coagulated milk. (17)
curdling. Formation of curds (coagulated proteins) that can happen when milk is overheated or an acid food, such as tomato juice, is added to milk incorrectly. (17)
curry. A type of Indian stew. (32)
custard. Mixture of milk (or cream), eggs, sugar, and a flavoring that is cooked until thickened. (18)

D

Daily Value. A dietary reference that appears on food labels. (12)
decaffeinated. Term describing a product, such as coffee or tea, made by removing most of the caffeine. (13)
decision-making process. A method for thinking about possible options and outcomes before making a choice. (1)

deficiency disease. An illness caused by the lack of a sufficient amount of a nutrient. (2)

dehydration. An abnormal loss of body fluids. (5) The process of drying; the removal of water from foods or other items. (13)

del pueblo. Term meaning of the people, which is used to describe Spanish cuisine. (30)

dendé oil. Palm oil that gives Brazilian dishes a bright yellow-orange color. (28)

diabetes mellitus. A body's lack of or inability to use the hormone insulin to maintain normal blood glucose levels. (4)

diet. All the food and drink a person regularly consumes. (4)

dietary antioxidant. A substance in foods that significantly reduces the harmful effects of oxygen on normal body functions. (2)

Dietary Guidelines for Americans. A set of science-based recommendations from the U.S. Departments of Agriculture and Health and Human Services that urge people to form healthful diet and activity habits in an effort to promote health and reduce disease risks. (3)

Dietary Reference Intakes (DRIs). Estimated nutrient intake levels used for planning and evaluating the diets of healthy people. (3)

dietary supplement. A purified nutrient or nonnutrient substance that is manufactured or extracted from natural sources. (2)

dietitian. A health care professional who has training in nutrition and diet planning. (7)

digestion. The bodily process of breaking food down into simpler compounds the body can use. (2)

dinnerware. Plates, cups, saucers, and bowls. (8)

discretionary calories. The calories left in a person's daily allowance after making nutrient-dense choices for all food group servings. (3)

double boiler. Small pan that fits into a larger pan. Food is put in the smaller pan, and water is placed in the larger pan. The food cooks by steam heat. (10)

dough. Flour-liquid mixture that is stiff enough to be shaped by hand. (23)

dovetail. To overlap tasks to use time more efficiently. (13)

downdraft vent. A vent used in some ranges in which a fan is mounted under the cooktop to draw cooking fumes away from food before they have a chance to rise through the room. (9)

drawn fish. Fish that has the entrails (insides) removed. (21)

dressed fish. Fish that has the entrails (insides), head, fins, and scales removed. (21)

drupes. Fruits, such as cherries, peaches, and plums, that have an outer skin covering a soft flesh that surrounds a single, hard pit. (16)

Dutch treat. A way of paying for a meal in a restaurant in which each person in a group pays for him- or herself. (25)

dynasty. A chain of rulers with the same ancestry. (32)

E

eating disorder. Abnormal eating behavior that endangers physical and mental health. (5)

eggplant. A fleshy, oval-shaped vegetable with a deep purple skin frequently used in Mediterranean dishes. (30)

elastin. Protein constituent of connective tissue in meat that is tough and elastic and cannot be softened by cooking. (19)

empanada. An Argentine appetizer. (28)

emulsion. Mixture that forms when oil and liquid are combined. (18)

endosperm. The largest part of a kernel of grain containing most of the starch and the protein of the kernel but few minerals and little fiber. (14)

EnergyGuide label. A yellow tag that shows an estimated yearly energy usage for the major appliance on which it appears. (9)

ENERGY STAR label. A label manufacturers voluntarily place on refrigerators, freezers, and dishwashers that exceed federal minimum energy standards by a certain amount. (9)

English service. Style of meal service in which the plates are served by the host and/or hostess and passed around the table until each guest has been served. (25)

enriched. Having added nutrients to replace those lost through processing. (14)

entree. Main course. (25)

entrepreneur. A person who sets up and runs his or her own business. (7)

environment. Interrelated factors, including air, water, soil, mineral resources, plants, and animals, that ultimately affect the survival of life on earth. (1)

enzymatic browning. Darkening process some fruits undergo when exposed to the air. (16)

enzyme. Complex protein produced by living cells that causes specific chemical reactions. (26)

escargot. A snail eaten as food. (29)

Estimated Average Requirement (EAR). A nutrient intake value that is based on research and estimated to meet the needs of half the healthy people in a group. (3)

etiquette. Rules set by society to guide social behavior. (25)

extension agent. Family and consumer sciences professional employed by the Cooperative Extension Service who works with adults and with young people involved in 4-H programs, offers classes, and/or writes educational materials that are published by the Department of Agriculture. (7)

F

fad. A practice that is very popular for a short time. (1)

fallacy. A mistaken belief. (1)

fasting. Denying oneself food. (1)

fat. One of the six basic types of nutrients that is an important energy source. (2)

fat fish. Fish having flesh that is fattier than the flesh of lean fish. (21)

fat replacer. A product that cuts the amount of fat in foods while keeping the flavors and textures fat provides. (1)

fat-soluble vitamin. A vitamin that dissolves in fats and can be stored in the fatty tissues of the body. (2)

fatty acid. A chemical chain containing carbon, hydrogen, and oxygen that is the basic component of all lipids. (2)

feijoada completa. Brazil's national dish, which is made with meat and black beans. (28)

felafel. A mixture of ground chickpeas, bulgur, and spices that is formed into balls and deep-fried. (31)

fermentation. Process that takes place when yeast cells act on sugars to produce carbon dioxide and alcohol; enzymatically controlled process in which a compound is broken down, such as a carbohydrate into carbon dioxide and ethyl alcohol. (23)

fiber. A form of complex carbohydrate from plants that humans cannot digest. (2)

filé. Flavoring and thickening agent made from the leaves of the sassafras tree, which have been dried and ground into a powder. (27)

fines herbes. A mixture of fresh chives, parsley, tarragon, and chervil used to flavor many French soups and stews. (29)

finfish. Fish that have fins and backbones. (21)

finished food. Convenience food that is ready for eating either immediately or after heating or thawing. (11)

fish and chips. Battered, deep-fried fish fillets served in England with a British version of French fries. (29)

fish fillet. The side of a fish cut lengthwise away from the backbone. (21)

fish steak. Cross-sectional slice taken from a dressed fish. (21)

fitness. The body's ability to meet physical demands. (5)

fixed expense. A regularly recurring cost in a set amount, such as rent, mortgage, or installment loan payments. (11)

flatware. Forks, knives, spoons, serving utensils, and specialty utensils used to serve and eat food. (8)

flavones. Pigments that make white vegetables, such as cauliflower, white. (15)

fleishig foods. Meat foods as described by Jewish dietary laws. (31)

flexible expense. A regularly recurring cost that varies in amount, such as food, clothing, or utility bills. (11)

food additive. A substance that is added to food for a specific purpose, such as preserving the food. (12)

food allergy. A response of the body's immune system to a food protein. (4)

Food and Drug Administration (FDA). The federal agency that ensures the safety and wholesomeness of all foods sold across state lines, except meat, poultry, and eggs. (1)

foodborne illness. A disease transmitted by food. (6)

food-drug interaction. An effect a drug has on the way the body absorbs or uses a nutrient or an effect a food has on the way the body absorbs or uses a drug. (4)

food intolerance. A negative physical reaction to a food substance that does not involve the body's immune system. (4)

fortified food. A food to which nutrients are added in amounts greater than what would naturally occur in the food. (2)

freeze-drying. A method of commercial food preservation in which water is removed from frozen food items. (26)

freezer burn. Dry, tough areas that occur on food surfaces that have become dehydrated due to exposure to dry air in a freezer. (26)

French knife. A versatile kitchen knife that is most often used to cut, chop, and dice fruits and vegetables. (10)

frijoles refritos. Refried beans, a popular Mexican dish. (28)

fritters. Fruits, vegetables, or meats that are dipped into a batter and fried in hot fat. (16)

functional food. A food that provides health benefits beyond the nutrients it contains. (1)

G

gaucho. Nomadic herders of the Pampas in South America during the eighteenth and nineteenth centuries. (28)

gazpacho. A Spanish soup made with coarsely pureed tomatoes, cucumbers, onions, garlic, green peppers, olive oil, and vinegar. (30)

gelatin. Gummy substance made from the bones and some connective tissues of animals. It may be flavored or unflavored for use as a food product. (17)

gelatin cream. Milk-based dessert thickened with unflavored gelatin. (17)

gelatinization. Swelling and subsequent thickening of starch granules when heated in water. (14)

generic product. A plain-labeled, no-brand grocery item. (12)

germ. The reproductive part of a kernel of grain, which is rich in vitamins, protein, and fat. (14)

ghee. Indian clarified butter. (32)

giblets. The edible internal organs of poultry. (20)

glucose. The form of sugar carried in the bloodstream for energy use throughout the body. (2)

gluten. A protein formed when wheat flour is moistened and thoroughly mixed that gives strength and elasticity to batters and doughs. (23)

goal. An aim a person tries to reach. (7)

gohan. The Japanese word for meal, which means rice. (32)

goiter. A visible enlargement of the thyroid gland resulting from an iodine deficiency. (2)

gourmet. A person who enjoys being able to distinguish the complex combinations of flavors that make up foods. (22)

grade. An indication of food quality. (12)

GRAS list. List of food additives that are "Generally Recognized as Safe" by the Food and Drug Administration (FDA). (12)

gratuity. Sum of money given to a waiter in a restaurant for service rendered. (25)

ground. To connect an appliance electrically with the earth. (8)

growth spurt. A period of rapid growth. (4)

guacamole. A spread made from mashed avocado, tomato, and onion that is popular in Mexico. (28)

gumbo. A Creole specialty that is a thick, souplike mixture containing a variety of seafood, poultry, meats, vegetables, and rice. (27)

H

haggis. A Scottish dish made from a sheep's stomach stuffed with a pudding made from oatmeal and the sheep's organs. (29)

Halal. Foods considered lawful for consumption according to the Islamic religion. (31)

Haram. Foods that are forbidden to be eaten according to the Islamic religion. (31)

haute cuisine. A style of French cooking characterized by elaborate preparations, fancy garnishes, and rich sauces. (29)

headspace. Space between the food and the closure of a food storage container. (26)

healthy weight. A body mass index of 18.5 to 24.9 in an adult. (5)

herb. A leaf of a plant usually grown in a temperate climate and used to season food. (22)

holloware. Tableware, such as bowls, tureens, and pitchers, used to serve food and liquids. (8)

homogenization. Mechanical process by which milkfat globules are broken into tiny particles and spread throughout milk or cream to keep the cream from rising to the surface of the milk. (17)

hors d'oeuvres. Small dishes designed to stimulate the appetite. (29)

hot pack. Process of packing vegetables or fruits that have been preheated in water or steam into canning jars and covering them with cooking liquid or boiling water. (26)

hot spot. An area of a food cooked in a microwave oven that reaches a higher temperature than surrounding areas due to receiving a greater concentration of microwave energy. (13)

hunger. The physical need for food. (1)

husmankost. The traditional, everyday style of cooking enjoyed in Swedish homes. (29)

hydrate. To cause a substance to absorb water. (17)

hydrogenation. A process by which hydrogen atoms are chemically added to unsaturated fatty acids in liquid oils to turn the oils into more highly saturated solid fats. (2)

hypertension. High blood pressure. (2)

I

immature fruit. Fruit that is small and has such characteristics as poor color, flavor, and texture, which will not improve with time. (16)

impulse buying. Making an unplanned purchase without much thought. (12)

imu. A pit lined with hot rocks used to roast a whole, young pig at a Hawaiian luau. (27)

Inca. A group of Native South Americans who built a large empire in the Andes mountains prior to the Spanish conquest. (28)
income. Money received. (11)
injera. Ethiopia's main dish, which is a large, sourdoughlike pancake made from a grain called teff. (31)
interview. A meeting between an employer and a job applicant held to discuss the applicant's qualifications for a job opening. (7)
irradiation. A commercial food preservation method that exposes food to low-level doses of gamma rays, electron beams, or X rays. (26)

J

jambalaya. A Creole specialty that is a mixture of rice; seasonings; and shellfish, poultry, and/or sausage. (27)

K

kaiseka. A delicate meal served after the Japanese tea ceremony. (32)
kartoffelpuffer. German potato pancakes. (29)
kasha. A Russian staple food made of buckwheat or other grains that are fried and then simmered until tender. (32)
kashrut. Jewish dietary laws. (31)
kernel. A whole seed of a cereal. (14)
kibbutzim. Cooperative farm villages in Israel. (31)
korma. A major Indian cooking technique in which foods are braised, usually in yogurt. (32)
kosher. Foods prepared according to Jewish dietary laws. (31)
kulich. A tall, cylindrical Russian yeast bread filled with fruits and nuts. (32)

L

lamb. The meat of sheep less than one year old. (19)
Latin America. The landmass that stretches southward from the Rio Grande to the tip of South America. (28)
leader. A person who has influence over others. (7)
lean fish. Fish that have very little fat in their flesh. (21)
leavening agent. An ingredient that produces gases in batters and doughs, causing baked products to rise and become light and porous. (23)
legumes. Peas, beans, and lentils. (15)
lifestyle. The way a person usually lives. (1)
lingonberry. A tart, red berry used in Swedish desserts. (29)
luau. Elaborate outdoor feast popular in the Hawaiian Islands. (27)
lutefisk. A traditional Norwegian fish dish made from dried cod that have been soaked in a lye solution before cooking. (29)

M

macromineral. A mineral needed in the diet in amounts of 100 or more milligrams each day. (2)
malnutrition. A lack of the right proportions of nutrients over an extended period, which can be caused by an inadequate diet or the body's inability to use the nutrients taken in. (2)
manioc. A starchy root plant eaten as a side dish and used in flour form in cooking and baking in South America. (28)
manners. Social behaviors. (25)
marbling. Flecks of fat found throughout the lean muscles of meat. (19)
masala. A mixture of spices used to make Indian curry. (32)
matzo. Unleavened bread that is part of Jewish cuisine. (31)
mazza. Arabian appetizers. (31)
meal manager. Someone who uses resources to reach goals related to preparing and serving food. (11)
meat. The edible portion of mammals. (19)
medical diet. An eating plan prescribed by a physician to address special needs of a person with a specific health problem. (4)
melons. Classification of fruits, including cantaloupe, honeydew, and watermelon, that are in the gourd family and are large and juicy and have thick skins and many seeds. (16)
menu. A list of the foods to be served at a meal. (11)
meringue. Fluffy white mixture of beaten egg whites and sugar, which may be soft or hard. (18)
metabolism. The chemical processes that take place in the cells after the body absorbs nutrients. (2)
mezedhes. Greek appetizers. (30)
microorganism. A living substance so small it can be seen only under a microscope. (6)
microwave. High-frequency energy wave used in microwave ovens to cook foods quickly. (9)
milchig foods. Dairy foods as described by Jewish dietary laws. (31)

milkfat. Fat portion of milk. (17)
milk solids. Nonfat portion of milk, which contains most of the vitamins, minerals, proteins, and sugar found in milk. (17)
mineral. One of the six basic types of nutrients that is an inorganic substance and becomes part of the bones, tissues, and body fluids. (2)
minestrone. A popular Italian vegetable soup thick with pasta. (30)
mold. Growth produced on damp or decaying organic matter or on living organisms. (26)
mole. A complex sauce used in Mexican cuisine. (28)
mollusk. Shellfish that has a soft body fully or partially covered by a hard shell. (21)

N

national brand. A brand that is advertised and sold throughout the country. (12)
natural light. Light that comes from the sun. (8)
new potatoes. Potatoes that are harvested and sent directly to market. (15)
night blindness. A condition resulting from a vitamin A deficiency, which is characterized by a reduced ability to see in dim light. (2)
nihon-cha. Japanese term for green teas. (32)
noncrystalline candy. Type of candy in which the sugar syrup is not allowed to form crystals; candy may be chewy or brittle. (24)
nonstick finish. Coating with nonstick properties used on some cookware and bakeware. (10)
nouvelle cuisine. A style of French cooking that emphasizes lightness and natural taste in foods. (29)
nutrient. A chemical substance in food that helps maintain the body. (2)
nutrient-dense food. A food that provides fairly large amounts of vitamins and minerals compared to the number of calories it supplies. (3)
nutrition. The study of how the body uses the nutrients in foods. (2)
nutrition labeling. An analysis of a food product's contributions to an average diet that appears on the product packaging. (12)

O

obesity. A condition characterized by excessive deposits of body fat. In an adult, obesity is defined as a body mass index of 30 or more. (5)
okra. Pod-shaped vegetable brought to the United States from Africa that is popular in the Deep South. (27)
omelet. A beaten egg mixture that is cooked without stirring and served folded in half. (18)
open dating. A system of putting dates on perishable and semiperishable foods to help consumers obtain products that are fresh and wholesome. (12)
open stock. A way of purchasing tableware in which each piece is purchased individually. (8)
organic food. A food produced without the use of synthetic fertilizers, pesticides, or growth stimulants. (12)
osteoporosis. A condition resulting from a calcium deficiency, which is characterized by porous, brittle bones. (2)
overweight. A condition characterized in an adult by a body mass index of 25 to 29.9. (5)

P

paella. A Spanish rice dish often containing chicken, shrimp, mussels, whitefish, peas, and rice and flavored with saffron, salt, pepper, and pimiento. (30)
pareve foods. Foods that contain neither meat nor milk as described by Jewish dietary laws. (31)
paskha. A rich cheesecake that is a popular Russian dessert. (32)
pasta. A paste made from wheat flour that is dried in various shapes, such as macaroni and spaghetti. (14)
pasteurization. Process by which milk and milk products are heated to destroy harmful bacteria. (17)
pastry. Tender, flaky baked product containing flour, fat, water, and salt, which is used as the base for pies, tarts, and other desserts. (24)
pectin. Carbohydrate found naturally in fruits that makes fruit juices jell. (26)
peer pressure. Influence that comes from people in a person's social group. (1)
pellagra. A disease resulting from a niacin deficiency, which is characterized by a raw and inflamed skin rash, abdominal pain, diarrhea, dementia, and paralysis. (2)
Pennsylvania Dutch. Group of German immigrants who settled in the southeast section of Pennsylvania. (27)
peristalsis. Waves of muscle contractions that push food through the digestive tract. (2)
permanent emulsion. Type of emulsion that will not separate on standing; type of emulsion that is formed when an emulsifying agent is added to a mixture of oil and a water-based liquid. (22)

pesticide. An agent used to kill insects, weeds, and fungi that attack crops. (12)
phyllo. A paper-thin pastry made with flour and water used to make many Greek desserts. (30)
phytochemical. A compound from plants that is active in the human body. (2)
pita bread. Flat, round, hollow bread common to the cuisines of Africa and the Middle East. (31)
pitting. Tiny indentations that mark the surface of some aluminum cookware due to a reaction with some foods and minerals. (10)
place setting. A set of all the dinnerware or flatware pieces used by one person. (8)
plantain. A green, starchy fruit that has a bland flavor and looks much like a large banana. (28)
pomes. Classification of fruits, including apples and pears, that have a central, seed-containing core surrounded by a thick layer of flesh. (16)
porcelain enamel. Glasslike material fused at very high temperatures to a base metal, such as the outer surfaces of cookware and bakeware. (10)
pork. The meat of swine. (19)
pot. A two-handled cooking utensil. (10)
potluck. A shared meal to which each person or family brings food for the whole group to eat. (27)
poultry. Any domesticated bird. (20)
precycling. Thinking about how packaging materials can be reused or recycled before buying a product. (12)
prepreparation. Any step done in advance to save time when getting a meal ready. (11)
pressure saucepan. Saucepan that cooks foods more quickly than a conventional pan because as pressure is increased, temperature also increases. (10)
process cheese. One of several types of products, including pasteurized process cheese, pasteurized process cheese food, pasteurized process cheese spread, coldpack cheese, and coldpack cheese food, made from various cheeses. (17)
processed food. A food that has undergone some preparation procedure, such as canning, freezing, drying, cooking, or fortification. (3)
processing time. The amount of time canned goods remain under heat (or under heat and pressure) in a canner. (26)
produce. Fresh fruits and vegetables. (12)
protein. One of the six basic types of nutrients that is required for growth, repair, and maintenance of every body cell. (2)
protein-energy malnutrition (PEM). A condition that may result from a diet that does not contain enough protein and calories. (2)
provincial cuisine. The style of French cooking practiced by most French families using locally grown foods and simple cooking methods. (29)
pudding basin. A deep, thick-rimmed bowl used to steam British puddings. (29)

Q

quiche. A French custard tart served in many variations as an appetizer and a main dish. (29)
quick-freezing. Process of subjecting foods to extremely low temperatures for a short time and then maintaining them at a normal freezing temperature. (26)

R

raw pack. Process of packing cold, raw vegetables in canning jars and covering them with boiling water or syrup. (26)
recipe. Instructions for preparing a particular food. (13)
Recommended Dietary Allowance (RDA). An average daily dietary intake level, based on an Estimated Average Requirement, that meets the nutrient needs of nearly all healthy people in a group. (3)
recycling. Processing a material so it can be used again. (11)
reference. A person an employer can call to ask about a job applicant's capabilities as a worker. (7)
refined. Term used to refer to cereal products made from grain that has had the bran and germ removed during processing and contains only the endosperm. (14)
reservation. An arrangement made with a restaurant to hold a table for a guest on a given date at a given time. (25)
retail cut. A smaller cut of meat taken from a larger wholesale cut and sold to consumers in retail stores. (19)
retort packaging. A commercial method of packaging food in which food is sealed in a foil pouch and then sterilized in a steam-pressure vessel known as a retort. (26)
rickets. A disease resulting from a vitamin D deficiency, which is characterized by crooked legs and misshapen breast bones in children. (2)
ripened cheese. Cheese in which controlled amounts of bacteria, mold, yeast, or enzymes were added and that was stored for a certain period at controlled temperatures. (17)

risotto. An Italian rice dish made with butter, chopped onion, stock or wine, and Parmesan cheese. Meats or seafood and vegetables may also be added. (30)

roux. Cooked paste of fat and flour used as the thickening agent in many sauces and gravies. (17)

RSVP. Letters often included on an invitation that stand for a French phrase meaning please respond. (25)

Russian (continental) service. Style of meal service in which no food is placed on the table; servants do all the serving and clearing. (25)

S

salad. Combination of raw and/or cooked ingredients, usually served cold with a dressing. (22)

saliva. A mucus- and enzyme-containing liquid secreted by the mouth that makes food easier to swallow and begins to break down starches. (2)

sangria. A Spanish punch made with red wine, fruit juice, and sparkling water. (30)

sanitation. Maintaining clean conditions to prevent disease and promote good health. (6)

saucepan. A one-handled cooking utensil. (10)

sauerkraut. Fermented or pickled cabbage. (29)

sauna. A steam bath in which water is poured on hot stones to create steam. (29)

schi. Russian cabbage soup. (32)

scorching. Burning that results in a color change. (17)

scum. Solid layer made up of milk solids and some fat that often forms on the surface of milk during heating. (17)

scurvy. A disease resulting from a vitamin C deficiency, which is characterized by bleeding gums, loss of teeth, and internal bleeding. (2)

semiprepared food. Convenience food that still needs to have some service performed. (11)

serrated blade. A sawtooth edge on a knife. (10)

service contract. An insurance policy for a major appliance that can be purchased from an appliance dealer to cover the cost of repairs for a period after the warranty on the appliance has expired. (9)

shelf life. The amount of time a food can be stored and remain wholesome. (26)

shellfish. Fish that have shells instead of backbones. (21)

shohet. A licensed slaughterer who butchers animals and fowl following methods described in Jewish dietary laws. (31)

shortened cake. Cake made with fat. (24)

siesta. A rest period that usually follows the midday meal in Mexico. (28)

slurry. A liquid mixture of milk and flour blended until smooth, which is used as a thickening agent in sauces and gravies. (17)

smörgåsbord. A Swedish buffet that includes a wide variety of hot and cold dishes. (29)

smørrebrød. Danish open-faced sandwiches usually made with thin, sour rye bread spread thickly with butter. (29)

soufflé. Fluffy baked preparation made with a starch-thickened sauce into which stiffly beaten egg whites are folded. (18)

soul food. A cuisine developed in the Southern United States that combines food customs of African slaves with food customs of Native Americans and European sharecroppers. (27)

sourdough. A dough containing active yeast plants that is used as a leavening agent. (27)

soybean. A legume with seeds that are rich in protein and oil, which is used in many different forms in Japanese and Chinese cooking. (32)

spätzle. Small dumplings made from wheat flour, which are a popular German side dish. (29)

spice. A dried root, stem, or seed of a plant grown mainly in the tropics and used to season food. (22)

springform pan. A round pan with a removable bottom that is held together by means of a spring or latch on the side of the pan. (10)

standing time. The time during which foods finish cooking by internal heat after being removed from a microwave oven. (13)

starch. Complex carbohydrates stored in plants. (14)

stemware. Glassware with three distinct parts: a bowl, a stem, and a base. (8)

stockinette. A cloth cover for a rolling pin used to keep dough from sticking to the rolling pin. (10)

stock soup. Soup made with a rich-flavored liquid in which meat, poultry, or fish; vegetables; and seasonings have been cooked. (22)

store brand. A brand sold only by a store or chain of stores. (12)

stress. Mental tension caused by change. (1)

strudel. A German dessert made with paper-thin layers of pastry filled with fruit. (29)

sugar syrup. A mixture of sugar and liquid that is cooked to a thick consistency. (24)

sukiyaki. A popular Japanese dish made of thinly sliced meat, bean curd, and vegetables cooked in a sauce. (32)

sulfuring. Antidarkening treatment used on some fruits before they are dried. (26)

syneresis. Leakage of liquid from a gel. (14)

T

table appointments. All the items needed at the table to serve and eat a meal. (8)
table d'hôte. Type of menu in which one price is given for an entire meal. (25)
table linens. Table coverings and napkins. (8)
tandoori. A simple Indian cooking technique, which requires a clay oven called a tandoor. (32)
tang. Prong that attaches a knife blade to the handle. (10)
tapas. Spanish appetizers. (30)
taste buds. Flavor sensors covering the surface of the tongue. (11)
taverna. A Greek cafe that serves as a public meeting place in small communities. (30)
tea. Leaves of a tropical evergreen or bush used to make a beverage, which is also called *tea* (13); the evening meal in rural areas or an afternoon snack in cities throughout the British Isles. (29)
technology. The use of knowledge to develop improved methods for doing tasks. (1)
teff. A milletlike grain grown only in Africa and the Middle East. (31)
temporary emulsion. Type of emulsion that forms when oil and a water-based liquid are agitated but breaks when the agitation stops. (22)
time-work schedule. A written plan listing actual times for doing specific tasks to prepare a meal or food product. (13)
tip. Sum of money given to a waiter in a restaurant for service rendered. (25)
tofu. A mild-flavored, custardlike cake made from soybeans. (32)
Tolerable Upper Intake Level (UL). The highest level of daily intake of a nutrient that is unlikely to pose risks of adverse health effects. (3)
tortilla. Flat, unleavened bread made from cornmeal and water used to make many Mexican dishes. (28)
toxin. Poison. (6)
trace element. A mineral needed in the diet in amounts less than 100 milligrams per day. (2)
trans fatty acid. A fatty acid with an odd molecular shape that is created when oils are partly hydrogenated. (2)
tropical fruits. Classification of fruits, including avocados, bananas, and pineapples, that are grown in warm climates and are considered to be somewhat exotic. (16)
truffles. A rare type of fungi that grow underground near oak trees and are used in many French recipes. (29)
tsukemono. Soaked foods, or lightly pickled pieces of daikon, cucumber, melon, eggplant, and other vegetables, which are a standard part of the main course at Japanese meals. (32)
tumbler. A piece of glassware without a stem. (8)

U

ultra-high temperature (UHT) processing. A preservation method that uses higher temperatures than regular pasteurization to increase the shelf life of foods like milk. (17)
underripe fruit. Fruit that has reached full size but has yet to ripen. (16)
underweight. A condition characterized by a body mass index of less than 18.5. (5)
United States Department of Agriculture (USDA). The federal agency that enforces standards for the quality and wholesomeness of meat, poultry, and eggs sold across state lines. (1)
unit pricing. A listing of a product's cost per standard unit, weight, or measure. (12)
universal design. Features of rooms, furnishings, and equipment that are usable by as many people as possible. (8)
universal product code (UPC). A series of lines, bars, and numbers that appears on the package of a food or nonfood item. This code is used by a computer scanner to identify a product, its manufacturer, and its size and form. (12)
unripened cheese. Cheese that is prepared for marketing as soon as the whey has been removed without being allowed to ripen or age. (17)
unshortened cake. Cake made without fat. (24)
USDA Food Guide. A science-based eating pattern that sorts foods of similar nutritive values into groups and subgroups and gives a recommended number of daily servings for each group. (3)

V

variety meats. Edible parts of animals other than muscle, such as liver, heart, and tongue. (19)
veal. The meat of cattle less than three months of age. (19)
vegetarian diet. A diet that is built partially or completely on fruits, vegetables, and other plant foods. (4)

vindaloo. A major Indian cooking technique in which foods have a hot, slightly sour flavor created by combining vinegar with spices. (32)

vitamin. One of the six basic types of nutrients that is a complex organic substance needed by the body in small amounts for normal growth, maintenance, and reproduction. (2)

W

waist-to-hip ratio. A mathematical relationship used to evaluate body shape that is calculated by dividing a person's waist measurement by his or her hip measurement. (5)

warranty. A seller's promise that a product will perform as specified or will be free from defects. (9)

wat. A spicy sauce or stew that is part of Ethiopian cuisine. (31)

water-soluble vitamin. A vitamin that dissolves in water and is not stored in the body to any great extent. (2)

watt. A unit of power; the cooking power of microwave ovens is measured and expressed in watts. (13)

wave pattern. The repeated cycle in which energy in a microwave oven is emitted by the magnetron tube. (9)

weeping. Layer of moisture that sometimes forms between a meringue and a filling. (18)

weight management. Using resources like food choices and physical activity to reach and/or maintain a healthy weight. (5)

wellness. A state of being in overall good physical, mental, and social health. (1)

whey. Liquid part of coagulated milk. (17)

whisk. A mixing tool made of loops of wire attached to a handle used to incorporate air into foods and to keep sauces from lumping. (10)

white sauce. A starch-thickened milk product used as a base for other sauces and as a component in many recipes. (17)

whole grain. Term used to refer to cereal products made from grain that contains all three parts of the kernel—bran, germ, and endosperm. (14)

wholesale cut. Large cut of meat shipped to a retail grocery store or meat market. (19)

wok. A versatile Chinese cooking utensil, which looks like a metal bowl with sloping sides. (32)

work center. Section in a kitchen that has been designed around a specific activity or activities. (8)

work simplification. Act of performing tasks in the simplest way possible in order to conserve time and energy. (11)

work triangle. Imaginary triangle formed by the focal points of the three major work centers found in a kitchen. (8)

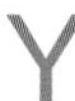

Y

yam. Dark orange tuber with moist flesh often confused with a sweet potato. (27)

yeast. Microscopic fungus that can cause fermentation in preserved foods resulting in spoilage. (26)

yield. The average amount or number of servings a given recipe will produce. (13)

Z

zakuska. Russian appetizers. (32)

Index

A

B

C

D

E

F

I

J

K

L

M

N

O

P

Q

R

S

T

U

V

W

Y

Z

Recipe Index

A

B

C

D

E

T

V

W

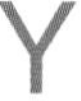